Technical Manual

20TH EDITION

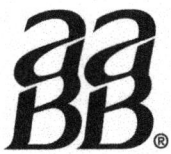

Other related publications available from the AABB:

Transfusion Therapy: Clinical Principles and Practice, 4th edition
Edited by Marisa Marques, MD; Joseph Schwartz, MD, MPH; and Yan Yun Wu, MD, PhD

Transfusion Medicine: Self-Assessment and Review, 3rd edition
By Douglas P. Blackall, MD, MPH, and Justin D. Kreuter, MD

Blood Transfusion Therapy: A Physician's Handbook, 12th edition
Edited by Nicholas Bandarenko, MD, and Karen King, MD

Judd's Methods in Immunohematology, 3rd edition
By John W. Judd, FIBMS; Susan T. Johnson, MSTM, MT(ASCP)SBB; and Jill Storry, PhD, FIBMS

Antibody Identification: Art or Science? A Case Study Approach
By Janis R. Hamilton, MS, MT(ASCP)SBB; Susan T. Johnson, MSTM, MT(ASCP)SBB;
and Sally V. Rudmann, PhD, MT(ASCP)SBB

To purchase books or to inquire about other book services, including digital downloads and large-quantity sales, please contact our sales department:
- 866.222.2498 (within the United States)
- +1 301.215.6499 (outside the United States)
- +1 301.951.7150 (fax)
- www.aabb.org>Resources>Marketplace

AABB customer service representatives are available by telephone from 8:30 am to 5:00 pm ET, Monday through Friday, excluding holidays.

Technical Manual

20TH EDITION

Edited by

Claudia S. Cohn, MD, PhD
Associate Professor/Director, Blood Bank Laboratory
University of Minnesota
Minneapolis, MN

Meghan Delaney, DO, MPH
Chief, Pathology and Laboratory Medicine Division, and
Director, Transfusion Medicine
Children's National Hospital
Washington, DC

Susan T. Johnson, MSTM, MT(ASCP)SBB
Director, Clinical Education
Versiti
Milwaukee, WI

Louis M. Katz, MD
Chief Medical Officer
Mississippi Valley Regional Blood Center
Davenport, IA

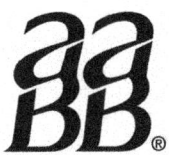

Mention of specific products or equipment by contributors to this AABB publication does not represent an endorsement of such products by the AABB nor does it indicate a preference for those products over other similar competitive products. Product listings, descriptions, and references are not intended to be comprehensive. Any forms and/or procedures in this book are examples. AABB does not imply or guarantee that the materials meet federal, state, or other applicable requirements. It is incumbent on the reader who intends to use any information, forms, policies, or procedures contained in this publication to evaluate such materials for use in light of particular circumstances associated with his or her institution.

AABB authors are requested to comply with a conflict of interest policy that includes disclosure of relationships with commercial firms. A copy of the policy is located at http://www.aabb.org.

Efforts are made to have publications of the AABB consistent in regard to acceptable practices. However, for several reasons, they may not be. First, as new developments in the practice of blood banking occur, changes may be recommended to the *Standards for Blood Banks and Transfusion Services*. It is not possible, however, to revise each publication at the time such a change is adopted. Thus, it is essential that the most recent edition of the *Standards* be consulted as a reference in regard to current acceptable practices. Second, the views expressed in this publication represent the opinions of authors. The publication of this book does not constitute an endorsement by the AABB of any view expressed herein, and the AABB expressly disclaims any liability arising from any inaccuracy or misstatement.

AABB
4550 Montgomery Avenue
Suite 700, North Tower
Bethesda, Maryland 20814-3304

ISBN No. 978-1-56395-370-5
Printed in the United States

Cataloging-in-Publication Data

Technical manual / editor, Claudia S. Cohn—20th ed.
        p. ; cm.
    Including bibliographic references and index.
    ISBN 978-1-56395-370-5
    1. Blood Banks—Handbooks, manuals, etc. I. Cohn, Claudia S. II. AABB.
    [DNLM: 1. Blood Banks-laboratory manuals. 2. Blood Transfusion-
    laboratory manuals. WH 25 T2548 2020]
    RM172.T43 2020
    615'.39—dc23
    DNLM/DLC

Technical Manual
Authors

Jason Acker, MBA, PhD

Caroline R. Alquist, MD, PhD

Chester Andrzejewski Jr, PhD, MD

J. Wade Atkins, MS, MT(ASCP)SBB, CQA(ASQ)

Debra J. Bailey, MT(ASCP)SBB

P. Dayand Borge Jr, MD, PhD

Colleen Bowman, MT(ASCP)SBB, CQA(ASQ)

Gwen Clarke, MD

Laura S. Connelly-Smith, MBBCh, DM

Lauren A. Crowder, MPH

Melissa M. Cushing, MD

Arthur B. Eisenbrey III, MD, PhD

Lay See Er, MSTM, SBB(ASCP)^{CM}, CQA(ASQ)

Richard O. Francis, MD, PhD

Steven M. Frank, MD

James D. Gorham, MD, PhD

Patricia C. Grace, RN, BSN

Nicole R. Guinn, MD

Sarah K. Harm, MD

Eldad A. Hod, MD

Jay Hudgins, DO

Orieji Illoh, MD

Melanie Jorgenson, RN, BSN, LSSGB

Cassandra D. Josephson, MD

Margaret A. Keller, PhD

James M. Kelley, MD, PhD

Debra A. Kessler, RN, MS

Patricia M. Kopko, MD

Kevin J. Land, MD

Lani Lieberman, MD

Michael L. Linenberger, MD, FACP

Paul M. Mansfield, MT(ASCP)^{CM}SBB

Irina Maramica, MD, PhD, MBA

Cami Melland, MLS(ASCP)^{CM}SBB

Yunchuan Delores Mo, MD

Sandra Nance, MS, MT(ASCP)SBB

Martin L. Olsson, MD, PhD

Thierry Peyrard, PharmD, PhD, EurSpLM

Rowena C. Punzalan, MD

Eva D. Quinley, MS, MT(ASCP)SBB, CQA(ASQ)

Fran Rabe, MS

Anna Razatos, PhD

Susan N. Rossmann, MD, PhD

Jeremy Ryan Peña, MD, PhD

Annette J. Schlueter, MD, PhD

Joseph Schwartz, MD, MPH

Nadine Shehata, MD, FRCP

Ira A. Shulman, MD

Whitney R. Steele, PhD, MPH

Sean R. Stowell, MD, PhD

Susan L. Stramer, PhD

David F. Stroncek, MD

Annika M. Svensson, MD, PhD

Yvette C. Tanhehco, PhD, MD, MS

Lynne Uhl, MD

Ralph R. Vassallo, MD, FACP

Franz F. Wagner, MD

Jennifer Webb, MD, MSCE

Julia S. Westman, PhD

Barbee I. Whitaker, PhD

Edward C.C. Wong, MD

Sandy Wortman, MT(ASCP)^{CM}SBB

Acknowledgments

THE 20TH EDITION OF the *AABB Technical Manual* is the collaborative result of many dedicated volunteers. My thanks go out to all the chapter authors, and my three Associate Editors for this edition—Meghan Delaney, Sue Johnson, and Lou Katz. They have been a "dream team" and I greatly appreciate their guidance in the subjects covered, and the many hours spent reviewing and revising each chapter with the authors.

We, in turn, would like to thank the many members of the following AABB committees and task forces who reviewed every word of the chapters, methods, and appendices in the 20th edition. Their participation makes this volume unique in the literature and contributes to its excellent reputation.

REVIEWING GROUPS

AABB Representative to ASFA

AABB Representative to ISBT Working Party for Transfusion Transmitted Infectious Disease

Cellular Therapy Section Coordinating Committee – Subgroup, Cellular Therapy Product Collection and Clinical Practices

Cellular Therapy Section Coordinating Committee – Subgroup, Product Manufacturing and Testing

Circular of Information Task Force

Clinical Transfusion Medicine Committee

Donor History Task Force

FDA Liaison Committee

Immunohematology Reference Laboratories Accreditation Program Unit

Immunohematology Reference Laboratories Standards Program Unit

Interorganizational Task Force on Domestic Disasters and Acts of Terrorism

Molecular Testing Laboratories Standards Program Unit

Patient Blood Management Education Committee

Patient Blood Management Standards Committee

Quality Systems Accreditation Committee

Relationship Testing Standards Program Unit

Transfusion Medicine Section Coordinating Committee – Subgroup, Donor and Blood Component Management

Transfusion Medicine Section Coordinating Committee – Subgroup, Pediatric Transfusion

Transfusion Medicine Section Coordinating Committee – Subgroup, Technical Practices and Serology

Transfusion Medicine Section Coordinating Committee – Subgroup, Transfusion Safety and Patient Blood Management

Transfusion-Transmitted Disease Committee

We would be remiss if we did not also mention the valuable material drafted by contributors to earlier editions that we included in this new edition. The selected tables, figures, methods, and narrative that we kept could not have been improved. Finally, we would like to thank AABB staff who supported our efforts.

Claudia S. Cohn, MD, PhD
Editor in Chief

Preface

ON BEHALF OF THE EDITORS, AUthors, and many reviewers I am pleased to introduce the 20th edition of the AABB *Technical Manual*. The *Technical Manual* conveys the latest information in blood banking/transfusion medicine along with well-established material. Using the model developed by previous editorial teams, when possible we paired new authors with seasoned veterans to bring a fresh perspective to the content. This also allows for continuity as new authors in the current edition move into the role of primary author for the next edition. I am grateful for the steady guidance and hard work of Associate Editors Meghan Delaney, DO, MPH; Sue Johnson, MSTM, MT(ASCP)SBB; and Louis Katz, MD. All of us were first-time editors of the *Technical Manual* and learned a great deal from AABB staff and the editors of past editions.

The *Technical Manual*'s excellence is ensured by a stringent peer-review process. Each chapter underwent an initial review by the editors for content and style, followed by reviews from numerous AABB committee members who provided focused expertise as well as comments on readability. Compliance experts then conducted a final check to make sure we provided the most up-to-date information on the standards, guidance, and regulations that help govern the activities readers engage in. These extra steps provide a high level of confidence that the *Technical Manual* is a reliable resource for our community.

The overall structure and content of the *Technical Manual* is adjusted periodically by survey responses and feedback from AABB membership. For the 19th edition several key measures were taken to focus the content and reduce redundancy. These measures were very successful and, as a result, few structural changes were necessary for this edition.

However, improvements in content continued unabated. Sue Johnson and the authors of the chapters on blood groups worked diligently to bring the book's terminology for blood group antigens more closely in line with official ISBT nomenclature. In fact, their work is already being used as an exemplar for other AABB publications. Chapters addressing topics that have evolved significantly since publication of the 19th edition underwent major revision. These expanded updates include content on massive transfusion, patient blood management, molecular testing, and relevant transfusion-transmitted disease. Other key updates involving several chapters resulted from the April 2020 release of new federal regulations on donor deferrals and subsequent revision of the donor history questionnaire.

The *Technical Manual* was in the final stages of production when the COVID-19 pandemic swept across the world. Not surprisingly, the pandemic had an impact on the book. First, we considered adding material about disaster preparedness, blood shortages, and convalescent plasma. However, the information was changing so rapidly that we felt pandemic-related content would be out of date by the time we went to press. Second, the final review meeting at the AABB office was converted to a virtual remote process. It took longer, but I believe the results are equal in quality of outcome. The third impact also relates to remote working. Our community as a whole has developed and improved ways to benefit from access to online resources. Accordingly, the methods and appendices are now posted online, rather than loaded onto a USB flash card in a pocket adhered to the inside back cover. Readers who turn to the table of contents page for the methods will find the access code there. We hope that the pandemic will be resolved well before publication of the 21st edition, and that informa-

tion on the virus, treatment, blood collection challenges, and lessons learned can be included in that edition.

It has been a privilege to work with the talented and dedicated staff at AABB and the transfusion medicine/blood banking community that helped to produce this edition. On behalf of the editors, authors, and reviewers we hope you enjoy using the 20th edition of the *Technical Manual* and find it a useful reference tool.

Claudia S. Cohn, MD, PhD
Editor in Chief

Contents in Print

Preface ix

QUALITY AND RELATED ISSUES

1. Quality Management Systems: Principles and Practice 1

Eva D. Quinley, MS, MT(ASCP)SBB, CQA(ASQ), and Patricia C. Grace, RN, BSN

Background 1
Concepts in Quality 2
Quality Management Systems Approach 4
Evaluation of the Quality Management System 5
The Quality Management System in Practice 5
Key Points 23
References 24
Appendix 1-1. Glossary of Commonly Used Quality Terms 26
Appendix 1-2. Code of Federal Regulations Quality-Related References 28
Appendix 1-3. Suggested Quality Control Performance Intervals for Equipment
    and Reagents 29

2. Facilities, Work Environment, and Safety 33

*J. Wade Atkins, MS, MT(ASCP)SBB, CQA(ASQ), and
    Colleen Bowman, MT(ASCP)SBB, CQA(ASQ)*

Safety Program 35
Fire Prevention 39
Electrical Safety 40
Biosafety 41
Chemical Safety 48
Radiation Safety 53
Shipping Hazardous Materials 56
General Waste Management 56
Key Points 57
References 57
Appendix 2-1. Safety Regulations and Recommendations Applicable to
    Health-Care Settings 61
Appendix 2-2. General Guidance for Safe Work Practices, Personal Protective
    Equipment, and Engineering Controls 63

Appendix 2-3. Biosafety Level 2 Precautions 66
Appendix 2-4. Sample List of Hazardous Chemicals That May Be Encountered
    in a Blood Bank 67
Appendix 2-5. Chemical Categories and How to Work Safely with Them 69
Appendix 2-6. Incidental Spill Response 71
Appendix 2-7. Managing Hazardous Chemical Spills 74

3.   Regulatory Considerations in Transfusion Medicine and Cellular Therapies 77

Joseph Schwartz, MD, MPH; Orieji Illoh, MD; and
    Yvette C. Tanhehco, PhD, MD, MS

FDA Oversight of Blood Establishments 78
Medical Laboratory Laws and Regulations 84
Local Laws, Hospital Regulations, and Accreditation 85
Human Cells, Tissues, and Cellular and Tissue-Based Products (HCT/PS) 86
Immune Effector Cells 89
Key Points 90
References 90

4.   National Hemovigilance: The Current State 95

Kevin J. Land, MD; Barbee I. Whitaker, PhD; and Lynne Uhl, MD

International Hemovigilance 96
US Hemovigilance 97
Recipient Hemovigilance in the United States 100
Blood Donor Hemovigilance in the United States 103
Next Steps in US Hemovigilance 106
Key Points 112
References 113
Appendix 4-1. Protocol for Hospital Reporting Adverse Events to Blood Suppliers . . 116
Appendix 4-2. Severity Grading Tool for Blood Donor Adverse Events 124

BLOOD COLLECTION AND TESTING

5.   Allogeneic and Autologous Blood Donor Selection 127

Debra A. Kessler, RN, MS, and Susan N. Rossmann, MD, PhD

Overview of Blood Donor Screening 127
Selection of Allogeneic Blood Donors 128
Abbreviated DHQ for Frequent Donors 132
Blood-Center-Defined Donor Eligibility Criteria 133
Recipient-Specific "Designated" or "Directed" Blood Donation 135
Key Points 137
References 137

6. Whole Blood and Apheresis Collection of Blood Components Intended for Transfusion................. 141

Jason Acker, MBA, PhD, and Anna Razatos, PhD

Donor Preparation and Care.. 141
Blood Collection 145
Blood Component Storage 153
Postcollection Processing/Blood Component Modification 158
Quarantine of Blood Components................................... 164
Labeling of Blood Components..................................... 164
Key Points 165
References 166

7. Infectious Disease Screening........................... 173

Lauren A. Crowder, MPH; Whitney R. Steele, PhD, MPH; and Susan L. Stramer, PhD

Historical Overview of Blood Donor Screening 173
Donor Screening Tests 177
Residual Infectious Risks of Transfusion 196
Screening for Specific Agents 199
Pathogen Inactivation Technology 215
Summary 217
Key Points 217
References 218

BLOOD GROUPS

8. Molecular Biology and Immunology in Transfusion Medicine 229

Sean R. Stowell, MD, PhD, and James D. Gorham, MD, PhD

Analysis of DNA 229
Analysis of Protein 238
Basic Immunology 243
Key Points 251
References 251

9. Blood Group Genetics 255

Margaret A. Keller, PhD, and Sandy Wortman, MT(ASCP)^{CM}SBB

Genomic Organization and Gene Regulation......................... 256
Genetic Variation... 262
Inheritance of Genetic Traits 266
Structural Variation 270
Chimerism... 273
Gene Position Effects 274

Genetic Modifiers of Blood Group Antigen Expression. 274
Population Genetics 275
Relationship Testing 278
Blood Group Gene Mapping 279
Gene, Protein, and Blood Group Terminology 280
Blood Group Genomics. 281
Summary 291
Key Points 292
References 293

10.   ABO and Other Carbohydrate Blood Group Systems 297

Martin L. Olsson, MD, PhD, and Julia S. Westman, PhD

The ABO system (001) 297
The H System (018) 310
The LE System (007) 313
I and i Antigens of the I Blood Group System (027) and I Blood Group Collection . . 315
P1PK (003) and GLOB (028) Blood Group Systems. 318
The FORS Blood Group System (031) 323
The SID Blood Group System (038). 323
Key Points 323
References 324

11.   The Rh System 329

Thierry Peyrard, PharmD, PhD, EurSpLM, and Franz F. Wagner, MD

Historical Perspective 329
Terminology. 332
Rh Locus 333
RHD Genotype 334
Antigens. 337
Rh Genotyping 346
Rh$_{null}$ Syndrome and the RhAG (030) Blood Group System 347
Antibodies to Rh Blood Group System Antigens. 347
Technical Considerations for Rh Typing. 348
Key Points 349
References 350

12.   Other Blood Group Systems and Antigens. 355

Cami Melland, MLS(ASCP)^{CM}SBB, and Sandra Nance, MS, MT(ASCP)SBB

The MNS System (002) 359
The LU System (005) 363
The KEL (006) and Xk (019) Systems 364
The FY System (008) 368
The JK System (009) 370
The DI System (010) 372
The YT System (011) 373
The XG System (012) 374

The SC System (013) 374
The DO System (014) 374
The CO System (015) 375
The LW System (016) 375
The CH/RG System (017) 377
The GE System (020) 377
The CROM System (021) 378
The KN System (022) 378
The IN System (023) 379
The OK System (024) 379
The RAPH System (025) 379
The JMH System (026) 379
The GIL System (029) 380
The RHAG System (030) 380
The JR System (032) 380
The LAN System (033) 380
The VEL System (034) 381
The CD59 System (035) 381
The AUG System (036) 381
The KANNO System (037) 382
The SID System (038) 382
The CTL2 System (039) 382
Antigens that Do Not Yet Belong to a Blood Group System 382
Erythroid Phenotypes Caused by Mutations in Transcription Factor Genes 384
Key Points 384
References 385

13.   Identification of Antibodies to Red Cell Antigens 389

*Lay See Er, MSTM, SBB(ASCP)^CM, CQA(ASQ), and
    Debra J. Bailey, MT(ASCP)SBB*

Basic Concepts in Red Cell Antigen Expression 390
Initial Antibody Identification Considerations 391
Basic Antibody Identification 394
Complex Antibody Identification 402
Selected Procedures 414
Considerations Following Antibody Identification 421
Immunohematology Reference Laboratories 424
Key Points 424
References 425
Suggested Readings 428

**14.   The Positive Direct Antiglobulin Test and Immune-
    Mediated Hemolysis 429**

P. Dayand Borge Jr, MD, PhD, and Paul M. Mansfield, MT(ASCP)^CM SBB

The DAT 430
Autoimmune Hemolytic Anemia 434
Drug-Induced Immune Hemolytic Anemia 445

Key Points 449
References 449
Appendix 14-1. Drugs Associated with Immune Hemolytic Anemia 452

15.   Platelet and Granulocyte Antigens and Antibodies 457

David F. Stroncek, MD, and Ralph R. Vassallo, MD, FACP

Platelet Antigens and Antibodies 457
Granulocyte Antigens and Antibodies 469
Key Points 473
References 473

16.   The HLA System. 479

*Jeremy Ryan Peña, MD, PhD; Arthur B. Eisenbrey III, MD, PhD; and
    Patricia M. Kopko, MD*

Biochemistry, Tissue Distribution, and Structure 479
Genetics of the MHC 484
HLA Typing 488
Other Non-HLA Histocompatibility Determinants 489
Crossmatching and Detection of HLA Antibodies. 490
The HLA System and Transfusion 491
HLA Testing and Transplantation 493
Other Clinically Significant Aspects of HLA 495
Clinical Consultation in HLA. 497
Regulatory Aspects of Clinical Histocompatibility 498
Future Directions 498
Summary 499
Key Points 499
References 499

ESSENTIALS OF TRANSFUSION PRACTICE

**17.   Transfusion-Service-Related Activities: Pretransfusion
        Testing and Storage, Monitoring, Processing,
        Distribution, and Inventory Management of
        Blood Components. 503**

Caroline R. Alquist, MD, PhD, and Sarah K. Harm, MD

Samples and Requests 503
Pretransfusion Testing of Recipient Blood 504
Blood and Blood Component Storage and Monitoring 509
Pretransfusion Processing 518
Distribution 522
Issuing of Components 523
Inventory Management 527
Key Points 529

References 530
Appendix 17-1. Sources of False-Positive Results in Antiglobulin Testing 533
Appendix 17-2. Sources of False-Negative Results in Antiglobulin Testing 534
Appendix 17-3. Causes of Positive Pretransfusion Test Results. 535

18. Administration of Blood Components **537**

Melanie Jorgenson, RN, BSN, LSSGB

Events and Considerations Before Dispensing Components 537
Blood Component Transportation and Dispensing 542
Blood Administration 543
Documentation of the Transfusion 547
Unique Transfusion Settings 548
Conclusion 549
Key Points 549
References 550

19. Hemotherapy Decisions and Their Outcomes **553**

Nadine Shehata, MD, FRCP, and Yunchuan Delores Mo, MD

Red Blood Cell Transfusion. 553
Platelet Transfusion 561
Plasma Transfusion 567
Cryoprecipitate Transfusion 569
Granulocyte Transfusion. 570
Massive Transfusion Protocols 571
Key Points 573
References 573

20. Patient Blood Management **583**

Steven M. Frank, MD, and Nicole R. Guinn, MD

Definition and Scope of Patient Blood Management 583
Resources to Support a PBM Program 584
Patient Blood Management Standards and Certification 585
Methods of Patient Blood Management 585
Data Collection 600
Extremes of Transfusion 605
Summary 606
Key Points 607
References 607

21. Approaches to Blood Utilization Auditing **613**

Ira A. Shulman, MD; Jay Hudgins, DO; and Irina Maramica, MD, PhD, MBA

The Auditing Process 614
Defining Audit Criteria 615
Types of Blood Utilization Review 617
Blood Utilization Review of Transfusions to High-Risk Patients 620

The Role of a Computerized Provider Order Entry System in Blood Utilization
  Review 620
Use of "Big Data" to Assess Performance and Progress Measures in
  Transfusion Medicine 621
Key Points 623
References 624

22. Noninfectious Complications of Blood Transfusion 627

Eldad A. Hod, MD, and Richard O. Francis, MD, PhD

Hemovigilance 627
Recognition and Evaluation of a Suspected Transfusion Reaction 627
Acute or Immediate Transfusion Reactions 634
Delayed Transfusion Reactions 648
Fatality Reporting Requirements 652
Key Points 653
References 653

SPECIAL PATIENTS AND SITUATIONS

23. Perinatal Issues in Transfusion Practice 659

Lani Lieberman, MD; Gwen Clarke, MD; and Annika M. Svensson, MD, PhD

Hemolytic Disease of the Fetus and Newborn 659
Pregnancy-Related Thrombocytopenia 665
Key Points 668
References 668

24. Neonatal and Pediatric Transfusion Practice 673

Edward C.C. Wong, MD, and Rowena C. Punzalan, MD

Hematopoiesis, Coagulation, and Physiology 673
RBC Transfusion in Neonates 675
RBC Transfusion in Infants Older than 4 Months and Children 682
Platelet Transfusion in Neonates and Children 685
Plasma and Cryoprecipitate Transfusion in Neonates and Children 687
Granulocyte Transfusion in Neonates and Children 688
Other Considerations Common to Transfusion of Neonates and Children 689
Adverse Effects and Prevention 694
Key Points 695
References 696

25. Therapeutic Apheresis 705

Jennifer Webb, MD, MSCE, and Chester Andrzejewski Jr, PhD, MD

General Principles 705
Device Modalities 706
Patient Evaluation and Management 707

Vascular Access 709
Anticoagulation 711
Adverse Effects 711
Pediatric Apheresis 713
Therapeutic Apheresis Indications 713
Therapeutic Apheresis Procedure Documentation, Payment, and Provider
    Credentialing 727
Key Points 729
References 730

26. The Collection and Processing of Hematopoietic Progenitor Cells 737

Laura S. Connelly-Smith, MBBCh, DM, and Michael L. Linenberger, MD, FACP

Clinical Utility 737
Histocompatibility, Donor Type, and Graft Source 741
HPC Collection 743
Processing Human Progenitor Cells 748
Specialized Cell-Processing Methods 750
Cryopreservation 751
Quality Control 752
Shipping and Transporting HPC Cellular Products 754
Patient Care 754
Regulatory and Accreditation Considerations 756
Conclusion 757
Key Points 757
References 758

27. Transfusion Support for Hematopoietic Stem Cell Transplant Recipients 767

James M. Kelley, MD, PhD, and Melissa M. Cushing, MD

ABO Compatibility for Blood Component Selection Following HSCT 768
Blood Component Support for HSCT Patients 772
Pediatric Considerations 773
Key Points 774
References 774

28. Human Tissue Allografts and the Hospital Transfusion Service 777

Annette J. Schlueter, MD, PhD; Fran Rabe, MS; and Cassandra D. Josephson, MD

Tissue Donation and Transplantation 777
Federal Regulations, State Laws, and Professional Standards 782
Hospital Tissue Services 784
Key Points 789
References 790

Index 793

Contents Online
www.aabb.org/methods

METHODS

1. General Laboratory Methods

Method 1-1. Shipping Hazardous Materials
Method 1-2. Monitoring Temperature During Shipment of Blood
Method 1-3. Treating Incompletely Clotted Specimens
Method 1-4. Solution Preparation Procedure
Method 1-5. Serum Dilution Procedure
Method 1-6. Dilution of Percentage Solutions Procedure
Method 1-7. Preparing a 3% Red Cell Suspension
Method 1-8. Preparing and Using Phosphate Buffer
Method 1-9. Reading and Grading Tube Agglutination

2. Red Cell Typing Methods

Method 2-1. Determining ABO Group of Red Cells—Slide Test
Method 2-2. Determining ABO Group of Red Cells and Serum—Tube Test
Method 2-3. Determining ABO Group of Red Cells and Serum—Microplate Test
Method 2-4. Initial Investigation of ABO Grouping Discrepancies Procedure
Method 2-5. Detecting Weak A and B Antigens and Antibodies by Cold Temperature Enhancement
Method 2-6. Confirming Weak A and B Antigens Using Enzyme-Treated Red Cells
Method 2-7. Confirming Weak A or B Subgroup by Adsorption and Elution
Method 2-8. Testing Saliva for A, B, H, Le^a, and Le^b Antigens
Method 2-9. Confirming Anti-A_1 in an A_2 or Weak A Subgroup
Method 2-10. Resolving ABO Discrepancies Caused by Unexpected Alloantibodies
Method 2-11. Determining Serum Group Without Centrifugation
Method 2-12. Determining Rh(D) Type—Slide Test
Method 2-13. Determining Rh(D) Type—Tube Test
Method 2-14. Determining Rh(D) Type—Microplate Test
Method 2-15. Testing for Weak D
Method 2-16. Preparing and Using Lectins
Method 2-17. Removing Autoantibody by Warm Saline Washes
Method 2-18. Using Sulfhydryl Reagents to Disperse Autoagglutination
Method 2-19. Using Gentle Heat Elution to Test Red Cells with a Positive DAT Result
Method 2-20. Dissociating IgG by Chloroquine for Antigen Testing of Red Cells with a Positive DAT Result
Method 2-21. Using Acid Glycine/EDTA to Remove Antibodies from Red Cells
Method 2-22. Separating Transfused from Autologous Red Cells by Simple Centrifugation
Method 2-23. Separating Transfused from Autologous Red Cells in Patients with Hemoglobin S Disease

3. Antibody Detection, Identification, and Compatibility Testing

Method 3-1. Using Immediate-Spin Compatibility Testing to Demonstrate ABO Incompatibility
Method 3-2. Saline Indirect Antiglobulin Test Procedure
Method 3-3. Albumin or LISS-Additive Indirect Antiglobulin Test Procedure
Method 3-4. LISS-Suspension Indirect Antiglobulin Test Procedure
Method 3-5. PEG Indirect Antiglobulin Test Procedure
Method 3-6. Prewarming Procedure
Method 3-7. Detecting Antibodies in the Presence of Rouleaux—Saline Replacement
Method 3-8. Preparing Ficin Enzyme Stock, 1% w/v
Method 3-9. Preparing Papain Enzyme Stock, 1% w/v
Method 3-10. Standardizing Enzyme Procedures
Method 3-11. Evaluating Enzyme-Treated Red Cells
Method 3-12. One-Stage Enzyme Procedure
Method 3-13. Two-Stage Enzyme Procedure
Method 3-14. Performing a Direct Antiglobulin Test
Method 3-15. Antibody Titration Procedure
Method 3-16. Using Sulfhydryl Reagents to Distinguish IgM from IgG Antibodies
Method 3-17. Using Plasma Inhibition to Distinguish Anti-Ch and -Rg from Other Antibodies with Similar Characteristics
Method 3-18. Treating Red Cells Using DTT or AET
Method 3-19. Neutralizing Anti-Sd^a with Urine
Method 3-20. Adsorption Procedure
Method 3-21. Using the American Rare Donor Program

4. Investigation of a Positive DAT Result

Method 4-1. Cold-Acid Elution Procedure
Method 4-2. Glycine-HCl/EDTA Elution Procedure
Method 4-3. Heat Elution Procedure
Method 4-4. Lui Freeze-Thaw Elution Procedure
Method 4-5. Cold Autoadsorption Procedure
Method 4-6. Determining the Specificity of Cold-Reactive Autoagglutinins
Method 4-7. Cold Agglutinin Titer Procedure
Method 4-8. Adsorbing Warm-Reactive Autoantibodies Using Autologous Red Cells
Method 4-9. Adsorbing Warm-Reactive Autoantibodies Using Allogeneic Red Cells
Method 4-10. Polyethylene Glycol Adsorption Procedure
Method 4-11. Performing the Donath-Landsteiner Test
Method 4-12. Detecting Drug Antibodies by Testing Drug-Treated Red Cells
Method 4-13. Detecting Drug Antibodies by Testing in the Presence of Drug

5. Hemolytic Disease of the Fetus and Newborn

Method 5-1. Testing for Fetomaternal Hemorrhage—The Rosette Test
Method 5-2. Testing for Fetomaternal Hemorrhage—Modified Kleihauer-Betke Test
Method 5-3. Using Antibody Titration Studies to Assist in Early Detection of Hemolytic Disease of the Fetus and Newborn

6.   Blood Collection, Component Preparation, and Storage

Method 6-1. Screening Female Donors for Acceptable Hemoglobin Level—Copper Sulfate
  Method
Method 6-2. Preparing the Donor's Arm for Blood Collection
Method 6-3. Collecting Blood and Samples for Processing and Testing
Method 6-4. Preparing Red Blood Cells from Whole Blood
Method 6-5. Preparing Prestorage Red Blood Cells Leukocytes Reduced from Whole Blood
Method 6-6. Using High-Concentration Glycerol to Cryopreserve Red Cells—Meryman
  Method
Method 6-7. Using High-Concentration Glycerol to Cryopreserve Red Cells—Valeri Method
Method 6-8. Checking the Adequacy of Deglycerolization of Red Blood Cells
Method 6-9. Preparing Fresh Frozen Plasma from Whole Blood
Method 6-10. Preparing Cryoprecipitated AHF from Whole Blood
Method 6-11. Thawing and Pooling Cryoprecipitated AHF
Method 6-12. Preparing Platelets from Whole Blood
Method 6-13. Removing Plasma from Platelets (Volume Reduction)

7.   Transplantation of Cells and Tissue

Method 7-1. Infusing Cryopreserved Hematopoietic Cells
Method 7-2. Processing Umbilical Cord Blood
Method 7-3. Investigating Adverse Events and Infections Following Tissue Allograft Use

8.   Quality Control Methods

Method 8-1. Validating Copper Sulfate Solution
Method 8-2. Calibrating Liquid-in-Glass Laboratory Thermometers
Method 8-3. Calibrating Electronic Oral Thermometers
Method 8-4. Testing Refrigerator Alarms
Method 8-5. Testing Freezer Alarms
Method 8-6. Calibrating Centrifuges for Platelet Separation
Method 8-7. Calibrating a Serologic Centrifuge for Immediate Agglutination
Method 8-8. Calibrating a Serologic Centrifuge for Washing and Antiglobulin Testing
Method 8-9. Testing Automatic Cell Washers
Method 8-10. Monitoring Cell Counts of Apheresis Components
Method 8-11. Counting Residual White Cells in Leukocyte-Reduced Blood and
  Components—Manual Method

APPENDICES

Appendix 1. Normal Values in Adults
Appendix 2. Selected Normal Values in Children
Appendix 3. Typical Normal Values in Tests of Hemostasis and Coagulation (Adults)
Appendix 4. Coagulation Factor Values in Platelet Concentrates
Appendix 5. Approximate Normal Values for Red Cell, Plasma, and Blood Volumes
Appendix 6. Blood Group Antigens Assigned to Systems

Appendix 7. Examples of Gene, Antigen, and Phenotype Symbols in Conventional and International Society of Blood Transfusion Terminology
Appendix 8. Examples of Correct and Incorrect Terminology
Appendix 9. Distribution of ABO/Rh Phenotypes by Race or Ethnicity
Appendix 10. Abbreviations Used in the *Technical Manual*, 20th Edition

---

A C K N O W L E D G M E N T

Special thanks to Maureen Beaton, MT(ASCP)BB, CQA(ASQ),
for review of the methods and appendices.

CHAPTER 1

Quality Management Systems: Principles and Practice

Eva D. Quinley, MS, MT(ASCP)SBB, CQA(ASQ), and Patricia C. Grace, RN, BSN

A QUALITY MANAGEMENT SYSTEM (QMS) is a collection of business processes focused on achieving quality while meeting customer requirements. It is expressed as the organizational structure, policies, procedures, processes, and resources needed to implement quality management. Why is this important in the fields of transfusion medicine and cellular therapies? The answer to this is simple—the customers served, whether they are other health-care providers or patients, depend on the assurance that the products and services produced and provided are safe and effective for their intended use. A QMS is the framework for continual improvement by enhancing customer satisfaction. In a QMS, customer requirements are defined, processes are designed to meet those requirements, and processes are in place to manage and improve the level of service that is provided.

It is also the expectation of regulators that organizations have processes in place to ensure that products and services are safe and successful in producing the desired results. The implementation of an effective QMS will help to ensure these outcomes.

Finally, with decreases in utilization and increased costs of operations, it is also important that organizations involved in transfusion medicine and cellular therapies operate in the most cost-effective manner possible. A good QMS will reduce rework, waste, and inefficiencies; thus,

an organization will spend fewer resources to achieve the same operational and quality outcomes. An effective QMS provides confidence to the customer, the organization, and other interested parties that the organization will provide products and services that consistently meet or exceed requirements or customer expectations, and it increases efficiencies, thus reducing costs.

BACKGROUND

Quality has been central to transfusion medicine from its inception, the opening of the first blood bank in the United States at the Cook County Hospital in Chicago in 1937. Continuous scientific progress in many aspects of transfusion medicine has contributed to the quality and safety of blood components and transfusion services, and now cellular therapies. During the 1990s, after the discovery of the human immunodeficiency virus (HIV) and the advent of AIDS, a very sensitized and informed public demanded that the highest level of quality be achieved and maintained in all processes involved in the provision of all blood components and services. The Food and Drug Administration (FDA) introduced the concept of a "zero risk blood supply" in an effort to decrease the inherent risk of the transmission of infectious agents and transfusion complications. Regulato-

Eva D. Quinley, MS, MT(ASCP)SBB, CQA(ASQ), Regional Director, Vitalant-Illinois, Chicago, Illinois; and Patricia C. Grace, RN, BSN, Senior Quality Director, Vitalant-California, Mather, California
The authors have disclosed no conflicts of interest.

ry agencies such as the FDA, the Centers for Medicare and Medicaid Services (CMS), and state departments of health, and accrediting organizations such as AABB, the College of American Pathologists (CAP), The Joint Commission, and the Foundation for the Accreditation of Cellular Therapies (FACT) require facilities operating in transfusion medicine and cellular therapies to establish and follow a quality assurance program, including quality control (QC) processes and procedures, as part of their licensing, certification, and/or accreditation programs. Every laboratory must comply with the Clinical Laboratory Improvement Amendments of 1988 (CLIA), quality requirements implemented by CMS that have a primary focus on laboratory quality. In 1995, the FDA released its *Guideline for Quality Assurance in Blood Establishments.* This guideline, along with other FDA-issued guidance, assists facilities in maintaining compliance with the current good manufacturing practice (cGMP) requirements found in the *Code of Federal Regulations* (CFR), Title 21, Parts 200 and 600. CFR Title 21, Part 820, formerly known as the GMP requirements for medical devices, provides regulations applicable to manufacturers of medical devices, including blood establishment computer systems (BECS).

AABB's Quality System Essentials (QSEs), minimum requirements for blood banking and cellular therapy operations, are based on all of these specifications and provide additional guidance in implementing practices that ensure quality and compliance with cGMP and current good tissue practice (cGTP) regulations. AABB and CAP are granted "deemed status" as accrediting organizations under the CLIA '88 program by CMS, as are The Joint Commission and some state regulatory bodies. The International Organization for Standardization (ISO) has established international standards in most fields, which represent minimal requirements. These standards are generic in content and can be applied to any organization, large or small, whatever its product may be. The United States is represented in ISO by the American National Standards Institute (ANSI). The Clinical and Laboratory Standards Institute (CLSI), formerly the National Committee for Clinical Laboratory Standards (NCCLS), a global organization headquartered in the United States, is a member of ANSI. The FDA and AABB incorporate many ISO principles into their regulations and standards. For example, AABB's QSEs are rooted in the 20 clauses of the ISO 9000 series and are compatible with ISO standards.

CONCEPTS IN QUALITY

Quality Assurance

The concept of quality assurance is broad, and the goals of quality assurance are to significantly decrease errors; ensure the credibility of results; implement safe and effective manufacturing processes and system controls; and ensure continued improvement in product safety and quality. A quality assurance program is defined as a system designed and implemented to ensure that manufacturing is consistently performed in such a way as to yield a product of consistent quality.[1] A good quality assurance program includes ways to detect, investigate, assess, prioritize, and correct errors, with the ultimate goal of error prevention. Quality assurance activities also include retrospective reviews and analyses of operational performance data to determine whether the overall process is in a state of control and to detect shifts or trends that require attention. Quality assurance provides information to process managers regarding levels of performance that can be used in setting priorities for process improvement.

Quality Control

QC is one aspect of a quality assurance program. Its purpose is to determine, through testing or observation, whether a process or particular task within a process is working as expected at a given time. QC involves sampling and testing. Historically, transfusion services and donor centers have used many QC measures as standard practices in their operations. Examples include reagent QC; product QC; clerical checks; visual inspections; and regular measurements, such as temperature readings on refrigerators and volume or cell counts on finished blood components. If QC is not within specifications, it may indicate a problem, either with the process itself or with how the process is being executed. Trends in QC may indicate the potential for a problem in the future.

Quality Management

Quality management considers interrelated processes in the context of the organization and its relations with customers and suppliers. It addresses the leadership role of executive management in creating a commitment to quality throughout the organization, the understanding of suppliers and customers as partners in quality, the management of human and other resources, and quality planning. An important goal in quality management is to establish a set of controls that ensure process and product quality but are not excessive. Controls that do not add value should be eliminated to conserve limited resources and allow staff to focus attention on those controls that are critical to the operation.

Statistical tools, such as process capability measurement and control charts, allow a facility to evaluate process performance during the planning stage and in operations. These tools help determine whether a process is stable (ie, in statistical control) and is capable of meeting product and service specifications.

Quality Systems

A system is defined as an organized, purposeful structure that consists of interrelated and interdependent elements (components, processes, entities, factors, members, parts, etc). These elements continually influence one another (directly or indirectly) to maintain their activity and the existence of the system, in order to achieve the goal of the system. The quality system is made up of a set of interrelated processes that work together to ensure quality. (See Fig 1-1.)

It is important to understand what a process is. Basically, a process can be defined as a set of activities that uses resources to transform inputs to outputs. The whole blood collection process, for example, has many inputs, such as a trained phlebotomist, an approved collection set, an approved arm-scrub solution, a calibrated scale, and phlebotomy standard operating procedures (SOPs), all working together to produce the output, a unit of whole blood. The quality of the output is determined by the quality and control that is in place with the inputs and with the process itself. Validation of a process is key in ensuring the process is consistent and produces the desired output. Validation is discussed more fully later in this chapter.

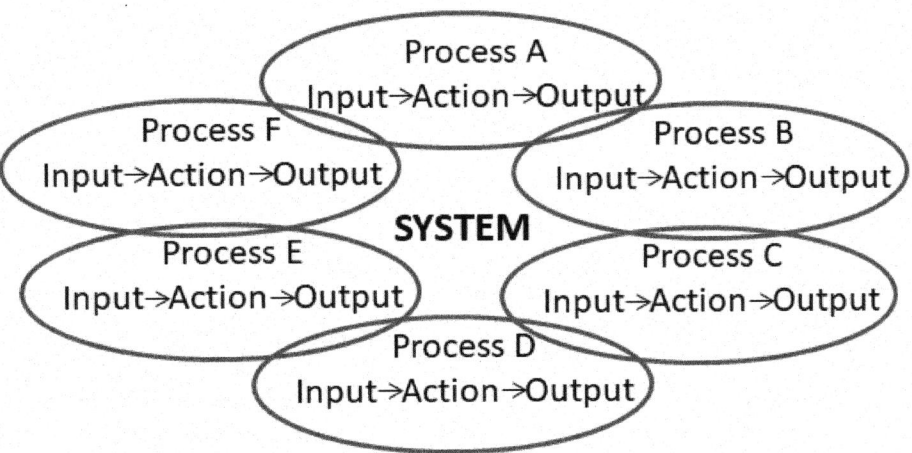

FIGURE 1-1. Systems and processes.

Control of the Process

Strategies for managing a process should address all of its components, including its interrelated activities, inputs, outputs, and resources. Supplier qualification, formal agreements, supply verification, and inventory control are strategies for ensuring that the inputs to a process meet specifications. Personnel training and competency assessment, equipment maintenance and control, management of documents and records, and implementation of appropriate in-process controls provide assurance that the process will operate as intended. End-product testing and inspection, outcome measurement, and customer feedback provide data to evaluate product quality and improve the process. These output measurements and quality indicators are used to evaluate the effectiveness of the process and process controls.

To manage a system of processes effectively, the facility must understand how its processes interact and what cause-and-effect relationships exist between them. As an example, the consequences of accepting a donor who is not eligible reach into almost every other process in the facility. If a donor with a history of high-risk behavior is not identified as such during the selection process, the donated unit(s) may return positive test results for one of the viral marker assays, triggering follow-up testing, look-back investigations, and donor deferral and notification procedures. Components must be quarantined and their discard documented. Personnel involved in collecting and processing the unit(s) are at risk of exposure to infectious agents. Part of quality planning is to identify these relationships so that quick and appropriate corrective action can be taken when process controls fail.

It is important to remember that operational processes include not only product manufacture or service creation but also the distribution of a product or service. Distribution generally involves interaction with the customer. The quality of that transaction is critical to customer satisfaction and should not be overlooked in the design and ongoing assessment of the QMS.

Quality Planning

A necessary activity to ensure success of the QMS is quality planning. This is defined as "a systematic process that translates quality policy into measurable objectives and requirements, and lays down a sequence of steps for realizing them within a specified timeframe."[2] A written quality plan provides the framework for implementing and maintaining an effective QMS. This should be a living document that is reviewed and edited as needed.

QUALITY MANAGEMENT SYSTEMS APPROACH

To develop and implement a QMS, it is important for organizations to follow a planned path. The steps of this path include:

1. Determining the needs and expectations of the customer and other interested parties.
2. Establishing a quality policy and quality objectives.
3. Determining the processes needed to obtain those quality objectives and who is responsible for those processes.
4. Ensuring adequate resources are available to execute those processes.
5. Determining and applying methods to evaluate those processes, including making a determination of the effectiveness and efficiency of each process.
6. Designing ways to prevent nonconformances and ways to correct nonconformances that are not prevented.
7. Establishing a process for continual improvement of the QMS.

Such an approach can be used to develop a QMS or to maintain and improve an existing QMS. The needs and expectations of the customer or interested parties must be defined and documented as fully as possible. The voice of the customer is critical to success. Once an organization understands what customers want, a quality policy and quality objectives should be developed with that information in mind. It is important to consider those who regulate or accredit the organization in the development of the policy and objectives. Although some do not consider these bodies as customers, they certainly have a vested interest in an organization that operates in transfusion medicine or cellular therapies. Resources to achieve the objectives must be determined, and then there must be a way to ensure that they are adequate. As described further in the next section, once the policy, objectives, and procedures are in place, methods to evaluate the effectiveness and efficiency of these are necessary. A major goal is to find ways to prevent nonconformances from happening in the first place, but because of the nature of the work, nonconformances will occur. When they do, it is imperative to have a method to detect and correct nonconformances and prevent them from happening again. Finally, because a quality system is somewhat dynamic, a philosophy of continual improvement needs to be developed and executed.

EVALUATION OF THE QUALITY MANAGEMENT SYSTEM

It is important to evaluate the QMS routinely to determine if it is working as expected. The evaluation should include the following items:

- Engagement of the stakeholders.
- Purpose of the evaluation.
- Audience for the evaluation.
- Information needed for the evaluation.
- Sources for information related to the evaluation.
- Tools.

Evaluation of the QMS begins with the engagement of those who have vested interest in the results of the evaluation. In blood establishments and cellular therapy facilities, stakeholders most often include quality, operations, and management but might include other areas such as recruitment and human resources, depending on what processes are being evaluated. The purpose of the evaluation should be aligned with issues of greatest concern. For example, one area of concern to blood establishments and to their customers is product availability. An evaluation of product availability would provide information as to whether the right product is available at the right time, and opportunities to improve where this falls short. The audience for the evaluation is determined by the stakeholders and usually would include senior management, inventory control, sales, and marketing.

Information needed for the evaluation depends on the purpose and the audience. Once these are decided, then information can be gathered to support decision-making or simply to inform. The information may come from a number of sources: production reports, error reports, audits or inspections, and customer feedback, to name a few.

A number of tools exist to evaluate the information. A tool is any chart, device, software, strategy, or technique that supports quality management efforts. Many of the tools are easy to use, but it is important that the audience be considered when choosing which tools to use. A number of software vendors produce software that is designed specifically to monitor and evaluate the QMS.

THE QUALITY MANAGEMENT SYSTEM IN PRACTICE

Several elements comprise a QMS, and the application of those elements in transfusion medicine and cellular therapies is described in the text that follows. Basic elements of the QMS include:

- Organization and leadership.
- Customer focus.
- Human resources.
- Equipment management.
- Suppliers and materials management.
- Process control and management.
- Documents and records.
- Information management.
- Management of nonconforming events.
- Monitoring and evaluation.
- Process improvement.
- Facilities, work environment, and safety.

Organization and Leadership

An organization must be structured such that the QMS can be well implemented. The structure should facilitate communication throughout the organization. It is also important that clear descriptions of authority and the responsibilities of each role are defined in writing. The role of senior management is fundamental to the success of any QMS. It is the responsibility of leadership to create an environment where individuals are fully engaged in the QMS and to monitor it to ensure that the system operates effectively. Specific duties assigned to top management include:

- Establishing, implementing, and maintaining a quality policy and associated quality goals and objectives.
- Providing adequate resources to carry out the operations of the facility and the QMS.
- Ensuring appropriate design and effective implementation of new or modified processes and procedures.
- Participating in the review and approval of policies, processes, and procedures.
- Enforcing adherence to operational and quality policies, processes, and procedures.
- Overseeing operations and regulatory and accreditation compliance.
- Periodically reviewing and assessing QMS effectiveness.
- Identifying designees and defining their responsibilities when assisting executive management in carrying out these duties.

The individual who is assigned to oversee an organization's quality activities should report to top management. This individual may perform some of the tasks but does not have to personally perform all the quality functions. It is desirable for this individual to operate totally separate from operations, although in smaller organizations the individual may be involved in operational activities as well. The key here is that the individual should never review his or her own work. Quality functions include the following:

- Review and approval of SOPs.
- Review and approval of training plans.

- Monitoring of training effectiveness and competency.
- Review and approval of validation protocols and results.
- Review, validation, and approval of QMS software.
- Development of evaluation criteria for systems.
- Review and approval of suppliers and maintenance of an approved supplier list.
- Review of product specifications.
- Determination of the suitability of products.
- Monitoring and trending.
- Review of reports of adverse reactions, error reports, and complaints.
- Audit of operational functions.
- Inspection oversight and management.
- Reporting to regulators, accrediting bodies, customers, or others as necessary.

Although traditionally the quality department has had responsibility for the majority of these activities, it may be wise to have operations participate in some of these activities, again with the caveat that one does not review one's own work. This reinforces the concept that quality is everyone's responsibility.

Customer Focus

To obtain true quality, it is imperative for an organization to understand the needs and requirements of the customer. Organizations that provide blood components or other cellular products and services have a variety of customers, and each should be considered. Processes and services should be designed and developed with the customer requirements in mind. Customer requirements need to be documented; oftentimes the documentation is contained in a supplier agreement or contract. Once the requirements are established, there should be a mechanism to receive feedback from the customer at regular intervals to determine if the requirements are being met. Such feedback may be obtained from an analysis of key metrics developed in conjunction with the customer (eg, fill rates, on-time delivery, customer complaint rates) or may be gleaned from customer surveys.

Human Resources

The human resources department is focused on activities relating to employees. These activities normally include recruiting, hiring, and training of new employees; training of current employees; employee benefits; management of employee concerns; oversight of performance reviews and necessary corrective actions; retention; and everyday staff needs. Staffing must be adequate to perform the work and to support the QMS.

Job Descriptions

Organizations should have well-written job descriptions for all personnel. The job descriptions should identify the key role and responsibilities of a particular position, as well as educational and experiential requirements. In some cases, the job description also contains physical requirements such as lifting a certain amount of weight or the ability to stand for long hours. Certain requirements in a job description may be the result of regulatory requirements or industry standards. For example, in some states individuals must have certain licenses to perform laboratory testing. Such requirements should be well defined within each job description. Job descriptions should be periodically reviewed to ensure that they are truly reflective of what an individual does in a particular job. Employees should review their job descriptions initially, following revision, and periodically to understand and acknowledge the responsibilities of the position. Often, regulators or accrediting agencies request to see current signed job descriptions during their inspections or assessments of an organization. An additional benefit of a well-written job description is that it serves as an aid to the development of a training curriculum.

Hiring

Human resources oversees the hiring process, which includes activities such as contacting candidates, setting up interviews, and ensuring new employees are oriented. It may also include pre-employment screening such as drug testing. During the hiring process, job qualifications are matched against applicant qualifications, and individuals are selected for hire based on their ability to meet those job qualifications, including training, education, and experience.

Orientation and Training

Orientation is critical for a new employee to get the right start. Each employee needs to understand his or her role, as well as how that role fits into the organization. Orientation training generally will include an overview of the organization and its customers, benefits training, an introduction to cGMP and/or cGTP regulations, privacy training, and safety training.

Specific training for tasks that are performed as part of an individual's actual job usually occurs in the operational department where the individual is hired. Training on SOPs that the individual will need to perform those tasks is required. Additionally, each employee needs to fully understand the cGMP/cGTP requirements applicable in the performance of a job. All training must be documented, and initial and ongoing assessments of competence are required.

Competency Assessments

To ensure that staff maintain the ability to perform their jobs well, routine competency assessments should be conducted to determine their level of competence in performing the work. Organizations need to have a written plan for conducting competency assessments, including what will be done if an individual does not pass. CMS has specific requirements for competency assessments of testing personnel. The minimal regulatory requirements for assessment of competency for such individuals include:

1. Direct observations of routine patient test performance, including patient preparation, if applicable, specimen handling, processing, and testing.
2. Monitoring the recording and reporting of test results.
3. Review of intermediate test results or worksheets, QC records, proficiency testing (PT) results, and preventive maintenance records.

4. Direct observations of the performance of instrument maintenance and function checks.

5. Assessment of test performance through testing previously analyzed specimens, internal blind testing samples, or external PT samples.

6. Assessment of problem-solving skills.

Competency assessment, which includes all six items, must be performed for testing personnel for each test the individual is approved to perform by the director of the CLIA-certified laboratory.[3]

The competency program should be documented and administered to all staff as required. There should be a defined schedule for the administration of the assessments. Documentation of the results of competency assessments should be available for inspection by regulatory or accrediting bodies.

Equipment Management

Equipment used in processes must be installed as directed by the manufacturer and qualified to ensure that it is working as intended. This qualification should be accomplished according to written procedures and documented. Installation qualification is necessary as part of validation activities and will be addressed later in this chapter. Organizations must ensure that they operate equipment in line with manufacturers' recommendations, which may include requirements for temperature, humidity, surrounding space, or other environmental conditions for operation.

Equipment must be maintained to ensure proper working conditions. Organizations should have written programs for equipment cleaning and maintenance in line with manufacturers' recommendations. Preventive maintenance should be established and well documented. Records of this work must be available for inspectors or assessors to view.

For equipment used in measurement, routine calibration is required. Calibration involves comparing a measurement device to a known standard and then adjusting it, if necessary, to measure the same as the standard. Routine calibration is a requirement for some equipment. An organization should have a written program

for calibration that lists what should be calibrated, the frequency of calibration, and procedures for performing the calibration. The manufacturer should recommend the frequency of calibration, and regulations can be found in the CFR.[4] However, if no guidance is available, the organization should follow standard practice in the industry or, if none exists, should establish a reasonable frequency based on the criticality of the measurement.

The actual performance of calibration can be outsourced to an approved outside vendor, but it is the organization's responsibility to maintain calibration records and to ensure that the vendor performs the activities in compliance with applicable regulations and standards. Calibration records and procedures need to be available during inspections and assessments.

Equipment QC, performed routinely, is also important in ensuring that equipment is operating as expected. Documentation of any QC that is performed should be evaluated in a timely manner, and the results should be evaluated to determine if there are trends over time that may indicate the equipment is beginning to drift. The frequency of QC is dependent on the criticality of the function of the equipment. Equipment used in donor eligibility determination and testing, for example, may require daily QC because of the criticality of its use. Review of QC records needs to be timely to limit the scope of investigation, should the review reveal a problem.

Selection of Equipment

Organizations should select equipment based on its ability to meet preestablished and documented specifications. Other factors that should be considered are cost, service, history with others in the industry, and support. Usually, organizations have several vendors from which to choose, and thus the additional factors become even more important. It is key that organizations establish criteria on the front end of the selection process; the equipment should fit the organization's needs. Workflow should be well defined before selection of equipment. The organization should not have to alter its process to fit the equipment unless there is only one supplier and no other choice. The manufacturer of the equipment should be qualified according to the organization's supplier qualification process.

Equipment Identification

Equipment should be uniquely identified, and a list of equipment should be maintained. This list should be kept up to date, and when equipment is moved from one location to another or removed from service, the action taken should be recorded. Because of the amount of equipment in an organization that performs blood banking, transfusion medicine, or cellular therapy activities, tracking equipment can be a daunting task. Software vendors have developed automated solutions to assist organizations with this, but even if it must be done manually, the tracking of equipment is necessary. Equipment that is out of service should be removed from operational areas, if at all possible, and clearly labeled as out of service so it will not be used in the manufacturing process.

Suppliers and Materials Management

Ensuring that a supplier can provide what is needed to perform the work and that the supplies meet preestablished specifications is a critical aspect of the QMS. Organizations must determine and document requirements and seek suppliers, through the process of supplier qualification, that meet those requirements.

Supplier Qualification

Supplier qualification is a process whereby an organization determines whether or not a supplier can meet its requirements. Such requirements usually include the ability to meet regulations, the availability of supply, the timeliness of delivery, responsiveness to issues and problems, cost, and support. Other requirements may be specific to the organization. It is a common practice for organizations to participate in buying groups that perform qualification of suppliers for those participating in the group.

Supplier qualification may include written surveys or on-site audits of the supplier and review of written surveys completed by current customers. Surveys may be more cost effective, but on-site audits are generally considered best if the supplier is providing materials or services that are critical to operations. In fact, the more critical the materials supplied, the more stringent the qualification should be. See Table 1-1 for a list of factors that may be considered during supplier qualification.

An organization should maintain a list of approved suppliers. This list should be reviewed routinely for each supplier's ability to consistently meet the needs of the organization. Suppliers

TABLE 1-1. Factors to Consider in Supplier Qualification

Factor	Examples
Licensure, certification, or accreditation	FDA, ISO, EU
Supplier-relevant quality documents	Quality manual, complaint-handling methodology
Results of audits or inspections	Previous FDA inspections, supplier qualification audit
Supply or product requirements	Ability to meet functional requirements
Cost of materials and services	Product cost, maintenance fees, parts costs
Delivery arrangements	Standing orders, turnaround time for stat
Financial security and market position	How long the organization has been in business, IRS 990
Support after sale	Training, validation guidance, contract/agreement review meetings

FDA = Food and Drug Administration; ISO = International Organization for Standardization; EU = European Union; IRS 990 = Internal Revenue Service Form 990.

can be added or removed from the list as necessary. Management of the list usually falls to the quality department, although it could be placed in an area such as purchasing, with quality oversight.

Contracts and Agreements

It is common practice to develop a written contract or agreement with a supplier that stipulates the organization's requirements and expectations. The document should define the role of both the organization and the supplier in the relationship and should also stipulate the manner in which the supplier will operate to meet the organization's needs. It is a good idea to establish and document metrics that can be monitored on a regular basis. If metrics indicate that there is a problem, corrective actions should be taken and documented. If the problem cannot be corrected, it may mean that the supplier should be removed from the approved list.

AABB standards stipulate that organizations should monitor their agreements. Other organizations have similar requirements. For example, The Joint Commission requires that hospital blood banks establish metrics with their blood suppliers that are evaluated routinely. The evaluation of metrics should be documented, as well as any corrective actions required of the supplier as a result of failure to meet the expectations.

Receipt and Inspection of Incoming Supplies

When supplies are initially received, it is important that they are physically separated from supplies that are in use until they can be inspected for suitability for use. Some organizations have caged areas where incoming supplies are quarantined until inspected; others use shelving and labeling, often with color coding, to quarantine incoming supplies. The incoming inspection and release is most commonly performed by the quality department, but in some instances, operations may conduct the inspection for quality.

Organizations should develop criteria for acceptance, and incoming supplies should be inspected against such criteria. Both external packaging and the contents of that packaging should be inspected for acceptance. If there is something wrong with the product or packag-

ing, the product must be quarantined, either physically or with clear labeling, until disposition is determined by the quality department. Supplies not meeting the preestablished criteria should remain in quarantine, and the supplier should be notified of the issue. The inspection should be conducted according to a written procedure, and there should be documentation of the suitability of the supplies or their disposition, if found unsuitable. Most often these supplies are returned to the supplier, but they may be discarded if the supplier does not need them for further investigation.

Process Control and Management

Process control is the sum of activities involved in ensuring a process is predictable, stable, and consistently operating at the target level of performance with only normal variation. Important aspects of process control include:

- SOPs.
- Process validation.
- Computer system validation.
- Test method validation.
- QC.
- Training.
- Tracking and trending.

Standard Operating Procedures

SOPs provide instruction on how to perform a task and are key to achieving consistency and control in operations. A full discussion of SOPs is provided in the "Documents and Records" section (further below).

Process Validation

One of the most important aspects of process control is the initial establishment that a process consistently works to produce a desired result; that is, the validation of the process. Process validation is defined as the collection and evaluation of data, from the process-design stage through commercial production, that establish scientific evidence that a process is capable of consistently delivering a high-quality product.[5] Validation establishes that a process has consistent results that meet predetermined requirements. Validations should be performed for all critical processes according to a written validation protocol. The protocol should contain the following:

- System description.
- Purpose of the validation.
- Risk assessment.
- Responsibilities.
- Test cases.
- Acceptance criteria.
- Problem-reporting mechanism.
- Approval signatures.
- Supporting documentation.

The system description identifies the components of the system used for the process and includes a description of how those components work together during the process. It should also include environmental conditions under which the system operates, as applicable, and any utility specifications.

The purpose of the validation is usually straightforward. Validations may be conducted because a process is new or something significant has changed within the process, and assurance is needed that the process still remains in a validated state. A process validation has three phases: installation qualification, operational qualification, and performance qualification. Installation qualification ensures that any equipment used within the process is installed appropriately and is qualified to perform as the manufacturer states. This evaluation should ensure that the environment, including utilities, is appropriate for its operation as defined by the manufacturer. It also ensures that necessary SOPs are written, training is developed, and staff are trained in the execution of related SOPs. Operational qualification demonstrates that the process operates as intended, and it focuses on the process capability (worst-case challenges). The final phase, performance qualification, demonstrates that the process works as expected in a normal working environment.

Although a manufacturer usually does a significant amount of validation work before bringing equipment or software to market, the end user still has to perform the user's own validation. For example, computer software vendors

do a tremendous amount of testing of the software to determine limitations, etc; yet, the user of that software must validate the software in the user's environment with the user's staff and SOPs. Consultants may be used to assist with validation, but final validation and the results of that validation are the responsibility of the end user. The amount of validation work needed is dependent on the process, its criticality, and the ability to test the end result 100% of the time or not. (See Fig 1-2.)

A risk assessment aids in the determination of how much testing must be done. The more risk a process introduces, the more testing an organization normally does. This is especially important when there is no way to test the end result of a process other than destructive testing. If the process is not a high-risk or critical process, then less testing may be done, as the organization is willing to accept the risk should the process not work as expected.

Within a validation there are multiple roles. The individual who writes the validation protocol is responsible for ensuring it is complete and contains all the necessary information and sufficient test cases to obtain the degree of assurance desired. Those who execute the validation protocol must have training in the process and may often be individuals who will perform the process routinely, although this is not always the case. The quality department and others, as appropriate, approve the validation protocol and the final results of the validation before a process is implemented.

Test cases should be developed to test the various parameters of the process and to challenge the process as much as reasonable. The more testing that is performed, the more assurance that the process works consistently, but it is not always possible to perform enough tests to get 100% assurance. Usually an organization seeks a comfort level of testing that is reasonable and in line with industry standards. Each test case should have expected results. If those results are not obtained, a problem report must be executed, and there should be a resolution before proceeding. Failure of a test case could be the result of improper installation qualification, a poorly written test case, an unrealistic expected result, or poor execution of the test case

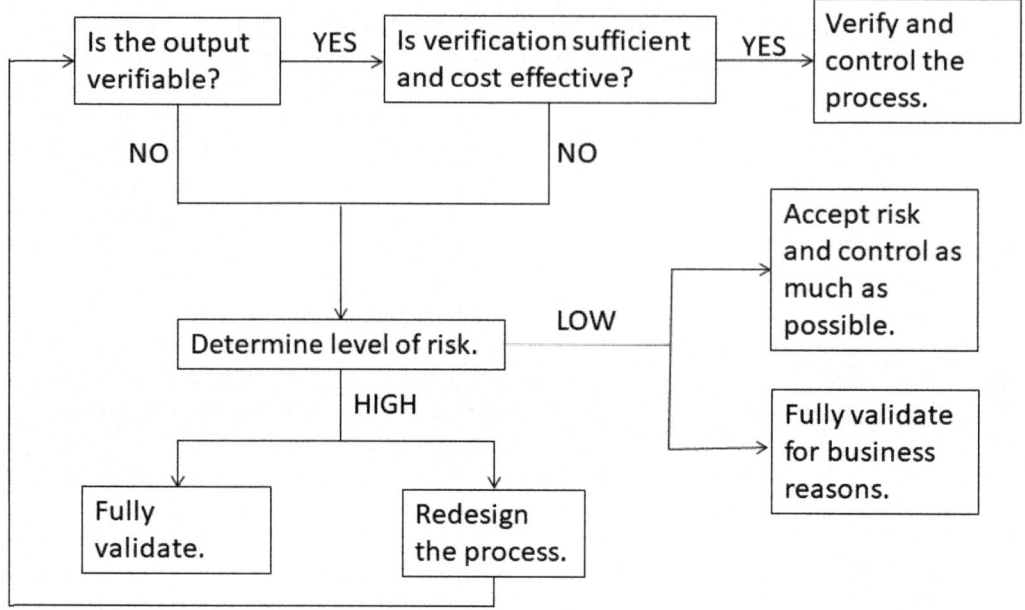

FIGURE 1-2. Process validation tree. Note: If low risk is not acceptable, a process design is usually required to remove residual risk.

itself. If investigation does not produce a cause and a resolution for the issue, then the process itself may have to be changed, or the process may be implemented with limitations that are documented within the validation summary.

The acceptance criteria for a validation must be documented before the validation work begins. This criteria should not be changed in the middle of a validation unless there is a good reason to change it. If change does occur, the validation protocol must be amended, and the amended protocol must be approved again.

Once the validation protocol is written, it needs approval from operations and quality, at a minimum. In a CLIA laboratory setting, the CLIA laboratory director must also approve validation work. Approval must occur before any execution of test cases. As stated above, if there is good reason to modify the protocol, it is necessary to amend it and have it approved again. The protocol may include supporting documentation such as user manuals or pertinent technical articles.

The validation proves the process is consistent and produces an end result that meets spec-

ifications. During the validation, an organization may uncover the following:

- Design flaws.
- Inadequate requirements.
- Errors in SOPs.
- Errors in user manuals.
- Training deficiencies.
- Incompatibilities with interfaces.
- Incompatibilities with the physical environment.
- Misconceptions about process capabilities.

Following completion of the test cases, a validation summary is normally written. This summary describes the expected and observed results and whether or not those results are acceptable. It also delineates any problems encountered during the validation and what was done to resolve those problems. It defines any process limitations, either known before beginning the validation or discovered during the validation. Finally, it contains a conclusion based on the results. Before implementing the process, the validation summary should be reviewed and approved, again by operations, quality, and the medical director, as appropriate. Supporting documentation may accompany the summary, as well as a timeline for implementation of the process, although this is often a separate document. It is important to remember that although a validation gives an organization confidence in its processes and significantly reduces the need for end-product testing, no validation, no matter how extensive, can test every possibility or control the human element. Continual process monitoring is needed to ensure the process remains in a validated state.

Computer System Validation

A computer system is composed of hardware, software, peripheral devices, networks, personnel, and documentation. Validation of the computer system in the environment where it will be used by those who will use it is required. This also includes validation of interfaces between systems. For example, a blood establishment would need to validate the interface between its BECS and a testing instrument. Although much work is done by the vendors who develop software, the end user must still perform a validation and may even repeat work that the vendor has already done to ensure that testing is performed under the environmental and process conditions experienced by the end user. An important part of validating a computer system is to ensure that the system can still operate when stressed. The FDA has issued guidance to assist organizations in the performance of computer system validation.[6]

Test Method Validation

When laboratories wish to implement a non-waived test using an FDA-approved or -cleared test system, CLIA requires that the performance specifications established by the manufacturer be verified by the laboratory before it reports patient results.[7] At a minimum, the laboratory must demonstrate that it can obtain performance specifications comparable to those of the manufacturer for accuracy, precision, reportable range, and reference intervals (normal values).

If the laboratory develops its own method, introduces a test system not subject to FDA approval or clearance, or makes modifications to an FDA-approved or -cleared test system, or if the manufacturer does not provide performance specifications, then the laboratory must establish the test system performance specifications before reporting patient results.[7] At a minimum, the following must be established for the test system:

- Accuracy.
- Precision.
- Reportable range of test results for the test system.
- Reference intervals (normal values).
- Analytical sensitivity.
- Analytical specificity, including interfering substances.
- Any other performance characteristic required for test performance (eg, specimen or reagent stability).

Based on performance specifications, the laboratory must also establish calibration and control procedures and document all activities for test method validation. Title 42 CFR, Part 493.1253 provides additional information on this.

Quality Control

QC is an important aspect of process control. It ensures the proper functioning of materials, reagents, equipment, and methods. QC is an event that is different from validation in that it is not repeated to gain assurance of consistency, but rather it is repeated at a given frequency to ensure results are within acceptable ranges, and also over time to determine if any trends are developing that might indicate something is eventually going to fail. The frequency of QC testing is usually determined by the criticality of what is being tested. Some QC frequency is dictated by regulatory or accrediting bodies such as the FDA.[4] Additional information on QC frequency is provided in Appendix 1-3. All QC should be well documented to include who did the testing, the date it was done, the results, and whether or not the testing was acceptable. Documentation should be concurrent with the performance of the testing, and records should be available for future inspections or assessments.

Unacceptable QC results should be evaluated, and the process should not continue until the issue is resolved. Corrective actions may be necessary before acceptable QC can be obtained. Items that fail QC should be marked "not for use" until the issue is resolved. Because QC is performed on a schedule, if a failure occurs, it may be necessary to assess product produced since the last acceptable QC result. This is clearly why determining the criticality of what is being tested is important; the more frequent the QC, the less product is involved in the evaluation.

Training

Orientation training is critical for new employees and is discussed along with specific job training and competency assessment in the "Human Resources" section. Workplace safety training is detailed in Chapter 2.

Tracking and Trending

Tracking is an integral part of record-keeping and is noted in the following section ("Documents and Records"). Trending is a concept embodied in many quality system activities.

Documents and Records

Documentation is important in that it provides evidence and details of what was done. Good documentation can provide full traceability (details) and trackability (a logical sequence of steps) in the execution of processes. Organizations involved in the production of blood and cellular products create many documents and records. These include:

- Quality manuals.
- Policies and process documents.
- SOPs.
- Work instructions.
- Job aids.
- Forms.
- Labels.

Document Creation

Documents should be created in a consistent manner. An SOP should be in place to define the format of documents as well as the review and approval process, both initially and at routine intervals. Documents should have unique identification (eg, numbering system), and changes to documents should be made in a controlled manner (change control). Document control is a key element of process control. Many organizations now have computerized document control systems that are validated for activities such as document development, routing for review and approval, controlled printing, revision, and archival. Most organizations are moving away from paper documentation as much as possible. Back-up documents are required, however, for those instances when computers are down.

Quality Manual

The quality manual is one of the most important documents in a blood or cellular therapy establishment. The quality manual describes the organization's quality policy, quality objectives, and overall approach to quality in all aspects of the business. It defines how the organization is structured (organization chart) to ensure implementation of the quality system and defines the roles of staff, including line staff all the way up to senior management. It points out how the quality system integrates with operational tasks and how those tasks are monitored to ensure quality outcomes.

Policies and Process Documents

Policies describe the manner in which an organization operates. They are high-level documents describing the position that an organization takes on a particular topic. Not all policies are regulated. For example, a dress code policy or a tobacco use policy is not required by any regulatory or accrediting bodies, but if an organization wants staff to dress a particular way or to avoid the use of tobacco in the work place, a policy is a good way to document and communicate the information. As necessary, policies are supported by other forms of documentation within an organization, such as SOPs and forms.

Process documents are also high level and describe the inputs for a process, the conversion that takes place, and the output of a process. A process document provides the big picture and may take the form of a flow chart. This is particularly helpful when trying to understand a process at a high level and when introducing concepts to personnel in training.

Standard Operating Procedures and Work Instructions

SOPs describe who does what and when (in sequence or order); they describe the steps of a process. Well-written SOPs provide the "how" in performing a process. They should be detailed enough for a trained individual to perform the task, but not so detailed that they are unnecessarily restrictive. SOPs should be written with input from subject-matter experts and should be validated to ensure that they are effective. SOP validation usually involves an individual performing the task using the SOP as written. The individual notes whether the steps in the SOP make sense, whether the steps can be performed as written, and if the desired outcome is achieved. Finalized SOPs should be reviewed and approved by the appropriate department personnel and the medical director, as appropriate, and then approved by quality before becoming effective and released. Staff should receive training on all SOPs applicable to their jobs, and SOPs must be accessible at all times to staff performing the work.

SOPs need to be periodically reviewed to ensure that they are current and are reflective of the work as it is being done. Some organizations review a portion of their SOPs each quarter to ensure that the entire collection of SOPs is reviewed at the required interval.

Work instructions provide step-by-step instructions for how a task is performed. They are more specific and more detailed than procedures. Not all organizations have work instructions; some organizations choose to just use the term *procedure* for all step-by-step documents. Whatever term an organization chooses, the documents describing how the work is done still need to be controlled and managed in a consistent manner. Changes to SOPs and/or work in-

structions need to be made in a controlled manner that allows for the changes to be approved, made, validated, and communicated to all stakeholders before implementation. Retraining may be necessary for significant SOP changes.

Job Aids

A job aid is an excerpt from an approved procedure or work instruction. These are often used when a portion of the SOP has a table or information that must be frequently referenced. Job aids must be controlled just as procedures and work instructions, and there should be a way to reference a job aid to the procedure it represents. Uncontrolled job aids should not be allowed. Job aids may be included as hyperlinks in computerized documents.

Forms

Blank forms provide templates for the capture of information. Once completed, a form becomes a record providing objective evidence of work performed and subject to record retention requirements. Forms should be managed within document control and should be designed by individuals with experience; it is not true that anyone can design a form. Often mistakes can be avoided by careful form design. If the form is not self-explanatory, instructions on how to complete it should be available, and individuals should receive training on completion of the form. This will reduce the likelihood of errors. Forms may be included as part of SOPs and may be hyperlinked in computerized documents.

Labels

Although not always thought of as a document, labels need to be created and maintained within the document control system to ensure that the label is correct, meets regulatory requirements, and is current. Changes to labels need to be managed just as changes to documents are: within a controlled system, reviewed for accuracy and compliance, and approved. Certain labels must be submitted to the FDA for approval.[8] Organizations must maintain a current master set of labels for reference.

Document Maintenance

As previously stated, documents should be created and maintained in a controlled manner. Version control is critical. Organizations also need to have a mechanism whereby changes to documents can be requested and communicated once those changes have occurred. A document history that records changes to a document should be developed and maintained. When a document is revised, and the revised copy is approved and released, an archived copy of the original version should be retained for future reference.

Organizations should prepare a master list of all the various types of documents in use. This list should define the most current version, how many copies are out, and where those copies are located. This aids in document control; when revisions occur, it helps to ensure that all old copies of the documents are removed and replaced with the revised version.

Records

Records are the evidence of what was done and prove that procedures were followed and documentation of the work performed was captured. Records should be created concurrently with the performance of the work, documenting each critical step. Good records provide the details (traceability—who, what, when, where, how) and a logical sequence of steps taken (trackability). It is also important that records are permanent, which means that indelible ink should be used. Any corrections should be made in a manner that allows one to see what the error was, who performed the correction, and when. Records should be managed so that the following aspects are addressed:

- Creation and identification of records.
- Confidentiality.
- Protection of the integrity of records.
- Protection from inadvertent destruction.
- Protection from damage from rodents, fire, and water.
- Storage and retrieval.
- Retention.
- Destruction.

Policies, process documents, procedures, and completed forms are also examples of records found in an organization involved in transfusion medicine and/or cellular therapy, and describe how the work was being performed at any particular time in the organization's history. The records may be in paper or electronic form and must be easily identified. There should also be information as to who created the record. Because organizations may use both signatures and initials, it is necessary to maintain a current signature sample and list of initials for all employees. If the identity of the record creator is captured electronically by entry into the computer system or by electronic badge swipe, this needs to be in compliance with electronic record-keeping rules.

Because of the nature of the records created by transfusion medicine or cellular therapy organizations, many records are confidential, especially those containing donor or patient information. Records should never be left where they can be viewed by individuals who have no need to view them. If records containing confidential information are made available to those outside the organization, any confidential information should be redacted.

Records, whether in paper or electronic form, must be protected from unauthorized changes, from inadvertent destruction, and from damage caused by rodents, fire, or water. Record storage should be designed to accomplish these goals. It also should allow the records to be retrieved easily. Access to records should be restricted, particularly if the records contain confidential information.

Organizations need to have a written record-retention policy that is compliant with regulations and standards; records should be retained in accordance with that policy. Once a record has reached its "end of life," it should be discarded in a manner that protects any confidential information. Such destruction methods include shredding, burning, and degaussing (a method to magnetically erase data from electronic storage media, eg, hard drives).

Many organizations outsource record storage, retrieval, retention, and destruction to offsite vendors. Such vendors should be qualified, and organizations need to ensure timely access to their records for inspections and assessments.

If records are stored electronically, an organization must ensure that the integrity of the electronic data is protected from unauthorized changes. Additionally, the data must be stored in a manner that would not cause inadvertent loss of data from overwriting, physical damage, or system crashes. Data integrity should be assessed periodically.

Organizations must have a documented mechanism for error correction for paper documents and for electronic documents. In both cases, it is important that the error is not obliterated. The common industry practice for correcting errors on paper documents is to draw a single line through the error, write the correction above it and then initial and date the correction. If an explanation for the correction is needed, this can be written alongside the correction. If there is insufficient room, an asterisk can be used and the explanation written elsewhere on the document, even on the back. Electronic document maintenance should allow an audit trail to show what the error was, what correction was made, who made it, and when it was made.

Information Management

Organizations have a tremendous amount of information that must be managed as part of the quality system, and much of that information, as previously stated, must be confidentially maintained. Access to information should be limited to those who need the information for work purposes. The integrity of data, both written and electronic, must be guarded. Unauthorized copying of information, whether paper or electronic, should not be allowed. If documents are maintained in a paper state and contain highly confidential information, they should be in locked file cabinets, and if stored electronically, they should be protected by access rights. Although the topic is not within the scope of this chapter, organizations that store protected health information must be compliant with the Health Insurance Portability and Accountability Act (HIPAA). More information on HIPAA may be found at www.hhs.gov/hipaa.

Backup of critical electronic information is important. Backups should be routinely run, and there should be written procedures to restore any data that may be inadvertently lost. Records should be retained according to written policies that ensure the timely destruction of documents that are no longer necessary.

Management of Nonconforming Events

Because nonconformances are inevitable in any system that involves human involvement, the QMS should contain processes and procedures to detect, document, investigate, correct, and follow up on nonconforming events such as the production of a product that does not meet specifications. Such processes and procedures must be in line with regulations and applicable standards and should include the following:

- Documentation of the event, either electronically or on paper, with some sort of classification, usually based on the severity of the risk.
- Determination of the effect, if any, on the quality of products or services.
- Evaluation of the effect on interrelated activities.
- Investigation and root cause analysis.
- Selection of appropriate corrective action.
- Implementation of corrective action, as appropriate.
- Notification and recall.
- Implementation of appropriate preventive action.
- Reporting to external agencies when required.
- Evaluation of the effectiveness of the corrective and preventive action (CAPA) taken.

Staff should be trained to find and report nonconformances, which include errors, accidents, and adverse reactions in donors and recipients. It is important to capture the facts of the event in sufficient detail to allow a complete and thorough investigation.

It is critically important, once a nonconformance is discovered, to determine the impact of that nonconformance on products and/or services. If the nonconformance has a negative impact on product quality, it may be necessary to quarantine the product(s) or to perform a recall if the product has been distributed. The sooner an organization can gain control of the affected product, the better. Organizations should always consider the impact on their products and/or services as soon as possible after discovery of a nonconformance.

It is also a good idea to determine if the nonconformance has impact on other areas of the organization's operations. It may be necessary to involve more than one department in the investigation to fully understand what occurred and its impact.

Not all nonconformances require a full investigation, but there is normally some level of investigation required for most nonconformances. A thorough investigation may involve interviewing staff, reviewing training records, direct observation of the process, and reviewing SOPs. Also, investigations may involve other record review or review of data to determine the extent of the nonconformance.

Root cause analysis is a collective term that describes a wide range of approaches, tools, and techniques used to uncover causes of problems. A root cause analysis to determine the cause or causes of the nonconformance is often necessary. It is important to continue to ask why, to determine the true root cause(s). Without finding the true cause of a nonconformance, it is possible that the problem will recur. If the root cause is fixed, the problem should not recur. Although there is substantial debate on the definition of *root cause*, the following are considered true[9]:

- Root causes are specific underlying causes.
- Root causes are those that can reasonably be identified.
- Root causes are those management has control to fix.
- Root causes are those for which effective recommendations for preventing recurrences can be generated.

There are several tools that are useful in performing a root cause analysis. These include brainstorming, useful in generating potential causes; a fishbone diagram, useful in determining causes and contributing factors; a failure mode effects analysis (FMEA), a step-by-step approach for identifying all possible failures in a design, a manufacturing or assembly process, or a product or service; and the five whys, useful for drilling down to the true cause. For the last one, there is no magic to the number five; one may ask fewer or more whys to get to the true cause of a nonconformance. (See Fig 1-3.)

Once the root cause has been identified, it is then important to select an appropriate corrective action. The action should fix the issue, but at the same time, the corrective action must be reasonable. For example, if the true fix for a problem is a new computer system to capture specific data accurately, this cannot be accomplished quickly, so a more reasonable alternative may need to be chosen until the new computer system can be implemented. Also, although it seems intuitive, it should be noted that an organization must ensure the corrective action actually addresses the true issue and is not merely addressing a symptom of the problem. In the example given, the organization may choose to implement a newly designed form to reduce the likelihood of error or may implement a second review for accuracy. A note of caution here, however, is that simply adding more review seldom fixes the problem. In fact additional review can sometimes make things worse.

As part of corrective action, notification of customers about the nonconformance may be necessary, and it may be necessary to recall additional product, depending on the scope of the issue and the results of the investigation. The organization should have a documented process for these actions.

Correcting the nonconformance is important, but equally important is determining if there are actions that can be taken to prevent the issue from recurring ever again. There are short-term corrective actions, which fix the problem temporarily, and long-term corrective actions, which normally include preventive action and permanently fix the problem. Finding the best way to minimize the likelihood of the problem recurring while maintaining the ability to operate within the constraints of limited resources is key.

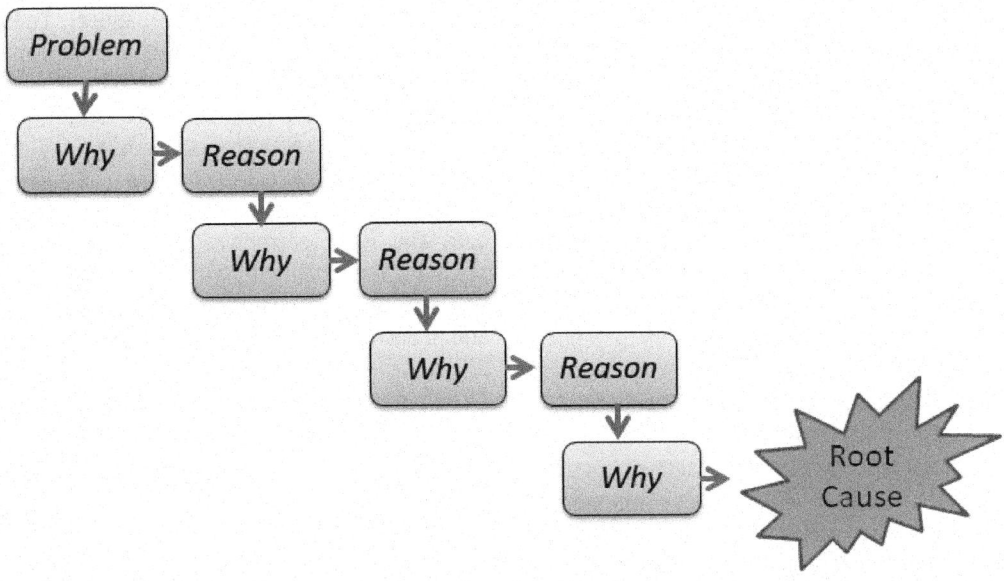

FIGURE 1-3. The five whys. Note: There is no magic to asking five times; it may take more or less to get to the root cause.

Preventive actions should be implemented whenever possible. For example, proper training might be considered a preventive action if it is determined that a nonconformance resulted from a lack of training. In this instance, training might be considered both a corrective and a preventive action. It fixes the current problem, and it prevents future occurrences at the same time.

Depending on the nature of the nonconformance, regulatory bodies or accrediting agencies may need notification as well. Processes and procedures should include information on whom to notify and when. A voluntary recall is instituted for nonconforming product that has been distributed. In-house products can be dealt with directly.

Fatalities related to blood collection or transfusion or to cellular therapy products must be reported as soon as possible to the FDA Center for Biologics Evaluation and Research (CBER). [See 21 CFR 606.170(b) and 1271.350(a)(i), respectively.] Instructions for reporting to CBER are available in published guidance[10] and on the FDA website.[11] A written follow-up report must be submitted within 7 days of the fatality and should include a description of any new procedures implemented to avoid recurrence. AABB *Association Bulletin #04-06* provides additional information on these reporting requirements, including a form for reporting donor fatalities.[12]

Regardless of their licensure and registration status with the FDA, all donor centers, blood banks, and transfusion services must promptly report biological product deviations (BPDs)—and information relevant to these events—to the FDA[13,14] using Form FDA 3486 when the event 1) is associated with manufacturing (ie, collecting, testing, processing, packing, labeling, storing, holding, or distributing); 2) represents a deviation from cGMP, established specifications, or applicable regulations or standards, or that is unexpected or unforeseen; 3) may affect the product's safety, purity, or potency; 4) occurs while the facility had control of, or was responsible for, the product; and 5) involves a product that has left the facility's control (ie, has been distributed).

Using the same form, facilities must also promptly report BPDs associated with a distributed cellular therapy product if the event represents a deviation from applicable regulations, standards, or established specifications that relate to the prevention of communicable disease transmission or contamination of the product. This requirement pertains to events that are unexpected or unforeseeable but may relate to the transmission or potential transmission of a communicable disease or may lead to product contamination.[15] More information concerning BPD reporting can be found on the FDA website.[16]

There must also be a mechanism to report medical device adverse events to the FDA and the device manufacturer.[17] The Joint Commission encourages reporting of sentinel events, including hemolytic transfusion reactions involving the administration of blood or components having major blood group incompatibilities.[18,19]

Hemovigilance reporting provides an opportunity to detect, investigate, and respond to adverse transfusion reactions and events that result in nonconformances. A number of organizations monitor such data, including FDA and the Centers for Disease Control and Prevention (CDC).

Monitoring and Evaluation

Organizations should have a system for monitoring and evaluating the effectiveness of the organization's processes. This system should be defined as part of the QMS. Monitoring can occur at various levels: the level of input to the process, the in-process activities, the results, or the process, or even the system in which the process resides. Although record review and analysis are ongoing forms of monitoring, the use of internal and external assessments of the processes is very useful. Assessments may include comparison of actual to expected results and can consist of quality assessments, peer reviews, self-assessments, and PT.

Organizations should have a process that describes how internal assessments are conducted. Each assessment should be well planned and conducted according to the plan. Assessors may look at data such as quality indicators and other quality records, observe processes as they are performed, or interview staff to determine if knowledge of processes and procedures is adequate, particularly for those events that are rare (eg, severe syncope or machine failure). The assessment should cover the QMS and, at a minimum, processes that are critical to the organization's operations. When issues are found during the assessment, the process should include a mechanism to respond to those issues, ensuring that important stakeholders are aware of the issues and what corrective actions, if any, are planned. The quality department should take responsibility for oversight of these assessments and to ensure that actions are taken as warranted.

Quality Indicators

Quality indicators are statistical measures that give an indication of output quality. They are useful in the evaluation of customer requirements, personnel, inventory management, and process control and stability (this list is not all inclusive). Quality indicators may be based on outcomes such as quantity-not-sufficient (QNS) rates, or they may be based on the process's ability to deliver an expected result consistently. As an example of a process quality indicator, if a customer requires stat deliveries to arrive within 1 hour, the percentage of deliveries that meet the customer's requirement is a measurement of the ability of the process to deliver within the required time frame. Organizations should establish alert limits for quality indicators; involving the customer is important in making sure that alert limits are appropriately set.

Organizations should communicate quality indicator results frequently so stakeholders are aware of how the organization is performing. Customers may want to be included in this reporting. Run charts, control charts, and bar charts are often useful in displaying quality indicator data. Control charts allow an organization to see if the process is operating as expected; if not, corrective actions are indicated.

Blood Utilization

In recent years, organizations have become even more focused on blood utilization patterns. This is driven by the desire to decrease costs and to provide better patient care. Patient blood management (PBM) as a discipline has come to the forefront; many organizations now have a staff member devoted to transfusion safety: the transfusion safety officer (TSO). Utilization committees review physician ordering and transfusion practices routinely. The committees also review sample collection and labeling, adverse events in patients, near-miss events, outdates, discard, appropriateness of use, and compliance. Many hospitals have set up order alerts in the hospital computer system to appear when physicians order outside of established guidelines. AABB has published clinical practice guidelines for red cell and platelet transfusion.[20,21]

Alternatives to red cell transfusion, such as preoperative anemia treatment, are under study or have been incorporated into routine practice in many health-care settings in efforts to decrease the need for transfusions. Physicians are asked to use data to determine if a second transfusion is warranted instead of issuing a blanket order for transfusion of 2 units, a common practice among transfusing physicians. (See Fig 1-4 for an example of this kind of improvement seen as a result of the implementation of a PBM program in a large teaching hospital.) The use of thromboelastography (TEG) or thromboelastometry (TEM) to guide physicians on when to transfuse to correct coagulation factor levels is now common practice. In addition to providing better patient care, PBM limits needless transfusions, thereby saving dollars and ensuring components are available for those who need them most.

External Assessments

External assessments are those that are conducted by agencies and organizations that are not affiliated with the facility being assessed. They may be voluntary, as in the case of AABB assessments, or mandatory, as in the case of FDA inspections. Organizations that assess or inspect blood banks, transfusion services, and cellular therapy facilities include the following:

- AABB.
- College of American Pathologists (CAP).
- Commission on Office Laboratory Accreditation (COLA).
- Centers for Medicare and Medicaid Services (CMS).
- The Joint Commission.
- Foundation for the Accreditation of Cellular Therapy (FACT).
- Food and Drug Administration (FDA).
- State health departments.

The list includes both accrediting organizations and regulatory entities. Other agencies such as the Department of Transportation (DOT) and the Nuclear Regulatory Commission (NRC) may assess the organization as well.

Accreditation is voluntary, whereas regulation is the law. The external assessments conducted by these entities are usually against standards or regulations promulgated by the organization that is performing the assessment. Although with any assessment or inspection there is some level of angst, these assessments

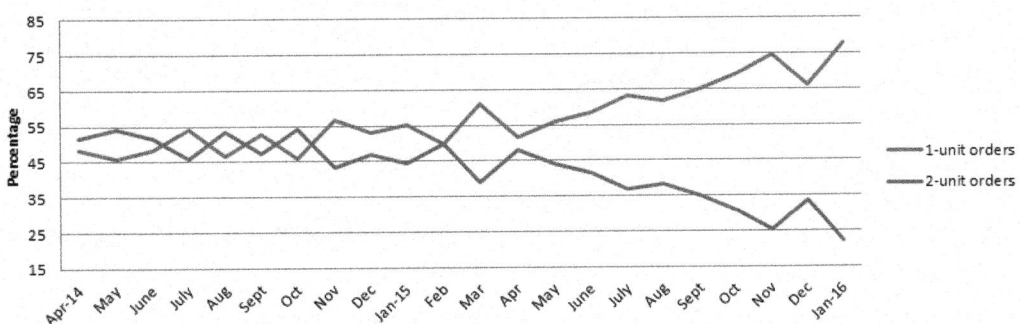

FIGURE 1-4. Results of patient blood management in reducing 2-unit blanket transfusions (lower line) at the University of Tennessee Medical Center Blood Bank, Knoxville, Tennessee. (Courtesy of Dr. Chris Clark and Anna Rains.)

are usually beneficial to the facility and are opportunities for learning and improving operations. It is important that staff are trained on how to conduct themselves during an assessment or inspection, both to decrease their anxiety and to ensure they understand the role and scope of authority for the assessor.

If issues are discovered during an external assessment or inspection, these are usually documented and provided to the facility in an exit meeting. The facility should perform root cause analysis and implement corrective actions as required. Normally the facility will submit a written response to the entity performing the external assessment. Just as with internal assessments, management needs to be well informed of the findings and corrective actions related to those findings.

Proficiency Testing

PT is the testing of samples previously unknown to a laboratory that are sent by a CMS-approved PT program. There are a number of organizations that provide PT samples; AABB, for example, provides PT for immunohematology reference laboratories. Normally a facility will perform at least three testing events each year. PT samples should be managed as any other samples that the laboratory tests, and the testing should be rotated among staff so that different individuals are tested. Submitted results are compared to other laboratories, and a pass/fail determination is assigned. Accrediting organizations monitor the PT results for facilities they accredit. When failures occur, it is expected that the facility will conduct an investigation, try to find the root cause of the issue, and implement any CAPA that is needed. Additionally, the accrediting body may require subsequent submission of one or more surveys following a failure to ensure the testing process remains in control and the CAPA was effective.

Process Improvement

Continuous improvement is a tenet of any quality program, and organizations that manufacture blood components or cellular therapy products should have processes in place that allow for continuous improvement in operations and in patient safety. Such processes should include a method to determine root causes of issues along with appropriate corrective and preventive actions and an evaluation of the effectiveness of those actions. Information gleaned from the nonconformance management system should be used to improve operations. This is a primary benefit of an effective nonconformance management process. Other sources of improvement opportunities include:

- Customer-supplier established metrics.
- Complaints.
- QC records.
- PT.
- Internal audits.
- Quality indicators.
- External assessments.
- Financial analysis of operations.

Many organizations combine the principles of Lean manufacturing and Six Sigma as part of their continuous improvement processes. Lean Six Sigma is "a managerial approach that combines Six Sigma methods and tools of the Lean manufacturing/lean enterprise philosophy, striving to eliminate waste of physical resources, time, effort, and talent, while ensuring quality in production and organizational processes."[22] Lean Six Sigma has two objectives: 1) a focus on eliminating non-value-added steps in processes and 2) eliminating defects and improving the overall process. Lean Six Sigma uses the define, measure, analyze, improve, and control (DMAIC) method—a five-step approach to process improvement. (See Table 1-2.) This approach can be used not only for problem-solving but also for process improvement. Organizations that have implemented Lean Six Sigma have made significant improvements in their processes while saving valuable resources.

Facilities, Work Environment, and Safety

Facilities must be adequate for the work performed and must be maintained to provide a safe environment for staff, patients, donors, and visitors. The facility itself must be clean and orderly so as not to jeopardize staff or product

TABLE 1-2. DMAIC Process

- **D**efine the problem, improvement activity, opportunity for improvement, project goals, and customer (internal and external) requirements

- **M**easure process performance

- **A**nalyze the process to determine root causes of variation, poor performance (defects)

- **I**mprove process performance by addressing and eliminating the root causes

- **C**ontrol the improved process and future process performance

safety. Sufficient space is necessary within the facility to prevent mix-ups during the performance of processes, and building utilities, ventilation, sanitation, trash, and hazardous substance disposal must support the organization's operations. Safety concerns include general safety components such as the use of nonslip surfaces and proper lifting techniques, as well as fire safety, biologic and chemical safety, radiation safety, and disaster preparedness, response, and recovery.

A written disaster plan that addresses both internal and external disasters is crucial for the organization, addressing what to do in the event of a disaster to maintain safety for staff and to maintain business continuity as much as possible. Staff must have training in safety and on the disaster plan itself. A routine test of the disaster plan, including the various scenarios that might produce disaster situations, needs to be exercised under the oversight of management.

KEY POINTS

1. **Organization and Leadership.** A defined organizational structure in addition to top management's support and commitment to the quality policy, goals, and objectives is key to ensuring the success of the quality management system.
2. **Customer Focus.** Quality organizations should understand and meet or exceed customer needs and expectations. These needs and expectations should be defined in a contract, agreement, or other document developed with regular feedback from the customer. Customer feedback is key to identifying process improvement opportunities.
3. **Human Resources.** Quality management of all personnel addresses adequate staffing levels and staff selection, orientation, training, and competency assessment, as well as specific regulatory requirements.
4. **Equipment Management.** Critical equipment may include instruments, measuring devices, and computer hardware and software. This equipment must be uniquely identified and operate within defined specifications, as ensured by qualification, calibration, maintenance, and monitoring.
5. **Suppliers and Materials Management.** Suppliers of critical materials and services (ie, those affecting quality) should be qualified, and these requirements should be defined in contracts or agreements. All critical materials should be qualified and then inspected and tested upon receipt to ensure that specifications are met. Unsuitable supplies should be identified, tracked, and reported to the supplier.
6. **Process Control and Management.** A systematic approach to developing new policies, processes, and procedures and controlling changes to them includes process validation, test method validation, computer system validation, equipment qualification, and QC. Validation must be planned and results reviewed and accepted. Validation plans are developed to provide a

high degree of confidence that processes are reliable and reproducible by ensuring appropriate installation qualification of equipment, operational qualification (including personnel training and SOP development), and performance qualification to achieve stated outcomes.

7. **Documents and Records.** Documents include policies, process descriptions, procedures, work instructions, job aids, forms, and labels. Records provide evidence that the process was performed as intended and allow assessment of product and service quality.

8. **Information Management.** Unauthorized access to, or modification or destruction of, data and information must be prevented, and confidentiality of patient and donor records maintained. Data integrity should be assessed periodically, and backup devices, alternative systems, and archived documents maintained.

9. **Management of Nonconforming Events.** Deviations from facility-defined requirements, standards, and regulations must be addressed by identifying, documenting, and classifying occurrences and assessing effects on quality. Root cause analysis is critical in determining appropriate corrective action. Nonconforming events that create potential risk for the public require reporting to external agencies.

10. **Monitoring and Evaluation.** Assessment of facility processes includes internal and external assessments, monitoring of quality indicators, blood utilization assessment, proficiency testing, and analysis of data.

11. **Process Improvement.** Opportunities for improvement may be identified from deviation reports, nonconforming products and services, customer complaints, QC records, proficiency testing results, internal audits, quality indicator monitoring, and external assessments. Process improvement includes determination of root causes, implementation of corrective and preventive actions, and evaluation of the effectiveness of these actions. The implementation of Lean Six Sigma can significantly increase efficiencies and reduce opportunities for error.

12. **Facilities, Work Environment, and Safety.** Procedures related to general safety; biologic, chemical, and radiation safety; fire safety; and disaster preparedness are required. Space allocation, building utilities, ventilation, sanitation, trash, and hazardous substance disposal must support the organization's operations.

REFERENCES

1. Food and Drug Administration. Guideline for quality assurance in blood establishments. (July 11, 1995) Silver Spring, MD: CBER Office of Communication, Outreach, and Development, 1995.

2. Business dictionary. Quality planning. Fairfax, VA: WebFinance, Inc, 2019. [Available at http://www.businessdictionary.com/definition/quality-planning.html (accessed September 8, 2019).]

3. Centers for Medicare and Medicaid Services. What do I need to do to assess personnel competency? Baltimore, MD: CMS, 2012. [Available at https://www.cms.gov/Regulations-and-Guidance/Legislation/CLIA/Downloads/CLIA_CompBrochure_508.pdf.]

4. Code of federal regulations. Title 21, CFR Part 606.60. Washington, DC: US Government Publishing Office, 2019 (revised annually).

5. Food and Drug Administration. Guidance for industry: Process validation: General principles and practices. (January 2011) Silver Spring, MD: CBER Office of Communication, Outreach, and Development, 2011.

6. Food and Drug Administration. General principles of software validation; final guidance for industry and FDA staff. (January 11, 2002) Silver Spring, MD: CBER Office of Communication, Outreach, and Development, 2002.

7. Code of federal regulations. Title 42, CFR Part 493. Washington, DC: US Government Publishing Office, 2019 (revised annually).

8. Food and Drug Administration. Guidance for industry: Changes to an approved application: Biological products: Human blood and blood components intended for transfusion or for further manufacture. (December 2014) Silver Spring,

MD: CBER Office of Communication, Outreach, and Development, 2014.

9. Rooney JJ, Vanden Heuvel LN. Root cause analysis for beginners. Quality Progress 2004;37:45-53.

10. Food and Drug Administration. Guidance for industry: Notifying FDA of fatalities related to blood collection or transfusion. (September 2003) Silver Spring, MD: CBER Office of Communication, Outreach, and Development, 2003.

11. Food and Drug Administration. Transfusion/donation fatalities: Notification process for transfusion related fatalities and donation related deaths. Silver Spring, MD: CBER Office of Communication, Outreach, and Development, 2019. [Available at https://www.fda.gov/vaccines-blood-biologics/report-problem-center-biologics-evaluation-research/transfusiondonation-fatalities.]

12. Reporting donor fatalities. Association bulletin #04-06. Bethesda, MD: AABB, 2004.

13. Code of federal regulations. Title 21, CFR Parts 606, 610, 630, and 640. Washington, DC: US Government Publishing Office, 2019 (revised annually).

14. Food and Drug Administration. Guidance for industry: Biological product deviation reporting for blood and plasma establishments. (March 2020) Silver Spring, MD: CBER Office of Communication, Outreach, and Development, 2020.

15. Code of federal regulations. Title 21, CFR Parts 1270 and 1271. Washington, DC: US Government Publishing Office, 2019 (revised annually).

16. Food and Drug Administration. Biological product deviations: Includes human tissue and cellular and tissue-based product (HCT/P) deviation reporting. Silver Spring, MD: CBER Office of Communication, Outreach, and Development, 2019. [Available at https://www.fda.gov/vaccines-blood-biologics/report-problem-center-biologics-evaluation-research/biological-product-deviations.]

17. Code of federal regulations. Title 21, CFR Part 803. Washington, DC: US Government Publishing Office, 2019 (revised annually).

18. Hospital accreditation standards. Oakbrook Terrace, IL: Joint Commission Resources, 2019.

19. Laboratory accreditation standards. Oakbrook Terrace, IL: Joint Commission Resources, 2017.

20. Carson JL, Grossman BJ, Kleinman S, et al. Red blood cell transfusion: A clinical practice guideline from AABB. Ann Intern Med 2012;157:49-58.

21. Kaufman M, Djulbegovic B, Gernsheimer T, et al. Platelet transfusion: A clinical practice guideline from the AABB. Ann Intern Med 2015;162:205-14.

22. Investopedia. Lean Six Sigma. New York: Investopedia LLC, 2018. [Available at http://www.investopedia.com/terms/l/lean-six-sigma.asp (accessed September 9, 2019).]

APPENDIX 1-1

Glossary of Commonly Used Quality Terms

Biovigilance	Collection and analysis of adverse-event data for the purpose of improving outcomes in the collection and use of blood components, organs, tissues, and cellular therapies.
Calibration	Comparison of measurements performed with an instrument to those made with a more accurate instrument or standard for the purpose of detecting, reporting, and eliminating errors in measurement.
Change control	Established procedures for planning, documenting, communicating, and executing changes to infrastructure, processes, products, or services. Such procedures include the submission, analysis, approval, implementation, and postimplementation review of the change and decisions made about the change. Formal change control provides a measure of stability and safety and avoids arbitrary changes that might affect quality.
Control chart	A graphic tool used to determine whether the distribution of data values generated by a process is stable over time. A control chart plots a statistic vs time and helps to determine whether a process is in control or out of control according to defined criteria (eg, a shift from a central line or a trend toward upper or lower acceptance limits).
End-product test and inspection	Verification through observation, examination, or testing (or a combination) that the finished product or service conforms to specified requirements.
Near-miss event	An unexpected occurrence that did not adversely affect the outcome but could have resulted in a serious adverse event.
Process	An action that takes input(s) and transforms it into output.
Process control	Activities intended to minimize variation within a process to produce a predictable output that meets specifications.
Qualification	Demonstration that an entity is capable of fulfilling specified requirements and verification of attributes that must be met or complied with for a person or thing to be considered fit to perform a particular function. For example, equipment may be qualified for an intended use by verifying performance characteristics, such as linearity, sensitivity, or ease of use. An employee may be qualified on the basis of technical, academic, and practical knowledge and skills developed through training, education, and on-the-job performance.
Quality assurance	Activities involving quality planning, control, assessment, reporting, and improvement necessary to ensure that a product or service meets defined quality standards and requirements.
Quality control	Operational techniques and activities used to monitor and eliminate causes of unsatisfactory performance at any stage of a process; involves sampling and testing.
Quality indicators	Measurable aspects of processes or outcomes that provide an indication of the condition or direction of performance over time. Quality indicators are used to monitor progress toward stated quality goals and objectives.
Quality management	The organizational structure, processes, and procedures necessary to ensure that the overall intentions and direction of an organization's quality program are met and that the quality of the product or service is ensured. Quality management includes strategic planning, allocation of resources, and other systematic activities, such as quality planning, implementation, and evaluation.

APPENDIX 1-1
Glossary of Commonly Used Quality Terms (Continued)

Quality planning	A systematic process that translates quality policy into measurable objectives and requirements, and lays down a sequence of steps for realizing them within a specified time frame.
Requirement	A stated or obligatory need or expectation that can be measured or observed and that is necessary to ensure quality, safety, effectiveness, or customer satisfaction. Requirements can include things that the system or product must do, characteristics that it must have, and levels of performance that it must attain.
Specification	Description of a set of requirements to be satisfied by a product, material, or process indicating, if appropriate, the procedures to be used to determine whether the requirements are satisfied. Specifications are often in the form of written descriptions, drawings, professional standards, and other descriptive references.
System	An organized, purposeful structure that consists of interrelated and interdependent elements (components, processes, entities, factors, members, parts, etc).
Validation	Demonstration through objective evidence that the requirements for a particular application or intended use have been met. Validation provides assurance that new or changed processes and procedures are capable of consistently meeting specified requirements before implementation.
Verification	Confirmation, by examination of objective evidence, that specified requirements have been met.

APPENDIX 1-2
Code of Federal Regulations Quality-Related References

Topic	Code of Federal Regulations, Title 21		
	Biologics, Blood	Drugs	Tissues, HCT/Ps
Personnel	600.10, 606.20	211.25, 211.28	1271.170
Facilities	600.11, 606.40	211.42-58	1271.190
Environmental control and monitoring		211.42	1271.195
Equipment	606.60	211.63-72, 211.105, 211.182	1271.200
Supplies and reagents	606.65	211.80	1271.210
Standard operating procedures	606.100	211.100-101	1270.31, 1271.180
Process changes and validation		211.100-101	1271.225, 1271.230
Quality assurance/quality control unit		211.22	
Label controls	610.60-68, 606.120-122	211.122-130	1271.250, 1271.370
Laboratory controls	606.140	211.160	
Records and record reviews	600.12, 606.160	211.192, 211.194, 211.196	1270.33, 1271.55, 1271.270
Receipt, predistribution, and distribution	606.165	211.142, 211.150	1271.265
Adverse reactions	606.170	211.198	1271.350
Tracking		211.188	1271.290
Complaints	606.170-171	211.198	1271.320
Reporting deviations	600.14, 606.171		1271.350
Storage	640.2, 640.11, 640.25, 640.34, 640.54, 640.69	211.142	1271.260

HCT/Ps = human cells, tissues, and cellular and tissue-based products.

APPENDIX 1-3
Suggested Quality Control Performance Intervals for Equipment and Reagents*

Equipment or Reagent	Frequency of Quality Control
Refrigerators/freezers/platelet storage	
Refrigerators	
• Recorder	Daily
• Manual temperature	Daily
• Alarm system board (if applicable)	Daily
• Temperature charts	Daily (review and change weekly)
• Alarm activation	Quarterly
Freezers	
• Recorder	Daily
• Manual temperature	Daily
• Alarm system board (if applicable)	Daily
• Temperature charts	Daily (review and change weekly)
• Alarm activation	Quarterly
Platelet Incubators	
• Recorder	Daily
• Manual temperature	Daily
• Temperature charts	Daily (review and change weekly)
• Alarm activation	Quarterly
• Ambient platelet storage	Every 4 hours
Laboratory equipment	
Centrifuges/cell washers	
• Speed	Quarterly
• Timer	Quarterly
• Function	Yearly
• Tube fill level (serologic)	Day of use
• Saline fill volume (serologic)	Weekly
• Volume of antihuman globulin dispensed (if applicable)	Monthly
• Temperature check (refrigerated centrifuge)	Day of use
• Temperature verification (refrigerated centrifuge)	Monthly

(Continued)

APPENDIX 1-3
Suggested Quality Control Performance Intervals for Equipment and Reagents*
(Continued)

Equipment or Reagent	Frequency of Quality Control
Heating blocks/waterbaths/view boxes	
● Temperature	Day of use
● Quadrant/area checks	Periodically
Component thawing devices	Day of use
pH meters	Day of use
Blood irradiators	
● Calibration	Yearly
● Turntable (visual check each time of use)	Yearly
● Timer	Monthly/quarterly
● Source decay	Dependent on source type
● Leak test	Twice yearly
● Dose delivery check (with indicator)	Each irradiator use
● Dose delivery verification	
− Cesium-137	Yearly
− Cobalt-60	Twice yearly
− Other source	As specified by manufacturer
Thermometers (vs NIST-certified or traceable thermometer)	
● Liquid-in-glass	Yearly
● Electronic	As specified by manufacturer
Timers/clocks	Twice yearly
Pipette recalibration	Quarterly
Sterile connection device	
● Weld check	Each use
● Function	Yearly
Blood warmers	
● Effluent temperature	Quarterly
● Heater temperature	Quarterly
● Alarm activation	Quarterly

APPENDIX 1-3
Suggested Quality Control Performance Intervals for Equipment and Reagents* (Continued)

Equipment or Reagent	Frequency of Quality Control
Blood collection equipment	
Whole blood equipment	
• Agitators	Day of use
• Balances/scales	Day of use
• Gram weight (vs NIST-certified)	Yearly
Microhematocrit centrifuge	
• Timer check	Quarterly
• Calibration	Quarterly
• Packed cell volume	Yearly
Cell counters/hemoglobinometers	Day of use
Blood pressure cuffs	Twice yearly
Apheresis equipment	
• Checklist requirements	As specified by manufacturer
Reagents	
Red cells	Day of use
Antisera	Day of use
Antiglobulin serum	Day of use
Transfusion-transmissible disease marker testing	Each test run
Miscellaneous	
Copper sulfate	Day of use
Shipping containers for blood and component transport (usually at temperature extremes)	Twice yearly

*The frequencies listed are suggested intervals, not requirements. For any new piece of equipment, installation, operational, and performance qualifications must be performed. After the equipment has been suitably qualified for use, ongoing QC testing should be performed. Depending on the operational and performance qualification methodology, the ongoing QC may initially be performed more often than the ultimately desired frequency. Once a record of appropriate in-range QC results has been established (during either equipment qualification or the ongoing QC), the frequency of testing can be reduced. At a minimum, the frequency must comply with the manufacturer's suggested intervals; if no such guidance is provided by the manufacturer, the intervals given in this table are appropriate to use. Recalibration of equipment may be required when there is reason to believe an unusual event might have affected calibration.

NIST = National Institute of Standards and Technology, QC = quality control.

CHAPTER 2
Facilities, Work Environment, and Safety

*J. Wade Atkins, MS, MT(ASCP)SBB, CQA(ASQ), and
Colleen Bowman, MT(ASCP)SBB, CQA(ASQ)*

THE PHYSICAL WORK ENVIRON-
ment can have a significant impact on the
safety, efficiency, and effectiveness of
work processes and on the quality of work. It
should be designed and managed in a way that
meets operational needs and provides for the
safety of staff and visitors. The layout of the
physical space; management of utilities; flow of
personnel, materials, and waste; and ergonomic
factors should all be considered in the facility
management plan.

In addition to providing adequate facilities,
the organization should develop and implement
a safety program that defines policies and procedures for safe work practices and emergency responses. Such a program also includes requirements for training, hazard communication, use
of engineering controls, and protective equipment. All employees are responsible for protecting their own safety and the safety of others by
adhering to policies and procedures set forth in
the facility safety program.

AABB requires its accredited facilities to plan,
implement, and maintain a program to minimize risks to the health and safety of donors, patients, volunteers, and employees from biological, chemical, and radiological hazards.[1,2] Other
professional and accrediting organizations, including the College of American Pathologists
(CAP), the Clinical and Laboratory Standards Institute, and The Joint Commission, have similar
or more detailed safety program requirements.[3-6]

US federal regulations and recommendations intended to protect the safety of workers
and the public in health-care settings are listed
in Appendix 2-1. Appendix 2-1 also lists relevant safety recommendations of trade and professional associations. The contents of these regulations and guidance are discussed in more
detail in each section of this chapter. US state
and local government regulations may have additional safety requirements, including architec-
tural and construction safety considerations.

FACILITIES

Facility Design and Workflow

Effective design and maintenance of facilities,
along with the physical organization of work activities, can help reduce or eliminate many potential hazards. Facility design, workflow, and
maintenance also affect process efficiency, productivity, error rates, employee and customer
satisfaction, and the quality of products and services.

During the design phase for a new or reno-
vated space, the location and flow of personnel,
materials, and equipment should be considered
in the context of the processes to be performed.

J. Wade Atkins, MS, MT(ASCP)SBB, CQA(ASQ), Quality Assurance Supervisor, and Colleen Bowman,
MT(ASCP)SBB, CQA(ASQ), Quality Assurance Specialist, National Institutes of Health, Bethesda, Maryland
The authors have disclosed no conflicts of interest.

Adequate space must be allotted for personnel movement, location of supplies and large equipment, and private or distraction-free zones for certain manufacturing tasks (eg, donor interviewing, record review, and blood component labeling). The facility must offer designated "clean" and "dirty" spaces and provide for controlled movement of materials and waste in and out of these areas. Chemical fume hoods and biological safety cabinets (BSCs) should be located away from drafts and high-traffic areas. The number and location of eyewash stations and emergency showers must also be considered in planning. In some cases, additional special water sources for reagent preparation must be provided. The location of very heavy equipment, such as irradiators, should be taken into account to ensure that the flooring has sufficient load-bearing capacity.

Laboratories must be designed with adequate illumination and electrical power and conveniently located electrical outlets. Emergency backup power sources, such as uninterruptible power supplies and backup generators, should be considered to ensure that blood components, cellular therapy products, and critical reagents are not compromised during power failures. The National Electrical Code is routinely used as a national guideline for the design of essential electrical distribution systems, with modifications approved by the local building authority that has jurisdiction.[7]

Heating, ventilation, and air handling must be adequate for the needs of the facility. Environmental monitoring systems should be considered for laboratories that require positive or negative air pressure differentials or where air filtration systems are used to control particle levels. The nationally accepted specifications for ventilation are published by the American Society of Heating, Refrigerating, and Air-Conditioning Engineers.[8]

Housekeeping

The workplace should be kept clean and free of clutter. Work surfaces and equipment should be regularly cleaned and disinfected. Items that may be hazardous or may accumulate dust and debris should not be stored above clean supplies or work-areas. Exits and fire safety equipment must not be blocked or obstructed in any way. Receptacles and disposal guidelines for nonhazardous solid waste and biohazard, chemical, and radiation waste should be clearly identified. Housekeeping responsibilities, methods, and schedules should be defined for every work area. Written procedures, initial training and continuing education of personnel, and ongoing monitoring of housekeeping effectiveness are essential to safe operations.

Clean Rooms

Sterile manufacturing by aseptic technique should be considered for open processing activities. Usually an ISO (International Standards Organization) Class 5 BSC can accommodate this requirement. Laboratories that process cellular therapy products may choose to adopt clean-room specifications and maintenance practices to meet the requirements of the Food and Drug Administration (FDA) current good tissue practice regulations.[9] International standards for clean rooms are published by ISO and provide specifications for general manufacturing applications to limit airborne particulates, contaminants, and pollutants.[10] These standards also provide guidance for pharmaceutical and biotechnology applications that include methods to assess, monitor, and control biocontamination.[11]

Restricted Areas

Hazardous areas should be clearly and uniformly identified with warning signs in accordance with federal Occupational Safety and Health Administration (OSHA) and Nuclear Regulatory Commission (NRC) standards so that personnel entering or working around them are aware of existing biological, chemical, or radiation dangers.[12-15] Adequate training must be provided for regular staff in these areas. Staff members not normally assigned to these areas should receive adequate training to avoid endangering themselves. Risk areas can be stratified. For example, high-risk areas might include those that contain chemical fume hoods, BSCs, and storage areas for volatile chemicals or radioisotopes. Technical work areas might be considered moderate risk and restricted to laboratory personnel. Administrative and clerical areas are generally considered low risk and not restricted. Guidance for restricted access based on biosafety levels is published by the US Department of Health and Human Services (DHHS).[16]

Organizations should consider establishing specific safety guidelines for visitors with business in restricted areas and verifying that safety guidelines have been reviewed before the visitors enter the area. Casual visitors should not be allowed in restricted areas. Children should not be allowed in areas where they could be exposed to hazards and should be closely supervised in those areas where their presence is permitted.

Mobile Sites

Mobile blood-collection operations can present special challenges. An advance safety survey of the proposed collection site helps ensure that hazards are minimized.

Responsibility for site safety should be assigned to an individual with adequate knowledge to recognize safety concerns and the authority to address them in a timely manner. All mobile personnel should be trained to recognize unsafe conditions and understand how to effectively implement infection-control policies and procedures in a variety of settings.

Hand-washing access is essential at collection sites. Carpeted or difficult-to-clean surfaces may be covered using an absorbent overlay with waterproof backing to protect them from possible blood spills. Portable screens and crowd-control ropes are helpful in directing traffic flow to maintain safe work areas. Food-service areas should be physically separated from areas for blood collection and storage. Blood-contaminated waste must be either returned to a central location for disposal or packaged and decontaminated in accordance with local regulations for medical waste.

Ergonomics

Consideration in physical design should be given to ergonomics and to accommodations for individuals covered under the Americans with Disabilities Act [42 United States Code (USC),

Sections 12101-12213, 1990]. Several factors may contribute to employee fatigue, musculoskeletal disorder syndromes, or injury, including the following[17]:

- Awkward postures—positions that place stress on the body, such as reaching overhead, twisting, bending, kneeling, or squatting.
- Repetition—performance of the same motions continuously or frequently.
- Force—the amount of physical effort used to perform work.
- Pressure points—pressing of the body against hard or sharp surfaces.
- Vibration—continuous or high-intensity hand/arm or whole-body vibration.
- Other environmental factors—extreme high or low temperatures or lighting that is too dark or too bright.

Actions to correct problems associated with ergonomics may include the following:

- Engineering improvements to reduce or eliminate the underlying cause, such as making changes to equipment, workstations, or materials.
- Administrative improvements, such as providing variety in tasks; adjusting work schedules and work pace; providing recovery or relaxation time; modifying work practices; ensuring regular housekeeping and maintenance of work spaces, tools, and equipment; and encouraging exercise.
- Provision of personal protective equipment (PPE), such as gloves, knee and elbow pads, protective footwear, and other items that employees wear to protect themselves against injury.

SAFETY PROGRAM

An effective safety program starts with a well-thought-out safety plan. This plan identifies the applicable regulatory requirements and describes how they will be met. A safety plan includes procedures to:

- Provide a workplace free of recognized hazards.
- Evaluate all procedures for potential exposure risks.
- Evaluate each job duty for potential exposure risks.
- Identify hazardous areas or materials with appropriate labels and signs.
- Educate staff, document training, and monitor compliance.
- Apply standard precautions (including universal and blood and body fluid precautions) to the handling of blood, body fluids, and tissues.
- Dispose of hazardous waste appropriately.
- Report incidents and accidents; provide treatment and follow-up.
- Provide ongoing review of safety policies, procedures, operations, and equipment.
- Prepare for and respond to disasters, including the testing of these facility-specific procedures at defined intervals.
- Prepare for and respond to threats to personal safety such as active shooters or bomb threats, at a facility-specific level.

Safety programs should consider the needs of all persons affected by the work environment. Most obvious is the safety of technical staff members, but potential risks for blood donors, ancillary personnel, volunteers, visitors, housekeeping staff, and maintenance and repair workers must also be evaluated. Laboratories should consider appointing a safety officer who can provide general guidance and expertise.[4] Typical duties of a safety officer are to develop the safety program, oversee orientation and training, perform safety audits, survey work sites, recommend changes, and serve on or direct the activities of safety committees. Facilities using hazardous chemicals and radioactive materials often assign specially trained individuals to oversee chemical and radiation protection programs as needed.[12,15] Five basic elements must be addressed for each type of hazard covered in the safety program:

- Training.
- Hazard identification and communication.
- Engineering controls and PPE.

- Safe work practices, including waste disposal.
- Emergency response plan.

Management controls should be established to ensure that these elements are implemented and maintained and that they are effective. Management is responsible for the following:

- Developing and communicating the written plan.
- Ensuring implementation and providing adequate resources.
- Providing access to employee health services related to prevention strategies and treatment of exposures.
- Monitoring compliance and effectiveness.
- Evaluating and improving the safety plan.

Basic Elements of a Safety Program

Training

Employees must be trained to recognize the hazards in their workplace and take appropriate precautions. Supervisors are responsible for assessing and documenting each employee's understanding of and ability to apply safety precautions before independent work is permitted. Safety training must precede even temporary work assignments if significant potential for exposure exists. Staff members who do not demonstrate the requisite understanding and skills must receive additional training. Training should be provided not only to laboratory staff but also to housekeeping and other personnel who may come into contact with hazardous substances or waste. Table 2-1 lists topics to cover in work safety training programs.

Hazard Identification and Communication

Employers are required to provide information about workplace hazards to their staff to help reduce the risk of occupational illnesses and injuries. Staff need to know what hazardous substances they are working with and where those materials are located in the facility. This communication is achieved by means of signage, labels on containers, written information, and training programs.

TABLE 2-1. Topics to Cover in a Work Safety Training Program

Work safety training programs should ensure that all personnel:

- Have access to a copy of pertinent regulatory texts and an explanation of the contents.

- Understand the employer's exposure control plan and how to obtain a copy of the written plan.

- Understand how hepatitis and human immunodeficiency virus (HIV) are transmitted and how often; and are familiar with the symptoms and consequences of hepatitis B virus (HBV), hepatitis C virus (HCV), and HIV infection.

- Know that they are offered vaccination against HBV.

- Recognize tasks that pose infectious risks and distinguish them from other duties.

- Know what protective clothing and equipment are appropriate for the procedures they will perform and how to use them.

- Know and understand the limitations of protective clothing and equipment (eg, different types of gloves are recommended according to the permeability of the hazardous material to be used).

- Know where protective clothing and equipment are kept.

- Become familiar with and understand all requirements for work practices specified in standard operating procedures for the tasks they perform, including the meaning of signs and labels.

- Know how to remove, handle, decontaminate, and dispose of contaminated material.

- Know the appropriate actions to take and the personnel to contact if exposed to blood or other biological, chemical, or radiologic hazards.

- Know the corrective actions to take in the event of spills or personal exposure to fluids, tissues, and contaminated sharp objects; know appropriate reporting procedures; and know what medical monitoring is recommended when parenteral exposure may have occurred.

- Know their right to access to medical treatment and medical records.

- Know fire safety procedures and evacuation plans.

- Recognize facility-specific verbal announcements and how to respond.

Engineering Controls and PPE

If the physical work space cannot be designed to eliminate the potential for exposure to hazards, appropriate protective gear must be provided. Engineering controls are physical plant controls or equipment, such as sprinkler systems, chemical fume hoods, and needleless systems that isolate or remove the hazard from the workplace.

PPE is specialized clothing or equipment, such as gloves, masks, and laboratory coats, worn by employees for protection against a hazard. Employees should remove their PPE, such as gloves and laboratory coats, and should wash their hands with soap and water when leaving a laboratory area. General guidance on the use of engineering controls and PPE is included in Appendix 2-2.

Safe Work Practices

Employees must be trained in how to work with hazardous materials in ways that protect themselves, their coworkers, and the environment. Safe work practices are defined as tasks performed in a manner that reduces the likelihood of exposure to workplace hazards. General recommendations for safe work practices are included in Appendix 2-2.

Emergency Response Plan

When engineering and work practice controls fail, employees must know how to respond promptly and appropriately. The purpose of advance planning is to control a hazardous situation as quickly and safely as possible. Regular testing of the emergency response plan identifies areas for improvement and builds staff confidence in their ability to respond effectively in a real emergency. OSHA requires facilities with more than 10 employees to have a written emergency response plan. Verbal communication of the plan is acceptable for facilities with 10 or fewer employees.[18]

Management Controls

Supervisory personnel must monitor safety practices in their areas of responsibility. Continuing attention to safety issues should be addressed in routine staff meetings and training sessions. Periodic audits performed by a safety professional increases safety awareness. Management should seek staff input on the design and improvement of the facility's safety plan.

The safety program policies, procedures, guidance, and supporting references should be documented in writing and made available to all personnel at risk. These documents should be reviewed on a regular basis and updated as technology evolves and new information becomes available. Risk mitigation studies should be conducted periodically. Strategies or other safety provisions should be updated or implemented with safety improvements. Work sites and safety equipment should be inspected regularly to ensure compliance and response readiness. Checklists may be helpful for documenting safety inspections and assessing safety preparedness.[3,4,19]

Employee Health Services

Hepatitis Prophylaxis

All employees routinely exposed to blood must be offered hepatitis B virus (HBV) vaccine if they do not already have HBV-protective antibodies (ie, antibodies to hepatitis B surface antigen). OSHA requires that the vaccine be offered at no cost to all employees and, if any employee refuses the vaccine, that the refusal be documented.[14]

Monitoring Programs

Employers must provide a system for monitoring exposure to certain substances as defined in the OSHA standard if there is reason to believe that exposure levels routinely exceed the recommended action level.[20]

Medical First Aid and Follow-Up

When requested by a worker who has sustained known or suspected blood exposure, monitoring for HBV, hepatitis C virus (HCV), and human immunodeficiency virus (HIV) infection should be provided with appropriate counseling. In some states, consent is required for this voluntary testing; rejection of offered testing must be documented. The usual schedule includes immediate tests of the worker and the source of the potentially infectious material, with follow-up testing of the worker at intervals after exposure.[13,14] All aspects of accident follow-up should be appropriately documented.

The Centers for Disease Control and Prevention (CDC) has published recommendations for both preexposure and postexposure prophylaxis if the contaminating material is HBV positive or if this information is unknown.[21] HBV immune globulin is usually given concurrently with HBV vaccine in cases of penetrating injuries. Postexposure prophylaxis for HIV is continually evolving; policies are generally based on Public Health Service recommendations and current standards of practice.

Reporting Accidents and Injuries

When an injury occurs, relevant information should be documented, including the date and time of injury and the place where it occurred; the nature of the injury; descriptions of what happened from the injured person and any witnesses; and the first aid or medical attention provided. The supervisor should complete any accident reports and investigation forms required by the institution's insurer and worker's compensation agencies. Employers must report fatalities and injuries resulting in the hospitalization of three or more employees to OSHA within 8 hours of the accident.[22]

OSHA requires health-service employers with 11 or more workers to maintain records of occupational injuries and illnesses requiring a level of care that exceeds the capabilities of a person trained in first aid.[23] Initial documentation must be completed within 6 days of the incident. Records of first aid provided by a non-physician for minor injuries, such as cuts or burns, do not need to be retained. All logs, summaries, and supplemental records must be preserved for at least 5 years beyond the calendar year of occurrence. Medical records of employees should be preserved for the duration of employment plus 30 years, with few exceptions.[24]

Latex Allergies

Adverse reactions associated with latex, powdered gloves, or both include contact dermatitis, allergic dermatitis, urticaria, and anaphylaxis. Medical devices that contain latex must bear a caution label. The National Institute for Occupational Safety and Health (NIOSH) offers recommendations to prevent these allergic reactions.[25] Most health-care facilities have adopted a latex-free glove policy to prevent latex allergy reactions.

FIRE PREVENTION

Fire prevention relies on a combination of facility design that is based on the National Fire Protection Association (NFPA) Life Safety Code, which identifies processes to maintain fire protection systems in good working order, and fire safe-work practices.[26] The Life Safety Code includes both active and passive fire-protection systems (eg, alarms, smoke detectors, sprinklers, exit lights in corridors, and fire-rated barriers).

Training

Fire safety training is recommended at the start of employment and at least annually thereafter. Training should emphasize prevention and an employee's awareness of the work environment, including how to recognize and report unsafe conditions, how to report fires, where the near-est alarm and fire-containment equipment are located and how to use it, and what the evacuation policies and routes are.

All staff members in facilities accredited by CAP or The Joint Commission are required to participate in fire drills at least annually.[3,5] In areas where patients are housed or treated, The Joint Commission requires quarterly drills on each shift. Staff participation and understanding should be documented.

Hazard Identification and Communication

Emergency exits must be clearly marked with an exit sign. Additional signage must be posted along the exit route to show the direction of travel if it is not immediately apparent. All flammable materials should be labeled with appropriate hazard warnings, and flammable storage cabinets should be clearly marked.

Engineering Controls and PPE

Laboratories storing large volumes of flammable chemicals are usually built with 2-hour fire separation walls, or with 1-hour separation walls if there is an automatic fire-extinguishing system.[4] Fire detection and alarm systems should be provided in accordance with federal, state, and local regulations. All fire equipment should be inspected on a regular basis to ensure that it is in good working order. Fire extinguishers should be readily available, and the staff should be trained to use them properly. Housekeeping and inventory management plans should be designed to control the accumulations of flammable and combustible materials stored in the facility. In areas where sprinkler systems are installed, all items should be stored at least 18 inches below the sprinkler heads. Facilities should consult local fire codes, which may require greater clearance.

Safe Work Practices

Emergency exit routes must be clear of anything that would obstruct evacuation efforts. Exit doors must not be locked in such a way as to impede egress. Permanent exit routes must be designed to allow free and unobstructed exit from all parts of the facility to an area of safety. Secondary exits may be required for areas larger than 1000 square feet; facilities should consult local safety authorities with jurisdiction, such as the local fire marshal and NFPA, for guidance on secondary exits.

Emergency Response Plan

The fire emergency response plan should encompass both facility-wide and area-specific situations. It should describe reporting and alarm systems; location and use of emergency equipment; roles and responsibilities of the staff during the response; "defend-in-place" strategies; and conditions for evacuation, evacuation procedures, and exit routes.[5,18]

When a fire occurs, the general sequence for immediate response should be to 1) rescue anyone in immediate danger; 2) activate the fire alarm system and alert others in the area; 3) confine the fire by closing doors and shutting off fans or other oxygen sources if possible; and 4) extinguish the fire with a portable extinguisher if the fire is small, or evacuate if it is too large to manage.

ELECTRICAL SAFETY

Electrical hazards, including fire and shock, may arise from the use of faulty electrical equipment; damaged receptacles, connectors, or cords; or unsafe work practices. Proper use of electrical equipment, periodic inspection and maintenance, and hazard recognition training are essential to help prevent accidents that may result in electric shock or electrocution. The severity of shock depends on the path that the electrical current takes through the body, the amount of current flowing through the body, and the length of time that current is flowing through the body. Even low-voltage exposures can lead to serious injury.[27]

Training

Safety training should be designed to make employees aware of electrical hazards associated with receptacles and connectors. This training should also help them recognize potential problems, such as broken receptacles and connectors, improper electrical connections, damaged cords, and inadequate grounding.

Hazard Identification and Communication

The safety plan should address the proper use of receptacles and connectors. Equipment that does not meet safety standards should be marked to prevent accidental use.

Engineering Controls and PPE

OSHA requires that electrical systems and equipment be constructed and installed in a way that minimizes the potential for workplace hazards. When purchasing equipment, the facility should verify that it bears the mark of an OSHA-approved independent testing laboratory, such as Underwriters Laboratories.[28] Adequate working space should be provided around equipment to allow easy access for safe operation and maintenance. Ground-fault circuit interrupters should be installed in damp or wet areas.

Safe Work Practices

Electrical safety practices focus on two factors: 1) proper use of electrical equipment and 2) proper maintenance and repair of this equipment. Staff should not plug equipment into or unplug equipment from an electrical source with wet hands. Overloading circuits with too many devices may cause the current to overheat the wiring and potentially generate a fire. Damaged receptacles and faulty electrical equipment must be tagged and removed from service until they have been repaired and checked for safety. Flexible cords should be secured to prevent tripping and should be protected from damage from heavy or sharp objects. Flexible cords should be kept slackened to prevent tension on electrical terminals, and cords should be checked regularly for cut, broken, or cracked insulation. Extension cords should not be used in lieu of permanent wiring.

Emergency Response Plan

In case of an emergency in which it is not possible to decrease the power or disconnect equipment, the power supply should be shut off from the circuit breaker. If it is not possible to interrupt the power supply, a nonconductive material, such as dry wood, should be used to pry a victim from the source of current.[27] Victims must not be touched directly. Emergency first aid for victims of electrical shock must be sought. Water-based fire extinguishers should not be used on electrical fires.

BIOSAFETY

The facility must define and enforce measures to minimize the risk of exposure to biohazard materials in the workplace. Requirements published by OSHA (Blood-Borne Pathogens Standard) and recommendations published by the US DHHS provide the basis for an effective biosafety plan.[13,14,16]

Blood-Borne Pathogens Standard

The OSHA Blood-Borne Pathogens Standard is intended to protect employees in all occupations where there is a risk of exposure to blood and other potentially infectious materials. It requires the facility to develop an exposure control plan and describes appropriate engineering controls, PPE, and work practice controls to minimize the risk of exposure. The standard also requires employers to provide HBV vaccinations to any staff members with occupational exposure, provide medical follow-up care in case of accidental exposure, and keep records related to accidents and exposures.

Standard Precautions

Standard precautions represent the most current recommendations by the CDC to reduce the risk of transmission of blood-borne pathogens and other pathogens in hospitals. Standard precautions apply to all patient-care activities, regardless of diagnosis, in which there is a risk of exposure to 1) blood; 2) any body fluids, secretions, and excretions, *except sweat*, regardless of whether or not they contain visible blood; 3) nonintact skin; or 4) mucous membranes.

The OSHA Blood-Borne Pathogens Standard refers to the use of universal precautions. However, OSHA recognizes the more recent guidelines from the CDC and, in Directive CPL 02-02-069, allows hospitals to use acceptable alternatives, including standard precautions, as long as all other requirements in the standard are met.[29]

Biosafety Levels

Recommendations for biosafety in laboratories are based on the potential hazards pertaining to specific infectious agents and the activities performed.[16] Biosafety recommendations include guidance on both engineering controls and safe work practices. The four biosafety levels are designated in ascending order, with increasing protection for personnel, the environment, and the community:

- Biosafety Level 1 (BSL-1) involves work with agents of no known or of minimal potential hazard to laboratory personnel and the environment. Activities are usually conducted on open surfaces, and no containment equipment is needed.
- BSL-2 work involves agents of moderate potential hazard to personnel and the environment, usually from contact-associated exposure. Most blood bank laboratory activities are considered BSL-2.
- BSL-3 includes work with indigenous or exotic agents that may cause serious or potentially lethal disease as a result of exposure to aerosols (eg, *Mycobacterium tuberculosis*) or by other routes (eg, HIV) that would result in grave consequences to the infected host. Recommendations for BSL-3 work are designed to contain aerosols and minimize the risk of surface contamination.
- BSL-4 applies to work with dangerous or exotic agents that pose high individual risk of life-threatening disease from aerosols (eg, agents of hemorrhagic fevers or filoviruses). BSL-4 is not applicable to routine blood-bank-related activities.

The precautions described in this section focus on BSL-2 requirements. Laboratories should consult the CDC or National Institutes of Health guidelines for precautions appropriate for higher levels of containment.

Training

OSHA requires annual training for all employees whose tasks increase their risk of infectious exposure.[14,29] Training programs must be tailored to the target group both in level and content. General background knowledge of biohazards, understanding of control procedures, or work experience cannot meet the requirement for specific training, although an assessment of such knowledge is a first step in planning program content. Workplace volunteers require at least as much safety training as paid staff members who perform similar functions.

Hazard Identification and Communication

The facility's exposure control plan communicates the risks present in the workplace and describes controls to minimize exposure. BSL-2 through BSL-4 facilities must have a biohazard sign posted at the entrance when infectious agents are in use. The sign notifies personnel and visitors of the presence of infectious agents, provides a point of contact for the area, and indicates any special protective equipment or work practices required.

Biohazard warning labels must be placed on containers of regulated waste; refrigerators and freezers containing blood or other potentially infectious material; and other containers used to store, transport, or ship blood or other potentially infectious materials. Blood components that are labeled to identify their contents and have been released for transfusion or other clinical use are exempted.

Engineering Controls and PPE

OSHA requires that hazards be controlled by engineering or work practices whenever possible.[14] Engineering controls for BSL-2 laboratories include limited access to the laboratory when work is in progress and BSCs or other containment equipment for work that may involve infectious aerosols or splashes. Handwashing sinks and eyewash stations must be available. The work space should be designed so that it can be easily cleaned, and bench tops should be impervious to water and resistant to chemicals and solvents.

To help prevent exposure or cross-contamination, work area telephones can be equipped with speakers to eliminate the need to pick up the receiver. Computer keyboards and telephones can be covered with plastic. Such equipment should be cleaned on a regular basis and when visibly soiled.

BSCs are primary containment devices for handling moderate-risk and high-risk organisms. There are three types—Classes I, II, and III—with Class III providing the highest protection to workers. In addition to protecting personnel during the handling of biohazard materials, a BSC may be used to prevent contamination of blood and cellular therapy products during open-processing steps. A comparison of the features and applications of the three classes of cabinets is provided in Table 2-2.

BSCs are not required by standard precautions, but centrifugation of open blood samples or manipulation of units known to be positive for HBV surface antigen or HIV are examples of blood bank procedures for which a BSC could be useful. The effectiveness of the BSC is a function of directional airflow inward and downward through a high-efficiency filter. Efficacy is reduced by anything that disrupts the airflow pattern. Care should be taken not to block the front intake and rear exhaust grills. BSC performance should be certified annually.[31]

In 2001, OSHA revised the Blood-Borne Pathogens Standard and required that employers implement appropriate control technologies and safer medical devices in exposure control plans and that employers solicit input from their employees to identify, evaluate, and select engineering and work practice controls. Examples of safer devices are needleless systems and self-sheathing needles in which the sheath is an integral part of the device.

TABLE 2-2.   Comparison of Classes I, II, and III Biological Safety Cabinets*

Category	Main Features	Intended Use	Common Applications
Class I	Unfiltered room air is drawn into the cabinet. Inward airflow protects personnel from exposure to materials inside the cabinet. Exhaust is high-efficiency particulate air (HEPA) filtered to protect the environment. It maintains airflow at a minimum velocity of 75 linear feet per minute (lfpm) across the front opening (face velocity).	Personal and environmental protection	To enclose equipment (eg, centrifuges) or procedures that may generate aerosols
Class II, general (applies to all types of Class II cabinets)	Laminar flow (air moving at a constant velocity in one direction along parallel lines) is used. Room air is drawn into the front grille. HEPA-filtered air is forced downward in a laminar flow to minimize cross-contamination of materials in the cabinet. Exhaust is HEPA filtered.	Personal, environmental, and product protection	Work with microorganisms assigned to Biosafety Levels 1, 2, or 3 Handling of products for which prevention of contamination is critical, such as cell culture propagation or manipulation of blood components in an open system
Class II, A	Approximately 75% of air is recirculated after passing through a HEPA filter. Face velocity = 75 lfpm.	See Class II, general	See Class II, general
Class II, B1	Approximately 70% of air exits through the rear grille, is HEPA filtered, and is then discharged from the building. The other 30% is drawn into the front grille, is HEPA filtered, and is recirculated. Face velocity = 100 lfpm.	See Class II, general	Allows for safe manipulation of small quantities of hazardous chemicals and biologics

(Continued)

TABLE 2-2. Comparison of Classes I, II, and III Biological Safety Cabinets* (Continued)

Category	Main Features	Intended Use	Common Applications
Class II, B2	All air is exhausted, and none is recirculated. A supply blower draws air from the room or outside and passes it through a HEPA filter to provide the downward laminar flow. Face velocity = 100 lfpm.	See Class II, general	Provides both chemical and biological containment; is more expensive to operate because of the volume of conditioned room air being exhausted
Class II, B3	Although similar in design to Type A, the system is ducted and includes a negative pressure system to keep any possible contamination within the cabinet. Face velocity = 100 lfpm.	See Class II, general	Allows for safe manipulation of small quantities of hazardous chemicals and biologics
Class III	Cabinet is airtight. Materials are handled with rubber gloves attached to the front of the cabinet. Supply air is HEPA filtered. Exhaust air is double HEPA filtered or may have one filter and an air incinerator. Materials are brought in and out of the cabinet either through a dunk tank or a double-door passthrough box that can be decontaminated. Cabinet is kept under negative pressure.	Maximum protection to personnel and environment	Work with Biosafety Level 4 microorganisms

*Data from the US Department of Health and Human Services.[30]

Disinfectants

The Environmental Protection Agency (EPA) maintains a list of chemical products that have been shown to be effective hospital antimicrobial disinfectants.[32] The Association for Professionals in Infection Control and Epidemiology also publishes a guidance to assist health-care professionals with decisions involving judicious selection and proper use of specific disinfectants.[33] For facilities covered under the Blood-Borne Pathogens Standard, OSHA allows the use of EPA-registered tuberculocidal disinfectants; EPA-registered disinfectants that are effective against both HIV and HBV; or, more commonly used, a diluted bleach solution, usually 10% by volume; or a combination of these, to decontaminate work surfaces.[29]

Before selecting a disinfectant product, several factors should be considered. Among them are the type of material or surface to be treated and the hazardous properties of the disinfectant product, such as corrosiveness and the level of disinfection required. After a product has been selected, procedures need to be written to ensure effective and consistent cleaning and treatment of work surfaces. Some factors to consider for effective decontamination include contact time, type of microorganisms, presence of organic matter, and concentration of the chemical agent. Laboratory personnel should review the basic information on decontamination and follow the manufacturer's instructions.

Decontamination

Reusable equipment and work surfaces that may be contaminated with blood require daily cleaning and decontamination. Obvious spills on equipment or work surfaces should be cleaned up immediately; routine wipe-downs with disinfectant should occur at the end of each shift or on a different frequency that provides equivalent safety. Equipment that is exposed to blood or other potentially infectious material must be decontaminated before it is serviced or shipped. When decontamination of all or a portion of the equipment is not feasible, a biohazard label stating which portions remain contaminated should be attached before the equipment is serviced or shipped.

Storage

Hazardous materials must be segregated, and areas for different types of storage must be clearly demarcated. Blood must be protected from unnecessary exposure to other materials and vice versa. If transfusion products cannot be stored in a separate refrigerator from reagents, specimens, and unrelated materials, areas within the refrigerator must be clearly labeled and extra care must be taken to reduce the likelihood of spills and other accidents. Storage areas must be kept clean and orderly; food or drink is never allowed where biohazard materials are stored.

PPE

When hazards cannot be eliminated, OSHA requires employers to provide appropriate PPE and clothing and to clean, launder, or dispose of PPE at no cost to their employees.[14] Standard PPE and clothing include uniforms, laboratory coats, gloves, face shields, masks, and safety goggles. Indications and guidance for their use are discussed in Appendix 2-2.

Safe Work Practices

Safe work practices appropriate for standard precautions include the following:

- Wash hands after touching blood, body fluids, secretions, excretions, and contaminated items, whether or not gloves are worn.
- Wear gloves when touching blood, body fluids, secretions, excretions, and contaminated items, and change gloves between tasks.
- Wear a mask and eye protection or a face shield during activities that are likely to generate splashes or sprays of blood, body fluids, secretions, and excretions.
- Wear a gown during activities that are likely to generate splashes or sprays of blood, body fluids, secretions, or excretions.
- Handle soiled patient-care equipment in a manner that prevents exposure; ensures that reusable equipment is not used for another patient until it has been cleaned and reprocessed appropriately; and ensures that single-use items are discarded properly.

- Ensure that adequate procedures are defined and followed for the routine care, cleaning, and disinfection of environmental surfaces and equipment.
- Handle soiled linen in a manner that prevents exposure.
- Handle needles, scalpels, and other sharp instruments or devices in a manner that minimizes the risk of exposure.
- Use mouthpieces, resuscitation bags, or other ventilation devices as an alternative to mouth-to-mouth resuscitation methods.

Laboratory Biosafety Precautions

Several factors need to be considered when assessing the risk of blood exposures among laboratory personnel. Some of these factors include the number of specimens processed, personnel behaviors, laboratory techniques, and types of equipment.[34] The laboratory director may wish to institute BSL-3 practices for procedures that are considered to be higher risk than BSL-2. When there is doubt whether an activity is BSL-2 or BSL-3, the safety precautions for BSL-3 should be followed. BSL-2 precautions that are applicable to the laboratory setting are summarized in Appendix 2-3.

Considerations for the Donor Room

The Blood-Borne Pathogens Standard acknowledges a difference between hospital patients and healthy donors, in whom the prevalence of infectious disease markers is significantly lower. The employer in a volunteer blood donation facility may determine that routine use of gloves is not required for phlebotomy as long as the following conditions exist[14]:

- Gloves are made available to those who want to use them, and their use is not discouraged.
- Gloves are required when an employee has cuts, scratches, or breaks in skin; when there is a likelihood that contamination will occur; while an employee is drawing autologous units; while an employee is performing therapeutic procedures; and during training in phlebotomy.
- The policy is periodically reevaluated.

Procedures should be assessed for risks of biohazard exposures and risks inherent in working with a donor or patient during the screening and donation processes. Some techniques or procedures are more likely to cause injury than others, such as using lancets for finger puncture, handling capillary tubes, crushing vials for arm cleaning, handling any unsheathed needles, cleaning scissors, and giving cardiopulmonary resuscitation.

In some instances, it may be necessary to collect blood from donors known to pose a high risk of infectivity (eg, collection of autologous blood or source plasma for the production of other products, such as vaccines). The FDA provides guidance on collecting blood from such "high-risk" donors.[35,36] The most recent regulations and guidance should be consulted for changes or additions.

Emergency Response Plan

Table 2-3 lists steps to take when a spill occurs. Facilities should be prepared to handle both small and large blood spills. Good preparation for spill cleanup includes several elements:

- Work areas designed so that cleanup is relatively simple.
- A spill kit or cart containing all necessary supplies and equipment with instructions for their use placed near areas where spills are anticipated.
- Responsibility assigned for kit or cart maintenance, spill handling, record-keeping, and review of significant incidents.
- Personnel trained in cleanup procedures and procedures for reporting significant incidents.

Biohazard Waste

Medical waste is defined as any waste (solid, semisolid, or liquid) generated in the diagnosis, treatment, or immunization of human beings or animals in related research, production, or testing of biologics. Infectious waste includes disposable equipment, articles, or substances that may harbor or transmit pathogenic organisms or their toxins. In general, infectious waste should

TABLE 2-3. Blood Spill Cleanup Steps

Evaluate the spill.
Wear appropriate protective clothing and gloves. If sharp objects are involved, gloves must be puncture resistant, and a broom or other instrument should be used during cleanup to avoid injury.
Remove clothing if it is contaminated.
Post warnings to keep the area clear.
Evacuate the area for 30 minutes if an aerosol has been created.
Contain the spill if possible.
If the spill occurs in the centrifuge, turn the power off immediately and leave the cover on for 30 minutes. The use of overwraps helps prevent aerosolization and contain the spill.
Use absorbent material to mop up most of the liquid contents.
Clean the spill area with detergent.
Flood the area with disinfectant and use it as described in the manufacturer's instructions. Allow adequate contact time with the disinfectant.
Wipe up residual disinfectant if necessary.
Dispose of all materials safely in accordance with biohazard guidelines. All blood-contaminated items must be autoclaved or incinerated.

be either incinerated or decontaminated before disposal in a sanitary landfill.

If state law allows, blood and components, suctioned fluids, excretions, and secretions may be carefully poured down a drain connected to a sanitary sewer. Sanitary sewers may also be used to dispose of other potentially infectious wastes that can be ground and flushed into the sewer. State and local health departments should be consulted about laws and regulations pertaining to disposal of biological waste into the sewer.

In the blood bank, all items contaminated with liquid or semi-liquid blood are to be considered hazardous materials. Items contaminated with dried blood are considered hazardous if there is potential for the dried material to flake off during handling. Contaminated sharp objects are always considered hazardous because of the risk for percutaneous injury. However, items such as used gloves, swabs, plastic pipettes with excess liquid removed, or gauze contaminated with small droplets of blood may be considered nonhazardous if the material is dried and will

not be released into the environment during handling.

Guidance for Biohazard Waste Disposal

Employees must be trained before handling or disposing of biohazard waste, even if it is packaged. The following disposal guidance are recommended[37]:

- Identify biohazard waste consistently; red seamless plastic bags (at least 2 mm thick) or containers carrying the biohazard symbol are recommended.
- Place bags in a protective container with closure upward to avoid breakage and leakage during storage or transport.
- Prepare and ship waste transported over public roads according to US Department of Transportation (DOT) regulations.
- Discard sharps (eg, needles, broken glass, glass slides, and wafers from sterile connection devices) in rigid, puncture-proof, leak-proof containers.

- Put liquids in leak-proof, unbreakable containers only.
- Do not compact waste materials.

Storage areas for infectious material must be secured to reduce accident risk. Infectious waste must never be placed in the public trash collection system. Most facilities hire private carriers to decontaminate and dispose of infectious or hazardous waste. The facility should disclose all risks associated with the waste in their contracts with private companies. The carrier is responsible for complying with all federal, state, and local laws for biohazard (medical) waste transport, treatment, and disposal.

Treating Infectious or Medical Waste

Facilities that incinerate hazardous waste must comply with EPA standards of performance for new stationary sources and emission guidelines for existing sources.[38] In this regulation, a hospital/medical/infectious waste incinerator is any device that combusts any amount of hospital waste or medical/infectious waste.

Autoclaving is another common method for decontamination of biohazard waste, used for blood samples and blood components. The following elements are considered in determining processing time for autoclaving:

- Size of load being autoclaved.
- Type of packaging of item(s) being autoclaved.
- Density of items being autoclaved.
- Number of items in a single autoclave load.
- Placement of items in the autoclave to allow for steam penetration.

It is useful to place a biological indicator in the center of loads that vary in size and contents to evaluate optimal steam penetration times. The EPA provides detailed information about choosing and operating such equipment.[37]

For decontamination, material should be autoclaved for a minimum of 1 hour. For sterilization, longer treatment times are needed. A general rule for decontamination is to process for 1 hour for every 10 pounds of waste. Usually, decontaminated laboratory wastes can be disposed of as nonhazardous solid wastes. The staff should check with the local solid-waste authority to ensure that the facility is in compliance with regulations for the area. Waste containing broken glass or other sharp items should be disposed of using a method consistent with policies for the disposal of other sharp or potentially dangerous materials.

CHEMICAL SAFETY

One of the most effective preventive measures that a facility can take to reduce hazardous chemical exposure is to choose alternative nonhazardous chemicals whenever possible. When the use of hazardous chemicals is required, purchasing these supplies in small quantities reduces the risks associated with storing excess chemicals and then dealing with their disposal.

OSHA requires that facilities using hazardous chemicals develop a written chemical hygiene plan (CHP) and that the plan be accessible to all employees. The CHP should outline procedures, equipment, PPE, and work practices that are capable of protecting employees from hazardous chemicals used in the facility.[15,20] The CHP must also provide assurance that equipment and protective devices are functioning properly and that criteria to determine implementation and maintenance of all aspects of the plan are in place. Employees must be informed of all chemical hazards in the workplace and be trained to recognize chemical hazards, protect themselves when working with these chemicals, and know where to find information about particular hazardous chemicals. Safety audits and annual reviews of the CHP are important control steps to help ensure that safety practices comply with the policies set forth in the CHP and that the CHP is up to date.

Establishing a clear definition of what constitutes hazardous chemicals is sometimes difficult. Generally, hazardous chemicals pose a significant health risk if an employee is exposed to them or a significant physical risk, such as fire or explosion, if handled or stored improperly. Categories of health and physical hazards are listed in Tables 2-4 and 2-5. The *NIOSH Pocket Guide*

TABLE 2-4. Categories of Health Hazards

Hazard	Definition
Carcinogens	Cancer-producing substances
Irritants	Agents causing irritation (eg, edema or burning) to skin or mucous membranes upon contact
Corrosives	Agents causing destruction of human tissue at the site of contact
Toxic or highly toxic agents	Substances causing serious biologic effects following inhalation, ingestion, or skin contact with relatively small amounts
Reproductive toxins	Chemicals that affect reproductive capabilities, including chromosomal damages and effects on fetuses
Other toxins	Hepatotoxins; nephrotoxins; neurotoxins; agents that act on the hematopoietic system; and agents that damage the lungs, skin, eyes, or mucous membranes

TABLE 2-5. Categories of Physical Hazards

Hazard	Definition
Combustible or flammable chemicals	Chemicals that can burn (including combustible and flammable liquids, solids, aerosols, and gases)
Compressed gases	Gases or mixtures of gases in a container under pressure
Explosives	Unstable or reactive chemicals that undergo violent chemical changes at normal temperatures and pressure
Unstable (reactive) chemicals	Chemicals that could be self-reactive under certain conditions (shocks, pressure, or temperature)
Water-reactive chemicals	Chemicals that react with water to release a gas that either is flammable or presents a health hazard

to Chemical Hazards provides a quick reference for many common chemicals.[39]

The facility should identify a qualified chemical hygiene officer to be responsible for developing guidelines for hazardous materials.[20] The chemical hygiene officer is also accountable for monitoring and documenting accidents and for initiating process change as needed.

Training

Employees who may be exposed to hazardous chemicals must be trained before they begin work in an area in which hazards exist. If a new employee has received prior training, it may not be necessary to retrain the individual, depending on the employer's evaluation of the new employee's level of knowledge. New employee training is likely to be necessary regarding such specifics as the location of each relevant safety data sheet (SDS), details on chemical labeling, PPE to be used, and site-specific emergency procedures.

Training must be provided for each new physical or health hazard when it is introduced into the workplace but not for each new chemical that falls within a particular hazard class.[15] For example, if a new solvent is brought into the workplace and the solvent has hazards similar to existing chemicals for which training has already been conducted, then the employer need only make employees aware of the new solvent's hazard category (eg, corrosive or irritant). However, if the newly introduced solvent is a suspected carcinogen and carcinogenic hazard training has not been provided, then new training must be conducted for employees with potential exposure. Retraining is advisable as often as necessary to ensure that employees understand the hazards linked to the materials with which they work, particularly any chronic and specific target-organ health hazards.

Hazard Identification and Communication

Hazard Communication

Employers must prepare a comprehensive hazard communication program for all areas in which hazardous chemicals are used to complement the CHP and "ensure that the hazards of all chemicals produced or imported are classified, and that information concerning the classified hazard is transmitted to employers and employees."[15] The program should include labeling of hazardous chemicals, instructions on when and how to post warning labels for chemicals, directions for managing SDS reports for hazardous chemicals in the facilities, and employee training. Safety materials made available to employees should include the following:

- The facility's written CHP.
- The facility's written program for hazard communication.
- Identification of work areas where hazardous chemicals are located.
- Required list of hazardous chemicals and the relevant SDSs. (It is the responsibility of the facility to determine which chemicals may present a hazard to employees. This determination should be based on the quantity of chemical used; physical properties, potency, and toxicity of the chemical; manner in which the chemical is used; and means available to control the release of, or exposure to, the chemical.)

Hazardous Chemical Labeling and Signs

The Hazard Communication Standard requires manufacturers of chemicals and hazardous materials to provide the user with basic information about the hazards of these materials through product labeling and the SDS.[15] Employers are required to provide employees who are expected to work with these hazardous materials with information about what the hazards of the materials are, how to read the labeling, how to interpret symbols and signs on the labels, and how to read and use the SDS.

At a minimum, hazardous-chemical container labels must include the name of the chemical, name and address of the manufacturer, hazard warnings, symbols, designs, and other forms of warning to provide visual reminders of specific hazards. The label may refer to any SDS for additional information. Labels applied by the manufacturer must remain on containers. The user may add storage requirements and dates of receipt, opening, and expiration. If chemicals are aliquoted into secondary containers, the secondary container must be labeled with the name of the chemical and appropriate hazard warnings. Additional information, such as precautionary measures, concentration if applicable, and date of preparation, are helpful but not mandatory.

It is a safe practice to label all containers with their content, even water. Transfer containers used for temporary storage need not be labeled if the person performing the transfer retains control and intends the containers to be used immediately. Information regarding acceptable standards for hazard communication labeling is provided by the NFPA[40] and the American Coatings Association.[41]

Signs meeting OSHA requirements must be posted in areas where hazardous chemicals are used. Decisions about where to post warning signs are based on the manufacturer's recommendations regarding the chemical hazards, the quantity of the chemical in the room or laboratory, and the potency and toxicity of the chemical.

Safety Data Sheet

The SDS identifies the physical and chemical properties of a hazardous chemical (eg, flash point or vapor pressure), its physical and health hazards (eg, potential for fire, explosion, and signs and symptoms of exposure), and precautions for the chemical's safe handling and use. Specific instructions in an individual SDS take precedence over generic information in the hazardous materials program.

Employers must maintain copies of each required SDS in the workplace for each hazardous chemical and ensure that SDS copies are readily accessible during each work shift to employees when they are in their work areas. When household consumer products are used in the workplace in the same manner that a consumer would use them (ie, when the duration and frequency of use, and therefore exposure, are not greater than those that the typical consumer would experience), OSHA does not require that an SDS be provided to purchasers. However, if exposure to such products exceeds that normally found in consumer applications, employees have a right to know about the properties of such hazardous chemicals. OSHA does not require or encourage employers to maintain an SDS for nonhazardous chemicals.

SDS forms typically include the following:

- Identification of properties.
- Hazard(s) identification.
- Composition/information on ingredients.
- First-aid measures.
- Fire-fighting measures.
- Accidental release measures.
- Handling and storage considerations.
- Exposure controls/personal protection information.
- Physical and chemical properties.
- Stability and reactivity.
- Toxicology information.
- Ecologic information.
- Disposal considerations.
- Transport information.
- Regulatory information.
- Other information.

Engineering Controls and PPE

Guidelines for laboratory areas in which hazardous chemicals are used or stored must be established. Physical facilities, and especially ventilation, must be adequate for the nature and volume of work conducted. Chemicals must be stored according to chemical compatibility (eg, corrosives, flammables, and oxidizers) and in minimal volumes. Bulk chemicals should be kept outside work areas. NFPA standards and others provide guidance for proper storage, sometimes in storage cabinets.[4,40,42]

Chemical fume hoods are recommended for use with organic solvents, volatile liquids, and dry chemicals with a significant inhalation hazard.[4] Although constructed with safety glass, most fume hood sashes are not designed to serve as safety shields. Hoods should be positioned in an area where there is minimal foot traffic to avoid disrupting the airflow and compromising the containment field.

PPE that may be provided, depending on the hazardous chemicals used, includes chemical-resistant gloves and aprons, shatter-proof safety goggles, and respirators.

Emergency showers should be accessible to areas where caustic, corrosive, toxic, flammable, or combustible chemicals are used.[4,43] There should be unobstructed access, within 10 seconds, to the showers from the areas where hazardous chemicals are used. Safety showers should be periodically flushed and tested for function, and associated floor drains should be checked to ensure that drain traps remain filled with water.

Safe Work Practices

Hazardous material should not be stored or transported in open containers. Containers and their lids or seals should be designed to prevent spills or leakage in all reasonably anticipated conditions. Containers should be able to safely store the maximum anticipated volume and be easy to clean. Surfaces should be kept clean and dry at all times.

When an employee is working with a chemical fume hood, all materials should be kept at least six inches behind the face opening. The vertical sliding sash should be positioned at the height specified on the certification sticker. The airfoil baffles and rear ventilation slots must not be blocked. Appendix 2-5 lists suggestions for working safely with specific chemicals.

Emergency Response Plan

The time to prepare for a chemical spill is before it occurs. A comprehensive employee training program should provide each employee with all tools necessary to act responsibly at the time of a chemical spill. The employee should know response procedures, be able to assess the severity of a chemical spill, know or be able to quickly look up the basic physical characteristics of the chemicals, and know where to find emergency response telephone numbers. The employee should be able to assess, stop, and confine the spill; either clean up the spill or call for a spill cleanup team; and follow procedures for reporting the spill. The employee must know when to ask for assistance, when to isolate the area, and where to find cleanup materials.

Chemical spills in the workplace can be categorized as follows[44]:

- *Incidental releases* are limited in quantity and toxicity and pose no significant safety or health hazard to employees. They may be safely cleaned up by employees familiar with the hazards of the chemical involved in the spill. Waste from the cleanup may be classified as hazardous and must be disposed of in the proper fashion. Appendix 2-6 describes appropriate responses to incidental spills.
- *Releases that may be incidental or may require an emergency response* may pose an exposure risk to employees depending on the circumstances. Considerations such as the hazardous substance properties, circumstances of release, and mitigating factors play a role in determining the appropriate response. The facility's emergency response plan should provide guidance on how to determine whether a spill is incidental or requires an emergency response.
- *Emergency response releases* pose a threat to health and safety regardless of the circumstances surrounding their release. These spills may require evacuation of the immedi-

ate area. The response typically comes from outside the immediate release area by personnel trained as emergency responders. These spills include those that involve immediate danger to life or health, serious threat of fire or explosion, and high levels of toxic substances.

Appendix 2-7 addresses the management of hazardous chemical spills. Spill cleanup kits or carts tailored to the specific hazards present should be available in each area. The kits or carts may contain rubber gloves and aprons, shoe covers, goggles, suitable aspirators, general absorbents, neutralizing agents, a broom, a dust pan, appropriate trash bags or cans for waste disposal, and cleanup directions. Chemical absorbents, such as clay absorbents or spill blankets, can be used for cleaning up a number of chemicals and thus may be advantageous for employees to use in spill situations.

With any spill of a hazardous chemical, but especially of a carcinogenic agent, it is essential to refer to the SDS and contact a designated supervisor or designee trained to handle these spills and hazardous waste disposal.[4] Facility environmental health and safety personnel can also offer assistance. The employer must assess the extent of the employee's exposure. After an exposure, an employee must be given an opportunity for medical consultation to determine the need for a medical examination.

Another source of workplace hazards is the unexpected release of hazardous vapors into the environment. OSHA has set limits for exposure to hazardous vapors from toxic and hazardous substances.[45] The potential risk associated with a chemical is determined by the manufacturer and listed on the SDS.

Chemical Waste Disposal

Most laboratory chemical waste is considered hazardous and is regulated by the EPA through the Resource Conservation and Recovery Act (42 USC §6901 et seq, 1976). This regulation specifies that hazardous waste can be legally disposed of only at an EPA-approved disposal facility. Disposal of chemical waste into a sanitary sewer is regulated by the Clean Water Act (33

USC §1251 et seq, 1977), and most US states have strict regulations concerning disposal of chemicals in the water system. Federal and applicable state regulations should be consulted when a facility is setting up and reviewing its waste disposal policies.

RADIATION SAFETY

Radiation can be defined as energy in the form of waves or particles emitted and propagated through space or a material medium. Gamma rays are electromagnetic radiation, whereas alpha and beta emitters are examples of particulate radiation. The presence of radiation in the blood bank, such as self-contained blood irradiators, requires additional precautions and training.[4,46]

Radiation Measurement Units

The measurement unit quantifying the amount of energy absorbed per unit mass of tissue is the gray (Gy) or radiation absorbed dose (rad); 1 Gy = 100 rad.

Dose equivalency measurements are more useful than simple energy measurements because dose equivalency measurements take into account the ability of different types of radiation to cause biological effects. The ability of radiation to cause damage is assigned a number, called a quality factor (QF). For example, exposure to a given amount of alpha particles (QF = 20) is far more damaging than exposure to an equivalent amount of gamma rays (QF = 1). The common unit of measurement for dose equivalency is the roentgen or rad equivalent man (rem). Rem is the dose from any type of radiation that produces biological effects in humans equivalent to 1 rad of x-rays, gamma rays, or beta rays. To obtain the dose from a particular type of radiation in rem, the number of rad should be multiplied by the QF (rad × QF = rem). Because the QF for gamma rays, x-rays, and most beta particles is 1, the dose in rad is equal to the dose in rem for these types of radiation.

Biological Effects of Radiation

Any harm to tissue begins with the absorption of radiation energy and subsequent disruption of chemical bonds. Molecules and atoms become ionized or excited (or both) by absorbing this energy. The direct action path leads to radiolysis or formation of free radicals that, in turn, alter the structure and function of molecules in the cell.

Molecular alterations can cause cellular or chromosomal changes, depending on the amount and type of radiation energy absorbed. Cellular changes can be manifested as a visible somatic effect (eg, erythema). Changes at the chromosome level may be manifested as leukemia or other cancers or possibly as germ-cell defects that are transmitted to future generations.

Several factors influence the level of biological damage from exposure, including the type of radiation, part of the body exposed, total absorbed dose, and dose rate. The total absorbed dose is the cumulative amount of radiation absorbed in the tissue. The greater the dose, the greater the potential for biological damage. Exposure can be acute or chronic. The low levels of ionizing radiation likely to occur in blood banks should not pose any detrimental risk.[47-50]

Regulations

The NRC controls the use of radioactive materials by establishing licensure requirements. States and municipalities may also have requirements for inspection, licensure, or both. The type of license for using radioisotopes or irradiators depends on the scope and magnitude of the use of radioactivity. US facilities should contact the NRC and appropriate state agencies for information on license requirements and applications as soon as such activities are proposed.

Each NRC-licensed establishment must have a qualified radiation safety officer who is responsible for establishing personnel protection requirements and for ensuring proper disposal and handling of radioactive materials. Specific radiation safety policies and procedures should address dose limits, employee training, warning signs and labels, shipping and handling guidance, radiation monitoring, and exposure management. Emergency procedures must be clearly defined and readily available to the staff.

In 2005, the NRC imposed additional security requirements for high-risk radioactive sources, including those used in blood irradiators.

The purpose of the increased controls is to reduce the risk of unauthorized use of radioactive materials that may pose a threat to public health and safety. These 2005 measures include controlled access, approval in writing of individuals deemed trustworthy and reliable to have unescorted access, a system of monitoring to immediately detect and respond to unauthorized access, and documentation of authorized personnel and monitoring activities.[51] In 2007, a requirement for fingerprinting was added.[52]

Exposure Limits

The NRC sets standards for protection against radiation hazards arising from licensed activities, including dose limits.[12] Such limits, or maximal permissible dose equivalents, are a measure of the radiation risk over time and serve as standards for exposure. The occupational total effective-dose-equivalent limit is 5 rem/year, the shallow dose equivalent limit (skin) is 50 rem/year, the extremity dose equivalent limit is 50 rem/year, and the eye dose equivalent limit is 15 rem/year.[12,47] Dose limits for an embryo or fetus must not exceed 0.5 rem during pregnancy.[12,47,53] Employers are expected not only to maintain radiation exposure below allowable limits, but also to keep exposure levels as far below these limits as can reasonably be achieved.

Radiation Monitoring

Monitoring is essential for early detection and prevention of problems resulting from radiation exposure. Monitoring is used to evaluate the facility's environment, work practices, and procedures and to comply with regulations and NRC licensing requirements. Monitoring is accomplished with the use of dosimeters, bioassays, survey meters, and wipe tests.[4]

Dosimeters, such as film or thermo-luminescent badges, rings, or both, measure personnel radiation doses. The need for dosimeters depends on the amount and type of radioactive materials in use; the facility radiation safety officer determines individual dosimeter needs. Film badges must be changed at least quarterly and in some instances monthly, be protected from high temperature and humidity, and be stored at work away from sources of radiation.

Bioassays, such as thyroid and whole body counting or urinalysis, may be used to determine whether there is radioactivity inside the body and if so, how much. If necessary, bioassays are usually performed quarterly and after an incident where accidental intake may have occurred.

Survey meters are sensitive to low levels of gamma or particulate radiation and provide a quantitative assessment of radiation hazard. Survey meters can be used to monitor storage areas for radioactive materials or wastes, testing areas during or after completion of a procedure, and packages or containers of radioactive materials. Survey meters must be calibrated annually by an authorized NRC licensee. Selection of appropriate meters should be discussed with the radiation safety officer.

In areas where radioactive materials are handled, all work surfaces, equipment, and floors that may be contaminated should be checked regularly with a wipe test. In the wipe test, a moistened absorbent material (the wipe) is passed over the surface and then measured for radiation.

Training

Personnel who handle radioactive materials or work with blood irradiators must receive radiation safety training before beginning work. This training should address the presence and potential hazards of radioactive materials in the employee's work area, general health protection issues, emergency procedures, and radiation warning signs and labels in use. Instruction in the following areas is also suggested:

- NRC regulations and license conditions.
- The importance of observing license conditions and regulations and of reporting violations or conditions of unnecessary exposure.
- Precautions to minimize exposure.
- Interpretation of results of monitoring devices.
- Requirements for pregnant workers.
- Employees' rights.
- Documentation and record-keeping requirements.

The need for refresher training is determined by the license agreement between the NRC and the facility.

Engineering Controls and PPE

Although self-contained blood irradiators present little risk to laboratory staff and film badges are not required for routine operation, blood establishments with irradiation programs must be licensed by the NRC.[48]

The manufacturer of the blood irradiator usually accepts responsibility for radiation safety requirements during transportation, installation, and validation of the unit as part of the purchase contract. The radiation safety officer can help oversee the installation and validation processes and should confirm that appropriate training, monitoring systems, procedures, and maintenance protocols are in place before use and that they reflect the manufacturer's recommendations. Suspected malfunctions must be reported immediately so that appropriate actions can be initiated.

Blood irradiators should be located in secure areas so that only trained individuals have access. Fire protection for the unit must also be considered. Automatic fire detection and control systems should be readily available in the immediate area. Blood components that have been irradiated are not radioactive and pose no threat to the staff or the general public.

Safe Work Practices

Each laboratory should establish policies and procedures for the safe use of radioactive materials. These policies and procedures should include requirements for following general laboratory safety principles, appropriate storage of radioactive solutions, and proper disposal of radioactive wastes. Radiation safety can be improved with the following procedures:

- Minimizing the time of exposure by working as efficiently as possible.
- Maximizing the distance from the source of the radiation by staying as far from the source as possible.
- Maximizing shielding (eg, by using a self-shielded irradiator or wearing a lead apron) when working with certain radioactive materials. These requirements are usually stipulated in the license conditions.
- Using appropriate shielding such as a lead barrier for gamma rays or plexiglass for beta particles.
- Using good housekeeping practices to minimize the spread of radioactivity to uncontrolled areas.

Emergency Response Plan

Radioactive contamination is the dispersal of radioactive material into or onto areas in which it is not intended—for example, the floor, work areas, equipment, personnel clothing, or personnel skin. The NRC regulations state that gamma or beta radioactive contamination cannot exceed 2200 disintegrations per minute (dpm) per 100 cm^2 in the posted (restricted) area or 220 dpm/100 cm^2 in an unrestricted area, such as a corridor. For alpha emitters, these values are 220 dpm/100 cm^2 and 22 dpm/100 cm^2, respectively.[54]

If a spill occurs, employees' contaminated skin surfaces must be washed several times, and the radiation safety officer must be notified immediately to provide further guidance. Others must not be allowed to enter the area until emergency response personnel arrive.

Radioactive Waste Management

Policies for the disposal of radioactive waste, whether liquid or solid, should be established with input from the radiation safety officer.

Liquid radioactive waste may be collected into large sturdy bottles labeled with an appropriate radiation waste tag. The rules for separation by chemical compatibility apply. Bottles must be carefully stored to protect against spillage or breakage. Dry or solid waste may be sealed in a plastic bag and tagged as radiation waste. The isotope, its activity, and the date on which the activity was measured should be recorded on the bag. Radioactive waste must never be discharged into the facility's drain system without prior approval by the radiation safety officer.

Radioisotopic Irradiator Removal and Replacement

Advances in technology have created alternatives to cesium irradiators that are comparable to, or even more effective than, those in use for blood irradiation. These non-radioisotopic irradiators mitigate security risks, eliminate liability risk, and provide longer lasting consistent throughput.

The Department of Energy's Office of Radiological Security offers a program to assist facilities that wish to make the switch from a cesium irradiator to a safer alternative. Financial incentives include no-cost removal and disposal of the cesium irradiator and partial payment toward a new non-radioisotopic device. Detailed information is available at ORSinfo@nnsa.doe.gov.

SHIPPING HAZARDOUS MATERIALS

Hazardous materials commonly shipped by transfusion medicine, cellular therapy, and clinical diagnostic services include infectious substances, biological substances, liquid nitrogen, and dry ice.

The US DOT regulations for transportation of hazardous materials are harmonized with the international standards published annually by the International Air Transport Association (IATA).[55,56] These regulations provide instructions for identifying, classifying, packaging, marking, labeling, and documenting hazardous materials to be offered for shipment on public roadways or by air.

Specimens are classified as Category A if they are known or likely to contain infectious substances in a form that is capable of causing permanent disability or life-threatening or fatal disease in otherwise healthy humans or animals when an exposure occurs. The proper shipping name for Category A specimens is "infectious substances, affecting humans" (UN2814) or "infectious substances, affecting animals only" (UN2900).

Specimens that may contain infectious substances but do not have the level of risk described above are classified as Category B, and the proper shipping name is "biological substance, Category B" (UN3373). HIV or HBV in culture is classified as a Category A infectious substance, but if these viruses are present in a specimen that is not an active culture, then they are still classified as Category B.

Patient specimens with minimal likelihood of containing pathogens are exempt from hazardous materials regulations if the specimens are properly packaged and marked. Blood components, cellular therapy products, and tissue for transfusion or transplantation are not subject to hazardous material regulations. Method 1-1 provides additional shipping instructions for safe transport of these materials. However, the most recent revision of the IATA or US DOT regulations should be consulted for the most current classification, packaging, and labeling requirements as well as for limitations on the volumes of hazardous materials that can be packaged together in one container.

GENERAL WASTE MANAGEMENT

Those responsible for safety at a facility must be concerned with protecting the environment as well as all staff members. Every effort should be made to establish facility-wide programs to reduce solid wastes, including nonhazardous and, especially, hazardous wastes (ie, biohazard, chemical, and radioactive wastes).[57]

A hazardous-waste-reduction program instituted at the point of use of the material achieves several goals. It reduces the institutional risk for occupational exposures to hazardous agents, reduces "cradle-to-grave" liability for disposal, and enhances compliance with environmental requirements to reduce pollution generated from daily operations of the laboratory.[37,58,59]

Facilities can minimize pollution of the environment by practicing the "three R's": reduce, reuse, and recycle. Seeking suitable alternatives to materials that create hazardous waste and separating hazardous waste from nonhazardous waste can reduce the volume of hazardous waste and decrease costs for its disposal.

Changes in techniques or materials to reduce the volume of infectious waste or render it less hazardous should be carefully considered, and employees should be encouraged to identify safer alternatives whenever possible.

Facilities should check with state and local health and environmental authorities about current requirements for storage and disposal of a particular multihazardous waste before creating that waste. If creating the multihazardous waste cannot be avoided, the volume of waste generated should be minimized. For example, in some states, copper sulfate contaminated with blood is considered a multihazardous waste. The disposal of this waste poses several problems with transportation from draw sites to a central facili-

ty for disposal of the final containers. State and local health departments must be involved in reviewing transportation and disposal practices where this is an issue, and procedures must be developed in accordance with state and local regulations as well as those of the US DOT. An example of a risk mitigation strategy would be implementing the use of approved devices to measure hemoglobin using a cuvette testing system. The cuvettes can then be discarded much like other sharps, therefore mitigating the risk of both chemical and blood-borne sources of exposure.

KEY POINTS

1. Facilities should be designed and maintained in a way that supports the work being done in the physical space. Designing the space to accommodate planned workflow, the need to restrict certain areas, the movement of materials and waste, equipment location, special air-handling requirements, and other critical aspects of the operation help ensure safety for staff and visitors, as well as the quality of products and services.
2. A facility's safety program should: a) strive to reduce hazards in the workplace; b) ensure that staff are trained to handle known hazards and potential risks; c) ensure that known hazards are clearly identified and marked; and d) describe policies and procedures for workplace safety and emergency response.
3. Safety programs should address fire, electrical, biological, chemical, and radioactive hazards that may be found in the facility.
4. For each type of hazard, five basic elements that must be covered are: a) training; b) hazard identification and communication; c) engineering controls and PPE; d) safe work practices, including waste disposal; and e) an emergency response plan.
5. Management controls ensure that the safety program is implemented, maintained, and effective. Management is responsible for: a) developing and communicating the written plan; b) ensuring implementation of the plan and providing adequate resources for this implementation; c) providing access to employee health services for prevention strategies and treatment of exposures; d) monitoring compliance and effectiveness; and e) evaluating and improving the safety plan.

REFERENCES

1. Gammon R, ed. Standards for blood banks and transfusion services. 32nd ed. Bethesda, MD: AABB, 2020.
2. Haspel RL, ed. Standards for cellular therapy services. 9th ed. Bethesda, MD: AABB, 2019.
3. Laboratory Accreditation Program laboratory general checklist. Northfield, IL: College of American Pathologists, 2018.
4. Clinical laboratory safety: Approved guideline. 3rd ed. NCCLS document GP17-A3. Wayne, PA: Clinical and Laboratory Standards Institute, 2012.
5. Hospital accreditation standards. Oakbrook Terrace, IL: The Joint Commission, 2019.
6. Laboratory accreditation standards. Oakbrook Terrace, IL: The Joint Commission, 2019.

7. NFPA 70—National electrical code. Quincy, MA: National Fire Protection Association, 2017.

8. ANSI/ASHRAE Standard 62.1-2016. Ventilation for acceptable indoor air quality. Atlanta, GA: American Society of Heating, Refrigerating, and Air-Conditioning Engineers, Inc, 2016.

9. Code of federal regulations. Title 21, CFR Part 1271.190. Washington, DC: US Government Publishing Office, 2019 (revised annually).

10. ISO-14644: Cleanrooms and associated controlled environments, Parts 1-9. ISO/TC 209. Geneva, Switzerland: International Organization for Standardization, 1999-2015.

11. ISO-14698: Cleanrooms and associated controlled environments—bio-contamination control, Part 1: General principles and methods. ISO/TC 209. Geneva, Switzerland: International Organization for Standardization, 2015.

12. Code of federal regulations. Title 10, CFR Part 20. Washington, DC: US Government Publishing Office, 2019 (revised annually).

13. Siegel JD, Rhinehart E, Jackson M, et al for the Healthcare Infection Control Practices Advisory Committee. 2007 Guideline for isolation precautions: Preventing transmission of infectious agents in healthcare settings. Atlanta, GA: Centers for Disease Control and Prevention, 2007. [Available at https://www.cdc.gov/infection control/guidelines/isolation/index.html.]

14. Code of federal regulations. Title 29, CFR Part 1910.1030. Washington, DC: US Government Publishing Office, 2019 (revised annually).

15. Code of federal regulations. Title 29, CFR Part 1910.1200. Washington, DC: US Government Publishing Office, 2019 (revised annually).

16. US Department of Health and Human Services. Biosafety in microbiological and biomedical laboratories. 5th ed. Washington, DC: US Government Publishing Office, 2009.

17. Bernard B, ed. Musculoskeletal disorders and workplace factors: A critical review of epidemiologic evidence for work-related musculoskeletal disorders of the neck, upper extremity, and low back. NIOSH publication no. 97-141. Washington, DC: National Institute for Occupational Safety and Health, 1997.

18. Code of federal regulations. Title 29, CFR Part 1910.38. Washington, DC: US Government Publishing Office, 2019 (revised annually).

19. Wagner KD, ed. Environmental management in healthcare facilities. Philadelphia: WB Saunders, 1998.

20. Code of federal regulations. Title 29, CFR Part 1910.1450. Washington, DC: US Government Publishing Office, 2019 (revised annually).

21. Centers for Disease Control and Prevention. Public Health Service guidelines for the management of occupational exposures to HBV, HCV, and HIV and recommendations for postexposure prophylaxis. MMWR Morb Mortal Wkly Rep 2001;50:1-52.

22. Code of federal regulations. Title 29, CFR Part 1904.39. Washington, DC: US Government Publishing Office, 2019 (revised annually).

23. Code of federal regulations. Title 29, CFR Parts 1904.1 and 1904.7. Washington, DC: US Government Publishing Office, 2019 (revised annually).

24. Code of federal regulations. Title 29, CFR Part 1910.1020. Washington, DC: US Government Publishing Office, 2019 (revised annually).

25. NIOSH Alert: Preventing allergic reactions to natural rubber latex in the workplace. (June 1997) NIOSH Publication No. 97-135. Washington, DC: National Institute for Occupational Safety and Health, 1997. [Available at http://www.cdc.gov/niosh/docs/97-135/.]

26. NFPA 101: Life safety code. Quincy, MA: National Fire Protection Association, 2018.

27. Fowler TW, Miles KK. Electrical safety: Safety and health for electrical trades student manual. (January 2009) NIOSH Publication No. 2009-113. Washington, DC: National Institute for Occupational Safety and Health, 2002.

28. OSHA technical manual: TED 1-0.15A. Washington, DC: US Department of Labor, 1999.

29. Enforcement procedures for the occupational exposure to bloodborne pathogens. Directive CPL 02-02-069. Washington, DC: US Department of Labor, 2001.

30. US Department of Health and Human Services. Appendix A: Primary containment for biohazards: Selection, installation, and use of biological safety cabinets. In: Biosafety in microbiological and biomedical laboratories. 5th ed. Washington, DC: US Government Publishing Office, 2009. [Available at http://www.cdc.gov/bio safety/publications.]

31. Richmond JY. Safe practices and procedures for working with human specimens in biomedical research laboratories. J Clin Immunoassay 1988;11:115-19.

32. US Environmental Protection Agency. Pesticide registration: Selected EPA-registered disinfectants. Washington, DC: EPA, 2016. [Available at

https://www.epa.gov/pesticide-registration/selected-epa-registered-disinfectants.]

33. Rutala WA. APIC guideline for selection and use of disinfectants. Am J Infect Control 1996;24:313-42.

34. Evans MR, Henderson DK, Bennett JE. Potential for laboratory exposures to biohazardous agents found in blood. Am J Public Health 1990;80:423-7.

35. Food and Drug Administration. Memorandum: Guideline for collection of blood or blood products from donors with positive tests for infectious disease markers ("high risk" donors). (September, 1989) Silver Spring, MD: CBER Office of Communication, Outreach, and Development, 1989.

36. Food and Drug Administration. Memorandum: Revision to 26 October 1989 guidelines for collection of blood or blood products from donors with positive tests for infectious disease markers ("high-risk" donors). (April 17, 1991) Silver Spring, MD: CBER Office of Communication, Outreach, and Development, 1991. [Available at https://www.fda.gov/vaccines-blood-biologics/other-recommendations-biologics-manufacturers/memoranda-blood-establishments.]

37. US Environmental Protection Agency. EPA guide for infectious waste management. EPA/530-SW-86-014. NTIS #PB86-199130. Washington, DC: National Technical Information Service, 1986.

38. Code of federal regulations. Title 40, CFR Part 264. Washington, DC: US Government Publishing Office, 2019 (revised annually).

39. NIOSH pocket guide to chemical hazards. Washington, DC: National Institute for Occupational Safety and Health, 2010. [Available at https://www.cdc.gov/niosh/npg.]

40. NFPA 704—Standard system for the identification of the hazards of materials for emergency response. Quincy, MA: National Fire Protection Association, 2017.

41. American Coatings Association. HMIS implementation manual. 4th ed. Neenah, WI: JJ Keller and Associates, Inc, 2014.

42. Lisella FS, Thomasston SW. Chemical safety in the microbiology laboratory. In: Fleming DO, Richardson JH, Tulis JJ, Vesley D, eds. Laboratory safety, principles, and practices. 2nd ed. Washington, DC: American Society for Microbiology Press, 1995:247-54.

43. American national standards for emergency eyewash and shower equipment. ANSI Z358.1-2014. New York: American National Standards Institute, 2014.

44. Inspection procedures for 29 CFR 1910.120 and 1926.65, paragraph (q): Emergency response to hazardous substance releases. OSHA Directive CPL 02-02-073. Washington, DC: Occupational Safety and Health Administration, 2007.

45. Code of federal regulations. Title 29, CFR Part 1910.1000. Washington, DC: US Government Publishing Office, 2019 (revised annually).

46. Cook SS. Selection and installation of self-contained irradiators. In: Butch S, Tiehen A, eds. Blood irradiation: A user's guide. Bethesda, MD: AABB Press, 1996:19-40.

47. Beir V. Health effects of exposure to low levels of ionizing radiation. Washington, DC: National Academy Press, 1990:1-8.

48. Regulatory guide 8.29: Instruction concerning risks from occupational radiation exposure. Washington, DC: Nuclear Regulatory Commission, 1996.

49. NCRP report no. 115: Risk estimates for radiation protection: Recommendations of the National Council on Radiation Protection and Measurements. Bethesda, MD: National Council on Radiation Protection and Measurements, 1993.

50. NCRP report no. 105: Radiation protection for medical and allied health personnel: Recommendations of the National Council on Radiation Protection and Measurements. Bethesda, MD: National Council on Radiation Protection and Measurements, 1989.

51. EA-05 090. Enforcement action: Order imposing increased controls (licensees authorized to possess radioactive material quantities of concern). (November 14, 2005) Rockville, MD: US Nuclear Regulatory Commission, 2005.

52. RIS 2007-14. Fingerprinting requirements for licensees implementing the increased control order. (June 5, 2007) Rockville, MD: US Nuclear Regulatory Commission, 2007.

53. US Nuclear Regulatory Commission regulatory guide 8.13: Instruction concerning prenatal radiation exposure. Washington, DC: NRC, 1999.

54. Nuclear Regulatory Commission regulatory guide 8.23: Radiation surveys at medical institutions. Washington, DC: NRC, 1981.

55. Code of federal regulations. Title 49, CFR Parts 171.22. Washington, DC: US Government Publishing Office, 2019 (revised annually).

56. Dangerous goods regulations manual. 54th ed. Montreal, PQ, Canada: International Air Transport Association, 2019 (revised annually).

57. United States Code. Pollution prevention act. 42 USC §§13101 and 13102 et seq.

58. Clinical laboratory waste management. Approved guideline. 3rd ed. GP05-A3. Wayne, PA: Clinical and Laboratory Standards Institute, 2011.

59. Code of federal regulations. Title 21, CFR Part 606.40(d)(1.) Washington, DC: US Government Publishing Office, 2019 (revised annually).

APPENDIX 2-1

Safety Regulations and Recommendations Applicable to Health-Care Settings

Agency/Organization	Reference	Title
Federal Regulations and Recommendations		
Nuclear Regulatory Commission	10 CFR 20	Standards for Protection Against Radiation
	10 CFR 36	Licenses and Radiation Safety Requirements for Irradiators
	Guide 8.29	Instructions Concerning Risks from Occupational Radiation Exposure
Occupational Safety and Health Administration	29 CFR 1910.1030	Occupational Exposure to Blood-borne Pathogens
	29 CFR 1910.1020	Access to Employee Exposure and Medical Records
	29 CFR 1910.1096	Ionizing Radiation
	29 CFR 1910.1200	Hazard Communication Standard
	29 CFR 1910.1450	Occupational Exposure to Hazardous Chemicals in Laboratories
Department of Transportation	49 CFR 171-180	Hazardous Materials Regulations
Environmental Protection Agency (EPA)		EPA Guide for Infectious Waste Management
Centers for Disease Control and Prevention		Guideline for Isolation Precautions in Hospitals
Food and Drug Administration	21 CFR 606.3-606.171	Current Good Manufacturing Practice for Blood and Blood Components
	21 CFR 630.40	General Requirements for Blood, Blood Components, and Blood Derivatives
	21 CFR 640.1-640.130	Additional Standards for Human Blood and Blood Products
	21 CFR 211.1-211.208	Current Good Manufacturing Practice for Finished Pharmaceuticals
	21 CFR 1270	Human Tissue Intended for Transplantation
	21 CFR 1271	Human Cells, Tissues, and Cellular and Tissue-Based Products

(Continued)

APPENDIX 2-1

Safety Regulations and Recommendations Applicable to Health-Care Settings
(Continued)

Agency/Organization	Reference	Title
Trade and Professional Organizations		
National Fire Protection Association (NFPA)	NFPA 70	National Electrical Code
	NFPA 70E	Electrical Safety Requirements for Employee Workplaces
	NFPA 101	Life Safety Code
	NFPA 99	Standards for Health Care Facilities
	NFPA 704	Standard for Identification of the Hazards of Materials for Emergency Response
National Paint and Coatings Association		Hazardous Materials Identification System Implementation Manual
International Air Transport Association		Dangerous Goods Regulations

CFR = Code of Federal Regulations.

APPENDIX 2-2
General Guidance for Safe Work Practices, Personal Protective Equipment, and Engineering Controls

UNIFORMS AND LABORATORY COATS

Personnel should wear closed laboratory coats or full aprons over long-sleeved uniforms or gowns when they are exposed to blood, corrosive chemicals, or carcinogens. The material of required coverings should be appropriate for the type and amount of hazard exposure. Plastic disposable aprons may be worn over cotton coats when there is a high probability of large spills or splashing of blood and body fluids; nitrile rubber aprons may be preferred when caustic chemicals are poured.

Protective coverings should be removed before the employee leaves the work area and should be discarded or stored away from heat sources and clean clothing. Contaminated clothing should be removed promptly, placed in a suitable container, and laundered or discarded as potentially infectious. Home laundering of garments worn in Biosafety Level 2 areas is not permitted because unpredictable methods of transportation and handling can spread contamination, and home laundering techniques may not be effective.[1]

GLOVES

Gloves or equivalent barriers should be used whenever tasks are likely to involve exposure to hazardous materials.

Types of Gloves

Glove type varies with the task:

- Sterile gloves: for procedures involving contact with normally sterile areas of the body.

- Examination gloves: for procedures involving contact with mucous membranes, unless otherwise indicated, and for other patient care or diagnostic procedures that do not require the use of sterile gloves.

- Rubber utility gloves: for housekeeping chores involving potential blood contact, instrument cleaning and decontamination procedures, and handling concentrated acids and organic solvents. Utility gloves may be decontaminated and reused but should be discarded if they show signs of deterioration (eg, peeling, cracks, or discoloration) or if they develop punctures or tears.

- Insulated gloves: for handling hot or frozen material.

The following situations require the use of gloves[1]:

The following guidelines should be used to determine when gloves are necessary[1]:

- For donor phlebotomy when the health-care worker has cuts, scratches, or other breaks in his or her skin.

- For phlebotomy of autologous donors or patients (eg, therapeutic apheresis procedures or intraoperative red cell collection).

- For persons who are receiving training in phlebotomy.

- When handling open blood containers or specimens.

- When collecting or handling blood or specimens from patients or donors known to be infected with a blood-borne pathogen.

- When examining mucous membranes or open skin lesions.

- When handling corrosive chemicals and radioactive materials.

(Continued)

APPENDIX 2-2
General Guidance for Safe Work Practices, Personal Protective Equipment, and Engineering Controls (Continued)

- When cleaning up spills or handling waste materials.

- When the likelihood of exposure cannot be assessed because of lack of experience with a procedure or situation.

The Occupational Safety and Health Administration (OSHA) does not require the routine use of gloves by phlebotomists working with healthy prescreened donors or the changing of unsoiled gloves between donors if gloves are worn.[1,2] Experience has shown that the phlebotomy process is low risk because donors typically have low rates of infectious disease markers. Also, exposure to blood is rare during routine phlebotomy, and other alternatives can be used to provide barrier protection, such as using a folded gauze pad to control any blood flow when the needle is removed from the donor's arm.

Employers whose policies and procedures do not require routine gloving should periodically reevaluate the potential need for gloves. Employees should never be discouraged from using gloves, and gloves should always be available.

Guidance on Use

The safe use of gloves by employees includes the following[3,4]:

- Securely bandage or cover open skin lesions on hands and arms before putting on gloves.

- Change gloves immediately if they are torn, punctured, or contaminated; after handling high-risk samples; or after performing a physical examination (eg, on an apheresis donor).

- Remove gloves by keeping their outside surfaces in contact only with outside and by turning the glove inside out while taking it off.

- Use gloves only when needed, and avoid touching clean surfaces such as telephones, doorknobs, or computer terminals with gloves.

- Change gloves between patient contacts. Unsoiled gloves need not be changed between donors.

- Wash hands with soap or other suitable disinfectant after removing gloves.

- Do not wash or disinfect surgical or examination gloves for reuse. Washing with surfactants may cause "wicking" (ie, enhanced penetration of liquids through undetected holes in the glove). Disinfecting agents may cause deterioration of gloves.

- Use only water-based hand lotions with gloves, if needed; oil-based products cause minute cracks in latex.

FACE SHIELDS, MASKS, AND SAFETY GOGGLES

Where there is a risk of blood or chemical splashes, the eyes and mucous membranes of the mouth and nose should be protected.[5] Permanent shields fixed as a part of equipment or bench design are preferred (eg, splash barriers attached to tubing sealers or centrifuge cabinets). All barriers should be cleaned and disinfected on a regular basis.

Safety glasses alone provide impact protection from projectiles but do not adequately protect eyes from biohazard or chemical splashes. Full-face shields or masks and safety goggles are recommended when permanent shields cannot be used. Many designs are commercially available; eliciting staff input on comfort and selection can increase use.

Masks should be worn whenever there is danger from inhalation. Simple, disposable dust masks are adequate for handling dry chemicals, but respirators with organic vapor filters are preferred for areas where noxious

APPENDIX 2-2

General Guidance for Safe Work Practices, Personal Protective Equipment, and Engineering Controls (Continued)

fumes are produced (eg, for cleaning up spills of noxious materials). Respirators should be fitted to their wearers and checked annually.

HAND WASHING

Frequent, thorough hand washing is the first line of defense in infection control. Blood-borne pathogens generally do not penetrate intact skin, so immediate removal reduces the likelihood of transfer to a mucous membrane or broken skin area or of transmission to others. Thorough washing of hands (and arms) also reduces the risks from exposure to hazardous chemicals and radioactive materials.

Employees should always wash their hands before leaving a restricted work area or using a biosafety cabinet, between medical examinations, immediately after becoming soiled with blood or hazardous materials, after removing gloves, or after using the toilet. Washing hands thoroughly before touching contact lenses or applying cosmetics is essential.

OSHA allows the use of waterless antiseptic solutions for hand washing as an interim method.[2] These solutions are useful for mobile donor collections or in areas where water is not readily available for cleanup purposes. If such methods are used, however, hands must be washed with soap and running water as soon as possible thereafter. Because there is no listing or registration of acceptable hand-wipe products similar to the one that the Environmental Protection Agency maintains for surface disinfectants, consumers should request data from the manufacturer to support advertising claims.

EYEWASHES

Laboratory areas that contain hazardous chemicals must be equipped with eyewash stations.[3,5] Unobstructed access within a 10-second walk from the location of chemical use must be provided for these stations. Eyewashes must operate so that both of the user's hands are free to hold open the eyes. Procedures and indications for use must be posted, and routine function checks must be performed. Testing eyewash fountains weekly helps ensure proper function and flushes out stagnant water. Portable eyewash systems are allowed only if they can deliver flushing fluid to the eyes at a rate of at least 1.5 liters per minute for 15 minutes. They should be monitored routinely to ensure the purity of their contents.

Employees should be trained in the proper use of eyewash devices, although prevention—through consistent and appropriate use of safety glasses or shields—is preferred. If a splash occurs, the employee should be directed to keep his or her eyelids open and to use the eyewash according to procedures, or the employee should go to the nearest sink and direct a steady, tepid stream of water into his or her eyes. Solutions other than water should be used only in accordance with a physician's direction.

After eyes are adequately flushed (many facilities recommend 15 minutes), follow-up medical care should be sought, especially if pain or redness develops. Whether washing the eyes is effective in preventing infection has not been demonstrated, but it is considered desirable when accidents occur.

1. Code of federal regulations. Title 29, CFR Part 1910.1030. Washington, DC: US Government Publishing Office, 2019 (revised annually).
2. Occupational Safety and Health Administration. Enforcement procedures for the occupational exposure to bloodborne pathogens. OSHA Instruction CPL 02-02-069. Washington, DC: US Government Publishing Office, 2001. [Available at https://www.osha.gov/enforcement/directives/cpl-02-02-069.]
3. Clinical laboratory safety: Approved guideline. 3rd ed (GP17-A3). Wayne, PA: Clinical and Laboratory Standards Institute, 2012.
4. CAP accreditation checklists: Laboratory general. Chicago: College of American Pathologists, 2018.
5. American national standards for emergency eyewash and shower equipment. ANSI Z358.1-2009. New York: American National Standards Institute, 2009.

APPENDIX 2-3
Biosafety Level 2 Precautions

Biosafety Level 2 precautions as applied in the blood establishment setting include at least the following[1,2]:

- High-risk activities are appropriately segregated from lower-risk activities, and the boundaries are clearly defined.

- Bench tops are easily cleaned and are decontaminated daily with a hospital disinfectant approved by the Environmental Protection Agency.

- Laboratory rooms have closable doors and sinks. An air system with no recirculation is preferred but not required.

- Workers are required to perform procedures that create aerosols (eg, opening evacuated tubes, centrifuging, mixing, or sonication) in a biological safety cabinet or equivalent or to wear masks and goggles in addition to gloves and gowns during such procedures. (Note: Open tubes of blood should not be centrifuged. If whole units of blood or plasma are centrifuged, overwrapping is recommended to contain leaks.)

- Gowns and gloves are used routinely and in accordance with general safety guidelines. Face shields or their equivalents are used where there is a risk from splashing.

- Mouth pipetting is prohibited.

- No eating, drinking, smoking, applying cosmetics, or manipulating contact lenses occurs in the work area. All food and drink are stored outside the restricted area, and laboratory glassware is never used for food or drink. Personnel are instructed to avoid touching their face, ears, mouth, eyes, or nose with their hands or other objects, such as pencils and telephones.

- Needles and syringes are used and disposed of in a safe manner. Needles must never be bent, broken, sheared, replaced in a sheath, or detached from a syringe before being placed in puncture-proof, leak-proof containers for controlled disposal. Procedures are designed to minimize exposure to sharp objects.

- All blood specimens are placed in well-constructed containers with secure lids to prevent leaking during transport. Blood is packaged for shipment in accordance with regulatory agency requirements for etiologic agents or clinical specimens, as appropriate.

- Infectious waste is not compacted and is decontaminated before its disposal in leak-proof containers. Proper packaging includes double, seamless, tear-resistant, orange or red bags that are enclosed in protective cartons. Both the cartons and the bags inside display the biohazard symbol. Throughout delivery to an incinerator or autoclave, waste is handled only by suitably trained persons. If a waste management contractor is used, the agreement should clearly define the respective responsibilities of the staff and the contractor.

- Equipment to be repaired or submitted for preventive maintenance, if potentially contaminated with blood, must be decontaminated before its release to a repair technician.

- Accidental exposure to suspected or actual hazardous material is reported to the laboratory director or responsible person immediately.

1. Clinical laboratory safety: Approved guideline. 3rd ed (GP17-A3). Wayne, PA: Clinical and Laboratory Standards Institute, 2012.
2. Fleming DO. Laboratory biosafety practices. In: Fleming DO, Richardson JH, Tulis JJ, Vesley DD, eds. Laboratory safety, principles, and practices. 2nd ed. Washington, DC: American Society for Microbiology Press, 1995:203-18.

APPENDIX 2-4
Sample List of Hazardous Chemicals That May Be Encountered in a Blood Bank

Chemical	Hazard
Ammonium chloride	Irritant
Bromelin	Irritant, sensitizer
Calcium chloride	Irritant
Carbon dioxide (frozen dry ice)	Caustic
Carbonyl iron powder	Oxidizer
Chloroform	Toxic, suspected carcinogen
Chloroquine	Irritant, corrosive
Chromium-111 chloride hexahydrate	Toxic, irritant, sensitizer
Citric acid	Irritant
Copper sulfate (cupric sulfate)	Toxic, irritant
Dichloromethane	Toxic, irritant
Digitonin	Toxic
Dimethyl sulfoxide	Irritant
Dry ice (carbon dioxide, frozen)	Caustic
Ethidium bromide	Carcinogen, irritant
Ethylenediaminetetraacetic acid	Irritant
Ethyl ether	Highly flammable and explosive, toxic, irritant
Ficin (powder)	Irritant, sensitizer
Formaldehyde solution (34.9%)	Suspected carcinogen, combustible, toxic
Glycerol	Irritant
Hydrochloric acid	Highly toxic, corrosive
Imidazole	Irritant
Isopropyl (rubbing) alcohol	Flammable, irritant
Liquid nitrogen	Caustic
Lyphogel	Corrosive
2-Mercaptoethanol	Toxic, stench
Mercury	Toxic
Mineral oil	Irritant, carcinogen, combustible
Papain	Irritant, sensitizer
Polybrene	Toxic
Sodium azide	Toxic, irritant, explosive when heated

(Continued)

APPENDIX 2-4

Sample List of Hazardous Chemicals That May Be Encountered in a Blood Bank (Continued)

Chemical	Hazard
Sodium ethylmercurithiosalicylate (thimerosal)	Highly toxic, irritant
Sodium hydrosulfite	Toxic, irritant
Sodium hydroxide	Corrosive, toxic
Sodium hypochlorite (bleach)	Corrosive
Sodium phosphate	Irritant, hygroscopic
Sulfosalicylic acid	Toxic, corrosive
Trichloroacetic acid	Corrosive, toxic
Trypsin	Irritant, sensitizer
Xylene	Highly flammable, toxic, irritant

APPENDIX 2-5

Chemical Categories and How to Work Safely with Them

Chemical Category	Hazard	Precautions	Special Treatment
Acids, alkalis, and corrosive compounds	Irritation, severe burns, tissue damage	During transport, protect large containers with plastic or rubber bucket carriers. During pouring, wear eye protection and chemical-resistant-rated gloves and gowns as recommended. Always add acid to water; never add water to acid. When working with large jugs, have one hand on the neck and the other hand at the base, and position them away from the face.	Store concentrated acids in acid safety cabinets. Limit volumes of concentrated acids to 1 liter per container. Post cautions for materials in the area. Report changes in appearance to chemical safety officer. (Perchloric acid may be explosive if it becomes yellowish or brown.)
Acrylamide	Neurotoxic, carcinogenic, absorbed through the skin	Wear chemically rated gloves. Wash hands immediately after exposure.	Store in a chemical cabinet.
Compressed gases	Explosive	Label contents. Leave valve safety covers on until use. Open valves slowly for use. Label empty tanks.	Transport using hand trucks or dollies. Place cylinders in a stand or secure them to prevent tipping over. Store in well-ventilated separate rooms. Do not store oxygen close to combustible gas or solvents. Check connections for leaks using soapy water.

(Continued)

APPENDIX 2-5

Chemical Categories and How to Work Safely with Them (Continued)

Chemical Category	Hazard	Precautions	Special Treatment
Flammable solvents	Classified according to flash point—see material safety data sheet, classified according to volatility	Use extreme caution when handling. Post "No Smoking" signs in working area. Keep a fire extinguisher and solvent cleanup kit in the room. Pour volatile solvents under a suitable hood. Use eye protection and chemical-resistant neoprene gloves when pouring. No flame or other source of possible ignition should be in or near areas where flammable solvents are being poured. Label as "flammable."	Make every attempt to replace hazardous materials with less hazardous materials. Store containers larger than 1 gallon in a flammable-solvent storage room or a fire safety cabinet. Ground metal containers by connecting the can to a water pipe or ground connection. If the recipient container is also metal, it should be electrically connected to the delivery container during pouring.
Liquid nitrogen	Freeze injury, severe burns to skin or eyes	Use heavy insulated gloves and goggles when working with liquid nitrogen.	The tanks should be securely supported to avoid being tipped over. The final container of liquid nitrogen (freezing unit) must be securely supported to avoid being tipped over.

APPENDIX 2-6
Incidental Spill Response*

Chemicals	Hazards	PPE	Control Materials

Acids
  Acetic
  Hydrochloric
  Nitric
  Perchloric
  Sulfuric
  Photographic
    chemicals (acidic)
	If inhaled, causes severe irritation.
	Contact causes burns to skin and eyes.
	Spills are corrosive.
	Fire or contact with metal may produce irritating or poisonous gas.
	Nitric, perchloric, and sulfuric acids are water-reactive oxidizers.
		Acid-resistant gloves
		Apron and coveralls
		Goggles and face shield
		Acid-resistant foot covers
			Acid neutralizers or absorbent material
			Absorbent boom
			Leak-proof containers
			Absorbent pillow
			Mat (cover drain)
			Shovel or paddle

Bases and caustics
  Potassium hydroxide
  Sodium hydroxide
  Photographic
    chemicals (basic)
	Spills are corrosive.
	Fire may produce irritating or poisonous gas.
		Gloves
		Impervious apron or coveralls
		Goggles or face shield
		Impervious foot covers
			Base control/neutralizer
			Absorbent pillow
			Absorbent boom
			Drain mat
			Leak-proof container
			Shovel or paddle

Chlorine
  Bleach
  Sodium hypochlorite
	Inhalation can cause respiratory irritation.
	Liquid contact can produce irritation of the eyes or skin.
	Toxicity is caused by alkalinity, possible chlorine gas generation, and oxidant properties.
		Gloves (double set of 4H undergloves and butyl or nitrile overgloves)
		Impervious apron or coveralls
		Goggles or face shield
		Impervious foot covers (neoprene boots for emergency response releases)
		Self-contained breathing apparatus (emergency response releases)
			Chlorine control powder
			Absorbent pillow
			Absorbent material
			Absorbent boom
			Drain mat
			Vapor barrier
			Leak-proof container
			Shovel or paddle

Cryogenic gases
  Carbon dioxide
  Nitrous oxide
  Liquid nitrogen
	Contact with liquid nitrogen can produce frostbite.
	Release can create an oxygen-deficient atmosphere.
	Nitrous oxide has anesthetic effects.
		Full face shield or goggles
		Neoprene boots
		Gloves (insulated to provide protection from the cold)
			Hand truck (to transport cylinder outdoors if necessary)
			Soap solution (to check for leaks)
			Putty (to stop minor pipe and line leaks)

(Continued)

APPENDIX 2-6

Incidental Spill Response* (Continued)

Chemicals	Hazards	PPE	Control Materials

Flammable gases
    Acetylene
    Oxygen gases
    Butane
    Propane
	Simple asphyxiant (displaces air).
	Inhaled vapors have an anesthetic potential.
	Flammable gases pose an extreme fire and explosion hazard.
	Release can create an oxygen-deficient atmosphere.
		Face shield and goggles
		Neoprene boots
		Double set of gloves
		Coveralls with hood and feet
			Hand truck (to transport cylinder outdoors if needed)
			Soap solution (to check for leaks)

Flammable liquids
    Acetone
    Xylene
    Methyl alcohol
        toluene
    Ethyl alcohol
    Other alcohols
	Vapors are harmful if inhaled (central nervous system depressants).
	Liquid is harmful if absorbed through the skin.
	Substances are extremely flammable.
	Liquid evaporates to form flammable vapors.
		Gloves (double set of 4H undergloves and butyl or nitrile overgloves)
		Impervious apron or coveralls
		Goggles or face shield
		Impervious foot covers
			Absorbent material
			Absorbent boom
			Absorbent pillow
			Shovel or paddle (nonmetal, nonsparking)
			Drain mat
			Leak-proof container

Formaldehyde and glutaraldehyde
    4% formaldehyde
    37% formaldehyde
    10% formalin
    2% glutaraldehyde
	Vapors are harmful if inhaled; liquids are harmful if absorbed through skin.
	Substances are irritants to skin, eyes, and respiratory tract.
	Formaldehyde is a suspected human carcinogen.
	37% formaldehyde should be kept away from heat, sparks, and flames.
		Gloves (double set of 4H undergloves and butyl or nitrile overgloves)
		Impervious apron or coveralls
		Goggles
		Impervious foot covers
			Aldehyde neutralizer or absorbent
			Absorbent boom
			Absorbent pillow
			Shovel or paddle (nonsparking)
			Drain mat
			Leak-proof container

APPENDIX 2-6
Incidental Spill Response* (Continued)

Chemicals	Hazards	PPE	Control Materials

Mercury
  Cantor tubes
  Thermometers
  Barometers
  Sphygmomanometers
  Mercuric chloride
	Mercury and mercury vapors are rapidly absorbed in respiratory tract, gastrointestinal (GI) tract, or skin.
	Short-term exposure may cause erosion of respiratory or GI tracts, nausea, vomiting, bloody diarrhea, shock, headache, or metallic taste.
	Inhalation of high concentrations can cause pneumonitis, chest pain, dyspnea, coughing, stomatitis, gingivitis, and salivation.
	Avoid evaporation of mercury from tiny globules by quick and thorough cleaning.
		Gloves (double set of 4H undergloves and butyl or nitrile overgloves)
		Impervious apron or coveralls
		Goggles
		Impervious foot covers
			Mercury vacuum or spill kit
			Scoop
			Aspirator
			Hazardous waste containers
			Mercury indicator powder
			Absorbent material
			Spatula
			Disposable towels
			Sponge with amalgam
			Vapor suppressor

*This list of physical and health hazards is not intended as a substitute for the material safety data sheet (SDS) information. In case of a spill or if any questions arise, always refer to the chemical-specific SDS for more complete information.

APPENDIX 2-7
Managing Hazardous Chemical Spills

Actions	Instructions for Hazardous Liquids, Gases, and Mercury
Deenergize.	Liquids: For 37% formaldehyde, deenergize and remove all sources of ignition within 10 feet of spilled hazardous material. For flammable liquids, remove all sources of ignition.
	Gases: Remove all sources of heat and ignition within 50 feet for flammable gases.
	Remove all sources of heat and ignition for nitrous oxide release.
Isolate, evacuate, and secure the area.	Isolate the spill area and evacuate everyone from the area surrounding the spill except those responsible for cleaning up the spill. (For mercury, evacuate within 10 feet for small spills or 20 feet for large spills.) Secure the area.
Have the appropriate personal protective equipment (PPE).	See Appendix 2-2 for recommended PPE.
Contain the spill.	Liquids or mercury: Stop the source of spill if possible.
	Gases: Assess the scene; consider the circumstances of the release (quantity, location, and ventilation). If circumstances indicate that it is an emergency response release, make appropriate notifications; if the release is determined to be incidental, contact the supplier for assistance.
Confine the spill.	Liquids: Confine the spill to the initial spill area using appropriate control equipment and material. For flammable liquids, dike off all drains.
	Gases: Follow the supplier's suggestions or request outside assistance.
	Mercury: Use appropriate materials to confine the spill (see Appendix 2-6). Expel mercury from the aspirator bulb into a leak-proof container, if applicable.
Neutralize the spill.	Liquids: Apply appropriate control materials to neutralize the chemical (see Appendix 2-6).
	Mercury: Use a mercury spill kit if needed.
Clean up the spill.	Liquids: Scoop up solidified materials, booms, pillows, and any other materials. Put used materials into a leak-proof container. Label the container with the name of the hazardous materials. Wipe up residual material. Wipe the spill area surface three times with a detergent solution. Rinse the areas with clean water. Collect the supplies used (eg, goggles or shovels) and remove gross contamination; place equipment to be washed and decontaminated into a separate container.
	Gases: Follow the supplier's suggestions or request outside assistance.
	Mercury: Vacuum up the spill using a mercury vacuum, or scoop up mercury paste after neutralization and collect the paste in a designated container. Use a sponge and detergent to wipe and clean the spill surface three times to remove absorbent. Collect all contaminated disposal equipment and put it into a hazardous waste container. Collect supplies and remove gross contamination; place equipment that will be thoroughly washed and decontaminated into a separate container.

APPENDIX 2-7

Managing Hazardous Chemical Spills (Continued)

Actions	Instructions for Hazardous Liquids, Gases, and Mercury
Dispose.	Liquids: Dispose of material that was neutralized as solid waste. Follow the facility's procedures for disposal. For flammable liquids, check with the facility safety officer for appropriate waste determination.
	Gases: The manufacturer or supplier will instruct the facility about disposal if applicable.
	Mercury: Label with appropriate hazardous waste label and Department of Transportation diamond label.
Report.	Follow appropriate spill documentation and reporting procedures. Investigate the spill; perform a root cause analysis if needed. Act on opportunities for improving safety.

CHAPTER 3

Regulatory Considerations in Transfusion Medicine and Cellular Therapies

Joseph Schwartz, MD, MPH; Orieji Illoh, MD; and Yvette C. Tanhehco, PhD, MD, MS

3

THE FIELDS OF TRANSFUSION MEDI-cine and cellular therapy are highly regulated disciplines. Over the years, different regulatory bodies have provided oversight at both the state and federal levels in the United States. The Food and Drug Administration (FDA) and the Centers for Medicare and Medicaid Services (CMS) are the primary regulatory agencies providing federal oversight. In addition, state health departments and other agencies may provide some degree of regulatory oversight. Individuals and establishments involved with transfusion medicine and cellular therapies should be familiar with the different requirements of these agencies.

It is important to distinguish between regulation and accreditation. Regulations have the force of law, while accreditation standards are not legally binding. Blood banks, transfusion services, and cellular therapy facilities must follow the rules set by regulatory agencies. In contrast, accreditation organizations such as AABB or The Joint Commission publish specific sets of standards that need to be met in order for accreditation to be granted. Some regulatory agencies will grant deeming authority to select accreditation organizations. For example, CMS regulates laboratory testing through the Clinical Laboratory Improvement Amendments (CLIA). CMS accepts certain accreditation organization inspections, meaning that the organizations have been approved by CMS as having standards and an inspection process that meet or exceed the CMS requirements. Table 3-1 summarizes agencies and organizations involved in regulation and accreditation of blood bank, transfusion medicine, and cellular therapy facilities. The scope of their regulatory oversight and/or accreditation is detailed on these organizations' respective websites. In addition, some states may have regulations pertaining to blood banks and cellular therapy facilities.

Joseph Schwartz, MD, MPH, Director, Transfusion Medicine and Cellular Therapy, Columbia University Medical Center and New York-Presbyterian Hospital, and Professor of Pathology and Cell Biology, Columbia University, New York, New York; Orieji Illoh, MD, Director, Division of Blood Components and Devices, Office of Blood Research and Review, Center for Biologics Evaluation and Research, Food and Drug Administration, Silver Spring, Maryland; and Yvette C. Tanhehco, PhD, MD, MS, Assistant Director, Transfusion Medicine, Director, Apheresis, and Director, Cellular Therapy Laboratory, Columbia University Irving Medical Center and New York-Presbyterian Hospital, and Assistant Professor of Pathology and Cell Biology, Columbia University, New York, New York

The authors have disclosed no conflicts of interest. This chapter reflects the views of the authors and should not be construed to represent their employers' views or policies.

TABLE 3-1. Regulatory and Accreditation Bodies Involved in Blood Banking and Cellular Therapies

Regulatory Agencies	Accreditation Organizations
Food and Drug Administration (FDA)	AABB
Centers for Medicare and Medicaid Services (CMS)	College of American Pathologists (CAP)
Department of Homeland Security	The Joint Commission
Nuclear Regulatory Commission (NRC)	Foundation for the Accreditation of Cellular Therapy (FACT)
Environmental Protection Agency (EPA)	National Marrow Donor Program (NMDP)
Occupational Safety and Health Administration (OSHA)	World Marrow Donor Association (WMDA)
Local state departments of health	American Association for Laboratory Accreditation (A2LA)
US Department of Transportation (US DOT)	
National Fire Protection Association (NFPA)	

FDA OVERSIGHT OF BLOOD ESTABLISHMENTS

In the United States, when federal laws are enacted by Congress, they are published as statutes and placed into the appropriate subject areas (titles) of the United States Code (USC).[1] Regulations created by federal agencies to enforce laws are placed (by title) in the *Code of Federal Regulations* (CFR). The FDA is the federal agency that enforces the federal laws related to drugs and biologics, which include blood and blood components, related devices, and manufacturing facilities.

Section 351 of the Public Health Service (PHS) Act (USC Title 42, Section 262) and the Food, Drug, and Cosmetic (FD&C) Act (21 USC 301 et seq) are two statutes that govern the regulation of blood and blood components. The PHS Act defines blood and blood components as biological products. This law was first established in 1944 as an expansion of the Biologics Control Act of 1902. In addition to requiring that biological products be manufactured in a manner to ensure the safety, purity, and potency of the product, the PHS Act requires a manufac-

turer to obtain a biologics license before placing a product in interstate commerce.[2] Furthermore, the US Department of Health and Human Services (DHHS) has broad authority to prevent communicable disease transmission under Section 361 of the PHS Act (42 USC 264).

The FDA regulates drugs and medical devices under the FD&C Act, which was first passed in 1938 and amended in 1976 to include medical devices. Under this act, blood and blood components are considered to be drugs because they are intended to cure, mitigate, treat, or prevent disease in humans. Manufacturers of drugs and certain devices must demonstrate to the FDA the safety and efficacy of a product before it can be marketed. The FD&C Act requires blood product manufacturers to register with the FDA, obtain biologics licenses to ship in interstate commerce, and follow current good manufacturing practice (cGMP) regulations. It also prohibits adulteration and misbranding of products, authorizes inspection of manufacturing facilities, and defines civil and criminal penalties for violations. The act establishes requirements for the use of unapproved drugs and devices in their investigational phases and in public health emergencies.[3]

Within the FDA, the Center for Biologics Evaluation and Research (CBER) regulates blood products and most other biological therapies.[4] CBER uses multiple overlapping safeguards to ensure that recipients of blood products or cellular therapies are protected. This FDA blood-safety system includes measures in the following areas: donor screening, donor testing, donor deferral records, product quarantine, and investigation of manufacturing deficiencies. The Center for Devices and Radiological Health (CDRH) regulates most medical devices, but CBER retains primary jurisdiction over medical devices used for blood donation, blood processing, transfusion, and cellular products. The FDA's Office of Regulatory Affairs (ORA) has responsibility for all field operations, which include inspections and investigations of blood and device manufacturers.[5]

The FDA promulgates applicable regulations for blood and blood components and related devices under both the PHS and FD&C Acts. Regulations for blood products are found in Parts 210, 211, and 600-680 of CFR Title 21.[6] These regulations are intended to ensure blood donor safety and the safety, purity, and potency of blood and blood components. In addition, blood establishments are required to report fatalities associated with blood donation or transfusion to the FDA. Table 3-2 provides a summarized list of relevant regulations applicable to blood establishments. On May 22, 2015, the FDA published a final rule, "Requirements for Blood and Blood Components Intended for Transfusion or for Further Manufacturing Use," revising 21 CFR Parts 606-660 and updating the FDA's previous requirements.[7] The new requirements include a determination of donor eligibility and donation suitability, as well as regulations to help protect donor health.

Manufacturers of blood and blood components may submit written requests to the FDA for approval of exceptions or alternative procedures to any requirement in the regulations [21 CFR 640.120 (a)]. When the FDA grants approvals of exceptions or alternative procedures, the circumstances for these approvals may not necessarily apply to other facilities. These approvals are periodically published on the FDA's website.[8]

In addition to regulations, which are legally binding, the FDA may publish recommendations in guidance documents. These guidance documents generally explain FDA's current thinking on an issue. The guidance may clarify or explain how manufacturers may comply with the statute or regulations, or establish good manufacturing standards for blood products. FDA guidance documents generally do not establish legally enforceable responsibilities unless specific regulatory or statutory requirements are cited. The FDA may consider requests for alternative approaches to the recommendations stated in guidance documents if such approaches satisfy the requirements of the applicable law or statute.[9]

As part of the development process for FDA regulations and guidance documents, several forums are offered for input from the public and regulated industry. Proposed rules and draft guidance documents are published in the *Federal Register* with an invitation for written comments, which are filed in public dockets. When final rules are published in the *Federal Register*, the accompanying preamble responds to key questions and comments submitted by the public. The FDA also receives petitions to write or change regulations. Expert opinions on current issues are sought from several advisory committees, including the FDA Blood Products Advisory Committee (BPAC); the FDA Cellular, Tissue, and Gene Therapies Advisory Committee (CTGTAC); and the DHHS Advisory Committee on Blood and Tissue Safety and Availability (ACBTSA). Public meetings and workshops hosted by the FDA on selected topics provide an additional opportunity for input. The FDA website provides links to relevant regulations and guidance documents.

Registration of Blood Establishments and Device Manufacturers

Blood establishments include blood and plasma donor centers, blood banks, transfusion services, other blood product manufacturers, and independent laboratories that engage in testing of donors and blood and blood components.[10]

TABLE 3-2. Regulations of Interest in Title 21 of the CFR (Food and Drugs)

Topic	Section	Topic	Section
FDA general		Donor eligibility	630.10, 630.15
Enforcement	1-19	Donation suitability	630.30
Research and development	50-58	Donor notification	630.40
cGMP for drugs	210-211	Blood product standards	640
Biological products	600-690	Blood collection	640.4
General	600	Blood testing	640.5, 610.40
Licensing	601	Red Blood Cells	640.10-.17
cGMP for blood components	606	Platelets	640.20-.25, 606.145
Personnel, resources	606.20-.65	Plasma	640.30-.34
Standard operating procedures	606.100	Cryoprecipitated AHF	640.50-.56
Labeling	606.120-.122	Exceptions, alternatives	640.120
Compatibility testing	606.151	Medical devices	800-898
Records	606.160-.165	Device adverse events	803
Adverse reactions	606.170	Hematology and pathology	864
Product deviations	606.171	Tissues	
Establishment registration	607	Human cells, tissues, and cellular and tissue-based products	1271*
General standards	610	General provisions	1271.1-.20
Donation testing	610.40	Procedures for registration and listing	1271.21-.37
Donor deferral	610.41, 630.10	Donor eligibility	1271.45-.90
Look-back	610.46-.47	cGTP	1271.145-.320
Dating periods	610.50, 610.53	Additional requirements and inspection and enforcement	1271.330-.440

*The following citations represent Subparts A, B, C, D, and E-F, respectively.
CFR = Code of Federal Regulations; FDA = Food and Drug Administration; cGMP = current good manufacturing practice; AHF = antihemophilic factor; cGTP = current good tissue practice.

The FDA has promulgated regulations that require blood establishments (21 CFR 607) and device manufacturers (21 CFR 807) to register their manufacturing facilities and list the products they manufacture. All establishments that manufacture blood products are required to register with the FDA, unless they are exempt under 21 CFR 607.65. Registrants must provide a list of every blood product manufactured, prepared, or processed for commercial distribution. Manufacturers must register and list their products within 5 days of beginning operations and annually.

Facilities that routinely collect and process blood (including autologous units) or perform such procedures as irradiation; washing; prestorage leukocyte reduction; pooling; or freezing, deglycerolization, and rejuvenation must register with the FDA. Transfusion services acting as depots that forward products to other hospitals must register as distribution centers. If blood irradiation is performed outside the blood bank or transfusion service, such as in a nuclear medicine department, that facility must register as well.

Transfusion services that do not collect or process blood and blood components are exempt (21 CFR 607.65) from the registration requirement in 21 CFR 607. In order to be exempt, they must be part of a facility certified under CLIA (1988; 42 USC 263a and 42 CFR 493) or certified for reimbursement by CMS.[11] Their manufacturing activities are basic, such as compatibility tests, preparing Red Blood Cells from whole blood, converting unused plasma to Recovered Plasma, pooling certain blood components immediately before transfusion, reducing leukocytes in blood components with bedside filters, or collecting blood only in emergency situations. Under the memorandum of understanding in 1980 between the FDA and CMS, the responsibility for routine inspections of these transfusion services was assigned to CMS.[12] The FDA, however, still has jurisdiction over transfusion services and may conduct its own inspections if warranted.

Licensure of Blood and Blood Component Manufacturers

Blood and blood component manufacturers who distribute blood products in interstate commerce must be registered and licensed. The blood establishment obtains approval for licensure by submitting a Biologics License Application (BLA) to the FDA. The FDA's evaluation of BLAs typically includes the review of supporting documents, such as standard operating procedures, labels, quality control data, and a prelicense facility inspection. Once a license is issued, the license number is placed on the label for those products approved to be distributed in interstate commerce. In addition, licensed manufacturers are required to inform the FDA of changes in the manufacturing process described in their approved BLA.[13] The reporting category for such changes depends on the potential of the change to adversely affect the safety, purity, and potency of the product.

The FDA has published specific guidance ("Changes to an Approved Application: Biological Products: Human Blood and Blood Components Intended for Transfusion or for Further Manufacture," December 2014) to assist blood establishments in determining the appropriate reporting mechanism.[14] As described in the guidance, the three reporting categories into which a change to an approved application may be placed are defined in 21 CFR 601.12 and are as follows:

- *Major Change:* A change that has a substantial potential to have an adverse effect on the safety or effectiveness of the product. Major changes require the submission of a Prior Approval Supplement (PAS) to the FDA, which the FDA must approve before the product is distributed in interstate commerce [21 CFR 601.12(b)].
- *Moderate Change:* A change that has a moderate potential to have an adverse effect on the safety or effectiveness of the product. Moderate changes require the submission of a Changes Being Effected in 30 Days Supplement (CBE30) to the FDA at least 30 days before interstate distribution of the product made using the change [21 CFR 601.12(c)].

In certain circumstances, the FDA may determine that the product made using the change may be distributed immediately upon receipt of the Changes Being Effected Supplement (CBE) by the FDA [21 CFR 601.12 (c)(5)].

- *Minor Change:* A change that has a minimal potential to have an adverse effect on the safety or effectiveness of the product. Minor changes do not need prior approval from the FDA but must be described by the manufacturer in an annual report [21 CFR 601.12(d)].

Blood-Related Devices

CBER has the lead responsibility for devices marketed for transfusion and the collection and processing of blood products and hematopoietic progenitor cells (HPCs). These devices include apheresis machines; devices and reagents used for compatibility testing; blood establishment computer software; and blood and human cells, tissues, and cellular and tissue-based product (HCT/P) screening tests for infectious diseases.

The medical device classifications are based on the risks the device poses to the patient and the user or on the level of controls that may be necessary to ensure the device can be operated safely and effectively[15]:

- Class I medical devices represent the lowest-level risks to the patient or user. Such devices are subject to a comprehensive set of regulatory authorities called general controls. General controls are applicable to all classes of devices. Examples of Class I devices include copper sulfate solutions for hemoglobin screening, blood grouping view boxes, and heat sealers.
- Class II medical devices carry greater patient or user risks than Class I devices. These are devices for which general controls alone are insufficient to provide reasonable assurance of the safety and effectiveness of the device, and for which there is sufficient information to establish special controls to provide such assurance. Most blood-related devices are in Class II and cleared through the 510(k) pathway, where a device is found to show equivalence to a predicate.
- Class III medical devices carry the greatest risk of the three device classifications. These are devices for which general controls, by themselves, are insufficient and for which there is insufficient information to establish special controls to provide reasonable assurance of their safety and efficacy. For example, tests used to determine red cell antigen type by molecular methods are regulated as Class III devices, requiring premarket approval (PMA).

The FDA approves some blood-related devices as biologics under the PHS Act and therefore requires the submission of BLAs or related supplements. These devices include reagents used for immunohematology testing by serologic methods and most donor-screening infectious disease assays [eg, tests for human immunodeficiency virus (HIV), hepatitis B virus (HBV), and hepatitis C virus (HCV)].

The FDA requires device manufacturers to register and list the products they manufacture (21 CFR 807). Each device category is assigned a code, and all cleared or approved manufacturers and products for that code are searchable in the Establishment Registration and Device Listing database on the CDRH website.[16]

Manufacturers and importers of medical devices must report deaths and serious injuries related to medical devices to the FDA (21 CFR 803).[17] User facilities must report deaths and serious injuries in which a device was or may have been a factor. Serious injury is defined as being life threatening, causing permanent impairment or damage, or needing medical or surgical intervention. For user facilities, reports of serious injuries are sent to the device manufacturer using FDA MedWatch Form 3500A within 10 working days of the event, or to the FDA if the device manufacturer is unknown. Deaths must be reported to both the manufacturer and the FDA. In years when a Form 3500A report is submitted, the user facility must send an annual user facility report (Form 3419) to the FDA by January 1 of the following year.[18] Users may voluntarily report other device-related adverse events or malfunctions to the FDA (Form 3500). All possible adverse events, whether reported or not, must be investigated, and these records must be kept on file for a minimum of 2 years.

FDA Inspections

The FDA inspects regulated facilities to determine compliance with regulations.[19] These inspections can be classified as one of the following:

- Prelicense or preapproval inspection after a manufacturer submits an application to the FDA for a biologics license or to market a new device or product.
- Routine inspection of a regulated facility.
- "For-cause" inspection, which involves investigation of a specific problem that has come to the FDA's attention, such as a complaint or fatality.

The FDA's ORA and CBER oversee inspection activities related to transfusion medicine and blood banking. The inspection of a blood establishment is to ensure manufacturers meet the standards described in applicable provisions of the regulations intended to protect donors and ensure the safety, purity, and potency of the products they make. These include regulations for blood components in Title 21 CFR Parts 600, 601, 606, 607, 610, 630, and 640, as well as the process and production controls, equipment regulations, and quality control requirements in 21 CFR 211. (See Table 3-2.) The licensed manufacturers must also meet any additional conditions of licensure incorporated in their approved BLA.[20]

When a blood establishment applies for a BLA, the facility is generally inspected by a team from CBER and ORA. Subsequent inspections may be performed by ORA.

ORA provides and publishes policies and instructions for FDA investigators. There is a specific *Compliance Program Guidance Manual (CPGM)* for inspections of licensed and unlicensed blood banks. The foundations for blood establishment inspections are in the general FDA regulations for cGMP and drugs, and the specific requirements for blood components. All inspections address the FDA's five layers of blood safety. Investigators review the following operational systems that are associated with the layers of safety: quality assurance, donor eligibility, product testing, quarantine/inventory management, and production and processing. Within each system, the investigators review standard operating procedures, personnel and training, facilities, equipment calibration and maintenance, and records. Specific requirements for individual systems and processes are discussed in detail in their respective chapters of the *CPGM*.[20]

Full inspections of all systems are designated Level I. After two favorable inspection profiles, facilities with only four or five systems sometimes have streamlined Level II inspections of three systems. Prelicense and preapproval inspections or for-cause investigations for complaints or fatalities need not follow these formats because they are more focused on a specific issue.

If the FDA investigator observes that significant objectionable practices, violations, or conditions are present that could result in a drug or device being adulterated or injurious to health, these observations are written and presented to the facility on FDA Form 483. The FDA Form 483 serves to notify the manufacturer of the objectionable conditions and does not constitute a final determination of whether a violation has occurred. Investigators are instructed to seek and record the manufacturer's intentions to make corrections. The investigator documents observations and discussions in an Establishment Inspection Report (EIR). The FDA reviews and considers all the information provided in a Form 483, EIR, and any responses from the manufacturer and then determines what further action, if any, is appropriate to protect public health.

The FDA can take a number of enforcement actions in response to a violation.[21] Enforcement actions are categorized as advisory, administrative, or judicial. Under advisory actions, the FDA issues a warning or an untitled letter, informing the manufacturer of noncompliant activities that could affect donor safety or result in the distribution of an unsafe biological product. The letters provide the facility with the opportunity for voluntary compliance. Administrative actions include product recalls, withdrawals of product approvals, formal citations of violation, and—for licensed facilities—suspension or revocation of a license. Judicial actions range from seizures of products to court injunctions, civil monetary penalties, and criminal prosecution.

Biological Product Deviation Reporting

When blood establishments discover after distribution that a blood product was manufactured in violation of rules, standards, or specifications, they must report the biological product deviation (BPD) to the FDA [21 CFR 606.171, 21 CFR 1271.350(b)]. BPD events are ones in which the safety, purity, or potency of a distributed blood product may be affected, and may involve any event associated with manufacturing a product, including collection, testing, processing, packing, labeling, or storing and distributing. Licensed and unlicensed manufacturers, registered blood establishments, and transfusion services that are exempt from registration are required to report BPDs in distributed products. Blood establishments must report a BPD as soon as possible, not to exceed 45 calendar days from the date the manufacturer became aware of the reportable event.[22] CBER publishes an annual summary of reported BPDs.[23] Most of the reports used to involve postdonation information. The FDA no longer considers postdonation information to require BPD reports. Blood establishments should have procedures to investigate a BPD and determine if the product should be recalled or withdrawn.

Managing Recalls and Withdrawals

The FDA's requirements for monitoring and investigating problems with drugs extend to the time after a product's release.

A recall is defined as the removal or correction of a marketed product that is in violation of the law (21 CFR 7.3 and 7.40). Recalls may be initiated by the manufacturers, requested by the FDA, or ordered by the FDA under statutory authority. The FDA classifies recalls by severity.[24] Recalls are classified as Class I, II, or III. Most blood component recalls are in Class III, not likely to cause adverse health consequences. Class II recalls are for products that may cause temporary adverse effects or remotely possible serious problems. Class I recalls involve a reasonable probability of serious or fatal adverse effects. All recalls are published by the FDA.[25,26]

Market withdrawals occur when a product has a minor violation that would not be subject to FDA legal action.[24] The manufacturer voluntarily removes the product from the market or corrects the violation. In collection establishments, problems such as postdonation information are often in this category. Withdrawals are not published.

In some blood guidance documents on infectious diseases, the FDA has included recommendations on whether to notify the recipient's physician about transfused units. In cases of possible recent infectious disease exposure in donors or transfusion recipients, the test-negative window periods for the agent and test kits should be consulted for scheduling prospective testing or reviewing retrospective results, such as for a donor who has been retested after an exposure.[27]

"Look-back" investigations on units from donors found after donation to have HIV or HCV are discussed in Chapter 7.

MEDICAL LABORATORY LAWS AND REGULATIONS

CMS regulates all US medical laboratories under CLIA [42 USC 263(a) and 42 CFR 493] and Section 353 of the PHS Act.[28,29] The law and regulations establish the requirements and procedures for laboratories to be certified under CLIA as both a general requirement and a prerequisite for receiving Medicare and Medicaid reimbursement. They provide minimal standards for facilities, equipment, and personnel. Furthermore, they require participation in a proficiency testing (PT) program.

To be certified, laboratories must have adequate facilities and equipment, supervisory and technical personnel with training and experience appropriate to the complexity of testing, a quality management system (see Chapter 1), and successful ongoing performance in CMS-approved PT.[30] All laboratories must register with CMS, submit to inspection by CMS or one of its "deemed status" partners, and obtain re-certification every 2 years.

All laboratory tests are rated for complexity by the FDA for CMS as waived or moderate or high complexity. Waived tests are simple and easily performed with limited technical training. Examples include over-the-counter tests, urinalysis dipsticks, copper sulfate specific-gravity hemoglobin screens, microhematocrits, and some simple devices for measuring hemoglobin. Laboratories that perform only waived tests register with CMS for a certificate of waiver. The Centers for Disease Control and Prevention provides technical and advisory support to CMS for laboratory regulation and has published good laboratory practice recommendations for waived-testing sites.[31]

Nonwaived tests are classified as being of moderate or high complexity based on a scoring system of needs for training, preparation, interpretive judgment, and other factors (42 CFR 493.17).[28] The "Medical Devices" section of the FDA website provides a searchable CLIA database that provides the complexity levels of specific tests.[32] Compatibility testing with manual reagents and infectious disease testing are generally considered high-complexity testing.

Blood banks and transfusion services have three pathways to obtain a CLIA certificate to perform testing: 1) certificate of compliance: approval via state health department inspections using CMS requirements; 2) certificate of accreditation: approval via a CMS-approved accrediting organization; and 3) CMS-exempt status: licensure programs for nonwaived laboratories in New York and Washington states that are accepted by CMS.[33]

The CLIA regulations delineate general requirements for facilities; quality systems, including quality assurance and quality control systems; and management and technical personnel qualifications. High-complexity tests require more stringent personnel qualifications. Immunohematology laboratories have standards for blood supply agreements, compatibility testing, blood storage and alarms, sample retention, positive identification of blood product recipients, investigation of transfusion reactions, and documentation (42 CFR 493.1103 and 493.1271).[28] Viral and syphilis serologic tests are part of the immunology requirements. CMS has also published guidance on conducting surveys (inspections).[34]

CMS has approved six laboratory accreditation organizations with requirements that meet CMS regulations: AABB, the American Osteopathic Association, the American Society for Histocompatibility and Immunogenetics (ASHI), the College of American Pathologists (CAP), COLA (formerly the Commission on Office Laboratory Accreditation), and The Joint Commission.[35] The Joint Commission has cooperative agreements with ASHI, CAP, and COLA to accept their laboratory accreditations in facility surveys.[36] CMS may perform its own follow-up surveys to validate those of the accreditation organizations.

CMS requires successful PT for ongoing laboratory certification of nonwaived testing. Within each laboratory section, CMS regulations specify tests and procedures (regulated analytes) that must pass approved PT if the laboratory performs them. The CMS website has a list of approved PT providers.[37] (PT is discussed in Chapter 1.) CMS can remove certification or impose fines for failure to comply with its regulations.

LOCAL LAWS, HOSPITAL REGULATIONS, AND ACCREDITATION

Facilities also should be familiar with all relevant state and local laws and regulations, including professional licensure requirements for medical and laboratory personnel, as many states have regulations that apply to blood banks and transfusion services. Furthermore, in some situations, facilities providing products or services in other states must comply with local regulations in the customer's location.

CMS approves hospitals for Medicare reimbursement through state surveys or accreditation programs from The Joint Commission, the American Osteopathic Association, and DNV Healthcare. These inspections cover CMS regulations for blood administration and the evaluation of transfusion reactions found within "Basic Hospital Functions" regulations [42 CFR 482.23(c)].[38] The Joint Commission has standards for preventing misidentification of laboratory specimens and transfusion recipients (National Patient Safety Goal section—NPSG.01.01.01, .01.03.01), checking blood products in the "Universal Protocol" preprocedure verification process ("time-out"—UP.01.01.01), and assessing transfusion appropriateness (MS.05.01.01).[39] The Joint Commission also addresses utilization review of blood components in the Performance Improvement (PI) section of the hospital accreditation requirements. Furthermore, in the same section of standards, The Joint Commission directs hospitals to collect data on all reported and confirmed transfusion reactions, and directs that these areas should "be measured regularly." The Joint Commission includes hemolytic transfusion reactions in its Sentinel Events reporting program.[40]

Both AABB and CAP have developed standards for transfusion services. The AABB *Standards for Blood Banks and Transfusion Services* is updated every 2 years.[41] The CAP transfusion medicine checklist TRM[42] is updated annually. AABB- and CAP-accredited facilities need to be physically surveyed every 2 years to receive reaccreditation. AABB and CAP can coordinate joint surveys of facilities seeking both types of accreditation.

HUMAN CELLS, TISSUES, AND CELLULAR AND TISSUE-BASED PRODUCTS (HCT/Ps)

HCT/Ps are defined as articles containing or consisting of human cells or tissues that are intended for implantation, transplantation, infu-sion, or transfer into a human recipient.[43] HCT/Ps can be derived from deceased or living donors (Table 3-3). The FDA has established a comprehensive, tiered, risk-based regulatory framework applicable to HCT/Ps. These regulations, which were published in three parts (referred to as the "tissue rules") and contained in 21 CFR Part 1271, became fully effective on May 25, 2005. They apply to all HCT/Ps, including HPCs, that were recovered on or after this date.[44,45]

Under this tiered, risk-based regulatory framework, some HCT/Ps (referred to as "361" HCT/Ps) are regulated solely under section 361 of the PHS Act (42 USC 264), which authorizes the FDA to establish and enforce regulations necessary to prevent the introduction, transmission, or spread of communicable diseases.[46] For an HCT/P to be regulated solely under section 361 of the PHS Act and the regulations in 21 CFR Part 1271, it must meet *all* of the following criteria in 21 CFR 1271.10(a):

1. The HCT/P is minimally manipulated (relates to the extent of processing).
2. The HCT/P is intended for homologous use only as reflected by the labeling, advertising, or other indications of the manufacturer's objective intent. (The product performs the same basic function or functions in the donor as in the recipient.)
3. The manufacture of the HCT/P does not involve the combination of the cells or tissues with another article, except for water, crystalloids, or a sterilizing, preserving, or storage agent, provided that the addition of water, crystalloids, or the sterilizing, preserving, or

TABLE 3-3. Examples of HCT/Ps

From Deceased Donors	From Living Donors
• Skin	• Hematopoietic stem/progenitor cells from peripheral or cord blood
• Dura mater	• Other cellular therapy products (eg, pancreatic islets, mesenchymal
• Cardiovascular tissues	stem/stromal cells, fibroblasts)
• Ocular tissues	• Reproductive cells and tissues
• Musculoskeletal tissues	

storage agent does not raise new clinical safety concerns with respect to the HCT/P.

4. The HCT/P either does not have a systemic effect and is not dependent on the metabolic activity of living cells for its primary function, or has a systemic effect or is dependent on the metabolic activity of living cells for its primary function, and is for autologous use; for allogeneic use in a first-degree or second-degree blood relative; or for reproductive use.

Manufacturers of 361 HCT/Ps must comply with the requirements in 21 CFR Part 1271, which include 1) establishment registration and product listing; 2) donor eligibility, including screening and testing for relevant communicable disease agents or diseases; and 3) current good tissue practice (cGTP); and are not subject to the requirements for premarket review and approval. FDA guidance documents related to these requirements can be found on the agency's website.[45]

If an HCT/P does not meet the criteria set out in 21 CFR 1271.10(a), and the establishment that manufactures the HCT/P does not qualify for any of the exceptions in 21 CFR 1271.15, the HCT/P will be regulated as a drug, device, and/or biological product under the FD&C Act and/or section 351 of the PHS Act (referred to as a "351" HCT/P) and applicable regulations, including 21 CFR 1271. For these HCT/Ps, premarket review and FDA approval will be required. During the development phase, an Investigational New Drug (IND) or Investigational Device Exemption (IDE) application must be submitted to the FDA before studies involving humans are initiated. Manufacturers are required to comply with the regulations in 21 CFR 1271 and all the regulations for drugs, devices, or biological products, as applicable (Table 3-4).

Peripheral blood stem cells (PBSCs), or cord blood for autologous use or for allogeneic use in a first- or second-degree blood relative, that meet all the other criteria in 21 CFR 1271.10(a) are regulated as 361 HCT/Ps. PBSCs from unrelated donors are regulated as 351 products; however, for some clinical indications of PBSCs, these regulations remain under a period of de-

layed implementation. For clarification on regulatory expectations for specific uses, it may be prudent to contact the agency directly. Minimally manipulated, unrelated umbilical cord blood intended for hematopoietic or immunologic reconstitution in patients with disorders affecting the hematopoietic system must be FDA licensed or used under an IND protocol. Minimally manipulated marrow that is not combined with another article (with some exceptions) and is intended for homologous use is not considered an HCT/P.

FDA regulations in 21 CFR Part 1271 require HCT/P manufacturers to have a tracking and labeling system that allows for tracking each product from the donor to the recipient and from the recipient back to the donor. HCT/P manufacturers are also required to inform the facilities that receive the products that they have established a tracking system. However, FDA's regulations for HCT/Ps, including the requirements for tracking, do not apply to facilities that receive, store, and administer cells or tissues but do not perform any manufacturing steps. The Joint Commission has hospital standards for receiving, handling, and tracing tissues and investigating adverse events (TS.03.01.01 to TS.03.03.01).[39] (See Chapter 28 for information on these standards.)

The Health Resources and Services Administration (HRSA) within DHHS oversees the CW Bill Young Cell Transplantation Program and the National Cord Blood Inventory for marrow and cord blood donations and transplant procedures coordinated by the National Marrow Donor Program (NMDP) in the United States.

The *Circular of Information for the Use of Cellular Therapy Products* is jointly written by AABB and multiple organizations involved in cellular therapy for users of certain minimally manipulated unlicensed cellular therapy products.[47] AABB and the Foundation for the Accreditation of Cellular Therapy (FACT) set voluntary standards covering the collection, processing, and administration of cellular therapy products.[48,49] AABB and FACT have standards review cycles of 2 and 3 years, respectively. (See Table 3-5.) The CAP transfusion medicine checklist[42] includes cellular therapy requirements. The World Marrow Donor Association

TABLE 3-4. US Regulations for Manufacturers of Hematopoietic Progenitor Cells

Type of HPC Product	Oversight/Regulatory Category	Key Regulations (21 CFR except as noted)	FDA Premarket Licensure, Approval, or Clearance?
Minimally manipulated marrow, not combined with another article (with some exceptions) and for homologous use	Health Resources and Services Administration oversight	42 US Code 274(k)	Not applicable
Autologous or allogeneic related-donor (first- or second-degree blood relative) HPCs	PHS Act Section 361: HCT/Ps*	1271.10(a)† (must meet all criteria); 1271 Subparts A-F	No
Minimally manipulated unrelated-donor peripheral blood HPCs, not combined with another article (with some exceptions) and for homologous use	PHS Act Sections 361 and 351: HCT/Ps regulated as drugs and/or biological products	1271 Subparts A-D Applicable biologics/drug regulations	Delayed implementation
Minimally manipulated unrelated-donor umbilical cord blood cells	PHS Sections 361 and 351: HCT/Ps regulated as drugs and/or biological products	1271 Subparts A-D	Yes (after October 20, 2011): BLA or IND application
HPCs that don't meet all the criteria in 21 CFR 1271.10(a)	PHS Sections 361 and 351: HCT/Ps regulated as drugs and/or biological products	1271 Subparts A-D Applicable drugs/biologics regulations	Yes: IND and BLA

*As defined by 2005 tissue regulations [21 CFR 1271.3(d)].

†21 CFR 1271.10(a) as applied to PHS Act Section 361 requires that HPCs be: 1) minimally manipulated, 2) for homologous use only, 3) not combined with another article (except water, crystalloids, or sterilizing, preserving, or storage agents with no new safety concerns), and 4) for autologous use or for allogeneic use in a first- or second-degree blood relative. (See full rule for details.)

HPC = hematopoietic progenitor cell; CFR = Code of Federal Regulations; FDA = Food and Drug Administration; PHS = Public Health Service; HCT/Ps = human cells, tissues, and cellular and tissue-based products; BLA = Biologics License Application; IND = Investigational New Drug.

(WMDA) fosters international collaboration to facilitate the exchange of high-quality hematopoietic stem cells for clinical transplantation worldwide and to promote the interests of donors. WMDA also accredits and qualifies donor registries that follow its global standards covering all aspects of unrelated hematopoietic stem cell registry operations. The NMDP standards set forth basic guidelines and requirements for programs working with the NMDP.

TABLE 3-5. Cellular Therapy Accreditation

Organization	Standards Review Cycle
AABB	2 years
FACT-JACIE (Foundation for the Accreditation of Cellular Therapy and the Joint Accreditation Committee of ISCT and EBMT)	3 years
National Marrow Donor Program (NMDP)	2 years
World Marrow Donor Association (WMDA)	5 years
College of American Pathologists (CAP)	Not set (publishes updated checklist annually)

The standards encompass network participation criteria with requirements for transplant centers, recruitment centers, and product collection centers. The NMDP standards are designed to ensure that donors and patients receive high-quality care and that government standards are met.

The Alliance for Harmonisation of Cellular Therapy Accreditation (AHCTA), which is under the umbrella of the Worldwide Network for Blood and Marrow Transplantation (WBMT), encompasses all the above-mentioned accreditation organizations. AHCTA is working to harmonize standards that cover all aspects of the process, from assessment of donor eligibility to transplantation and clinical outcome for hematopoietic stem cells and related cellular therapies. AHCTA provides helpful documents to navigate the different sets of participating organizations' standards. Moreover, crosswalk documents comparing the different sets of cellular therapy standards were created and are available on the WBMT website.[50]

IMMUNE EFFECTOR CELLS

The FDA approved the first gene therapy in the United States in 2017. Kymriah (tisagenlecleucel), indicated for pediatric and young adult patients with relapsed/refractory acute lymphoblastic leukemia (ALL), was approved using the FDA's risk evaluation and mitigation strategy (REMS).[51] Several months later, the FDA approved a second gene therapy, Yescarta (axicabtagene ciloleucel), for the treatment of relapsed/refractory large B-cell lymphoma in adults with REMS. The FDA Amendments Act (FDAAA) in 2007 gave FDA the authority to require REMS from drug manufacturers to ensure that the benefits of a drug or biological product outweigh its risks. REMS is a safety strategy to manage a known or potential serious risk associated with a drug and to enable patients to have continued access to such drugs by managing their safe use.[52]

Following the approval of the first gene therapy, FACT published standards for immune effector cells (IECs) in March 2018. The main objective of these standards is to promote quality practice in IEC administration. IECs include genetically engineered cells and therapeutic vaccines made from dendritic cells, natural killer cells, T cells, and B cells and are used to modulate an immune response for therapeutic intent.[53] The IEC Standards and Accreditation Program was created by a task force representing FACT, the International Society for Cellular Therapy (ISCT), the American Society for Gene and Cellular Therapy (ASGCT), and the Society for Immunotherapy of Cancer (SITC) leadership, as well as academicians and cellular therapists from 10 cancer centers.[54]

KEY POINTS

1. The fields of transfusion medicine and cellular therapy are highly regulated, involving multiple regulatory agencies and accreditation organizations.
2. The FDA regulates biological products, including blood and blood components, HCT/Ps, and related devices through established laws and regulations. In addition to the legally binding regulations, the FDA periodically publishes recommendations in guidance documents. The FDA website provides links to blood- and HCT/P-related regulations and relevant guidance documents.
3. Blood establishments and device manufacturers must register their manufacturing facilities and list the products they manufacture. Some blood establishments (eg, transfusion services that do not collect or process blood and blood components) are exempt from registration but must be CLIA certified.
4. Blood establishments that manufacture or participate in the manufacture of blood and blood components are inspected by the FDA to determine compliance with regulations. Observations of significant noncompliance are reported to the facility in writing for its response and correction. The FDA determines if further enforcement action is appropriate.
5. The FDA requires drug (and blood) manufacturers to conduct recalls or market withdrawals when noncompliance is found after products are distributed, such as when postdonation information is received.
6. CMS regulates all US medical laboratories under CLIA. CLIA regulations establish requirements for certification. This includes the use of adequate facilities, qualified personnel commensurate with the complexity of testing, and ongoing successful performance in proficiency testing by CMS-approved vendors. Laboratory approval by CMS is granted via inspections performed by CMS-approved accrediting organizations or state health departments.
7. Health-care facilities also have CMS regulations for their activities, and The Joint Commission and other organizations accredit many hospitals for CMS compliance. CMS and The Joint Commission have requirements for monitoring transfusion practices, evaluating adverse transfusion reactions, and preventing mistransfusions.
8. HCT/Ps are regulated by the FDA under a tiered risk-based framework. The FDA website provides links to HCT/P-related regulations and relevant guidance documents.

REFERENCES

1. Office of the Law Revision Council. United States Code. Washington, DC: US House of Representatives, 2019. [Available at http://uscode.house.gov/.]
2. Food and Drug Administration. Frequently asked questions about therapeutic biological products. Silver Spring, MD: FDA, 2015. [Available at https://www.fda.gov/drugs/therapeutic-biologics-appli cations-bla/frequently-asked-questions-about-therapeutic-biological-products.]
3. Food and Drug Administration. Federal Food, Drug, and Cosmetic Act (FD&C Act). Silver Spring, MD: FDA, 2018. [Available at https://www.fda.gov/regulatory-information/laws-enforced-fda/federal-food-drug-and-cosmetic-act-fdc-act.]
4. Food and Drug Administration. Blood and blood products. Silver Spring, MD: CBER Office of Communication, Outreach, and Development, 2019. [Available at https://www.fda.gov/vaccines-blood-biologics/blood-blood-products.]
5. Food and Drug Administration. Office of Regulatory Affairs. Silver Spring, MD: FDA, 2019. [Available at https://www.fda.gov/about-fda/office-global-regulatory-operations-and-policy/office-regulatory-affairs.]
6. Electronic code of federal regulations. Washington, DC: US Government Publishing Office, 2019. [Available at https://gov.ecfr.io/cgi-bin/ECFR.]
7. Food and Drug Administration. Requirements for blood and blood components intended for

transfusion or for further manufacturing use; final rule. (May 22, 2015) Fed Regist 2015; 80:29841-906. [Available at https://www.fed eralregister.gov/articles/2015/05/22/2015-12228/requirements-for-blood-and-blood-com ponents-intended-for-transfusion-or-for-further-manufacturing.]

8. Food and Drug Administration. Exceptions and alternative procedures approved under 21 CFR 640.120. Silver Spring, MD: CBER Office of Communication, Outreach, and Development, 2019. [Available at https://www.fda.gov/vaccines-blood-biolog ics/regulation-blood-supply/exceptions-and-alternative-procedures-approved-under-21-cfr-640120.]

9. Food and Drug Administration. Guidance, compliance and regulatory information (biologics). Silver Spring, MD: CBER Office of Communication, Outreach, and Development, 2019. [Available at https://www.fda.gov/vaccines-blood-biologics/guidance-compliance-regulatory-infor mation-biologics.]

10. Code of federal regulations. Title 21, CFR Part 607.3. Washington, DC: US Government Publishing Office, 2019 (revised annually).

11. Code of federal regulations. Title 21, CFR Part 607.65. Washington, DC: US Government Publishing Office, 2019 (revised annually).

12. MOU 225-80-4000. Memorandum of understanding between the Health Care Financing Administration and the Food and Drug Administration. (June 6, 1983) Silver Spring, MD: FDA, 1983. [Available at https://www.fda.gov/about-fda/domestic-mous/mou-225-80-4000.]

13. Code of federal regulations. Title 21, CFR Part 601.12. Changes to an approved application. Washington, DC: US Government Publishing Office, 2019 (revised annually).

14. Food and Drug Administration. Guidance for industry: Changes to an approved application: Biological products: Human blood and blood components intended for transfusion or for further manufacture. (December 2014) Silver Spring, MD: CBER Office of Communication, Outreach, and Development, 2014. [Available at https://www.fda.gov/media/86137/down load.]

15. Food and Drug Administration. Classify your medical device. Silver Spring, MD: CDRH, 2018. [Available at https://www.fda.gov/medi cal-devices/overview-device-regulation/classify-your-medical-device.]

16. Food and Drug Administration. Device registration and listing: Search registration and listing. Silver Spring, MD: CDRH, 2017. [Available at https://www.fda.gov/medical-devices/device-registration-and-listing/search-registration-and-listing.]

17. Code of federal regulations. Title 21, CFR Part 803. Washington, DC: US Government Publishing Office, 2019 (revised annually).

18. Food and Drug Administration. Mandatory reporting requirements: Manufacturers, importers and device user facilities. Silver Spring, MD: CDRH, 2019. [Available at https://www.fda.gov/medical-devices/postmarket-requirements-devices/mandatory-reporting-requirements-manufacturers-importers-and-device-user-facili ties#1.]

19. Food and Drug Administration. What does FDA inspect? Silver Spring, MD: FDA, 2018. [Available at https://www.fda.gov/about-fda/fda-basics/what-does-fda-inspect.]

20. Food and Drug Administration. Blood and blood components. Inspection of licensed and unlicensed blood banks, brokers, reference laboratories, and contractors—7342.001. In: Compliance Program guidance manual. Silver Spring, MD: CBER Office of Compliance and Biologics Quality, 2016. [Available at https://www.fda.gov/media/84887/download.]

21. Food and Drug Administration. Inspections, compliance, enforcement, and criminal investigations. Regulatory procedures manual. Silver Spring, MD: FDA, 2017. [Available at https://www.fda.gov/inspections-compliance-enforce ment-and-criminal-investigations/compliance-manuals/regulatory-procedures-manual#_top.]

22. Code of federal regulations. Title 21, CFR Part 606.171. Washington, DC: US Government Publishing Office, 2019 (revised annually).

23. Food and Drug Administration. Biological product deviation reports annual summaries. Silver Spring, MD: CBER Office of Communication, Outreach, and Development, 2019. [Available at https://www.fda.gov/vaccines-blood-biolog ics/report-problem-center-biologics-evaluation-research/biological-product-deviation-reports-annual-summaries.]

24. Food and Drug Administration. Recalls, market withdrawals, and safety alerts. Silver Spring, MD: FDA, 2019. [Available at https://www.fda.gov/safety/recalls-market-withdrawals-safety-alerts.]

25. Food and Drug Administration. Recalls (biologics). Silver Spring, MD: CBER Office of Communication, Outreach, and Development, 2019. [Available at https://www.fda.gov/vaccines-

blood-biologics/safety-availability-biologics/re-calls-biologics.]

26. Food and Drug Administration. Enforcement reports. Silver Spring, MD: FDA, 2019. [Available at https://www.fda.gov/safety/recalls-market-withdrawals-safety-alerts/enforcement-reports.]

27. Food and Drug Administration. Blood guidances. Silver Spring, MD: CBER Office of Communication, Outreach, and Development, 2018. [Available at https://www.fda.gov/vaccines-blood-biologics/biologics-guidances/blood-guidances.]

28. Code of federal regulations. Laboratory requirements. Title 42, CFR Part 493. Washington, DC: US Government Publishing Office, 2019 (revised annually).

29. United States code. Certification of laboratories. Title 42, USC Part 263a.

30. Rauch CA, Nichols JH. Laboratory accreditation and inspection. Clin Lab Med 2007;27:845-58.

31. Howerton D, Anderson N, Bosse D, et al. Good laboratory practices for waived testing sites: Survey findings from testing sites holding a certificate of waiver under the Clinical Laboratory Improvement Amendments of 1988 and recommendations for promoting quality testing. MMWR Recomm Rep 2005;54(RR-13):1-25.

32. Food and Drug Administration. Medical device databases. Silver Spring, MD: CDRH, 2019. [Available at https://www.fda.gov/medical-devices/device-advice-comprehensive-regulatory-assistance/medical-device-databases.]

33. Clinical Laboratory Improvement Amendments (CLIA): How to obtain a CLIA certificate. (March 2006) Baltimore, MD: Centers for Medicare and Medicaid Services, 2006. [Available at https://www.cms.gov/Regulations-and-Guidance/Legislation/CLIA/downloads/howobtaincliacertificate.pdf.]

34. Interpretive guidelines for laboratories. Appendix C. Survey procedures and interpretive guidelines for laboratories and laboratory services. Baltimore, MD: Centers for Medicare and Medicaid Services, 2018. [Available at https://www.cms.gov/Regulations-and-Guidance/Legislation/CLIA/Interpretive_Guidelines_for_Laboratories.html.]

35. List of approved accreditation organizations under the Clinical Laboratory Improvement Amendments (CLIA). Baltimore, MD: Centers for Medicare and Medicaid Services, 2017. [Available at https://www.cms.gov/Regulations-and-Guidance/Legislation/CLIA/Accreditation_Organizations_and_Exempt_States.html.]

36. Laboratory services. Facts about the cooperative accreditation initiative. Oakbrook Terrace, IL: The Joint Commission, 2019. [Available at http://www.jointcommission.org/facts_about_the_cooperative_accreditation_initiative/ (accessed March 3, 2020).]

37. CLIA approved proficiency testing programs - 2019. Baltimore, MD: Centers for Medicare and Medicaid Services, 2019. [Available at https://www.cms.gov/Regulations-and-Guidance/Legislation/CLIA/downloads/ptlist.pdf.]

38. Code of federal regulations. Condition of participation: Nursing services. Title 42, CFR Part 482.23(c). Washington, DC: US Government Publishing Office, 2019 (revised annually).

39. 2019 Hospital accreditation standards. Oakbrook Terrace, IL: The Joint Commission Resources, 2018.

40. Sentinel event. Oakbrook Terrace, IL: The Joint Commission, 2017. [Available at https://www.jointcommission.org/sentinel_event_policy_and_procedures/ (accessed March 3, 2020).]

41. Gammon R, ed. Standards for blood banks and transfusion services. 32nd ed. Bethesda, MD: AABB, 2020.

42. College of American Pathologists, Commission on Laboratory Accreditation. Transfusion medicine checklist. 2019 ed. Northfield, IL: CAP, 2019.

43. Code of federal regulations. Title 21, CFR Part 1271.3(d). Washington, DC: US Government Publishing Office, 2019 (revised annually).

44. Code of federal regulations. Title 21, CFR Part 1271. Washington, DC: US Government Publishing Office, 2019 (revised annually).

45. Food and Drug Administration. Tissue guidances. Silver Spring, MD: CBER Office of Communication, Outreach, and Development, 2019. [Available at https://www.fda.gov/vaccines-blood-biologics/biologics-guidances/tissue-guidances.]

46. United States code. Regulations to control communicable diseases. Title 42, USC Part 264.

47. AABB, America's Blood Centers, American Red Cross, American Society for Apheresis, American Society for Blood and Marrow Transplantation, College of American Pathologists, Cord Blood Association, Foundation for the Accreditation of Cellular Therapy, ICCBBA, International Society for Cellular Therapy, Joint Accreditation Committee of ISCT and EBMT, National Marrow Donor Program, World Marrow Donor Association. Circular of information for the use of cellular therapy products. Bethesda, MD: AABB,

2018. [Available at http://www.aabb.org/aabb cct/coi/Documents/CT-Circular-of-Informa tion.pdf (accessed September 14, 2019).]

48. Haspel RL, ed. Standards for cellular therapy services. 9th ed. Bethesda, MD: AABB, 2019.

49. FACT-JACIE International standards for hematopoietic cellular therapy product collection, processing and administration. 6th ed. Omaha, NE: Foundation for the Accreditation of Cellular Therapy, 2018.

50. Alliance for Harmonisation of Cellular Therapy Accreditation. Comparison of cellular therapy standards: Crosswalk documents. AHCTA, 2016-2017. [Available at https://www.wbmt. org/ahcta/documents/ (accessed September 14, 2019).]

51. FDA News Release: FDA approval brings first gene therapy to the United States. (August 30, 2017) Silver Spring, MD: Food and Drug Administration, 2017. [Available at https://www.

fda.gov/news-events/press-announcements/ fda-approval-brings-first-gene-therapy-united-states.]

52. Food and Drug Administration. REMS integration initiative. Silver Spring, MD: FDA, 2018. [Available at https://www.fda.gov/industry/ prescription-drug-user-fee-amendments/rems-integration-initiative.]

53. Foundation for the Accreditation of Cellular Therapy. FACT standards for immune effector cells. 1st ed, version 1.1. Omaha, NE: FACT, 2018. [Available at http://www.factwebsite. org/iecstandards/ (accessed September 14, 2019).]

54. Maus MV, Nikiforow S. The why, what, and how of the new FACT standards for immune effector cells. J Immunother Cancer 2017;5:36-40.

CHAPTER 4

National Hemovigilance: The Current State

Kevin J. Land, MD; Barbee I. Whitaker, PhD; and Lynne Uhl, MD

THE CONCEPT OF VIGILANCE IN RELAtion to donor and recipient safety within AABB and its membership has existed for a number of years.[1-4] The term *hemovigilance* has been defined as "[a] set of surveillance procedures of the whole transfusion chain intended to minimize adverse events or reactions in donors and recipients and to promote safe and effective use of blood components."[5] Hemovigilance, however, will have limited utility if used only to monitor events rather than implement changes or if data are shared and compared only within a single institution. Also important are incidents and mistakes (errors) that do not result in harm (near-misses). Identification of these can enhance awareness of potential risks and lead to a safer environment for transfusion.

As implied by the phrase "the whole transfusion chain," hemovigilance is considered to be a national-level activity and has been since inception, when countries were struggling with the (primarily infectious) complications of blood component therapy. Today, hemovigilance increasingly includes not merely the collection of data across many institutions and geopolitical entities at state, regional, national, and international levels, but also the analysis of shared data and best practices. This is encouraging progress, for donor and recipient safety are global concerns and benefit most from lessons learned next door, across the country, and around the world.

Hemovigilance structures the data and subsequent analysis using standardized definitions and conventions, allowing data to be widely shared and compared in order to identify and influence best practices across institutions. Hemovigilance is the ultimate benchtop-to-bedside collaboration where stakeholders (donors, recipients, researchers, policy makers, blood establishments, and hospitals) share data and ideas, design interventions to address gaps and failures, then implement potential solutions, evaluate the results, and further refine hypotheses based on real-world data.

Within the United States, public and private organizations have been encouraged to collaborate to improve donor and patient outcomes. Although much work remains toward a comprehensive hemovigilance system, the combined efforts of governmental, public, and private organizations have helped close the gap between US hemovigilance and that of other nations.

Kevin J. Land, MD, Adjunct Professor of Pathology, UT Health Science Center at San Antonio, San Antonio, Texas, and Vice President of Clinical Services, Vitalant, Tempe, Arizona; Barbee I. Whitaker, PhD, Lead General Health Scientist, Office of Biostatistics and Epidemiology, Center for Biologics Evaluation and Research, US Food and Drug Administration, Silver Spring, Maryland; and Lynne Uhl, MD, Vice Chair for Laboratory and Transfusion Medicine, Beth Israel Deaconess Medical Center, Division Director, Laboratory and Transfusion Medicine, Beth Israel Deaconess Medical Center, and Associate Professor of Pathology, Harvard Medical School, Boston, Massachusetts
The authors have disclosed no conflicts of interest. This chapter reflects the views of the authors and should not be construed to represent their employers' views or policies.

This chapter focuses on what is being done in other countries and what is being done with the increased transparency and collaboration across the United States to improve donor and recipient outcomes.

INTERNATIONAL HEMOVIGILANCE

Hemovigilance has more than two decades of history in the international arena, with so many programs being established as a consequence of concern over transfusion-transmitted viral infections and their sequelae [eg, transfusion-transmitted human immunodeficiency virus (HIV), hepatitis B, and hepatitis C]. The architecture and oversight of these hemovigilance programs vary widely, with management and control by various organizations, including blood establishments, governmental regulators, national medical societies, and public health agencies.[6,7] Hemovigilance has been implemented on a country-by-country basis, with early adopters now having the more robust systems, as expected with experience. In January of 1993, the Japanese Red Cross Society began aggregating information on adverse reactions and infectious diseases at a national level.[8] In 1994, France became the first European country to develop a formal national hemovigilance system in response to HIV transfusion transmissions in that country. Since then, many other hemovigilance systems have been developed and regularly provide annual reports. References at the end of the chapter may be consulted for a more thorough review of international hemovigilance efforts or a treatise on how to set up a national hemovigilance system.[5,8]

The Serious Hazards of Transfusion (SHOT) reporting system in the United Kingdom is considered a very successful hemovigilance system. As shown in Fig 4-1, the increased involvement by stakeholders and the maturity of the program resulted in more reports but fewer fatalities. The most notable achievement of the SHOT program is reporting of the association of plasma and platelet transfusions derived from female donors and the incidence of transfusion-related acute lung injury (TRALI) in the early 2000s[9] that led to changes in the management of donor collections and product manufacturing around the world.[10] Equally important are the SHOT data on lapses in safe transfusion practice, including inadequate patient identification at the time of specimen acquisition and blood product

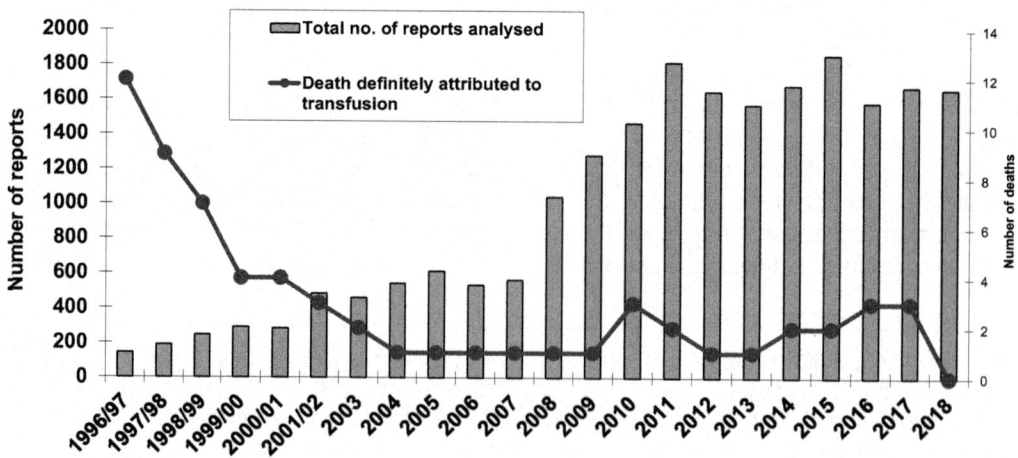

FIGURE 4-1. Total reports submitted to the UK's Serious Hazards of Transfusion program between 1996 and 2018, and total deaths determined as definitely caused by transfusion. (Graphic provided courtesy of Debbi Poles and Shruthi Narayan from SHOT.)

administration.[11] These data have prompted public campaigns engaging patients to actively participate in their care as a means to mitigate risks of misidentification and transfusion errors. More resources can be found on the Joint UK Blood Transfusion and Tissue Transplantation Services Professional Advisory Committee website.[12] Increasingly, other countries such as Australia, are providing free and comprehensive resources to the international transfusion medicine community on their websites.

In 1998, those practicing hemovigilance in Europe established the European Haemovigilance Network (EHN) to bring practitioners together to exchange ideas for improving patient safety and hemovigilance reporting. Eventually, national hemovigilance programs were required by the 2002 and 2005 European Blood Directives (2002/98/EC, 2005/61/EC),[13,14] which mandated implementation of hemovigilance systems with a set of minimum common donor and recipient data elements in all European Union (EU) member states, and subsequent reporting of results to EU authorities. The EHN was reinvented as the International Haemovigilance Network (IHN) in 2009, when the interest and membership of non-EU countries made it clear that the desire to develop robust hemovigilance systems and share critical experiences was truly global. Information on hemovigilance systems participating in the IHN is available (https://www.ihn-org.com/membership/current-members/). International efforts for hemovigilance data- and knowledge-sharing include, but are not limited to: the International Surveillance of Transfusion-Associated Reactions and Events (ISTARE) database from IHN[15] and Project Notify Library (http://www.notifylibrary.org) from the World Health Organization (WHO).[16]

The historical focus of hemovigilance systems has been on hospital surveillance and the reporting of transfusion-associated adverse events into a central data repository. Interest in donor hemovigilance is more recent, enhanced with studies showing higher reaction rates among young donors.[17-18] The goal of hemovigilance systems should be acquiring and trending high-quality, representative, and validated surveillance data, not on capturing *all* potential data. Separating

surveillance from clinical data is important. Although the two types of data are very similar, clinical decision-making asks and answers fundamentally different questions about an individual's health and subsequent care. Surveillance data focus more on trending summary data that may or may not be ultimately classified in a manner suited for the clinician-patient relationship.

Eventually, as hemovigilance programs have evolved, it has become increasingly clear that proper analysis of hemovigilance events requires standardization of data structures and harmonization of terminology with simple and objective definitions that lend themselves to comparison (eg, expressing adverse events per transfusion or per 1000 donations, etc), as well as extensive use of subject matter experts to aid in interpretation and validation of the data.[17,18]

US HEMOVIGILANCE

In 2009, US hemovigilance was described as a "patchwork of reporting processes"[19] with significant but limited programs to collect specific donor and recipient data and where only fatal transfusion reactions, donation-related deaths, and product deviations were reported at a national level to the US Food and Drug Administration (FDA). These programs capture a subset of hemovigilance data, but do not comprise a complete system meeting all the criteria for "mature" hemovigilance. In 2003, the FDA took initial steps toward mandating more comprehensive US hemovigilance through the proposed rule "Safety Reporting Requirements for Human Drug and Biological Products"; however, at the time of this writing, this remains in draft status.[20]

Hospitals and transfusion services are required to perform an investigation of all serious adverse reactions associated with blood transfusion and to report complications that may be related to the blood donor or to the manufacture of the blood components to the collection facility [Title 21, Code of Federal Regulations (CFR), Part 606.170]. Transfusion- and donation-related fatalities must also be reported directly to the FDA by the transfusing or collecting facility. The FDA publishes an annual report of the reported fatalities (https://www.fda.gov/vaccines-blood-

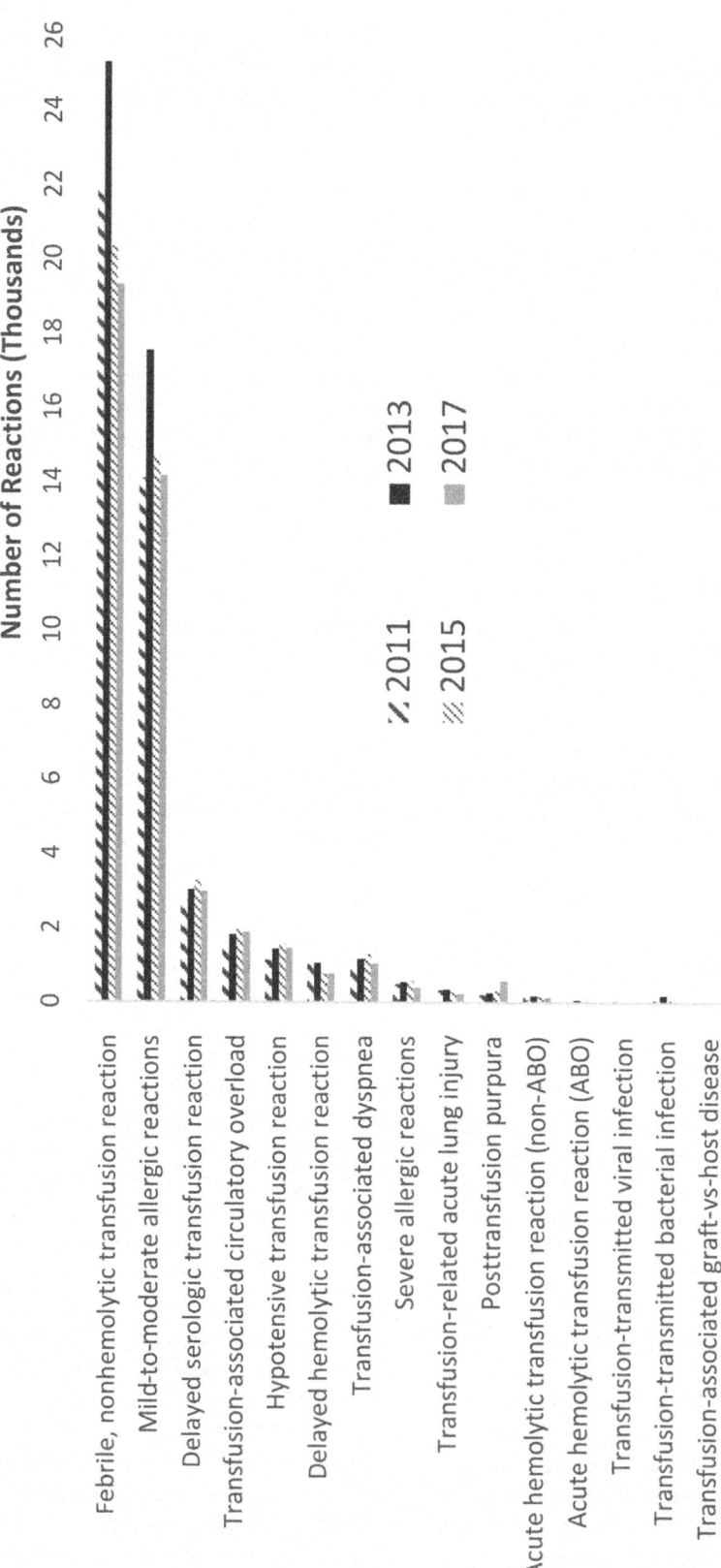

FIGURE 4-2. Transfusion-related adverse reactions reported in National Blood Collection and Utilization Survey (NBCUS).[21]

biologics/report-problem-center-biologics-evalua tion-research/transfusiondonation-fatalities). Mandatory reporting of product deviations by licensed manufacturers, unlicensed registered blood establishments, and transfusion services has also been defined by the FDA (21 CFR 606.171). These requirements will likely continue even if a more formal US national hemovigilance system is eventually required, because hemovigilance reports are retrospective, whereas reporting to the FDA following an adverse event or for product deviations must occur in near-real time, as outlined in the CFR.

There is no mandatory nationwide, systematic assessment of transfusion reactions that were not fatal, nor of nonfatal donation-related reactions, in the United States. However, a few investigator-led or collaborative research initatives [American Red Cross (ARC), Vitalant Research Institute, and collaborations sponsored by the National Heart, Lung, and Blood Institute (NHLBI) such as the Retrovirus Epidemiology Donor Study (REDS), REDS-II, and the Recipient Epidemiology and Donor Evaluation Study-III (REDS-III)] have generated extensive results in the areas of emerging infectious diseases, noninfectious complications of transfusion, and donation-related reactions.

In parallel, Drs. Harold Kaplan and James Battles developed the impactful medical event (incident) reporting system for transfusion medicine (MERS-TM) in hospitals in the mid-1990s.[22] In addition, National Blood Collection and Utilization Survey Reports have included summary reports of transfusion reactions and serious donation-related adverse events since 2007 (Fig 4-2).[21] The launch of a voluntary system of hemovigilance in the United States has required collaboration among all stakeholders and many organizations. Specific acknowledgement is given to the strategic partnership, resources, financial support, and guidance provided by the US Department of Health and Human Services (DHHS), including the FDA and Centers for Disease Control and Prevention (CDC).

Task Force on Biovigilance

In early 2006, a number of prominent individuals in transfusion medicine recognized the need for a broader, more cohesive and coordinated approach, termed *biovigilance*, that encompassed not only blood recipient and blood donor hemovigilance but also tissues and organs, and cellular therapy (CT) components.[23] AABB established an Interorganizational Task Force on Biovigilance, inviting key governmental thought leaders and representatives from the private sector to initiate the development of a national biovigilance program. Amid concerns of additional oversight by government agencies, including a perception that such oversight could result in punitive actions that might interfere with patient care, hemovigilance was established in the United States within a framework of a public-private partnership.[24] Through the efforts of the task force and an international working group of advisors representing established hemovigilance systems, recipient and donor hemovigilance programs were designed based on the important tenets of voluntary reporting: confidentiality, a just culture (nonpunitive data analysis), and efficient data reporting with a focus on improvements to patient and donor safety. The task force was also critical in the development of case definitions and data requirements for the national recipient hemovigilance system, described below.

Elements of Biovigilance

Efficient reporting for recipient hemovigilance was achieved through leveraging an existing hospital event reporting system, the CDC's National Healthcare Safety Network (NHSN) (see Recipient Hemovigilance, below). Donor hemovigilance required building a new infrastructure to capture national reporting by US blood establishments (see Blood Donor Hemovigilance, below). Other areas essential to comprehensive biovigilance in the United States include tissue and organ surveillance and cellular therapies (CT) biovigilance. CT adverse event and outcome monitoring occurs through national and international registries, including the Center for International Blood and Marrow Transplant Research (CIBMTR), the National Marrow Donor Program (NMDP), and the World Marrow Donor Association (WMDA). In ongoing efforts to promote hemovigilance ideals, AABB *Standards for Blood Banks and Transfusion Services (Standards)* requires accredited blood banks, transfusion services, and blood centers to adopt nationally recognized classifications [or internationally recognized, such as defined by the International Society of Blood Transfusion (ISBT), for countries lacking their own such classifications] for adverse reactions associated with blood donation and the transfusion of blood and blood components.[25(p89)]

RECIPIENT HEMOVIGILANCE IN THE UNITED STATES

CDC's NHSN is a secure, web-based surveillance system. Originally developed to capture data on hospital-acquired infections (HAI), it is now used by over 12,000 US health-care facilities to report on a variety of infection-related and other patient safety issues.[26] The hemovigilance module of the NHSN, which began national data collection in 2010, allows hospitals to monitor their own transfusion activity as well as to share data with external groups (governmental and nongovernmental; described below) at the individual hospital's discretion, for mandatory or voluntary reporting activities.[27]

The NHSN modules were established as data repositories for surveillance of adverse events and reactions of interest. To be comparable between hospitals, data must be reported using standard definitions for all aspects of data element reporting. Ideally, reporting thresholds would be as similar as possible between different hospitals. The components of the NHSN hemovigilance module and the terms and definitions employed were developed and thoroughly vetted by subject matter experts. The major components of the module include: 1) demographic and utilization data, which permit classification of facilities for comparisons in aggregate data analyses; 2) reports on transfusion-related adverse reactions in accordance with case definition criteria, as well as severity and imputability grading (Table 4-1); and 3) incident reporting (ie, mistakes, errors, or adverse events associated with transfusion). Reporting of incidents is not mandatory for participation unless associated with patient harm. As of 2018, 359 transfusion services have enrolled in the NHSN hemovigilance module, of which 133 are actively reporting data to NHSN (Kracalik I, CDC personal communication, April 8, 2020). At this time, hemovigilance reporting into the CDC NHSN requires manual data entry, although a mechanism exists for reporting monthly denominators through clinical documentation architecture (CDA).

Tools to integrate hospital reporting of product-related adverse events, such as transfusion-associated circulatory overload (TACO), TRALI, or suspected transfusion-transmitted infection (TTI), with blood center investigations can facilitate comprehensive understanding of adverse reactions. An example of this is the recently completed harmonized form for reporting adverse transfusion reactions to blood suppliers, developed by members of the AABB Hemovigilance Committee, Hemovigilance Education and Analytics Committee, and Donor Hemovigilance Working Group (see Appendix 4-1).[28] Complex case definitions for entities such as TACO and TRALI need periodic reevaluation as new information and technology are used to diagnose and treat transfusion complications. Such exercises need to reflect the potentially different needs of the clinical, research, and surveillance communities. Ideally, changes to these definitions should be validated by each community.[29,30]

Collaborative efforts between the CDC and state departments of public health continue to promote statewide reporting into the NHSN hemovigilance network. For example, in 2014, the state of Massachusetts implemented mandatory reporting into the NHSN hemovigilance module as a means to comply with state regulatory requirements on transfusion activity and transfusion-related adverse events.[27,31] Statewide participation provided insight into varying transfusion practices and utilization, and a more informed picture of transfusion-related adverse events has emerged, including events related to TTI and TACO.[32,33] Additionally, statewide participation affords the opportunity to track trends in practice changes (eg, mitigation strategies for TTI, adoption of new blood component

TABLE 4-1. NHSN Hemovigilance Module Adverse Reaction Codes, Severity Codes, and Imputability*†

Case Definition	Severity	Imputability
Definitive: The adverse reaction fulfills all of the case definition criteria. *Probable:* The adverse reaction meets some of the clinical signs of symptoms or radiologic, laboratory evidence, and/or available information but does not meet all definitive case definition criteria.	*Nonsevere:* Medical intervention (eg, symptomatic treatment) is required but there is minimal risk of permanent damage to the transfusion recipient. *Severe:* Inpatient hospitalization or prolonged hospitalization is directly attributable to the transfusion reaction, persistent or significant disability or incapacity of the patient as a result of the reaction, or a medical or surgical intervention is necessary to preclude permanent damage or impairment of a body function. *Life-threatening:* Major intervention was required after the transfusion reaction (eg, vasopressors, intubation, transfer to intensive care) to prevent death. *Death:* The recipient died as a result of the transfusion reaction. *Not determined:* The severity of the adverse reaction is unknown or not stated.	*Definite:* There is conclusive evidence that the reaction can be attributed to the transfusion. *Probable:* There are other potential causes present that could explain the recipient's symptoms, but transfusion is the most likely cause of the reaction. *Possible:* There are other potential causes that are most likely; however, transfusion cannot be ruled out.

(Continued)

TABLE 4-1. NHSN Hemovigilance Module Adverse Reaction Codes, Severity Codes, and Imputability*† (Continued)

Optional	Optional	Optional
Possible: The reported clinical signs or symptoms, radiologic or laboratory evidence, and available information are not sufficient to meet definitive or probable case definition criteria.		*Doubtful:* There is evidence clearly in favor of a cause other than the transfusion, but transfusion cannot be excluded. *Ruled out:* There is conclusive evidence beyond reasonable doubt of a cause other than the transfusion. *Not determined:* The relationship between the reaction and transfusion is unknown or not stated.

*Used with permission from Chung et al.[27]

†The **NHSN** Hemovigilance Module protocol specifies the case definition for 12 adverse transfusion reactions based on the presence of signs, symptoms, and laboratory and radiologic data. Reactions are reported with a severity designation based on clinical outcomes. Imputability designations that specify the likelihood that reaction was associated with the transfusion event are also reported.

offerings such as whole blood) by transfusion services.[33]

Getting Connected

CDC's NHSN Hemovigilance Module website provides resources and training materials for facilities to get access and start reporting into the system (https://www.cdc.gov/nhsn/acute-care-hospital/bio-hemo/setup.html). Once access to the module has been attained, the hospital must complete the Annual Hospital Survey before any data submission may begin. This survey includes a significant number of data elements that describe the demographics of the hospital. Following its completion, the hospital can submit data using web forms to complete monthly reporting plans and then report monthly denominators, adverse reactions, and incidents. Monthly denominator reports include the components transfused each month and are provided in the month following the reporting month. Adverse events (reactions and incidents) should be reported upon completion of their investigation.

Transfusion-Related Adverse Reaction Reporting

Adverse reactions should be investigated and categorized according to the CDC protocol[26] into 12 different reaction types and coded according to the degree to which each reaction conforms to the surveillance definition (criteria), the severity or grade of the reaction, and the reaction's imputability to the transfusion (Table 4-1). Imputability is an important concept for hemovigilance; it is the degree to which the reaction was caused by the transfusion. With the January 2017 release of the NHSN Hemovigilance Module, CDC instituted a function to collect specific data related to case imputability and propose an imputability score. More recent developments (January 2018) allow the reporting organization the ability to indicate its agreement with that computer-based assessment. As the formal definitions of imputability and severity continue to mature, hemovigilance systems around the world are beginning to incorporate them into their reports.

Transfusion Incident Reporting

Mistakes or incidents associated with transfusion can be reported on a detailed incident form or summarized on a monthly incident summary report. The CDC requires detailed incident form use for those incidents that result in a transfusion reaction. However, nonharmful incident review and more detailed reporting can be a valuable activity if conducted regularly and compared with other transfusion services that use the CDC standardized event codes that are based on the adverse event coding system developed in MERS-TM (Fig 4-3).[34]

Using Recipient Data via NHSN Group Function

Hospitals participating in the NHSN Hemovigilance Module can share their data with external partners (groups) through the group function built into the NHSN system. This eliminates the need to enter data into multiple systems. Although group users (managers) can access data from all participating hospitals, hospitals cannot access any data from other hospitals in their group. Hospitals and blood centers in Massachusetts comply with the state's regulatory requirement by sharing their data with the NHSN group maintained by the state (Fig 4-4). Data can also be shared with a NHSN group maintained by a Patient Safety Organization (PSO) developed under the Patient Safety and Quality Improvement Act of 2005 (PSQIA).[35,36]

BLOOD DONOR HEMOVIGILANCE IN THE UNITED STATES

Part of maintaining a safe and adequate blood supply involves vigilance over donor safety and well-being. Blood establishments must be the stewards of safety that donors expect them to be. This commitment to the donor requires attention to continuous improvement in donor recruitment, donor management, the process of blood collection, and donor safety; hence, the need for a donor hemovigilance system.

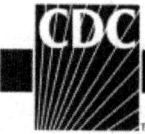

NHSN Biovigilance Component
Hemovigilance Module Surveillance Protocol v2.5.2
www.cdc.gov/nhsn

Incident Codes

Note: Incident codes are based on MERS TM (US) and TESS (Canada) incident classification schemes.

Product Check-In
(Transfusion Service)
Events that occur during the shipment and receipt of products into the transfusion service from the supplier, another hospital site, satellite storage, or clinical area.
PC 00 Detail not specified
PC 01 Data entry incomplete/incorrect/not performed
PC 02 Shipment incomplete/incorrect
PC 03 Products and paperwork do not match
PC 04 Shipped/transported under inappropriate conditions
PC 05 Inappropriate return to inventory
PC 06 Product confirmation incorrect/not performed
PC 07 Administrative check not incorrect/not performed (record review/audit)
PC 08 Product label incorrect/missing

Product Storage
(Transfusion Service)
Events that occur during product storage by the transfusion service.
US 00 Detail not specified
US 01 Incorrect storage conditions
US 03 Inappropriate monitoring of storage device
US 04 Unit stored on incorrect shelf (e.g., ABO/autologous s/directed)
US 05 Incorrect storage location

Inventory Management
(Transfusion Service)
Events that involve quality management of the blood product inventory.
IM 00 Detail not specified
IM 01 Inventory audit incorrect/not performed
IM 02 Product status incorrectly/not updated online (e.g., available/discarded)
IM 03 Supplier recall/traceback not appropriately addressed/not performed
IM 04 Product order incorrectly/not submitted to supplier
IM 05 Outdated product in available inventory
IM 06 Recalled/quarantined product in available inventory

Product/Test Request
(Clinical Service)
Events that occur when the clinical service orders patient tests or blood products for transfusion.
PR 00 Detail not specified
PR 01 Order for wrong patient
PR 02 Order incompletely/incorrectly ordered (online order entry)
PR 03 Special processing needs not indicated (e.g., CMV negative, autologous)
PR 04 Order not done
PR 05 Inappropriate/unnecessary (intended) test ordered
PR 06 Inappropriate/unnecessary (intended) blood product ordered
PR 07 Incorrect (unintended) test ordered
PR 08 Incorrect (unintended) blood product ordered

Product/Test Order Entry
(Transfusion Service)
Events that occur when the transfusion service receives a patient order. This process may be excluded if clinical service uses online ordering.
OE 00 Detail not specified
OE 01 Order entered for wrong patient
OE 02 Order incompletely/incorrectly entered online
OE 03 Special processing needs not entered (e.g., CMV-, autologous)
OE 04 Order entry not done
OE 05 Inappropriate/unnecessary (intended) test order entered
OE 06 Inappropriate/unnecessary (intended) blood product order entered
OE 07 Incorrect (unintended) test ordered
OE 08 Incorrect (unintended) blood product ordered

Sample Collection
(Service collecting the samples)
Events that occur during patient sample collection.
SC 00 Detail not specified
SC 01 Sample labeled with incorrect patient name
SC 02 Not labeled
SC 03 Wrong patient collected
SC 04 Collected in wrong tube type
SC 05 Sample QNS
SC 06 Sample hemolyzed
SC 07 Label incomplete/illegible/incorrect (other than patient name)
SC 08 Sample collected in error
SC 09 Requisition arrived without samples
SC 10 Wristband incorrect/not available
SC 11 Sample contaminated

FIGURE 4-3. NHSN Hemovigilance Module incident codes. [Reprinted from NHSN Manual: Biovigilance Component Protocol April 2018 (page 1 of 3).[26]]

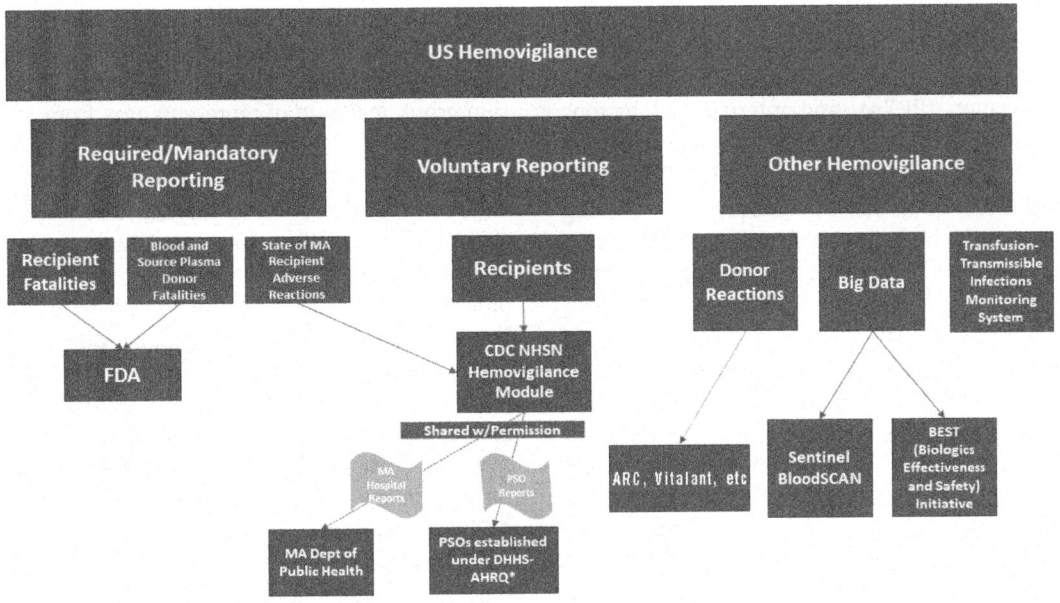

FIGURE 4-4. Hemovigilance in the United States.
*Regulated by HHS Agency for Healthcare Research and Quality (AHRQ), authorized by the Patient Safety and Quality Improvement Act of 2005 (PSQIA).
FDA = Food and Drug Administration; CDC = Centers for Disease Control and Prevention; NHSN = National Healthcare Safety Network; PSO = patient safety organization; ARC = American Red Cross; BloodSCAN = Blood Safety Continuous Active Surveillance Network.

Blood establishments collect a wealth of data every day centered on donor-related activities. They are driven to maximize the efficiency of collecting each donation type while also reducing the risk of donor harm. Blood-center-based donor hemovigilance systems and collaborative research have evolved primarily to capture adverse reaction rates and have been used in donor safety studies to mitigate adverse events.[34,37-39] Donor hemovigilance programs within large blood systems have demonstrated their utility in identifying and implementing measures that improve donation safety for young donors.[34,40] Blood center data have also been analyzed to help identify donation deterrents and motivators and to increase overall donor satisfaction.[41-42] Improvements in donor safety can occur through a variety of methods, such as avoiding donors at high risk for vasovagal reactions (eg, potential donors with low estimated blood volume), educating donors and

staff on donor hydration and salt loading of donors, improving the ability to predict donors at risk for vasovagal reactions with loss of consciousness (especially off-site), and developing strategies to decrease deferrals (eg, monitoring iron stores and iron replacement) and increase donor return rates. Blood establishments, through a mature donor hemovigilance system, use collected data not only to improve donor safety and satisfaction but also to inform decisions about complex business and operational issues.

Background

As with the recipient hemovigilance system in the United States, US donor hemovigilance was developed through the AABB Interorganizational Task Force on Biovigilance. A donor hemovigilance working group was established with representation from US blood establishments, hospital-based blood collection programs, the US Armed Services Blood Program, Canadian Blood Services, the Plasma Protein Therapeutics Association (PPTA), and international liaisons from the ISBT and the International Haemogilance Network (IHN), in partnership with representatives from the US DHHS. The working group was charged to develop and implement a national monitoring program on donor safety issues. Tasks included developing a set of common definitions for US donor hemovigilance based on existing models and providing subject matter expertise for the development of software, funded by DHHS, that would gather donor data and provide a systematic and standard mechanism to calculate and compare rates. This yielded the Donor Hemovigilance Analysis and Reporting Tool (DonorHART), which offered a robust set of reporting and graphing tools designed to simplify initial data reporting and aggregate data analysis.

Observed variation in reaction rates, reported to DonorHART, led to changes in practice in one blood center that likely reduced reaction rates among donors younger than 30 years old.[43,44] Donor hemovigilance reports have been published based on data from the small number of participating blood collectors (Fig 4-5 and Table 4-2).[45-47] These generally confirm findings reported in the literature by large proprietary donor hemovigilance programs (ARC, Vitalant). US donor hemovigilance is still active, with organizations such as ARC and Vitalant Research Institute contributing significantly. However, use of the DonorHART program ended September 25, 2018, as a result of system maintenance costs. Ongoing efforts to standardize donor hemovigilance continue, as evidenced by the recent requirement in AABB *Standards* to use standardized classifications. In addition, there was an international project in which members from the AABB Donor Hemovigilance Working Group along with ISBT and PPTA representatives collaborated to standardize the severity grading of donor adverse reactions (see below and Appendix 4-2).

A Global Standard

Over the years, many organizations (ISBT, IHN, ARC, America's Blood Centers, Vitalant, and others) have worked together to make well-accepted and universal definitions, terms, and ideas for donor hemovigilance. A formal revision group made up of representatives from the ISBT Hemovigilance Working Party, the IHN, and the AABB Donor Hemovigilance Working Group collaborated to revise the 2008 ISBT standard for surveillance of complications related to blood donation. The group reconciled the differences between the AABB and ISBT surveillance terms and, in December 2014, published the first internationally harmonized AABB-ISBT standard definitions for complications related to blood donation. The Alliance of Blood Operators, the European Blood Alliance, and the IHN have formally endorsed these definitions.[40,45,48] Additional validation of this standard has resulted in confirmation of its applicability and recommendations for the additional development of a harmonized structure for the severity and imputability assessments of donor reactions. Between January 2018 and June 2019, an international hemovigilance working group involving AABB, ISBT, and PPTA representatives developed and validated a Donor Adverse Reaction Severity Grading Tool,[49,50] which is designed to be used along with the 2014 AABB-ISBT standard definitions for complications related to blood donation (see Appendix 4-2). The tool provides a standardized, objective framework for grading severity and addresses the lack of consistency in severity grading seen during validation of the 2014 definitions. This harmonization of definitions facilitates easy national and international comparison between blood centers and systems. The tool is patterned after Common Terminology Criteria for Adverse Events (CTCAE1), a well-known clinical severity scale. CTCAE1 rates severity from Grades 1 through 5, roughly associated with mild, moderate, severe, life-threatening, and fatal levels, respectively.[50]

NEXT STEPS IN US HEMOVIGILANCE

In a 2009 DHHS report on the critical gaps in US biovigilance,[19] Sixteen gaps were identified for blood, tissue, and organ national vigilance

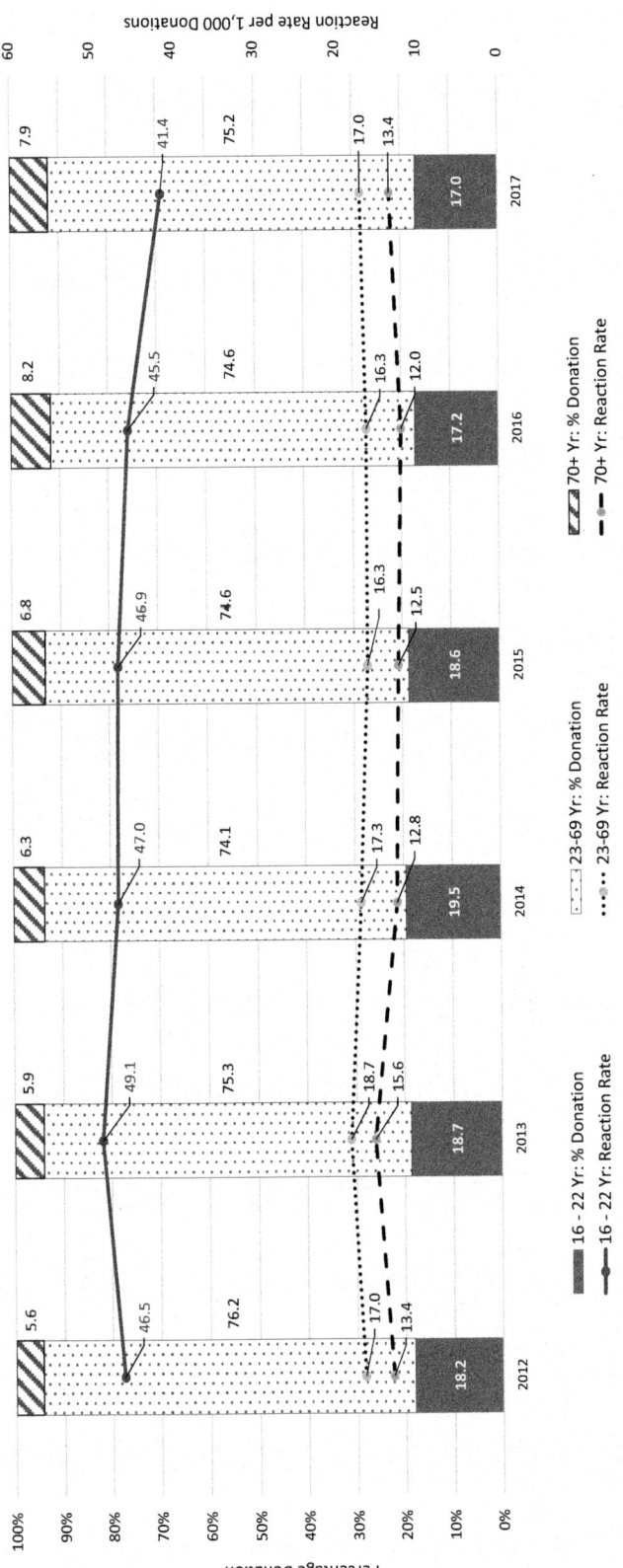

FIGURE 4-5. Percentage donation and donor reaction rate by donor age (2012-2017 AABB Donor Hemovigilance Highlights).[47]

TABLE 4-2. Reaction Rates per 1,000 Donations by donor reaction types (2012-2017 AABB Donor Hemovigilance Highlights)[47]

Reaction Type	2012 (n=5)	2013 (n=6)	2014 (n=10)	2015 (n=10)	2016 (n=11)	2017 (n=7)
Overall Reactions	22.2	24.3	22.8	21.9	22.2	20.8
Vasovagal	15.9	17.4	16.3	14.8	14.4	13.2
Prefaint, no LOC (uncomplicated or minor)	13.6	14.9	14.0	12.2	12.1	10.8
LOC	2.3	2.5	2.3	2.6	2.4	2.3
Local Injury Related to needle	3.0	3.3	3.1	3.5	4.5	3.7
Nerve Irritation	0.2	0.2	0.2	0.2	0.2	0.2
Hematoma / Bruise	2.7	3.0	2.8	3.1	4.0	3.0
Arterial Puncture	0.03	0.03	0.03	0.04	0.05	0.05
Painful Arm	0.1	0.1	0.1	0.2	0.2	0.4
Delayed bleeding	-	-	-	-	0.002	0.01
Infection	-	-	-	0.01	0.003	0.01
Major Blood Vessel Injury	-	-	-	-	-	-
Injury	0.1	0.1	0.1	0.1	0.06	0.06
Major Injury	0.01	0.01	0.01	0.1	0.03	0.02
Minor Injury	0.1	0.1	0.1	0.02	0.03	0.04

Apheresis-related	2.8	3.1	2.9	3.3	3.0	3.8
Citrate	0.2	0.2	0.2	0.2	0.2	0.3
Hemolysis	0.004	0.005	0.004	0.005	0.006	0.001
Air Embolus	0.001	0.001	0.001	-	0.001	-
Infiltration	2.6	2.8	2.7	3.1	2.7	3.6
Allergic	0.2	0.2	0.2	0.04	0.04	0.03
Local	0.2	0.2	0.2	0.03	0.03	0.03
Systemic	0.04	0.04	C.04	0.01	0.004	0.004
Anaphylaxis	-	-	-	-	0.001	-
Major Cardiovascular Event	0.001	0.001	0.001	0.001	-	-
Angina pectoris within 24 hours	0.001	0.001	0.001	-	-	-
Cardiac arrest	-	-	-	-	-	-
Cerebrovascular accident	-	-	-	0.001	-	-
Myocardial infarction within 24 hours	-	-	-	-	-	-
Transient Ischemic Attack within 24 hours (TIA)	-	-	-	-	-	-
Other	0.2	0.3	0.2	0.2	0.2	0.02

n = number of blood collection facilities that participated in the DonorHART system.

programs, eight of which were focused on blood-related activities (Table 4-3). Ten years later, many of the gaps have been addressed, while others persist. Gaps 4 and 6 are largely closed, with precise recipient and donor definitions and identified denominator data; however, the system is still very fragmented (Gap 1) and lacking in comprehensive national reporting, with only a small number of hosptials participating in the CDC NHSN Hemovigilance Module and a few blood collectors voluntarily providing detailed data on donor adverse events (Gap 5), beyond the FDA-required fatality reporting. Unfortunately, tissue and organ biovigilance efforts worldwide (not just the United States) lag behind blood donor and recipient hemovigilance efforts, meaning that Gaps 9 through 16 are still relevant today. Project Notify, however, is an example of how international experts are working together to address tissue and organ biovigilance.

TABLE 4-3. Gaps Identified in US Biovigilance, 2009[18]

Blood	Gap 1	Patchwork and sometimes fragmented system of various adverse event reporting.
	Gap 2	Likely underreporting of transfusion adverse events.
	Gap 3	Challenges with FDA-required reporting.
	Gap 4	Need for accurate recipient denominator data, precise definitions, and training.
	Gap 5	No national surveillance of donor serious adverse events other than fatalities.
	Gap 6	Need for accurate donor denominator data, precise definitions, and training.
	Gap 7	Need for accurate tracking of all donor infectious disease test data.
	Gap 8	Need for timely analysis of reported data.
Tissues	Gap 9	Limited information on the potential for HCT/Ps to transmit infectious disease.
	Gap 10	Ability to ascertain that reported infections in HCT/P recipients can be attributed to the tissue is limited.
	Gap 11	Regulations concerning HCT/P adverse reaction reporting do not extend to the level of the health-care facility or health-care provider.
	Gap 12	Current mechanisms for tracking HCT/P grafts to the level of the recipient are limited.
	Gap 13	Adverse reaction reporting for HCT/Ps regulated solely under Section 361 of the PHS Act is limited to infectious diseases.
	Gap 14	Information about adverse reactions in other recipients of HCT/Ps from an implicated donor may not be readily available.
Organs	Gap 15	Lack of nationwide common organ/tissue donor network system for real-time reporting, data collection, communication, and analysis of donor transmitted diseases in organ and tissue transplant recipients, including a common donor identifier necessary for linkage back to implicated donors of both organs and tissues.
	Gap 16	No requirement to retain donor and recipient samples.

FDA = Food and Drug Administration; HCT/Ps = human cells, tissues, and cellular and tissue-based products; PHS = Public Health Service.

Although reporting institutions technically should have always had access to their own data, the complexities of hospital information systems and blood establishment computer systems (BECS) have not lent themselves to easy accessibility to and analysis of data. Fortunately, this is beginning to be addressed in broad terms with the successful completion of national repository databases [eg, the Transfusion-Transmissible Infections Monitoring System (TTIMS)], the publishing of annual reports, and (limited) access to composite data for researchers and analysts. Short of a formal revamping of the current reporting system and increasing what is required to be reported, Gaps 2, 3, and 5 will likely remain, at least at the national level. It is encouraging that some progress is being seen in addressing these gaps at the state level (ie, Massachusetts), which eventually may be seen as the necessary next step to integrate reporting at the national level. Real-time data availability (Gap 8) is also a difficult issue, but steps are being made to shorten the reporting window.

As the blood banking industry and threats to blood and transfusion safety continue to evolve, so do the tools needed to evaluate the risk and the impact of professionals' decisions. Because of ongoing concerns about the need for real-time assessment of postmarket recipient risk and as a result of a congressional mandate (Food and Drug Administration Amendments Act of 2007), the FDA developed the Sentinel Blood Safety Continuous Active Surveillance Network (BloodSCAN) Program in 2011 as an active surveillance system to monitor the safety of FDA-regulated medical products, including blood components (see www.sentinelinitiative.org for more information).[51,52] It is a distributed database composed of data from 18 data partners, covering over 300 million person-years of health data. The project's aim is to help the FDA work with public, academic, and private entities to collect quality data, provide a rapid response (days to weeks) to safety questions, and make the results accessible to the public domain.

More recently, in 2017 the Biologics Effectiveness and Safety (BEST) initiative expanded use of the common data models (a way of organizing data from different primary sources into a standard secondary structure for analysis) to ap-

ply active surveillance and advanced technical tools, including artificial intelligence and natural language processing to hemovigilance questions. Such nonstructured data investigations show promise for linking textual data from the electronic health record (EHR) with transfusion exposure. These projects go a long way toward addressing several of the key hemovigilance deficiencies, including real-time data availability. Although such data mining may speed up discovery of emerging events, there is also the inherent risk of inaccurate and/or incomplete data, resulting in false signals.

The Observational Health Data Sciences and Informatics (OHDSI, pronounced "Odyssey"; ohdsi.org) program is another example of how people are collecting and analyzing health-care data in new and powerful ways. ODHSI is a multi-stakeolder, international, interdisciplinary collaborative creating open-source solutions to large-scale analytics or observational health data. The mission of OHDSI is "to improve health by empowering a community to collaboratively generate the evidence that promotes better health decisions and better care."

With the constant threat of existing (eg, HIV) and emerging infectious diseases (EIDs; eg, West Nile virus, Zika virus, and Chagas disease), improved infectious disease surveillance and rapid alert systems are still considered primary parts of any national hemovigilance program (Gap 7). AABB maintains a stand-alone online network specifically designed for reporting of West Nile virus and Zika virus testing results (see http://www.aabb.org/research/hemovigilance). This system tracks donor screening data—including confirmatory testing data to differentiate true from false positives—on a real-time basis for each EID and includes the ability to produce reports by geographic location and time period.

In early 2015, the FDA's Center for Biologics Evaluation and Research (CBER) and NHLBI announced a joint program to develop TTIMS, by leveraging existing and successful programs (REDS-II) to establish a framework for TTI surveillance to include known pathogens and EIDs. Such programs are invaluable to objectively assess the value of new blood safety initiatives, such as the FDA's changes in policy for male-to-male (MSM) sexual contact from lifetime deferral to a deferral of 1 year, and further to 3 months, since the last MSM sexual contact. Programs such as Sentinel BloodSCAN, BEST, and TTIMS are needed for the FDA to have the objective national data necessary for other potential policy changes, such as discontinuing certain required tests or changing other identification testing requirements for components modified with pathogen reduction technology.

Given the privatized, competitive nature of the US health-care system, the United States may never have a hemovigilance program like SHOT or other programs in countries with single-payer health-care systems. Although the availability of long-term funding for private-sector programs may be concerning (DonorHART and the AABB Center for Patient Safety programs are no longer active), most of the other national programs described above have more stable funding commitments in place. To be successful, systems must continue to provide stakeholders with quality data to drive new safety hypotheses and objective analytics to demonstrate outcomes.

Instead of an ineffective "patchwork," as once described, perhaps it is better to describe the current US biovigilance system as a true "network" of independent and interdependent solutions, each built by committed stakeholders from a variety of disciplines and interests, nationally and increasingly internationally, with an overarching common goal of improving donor and patient safety. Countries like the United States no longer have to rely soley on their own resources. If a country's hemovigilance system can be considered a network, then globally, hemovigilance is best imagined as a network of networks currently being woven together alongside a variety of research, public, and private hemovigilance programs whose net goal is the optimal care of blood donors and patients receiving transfusions worldwide.

ACKNOWLEDGMENT

The authors thank Srijana Rajbhandary for her assistance in updating the chapter.

KEY POINTS

1. Hemovigilance is surveillance of the whole transfusion chain to minimize adverse events or reactions in donors and recipients and promote safe and effective use of blood components. It is a collaboration where stakeholders (researchers, policy makers, blood establishments, and hospitals) share data and ideas, implement potential solutions, evaluate the results, and further refine them based on real-world data.

2. The earliest hemovigilance efforts arose out of concerns over transfusion-transmitted viral infections and their sequelae for blood recipients.

3. In the United States, national hemovigilance has lagged. Currently, it consists of independent and interdependent programs functioning as a loose network collecting specific, high-level donor and recipient data at national or near-national levels. Some individual programs, however, although not national in scale, are very robust in their ability to capture and validate their data.

4. Surveillance and clinical decision-making are overlapping but separate concepts. Clinical decision-making asks and answers questions important to the health and care of an individual patient, whereas surveillance focuses more on trending summary data that may or may not ultimately be classified similarly to the clinical findings.

5. Patient safety organizations (PSOs) were formed to improve health safety by providing a confidential environment for voluntary reporting and analysis of patient safety events.

6. Blood establishments have an obligation to minimize the risks of blood collection. The rise in formal donor hemovigilance efforts over the past decade resulted in internationally harmonized AABB-ISBT standard definitions for complications related to blood donation.

7. There are challenges common to all newly introduced surveillance programs, including 1) delays between data submission and release of reports; 2) the lack of sufficiently granular data to explain many observations; 3) the concern that systems may not adequately capture new, rapidly evolving, or unusual events and that resources are insufficient for modifications needed to improve analyses and to respond to new threats; 4) the reality that systems do not capture all events from all potential institutions; 5) the lack of consistency in use and definitions of terms across institutions; and 6) that financial pressures constantly expect systems to provide more and increasingly sophisticated results with fewer resources.

8. Ongoing efforts are underway to help standardize terminology, which will continue to help hemovigilance programs share data and improve outcomes.

REFERENCES

1. Busch MP, Lee LL, Satten GA, et al. Time course of detection of viral and serological markers preceding human immunodeficiency virus type 1 seroconversion: Implications for screening of blood and tissue donors. Transfusion 1995;35(2):91-7.

2. Jennings ER, Hindman WM, Zak B, et al. The thymol turbidity test in screening of blood donors. Am J Clin Pathol 1957;27(5):489-502.

3. Keating LJ, Gorman R, Moore R. Hemoglobin and hematocrit values of blood donors. Transfusion 1967;7(6):420-4.

4. AuBuchon JP, Whitaker BI. America finds hemovigilance! Transfusion 2007;47:1937-42.

5. De Vries RRP, Faver J-C, eds. Hemovigilance: An effective tool for improving transfusion safety. West Sussex, UK: Wiley-Blackwell, 2012.

6. Strengers PFW. Haemovigilance – Why? [Available at http://www.ztm.si/uploads/publication/990/1009.pdf (accessed September 16, 2019).]

7. DHHS Advisory Committee on Blood and Tissue Safety and Availability meeting minutes, April 30-May 1 and November 19-20, 2009 transcripts. Silver Spring, MD: Department of Health and Human Services, 2009.

8. Japanese Red Cross Society. Haemovigilance annual report 1993-2001. Tokyo: Japanese Red Cross Central Blood Center, 2003. [Available at http://www.jrc.or.jp/mr/english/ (accessed September 6, 2018).]

9. Serious Hazards of Transfusion. TRALI tables. Manchester, UK: SHOT, 2010. [Available at www.shotuk.org/shot-reports/trali-tables/ (accessed April 8, 2020).]

10. Bolton-Maggs PHB, Cohen H. SHOT haemovigilance and progress in improving transfusion safety. Br J Haematol 2013;163(3):303-14.

11. PHB Bolton-Maggs, Poles D, et al for the Serious Hazards of Transfusion (SHOT) Steering Group. The 2017 Annual SHOT Report. Manchester, UK: SHOT, 2018. [Available at https://www.shotuk.org/shot-reports/ (accessed April 8, 2020).]

12. Joint United Kingdom (UK) Blood Transfusion and Tissue Transplantation Services Professional Advisory Committee. Welcome to the National Blood Transfusion Committee. [Available at https://www.transfusionguidelines.org/uk-transfusion-committees/national-bloodtransfusion-committee (accessed April 8, 2020).]

13. European Union. Directive 2002/98/EC of the European Parliament and of the Council of 27 January 2003 setting standards of quality and safety for the collection, testing, processing, storage and distribution of human blood and blood components and amending Directive 2001/83/EC. Official Journal of the European Union 2003;L33:30-40. [Available at http://eur-lex.europa.eu/legal-content/EN/TXT/?uri=CELEX%3A32002L0098.]

14. European Commission. Commission Directive 2005/61/EC of 30 September 2005 implementing Directive 2002/98/EC of the European Parliament and of the Council as regards traceability requirements and notification of serious adverse reactions and events (text with EEA relevance). Official Journal of the European Union 2005;L256:350-8. [Available at http://eur-lex.europa.eu/legal-content/EN/ALL/?uri=CELEX%3A32005L0061.]

15. Politis C, Wiersum JC, Richardson C, et al. The International Haemovigilance Network Database for the Surveillance of Adverse Reactions and Events in Donors and Recipients of Blood Components: Technical issues and results. Vox Sang 2016 Nov;111(4):409-17.

16. World Health Organization. Blood transfusion safety. Haemovigilance. Geneva: WHO, 2019. [Available at http://www.who.int/bloodsafety/haemovigilance/en/ (accessed September 6, 2018).]

17. Zins C. Conceptual approaches for defining data, information, and knowledge. J Am Soc Inform Sci Tech 2007;58(4):479-93.

18. Strehlow RA. Content analysis of definitions. In: Wright SE, Strehlow RA, eds. Standardizing and harmonizing terminology: Theory and practice. ASTM STP 1223. Philadelphia: American Society for Testing and Materials, 1994:53-62.

19. Public Health Service Biovigilance Task Group. Biovigilance in the United States: Efforts to bridge a critical gap in patient safety and donor health. Washington, DC: DHHS, 2009. [Available at https://wayback.archive-it.org/3922/20140403203201/http://www.hhs.gov/ash/bloodsafety/biovigilance/ash_to_acbsa_oct_2009.pdf.]

20. Food and Drug Administration. Safety reporting requirements for human drug and biological products; proposed rule. (March 14, 2003) Fed Regist 2003;68:12405-97. [Available at https://www.federalregister.gov/documents/2003/03/14/03-5204/safety-reporting-requirements-for-human-drug-and-biological-products.]

21. US Department of Health and Human Services. National Blood Collection and Utilization Survey (website). Washington, DC: Office of Infectious Disease and HIV/AIDS Policy, 2020. [Available at https://www.hhs.gov/oidp/topics/blood-tissue-safety/surveys/national-blood-collection-and-utilization-survey/index.html.]

22. Kaplan HS, Battles JB, Van der Schaaf TW, et al. Identification and classification of the causes of events in transfusion medicine. Transfusion 1998;38(11-12):1071-81.

23. Strong DM, AuBuchon J, Whitaker B, Kuehnert MJ. Biovigilance initiatives. ISBT Science Series 2008;3:77-84.

24. AuBuchon JP, Whitaker BI. America finds hemovigilance! Transfusion 2007;47:1937-42.

25. Gammon R, ed. Standards for blood banks and transfusion services. 32nd ed. Bethesda, MD: AABB, 2020.

26. National Healthcare Safety Network. Blood safety surveillance. Atlanta, GA: Centers for Disease Control and Prevention, 2018. [Available at http://www.cdc.gov/nhsn/acute-care-hospital/bio-hemo/.]

27. Chung KW, Harvey A, Basavaraju SV, Kuehnert, MJ. How is national recipient hemovigilance conducted in the United States? Transfusion 2015;55(4):703-7.

28. AABB. Common transfusion reaction reporting form (report of adverse transfusion reaction to blood suppliers). Bethesda, MD: AABB, 2019. [Available at http://www.aabb.org/research/hemovigilance/Documents/AABB-Transfusion-Adverse-Reaction-Form.pdf (accessed September 16, 2019).]

29. Wiersum-Osselton JC, Whitaker B, Grey S, et al. Revised international surveillance case definition of transfusion-associated circulatory overload: A classification agreement validation study. Lancet Haematol 2019;6(7):e350-8.

30. Vlaar APJ, Toy P, Fung M, et al. A consensus redefinition of transfusion-related acute lung injury. Transfusion 2019;59(7):2465-76.

31. Cumming M, Osinski A, O'Hearn L, et al. Hemovigilance in Massachusetts and the adoption of statewide hospital blood bank reporting using the National Healthcare Safety Network. Transfusion 2017;57(2):478-83.

32. Haass KA, Sapiano MRP, Savinkina A, et al. Transfusion-transmitted infections reported to the National Healthcare Safety Network Hemovigilance Module. Transfus Med Rev 2019; 33(2):84-91.

33. Massachusetts Department of Public Health. Hemovigilance program data summary January – December 31, 2017. Jamaica Plain, MA: Bureau of Infectious Disease and Laboratory Sciences, 2018. [Available at https://www.mass.gov/service-details/reporting-requirements-for-blood-banks-and-hemovigilance-in-massachusetts.]

34. Eder AF, Dy BA, Kennedy JM, et al. Improved safety for young whole blood donors with new selection criteria for total estimated blood volume. Transfusion 2011;51:1522-31.

35. Patient Safety and Quality Improvement Act of 2005. Pub. L. No.109-41, §§ 921-26, 119 Stat.424 (2005). Rockville, MD: Agency for Healthcare Research and Quality, 2005. [Available at http://www.gpo.gov/fdsys/pkg/PLAW-109publ41/pdf/PLAW-109publ41.pdf.]

36. PSO Privacy Protection Center. Common formats background. Rockville, MD: Agency for Healthcare Research and Quality, 2005. [Available at https://www.psoppc.org/psoppc_web/publicpages/commonFormatsOverview (accessed April 12, 2020).]

37. Custer B, Bravo M, Bruhn R, et al. Predictors of hemoglobin recovery or deferral in blood donors with an initial successful donation. Transfusion 2014;54(9):2267-75.

38. Wieling W, France CR, van Dijk N, et al. Physiologic strategies to prevent fainting responses during or after whole blood donation. Transfusion 2011;51(12);2727-38.

39. Eder AF. Current efforts to reduce the risk of syncope among young blood donors. Curr Opin Hematol 2012;19(6):480-5.

40. Tomasulo P, Kamel H, Bravo M, et al. Interventions to reduce the vasovagal reaction rate in young whole blood donors. Transfusion 2011; 51:1511-21.

41. Kamel HT, Bassett MB, Custer B, et al. Safety and donor acceptance of an abbreviated donor history questionnaire. Transfusion 2006;46(10): 1745-53.

42. Bednall TC, Bove LL. Donating blood: A meta-analytic review of self-reported motivators and deterrents. Transfus Med Rev 2011;25(4):317-34.

43. Townsend M, Land KJ, Whitaker B, et al. US donor hemovigilance system: Mechanism for nationwide reporting (abstract 3A-S1-02). Vox Sang 2001;101(Suppl 1):11-12.

44. Land KJ. Update on donor hemovigilance. Presented at DHHS Advisory Committee on Blood Safety and Availability, November 4-5, 2010.

45. Land KJ, Whitaker BI, for the AABB US Donor Hemovigilance Working Group. The 2012 AABB donor hemovigilance report. Bethesda, MD: AABB, 2013. [Available at http://www. aabb.org/research/hemovigilance/Pages/ donor-hemovigilance.aspx (accessed September 6, 2018).]

46. Rajbhandary S, Stubbs J, Land KJ, Whitaker BI, for the AABB US Donor Hemovigilance Working Group. The 2012-2014 AABB donor hemovigilance report. Bethesda, MD: AABB, 2016. [Available at http://www.aabb.org/ research/hemovigilance/Pages/donor-hemovig ilance.aspx (accessed September 6, 2018).]

47. AABB. 2012-2017 Donor hemovigilance highlights. Bethesda, MD: AABB, 2019. [Available at: http://www.aabb.org/research/hemovigi lance/Documents/2012-2017-AABB-Donor-Hemovigilance-Highlights.pdf (accessed April 8, 2020).]

48. Goldman M, Land K, Wiersum-Osselton J. Development of standard definitions for surveillance of complications related to blood donation. Vox Sang 2016;110:185-8.

49. Donor hemovigilance. Bethesda, MD: AABB, 2019. [Available at http://www.aabb.org/ research/hemovigilance/Pages/donor-hemovig ilance.aspx (accessed September 17, 2019).]

50. Townsend M, Kamel HT, Van Buren N, et al. Development and validation of donor adverse reaction severity grading tool: Enhancing objective grade assignment to donor adverse events. Transfusion 2020 (in press).

51. Menis M, Izurieta HS, Anderson SA, et al. Outpatient transfusions and occurrence of serious noninfectious transfusion-related complications among US elderly, 2007-2008: Utility of large administrative databases in blood safety research. Transfusion 2012;52:1968-76.

52. Menis M, Anderson SA, Forshee RA, et al. Transfusion-related acute lung injury and potential risk factors among the inpatient US elderly as recorded in Medicare claims data, during 2007 through 2011. Transfusion 2014;54: 2182-93.

APPENDIX 4-1.
Protocol for Hospital Reporting Adverse Events to Blood Suppliers

REPORT OF ADVERSE TRANSFUSION REACTION TO BLOOD SUPPLIERS

INSTRUCTIONS: Send the form to <u>ALL</u> blood suppliers that provided blood components to this patient. Timely reporting is important, so that, if appropriate, the blood supplier may prevent the transfusion of other products from the same donor(s). [Complete areas which are not included in your internal hospital work-up and attach work-up.]

Do you suspect this reaction is the result of an attribute specific to the donor or the blood product?

☐ **Yes or suspected:**

Reaction did not result in fatality: Complete this form and forward to the blood supplier(s).

Reaction resulted in fatality: Complete this form, forward to the blood supplier(s), AND report fatality to FDA.

☐ **No:** Stop, do not report to the blood supplier.

☐ **Other:** Consult with the blood supplier physician.

Additional Blood Supplier Instructions for the Hospital Transfusion Service, as applicable:

GENERAL INSTRUCTIONS

Please attach the following:

- Copy of completed hospital internal Transfusion Reaction Work-up Form
- Copy of Pre- and Post- transfusion chest x-ray reports for suspected TRALI reactions
- Copy of Culture and pending tests *(when available)* for suspected sepsis cases
- Copy of applicable Admission Note, Physician notes regarding reaction, Discharge Note
- Copy of allergy and medication list for suspected allergy reactions

For blood supplier use only:	Case Identification #		Date Received / / **(mm/dd/yy)**

1

APPENDIX 4-1.
Protocol for Hospital Reporting Adverse Events to Blood Suppliers (Continued)

REPORTING FACILITY INFORMATION

Date Submitted / / **(mm/dd/yy)**	Reporting Facility

Name of Person Filling Out Form	Title

Facility Addrress

Telephone Number	Fax #	Email

Transfusion Services Medical Director

Transfusion Services Medical Director Email	Phone #

Blood Bank Medical Director

Blood Bank Medical Director Email	Phone #

PATIENT/RECIPIENT INFORMATION

Medical Record #	Name *(optional)*
Age	Date of Birth / / **(mm/dd/yy)** *(optional)*
Weight	Sex
Attending Physician *(optional)*	Attending's Phone # *(optional)*

Admitting or Primary Diagnosis

Indication for Transfusion

Relevant Severe Co-morbidities *(if applicable)*

Pertinent Medications

List transfusion history within 24 Hours **PRIOR** to reaction *(Attach additional sheets if necessary.)*

List transfusion history within 24 hours **AFTER** reaction

Any prior history of transfusion reactions *(type and date)*

Current Status at Time of Reporting:

☐ Returned to pre-transfusion status.	☐ Expired *(Transfusion related fatality)*** / / **(mm/dd/yy)** *(if available)*
☐ Still requires support related to transfusion reaction.	☐ Expired *(Not transfusion related)* / / **(mm/dd/yy)** *(if available)*

☐ Other/Unknown, Specify:

* *Report to FDA within 24 hours.*

2

APPENDIX 4-1.
Protocol for Hospital Reporting Adverse Events to Blood Suppliers (Continued)

BLOOD COMPONENT(S) INFORMATION

* Please list all components that were transfused **within the 24 hours prior to the transfusion reaction.** *(Attach additional sheets if necessary.)*
* For transfusion under massive transfusion protocol or rapid multiple transfusions, please give best estimate of date and time of each unit. *(Attach anesthesiology record if possible.)*

Blood Supplier	Unit Number	Component Type or Code	Volume Transfused *(approximate in mL.)*	Date/Time Transfusion Start	Date/Time Transfusion Stop	Was Product Modified by Hospital?
				___/___/___ (mm/dd/yy) ___:___ (hh:mm) ☐ am ☐ pm	___/___/___ (mm/dd/yy) ___:___ (hh:mm) ☐ am ☐ pm	☐ No ☐ Yes, Specify:
				___/___/___ (mm/dd/yy) ___:___ (hh:mm) ☐ am ☐ pm	___/___/___ (mm/dd/yy) ___:___ (hh:mm) ☐ am ☐ pm	☐ No ☐ Yes, Specify:
				___/___/___ (mm/dd/yy) ___:___ (hh:mm) ☐ am ☐ pm	___/___/___ (mm/dd/yy) ___:___ (hh:mm) ☐ am ☐ pm	☐ No ☐ Yes, Specify:
				___/___/___ (mm/dd/yy) ___:___ (hh:mm) ☐ am ☐ pm	___/___/___ (mm/dd/yy) ___:___ (hh:mm) ☐ am ☐ pm	☐ No ☐ Yes, Specify:
				___/___/___ (mm/dd/yy) ___:___ (hh:mm) ☐ am ☐ pm	___/___/___ (mm/dd/yy) ___:___ (hh:mm) ☐ am ☐ pm	☐ No ☐ Yes, Specify:
				___/___/___ (mm/dd/yy) ___:___ (hh:mm) ☐ am ☐ pm	___/___/___ (mm/dd/yy) ___:___ (hh:mm) ☐ am ☐ pm	☐ No ☐ Yes, Specify:
				___/___/___ (mm/dd/yy) ___:___ (hh:mm) ☐ am ☐ pm	___/___/___ (mm/dd/yy) ___:___ (hh:mm) ☐ am ☐ pm	☐ No ☐ Yes, Specify:
				___/___/___ (mm/dd/yy) ___:___ (hh:mm) ☐ am ☐ pm	___/___/___ (mm/dd/yy) ___:___ (hh:mm) ☐ am ☐ pm	☐ No ☐ Yes, Specify:
				___/___/___ (mm/dd/yy) ___:___ (hh:mm) ☐ am ☐ pm	___/___/___ (mm/dd/yy) ___:___ (hh:mm) ☐ am ☐ pm	☐ No ☐ Yes, Specify:

3

APPENDIX 4-1.
Protocol for Hospital Reporting Adverse Events to Blood Suppliers (Continued)

REACTION INFORMATION

Date/Time Transfusion Started: / / (mm/dd/yy) : (hh:mm) ☐ am ☐ pm
Date/Time Reaction Started: / / (mm/dd/yy) : (hh:mm) ☐ am ☐ pm
Date/Time Transfusion Stopped: / / (mm/dd/yy) : (hh:mm) ☐ am ☐ pm

Reaction Vital Signs

	Pre-Transfusion	During Reaction	Post-Reaction
Date/Time	/ / (mm/dd/yy) : (hh:mm) ☐ am ☐ pm	/ / (mm/dd/yy) : (hh:mm) ☐ am ☐ pm	/ / (mm/dd/yy) : (hh:mm) ☐ am ☐ pm
Temperature	°C/°F	°C/°F	°C/°F
Blood Pressure (Systolic)	mm Hg	mm Hg	mm Hg
Blood Pressure (Diastolic)	mm Hg	mm Hg	mm Hg
Pulse	bpm	bpm	bpm
Respiratory Rate	rpm	rpm	rpm
O$_2$ Sat	%	%	%

Symptoms/Signs at Time of Reaction – Check all that apply.

☐ **Abdominal pain/cramps** [1,4]
☐ **Angioedema** [1]
☐ **Anxiety** [1]
☐ **Arrythmia** [1]
☐ **Back pain** [4]
☐ **Cardiac arrest** [1]
☐ **Chest pain** [4]
☐ **Chest tightness** [1, 3]
☐ **Chills/Rigors** [4]
☐ **Cough** [3, 4]
☐ **Cyanosis** [1, 2, 3]
☐ **Diarrhea** [1]
☐ **DIC** [4]

☐ **Dyspnea** [1, 2, 3, 4]
☐ **Edema – pulmonary** [2,3]
☐ **Edema – Pedal** [3]
☐ **Erythema** [1]
☐ **Fever** [2, 4]
☐ **Flushing** [1]
☐ **Headache** [3, 4]
☐ **Hoarseness/Stridor** [1]
☐ **Hypertension** [2, 3]
☐ **Hypotension** [1, 2, 4]
☐ **Hypoxemia** [2, 3]
☐ **Impending doom** [1]
☐ **Jugular venous distension** [3]

☐ **Loss of consciousness** [1]
☐ **Nausea/Vomiting** [1, 4]
☐ **Oliguria** [4]
☐ **Orthopnea** [3]
☐ **Pain at infusion site** [4]
☐ **Pruritis** [1]
☐ **Shock** [1, 4]
☐ **Substernal pain** [1]
☐ **Tachycardia** [1, 2, 3, 4]
☐ **Tachypnea** [2,3]
☐ **Urticaria** [1]
☐ **Wheezing** [1, 4]
☐ **Widened pulse pressure** [3]

Allergic/Anaphylactic [1] | **TRALI** [2] | **TACO** [3] | **Septic Transfusion Reaction** [4]

Suspected Adverse Reaction: Assign priority if more than one possibility*

☐ Allergic/Anaphylaxis[†]	☐ Transfusion-related acute lung injury (TRALI)[‡]	☐ Septic transfusion reaction[§]

☐ Other, specify:

Additional information:
(If more than one possibility, assign priority.)

* Please refer to the | **National Healthcare Safety Network Biovigilance Component Hemovigilance Module Surveillance Protocol** | for complete definitions.

[†] Attach allergy and medication list
[‡] Attach Chest x-ray
[§] Please forward results of culture and pending tests when available

AABB. Advancing Transfusion and Cellular Therapy Worldwide

4

(Continued)

APPENDIX 4-1.
Protocol for Hospital Reporting Adverse Events to Blood Suppliers (Continued)

PULMONARY-ALLERGIC-ANAPHYLACTIC REACTION INFORMATION

Risk Factors for Acute Lung Injury – Check all that apply.

☐ Acute Respiratory Distress Syndrome (ARDS)
☐ Aspiration
☐ Pneumonia
☐ Toxic inhalation
☐ Lung contusion
☐ Near drowning
☐ Pulmonary hemorrhage

☐ Severe sepsis
☐ Shock
☐ Multiple trauma
☐ Burn
☐ Acute pancreatitis
☐ Cardiopulmonary bypass
☐ Drug overdose
☐ Volume overload
☐ Renal failure

☐ Upper airway obstruction
☐ Diffuse alveolar damage
☐ Chemotherapy
☐ Amiodarone
☐ Disseminated intravascular coagulation
☐ Radiation to thorax
☐ Massive blood transfusion

Additional comments *(Other risk factors)*

Diagnostics – Check box and/or enter values.

	Pre-Transfusion				Post-Transfusion			
	Date and Time	Yes/No/ Not Done		Pre-Tx Values	Date and Time	Yes/No/ Not Done		Post-Tx Values
O₂ sat $\leq$ 90% on room air	/ / (mm/dd/yy) : (hh:mm) ☐ am ☐ pm	☐ Yes	☐ No	☐ Not Done		/ / (mm/dd/yy) : (hh:mm) ☐ am ☐ pm	☐ Yes	☐ No	☐ Not Done	
PaO₂/FiO₂ $\leq$ 300 mm Hg	/ / (mm/dd/yy) : (hh:mm) ☐ am ☐ pm	☐ Yes	☐ No	☐ Not Done		/ / (mm/dd/yy) : (hh:mm) ☐ am ☐ pm	☐ Yes	☐ No	☐ Not Done	
Chest X-ray: Bilateral infiltrates *(Attach chest x-ray if available)*	/ / (mm/dd/yy) : (hh:mm) ☐ am ☐ pm	☐ Yes	☐ No	☐ Not Done		/ / (mm/dd/yy) : (hh:mm) ☐ am ☐ pm	☐ Yes	☐ No	☐ Not Done	
Chest X-ray: Widened cardiac silhouette (cardiomegaly)	/ / (mm/dd/yy) : (hh:mm) ☐ am ☐ pm	☐ Yes	☐ No	☐ Not Done		/ / (mm/dd/yy) : (hh:mm) ☐ am ☐ pm	☐ Yes	☐ No	☐ Not Done	
Elevated **BNP** *(Provide value in pg/mL.)* ☐ BNP ☐ NT-proBNP	/ / (mm/dd/yy) : (hh:mm) ☐ am ☐ pm	☐ Yes	☐ No	☐ Not Done		/ / (mm/dd/yy) : (hh:mm) ☐ am ☐ pm	☐ Yes	☐ No	☐ Not Done	
Elevated **Central Venous Pressure** greater than 12 mm Hg *(Provide values.)*	/ / (mm/dd/yy) : (hh:mm) ☐ am ☐ pm	☐ Yes	☐ No	☐ Not Done		/ / (mm/dd/yy) : (hh:mm) ☐ am ☐ pm	☐ Yes	☐ No	☐ Not Done	
Positive Fluid Balance *(in mL) (Attach patient I/O report if available.)*	/ / (mm/dd/yy) : (hh:mm) ☐ am ☐ pm	☐ Yes	☐ No	☐ Not Done		/ / (mm/dd/yy) : (hh:mm) ☐ am ☐ pm	☐ Yes	☐ No	☐ Not Done	
Transient decrease **White Blood Cell Count**	/ / (mm/dd/yy) : (hh:mm) ☐ am ☐ pm	☐ Yes	☐ No	☐ Not Done		/ / (mm/dd/yy) : (hh:mm) ☐ am ☐ pm	☐ Yes	☐ No	☐ Not Done	

Advancing Transfusion and
Cellular Therapies Worldwide

APPENDIX 4-1.
Protocol for Hospital Reporting Adverse Events to Blood Suppliers (Continued)

Treatment and Clinical Course		
	Treatment *(Check yes, if treatment was administered.)*	**Response to Treatment** *(Check yes, if patient improved following treatment.)*
Acetaminophen	☐ Yes	☐ Yes
Antihistamines	☐ Yes	☐ Yes
Bronchodilators	☐ Yes	☐ Yes
Diuretics	☐ Yes	☐ Yes
Epinephrine	☐ Yes	☐ Yes
Intubation/Ventilatory support	☐ Yes	☐ Yes
Oxygen supplementation	☐ Yes	☐ Yes
Steroids	☐ Yes	☐ Yes
Vasopressors	☐ Yes	☐ Yes
Other (specify):	☐ Yes	☐ Yes

Additional comments *(Attach additional clinical information if available.)*

If TRALI is suspected, please save an EDTA (purple-top) patient sample.
Recipient HLA type:
Recipient HNA type:
Recipient HLA/HNA antibody status:
Donor HLA/HNA antibody result (if performed on unit):
Donor HLA type (if available):

Advancing Transfusion and
Cellular Therapies Worldwide

6

(Continued)

APPENDIX 4-1.
Protocol for Hospital Reporting Adverse Events to Blood Suppliers (Continued)

SUSPECTED BACTERIAL CONTAMINATION

Were the suspect components returned to the blood bank? ☐ No ☐ Yes

On repeat visual inspection, does the component reveal any abnormalities *(e.g. clumps,discoloration, hemolysis)***?**
☐ No ☐ Yes: Describe: ☐ Unevaluable

Suspect component – Source used: ☐ Bag ☐ Segment ☐ Not done

Gram stain performed: ☐ Negative ☐ Positive ☐ Not done	**Result** *(organism identified, if positive)***:**
Culture performed: ☐ Negative ☐ Positive ☐ Pending ☐ Not done	**Result** *(organism identified, if positive)***:**

Was a secondary test performed by the hospital for this component (PGD or equivalent)?
☐ No ☐ Yes, Specify:

Patient's pre-transfusion blood culture: ☐ Negative ☐ Positive ☐ Pending ☐ Not done

Date/Time: / / (mm/dd/yy) : (hh:mm) ☐ am ☐ pm	**Result** *(organism identified, if positive)***:**

Patient's post-transfusion blood culture result: ☐ Negative ☐ Positive ☐ Pending ☐ Not done

Date/Time: / / (mm/dd/yy) : (hh:mm) ☐ am ☐ pm	**Result** *(organism identified, if positive)***:**

Does the patient have history of fever or other infection related to his/her underlying medical condition? ☐ No ☐ Yes

Was the patient on antibiotics at the time of transfusion? ☐ No ☐ Yes, Name:

Is the patient currently being treated with antibiotics? ☐ No ☐ Yes, Name:

Did the patient have an absolute neutropenia (neutrophil count less than 500 per µl) prior to transfusion? ☐ No ☐ Yes

Comments:

FOR TRANSFUSION MEDICAL DIRECTOR REVIEW

Provisional Interpretation and Classification*

Reaction	☐ Allergic/Anaphylactic ☐ TRALI ☐ TACO ☐ Septic Transfusion Reaction ☐ Other:
Case definition criteria	☐ Definitive ☐ Probable ☐ Possible
Severity	☐ Non-severe ☐ Severe ☐ Life Threatening ☐ Death
Imputability	☐ Definite ☐ Probable ☐ Possible ☐ Doubtful ☐ Ruled out ☐ Not Determined
Notes	

Tranfusion Medical Director contact/phone/email

Tranfusion Medical Director (or designee) signature

* Please refer to the | **National Healthcare Safety Network Biovigilance Component Hemovigilance Module Surveillance Protocol** | for complete definitions.

APPENDIX 4-1.
Protocol for Hospital Reporting Adverse Events to Blood Suppliers (Continued)

FOR BLOOD SUPPLIER USE	
Interpretation and Classification*	
Reaction	☐ Allergic/Anaphylactic ☐ TRALI ☐ TACO ☐ Septic Transfusion Reaction ☐ Other:
Case definition criteria	☐ Definitive ☐ Probable ☐ Possible
Severity	☐ Non-severe ☐ Severe ☐ Life Threatening ☐ Death
Imputability	☐ Definite ☐ Probable ☐ Possible ☐ Doubtful ☐ Ruled out ☐ Not Determined

Notes *(Attach additional reports, if available.)*

Blood Supplier contact/phone/email

* Please refer to the | **National Healthcare Safety Network Biovigilance Component Hemovigilance Module Surveillance Protocol** | for complete definitions.

8

APPENDIX 4-2.
Severity Grading Tool for Blood Donor Adverse Events

A User Brochure
Introduction:

The severity assignment tool is designed to be used with the Standard for Surveillance of Complications Related to Blood Donation published in 2014 by ISBT/AABB/IHN. Severity assignment can be hampered by subjectivity; this tool was created to enhance objective assignment of severity. The Severity assignment is patterned after an established clinical severity scale, Common Terminology Criteria for Adverse Events (CTCAE1) v 5.0, which rates severity by Grades 1-5, with 1 through 5 being roughly associated with mild, moderate, severe, life-threatening and death. Definitions and general considerations for severity grading include:

Severity Grade	General factors to consider in assigning severity Donor Adverse Event (DAE) Severity Tool	(DAE) Examples
Grade 1	No Outside Medical Care (OMC) **AND** Short duration ≤ 2 weeks **AND** No limitation on Activities of Daily Living (ADL) **AND** Resolved with no or minimal intervention	Arterial puncture, pressure bandage applied, resolved without intervention or sequelae Vasovagal event that resolves with comfort care and/or oral hydration Citrate reaction resolved with oral calcium or reduction in infusion rate
Grade 2	OMC, no hospitalization **OR** Duration >2 weeks- ≤ 6 months **OR** Limitations on ADL for ≤2 weeks	Superficial thrombophlebitis resolved with oral antibiotics, no sequelae Vasovagal event that requires transport to ER for IV hydration Lacerations requiring sutures
Grade 3	Not life-threatening **AND any of the following** Hospitalization **OR** Duration >6 months **OR** Limitations on ADL >2 weeks **OR** Require surgery **OR** Other serious complications (Category E)	Arteriovenous fistula requiring surgical repair Fracture, dental injury, or concussion TIA and other cardiovascular events, which are not life-threatening
Grade 4*	Immediate medical intervention required to prevent death	LOC with fall and intracranial bleed Anaphylaxis requiring intubation or tracheostomy
Grade 5*	Death	Death

* Grade 4 and Grade 5 are not shown in the Severity Grading Tool of Blood Donor Adverse Events .

CTCAE v 5: Common Terminology for Adverse Events Version 5.0; published November 27, 2017; US Department of Health and Human Services, National Institutes of Health, National Cancer Institute

AABB Donor Hemovigilance Working Group

APPENDIX 4-2.
Severity Grading Tool for Blood Donor Adverse Events (Continued)

Instructions for Use

- Determine category of Donor Adverse Event (DAE) using ISBT/AABB/IHN Standard for Surveillance of Complications Related to Blood Donation, December 2014.

- For Grade 1, the reaction must satisfy all criteria listed

- Select the **highest applicable grade** of severity; for example, if a vasovagal reaction resulted in a fall and the donor was seen in the emergency room where she required sutures (Grade 2) to repair a laceration on her arm and was also diagnosed with a concussion (Grade 3), the final severity assignment would be **Grade 3.**

- Occasionally a donor may experience multiple adverse events. Assigning a severity grade in such cases requires judgement.

  * If the reactions are distinct, with more than one type DAE classification, assign each DAE a separate Severity Score based on the Grading Tool. (Example, citrate reaction that resolves with oral calcium **[Gr1]** plus a nerve injury that impacts ADL for more than 2 weeks **[Gr3]**).

  — If the DAEs are related or difficult to distinguish , then assign a single Severity Grade based on the highest applicable Severity Grade.

- Not all Grades are applicable for all DAE; for instance, all DAE involving major blood vessel injury, cardiac and cerebrovascular incidents are graded at least Grade 3 ; no option for Grade 1 or 2 is given. Likewise, DAEs involving arm pain are not life-threatening and are limited to Grades 1, 2 or 3.

- Grades 4 (Life-threatening) and 5 (Death) are very rare. **Neither Grade 4 nor Grade 5 is shown in the Severity Assessment Table/Tool,** and should only be selected when the final diagnosis is confirmed in consultation with appropriate medical personnel. (See definition of Life-threatening).

- Death due to a blood donation or if donation was a contributing factor should be reported to the competent authority as required by law.

- Imputability: This grading tool is developed to assist with assignment of severity. Imputability must be assessed separately for determination of the relationship of the donation to severe DAEs, as required for fatality reporting. Please refer to Standard for Surveillance of Complications Related to Blood Donation 2014 — ISBT/AABB/IHN.

Working Definitions and Abbreviations for Use in Grading Reactions:

- ***Outside Medical Care (OMC):*** donor is evaluated and/or treated by Emergency Medical Response (EMR), Health Care Professional (HCP), urgent care, hospital emergency room (ER) without admission to the hospital. Please note that if EMR is called (an ambulance) and the donor is evaluated but not transported, then it is still considered OMC.

- ***Hospitalization:*** admission to the hospital; does NOT include being seen and discharged from urgent care or hospital emergency department.

- ***Life-threatening***: any adverse event that places the subject at ***immediate*** risk of death without intervention.

  * A DAE should be graded as life-threatening, ***Grade 4,*** only if the situation required immediate action to prevent death. For instance, the following interventions would suggest a life-threatening DAE: intubation or tracheostomy for stridor, wheezing, bronchospasm or laryngeal edema (anaphylactic shock).

  * A situation that is ***potentially*** life-threatening should NOT be given a ***Grade 4*; *Grade 4*** is reserved for only those DAE that actually required intervention to prevent death.

- ***Surgery:*** Any procedure that required regional (spinal, block), inhalation or general anesthesia. The following are NOT considered surgery: simple sutures, staples, butterfly closure.

- ***Activities of Daily Living (ADL)*:** Include everyday household chores, doing necessary business, shopping, going to work or school, or getting around for other purposes. ADL are impacted if the donor

  * Needs the help of other persons with bathing or showering, dressing, eating, getting in or out of bed or chairs, using the toilet, and getting around the home (Self-care ADL)

  * Cannot work, attend school or manage routine personal/family activities because of the Donor Adverse Event (Instrumental ADL).

(Continued)

APPENDIX 4-2.
Severity Grading Tool for Blood Donor Adverse Events (Continued)

Severity Grading Tool of Blood Donor Adverse Events

Category	Grade 1	Grade 2	Grade 3
A.1. Blood outside vessel --Haematoma --Arterial puncture --Delayed bleeding	• No OMC • Localized to venipuncture site	• OMC (EMR, ER, PCP, Urgent care), no hospitalization, or • ADL ≤2 weeks, or • Generalized beyond venipuncture site	• Hospitalization, or • ADL >2 weeks, or • Severe sequelae, or • Surgical intervention
A.2. Arm Pain --Nerve injury/irritation --Other arm pain	• No OMC • Duration ≤2 weeks	• OMC (EMR, ER, PCP, Urgent care), no hospitalization, or • Duration >2 weeks to ≤6 months, or • ADL ≤2 weeks	• Duration > 6 months, or • ADL >2 weeks
A.3. Localized infection/inflammation of vein or soft tissue --Superficial thrombophlebitis --Cellulitis	• No OMC	• OMC (EMR, ER, PCP, Urgent care), no hospitalization, or • ADL ≤2 weeks, or • Resolved with oral antibiotics	• Hospitalization, or • ADL >2 weeks, or • Resolved with IV treatment
A.4. Other major blood vessel injury --Deep venous thrombosis --Arteriovenous fistula --Compartment syndrome --Brachial artery pseudoaneurysm			• Diagnoses medically confirmed, or • Treated with antioagulant therapy, or • Required surgical intervention
B. Vasovagal reactions --Vasovagal reaction, no loss of consciousness (LOC) --Vasovagal reaction, loss of consciousness (LOC)	• No OMC	• OMC (EMR, ER, PCP, Urgent care), no hospitalization, or • ADL ≤2 weeks, or • Suture of laceration(s), or • IV rehydration	• Hospitalization, or • ADL >2 weeks, or • Fracture(s), medically confirmed concussion, dental injury requiring dental procedure, e.g. cap/crown, dental implant, bridge, tooth extraction, dentures
C. Related to apheresis --Citrate reaction --Haemolysis --Air embolism --Infiltration	• No OMC • Citrate toxicity (including carpopedal spasm) resolved with or without oral calcium	• OMC (EMR, ER, PCP, Urgent care), no hospitalization, or • ADL ≤2 weeks, or • Citrate toxicity requiring intravenous calcium	• Hospitalization, or • ADL >2 weeks, or • Abnormal cardiac rhythm medically diagnosed
D. Allergic Reaction --Local allergic reaction --Generalized (anaphylactic) reaction	• No OMC • Managed with over-the-counter medications--topical steroids, antihistamine	• OMC (EMR, ER, PCP, Urgent care), no hospitalization, or • Generalized reaction including bronchospasm, laryngospasm managed with inhalation or oral bronchodilator and/or auto-injector (EpiPen)	• Hospitalization, or • Generalized reaction, including bronchospasm, laryngospasm or anaphylaxis, requiring management with intravenous steroids and/or epinephrine, but NOT intubation or tracheostomy
E. Other serious complication --Acute cardiac symptoms --Myocardial infarction --Cardiac arrest --Transient ischemic attack --Cerebrovascular accident (Stroke)			• Diagnoses medically confirmed
F. Other	• No OMC • No injury	• OMC (EMR, ER, PCP, Urgent care), no hospitalization, or • Duration >2 weeks to ≤6 months, or • ADL ≤2 weeks	• Hospitalization, or • Duration > 6 months, or • ADL >2 weeks, or • Surgical intervention

CHAPTER 5

Allogeneic and Autologous Blood Donor Selection

Debra A. Kessler, RN, MS, and Susan N. Rossmann, MD, PhD

THE FOREMOST RESPONSIBILITY OF BLOOD collection facilities is to maintain a safe and adequate blood supply. The selection of appropriate blood donors is essential to protect donors' health during and following donation and to ensure the safety, quality, identity, purity, and potency of the donated blood components to protect the transfusion recipient. Key elements of the selection process, as part of the overall approach to blood safety, are donor education, use of a Food and Drug Administration (FDA)-accepted donor history questionnaire and materials, a focused physical examination, and the results of infectious disease testing (see Chapter 7); management of all information about the donation, including subsequent postdonation information, and the donation process itself must be completed in accordance with current good manufacturing practice.

This chapter describes the current federal regulations, accreditation requirements, and medical considerations related to both screening blood donors before their blood is collected and donor testing for relevant transfusion-transmitted infections (RTTIs), as defined by the FDA in the *Code of Federal Regulations* (CFR), Title 21, Part 630.3(h).[1-3]

OVERVIEW OF BLOOD DONOR SCREENING

The blood collection facility must determine donor eligibility in accordance with federal and state regulations and AABB's voluntary accreditation standards. Specific criteria used to select donors are established by FDA regulations and recommendations in guidance and memoranda. In addition, AABB has developed professional standards for donor selection with which accredited blood collection facilities must comply.[1]

Blood collection facilities provide prospective blood donors with information on the donation process and potential donation-related adverse effects and instruct them not to donate if they have risk factors associated with an RTTI. The donor screening process includes a focused physical examination and direct questioning about specific risk behaviors, medications, travel, and other factors that potentially affect transfusion recipient or donor safety. The donor screening questions address risks related to RTTIs for which sensitive tests are currently performed [eg, human immunodeficiency virus (HIV)], for which tests are not universally used (eg, *Babesia*), and for which licensed screening

Debra A. Kessler, RN, MS, Vice President, Medical Programs and Services, New York Blood Center, New York, New York; and Susan N. Rossmann, MD, PhD, Chief Medical Officer, Gulf Coast Regional Blood Center, Houston, Texas

The authors have disclosed no conflicts of interest.

tests are not yet available (eg, sporadic and variant Creutzfeldt-Jakob diseases (CJD) and malaria). In addition, centers may ask donors questions about a history of pregnancies to determine whether testing for HLA antibodies is necessary, as part of a risk reduction strategy for transfusion-related acute lung injury (TRALI). Facilities must establish donor eligibility on the day of donation and before collection. If a donor's responses to the screening questions are incomplete or unclear, the blood collection establishment may clarify the responses within 24 hours of donation and remain compliant with the "day of collection" requirement [21 CFR 630.10(c)].

If individuals are instructed not to donate blood for others because of their health history, reactive test results, behavioral risks, or medical reasons, they must be added to a confidential deferral list at the blood center to prevent future donations [21 CFR 606.160(e)(1) and (2), and 630.10(d)(1)]. Depending on the causative reason, deferrals may be for a defined interval of time, for an indefinite period (for which there may be the possibility of reinstatement to the donor pool), or permanent with no potential for reinstatement as a blood donor in the future.[1] In addition, collection facilities are required to manage postdonation information that could affect the safety, purity, and potency of the blood components from the current donation and any previous donations, and affect the future eligibility of the donor.[2]

The criteria to evaluate individuals who are donating blood for their own use (autologous donation) may be less stringent than those for people who donate for use by others (allogeneic donation). However, the focus remains on providing the safest possible blood for transfusion to the donor-patient and on evaluating the risks that the collection procedure poses to his or her health.[3]

The AABB Donor History Questionnaire (DHQ) is currently used by most blood collection facilities in the United States.[4-7] The references in this chapter are to DHQ version 2.1, which at the time of writing was still under review by the FDA. The v2.1 DHQ incorporates the recommendations of the April 2020 FDA guidances for CJD, HIV, and malaria.[8-10] The April 2020 CJD guidance was issued as final, but those for HIV and malaria were implemented without prior public comment. The FDA intends to revise and replace the HIV and malaria guidances after considering feedback from the comment period. However, the agency expects that the recommendations set forth in the guidances will continue to apply.

A precautionary approach attempts to reduce the risk of known or potential RTTIs but also results in the deferral of many healthy donors. Medical directors of blood collection facilities are responsible for determining donor eligibility policies on issues that are not covered by regulations or standards.[3,11-14] Consequently, medical decisions regarding the same issue may differ among facilities or even among physicians at the same facility. Considerable variability exists in national and international practices for determining donor eligibility, which reveals the inherent uncertainty in risk assessment.[12] The facility's collection staff should be able to explain to donors the intended purpose of AABB and FDA requirements, as well as their center-specific eligibility screening practices.

Answers to the most frequently asked questions about federal regulations defining blood donor eligibility are available to the public in the "Questions about Blood" section of the FDA website.[15] Frequently asked questions about the interpretation or underlying rationale of AABB *Standards for Blood Banks and Transfusion Services (Standards)* can be found through the AABB Standards Portal,[16] or questions may be directed to the AABB Standards Department (standards@aabb.org); responses and discussion of selected issues are posted on the AABB website.

SELECTION OF ALLOGENEIC BLOOD DONORS

Registration and Donor Identification

In the United States, blood components for allogeneic transfusion are typically collected from volunteer, nonremunerated donors; otherwise, components must be labeled as being from paid donors [21 CFR 606.121(c)(8)(v)].

Prospective blood donors should provide an acceptable form of identification. Acceptable forms of identification include government-issued documents, such as a driver's license or passport, or a blood-center-issued donor card with a unique numeric or alphanumeric code, or other forms of identification as determined by the blood collection facility. Most facilities no longer use Social Security numbers for donor identification because of donor privacy concerns.

Accurate records are essential to identify all prior donations from any given donor, including whether the donor has ever given blood under a different name, so that the link with all prior donations within the blood system is maintained. Accurate records are also essential to ensure that the donor can be contacted following the donation and informed of test results or other relevant information from the current donation, if necessary. Facilities must make reasonable attempts to notify the donor within 8 weeks of the donation if any test results disqualify the individual from continued donation.[2] FDA regulations published in the CFR require facilities to ask donors to provide a postal address where they can be reached during this interval for counseling or other follow-up, if necessary [21 CFR 630.10(g)(1)]. Accurate donation records must be kept by the facility for the requisite amount of time, according to current regulations and standards [21 CFR 606.160; AABB Reference Standard 6.2A[1(pp73-75)]].

Individual blood collection facilities or systems must maintain a list of deferred donors, but, notably, there is currently no national registry of deferred blood donors in the United States. Individuals who are deferred by one blood center may be eligible in another blood system. The available evidence suggests that national deferral registries are not necessary or useful because they do not contribute to blood safety and do not prevent the release of unsuitable components.[17] In addition, national registries have raised privacy concerns.

Educational Materials and Donor Acknowledgment and Consent

US blood collection facilities provide all prospective blood donors with information about blood donation via educational materials, donor acknowledgment, and informed consent. The AABB DHQ Blood Donor Educational Material incorporates all necessary elements required by federal regulations and AABB *Standards*, and facilities may add elements to protect both blood donors and transfusion recipients.[1,2,4] At each encounter, the donor must be informed about the collection procedure in terms that the donor understands, and the donor's consent and/or acknowledgment must be documented. It must also be documented that the donor has read the educational material, has had an opportunity to ask questions, agrees not to donate if the donation could result in a risk to recipients as outlined in the educational material, and may withdraw from the donation procedure.[1] The setting used for the donor screening process should provide adequate privacy for donors to be comfortable discussing confidential information. The donor should be informed about possible adverse reactions to the collection procedure and the tests that will be performed for RTTIs on his or her donated blood. The donor must also be informed of the notification process for positive test results, any reporting requirements to public health authorities, and the possibility of inclusion in the facility's deferral registry and subsequent deferral from future donation. Donors should also be informed if investigational tests or other research may be performed on samples or information collected during the blood donation. Finally, the limitations of the tests to detect early infections and the possibility that a test may not be performed if samples are not adequate should be explained to the donor. The Blood Donor Educational Material instructs the donor not to donate blood for the purpose of receiving free infectious disease testing. Blood collection facilities must comply with applicable state laws to obtain permission from parents or guardians for minors (ie, 16- or 17-year-olds).[1] Moreover, AABB Standard 5.2.2 requires that blood collection facilities have a process to provide information about the donation process to parents or legally authorized representatives of donors when parental permission is required.[1(p16)]

Blood collection facilities should also establish policies on accommodating individuals who are not fluent in English or are illiterate, are vision or hearing impaired, or have other physical disabilities. Many facilities try to make reasonable accommodations for donors' special needs. However, facilities must also ensure that the collection procedure does not pose undue risk to donors or staff members, that an accurate health history can be obtained, and that the acknowledgment/consent process is not compromised. The final authority for decisions on such issues rests with the facility's medical director who is responsible for all aspects of donor qualification and phlebotomy.[1]

Donor Qualification by Focused Physical Examination and Hemoglobin or Hematocrit Measurement

Qualification screening procedures for blood donation include a focused physical examination and a hemoglobin or hematocrit measurement.[1,2] The donor eligibility regulations define not only the specific physical requirements but also the level of medical supervision required for the assessment (21 CFR 630.5; 21 CFR 630.10). This evaluation has potential implications for the potency or safety of the collected component and/or the well-being of the donor. Additional requirements apply to apheresis donors, who must meet the height, weight, and hemoglobin or hematocrit requirements approved by the FDA for the automated collection device. The collector must weigh the donor and not rely on self-reported weight for donation of any plasma product collected by apheresis.

The donor must have his or her blood pressure measured and is eligible to donate only if it falls within the range of 90 to 180 mm Hg for systolic and 50 to 100 mm Hg for diastolic pressures. If the measurement falls outside of these ranges, the donor must be deferred unless seen in person by a physician to assess the safety of performing a collection. For pulse, the rate must be between 50 and 100 beats per minute without irregularities in rhythm. A physician may approve donation for rates outside this range or irregularities in rhythm, using his or her judgment. This approval may be in person or by telephone. Approval for blood pressure or pulse outside the stated ranges cannot be delegated to a nonphysician nor defined by a standard operating procedure (SOP).

In general, neither the FDA nor AABB specifies the test method, specimen type [capillary (finger stick) or venous blood], or acceptable performance characteristics for tests used for hemoglobin/hematocrit screening. One exception is that a capillary sample collected from an earlobe puncture is not an acceptable specimen for hemoglobin/hematocrit screening for allogeneic or autologous donors because of its poor accuracy.[1] Most US blood collection facilities use finger stick samples for hemoglobin/hematocrit determination. These samples tend to give slightly higher values than venous samples.[18]

The methods to measure hemoglobin or hematocrit are generally selected for their ease of use in the mobile blood collection setting. The copper sulfate density method (Method 6-1) is still an acceptable screening tool in blood centers in the United States but has been largely replaced by methods such as spectrophotometric measurement of hemoglobin with portable devices or hematology analyzers to measure hematocrit. The point-of-care methods that use portable devices yield quantitative hemoglobin results, with a coefficient of variation (CV) of 1.3%.[19] A typical automated analyzer measures hemoglobin levels in a venous sample with a CV $\leq 1.2\%$.[19] Most quantitative methods currently in use reliably measure hemoglobin levels within approximately 0.2 to 0.5 g/dL, and the vast majority of donors deferred for hemoglobin or hematocrit have values near the cutoff. For capillary-sample-based methods, the most likely source of preanalytical error is the sampling technique, and testing must be performed in compliance with the manufacturer's instructions. A noninvasive measurement, not involving a blood sample but using measurements through the skin, has recently been approved.

Donor hemoglobin screening may help ensure a minimum content of hemoglobin in a unit of Red Blood Cells (RBCs), but currently neither the FDA nor AABB define potency standards for RBC units prepared from whole blood collection. If a donor's hemoglobin level is 12.5 g/dL, a 500-mL whole blood collection is expected to yield about 62.5 g of hemoglobin per unit of RBCs, but determining the final content of hemoglobin in an RBC unit prepared from whole blood is not required. AABB *Stan-*

dards requires apheresis RBC units to be prepared using a method known to ensure a final component containing a mean hemoglobin level of 60 g, with 95% of the units sampled containing >50 g of hemoglobin.[1(p27)]

As of May 2016, FDA regulations define the minimum acceptable hemoglobin concentration for male donors as 13.0 g/dL or the essentially equivalent hematocrit of 39% [21 CFR 630.10(f)(3)(i)(B)]. For females, the acceptable hemoglobin concentration is 12.5 g/dL or 38% hematocrit [21 CFR 630.10(f)(3)(i)(A)]. Hemoglobin or hematocrit screening may help prevent collection of blood from a donor with significant anemia, but it is clear that many donors do not have adequate iron stores even though they meet donor hemoglobin requirements.[20] This could have implications for the health of the donor as well as the potency of the collected component. If the organization wishes to collect blood from female donors with hemoglobin levels of 12.0 to 12.5 g/dL, or 36% to 38% hematocrit, they may do so if additional steps are followed to ensure that the health of the donor will not be adversely affected by the donation, in accordance with a procedure that has been found acceptable for this purpose by the FDA [21 CFR 630.10(f)(3)(i)(A)]. At the time of this writing, the procedures the FDA will approve to accept female donors with hemoglobin values of 12.0 to 12.5 g/dL are not clear. The strategies might involve extended intervals between donations, iron supplementation, and/or ferritin testing (using a predonation sample). Unfortunately, no point-of-care tests for assessing iron stores are available at this time.

Low hemoglobin/hematocrit is the most common reason for blood donor deferral at most donor centers. The various strategies to mitigate nonanemic iron deficiency in blood donors address the concern that has arisen about possible health effects of low iron, particularly among teens, females of childbearing potential, and frequent donors of either gender.[21-25] Both physical issues and impaired cognitive functions have been suggested in individuals with low iron stores, even in the absence of anemia.[26] Donors, particularly frequent donors, may develop iron-deficient erythropoiesis or advance to frank absence of iron stores.[23] Without iron supplementation, two-thirds of donors may not recover iron stores even after 168 days (24 weeks).[27] Recent studies have shown the benefit of iron supplementation in improving iron stores and hemoglobin in these donors. The amount of elemental iron found in an over-the-counter daily multivitamin is typically 19 mg; iron tablets available over the counter may contain 38 mg of elemental iron. Either can be an effective supplement for blood donors with adverse effects indistinguishable from placebo.[28] Another successful approach is to perform ferritin testing and to notify donors who have low levels, offering them the option of iron supplementation or delaying further donation.[23-28] Simple notification of donors of their low iron status was shown to be essentially as effective as providing iron supplements.[28] Various methods can be used to encourage iron replacement with blood donors, including providing iron tablets to the donor at the donation site, providing coupons for iron products, and/or informing donors of the need for supplemental iron. Low ferritin levels can also serve as the basis for an extended deferral from donations that include red cell components. Extended deferrals without providing information about ferritin or iron supplementation will not restore iron levels in a reasonable time. Donors with an abnormally low or high ferritin level should be referred to their health-care provider for evaluation, as appropriate.

Finally, before phlebotomy, the collection staff inspect the donor's antecubital skin to determine that it is free of lesions and evidence of injection drug use, such as multiple needle punctures (eg, small scars lined up in "tracks") and that the veins are adequate for donation. Scars or pitting on the forearm associated with frequent blood donation should not be mistaken for evidence of injection drug use. Common and mild skin disorders (eg, poison ivy rash) are not a cause for deferral unless there are signs of localized bacterial superinfection or the condition interferes with proper skin disinfection in the antecubital site before phlebotomy.

Health History Assessment—AABB DHQ

The AABB DHQ is now used by most blood centers in the United States. The DHQ includes the information required for compliance with both AABB *Standards* and the FDA. Its use is not mandated by the FDA,[6,7] but alternative procedures for collecting required information from blood donors must be submitted for FDA approval in a Prior Approval Supplement under 21 CFR 601.12(b) before implementation. In addition, the FDA acknowledges that the DHQ documents contain questions related to the following issues not addressed by any FDA regulations or recommendations: cancer; certain organ, tissue, or marrow transplants; and bone or skin grafts. However, AABB recommends that blood collection facilities implement the DHQ materials, including the following documents, as accepted by the FDA and in their entirety:

- Blood Donor Educational Material.
- Full-Length DHQ.
- User Brochure, including glossary and references.
- Medication Deferral List.

The use of the DHQ flowcharts as a resource is optional, and facilities may implement an equivalent method to evaluate responses to the DHQ. The current FDA-recognized DHQ and accompanying materials, Version 2.0, materials are available to the public on the AABB website.[6]

The wording, order, and text of the DHQ questions must not be changed because FDA has accepted the current DHQ as presented. The User Brochure for the DHQ details the purpose and limitations for the use of the DHQ and related materials. Changes to the DHQ questions, even minor, are not permitted. Once revised, the documents are no longer recognized by FDA as the accepted AABB documents. Facilities may choose to include additional questions as long as they are 1) in the designated area for additional questions at the end of the DHQ, and 2) more restrictive. The DHQ documents are intended to be self-administered by the donor, but facilities may choose to use direct oral questioning or a combination of both methods to administer the DHQ.

If AABB standards or FDA regulations do not address specific medical conditions that a blood collection facility has chosen to include in the DHQ, the facility must develop SOPs for determining the criteria for acceptance or deferral of a donor. A rational approach to donor health history assessment should attempt to balance the need to take appropriate precautions to protect the blood supply with avoiding unnecessarily restrictive policies that disqualify large segments of the population without contributing to either recipient or donor safety.[3] Decisions about donor eligibility should be based on available evidence regarding the risk that the medical condition or history poses to the blood donor and the transfusion recipient.

If a potential risk exists for the transfusion recipient or donor, the effectiveness and incremental benefit of screening donors by questioning should be evaluated, especially in light of other safeguards that protect the donor or other transfusion practices that mitigate potential risks to the recipient. If the facility receives postdonation information that should have been cause for deferral had it been reported at the time of donation, then any subsequent actions, such as product quarantine, retrieval, market withdrawal, or consignee notification, should be commensurate with the potential hazard and likelihood of possible harm to the recipient. The facility's approach to developing donor deferral criteria should take into account evidence as it becomes available to modify those decisions. Issues that allow for medical judgment and for which questions exist in the DHQ can be explored further with the donor, but each donor center must develop and follow its own procedures.[3]

ABBREVIATED DHQ FOR FREQUENT DONORS

Blood collection facilities have recognized for years that frequent and repeat donors, notably platelet and plasma donors, must answer the same questions at every donation about remote risk factors that are not likely to change—a situation that leaves many dedicated donors dissatisfied with the donation experience. An abbreviated questionnaire for frequent donors may improve their experience. The FDA allows the administration of AABB's abbreviated DHQ (aDHQ) for frequent donors who qualify by successfully completing the full-length DHQ on at least two separate occasions, with one or more donations within the past 6 months. The User Brochure for the aDHQ details the purpose and limitations on the use of the aDHQ. The AABB aDHQ, which was developed and validated by the Donor History Task Force (DHTF) along with the full-length DHQ, has been officially recognized in FDA guidance as "acceptable" and can be implemented by blood collection facilities using the corresponding full-length DHQ.[7] In the aDHQ, two "capture questions" about new diagnoses or treatments since the last donation replace 14 previous questions about remote risks (eg, blood transfusion and babesiosis).

In some cases, measures must be immediately taken to reduce risk from an emerging or re-emerging RTTI. Donor screening may play a particularly important role if testing is not available or used, or if the agent has not been shown to be reduced by available pathogen-inactivation measures. Donor information and/or education materials requesting self-deferral can be implemented quickly, asking prospective donors not to donate if, for example, they have traveled to certain regions where the RTTI is common or there is an outbreak. Donor screening questions may also be added to the end of the DHQ, assessing travel risks or exposure to others who may have been infected. The interval before such screening questions are implemented will vary with the length of time it takes to modify a blood collection facility's operational methods involved in donor screening. This may include its blood establishment computer system (BECS), SOPs, and staff training. It may be necessary to temporarily stop collections entirely in locations where the risk otherwise cannot be effectively managed. The FDA, other authorities, and/or AABB will provide guidance in emergency situations, to which blood collection facilities should remain alert and flexible to meet such emergencies. Depending on the situation, measures such as donor education information and

screening questions may become a permanent part of donor screening or may be discontinued as the risk recedes.

BLOOD-CENTER-DEFINED DONOR ELIGIBILITY CRITERIA

Unlike questions about potential risks to transfusion recipients, most selection criteria directed primarily at protecting donor safety are left to the discretion of the blood center's medical director. Consequently, practice varies at different blood centers.[3,12] AABB *Standards* requires that prospective donors appear to be in good health and be free of major organ disease (eg, diseases of the heart, liver, or lungs), cancer, or abnormal bleeding tendency, unless determined eligible by the medical director.[1(p64)] The rationale for each deferral for medical conditions should be carefully considered because even temporary deferrals adversely affect the likelihood that individuals will return to donate blood.[29]

Cancer

Each year in the United States, blood collection facilities receive hundreds of reports of cancer in individuals who had donated blood. Direct transmission of cancer through blood transfusion—although biologically plausible—has not yet been documented to occur even though people with cancer frequently donate blood before discovering their diagnosis.[30] A retrospective study examined the incidence of cancer among patients in Denmark and Sweden who received blood from donors with subclinical cancer at the time of donation. Of the 354,094 transfusion recipients, 12,012 (3%) were exposed to blood components from precancerous donors, yet there was no excess risk of cancer among these recipients compared with recipients of blood from donors without cancer.[31] A similar study indicated no risk for recipients of blood from donors who were later demonstrated to have chronic lymphocytic leukemia.[32] These data indicate that cancer transmission by blood collected from blood donors with incident cancer, if it occurs at all, is so rare that it could not be detected in a large cohort of transfusion recipients that included the total blood experience of two countries over several years.

In considering the future eligibility of donors with cancer, some degree of caution is warranted to allow sufficient time for donors to recover after chemotherapy or other treatment. There are currently no US federal regulations or professional standards regarding the criteria that should be used to evaluate donors with a history of cancer. For this reason, a blood center's medical director has considerable flexibility in determining donor eligibility policies.

Almost all licensed blood collection facilities currently accept donors who report localized cancers after treatment, with no deferral period. These cancers include skin cancer (eg, basal cell or superficial squamous cell carcinoma) and carcinoma in situ (eg, cervical) that have been fully excised and are considered cured. Most facilities defer individuals with a history of a solid organ or nonhematologic malignancy for a defined period after completion of treatment, provided that the donor remains symptom free without recurrence. The deferral period following completion of treatment for cancer ranges from 1 to 5 years.[31] Centers vary in approach to deferrals for donors with hematologic malignancies and invasive melanoma. These various deferral policies are currently defensible but should be reevaluated if new information becomes available about the potential for cancer transmission through blood transfusion.

Bleeding Conditions or Blood Diseases

Bleeding conditions and blood diseases have the potential to affect donor safety, as well as product potency, and blood collection facilities must define SOPs for handling donors with hematologic disorders. In general, prospective donors should be evaluated for bleeding conditions or blood diseases that 1) place the donors at risk of bleeding or thrombosis as a result of the collection procedure or 2) may affect the hemostatic efficacy of their blood and its suitability for transfusion to others.[3]

Plasma components and Cryoprecipitated Antihemophilic Factor should contain adequate amounts of functional coagulation factors and should not contain significant inhibitory or prothrombotic factors. Similarly, platelet components intended as the sole source for patients should contain platelets that have adequate function and are not irreversibly impaired by the presence of inhibitors.

Individuals with a history of a significant bleeding diathesis are usually counseled to avoid blood donation. However, screening donors for such a history does not prevent the rare but serious thrombotic or hemorrhagic complications in otherwise healthy blood donors. Individuals with hemophilia, clotting factor deficiencies, or clinically significant inhibitors—all of which are manifested by variable bleeding tendencies—require deferral for both donor safety and product potency considerations. The exception is Factor XII deficiency, which is not associated with either bleeding or thrombosis.

Carriers of autosomal-recessive or sex-linked recessive mutations in clotting factors usually are not at risk of bleeding. They typically have decreased factor levels but are accepted by most facilities because of the normal, wide variability in clotting factor activity levels (50% to 150%) compared to the much lower relative activity that is necessary to maintain hemostasis (5% to 30%).[3] Individuals with von Willebrand disease are typically deferred by most facilities, although some may allow individuals with mild disease and no history of bleeding to donate red cells. Antithrombotic medications are discussed below.

Heart and Lung Conditions

Cardiovascular disease is common in the United States, affecting an estimated 86 million (more than 1 in 3) adults.[33] Prospective blood donors are asked if they have ever had problems with their heart or lungs as a donor safety measure, but the criteria for accepting donors with a history of heart or lung disease are defined by each blood center.

The collective, published experience with autologous donation by patients scheduled for cardiac procedures has demonstrated that adverse effects are not more frequent than in donors without a history of cardiac disease.[34-38] Despite the relative frequency of cardiovascular disease in the adult population, vasovagal reactions occur in only about 2% to 5% of whole blood donations by healthy donors and are actually more likely to occur among young, healthy adolescents than older adults at greater risk for cardiac conditions.[39,40]

A rational approach to screening donors with a history of cardiac disease allows the acceptance of donors who are asymptomatic on the day of donation, have been medically evaluated, and report no functional impairment or limitations on daily activity after being diagnosed or treated for cardiac disease. Some donor centers advise individuals to wait at least 6 months after a cardiac event, procedure, or diagnosis. These centers then allow these individuals to donate if they have been asymptomatic and able to perform their usual daily activities during this interval. Indications for deferral may include recent symptoms, limitations on activity or functional impairment resulting from unstable angina, recent myocardial infarction, left main coronary disease, ongoing congestive heart failure, or severe aortic stenosis.[3]

Medications

The DHQ and Medication Deferral List contain the requirements for deferrals for specific medications as stipulated by the FDA and AABB. These requisite medication deferrals fall into five broad categories:

- Potent teratogens that pose potential harm to unborn children (although there have been no documented cases of adverse fetal outcomes related to transfusions from donors taking these medications).
- Antibiotics or antimicrobials to treat an infection that could be transmitted through blood transfusion (excluding preventive antibiotics for acne, rosacea, and other chronic conditions with a low risk of bacteremia).
- Anticoagulants and antiplatelet agents that affect component potency (plasma or platelet components only).

Although blood collection facilities may add medications whose use requires local donor deferral to the Medication Deferral List, many have chosen to use the Medication Deferral List as developed by AABB and reviewed by the FDA or have added only a few drugs. The DHTF has encouraged facilities to fully consider the reasons behind each local deferral and avoid unnecessary deferral practices.[3] The recent explosion in the number of drugs affecting platelet function or clotting, such as the direct Factor X inhibitors, which are increasingly used instead of warfarin, are often encountered as a cause for deferral [21 CFR 630.10(e); 21 CFR 640.21(b) and (c)].

FDA's older pregnancy-risk categories, which are designed to assess the benefit-vs-risk ratio if drugs are taken during pregnancy, are often inappropriately used for blood donor selection. For example, categories D and X include some commonly used drugs (eg, oral contraceptives and anticholesterol agents) that may be contraindicated in pregnancy but pose negligible, if any, risk to any transfusion recipient. In 2016, FDA eliminated the risk categories and introduced a new descriptive approach to prescription drug labeling for risk to pregnant or breastfeeding women, which may also make the inappropriate application to blood donor eligibility less of a problem.[41]

Local medication deferrals are often based on concerns about the reason for the potential donor's use of the medication and his or her underlying medical condition rather than on any inherent threat posed by residual medication in the collected blood component. Most drugs used by donors pose no harm to recipients, and many factors should be considered when evaluating the potential risk of a drug's use by a donor (eg, the medication's half-life, mean and peak plasma concentration, residual concentration in a blood component, and dilution when transfused to a recipient).

RECIPIENT-SPECIFIC "DESIGNATED" OR "DIRECTED" BLOOD DONATION

Exceptional Medical Need

In certain limited clinical circumstances, a recipient may benefit from blood components collected from a specific donor. Such a recipient might be a patient with multiple antibodies or with antibodies to high-prevalence antigens who requires units from donors whose red cells are negative for the corresponding antigens. Frequent donation by a specific donor for a specific patient with a medical need requires that the blood collection facility have a procedure that typically calls for both a request from the patient's physician and approval by the donor center's physician. The donor must meet all allogeneic donor selection requirements, with the exception of donation frequency, provided that he or she is examined and certified by a physician [21 CFR 630.15(a)(1)(ii)(B)]. In emergency medical situations, blood components can be released before test results for RTTIs are available provided that the units are labeled and managed in accordance with the CFR. Granulocyte components are generally released this way, as they expire in 24 hours. Testing on the units must be completed as soon as possible after release or shipment, and results must be promptly reported to the hospital or transfusion service.[2]

Directed Blood Donations

The use of directed donors, that is, when patients ask the blood center if they can designate their own blood donors (usually relatives or friends) for their anticipated transfusion needs, has decreased in recent years, but there is still ongoing demand. The concern likely reflects an inaccurate perception continuing among the general public of the risk for RTTIs associated with blood transfusion from the general inventory. Most facilities and hospitals accommodate the associated collection, storage, tracking, payment, and logistical difficulties to provide a directed donation service.

Directed donations have higher viral marker rates than volunteer donations, mostly but not entirely reflecting the higher prevalence of first-time donors among the former group.[42] There is no evidence that directed donations are safer to use than donations from volunteer community donors. On the contrary, some concerns persist that directed donors may feel unduly pressured to give blood, which could compromise blood safety. The confidentiality of directed donors

with positive test results may be difficult to maintain. Nevertheless, directed donations are sometimes sought by patients and their families, particularly for neonatal and other pediatric patients.

Directed donors must meet the same criteria as voluntary donors, and their blood can be used for other patients if not needed by the individual for whom the donations were initially intended. The facility should clearly communicate its directed-donation procedures so that the expectations regarding availability of directed-donor units are known to the hospital, ordering physician, and patient. The communication required includes defining the mandated interval between collection of the blood and its availability to the patient, mentioning the possibility that the patient will identify donors who are not ABO compatible or not otherwise acceptable blood donors, and defining the policy for release of donor-directed units for transfusion to other patients.

Autologous Blood Donations

Autologous donations have declined dramatically in the United States since the 1990s. Waning interest in autologous donations may reflect the decline in viral risk associated with allogeneic blood transfusion, the lower rate of surgical transfusion generally, and, consequently, the minimal medical benefit and increased cost of autologous blood.[43-45] The most appropriate candidates are alloimmunized donors for whom compatible blood is hard to collect, who are undergoing elective surgery for which transfusion will likely be required, and who have adequate time before the procedure to replace the hemoglobin lost via phlebotomy.

In general, the use of preoperative autologous blood donation alone provides only a relatively small benefit in reducing the probability of allogeneic transfusion and may actually increase the risk of lower postoperative hematocrits. Preoperative autologous donations may still be used in conjunction with other blood conservation methods, such as acute normovolemic hemodilution, perioperative blood recovery, and pharmacologic strategies (see further discussion in Chapter 20).

Patients identified as candidates for autologous donation are evaluated by the donor center as well as the referring physician. The following criteria for autologous donations are specified by the FDA, AABB, or both:

- A prescription or order from the patient's physician.
- Minimum hemoglobin concentration of 11 g/dL or hematocrit of 33%.
- Collection at least 72 hours before the anticipated surgery or transfusion.
- Absence of conditions presenting a risk of bacteremia.
- Use only for the donor-patient if labeled "autologous use only."

Contraindications to autologous blood donation should be defined by the blood center and may include medical conditions associated with the greatest risk from blood donation, such as 1) unstable angina, 2) recent myocardial infarction or cerebrovascular accident, 3) significant cardiac or pulmonary disease with ongoing symptoms but without an evaluation by the treating physician, or 4) untreated aortic stenosis.[45] Both the ordering physician and the donor center physician need to carefully balance the risks of the collection procedure against any perceived benefit to the patient-donor. The FDA has issued guidance on the process by which autologous donations may be collected, making it clear that rules for allogeneic donors may not necessarily be applied.[46]

KEY POINTS

1. The AABB DHQ and associated documents, including an abbreviated form for frequent donors, were developed by AABB's DHTF, and their use is recognized by the FDA as an adequate process to determine the eligibility of volunteers for allogeneic blood donation.
2. The current version of the DHQ and associated documents, Version 2.0, are available on the AABB website, and the May 2016 FDA guidance formally recognizing all DHQ documents is available on the FDA website.[6,7]
3. Prospective blood donors are informed of the risks of blood donation, clinical signs and symptoms associated with HIV infection, behavioral risk factors for transmission of RTTIs, and importance of refraining from blood donation if they are at increased risk of carrying an RTTI.
4. There are possible negative health effects of low iron levels (even in the absence of anemia) in donors who are in their teens, who are females of childbearing potential, or who are repeat donors (of either gender).
5. To be accepted for allogeneic blood donation, individuals must feel healthy and well on the day of donation and must meet all AABB and FDA requirements, as well as medical criteria defined by the blood collection facility.
6. The ongoing demand from patients to choose specific donors to provide blood for their transfusions during scheduled surgeries in the absence of a defined medical need has dramatically decreased in recent years but persists despite the lack of evidence of improved safety with directed donations.

REFERENCES

1. Gammon R, ed. Standards for blood banks and transfusion services. 32nd ed. Bethesda, MD: AABB, 2020.
2. Code of federal regulations. Title 21, CFR Parts 600 to 799. Washington, DC: US Government Publishing Office, 2019 (revised annually).
3. Eder AF, Goldman M, eds. Screening blood donors with the donor history questionnaire. Bethesda, MD: AABB Press, 2019.
4. Zou S, Eder AF, Musavi F, et al. ARCNET Study Group. Implementation of the uniform donor history questionnaire across the American

Red Cross Blood Services: Increased deferral among repeat presenters but no measurable impact on blood safety. Transfusion 2007;47:1990-8.

5. Fridey JL, Townsend M, Kessler D, Gregory K. A question of clarity: Redesigning the AABB blood donor history questionnaire—a chronology and model for donor screening. Transfus Med Rev 2007;21:181-204.

6. Blood donor history questionnaires. Version 2.0. Bethesda, MD: AABB, 2016. [Available at http://www.aabb.org/tm/questionnaires/Pages/dhqaabb.aspx (accessed August 24, 2018).]

7. Food and Drug Administration. Guidance for industry: Implementation of acceptable full-length and abbreviated donor history questionnaires and accompanying materials for use in screening donors of blood and blood components. (May 2016) Silver Spring, MD: CBER Office of Communication, Outreach, and Development, 2016. [Available at https://www.fda.gov/downloads/BiologicsBloodVaccines/GuidanceComplianceRegulatoryInformation/Guidances/Blood/UCM273685.pdf.]

8. Food and Drug Administration. Guidance for Industry: Revised recommendations to reduce the risk of transfusion-transmitted malaria. (April 2020) Silver Spring, MD: CBER Office of Communication, Outreach, and Development, 2020. [Available at https://www.fda.gov/regulatory-information/search-fda-guidance-documents/revised-recommendations-reduce-risk-transfusion-transmitted-malaria.]

9. Food and Drug Administration. Guidance for Industry: Revised recommendations to reduce the risk of human immunodeficiency virus transmission by blood and blood products. (April 2020) Silver Spring, MD: CBER Office of Communication, Outreach, and Development, 2020. [Available at https://www.fda.gov/regulatory-information/search-fda-guidance-documents/revised-recommendations-reducing-risk-human-immunodeficiency-virus-transmission-blood-and-blood.]

10. Food and Drug Administration. Guidance for Industry: Revised recommendations to reduce the risk of transmission of Creutzfeldt-Jakob disease and variant Creutzfeldt-Jakob disease by blood and blood components. (April 2020) Silver Spring, MD: CBER Office of Communication, Outreach, and Development, 2020. [Available at https://www.fda.gov/regulatory-information/search-fda-guidance-documents/recommendations-reduce-possible-risk-transmission-creutzfeldt-jakob-disease-and-variant-creutzfeldt.]

11. Eder AF. Evidence-based selection criteria to protect the blood donor. J Clin Apher 2010;25:331-7.

12. Eder AF, Goldman M, Rossmann S, et al. Selection criteria to protect the blood donor in North America and Europe: Past (dogma), present (evidence), and future (hemovigilance). Transfus Med Rev 2009;23:205-20.

13. Strauss RG. Rationale for medical director acceptance or rejection of allogeneic plateletpheresis donors with underlying medical disorders. J Clin Apher 2002;17:111-17.

14. Reik RA, Burch JW, Vassallo RR, Trainor L. Unique donor suitability issues. Vox Sang 2006;90:255-64.

15. Food and Drug Administration. Questions about blood. Silver Spring, MD: CBER Office of Communication, Outreach, and Development, 2016. [Available at https://www.fda.gov/vaccines-blood-biologics/blood-blood-products/questions-about-blood.]

16. Standards portal. Bethesda, MD: AABB, 2019. [Available at http://www.aabb.org/sa/Pages/Standards-Portal.aspx (accessed September 18, 2019).]

17. Cable R, Musavi F, Notari E, Zou S. ARCNET Research Group. Limited effectiveness of donor deferral registries for transfusion-transmitted disease markers. Transfusion 2008;48:34-42.

18. Cable RG, Steele WR, Melmed RS, et al for the NHLBI Retrovirus Epidemiology Donor Study-II (REDS-II). The difference between fingerstick and venous hemoglobin and hematocrit varies by sex and iron stores. Transfusion 2012;52:1031-40.

19. Cable RG. Hemoglobin determination in blood donors. Transfus Med Rev 1995;9:131-44.

20. Cable RG, Glynn SA, Kiss JE, et al, for the NHLBI Retrovirus Epidemiology Donor Study-II (REDS-II). Iron deficiency in blood donors: Analysis of enrollment data from the REDS-II Donor Iron Status Evaluation (RISE) study. Transfusion 2011;51:511-22.

21. Beutler E, Waalen J. The definition of anemia: What is the lower limit of normal of the blood hemoglobin concentration? Blood 2006;107:1747-50.

22. Simon TL, Garry PJ, Hooper EM. Iron stores in blood donors. JAMA 1981;245:2038-43.

23. Cable RG, Glynn SA, Kiss JE, et al. Iron deficiency in blood donors: The REDS-II Donor Iron Sta-

tus Evaluation (RISE) study. Transfusion 2012;
52:702-11.

24. Updated strategies to limit or prevent iron deficiency in blood donors. Association bulletin
#17-02. Bethesda, MD: AABB, 2017. [Available
at http://www.aabb.org/programs/publica
tions/bulletins/Docs/ab17-02.pdf#search=as
sociation%20bulletin%20iron (accessed August
24, 2018).]

25. Bialkowski W, Bryant BJ, Schlumpf KS, et al.
The strategies to reduce iron deficiency in blood
donors randomized trial: Design, enrollment
and early retention. Vox Sang 2015;108:178-
85.

26. Eder AF, Kiss JE. Adverse reactions and iron deficiency after blood donation. In: Simon TL, Mc-
Cullough J, Snyder EL, et al, eds. Rossi's principles of transfusion medicine. 5th ed. Chichester,
UK: John Wiley and Sons, 2016:43-57.

27. Kiss JE, Brambilla D, Glynn SA, et al, for the National Heart, Lung, and Blood Institute (NHLBI)
Recipient Epidemiology and Donor Evaluation
Study–III (REDS-III). Oral iron supplementation
after blood donation: A randomized clinical trial. JAMA 2015;313:575-83.

28. Mast AE, Bialkowski W, Bryant BJ, et al. A randomized, blinded, placebo-controlled trial of education and iron supplementation for mitigation
of iron deficiency in regular blood donors.
Transfusion 2016;56:1588-97.

29. Custer B, Schlumpf KS, Wright D, et al. NHLBI
Retrovirus Epidemiology Donor Study-II. Donor
return after temporary deferral. Transfusion
2011;51:1188-96.

30. Eder AF. Blood donors with a history of cancer.
In: Eder AF, Goldman M, eds. Screening blood
donors with the donor history questionnaire.
Bethesda, MD: AABB Press, 2019:63-78.

31. Edgren G, Hjalgrim H, Reilly M, et al. Risk of
cancer after blood transfusion from donors with
subclinical cancer: A retrospective cohort study.
Lancet 2007;369:1724-30.

32. Hjalgrim H, Rostgaard K, Vasan SK, et al. No evidence of transmission of chronic lymphocytic
leukemia through blood transfusion. Blood
2015;126:2059-61.

33. AHA Statistics Committee and Stroke Statistics
Subcommittee. Heart disease and stroke statistics—2016 update: A report from the American
Heart Association. Circulation 2016;133:e38-
360.

34. Kasper SM, Ellering J, Stachwitz P, et al. All adverse events in autologous blood donors with

cardiac disease are not necessarily caused by
blood donation. Transfusion 1998;38:669-73.

35. Mann M, Sacks HJ, Goldfinger D. Safety of autologous blood donation prior to elective surgery for a variety of potentially high risk patients. Transfusion 1983;23:229-32.

36. Klapper E, Pepkowitz SH, Czer L, et al. Confirmation of the safety of autologous blood
donation by patients awaiting heart or lung
transplantation: A controlled study using hemodynamic monitoring. J Thorac Cardiovasc Surg
1995;110:1594-9.

37. Dzik WH, Fleisher AG, Ciavarella D, et al. Safety and efficacy of autologous blood donation before elective aortic valve operation. Ann Thorac
Surg 1992;54:1177-80.

38. Popovsky MA, Whitaker B, Arnold NL. Severe
outcomes of allogeneic and autologous blood
donation: Frequency and characterization.
Transfusion 1995;35:734-7.

39. Eder AF, Dy BA, Kennedy J, et al. The American
Red Cross donor hemovigilance program: Com-
plications of blood donation reported in 2006.
Transfusion 2008;48:1809-19.

40. Wiltbank TB, Giordano GF, Kamel H, et al. Faint
and prefaint reactions in whole-blood donors:
An analysis of predonation measurements and
their predictive value. Transfusion 2008;48:
1799-808.

41. Food and Drug Administration. Content and format of labeling for human prescription drug and
biological products; requirements for pregnancy
and lactation labeling; final rule. Title 21, CFR
Part 201. (December 4, 2014) Fed Regist 2014;
79:72063-103. [Available at https://www.fed
eralregister.gov/documents/2014/12/04/
2014-28241/content-and-format-of-labeling-for-
human-prescription-drug-and-biological-prod
ucts-requirements-for.]

42. Dorsey KA, Moritz ED, Steele WR, et al. A comparison of human immunodeficiency virus,
hepatitis C virus, hepatitis B virus and human
T-lymphotropic virus marker rates for directed
versus volunteer blood donations to the American Red Cross during 2005 to 2010. Transfusion 2013;53:1250-6.

43. Brecher ME, Goodnough LT. The rise and fall of
preoperative autologous blood donation. Transfusion 2002;42:1618-22.

44. Schved JF. Preoperative autologous blood donation: A therapy that needs to be scientifically
evaluated. Transfus Clin Biol 2005;12:365-9.

45. Goodnough LT. Autologous blood donation. Anesthesiol Clin North Am 2005;23:263-70.

46. Food and Drug Administration. Guidance for industry: Determining donor eligibility for autologous donors of blood and blood components intended solely for autologous use—compliance policy. (August 2016) Silver Spring, MD: CBER Office of Communication, Outreach, and Development, 2016.

CHAPTER 6

Whole Blood and Apheresis Collection of Blood Components Intended for Transfusion

Jason Acker, MBA, PhD, and Anna Razatos, PhD

B LOOD HAS BEEN COLLECTED AND transfused for over 100 years.[1] This chapter describes current methods available for collecting, preparing, storing, and modifying blood components, specifically Red Blood Cells (RBCs), platelets, and plasma, for transfusion according to AABB and international standards. Detailed descriptions of the various blood components can be found in the *Circular of Information for the Use of Human Blood and Blood Components*.[2] Blood components can be manually separated in the laboratory from whole blood (WB) collected from blood donors. Recent technological advances have introduced automated methods to separate blood components from WB in the laboratory. Apheresis devices can also be used to separate and collect blood components directly from the donor and return the remaining portions. "Hemapheresis" or "apheresis" refers to automated blood component collection procedures and is derived from the Greek word "aphairos," meaning "to take from." Blood centers use a combination of WB collections and apheresis to meet transfusion demands.

DONOR PREPARATION AND CARE

Donor Consent

Potential donors must be provided with predonation education, counseling about the blood donation process, and an opportunity to have their questions answered before every blood donation. Per AABB *Standards for Blood Banks and Transfusion Services* (*Standards*) and the *Code of Federal Regulations* (CFR), blood centers are required to obtain donors' written acknowledgment of the following elements [AABB Standards 5.2-5.4 and Title 21 CFR, Part 630.10(g)][3,4(pp15-17)]:

- The donor has been provided and has reviewed information regarding the risks and hazards of the specific donation procedure.
- The donor has reviewed the educational material regarding relevant transfusion-transmitted infections.
- A sample of the donor's blood is tested for specified transfusion-transmitted pathogens.

Jason Acker, MBA, PhD, Senior Research Scientist, Canadian Blood Services, and Professor, Laboratory Medicine and Pathology, University of Alberta, Edmonton, Alberta, Canada; and Anna Razatos, PhD, Senior Medical Science Liaison, Terumo BCT, Lakewood, Colorado
The authors have disclosed no conflicts of interest.

- If the donation is determined to be unsuitable or if the donor is deferred from donation, the donor's record will identify the donor as ineligible to donate, and the donor will be notified of the basis for the deferral and the period of deferral.
- The donor has the opportunity to ask questions and withdraw from the donation procedure.

In addition, the CFR requires the blood center's responsible physician or appropriate designee to obtain donors' informed consent for plasmapheresis and plateletpheresis collections. The physician or appropriate designee should explain the risk of the procedure to the donor, provide an opportunity for the donor to ask questions, and give the donor a chance to refuse to donate. The informed consent process for plateletpheresis must be performed before the first donation and annually thereafter [21 CFR Parts 640.21(g) and 630.5]. Likewise, the informed consent process for plasmapheresis stipulates these requirements, and that the process be repeated if more than 6 months elapse between plasmapheresis collections (21 CFR 630.15).

Donor Eligibility and Identification

Phlebotomy must be performed only after the donor has been found to be eligible for blood donation. Identification of blood components and maintaining test results linked to the donor are critical to ensure recipient safety and to permit look-back investigations and product withdrawals if indicated. The blood component identification process uses both a bar-coded and an eye-readable unique donation identification number (DIN) that is assigned to the donation record, donor history questionnaire, each sample tube, and each component prepared from the donation. Electronic records of the donation are assigned the same number. The DIN should be verified on the donation record, collection primary and secondary containers, and sample tubes before the blood collection can proceed. A final check of appropriate labeling before phlebotomy helps to ensure that the donor history data, laboratory data, and other manufacturing data are associated with the correct DIN and blood components.

Vein Selection and Disinfection Methods for the Venipuncture Site

The phlebotomist inspects both arms of the donor to select a prominent, large, firm vein in the antecubital fossa to permit a single, readily accessible phlebotomy site that is devoid of scarring or skin lesions.

Specific instructions in the package insert for the use of approved agents should be followed for phlebotomy site disinfection. These methods provide surgical cleanliness, but none of the methods can achieve an absolutely aseptic site. Approximately 50% of donors had no bacterial colonies in studies using a contact plate culture of the venipuncture site after disinfection with povidone iodine or isopropyl alcohol plus iodine tincture, whereas the remaining donors had low colony numbers (1 to 100).[5] Rarely (1%) did donors have more than 100 colonies after arm disinfection.[5] Bacteria residing deep within skin layers are not accessible to disinfectants and may contribute to product contamination. In one study, pigskin epidermal cells were detectable in the lavage fluid in 1 out of 150 punctures.[6] Diversion of at least the first 10 milliliters of blood into a special diversion pouch can capture skin debris and has been shown to reduce the proportion of platelet components containing viable bacteria.[4(p22),7-9] Blood in this pouch can be used for laboratory testing.

Donor Care after Phlebotomy

Immediately after collection, the needle is withdrawn into a protective sleeve to prevent accidental injuries. Local pressure is applied by hand to the gauze placed directly over the venipuncture site while the donor's arm is kept elevated. Pressure is applied until hemostasis is achieved and a bandage or tape may be applied.

AABB Standard 5.3.3 requires blood centers to provide donors with written instructions about care after donation.[4(p17)] Postphlebotomy care includes observing the donor for signs or symptoms of reactions. If donors tolerate a sitting position without problems, they may proceed to a recovery area and should be encouraged to drink fluids and have light snacks and remain in the recovery area for about 15 minutes or until they feel comfortable to leave. In addition, blood centers may encourage the donor to drink more fluid and refrain from heavy lifting or vigorous exercise or activities that might put the donor or others at risk for several hours after blood donation. The donor is also instructed to apply local pressure to the phlebotomy site if any bleeding recurs and to call the blood center if the bleeding does not stop with pressure. Appropriate contact information is provided so that the donor can report if he or she feels that the donated unit should not be used, has any reactions, or experiences any signs or symptoms of infection.

Adverse Donor Reactions

Adverse reactions can occur at the time of donation or after the donor has left the blood center. In a comprehensive donor hemovigilance program reported by the American Red Cross, adverse reactions were reported for WB collections (349 in 10,000), plateletpheresis (578 in 10,000), and double RBC unit collections (538 in 10,000), the vast majority of which were minor presyncopal reactions and small hematomas.[10] Serious adverse reactions were slightly more common for WB collections (7.4 in 10,000) compared with plateletpheresis (5.2 in 10,000) and double RBC unit collections (3.3 in 10,000).[10] Reactions that needed medical care after the donor left the donation site occurred in roughly 3 in 10,000 donations.[11] A population-based European study found the rate of complications leading to long-term morbidity or disablement to be 0.5 in 10,000 donations and 0.23 in 10,000, respectively.[12] All adverse reactions occurring during collection procedures must be documented along with the results of thorough investigations.

Needle-Related Injuries

Bruise or Hematoma. Bruises are the most common adverse event after phlebotomy, occurring in 23% of donors based on postdonation interviews.[11] Hematomas, defined as the accumulation of blood under the skin, are less common

than bruises, occurring in 1.7% of donors.[11] Bruises and minor hematomas (less than 2 by 2 inches) generally do not prevent donors from donating again.[11]

Local Nerve Injury. Phlebotomy-related nerve injuries are relatively uncommon but still inevitably occur even with good phlebotomy technique because of anatomic variation and the close association of nerves with veins. Donors may complain of sensory changes away from the phlebotomy site, such as in the forearm, wrist, hand, upper arm, or shoulder. These injuries are usually transient, followed by full recovery.[11] However, in 7% of injured donors, recovery may take 3 to 9 months.[11] In severe cases, referral to a neurologist may be indicated.

Arterial Puncture. Arterial puncture is a rare event occurring in less than 1 in 10,000 donations.[11] Presence of bright red blood, rapid collection (within 4 minutes), and a pulsating needle suggest arterial puncture, although not all signs might be present.[11] Hematomas are more likely to occur with arterial punctures. When puncture is recognized early, the needle should be pulled out immediately, and local pressure should be applied for an extended period. Most donors recover quickly, but some might present with waxing and waning hematomas, a mass that should be evaluated, or a pseudoaneurysm.

Systemic Reactions

Vasovagal Reactions. Vasovagal reactions (also referred to as pre-faint or presyncope) include dizziness, sweating, nausea, vomiting, weakness, apprehension, pallor, hypotension, and bradycardia.[11] The reaction might progress to syncope (loss of consciousness); convulsions and loss of bladder and bowel function might also occur. Syncope can also result from orthostatic blood pressure changes after donation. Vasovagal reactions are distinguished by a low pulse rate, whereas reactions related to volume depletion are associated with an increased pulse rate. This difference, however, has no practical value, as both mechanisms are treated similarly. In case of vasovagal reaction, phlebotomy should be stopped, and the donor should be placed in a recumbent position. Applying cold wet towels to the donor's neck and shoulders and loosening the donor's clothes can assist in symptom management. Some donors with severe reactions or with prolonged recovery times may need short-term observation or intravenous fluid administration in an emergency room. Telephone follow-up for donors who have experienced severe reactions is helpful to assess the donors for any residual symptoms. Donor reactions after WB donation do not accurately predict the possibility of recurrent syncope in returning donors, although they reduce the likelihood of future donations.[13]

Most reactions occur at the collection site, either in the donation chair or the recovery area.[14] The main predictors of immediate and delayed vasovagal and presyncopal reactions are young age, low estimated blood volume (<3.5 L), fear, and first-time donation status.[14-17] In donors experiencing a reaction, loss of consciousness is most concerning as it can lead to injury, especially if the donor has left the donation site.[14] Blood Systems, Inc, reported a rate of syncope during and after phlebotomy as 27 per 10,000 WB donations, with an associated injury rate of 1.3 per 10,000 WB donations.[14] Approximately 10% of loss of consciousness reactions occur after the donor leaves the donation site.[14] Deferral strategies for young donors with estimated low blood volume and physiologic strategies to minimize donor reactions are aimed at improving donor safety.[15,18] Donor education, environmental controls, instructions to donors to drink fluid before and after donation, distraction, and muscle tension have been identified as strategies to reduce reactions in young donors.[18,19] Deferral of low-blood-volume (less than 3.5 L) donors may be helpful in reducing the risk of reactions, especially in young donors.

Citrate Reactions. During apheresis, blood that is anticoagulated with citrate in the apheresis systems is returned to the donor at an acceptable rate.[20] In healthy individuals, citrate is rapidly metabolized, but some donors can experience mild citrate reactions (paresthesias or tingling sensations).[20] Oral calcium supplementation is advised for symptomatic management of hypocalcemia.[20]

Fatalities Due to Blood Donation

The Food and Drug Administration (FDA) requires blood establishments to report deaths associated with blood donation. According to the FDA, in 2015, allogeneic blood donations accounted for 12.0 million WB-derived and apheresis RBC components, 2.4 million platelet components, and 3.7 million plasma components, whereas in 2016, there were 38.3 million source plasma donations.[21] Fatalities associated with blood donation are extremely rare. Over the 5-year reporting period of 2013 to 2017, there were 47 reported donation-associated fatalities, with seven cases since 2014 having an imputability of definite/certain, probable/likely, or possible.[21]

Therapeutic Phlebotomy

Therapeutic phlebotomy is a treatment for blood disorders, such as hemochromatosis, polycythemia vera and other conditions associated with erythrocytosis such as testosterone supplementation,[22] and certain porphyrias, in which the removal of red cells or reduction of iron stores is an effective method for managing the disease.[23,24] The CFR [21 CFR 630.15(a)(2)] and AABB Standard 5.6.7.1 specify that units collected as therapeutic phlebotomies can be used for allogeneic transfusion when the individual donor meets other allogeneic blood donor criteria.[4(p24)] Generally, units from therapeutic donors intended for allogeneic transfusion must be labeled with the disease or condition requiring therapeutic phlebotomy. However, allogeneic blood donation is accepted, for example from individuals with hereditary hemochromatosis or individuals with erythrocytosis from testosterone therapy, if the FDA has approved an "exception or alternative procedure" under 21 CFR 640.120. Such variances can waive both the labeling requirement and limitations on the frequency of donation.

Treatment by phlebotomy primarily consists of donating 500 mL of WB, although donation of RBCs by apheresis can also be considered.[25] Several studies have demonstrated that blood collected from stable or uncomplicated hemochromatosis patients is safe for transfusion in terms of transfusion-transmitted infections.[26-28]

Hemochromatosis is a genetic disorder characterized by absorption of excess iron that can accumulate in tissues and organs, potentially resulting in toxicity and organ damage.[24,29] Treatment of hemochromatosis by regular phlebotomy involves an iron depletion phase to lower serum ferritin concentration to an acceptable level, followed by a maintenance phase to keep serum ferritin levels low.[29,30] In polycythemia vera and other conditions associated with erythrocytosis, phlebotomy is used to reduce the risk of venous thromboembolism that is associated with hyperviscosity. The frequency required is titrated to the hematocrit of the patient, attempting to maintain levels ≤52% and ≤48% in males and females, respectively.[31]

BLOOD COLLECTION

Whole Blood Collection

AABB Reference Standard 5.4.1A permits collection of 10.5 mL of blood per kilogram of the donor's weight for each donation, including the blood unit and all samples for testing.[4(pp62-69)] In North America and Europe, the volume of WB collected during routine phlebotomy is typically either 450 ± 10% (405-495 mL) or 500 mL ± 10% (450-550 mL). The volume may be different in other regions and may be as low as 200 to 250 mL. For general blood banking applications, the volume of WB collected can be determined from the net weight in grams collected divided by the density of WB (1.053 g/mL).[32] Donors in the United States must weigh a minimum of 50 kg (110 lb) with a minimum hemoglobin (or hematocrit) of 12.5 g/dL (38%) for women and 13.0 g/dL (39%) for men (AABB Standard 5.4.1A).[4(pp62-69)] The CFR allows blood collection from females with hemoglobin (or hematocrit) of 12.0 to 12.5 g/dL (36-38%), provided blood centers take additional steps to ensure that the health of the donor is not adversely affected [21 CFR 630.10(f)(3)(i)(A)]. Donor qualification criteria vary around the world depending on local regulatory requirements.

Collection volumes must be within the manufacturer's specified range to ensure the correct anticoagulant-to-WB ratio. Volumes exceeding the manufacturer's specifications for allogeneic collections should be discarded. Low-volume allogeneic collections should be relabeled as "RBCs Low Volume." WB-derived RBCs that are labeled as low-volume units are made available for transfusion when 300 to 404 mL of WB is collected into an anticoagulant volume calculated for 450 ± 45 mL, or when 333 to 449 mL of WB is collected into an anticoagulant volume calculated for 500 ± 50 mL (AABB Standard 5.7.4.7).[4(p27)] Evidence indicates that the volume in undercollected and overcollected units (275-600 g) does not affect in-vivo red cell recovery even after 21 to 35 days of storage.[33,34] Plasma and platelets from low-volume units should be discarded.

The average time to collect 500 mL of WB is less than 10 minutes. A draw time longer than 15 to 20 minutes may not be suitable for collecting platelets or plasma for transfusions, as determined by blood center policy. The collection bag should be periodically mixed during the collection to ensure uniform distribution of anticoagulant.

WB is collected into sterile, plastic bags containing anticoagulant. Bags are typically plasticized polyvinyl chloride (PVC).[35] Typical anticoagulants would include citrate-phosphate-dextrose (CPD), citrate-phosphate-dextrose-dextrose (CP2D), or citrate-phosphate-dextrose-adenine (CPDA-1). WB in acid-citrate-dextrose (ACD), CPD, or CP2D has an expiration date of 21 days when stored at 1 to 6 C; the maximum storage time for units in CPDA-1 is 35 days (AABB Reference Standard 5.1.8A).[4(pp52-61)]

Blood bags should list an expiry date and include label data required by regulatory authorities. Sterile collection systems can contain integrally attached tubing to allow aseptic fluid transfer to satellite containers for component preparation, as well as integral access ports for open connection of infusion sets or other spiked entry. Open spiked access reduces the expiration from the time of entry to reduce the risk of bacterial sepsis. Innovations in WB collection include scales for monitoring the collection volume with automatic mixing and devices to add anticoagulant at a fixed ratio as the blood is withdrawn from the vein.

The acceptable temperature during short-term storage, transport, and handling of WB immediately after collection is determined by processing requirements for component preparation. In some cases, this may mean that collections at mobile blood drives or fixed collection sites should be transported as soon as possible to the central component preparation laboratory. With other processing methods, transportation may not be as urgent. Requirements for cooling and transportation methods are quite variable, and the specifications of the appropriate device manufacturer should be carefully followed. WB destined for platelet preparation should not be cooled to less than 20 C. In the United States, platelets must be separated from WB within 8 hours of collection (AABB Reference Standard 5.1.8A).[4(pp52-61)] It can take 10-16 hours from time of collection for a unit of blood to reach 20 C when packed in a crate at 20-24 C.[36] To cool blood more rapidly, units are typically placed in specific storage environments, or some centers use cooling plates that provide rate-controlled cooling toward 20 C. These cooling plates contain 1,4-butanediol, which has a melting temperature of 20 C and serves as a heat absorber. With the cooling plates, about 2 hours are needed for the collected blood to reach 20 C.[36] WB that will not be used to prepare platelets should be cooled to refrigerator temperature as soon as possible; this is often accomplished by placing the unit on wet ice or other appropriate cooling media.

Tests for ABO group, Rh type, unexpected alloantibodies, and transfusion-transmitted infections are performed. Each collection must be tested unless the donor is undergoing repeated procedures to support a specific patient—for example, for some apheresis procedures, testing for infectious disease markers may be required only at 30-day intervals [21 CFR 610.40(c)].

Component Preparation Methods from Whole Blood

Blood collection and component separation systems may be designed in different configurations depending on the needs of the blood manufacturer (Fig 6-1).[37] Satellite bags and integrally attached tubing that are hermetically sealed allow component manufacturing to take place in a closed system. The blood container should not be entered before issue except for the purposes of sample collection, postcollection processing, or transfer of components to a different container. Components prepared with an open system require a reduction in their expiration time from the time that the system was opened to reduce the risk of bacterial contamination. The expiration period of an open system is 24 hours for RBCs stored at 1 to 6 C; 4 hours for WB, RBCs, and platelets held at room temperature; or 4 hours for thawed cryoprecipitate and plasma (AABB Reference Standard 5.1.8A).[4(pp52-61)] The use of approved sterile connection devices maintains a functionally closed system when various connections are performed, such as pooling or sampling, thereby maintaining the component's original expiry date (AABB Standard 5.7.2).[4(p24)]

All current methods for separation and preparation of the three major blood components—RBCs, platelets, and plasma—rely on one or more centrifugation and expression steps. Centrifuges and both manual and automated expression devices should be properly validated, maintained, and calibrated, or checked in a systematic manner to verify the processing conditions (AABB Standard 3.5.1).[4(p5)]

Following separation by centrifugation, components must be carefully divided into separate containers for further processing. Many laboratories use manual extractors for this purpose, in which case the component laboratory staff identifies when the red cell interface approaches the tubing and stops expression using a hemostat. Blood component extractors are available for automating the separation of WB components by detecting the component interfaces and automatically stopping the extraction process. After primary centrifugation, WB is placed in the extractor, and a pressure plate creates an outflow of components from the container. Outflow can occur from the top and/or bottom of the container, depending on the method of manufacturing that is used at the blood center.

Component processing methods from WB are typically defined based on the method used to separate the platelets from the WB.[37,38] For preparation of platelets from WB, two primary methods are available: preparation from platelet-

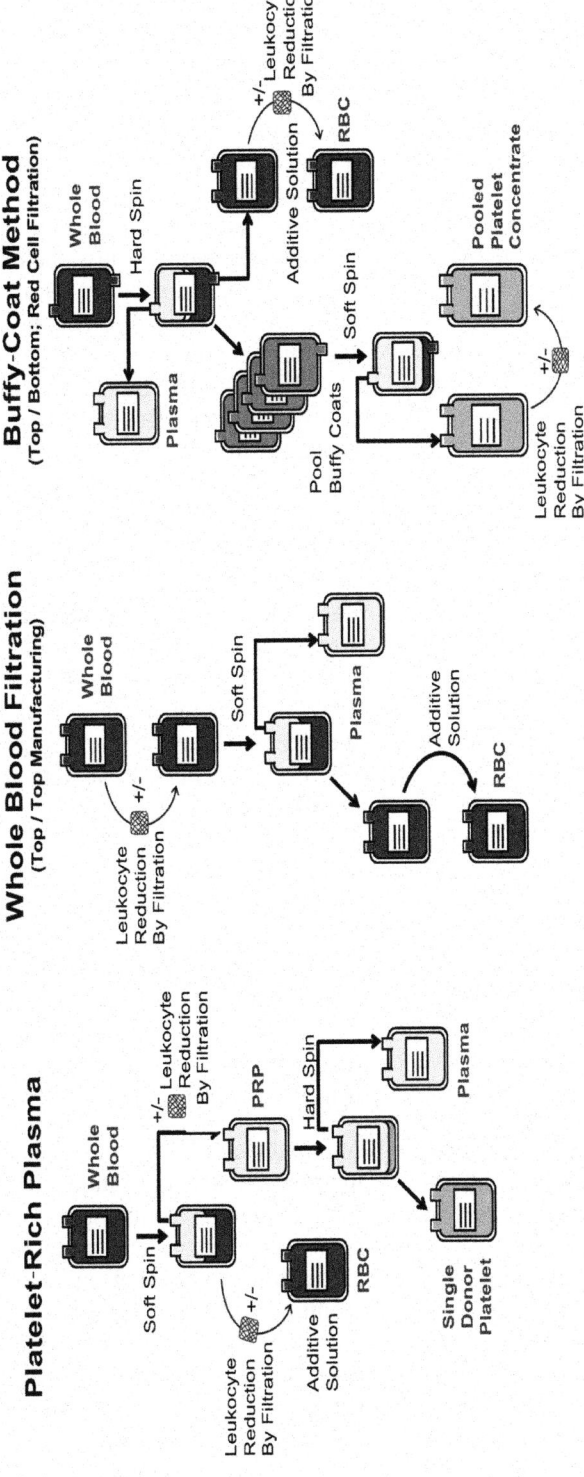

FIGURE 6-1. Representative schematic of the various methods used to produce red cell, platelet, and plasma components from whole blood.

rich plasma (PRP) or preparation from a buffy coat. Both methods involve centrifugation, and parameters must be tailored for the blood bag system and the method of platelet preparation to ensure that safe, high-quality products are produced.

Platelet-Rich Plasma Manufacturing Method. Preparation of components from PRP begins with a "soft spin" of the WB to separate red cells from the PRP and is followed by expression and hard spin of the PRP to concentrate platelets. This is done either manually, using semiautomated extractors, or with fully automated systems. Plasma for further processing is removed from the platelet pellet, which is held undisturbed for 0.5 to 2 hours before being resuspended in the residual plasma.[37,39] The red cell concentrate from the PRP method can be further leukocyte-reduced by inline filtration and stored in an approved red cell additive solution.

Single whole-blood-derived platelet units prepared using the PRP must contain $\geq 5.5 \times 10^{10}$ platelets in 90% of units sampled, must have a pH ≥ 6.2 (AABB Standard 5.7.4.20) at outdate,[4(p29)] and are usually suspended in 40 to 70 mL of plasma. Studies have shown acceptable recovery and survival rates when platelets are stored in plasma volumes of 35 to 40 mL.[40,41] Four to 6 units of platelets are typically pooled to create one therapeutic dose, which is labeled and stored in plasma in an approved container. Pools must be transfused within 4 hours (AABB Reference Standard 5.1.8A).[4(pp52-61)] Platelets prepared by the PRP method can be filtered to reduce leukocytes as single PRP units or as a pooled platelet concentrate using a leukocyte reduction filter. Leukocyte-reduced pooled platelets must have a residual leukocyte count of $<5 \times 10^6$ per transfusable dose in the United States or $<1 \times 10^6$ in Canada and Europe, as well as a pH of ≥ 6.2 at the end of storage (AABB Standard 5.7.4.20).[4(p30)]

Buffy-Coat Manufacturing Method. The buffy-coat method is employed in many countries but is not approved for use in the United States. In short, non-leukocyte-reduced WB units are first centrifuged under a high g-force (ie, hard or heavy spin), and plasma, red cells, and buffy coats are separated for further processing. Individual buffy coats from 4 or 5 units are

pooled with 1 unit of plasma and then centrifuged under a low g-force (ie, soft or light spin) to separate the platelet concentrate for additional processing, such as leukocyte reduction. These processes are often associated with extended holding of the WB and buffy coats for 8 to 24 hours at 20 to 24 C.[42,43] Hold times are generally adjusted to ease the operational logistics for the blood center. Compared to the PRP preparation method, the buffy-coat method yields more plasma, greater red cell loss, better initial white blood cell reduction before filtration, and moderate reduction in viable bacteria in the platelets that interact with leukocytes.[39,44]

Whole-Blood Filtration Manufacturing Method. When platelet components cannot be produced from a WB unit due to logistical reasons or product demand, the WB unit may be cooled to 1 to 6 C within 8 hours of collection and subsequently processed into red cell and plasma components. Leukocyte reduction by filtration of the anticoagulated WB can be performed before centrifugation, followed by manual or semiautomated separation of the red cell and plasma components. Methods to separate the red cells from the plasma should result in an RBC component with a hematocrit of $\leq 80\%$ (AABB Standard 5.7.4.1.1).[4(p26)] Additive solutions may be used to extend the storage of the RBCs. Prestorage leukocyte reduction by filtration of WB using platelet-sparing filters has been used to produce leukocyte-reduced RBC, platelet, and plasma components that meet FDA criteria for product quality.[45]

Automated Production of Components from Whole Blood

Automated production of blood components can improve the standardization of components. Automated devices control the rate of extraction, detect an interface with an optical sensing device, provide clamping and sealing of tubing, monitor component weights, add storage solutions, and perform other useful functions that assist in the consistent preparation of blood components. Some systems combine all of these functions, including centrifugation, without relying on operator interventions. These fully automated systems for the preparation of RBCs and plasma and platelet concentrates from WB are used in Europe and other international sites and was recently approved for use in the United States. The quality of RBC, platelet, and plasma components produced using automated production systems have been shown to meet quality specifications.[46-48]

Apheresis Collection of Blood Components

Apheresis devices are continuous systems that remove blood from a donor, separate the blood into the desired components, and return the remaining blood back to the donor. Apheresis allows for the concurrent collection of RBCs, platelets, and plasma from a single donor, depending on the regulatory approval of each individual device. The type or combination of components that can be collected by an apheresis device from a single donor is dependent on donor characteristics such as height, weight, sex, platelet count, and hematocrit or hemoglobin. Apheresis devices employ software algorithms that determine donor eligibility while maintaining donor safety.

The collection of components by apheresis follows many of the same rules and standards that apply to WB donation. Anticoagulants approved for use with apheresis devices include ACD formula A (ACD-A) or ACD formula B (ACD-B). Although the apheresis collection and preparation processes differ from WB-derived components, the storage and transportation requirements and several quality-control steps are the same for both processes.

Red Cell Apheresis

Roughly 15% of RBCs in the United States are collected by apheresis vs WB.[49] RBCs collected by apheresis contain at least 60 g of hemoglobin or 180 mL red cell volume per unit (AABB Standard 5.7.4.8).[4(p27)] Apheresis devices are approved to collect RBCs in the following combinations[50]:

- Single RBC unit.
- Single RBC unit in combination with platelets and/or plasma.
- Double RBC units only.

Similar to WB, RBCs collected by apheresis can be stored in additive solutions to extend the shelf life of the components. Storage solutions can be added manually or by the apheresis device after RBC collection.

Platelet Apheresis

In the United States, the use of apheresis platelets has been steadily increasing over the past 25 years. It is estimated that 92% of platelets transfused in the United States are apheresis platelets.[49] Apheresis devices are designed to collect single, double, or triple units of platelets from individual donors depending on donor characteristics. Apheresis platelets can be collected concurrently with single RBC units and/or plasma.

AABB Standard 5.7.4.21 requires that platelets collected by apheresis contain at least 3×10^{11} platelets in 90% of units tested.[4(p30)] Units containing less than 3.0×10^{11} platelets should be labeled with the actual platelet count.[51]

Apheresis platelet donors may donate more frequently than WB donors but must meet all other criteria for WB donation. The interval between donations should be at least 2 days, and donors should not undergo plateletpheresis more than twice in a week or 24 times in a rolling 12-month period (AABB Standard 5.5.3.1).[4(p20)] If a unit of WB is collected or if it becomes impossible to return the donor's red cells during plateletpheresis, at least 8 weeks should elapse before a subsequent plateletpheresis procedure unless the red cell extracorporeal volume is less than 100 mL (AABB Standard 5.5.3.2).[4(p20)] Platelets may be collected more frequently from donors if there is exceptional medical need for a specific recipient and the blood center's responsible physician determines that the health of the donor will not be adversely affected by the collection. Donors who have taken antiplatelet medications that irreversibly inhibit platelet function are deferred for specific intervals before donation (48 hours for aspirin/ aspirin-containing medications and piroxicam; 14 days for clopidogrel and ticlopidine) because apheresis platelets are often the sole source of platelets given to a patient (AABB Standard 5.4.1A).[4(pp62-69)]

AABB Standard 5.5.3.4 permits qualification of a donor with a platelet count from a sample collected immediately before the procedure or one obtained either before or after the previous procedure.[4(p21)] Triple collections from first-time donors require a qualifying platelet count from a sample collected before the donation (AABB Standard 5.5.3.4.1).[4(p21)] Exceptions to these laboratory criteria should be approved in writing by the apheresis program physician based on documented medical need. For apheresis collections, FDA guidelines require a periodic review of donor records to monitor platelet counts.[51]

Apheresis devices are capable of collecting platelets in less plasma volume, in a volume-reduced or hyperconcentrated state. Hyperconcentrated platelets must be diluted with platelet additive solution (PAS) to support storage up to either 5 or 7 days depending on local regulatory approvals.[52-54]

Plasma Apheresis

Plasma collected by apheresis represents 12% of plasma intended for transfusion in the United States.[49] Apheresis devices can collect plasma alone or in combination with single RBC units and/or platelets. The total volume of plasma collected is based on the physical characteristics of donors and limited by the labeling of the apheresis devices. Plasma collected by apheresis devices is typically leukocyte reduced.

A distinction is made between infrequent plasmapheresis, in which the donor undergoes plasmapheresis no more frequently than once every 4 weeks, and serial plasmapheresis or source plasma collection. The latter is the process to collect plasma for fractionation into plasma derivatives, in which the donation is more frequent than once every 4 weeks. For donors in infrequent plasmapheresis programs, donor selection and monitoring requirements are the same as those for WB donation.

Apheresis Devices

The Trima Accel System (Terumo BCT)

The Trima Accel Automated Blood Collection System (Trima Accel) is a continuous-flow, single-stage system that uses centrifugal force to separate blood into components while the donor is connected to the device. The Trima Accel system consists of the device, software, and sterile, single-use, disposable tubing sets with integrated blood storage bags. WB is drawn from the donor and mixed with anticoagulant in the disposable tubing set. The Trima Accel is cleared for use with the anticoagulant ACD-A. The blood and anticoagulant are pumped into the separation channel, which is spun in the centrifuge to separate the blood into its components. Blood that is not collected is returned to the donor during the procedure. Plasma is leukocyte reduced in the separation channel. Platelets and WBCs flow out of the separation channel and into the leukocyte reduction system chamber, which separates the platelets from the white cells based on size; leukocyte-reduced platelets flow out of the chamber into the final platelet storage bag. The Trima Accel system can leukocyte-reduce red cells via in-line filtration as well as automate the addition of the appropriate volume of RBC storage solution, or these steps can be completed manually after the collection. The Trima Accel is cleared for use with the red cell storage solution AS-3 in the United States, and SAGM (saline, adenine, glucose, and mannitol) in Europe. It can also collect plasma-reduced platelets concentrates with automated addition of the appropriate volume of PAS.

The Trima Accel system can be used to collect the following components alone or in combination depending on donor size, sex, platelet count, and hematocrit:

- Single, double, or triple units of platelets stored in plasma or PAS.
- Plasma that can be prepared into Fresh Frozen Plasma (FFP), Plasma Frozen Within 24 Hours After Phlebotomy (PF24), and Plasma Frozen Within 24 Hours After Phlebotomy Held At Room Temperature Up To 24 Hours After Phlebotomy (PF24RT24).
- Single or double units of leukocyte-reduced RBCs stored in RBC storage solution.
- Single or double units of RBCs stored in RBC storage solution.

In the United States, the Trima Accel Extended Life Platelet (ELP) storage bag is cleared to store leukocyte-reduced platelets in 100% plasma for up to 7 days and in PAS up to 5 days. Platelet storage duration outside of the United States is dependent on local regulations and/or regulatory approvals.

The Amicus Separator System (Fresenius Kabi)

The Amicus Separator System is an automated blood cell separator intended for the collection of blood components and mononuclear cells. The separator can be configured to collect red cells and plasma concurrently with platelets. The Amicus Separator System is composed of the Amicus separator instrument and a disposable apheresis kit specific to the procedure being performed. The instrument is a continuous-flow, centrifugal device that draws WB from a donor, separates the blood into its components, collects one or more of the blood components, and returns the remainder of the blood components to the donor along with saline for fluid replacement. Amicus is cleared for use with the anticoagulant ACD-A. The first stage employs a soft spin to separate the heaviest cells—red cells and white cells—from the platelets and plasma, resulting in leukocyte reduction of the platelets. In the second stage, the PRP is pumped into the collection chamber, where the platelets are concentrated.

The Amicus separator allows for the use of a single- or double-needle configuration. Single-needle platelet collection procedures provide an optional concurrent red cell collection. Both single-needle and double-needle procedures provide for optional concurrent plasma collection.

The Amicus platelet storage container is cleared to store platelets in 100% plasma for up to 7 days and to store platelets in a mixture of 35% plasma, 65% PAS-3 up to 5 days. The Amicus is cleared for use with the RBC storage solution (additive solution) AS-1 in the US market, and SAGM in the European market.

Amicus can be used to collect the following components alone or in combination depending on donor weight, height, platelet count, and hematocrit:

- Single, double, or triple units of platelets stored in plasma or a mixture of 35% plasma, 65% PAS-3.

- Plasma that can be prepared into FFP, PF24, and PF24RT24.
- Single units of leukocyte-reduced RBCs stored in RBC storage solution.

The Amicus device is also capable of performing mononuclear cell collections and therapeutic apheresis procedures such as therapeutic plasma exchange.

Alyx Component Collection System (Fresenius Kabi)

The Alyx Component Collection System (Alyx) is an automated device designed to collect and separate WB from donors. The WB is centrifugally separated into its cellular and plasma components. Cellular and/or plasma components are retained in collection containers or returned to the donor according to the predetermined collection procedures. Alyx uses a rigid, cylinder-shaped chamber in the centrifuge to separate the plasma from the cells. During reinfusion, the plasma and saline are returned to the donor. When the collection is complete, Alyx automatically adds the preservative solution and pumps the red cells through an in-line leukocyte reduction filter into the final storage bags.

Alyx has a closed, disposable kit which has all solutions and containers preattached. It is cleared for use with the anticoagulant ACD-A and AS-1 in the United States, or SAGM (in Europe) as the red cell preservation solution.

Alyx can be used to collect the following components depending on donor weight and hematocrit/hemoglobin:

- Double units of leukocyte-reduced RBCs.
- Single units of leukocyte-reduced RBCs and 2 or 3 units of plasma.
- Up to 4 units of plasma.

Plasma can be prepared into FFP, PF24, and PF24RT24.

Aurora Plasmapheresis System (Fresenius Kabi)

The Aurora Plasmapheresis System, consisting of the instrument (hardware and software) and a single-use disposable set, is an automated plasmapheresis system intended for routine collection of source plasma. The Aurora system uses 4% sodium-citrate anticoagulant and allows for a saline replacement option. The collection of plasma by the Aurora Xi System is a fully automated procedure with the donor connected to the PLASMACELL Xi disposable set. The Aurora Xi System is based on a rapidly rotating separator (membrane filter) to separate plasma from WB. The collection procedure requires a single venipuncture, which means that one access site is used to draw WB and return concentrated cellular components. The procedure involves alternating cycles, in which blood is drawn and plasma is separated and collected, followed by return of residual cellular components. Venous pressure is continuously monitored to avoid exceeding the flow capacity of the donor's vein.

The MCS+ LN8150 Device (Haemonetics)

The Haemonetics MCS+ LN8150 system consists of a device, protocol software, and single-use, disposable set components. Using a single-access, functionally closed kit, the device draws WB from the donor's vein and proportionally mixes it with anticoagulant solution. Using the blow-molded bowl technology, it separates donor WB into its components.

Depending on donor size and hematocrit, the MCS+ LN8150 is capable of collecting single or double units of RBCs with or without concurrent plasma collection, depending on donor size and hematocrit. Blood components that are not collected are returned to the donor, optionally with a configurable volume of saline to compensate for the volume loss. The device automatically administers the appropriate volume of red cell preservative solution to the collected unit(s). Disposable sets are offered with an integrated leukocyte reduction filter. The filtration of RBC units by gravity is performed off-line after the collection is complete.

The MCS+ LN9000 Device (Haemonetics)

The Haemonetics MCS+ LN9000 system consists of a device, protocol software, and single-use, disposable set components. Using a single-access, functionally closed kit, the device draws WB from the donor's vein and proportionally

mixes it with anticoagulant solution. WB is separated into its components using the Latham bowl separation technology. The buffy-coat layer containing platelets and WBCs is formed within the bowl, supported by plasma-controlled management of the hematocrit (critical flow). Platelets are elutriated from the bowl and collected by using rapid plasma flow through the cellular layers (surge technique). Blood components that are not collected are returned to the donor, optionally with a configurable volume of saline to compensate for the volume loss.

Depending on donor size and platelet count, the MCS+ LN9000 is capable of collecting single, double, or triple units of apheresis platelets with or without concurrent plasma collection. Disposable sets are offered with an integrated leukocyte reduction filter. The filtration of platelet units by gravity is automatically performed during the collection procedure, making final leukocyte-reduced platelet components available at the end of the procedure.

The PCS2 Device (Haemonetics)

The Haemonetics PCS2 system consists of a collection device, protocol software, and a compatible single-use, disposable set optimized for the collection of source plasma and plasma for transfusion. With the Haemonetics single-use, single venous access component set, the PCS2 device draws WB from the donor's vein and proportionally mixes it with anticoagulant solution. Using blow-molded bowl technology, the PCS2 separates WB from a donor into its components and collects a user-configurable volume of plasma based on the donor profile into a collection container. Blood components that are not collected are returned to the donor, optionally with a configurable volume of saline to compensate for the volume loss.

The NexSys PCS Device with YES Technology (Haemonetics)

NexSys PCS with embedded yield-enhancing solution (YES) technology is a collection device that uses a disposable, single-use, single venous access component set to draw WB from the donor's vein and proportionally mix it with anticoagulant solution. Using blow-molded bowl technology, the NexSys PCS system separates WB from a donor into its components and collects an operator-configurable volume of source plasma and deposits it into a collection container. Blood components that are not collected are returned to the donor, optionally with a configurable volume of saline to compensate for the volume loss.

BLOOD COMPONENT STORAGE

Cold-Stored Whole Blood for Transfusion

WB is most often separated into components; however, it can be stored as WB for transfusion for up to 35 days in approved anticoagulant/storage solutions (AABB Reference Standard 5.1.8A).[4(pp52-61)] WB can be stored non-leukocyte-reduced or can be leukocyte-reduced using a platelet-sparing filter. Recently, successful use of low-titer anti-A/anti-B, group O WB in military trauma resuscitation has renewed interest in use of stored WB by the civilian trauma medicine community.[1,55-57] WB and RBCs have similar volume and identical storage and transportation temperature requirements. WB offers operational simplicity compared to balanced component therapy (delivery of a balanced ratio of RBCs, plasma, and platelets) for massively bleeding patients.[55] WB contains cold-stored platelets that appear to have equivalent or better hemostatic effect than platelets stored at room temperature.[56,58] Transfusion of WB has the advantage of providing a balanced resuscitation fluid in one bag rather than up to four bags of RBCs, platelets, and plasma.[56]

Red Blood Cell Component Storage

Containers for WB and RBC storage often are composed of PVC plasticized with di(2-ethylhexyl) phthalate (DEHP). DEHP not only imparts flexibility to the PVC but also has been shown to protect red cells against hemolysis during storage. Because of concerns over the possible toxicity of DEHP, alternative plasticizers

such as butyryl-trihexyl-citrate (BTHC), 1,2-cyclohexane dicarboxylic acid diisononyl ester (DINCH), and di(2-ethylhexyl) terephthalate (DEHT) have been explored as alternatives to DEHP.[59] The protective effect of DEHP on red cells has made finding an equally effective substitute for DEHP challenging. In the absence of DEHP to stabilize the red cell membrane, it has been suggested that next-generation additive solutions might be able to compensate for this lack of stabilization when alternate plasticizers are employed.[60] PAGGSM (phosphate-adenine-glucose-guanosine-saline-mannitol), AS-3, or PAGGGM (phosphate-adenine-glucose-guanosine-gluconate-mannitol) in DINCH- or DEHT-plasticized collection and storage systems perform similarly to DEHP-PVC containers with AS-1 or SAGM.[60,61]

RBCs from WB in anticoagulant-preservative CPD or CP2D have a shelf life of 21 days at 1 to 6 C with a hematocrit of 65% to 85%, or 35 days in CPDA-1 with a hematocrit of <80% (AABB Reference Standard 5.1.8A).[4(pp52-61)] The use of additive solutions enables extension of RBC shelf life up to 42 days in the United States and to 56 days in some other jurisdictions. Additive solutions reduce the hematocrit to approximately 55% to 65%. RBCs stored for less than 7 to 10 days are often issued for neonatal or pediatric transfusions, although practice varies both with regard to length of storage and preferred anticoagulant or additive solution at different institutions, with sparse evidence to suggest an optimal approach. For RBCs collected either from WB or apheresis, hemolysis at the end of storage should be less than 1% in the United States or less than 0.8% in the European Union (EU) and other sites outside the United States.[62,63]

Visual inspection of RBC units can detect abnormal color or appearance caused by hemolysis, or clots. Abnormal color in the bag can also be caused by bacterial contamination.[64] An abnormal-appearing unit can be centrifuged to facilitate inspection of the supernatant for hemolysis. In the case of suspected bacterial contamination, visual inspection of the supernatant may reveal murky, brown, or red fluid.[64] However, visual inspection will not detect all contaminated units. Blood clots in RBC units are often too small to be detected visually and are revealed during transfusion when they clog the transfusion filter, or in the component laboratory when the units fail to pass through a leukocyte reduction filter. Units that fail visual inspection or are otherwise found to contain clots should not be released for transfusion.

Hemoglobin content and hematocrit per RBC unit vary because of differences between donors and between blood component manufacturing methods.[44,65,66] For example, more hemoglobin is generally lost and there is a resulting lower hematocrit in the RBC unit produced when platelets are manufactured by buffy-coat preparation methods than with PRP-type methods. Hemoglobin content per unit and the final hematocrit may be more precisely controlled with apheresis collections. Total hemoglobin content is not directly regulated but has a lower limit of 45 g per unit in the United States or 40 g per unit for leukocyte-reduced RBCs in Europe.[62] Some experts have advocated for tighter standardizing of hemoglobin and hematocrit in RBC units.[67,68]

Segments are made from tubing from the RBC container, marked with repeating serial numbers, and may be sealed at several locations with either a dielectric (heat) sealer or a metal clip (grommet) to prepare approximately 13 to 15 segments with the unique number. These segments may be used later for ABO/Rh typing, crossmatching, antigen typing, investigation of adverse transfusion reactions (with the exception of bacterial contamination), or other laboratory tests. However, care should be taken in using segments to evaluate the quality of the RBC component, as significant differences between measurements of hemoglobin, hemolysis, and hematocrit have been shown to exist.[69,70]

Platelet Component Storage

Platelets are stored and shipped at 20 to 24 C in plastic containers that have greater gas permeability than those for RBCs or plasma and must be continuously agitated during storage to support platelet metabolism and ensure adequate in-vivo recovery (AABB Reference Standard 5.1.8A).[4(pp52-61),51,71] Modern platelet containers with high gas permeability are composed of PVC plasticized with either BTHC or tri(2-ethylhexyl) trimellitate or, alternatively, are composed of ethylvinyl acetate, polyolefins (polyethylene or polypropylene), or fluoropolymers.[35] Agitation supports platelet metabolism by ensuring effective exchange of oxygen, carbon dioxide, and lactic acid between the platelets and the suspending media. Long periods of static storage of platelets disrupt oxidative metabolism and enhance glycolysis, resulting in increased lactic acid production and consequently a decline in pH.[72] If pH levels decline to less than 6.2, platelets will have unacceptably low in-vivo recoveries.[73] During transport from blood centers to hospitals or to other blood centers or during long-distance air transport, platelets are not agitated. In-vitro studies have shown minimal platelet damage when they are stored without agitation for up to 24 hours.[72,74,75] However, longer periods without agitation can lead to unacceptable pH decline.[74]

With 20 to 24 C storage, contaminating bacteria can proliferate during storage and result in septic transfusion reactions, some of which are fatal. Platelet storage containers can support shelf life up to 5 or 7 days; however, platelet storage is limited by local regulations to minimize the risk of septic transfusion reactions. These limits are determined by the different mitigation strategies implemented in the various world regions. Mitigation strategies include donor screening, skin disinfection, blood diversion, component testing by culture, point-of-issue testing, and pathogen inactivation. In the United States, according to the September 2019 guidance for industry from the FDA,[76] platelet shelf life can be extended to 5 days if pathogen inactivation is used, or up to 7 days with secondary bacteria testing (reculture or rapid testing) or large-volume, delayed sampling using approved devices. Platelet shelf life will be limited to either 5 days, with primary culture plus secondary testing cleared as a safety measure or pathogen inactivation, or 7 days, in an approved container, with the addition of secondary testing by culture or point-of-issue testing. Other countries already allow up to 7-day platelet shelf life with pathogen inactivation (eg, Switzerland) or large-volume, delayed sampling (eg, Canada and the United Kingdom).[77]

Visual inspections of platelets after they are prepared show an absence of visible red cells in the vast majority of units, which implies that the units contain fewer than 0.4×10^9 red cells. Generally, the number of red cells in a standard transfusable unit of platelets does not exceed 1.0×10^9, although occasionally WB-derived platelets contain more red cells.[78] If red cells are visible in a component, the hematocrit should be measured. AABB Standard 5.15.5 states that if the component contains greater than 2 mL of red cells, the red cells must be ABO compatible with the recipient's plasma and be cross-matched. In such cases, a sample of donor blood is attached to the container for compatibility testing.[4(p38)]

On the day of preparation, some WB-derived platelet units, as well as apheresis platelet units, may contain clumps composed of platelet aggregates.[78,79] In routine practice, visual inspection is adequate to determine the degree of clumping subjectively and ensure that units with excessive clumping are not labeled for distribution and transfusion. Most of the clumps seen on day 0 dissipate on day 1 of storage with continuous agitation, particularly those units showing light to moderate clumping.[78] The temperature, centrifugation speed used in the production of WB platelets, and leukocyte reduction by filtration may influence the presence of platelet aggregates.[79,80] Some blood centers have also reported donor dependence, where platelet aggregates are observed in multiple donations from the same donor.[81]

Occasionally, because of adverse shipping conditions, temporary equipment failures, or power outages, platelets cannot be maintained at 20 to 24 C. One study indicated that platelets can maintain their in-vitro properties after exposure to 37 C for 6 hours, followed by room-temperature storage without agitation for an additional 18 hours.[82] However, negative effects on in-vivo platelet recovery and survival when platelets are stored at temperatures less than 20 C have been reported.[83,84] Thus, proper steps should be taken to maintain the required range of temperatures during storage at the blood center and during transport.

In Europe, apheresis and WB-derived platelets can be stored in either plasma or PAS. Com-mercially available PAS formulations support platelet storage with 30% to 40% plasma carry-over.[52] Lower plasma carryover requires investigational PAS formulations that contain bicarbonate and glucose to maintain platelet metabolism and viability. Benefits of PAS-stored platelets include fewer adverse transfusion reactions, lower titers of anti-A and B antibodies, as well as increased availability of plasma for further manufacturing.[52] The negative effect of platelets stored in PAS is lower posttransfusion count increments.[52] In the United States, current PAS formulations are approved for storage of apheresis platelets only and cannot be used for the storage of platelets prepared from WB.

Plasma Component Storage

Plasma preparations are defined and regulated through extensive combinations of differences in collection methods, storage temperatures, freezing methods, secondary processing, timing, and storage after thawing. These specifications are covered in an array of standards, rules, and guidelines overlaid with various requirements of the country where the plasma is prepared and/or used. Major, although not exclusive, sources of this information include the US CFR, FDA guidance documents, the US *Circular of Information*, AABB *Standards*, and EU directives. The definitions and requirements of the country where the plasma is prepared should always be consulted.

Plasma from WB and apheresis collections is generally frozen to maintain factor activity and provide an extended shelf life. Delayed freezing of fresh plasma can result in lower levels of Factors V and VIII.[85,86] Frozen plasma is thawed for clinical use and may be maintained at 1 to 6 C for some time before use. Frozen plasma is also the source of cryoprecipitate and cryoprecipitate-reduced plasma. Plasma may be used for transfusion or for the preparation of specific plasma protein products through fractionation processes.

Fresh Frozen Plasma

In the United States, FFP can be prepared from plasma collected either from WB or by apheresis. A plasma unit derived from WB contains, on average, 300 mL, but apheresis units may contain as much as 400 to 600 mL of plasma. FFP contains acceptable levels of all coagulation factors, antithrombin, and ADAMTS13.[86] FFP must be placed in the freezer within 8 hours of collection (AABB Reference Standard 5.1.8A) or as directed by the manufacturer's instructions for use of the blood collection, processing, and storage system (AABB Standards 5.1.8A and 5.7.4.9).[4(pp28,52-61)] FFP has a shelf life of 12 months when stored at −18 C or colder and, with FDA approval, may be stored for up to 7 years from collection at −65 C (AABB Reference Standard 5.1.8A).[4(pp52-61)]

The Council of Europe, somewhat more stringently, defines "plasma, fresh frozen" as prepared from either WB or plasma collected by apheresis. Plasma freezing must be initiated within 6 hours, or within 24 hours if WB is rapidly cooled to 20 to 24 C following collection.[62] Freezing must be completed within 1 hour and achieve a temperature of less than −25 C. Rapid freezing of plasma can be accomplished using a blast freezer, dry ice, or a mixture of dry ice with either ethanol or antifreeze. Plasma, fresh frozen has an expiry time of 36 months if held at less than −25 C, or 3 months if held at −18 C to −25 C.[62] The Council of Europe does not stipulate specific thawing methods—only that thawing be performed in a properly controlled environment with no insoluble cryoprecipitate visible upon completion of the thaw procedure.[62]

Plasma should be thawed immediately after removal from storage at 30 to 37 C in a waterbath or by using an FDA-cleared dry-thawing device. When a waterbath is used, the component must be placed in a protective plastic overwrap (AABB Standard 5.7.4.9.1).[4(p28)] Thawing of larger units of FFP collected by apheresis may require more time. FFP, once thawed, has a shelf life of 24 hours at 1 to 6 C. Thawed plasma held longer than 24 hours must be relabeled as Thawed Plasma and can be stored for an additional 4 days at 1 to 6 C if prepared in a closed system (AABB Standards 5.7.4.13 and 5.1.8A).[4(pp29,52-61)]

The glass-transition temperature of plasma storage bags is dependent on the material composition, but for PVC containers it is between −20 C and −35 C.[87] At and below these temperatures, the container is brittle and is fragile enough to break during transport and handling. Leaky containers should not be used for transfusion and should be discarded.

AABB requires interventions to reduce the risk of transfusion-related acute lung injury (TRALI) from plasma-containing components. Current approaches for apheresis platelets, plasma, and WB for transfusion include collection from males, never-pregnant females, or parous females who test negative for HLA antibodies, to minimize the risk of exposing patients to HLA alloantibodies that could cause TRALI (AABB Standard 5.4.1.3).[4(p18)]

Quarantined plasma is held in storage until the donor returns for a subsequent donation. It was introduced to increase the viral safety of plasma. The Council of Europe permits the release of FFP from quarantine after the donor returns to the blood center after a minimum quarantine period that is greater than the diagnostic window period for viral infection (typically 6 months). Donors must have negative test results for at least hepatitis B surface antigen, antibodies to human immunodeficiency virus, and antibodies to hepatitis C virus. With the use of nucleic acid tests for viral screening, this window period for quarantined FFP may be reduced.[88]

Plasma Frozen Within 24 Hours After Phlebotomy

The FDA defines plasma that is frozen to less than −18 C within 24 hours of collection as PF24. PF24 can be prepared from plasma collected either from WB or by apheresis. PF24 is prepared when WB or plasma cannot be transported, processed, and frozen within 8 hours after phlebotomy due to geographic or logistical constraints. PF24 is equivalent to FFP with the exception of Factor V, Factor VIII, and protein C levels.[2] The component prepared from apheresis collections must be stored at 1 to 6 C within 8 hours of collection and frozen within 24 hours (AABB Standard 5.7.4.10).[4(p28)] Once thawed, PF24 has a shelf life of 24 hours at 1 to 6 C (AABB Reference Standard 5.1.8A).[4(pp52-61)] Thawed plasma held longer than 24 hours must be relabeled as Thawed Plasma, which can be stored for an additional 4 days at 1 to 6 C (AABB Standards 5.7.4.13 and 5.1.8A).[4(pp29,52-61)]

Plasma Frozen Within 24 Hours After Phlebotomy Held At Room Temperature Up To 24 Hours After Phlebotomy

Plasma held for up to 24 hours after collection at room temperature and then stored at less than −18 C is PF24RT24 (AABB Standard 5.7.4.11).[4(p28)] PF24RT24 can be prepared from plasma collected either from WB or by apheresis. PF24RT24 is prepared when WB or plasma cannot be transported, processed, and frozen within 8 hours after phlebotomy due to geographic or logistical constraints. PF24RT24 is equivalent to FFP, with the exception of Factor V, Factor VIII, and protein S levels.[2] Once thawed, PF24RT24 has a shelf life of 24 hours at 1 to 6 C (AABB Reference Standard 5.1.8A).[4(pp52-61)] Thawed plasma held for longer than 24 hours must be relabeled as Thawed Plasma and can be stored for an additional 4 days at 1 to 6 C (AABB Standards 5.7.4.13 and 5.1.8A).[4(pp29,52-61)]

Thawed Plasma

Thawed Plasma is FFP, PF24, or PF24RT24 that has been thawed and held at 1 to 6 C for >24 hours (AABB Standard 5.7.4.13).[4(p29)] Thawed Plasma may be held at 1 to 6 C for up to 4 days after the initial 24-hour postthaw period has elapsed. Stable Factor II and fibrinogen and reduced amounts of other factors (especially Factors V and VIII, for which transfusion of plasma is rarely indicated) have been observed in Thawed Plasma. Thawed Plasma prepared from FFP and stored for up to 5 days after thawing has reduced levels of Factor V, Factor VII, and Factor VIII.[89-91] Storage of thawed Plasma Cryoprecipitate Reduced for up to 5 days does not affect levels of fibrinogen, Factor VIII, or von Willebrand factor (vWF) but can result in reductions in ADAMTS13, Factor V, and Factor VII.[92] Thawed plasma has acceptable factor levels, with the exception of Factor V and Factor VIII, and is typically used to avoid delays associated with thawing in emergency situations.

Liquid Plasma

In the United States, liquid plasma for transfusion can be separated from WB at any time during the WB storage period and stored at 1 to 6 C for up to 5 days after the WB expiration date [AABB Reference Standard 5.1.8A and 21 CFR 610.53(b)].[4(pp52-61)] For WB stored in ACD/CPD or CP2D, the expiration for Liquid Plasma is 26 days. If WB is stored in CPDA-1, the Liquid Plasma expiration date is 40 days following collection. Liquid Plasma has acceptable factor levels, with the exception of Factor V and Factor VIII, and is typically used to avoid delays associated with thawing in emergency situations.

Cryoprecipitated AHF

Cryoprecipitated Antihemophilic Factor (AHF), or simply "cryoprecipitate" in Europe, is a concentrated cryoglobulin fraction that is prepared from FFP. FFP can be thawed to prepare Cryoprecipitated AHF by placing the FFP in a refrigerator (at 1 to 6 C) overnight or in a circulating waterbath at 1 to 6 C. Cold-insoluble protein that precipitates when FFP is thawed to 1 to 6 C is collected by centrifugation, and the supernatant plasma is transferred into a satellite container. The precipitate is resuspended in a small amount of residual plasma, generally 15 mL, and the precipitate is refrozen. The Cryoprecipitated AHF is placed in a freezer within an hour of removal from the refrigerated centrifuge and can be stored at −18 C for 12 months from the original collection date (AABB Reference Standard 5.1.8A).[4(pp52-61)] In Europe, thawing is to be performed at 2 to 6 C, and the component can be stored for up to 3 months at −18 to −25 C or for 36 months below −25 C.[62]

AABB Standard 5.7.4.15 requires that Cryoprecipitated AHF contain at least 80 international units (IU) of Factor VIII and 150 mg of fibrinogen per unit,[4(p29)] although the average fibrinogen content is generally 250 mg.[93] European standards require at least 70 IU of Factor VIII, 140 mg of fibrinogen, and 100 IU of vWF per unit.[62] Current preparations are reported to have much higher amounts of fibrinogen (median: 388 mg/unit).[94] Rapid freezing of FFP is found to increase the Factor VIII yield in Cryoprecipitated AHF.[95] Anti-A and anti-B are known to be present in Cryoprecipitated AHF, but the combined amount of these antibodies from the unit of plasma is only 1.15% of the total.[96]

Thawed Cryoprecipitated AHF should be used as soon as possible but may be held at room temperature (20-24 C) for 6 hours as a single unit or as a pool prepared in a closed system using an approved sterile connection device, or conversely for 4 hours if pooling was with an open system (AABB Reference Standard 5.1.8A).[4(pp52-61)] Pooling may be accomplished with the aid of a diluent, such as 0.9% sodium chloride (USP), to facilitate removal of material from individual bags.

At room temperature, the mean declines in Factor VIII levels at 2, 4, and 6 hours are approximately 10%, 20%, and 30%, respectively.[97] Cryoprecipitated AHF from blood groups A and B has higher levels of Factor VIII compared to that derived from blood group O donors (about 120 vs 80 IU per bag, respectively).[98] Thawed cryoprecipitate should not be refrozen.[62]

Plasma Cryoprecipitate Reduced

Plasma Cryoprecipitate Reduced (United States) or Plasma, Fresh Frozen Cryoprecipitate-Depleted (Europe) is the residual fluid after removal of Cryoprecipitated AHF. If prepared using a closed system, Plasma Cryoprecipitate Reduced must be refrozen with 24 hours of thawing the FFP from which it is derived, and stored at less than −18 C (AABB Reference Standard 5.1.8A).[4(pp52-61)] The storage temperatures and expirations stipulated in US and European regulations that apply to FFP also apply to this component. The component contains a normal level of Factor V (85%), Factor I, Factor VII, Factor X, antiplasmin, antithrombin, protein C, and protein S. Even after the removal of cryoprecipitate, the component has a fibrinogen level of about 200 mg/dL.[99] Levels of Factor VIII, the vWF antigen, vWF activity, fibrinogen, and Factor XIII are decreased.[92,100] Plasma Cryoprecipitate Reduced is used almost exclusively for plasma exchange or transfusion in patients with thrombotic thrombocytopenic purpura.[2]

Recovered and Source Plasma

Blood centers often convert plasma and Liquid Plasma to an unlicensed Recovered Plasma or "plasma for manufacture" component, which is usually shipped to a fractionator and processed into derivatives, such as albumin, coagulation factors, and/or immune globulins. To ship Recovered Plasma, the collecting facility must have a "short supply agreement" with the manufacturer (21 CFR 601.22). Because Recovered Plasma has no expiration date, records for this component should be retained indefinitely. Storage conditions and expiry dates for Recovered Plasma are established by the plasma fractionator. FFP used as human plasma for fractionation in Europe must comply with the applicable European Pharmacopoeia guidelines.

Source Plasma is collected by apheresis and stored at the appropriate temperature required for further manufacturing of plasma protein products. Source Plasma donors are typically paid and have different donor qualification criteria compared to infrequent plasmapheresis donors (AABB Standard 5.5.2).[4(p19)] Source Plasma donors can donate a maximum of two times in a 7-day period, and the interval between two collections must be at least 2 days (AABB Standard 5.5.2.2.1).[4(p20)] In addition to required testing for infectious agents on each donation, Source Plasma donors require physical examination and testing to determine total plasma or serum protein and immunoglobulin composition on the day of initial plasmapheresis and at least every 4 months thereafter [21 CFR 640.65(b)(1)].

POSTCOLLECTION PROCESSING/BLOOD COMPONENT MODIFICATION

Prestorage Leukocyte Reduction by Filtration

Blood collection systems can include in-line filters for removal of leukocytes from WB, RBC units, and/or platelets. Many WB leukocyte reduction systems allow filtration at ambient temperature for up to 24 hours after collection. WB and RBC filtration may also be started and/or completed at refrigerator temperatures. The residual number of leukocytes in 95% of leukocyte-reduced, WB-derived, single-donor platelet units tested must be less than 8.3×10^5 per unit (AABB Standard 5.7.4.19).[4(p30)] The Council of Europe requires that the residual number of leukocytes be less than 1×10^6 per unit in 90% of RBCs and pooled platelet and apheresis platelet components tested.[62] The FDA requires that the residual number of leukocytes be less than 5×10^6 per unit in 95% of RBCs and pooled platelet and apheresis platelet components tested, with 95% confidence.[35,36]

In the United States, leukocyte reduction by filtration of RBCs must result in a component that contains at least 85% of the original red cell (AABB Standard 5.7.4.6) or platelet content.[4(p27),101] After filtration, single-donor platelet units must have $>5.5 \times 10^{10}$ platelets per unit in 75% of units tested, with 90% of units having a pH ≥ 6.2 at the end of allowable storage (AABB Standard 5.7.4.19).[4(p30)] Also, 95% of leukocyte-reduced apheresis platelets must contain $\geq 3.0 \times 10^{11}$ platelets per unit and have a pH ≥ 6.2, with 95% confidence, at the end of allowable storage.[36] The Council of Europe's standards require that 90% of units tested have a minimum of 40 g of hemoglobin in each RBC unit and $>2 \times 10^{11}$ platelets in each platelet unit after leukocyte reduction.[62]

Prestorage leukocyte reduction is generally performed soon after WB collection and is always performed within 5 days of collection. In-line WB filters that remove both WBCs and platelets permit preparation of leukocyte-reduced RBCs and FFP. In-line WB filters that spare platelets permit preparation of leukocyte-reduced RBCs, FFP, and platelets. If WB is collected without the in-line leukocyte reduction filter, a filter can be attached to the tubing using an FDA-cleared sterile connection device.[101] Apheresis devices are designed to leukocyte-reduce plasma and platelets during the collection such that the components do not require postcollection leukocyte reduction.

Sickle cell trait in red cells is the most common cause of WBC filtration failure. Approximately 50% of the RBC units with sickle cell trait fail to filter. Although the other 50% pass through the filter, the residual leukocyte content may be higher than allowable limits.[102]

Because levels of residual leukocytes in leukocyte-reduced components are below the level of detection for most standard hematology analyzers, Nageotte hemocytometry and flow cytometry have historically been used to quantify white cell content in blood components. A Nageotte hemocytometer is a fixed-volume (50-μL) device that contains an etched grid to facilitate manual counting of cells under a microscope.[103] Flow-cytometry methods involve labeling of fresh or fixed cells with a fluorescent DNA-binding dye such that the leukocytes can be counted relative to an internal calibration bead. In a multicenter study, flow cytometry gave more precise results than Nageotte hemocytometry when freshly prepared samples (within 24 hours) were tested.[104] In general, Nageotte hemocytometry tends to underestimate the number of white cells compared to flow cytometry. Automated optical systems using image analysis are now available to measure white cell counts, reducing the technical burdens associated with both Nageotte and flow cytometry.[105]

Pooling of Blood Components

Pooling of platelet or plasma components from multiple blood donors can be used to increase the therapeutic dose of cell or plasma protein components in a product. When pooled by the component manufacturer or hospital service and the connections are performed using a sterile connection device, the component sterility and expiry time are not compromised (AABB Standard 5.7.2.1.1).[4(p24)]

For open systems, pooled platelets have an expiration time of 4 hours from when the system was opened for pooling (Reference Standard 5.1.8A).[4(pp52-61)] Closed systems for prestorage pooling of platelets licensed by the FDA permit storage of pooled platelets for up to 5 days from collection of the oldest units in the pool (Reference Standard 5.1.8A).[4(pp52-61)] Four to 6 leukocyte-reduced or non-leukocyte-reduced platelet units (generally, from ABO-identical units) are pooled using a set consisting of a multi-lead tubing manifold for sterile connection. If non-leukocyte-reduced units are pooled, they can be leukocyte-reduced by filtration as part of the pooling process. The shortest expiration date of the pooled units determines the expiration date of the pool [21 CFR 610.53(B)].

In the United States, each pool prepared from leukocyte-reduced platelets must have <5.0 × 10^6 residual leukocytes. Approved pooling sets must also allow sampling of the pool for bacteria detection. A record of the ABO/Rh type, DIN, and collecting facility for each unit in the pool must be maintained by the component manufacturer (Standard 5.7.3.3).[4(p25)]

Many international blood manufacturers prepare prestorage pools of buffy-coat platelets that are preserved in PAS or in the plasma from one of the units from which platelets are prepared.[106] Instruments that automate the pooling process are being used globally to improve efficiency in the blood component laboratory. Outside of the United States, systems for prestorage pooling of buffy-coat-derived platelets can be followed by pathogen inactivation treatment.

Cryoprecipitated AHF units pooled immediately before transfusion in an open system have an expiration time of 4 hours at 20 to 24 C storage (AABB Reference Standard 5.1.8A).[4(pp52-61)] Prestorage pools can also be prepared in an open system and stored for 12 months at −18 C (AABB Reference Standard 5.1.8A).[4(pp52-61)] After thawing, the component expires in 4 hours (AABB Reference Standard 5.1.8A).[4(pp52-61)] Prestorage pools prepared using an FDA-cleared sterile connection device can be stored for 12 months at −18 C and have a postthaw expiration time of 6 hours (AABB Reference Standard 5.1.8A).[4(pp52-61)] The number of units pooled may vary and can consist of 4, 5, 6, 8, or 10 units. Prestorage pools must be placed in a freezer within 1 hour after removal from a refrigerated centrifuge (AABB Reference Standard 5.1.8A).[4(pp52-61)] The potency of the pool is calculated by assuming that each unit in the pool contains 80 IU of coagulation Factor VIII and 150 mg of fibrinogen multiplied by the number of units in the pool (AABB Standard 5.7.4.15).[4(p29)]

Cryopreservation of Red Blood Cells

Currently, there are two methods used for the cryopreservation of RBC components: low glycerol/rapid cooling[107] and high-glycerol/slow cooling.[108,109] A less commonly used method involves low concentrations (15-20%) of glycerol, rapid cooling (>100 C/minute), storage in liquid nitrogen (−196 C) or nitrogen vapor (−165 C), and rapid thawing in a 42 to 45 C waterbath. The more common cryopreservation method found in the United States and most international blood centers is the use of a high concentration of glycerol (40%) in conjunction with slow cooling (? 1 C/min), storage at ≤−65 C, and rapid thawing in a 37 C waterbath. In each method, controlled addition and removal of glycerol are required to prevent osmotic lysis of the red cells and to minimize the transfusion recipient's exposure to the chemical cryoprotectant. RBC components must be cryopreserved within 6 days of collection unless they have been biochemically rejuvenated or are rare RBC units, which can be cryopreserved without rejuvenation up to the date of expiration (AABB Standard 5.7.4.2.1).[4(p26)]

Cryopreserved RBCs must be stored at temperatures equal to or less than −65 C and expire after 10 years. Rare frozen units may be used beyond the expiration date, but a policy must be in place for release of these units (AABB Reference Standard 5.1.8A).[4(pp52-61)] European regulations permit the cryogenic storage of cryopreserved RBCs for up to 30 years.[62] Cryopreserved RBC units should be handled with care because the PVC or polyolefin freezing storage containers may crack during shipment or if handled roughly. Rare RBC components that were thawed and deglycerolized can be refrozen and rethawed when needed without adversely affecting the recovery of the components.[110]

Glycerol must be removed after thawing by a method that allows for the addition and removal of sodium chloride solutions. Addition and removal of glycerol (deglycerolization) can be performed in an open system, with postthaw storage limited to 24 hours at 1 to 6 C (AABB Reference Standard 5.1.8A).[4(pp52-61)] With open system processing, the final solution in which cells are suspended is 0.9% sodium chloride and 0.2% dextrose. Dextrose provides nutrients and has been shown to support satisfactory posttransfusion viability for 4 days of storage after deglycerolization.[111]

The commercial availability of automated, closed-system cell processors for the addition and removal of glycerol allows extended post-thaw storage of cryopreserved red cells. Glycerol is added within 6 days of WB collection, and the postthaw storage can be for up to 14 days at 1 to 6 C in AS-3 in the United States or 7 days in SAGM in Europe.[111,112] Non-leukocyte-reduced RBC components processed using a closed-system cell processor and cryopreserved have a hematocrit of 51% to 53% and contain a mean 9.0 × 10^6 leukocytes per unit.[113] European standards require that cryopreserved red cell products have a minimum of 36 g of hemoglobin per unit, a hematocrit of 35% to 70%, and a supernatant hemoglobin level <0.2 g per unit.[62]

Cryopreservation and Cold Storage of Platelets

Cryopreserved platelets treated with 4% to 6% dimethyl sulfoxide (DMSO) and stored at less than −80 C for 2 to 4 years have been shown to maintain hemostatic function.[114-116] Removal of DMSO before freezing allows platelets to be thawed and reconstituted immediately with plasma, making these units suitable for military and civilian trauma use.[116,117] Platelet cryopreservation and the subsequent thawing processes are, however, time-consuming and more expensive than standard room-temperature storage. Clinical trials are underway to support cryopreservation of platelets.[118-120]

Cold storage of platelets at 1 to 6 C has a number of advantages over room-temperature storage, including prolonged shelf life due to reduced metabolism, enhanced hemostatic activity, improved bacteriologic safety, and ease of storage and transport.[121] Storage of platelets at 1 to 6 C can result in increased cell activation and procoagulant function, which has raised interest in using this product to treat actively bleeding patients.[58] In the United States, apheresis platelets can be stored at 1 to 6 C without agitation for up to 3 days (21 CFR 640.24 and 21 CFR 640.25). Cold storage of platelets can result in reduced in-vivo recovery and survival compared with room-temperature-stored platelets.[71,122]

Irradiation of Blood Components

Cellular blood components can be irradiated to reduce the risk of transfusion-associated graft-vs-host disease (GVHD).[123] Irradiation sources include gamma rays—from either cesium-137 blood component irradiators or cobalt-60 sources—or x-rays produced by radiation therapy linear accelerators or stand-alone units. Both sources achieve satisfactory results in inactivating T lymphocytes. Free-standing irradiators are commercially available for blood bank use.

In the United States, the radiation dose targeted to the midplane of the container must be at least 25 gray (Gy) [2500 centigray (cGy)] and no more than 50 Gy (5000 cGy).[62,124] Moreover, the minimum delivered dose to any portion of the blood components must be at least 15 Gy in a fully loaded canister (AABB Standard 5.7.3.2).[4(p25)] The European standard requires a higher dose, with no part of the component receiving <25 Gy and a maximum dose to any part of the component of 50 Gy.[62] Both US and European standards are effective for prevention of GVHD.

Each instrument must be routinely monitored to ensure that an adequate dose is delivered to the blood container during irradiation (AABB Standard 5.7.3.2.1).[4(p25)] Dose mapping using irradiation-sensitive films or badges that monitor the delivered dose are used for quality control of the irradiators.[124] Irradiation-sensitive labels are a requirement in Europe.[62] FDA regulations require verification of the delivered dose annually for the cesium-137 source and semiannually for the cobalt-60 source (AABB Standard 5.7.3.2.1).[4(p25)] For x-ray irradiators, the dosimetry should be performed in accordance with the manufacturer's recommendations (AABB Standard 5.7.3.2.1).[4(p25)] Dose verification is also required after major repairs or relocation of the irradiator (AABB Standard 5.7.3.2.1).[4(p25)] For gamma irradiators, the turntable operation, timing device, and lengthening of irradiation time caused by source decay should also be monitored periodically.

In the United States, RBCs may be irradiated up to the end of their storage shelf life. The postirradiation expiration date is 28 days from the date of irradiation or the original expiration date, whichever is earlier (AABB Reference Standard 5.1.8A).[4(pp52-61)] In Europe, RBCs may be irradiated only up to day 28 following collection, and irradiated cells may not be stored longer than the earlier of 14 days after irradiation or 28 days after collection.[62] Platelets may be irradiated until their expiration date, and their postirradiation expiration date is the same as the original expiration date (AABB Reference Standard 5.1.8A).[4(pp52-61)]

Irradiation of RBCs followed by storage results in a decrease in the in-vitro quality of the blood components. The pre- and postirradiation storage period has been shown to affect the level of hemolysis and supernatant potassium level in RBCs, which may pose a risk to certain patient populations.[125,126] For example, in neonates and in rapid transfusions to small children, high potassium levels may cause cardiac complications,[127] prompting the use of a shorter expiry for irradiated RBCs or washing of components before transfusion. Platelets are not damaged by an irradiation dose as high as 50 Gy.[128]

Washing of Red Cell and Platelet Components

Washed RBCs are recommended for large-volume transfusions to potassium-sensitive patients, particularly neonates when fresh units are not available,[129] for recipients who have a history of plasma-related transfusion reactions,[130] and to mitigate TRALI.[131] The use of washed RBCs has been proposed as a means to remove the accumulation of proinflammatory cells and molecules in stored RBCs to reduce the bioactivity of the component[132] and may be an effective means to address red cell degradation during storage.[133]

RBCs can be washed in the blood bank using manual methods, semiautomated cell processors, or blood recovery devices just before transfusion to reduce the concentration of plasma or immunoglobulins.[129,134,135] Methods must ensure RBCs are washed with a volume of compatible solution that will remove almost all of the plasma (AABB Standard 5.7.4.5).[4(p27)] Because of the potential for bacterial contamination during washing of RBCs using an open processing system and decreased red cell viability when resus-

pended in saline rather than an additive solution in the postwash period, a 24-hour expiry is applied to these components (AABB Reference Standard 5.1.8A).[4(pp52-61)] The use of closed-system, semiautomated cell processors and modern additive solutions can extend the postwash storage solution.[134] European standards require washed components to have a minimum of 40 g of hemoglobin per unit, a hematocrit of 0.50 to 0.70, less than 0.8% hemolysis, and less than 0.5 g of supernatant protein per unit.[62]

Volume Reduction of Blood Components

Volume-reduced platelets may be needed to reduce the amount of plasma transfused to prevent cardiac overload, to minimize ABO antibody infusion, for intrauterine transfusion, or to minimize the risk of repeated transfusion reactions. The volume of a platelet unit (single-donor, WB-derived) can be reduced to 10 to 15 mL/unit by centrifugation just before transfusion. In-vitro characteristics such as platelet morphology, mean volume, hypotonic shock response, synergistic aggregation, and platelet factor 3 activity appear to be maintained when volume reduction is performed on storage day 5, and platelet increments after transfusion have been satisfactory.[136] The in-vitro recovery rate of platelets is roughly 85% after volume reduction. Prepooled single-donor platelets from WB that are volume reduced by centrifugation ($580 \times g$ for 20 minutes) from an approximate volume of 60 mL to between 35 and 40 mL yield a high platelet count ($>2.3 \times 10^9$/L).[137] Lowering the pH of platelets prepared from WB avoids platelet aggregates visible to the unaided eye (macroaggregates).[138] The addition of 10% ACD-A to platelets to lower the pH before centrifugation can help with resuspension of high-concentration platelets and avoid aggregation.[138] If an open system is used, the maximum allowable storage time is 4 hours.

Pathogen Inactivation

Blood is the safest it has ever been. However, despite extensive blood donor history screening and testing, the risk of transfusion-transmitted infection from both known and emerging pathogens persists.[139] Blood components can be treated with pathogen inactivation technologies to inactivate pathogens such as viruses, bacteria, and parasites and hence reduce the risk of transfusion-transmitted infections.[139] The majority of pathogen inactivation methods damage the nucleic acids of viruses, bacteria, and parasites, preventing their replication.[139] These methods are also known to inactivate residual white cells and hence can be used to replace gamma or x-ray irradiation to prevent GVHD. Because platelets, plasma, and RBCs do not contain genomic nucleic acids, they are relatively unaffected by pathogen inactivation treatment.[139]

INTERCEPT (Cerus Corporation) employs amotosalen and ultraviolet A (UVA) light to damage nucleic acids of pathogens. It has regulatory approval in Europe (CE mark), Canada (Health Canada), and the United States (FDA) for treatment of platelets and plasma. Treatment consists of the addition of 150 μM amotosalen followed by illumination with 3.0 Joules/cm^2 UVA light (λ = 320-400 nm). After illumination, amotosalen is removed using the integral chemical adsorption device (residual concentration of amotosalen plus photoproducts: 0.02 mg/mL for platelets and 0.01 mg/mL for plasma).[140] Average activity values for coagulation and antithrombotic factors are reported to be within reference ranges for treated plasma.[141] In-vitro studies have reported some loss in platelet properties and function.[142]

The *Mirasol PRT System* (Terumo BCT) employs riboflavin (vitamin B2) and UV light to damage nucleic acids of pathogens. It has a regulatory CE mark for the treatment of platelets and plasma. Treatment consists of adding 35 mL of riboflavin followed by illumination for 6 to 10 minutes with 6.24 Joules/mL UV light (λ = 280-400 nm). Riboflavin is a naturally occurring vitamin that does not require removal. The platelet or plasma product does not require any posttreatment processing and hence is ready for transfusion. Coagulation and anticoagulant proteins are well preserved in plasma treated with the Mirasol system.[143,144] In-vitro studies have reported some loss in platelet properties and function.[142] The Mirasol PRT System is also approved under CE mark for treatment of WB for

transfusion, with the same platform used to treat platelets and plasma.

The *THERAFLEX UV-Platelet System* (Maco-Pharma and German Red Cross) is CE marked for treatment of platelets. It is based on application of UVC light (λ = 254 nm) to damage nucleic acids of pathogens, combined with intense agitation of the platelet unit to ensure a uniform treatment of the entire volume of the unit.[145] No photoactive compounds are added to the blood components; therefore, there is no chemical removal step.[145]

The *THERAFLEX MB-Plasma System* (Maco-Pharma) is CE marked for treatment of plasma. Methylene blue (MB) has been shown to inactivate pathogens by damaging nucleic acids.[146] MB is added to thawed FFP in pill form (85 μg anhydrous MB chloride) followed by activation using white light. Thawing of frozen plasma is a precursor step for MB treatment in order to lyse white cells that may harbor viral particles.[146] After activation, MB is removed with a filter (residual concentration: 0.3 μM), and plasma can be refrozen.[146] MB-treated plasma contains 10% to 35% less Factor VIII and fibrinogen than untreated plasma, depending on varying analytical procedures and laboratories.[146]

Octaplas (Octapharma AG) is solvent/detergent (SD)-treated, pooled human plasma approved in Europe (CE mark), Canada (Health Canada), and the United States (FDA). SD plasma does not damage nucleic acids; rather, it disrupts viral envelopes, cells, and most protozoa. It is not effective against nonenveloped viruses.[147] SD plasma is prepared from plasma pooled from many donors that is tested for standard transfusion-transmitted agents and (nonenveloped) parvovirus B19 DNA, hepatitis A, and hepatitis E virus RNA. It undergoes treatment with the solvent 1% tri-n-butyl phosphate and the detergent 1% Triton X-100 to disrupt viral lipid envelopes.[147] SD plasma is manufactured in facilities that can manage large-scale production, rather than in blood centers. Final transfusable units consist of 200 mL of ABO-group-specific plasma that is stored frozen at −18 C with an expiration date of 12 months.[148] Most coagulation factors are reduced by approximately 10% in SD plasma, except for Factor VIII, which is reduced by 20%.[149] Also, levels of protein S and alpha$_2$-

antiplasmin, which are labile to SD treatment, are controlled to ensure levels within the range of normal human plasma (>0.4 IU/mL).[150] The component is labeled with the ABO blood group and, once thawed, should be used within 24 hours.

QUARANTINE OF BLOOD COMPONENTS

All units of blood collected should be immediately placed in quarantine in a designated area until donor information and donation records have been reviewed, the current donor information has been compared to the previous information, the donor's previous deferrals have been examined, and all laboratory testing has been completed (21 CFR 606.100). Because of the limited amount of time after collection that is available for component separation, WB units may be separated into components before all of the aforementioned processes have been completed. Separated components are quarantined at the appropriate temperature until all of the suitability processes have been completed and reviewed. Often, physical and electronic quarantine are used simultaneously.

Certain blood components from previous donations by donors whose more recent donations test positive for infectious agents also require quarantine and appropriate disposition, as do units identified as unsuitable for transfusion because of postdonation information. Other components may need to be quarantined so that QC samples can be taken and analyzed. For instance, if a sample is obtained for bacteria detection, the component is held in quarantine for some predetermined time and then released if the test result is negative.

A thorough understanding of the quarantine process is needed to prevent erroneous release of unsuitable blood components. Components may be removed from the quarantine area, labeled, and released for distribution if all of the donor information, previous donor records, and current test results are satisfactory. Optimally, labeling and release from quarantine are tightly controlled using the blood establishment computer system to prevent distribution of any component for which any disqualifying information has been generated.

Some blood components require emergency release because they have a very short storage time. Emergency release requires physician approval and a label or tie tag to indicate that testing was incomplete at the time of release (AABB Standard 5.27.3).[4(p44)]

Despite the widespread use of software to control manufacturing processes, instances of failure resulting in the distribution of unsuitable components continue to be reported to the FDA, the majority of which are due to human error or process control failures.[151]

LABELING OF BLOOD COMPONENTS

The FDA requirements for labeling of blood and components are available in several publications. The "Guideline for the Uniform Labeling of Blood and Blood Components" was published in 1985.[152] Detailed requirements for the labeling of blood components are described in the CFR (21 CFR 606.120, 606.121, and 606.122). AABB *Standards* requires that accredited facilities label blood and blood component containers in accordance with the most recent version of the "United States Industry Consensus Standard for the Uniform Labeling of Blood and Blood Components Using ISBT 128" (AABB Standard 5.1.6.3.1).[4(p12)] This document outlines the information that must appear in the text of blood bag labels. Specifically, it defines the data identifiers use in transfusion and transplant settings, including the layout and precise placement of bar codes.

Base labels and any additional labels that are placed directly on the container must use approved adhesives. In accordance with the 1985 FDA guideline, only those substances that are FDA approved as "indirect food additives" may be used in adhesives and coating components for labels placed over the base label.[152] The FDA has additional standards for labels that are applied directly on plastic blood containers. Tie tags may be used as an extension of the label if there is insufficient label space, particularly for informational items that do not have to be directly affixed to the container. National regulatory requirements should be verified when selecting labels and establishing labeling policies.

The FDA rule that requires all blood components to be labeled with a bar-coded label became effective on April 26, 2006. The rule requires that, at a minimum, the label contain the following bar-coded information: 1) the unique facility identifier (ie, registration number), 2) lot number relating to the donor, 3) product code, and 4) ABO group and Rh type of the donor. These pieces of information must be present in eye-readable and machine-readable format. The rule applies to blood establishments that collect and prepare blood components, including hospital transfusion services that perform manufacturing steps such as preparation of pooled cryoprecipitate and/or divided units or aliquots of RBCs, platelets, and plasma for pediatric use.

Another major part of labeling in the United States is the *Circular of Information,*[2] which must be made available to everyone involved in the transfusion of blood components. The *Circular* is produced by AABB, the American Red Cross, America's Blood Centers, and the Armed Services Blood Program and is recognized as acceptable by the FDA. It provides important information about each blood component and should be consulted for information not included in this chapter.

Special message labels may also be affixed to blood component containers. The labels may include one or more of the following indications: 1) hold for further manufacturing, 2) for emergency use only, 3) for autologous use only, 4) not for transfusion, 5) irradiated, 6) biohazard, 7) from a therapeutic phlebotomy, and 8) screened for special factors [eg, HLA type or cytomegalovirus (CMV) antibody status]. ISBT 128 allows incorporation of special attributes of the component, such as CMV antibody status, from the previous donation.

As mentioned above, additional information on the container can be conveyed using a tie tag. Tie tags are especially useful for autologous and directed donations. Tie tags include the patient's identifying information, name of the hospital where the patient will be admitted for surgery, date of surgery, and other information that may be helpful to the hospital transfusion service.

Each component must also bear a unique DIN that can be traced back to the blood donor. If components are pooled, a pool number must allow tracing to the individual units within a pool.

An important source of information is ICCBBA (formerly known as the International Council for Commonality in Blood Banking Automation). The ICCBBA website (www.iccbba.org) features updates and a revised list of product codes. ISBT 128 technical specifications support the use of radiofrequency ID tags and other means of electronic data transmission.[153,154]

KEY POINTS

1. Potential donors must be provided with predonation education, counseling about the blood donation process, and an opportunity to have their questions answered before every blood donation.

2. Adverse reactions can occur at the time of donation or after the donor has left the blood center. All adverse reactions occurring during collection procedures must be documented along with the results of thorough investigations.

3. Most adverse donor reactions are mild and require no further medical care. These reactions can be systemic (eg, fainting) or local (eg, hematoma). Deferral of low-blood-volume (<3.5 L) donors may be helpful in reducing the risk of vasovagal reactions, especially in young donors.

4. Therapeutic phlebotomy is a treatment for blood disorders in which the removal of red cells or reduction of iron stores is an effective method for managing the disease.

5. Blood collection and component separation systems may be designed in different configurations depending on the needs of the blood manufacturer. Component processing methods from

whole blood are typically defined based on the method used to separate the platelets from the whole blood.

6. Apheresis devices are continuous systems that remove blood from a donor, separate the blood into the desired components, and return the remaining blood to the donor. Blood component combinations are dependent on regulatory approval for each of the apheresis devices and individual donor data.

7. Plasma preparations are defined and regulated through extensive combinations of differences in collection methods, storage temperatures, freezing methods, secondary processing, timing, and storage after thawing.

8. Postcollection modification to blood components may include prestorage leukocyte reduction by filtration, pooling, cryopreservation, irradiation, washing, volume reduction, or pathogen inactivation.

9. All units of blood collected should be immediately placed in quarantine in a designated area until donor information and donation records have been reviewed, the current donor information has been compared to the previous information, the donor's previous deferrals have been examined, and all laboratory testing has been completed.

10. The blood component identification process uniformly uses both a bar-coded and an eye-readable, unique DIN that is assigned to each sample tube and each component prepared from the donation.

11. Bar-coded and eye-readable container labels follow the ISBT symbology (ISBT 128), which allows identification of the manufacturer throughout the world, more product codes, better accuracy as a result of reduced misreads during scanning, and enhanced conveyance of other labeling information.

REFERENCES

1. Chandler MH, Roberts M, Sawyer M, Myers G. The US military experience with fresh whole blood during the conflicts in Iraq and Afghanistan. Semin Cardiothorac Vasc Anesth 2012; 16(3):153-9.

2. AABB, American Red Cross, America's Blood Centers, Armed Services Blood Program. Circular of information for the use of human blood and blood components. (October 2017) Bethesda, MD: AABB, 2017. [Available at https://www.aabb.org/tm/coi/Documents/coi1017.pdf (accessed October 1, 2019).]

3. Code of federal regulations. Title 21, Food and Drugs: Part 606, Current good manufacturing practice for blood and blood components; Part 610, General biological products standards; Part 630, Requirements for blood and blood components intended for transfusion or for further manufacturing use; Part 640, Additional standards for human blood and blood products. Washington, DC: US Government Publishing Office, 2019. (revised annually).

4. Gammon R, ed. Standards for blood banks and transfusion services. 32nd ed. Bethesda, MD: AABB, 2020.

5. Goldman M, Roy G, Frechette N, et al. Evaluation of donor skin disinfection methods. Transfusion 1997;37(3):309-12.

6. Buchta C, Nedorost N, Regele H, et al. Skin plugs in phlebotomy puncture for blood donation. Wiener klinische Wochenschrift 2005; 117(4):141-4.

7. de Korte D, Curvers J, de Kort WL, et al. Effects of skin disinfection method, deviation bag, and bacterial screening on clinical safety of platelet transfusions in the Netherlands. Transfusion 2006;46(3):476-85.

8. McDonald CP, Roy A, Mahajan P, et al. Relative values of the interventions of diversion and improved donor-arm disinfection to reduce the bacterial risk from blood transfusion. Vox Sang 2004;86(3):178-82.

9. de Korte D, Marcelis JH, Verhoeven AJ, Soeterboek AM. Diversion of first blood volume results in a reduction of bacterial contamination for whole-blood collections. Vox Sang 2002; 83(1):13-16.

10. Eder AF, Dy BA, Kennedy JM, et al. The American Red Cross donor hemovigilance program:

Complications of blood donation reported in 2006. Transfusion 2008;48(9):1809-19.

11. Newman BH. Blood donor complications after whole-blood donation. Curr Opin Hematol 2004;11(5):339-45.

12. Sorensen BS, Johnsen SP, Jorgensen J. Complications related to blood donation: A population-based study. Vox Sang 2008;94(2):132-7.

13. Eder AF, Notari EP 4th, Dodd RY. Do reactions after whole blood donation predict syncope on return donation? Transfusion 2012;52(12):2570-6.

14. Bravo M, Kamel H, Custer B, Tomasulo P. Factors associated with fainting: Before, during and after whole blood donation. Vox Sang 2011;101(4):303-12.

15. Rios JA, Fang J, Tu Y, et al. The potential impact of selective donor deferrals based on estimated blood volume on vasovagal reactions and donor deferral rates. Transfusion 2010;50(6):1265-75.

16. Kamel H, Tomasulo P, Bravo M, et al. Delayed adverse reactions to blood donation. Transfusion 2010;50(3):556-65.

17. France CR, France JL, Kowalsky JM, et al. Assessment of donor fear enhances prediction of presyncopal symptoms among volunteer blood donors. Transfusion 2012;52(2):375-80.

18. Tomasulo P, Kamel H, Bravo M, et al. Interventions to reduce the vasovagal reaction rate in young whole blood donors. Transfusion 2011;51(7):1511-21.

19. Eder AF, Kiss JE. Adverse reactions and iron deficiency after blood donation. In: Simon TL, McCullough J, Snyder EL, et al, eds. Rossi's principles of transfusion medicine. 5th ed. Chichester, UK: John Wiley and Sons, 2016:43-57.

20. Lee G, Arepally GM. Anticoagulation techniques in apheresis: From heparin to citrate and beyond. J Clin Apher 2012;27(3):117-25.

21. Food and Drug Administration. Fatalities reported to FDA following blood collection and transfusion - Annual summary for fiscal year 2016. Silver Spring, MD: CBER Office of Communication, Outreach, and Development, 2016. [Available at https://www.fda.gov/media/111226/download.]

22. Chin-Yee B, Lazo-Langner A, Butler-Foster T, et al. Blood donation and testosterone replacement therapy. Transfusion 2017;57(3):578-81.

23. Kim KH, Oh KY. Clinical applications of therapeutic phlebotomy. J Blood Med 2016;7:139-44.

24. Marrow B, Clarkson J, Chapman CE, Masson S. Facilitation of blood donation amongst haemo-

chromatosis patients. Transfus Med 2015;25(4):239-42.

25. Evers D, Kerkhoffs JL, Van Egmond L, et al. The efficiency of therapeutic erythrocytapheresis compared to phlebotomy: A mathematical tool for predicting response in hereditary hemochromatosis, polycythemia vera, and secondary erythrocytosis. J Clin Apher 2014;29(3):133-8.

26. Jolivet-Gougeon A, Ingels A, Danic B, et al. No increased seroprevalence of anti-Yersinia antibodies in patients with type 1 (C282Y/C282Y) hemochromatosis. Scand J Gastroenterol 2007;42(11):1388-9.

27. Sanchez AM, Schreiber GB, Bethel J, et al. Prevalence, donation practices, and risk assessment of blood donors with hemochromatosis. JAMA 2001;286(12):1475-81.

28. Leitman SF, Browning JN, Yau YY, et al. Hemochromatosis subjects as allogeneic blood donors: A prospective study. Transfusion 2003;43(11):1538-44.

29. McDonnell SM, Grindon AJ, Preston BL, et al. A survey of phlebotomy among persons with hemochromatosis. Transfusion 1999;39(6):651-6.

30. Phlebotomy guidelines for patients with hereditary hemochromatosis. Greenville, SC: Iron Disorders Institute, 2011. [Available at http://www.irondisorders.org/Websites/idi/files/Content/854256/Physician%20Chart%20phlebotomy%20detail2011.pdf (accessed October 1, 2019).]

31. Keohane C, McMullin MF, Harrison C. The diagnosis and management of erythrocytosis. BMJ 2013;347:f6667.

32. Wagner SJ. Whole blood and apheresis collections for blood components intended for transfusion. In: Fung MK, Eder AF, Spitalnik SL, Westhoff CM, eds. Technical manual. 19th ed. Bethesda, MD: AABB; 2017:125-60.

33. Button LN, Orlina AR, Kevy SV, Josephson AM. The quality of over- and undercollected blood for transfusion. Transfusion 1976;16(2):148-54.

34. Davey RJ, Lenes BL, Casper AJ, Demets DL. Adequate survival of red cells from units "undercollected" in citrate-phosphate-dextrose-adenine-one. Transfusion 1984;24(4):319-22.

35. Prowse CV, de Korte D, Hess JR, van der Meer PF. Commercially available blood storage containers. Vox Sang 2014;106(1):1-13.

36. Pietersz RN, de Korte D, Reesink HW, et al. Storage of whole blood for up to 24 hours at ambient temperature prior to component preparation. Vox Sang 1989;56(3):145-50.

37. Hardwick J. Blood processing. ISBT Science Series 2008;3:148-76.

38. Devine DV, Howe D. Processing of whole blood into cellular components and plasma. ISBT Science Series 2010;5:78-82.

39. Levin E, Culibrk B, Gyongyossy-Issa M, et al. Implementation of buffy coat platelet component production: Comparison to platelet-rich plasma platelet production. Transfusion 2008; 48(11):2331-7.

40. Holme S, Heaton WA, Moroff G. Evaluation of platelet concentrates stored for 5 days with reduced plasma volume. Transfusion 1994; 34(1):39-43.

41. Ali AM, Warkentin TE, Bardossy L, et al. Platelet concentrates stored for 5 days in a reduced volume of plasma maintain hemostatic function and viability. Transfusion 1994;34(1):44-7.

42. van der Meer PF, Cancelas JA, Cardigan R, et al. Evaluation of overnight hold of whole blood at room temperature before component processing: Effect of red blood cell (RBC) additive solutions on in vitro RBC measures. Transfusion 2011;51(Suppl 1):15s-24s.

43. Perez-Pujol S, Lozano M, Perea D, et al. Effect of holding buffy coats 4 or 18 hours before preparing pooled filtered PLT concentrates in plasma. Transfusion 2004;44(2):202-9.

44. Acker JP, Hansen AL, Kurach JD, et al. A quality monitoring program for red blood cell components: In vitro quality indicators before and after implementation of semiautomated processing. Transfusion 2014;54(10):2534-43.

45. Snyder EL, Whitley P, Kingsbury T, et al. In vitro and in vivo evaluation of a whole blood platelet-sparing leukoreduction filtration system. Transfusion 2010;50(10):2145-51.

46. Plaza EM, Cespedes P, Fernandez H, et al. Quality assessment of buffy-coat-derived leucodepleted platelet concentrates in PAS-plasma, prepared by the OrbiSac or TACSI automated system. Vox Sang 2014;106(1):38-44.

47. Lagerberg JW, Salado-Jimena JA, Lof H, et al. Evaluation of the quality of blood components obtained after automated separation of whole blood by a new multiunit processor. Transfusion 2013;53(8):1798-807.

48. Johnson L, Winter KM, Kwok M, et al. Evaluation of the quality of blood components prepared using the Reveos automated blood processing system. Vox Sang 2013;105(3):225-35.

49. Rajbhandary S, Whitaker BI, Perez GE. The 2014-2015 AABB Blood Collection and Utilization Survey report. Bethesda, MD: AABB, 2018.

50. Food and Drug Administration. Guidance for industry: Recommendations for collecting red blood cells by automated apheresis methods - technical correction February 2001. Silver Spring, MD: CBER Office of Communication, Outreach, and Development, 2001. [Available at https://www.fda.gov/vaccines-blood-biologics/biologics-guidances/blood-guidances.]

51. Food and Drug Administration. Guidance for industry and FDA review staff: Collection of platelets by automated methods. (December 2007) Silver Spring, MD: CBER Office of Communication, Outreach, and Development, 2007. [Available at https://www.fda.gov/vaccines-blood-biologics/biologics-guidances/blood-guidances.]

52. van der Meer PF, de Korte D. Platelet additive solutions: A review of the latest developments and their clinical implications. Transfus Med Hemother 2018;45(2):98-102.

53. Slichter SJ, Corson J, Jones MK, et al. Exploratory studies of extended storage of apheresis platelets in a platelet additive solution (PAS). Blood 2014;123(2):271-80.

54. Ringwald J, Walz S, Zimmermann R, et al. Hyperconcentrated platelets stored in additive solution: Aspects on productivity and in vitro quality. Vox Sang 2005;89(1):11-18.

55. Cap AP, Beckett A, Benov A, et al. Whole blood transfusion. Mil Med 2018;183(Suppl 2):44-51.

56. Yazer MH, Cap AP, Spinella PC, et al. How do I implement a whole blood program for massively bleeding patients? Transfusion 2018;58(3):622-8.

57. Yazer MH, Spinella PC. The use of low-titer group O whole blood for the resuscitation of civilian trauma patients in 2018. Transfusion 2018;58(11):2744-6.

58. Nair PM, Pidcoke HF, Cap AP, Ramasubramanian AK. Effect of cold storage on shear-induced platelet aggregation and clot strength. J Trauma Acute Care Surg 2014;77(3 Suppl 2):S88-93.

59. van der Meer PF, Reesink HW, Panzer S, et al. Should DEHP be eliminated in blood bags? Vox Sang 2014;106(2):176-95.

60. Lagerberg JW, Gouwerok E, Vlaar R, et al. In vitro evaluation of the quality of blood products collected and stored in systems completely free of di(2-ethylhexyl)phthalate-plasticized materials. Transfusion 2015;55(3):522-31.

61. Graminske S, Puca K, Schmidt A, et al. In vitro evaluation of di(2-ethylhexyl) terephthalate plasticized polyvinyl chloride blood bags for red blood cell storage in AS-1 and PAGGSM additive solutions. Transfusion 2018;58(5):1100-7.

62. European Directorate for the Quality of Medicines and HealthCare. Guide to the preparation, use and quality assurance of blood components. Strasbourg, France: Council of Europe, 2017.

63. Hess JR. Measures of stored red blood cell quality. Vox Sang 2014;107(1):1-9.

64. Kim DM, Brecher ME, Bland LA, et al. Visual identification of bacterially contaminated red cells. Transfusion 1992;32(3):221-5.

65. Jordan A, Chen D, Yi Q-L, Acker JP. Assessing the influence of component processing and donor characteristics on red cell concentrates using quality control data. Vox Sang 2016;111(1): 8-15.

66. Hansen AL, Kurach JD, Turner TR, et al. The effect of processing method on the in vitro characteristics of red blood cell products. Vox Sang 2015;108(4):350-8.

67. Sweeney JD. Standardization of the red cell product. Transfus Apher Sci 2006;34:213-18.

68. Hogman CF, Mcryman HT. Red blood cells intended for transfusion: Quality criteria revisited. Transfusion 2006;46:137-42.

69. Janatpour KA, Paglieroni TG, Crocker VL, et al. Visual assessment of hemolysis in red blood cell units and segments can be deceptive. Transfusion 2004;44(7):984-9.

70. Kurach JD, Hansen AL, Turner TR, et al. Segments from red blood cell units should not be used for quality testing. Transfusion 2014; 54(2):451-5.

71. Murphy S, Gardner FH. Effect of storage temperature on maintenance of platelet viability—deleterious effect of refrigerated storage. N Engl J Med 1969;280(20):1094-8.

72. Dumont LJ, Gulliksson H, van der Meer PF, et al. Interruption of agitation of platelet concentrates: A multicenter in vitro study by the BEST Collaborative on the effects of shipping platelets. Transfusion 2007;47(9):1666-73.

73. Dumont LJ, AuBuchon JP, Gulliksson H, et al. In vitro pH effects on in vivo recovery and survival of platelets: An analysis by the BEST Collaborative. Transfusion 2006;46(8):1300-5.

74. Wagner SJ, Vassallo R, Skripchenko A, et al. The influence of simulated shipping conditions (24- or 30-hr interruption of agitation) on the in vitro properties of apheresis platelets during 7-day storage. Transfusion 2008;48(6):1072-80.

75. Vassallo RR, Wagner SJ, Einarson M, et al. Maintenance of in vitro properties of leukoreduced whole blood-derived pooled platelets after a 24-hour interruption of agitation. Transfusion 2009; 49(10):2131-5.

76. Food and Drug Administration. Guidance for industry: Bacterial risk control strategies for blood collection establishments and transfusion services to enhance the safety and availability of platelets for transfusion. Silver Spring, MD: CBER Office of Communication, Outreach, and Development, September 2019. [Available at: https://www.fda.gov/regulatory-information/search-fda-guidance-documents/]

77. McDonald C, Allen J, Brailsford S, et al. Bacterial screening of platelet components by National Health Service Blood and Transplant, an effective risk reduction measure. Transfusion 2017; 57(5):1122-31.

78. Berseus O, Hogman CF, Johansson A. Simple method of improving the quality of platelet concentrates and the importance of production control. Transfusion 1978;18(3):333-8.

79. McCullough J, Dodd R, Gilcher R, et al. White particulate matter: Report of the ad hoc industry review group. Transfusion 2004;44(7):1112-18.

80. Welch M, Champion AB. The effect of temperature and mode of agitation on the resuspension of platelets during preparation of platelet concentrates. Transfusion 1985;25(3):283-5.

81. van der Meer PF, Dumont LJ, Lozano M, et al. Aggregates in platelet concentrates. Vox Sang 2015;108(1):96-100.

82. Moroff G, George VM. The maintenance of platelet properties upon limited discontinuation of agitation during storage. Transfusion 1990; 30(5):427-30.

83. Moroff G, Holme S, George VM, Heaton WA. Effect on platelet properties of exposure to temperatures below 20 degrees C for short periods during storage at 20 to 24 degrees C. Transfusion 1994;34(4):317-21.

84. Gottschall JL, Rzad L, Aster RH. Studies of the minimum temperature at which human platelets can be stored with full maintenance of viability. Transfusion 1986;26(5):460-2.

85. Smith JF, Ness PM, Moroff G, Luban NL. Retention of coagulation factors in plasma frozen after extended holding at 1-6 degrees C. Vox Sang 2000;78(1):28-30.

86. Dumont LJ, Cancelas JA, Maes LA, et al. The bioequivalence of frozen plasma prepared from whole blood held overnight at room temperature compared to fresh-frozen plasma prepared within eight hours of collection. Transfusion 2015;55(3):476-84.

87. Hmel PJ, Kennedy A, Quiles JG, et al. Physical and thermal properties of blood storage bags:

Implications for shipping frozen components on dry ice. Transfusion 2002;42(7):836-46.

88. Roth WK. Quarantine plasma: Quo vadis? Transfus Med Hemother 2010;37(3):118-22.

89. Scott E, Puca K, Heraly J, et al. Evaluation and comparison of coagulation factor activity in fresh-frozen plasma and 24-hour plasma at thaw and after 120 hours of 1 to 6 degrees C storage. Transfusion 2009;49(8):1584-91.

90. Sheffield WP, Bhakta V, Mastronardi C, et al. Changes in coagulation factor activity and content of di(2-ethylhexyl)phthalate in frozen plasma units during refrigerated storage for up to five days after thawing. Transfusion 2012; 52(3):493-502.

91. Sheffield WP, Bhakta V, Yi QL, Jenkins C. Stability of thawed apheresis fresh-frozen plasma stored for up to 120 hours at 1 degrees C to 6 degrees C. J Blood Transfus 2016;2016: 6260792.

92. Bhakta V, Jenkins C, Ramirez-Arcos S, Sheffield WP. Stability of relevant plasma protein activities in cryosupernatant plasma units during refrigerated storage for up to 5 days postthaw. Transfusion 2014;54(2):418-25.

93. Ness PM, Perkins HA. Fibrinogen in cryoprecipitate and its relationship to factor VIII (AHF) levels. Transfusion 1980;20(1):93-6.

94. Callum JL, Karkouti K, Lin Y. Cryoprecipitate: The current state of knowledge. Transfus Med Rev 2009;23(3):177-88.

95. Farrugia A, Prowse C. Studies on the procurement of blood coagulation factor VIII: Effects of plasma freezing rate and storage conditions on cryoprecipitate quality. J Clin Pathol 1985; 38(4):433-7.

96. Smith JK, Bowell PJ, Bidwell E, Gunson HH. Anti-A haemagglutinins in factor VIII concentrates. J Clin Pathol 1980;33(10):954-7.

97. Pesquera-Lepatan LM, Hernandez FG, Lim RD, Chua MN. Thawed cryoprecipitate stored for 6 h at room temperature: A potential alternative to factor VIII concentrate for continuous infusion. Haemophilia 2004;10(6):684-8.

98. Gunson HH. Variables involved in cryoprecipitate production and their effect on factor VIII activity. Report of a working party of the Regional Transfusion Directors Committee. Br J Haematol 1979;43(2):287-95.

99. Smak Gregoor PJ, Harvey MS, Briet E, Brand A. Coagulation parameters of CPD fresh-frozen plasma and CPD cryoprecipitate-poor plasma after storage at 4 degrees C for 28 days. Transfusion 1993;33(9):735-8.

100. Yarranton H, Lawrie AS, Mackie IJ, et al. Coagulation factor levels in cryosupernatant prepared from plasma treated with amotosalen hydrochloride (S-59) and ultraviolet A light. Transfusion 2005;45(9):1453-8.

101. Food and Drug Administration. Guidance for industry: Pre-storage leukocyte reduction of whole blood and blood components intended for transfusion. (September 2012) Silver Spring, MD: CBER Office of Communication, Outreach, and Development, 2012. [Available at https://www.fda.gov/downloads/Biologics-BloodVaccines/GuidanceComplianceRegulatoryInformation/Guidances/Blood/UCM3206 41.pdf.]

102. Schuetz AN, Hillyer KL, Roback JD, Hillyer CD. Leukoreduction filtration of blood with sickle cell trait. Transfus Med Rev 2004;18(3):168-76.

103. Lutz P, Dzik WH. Large-volume hemocytometer chamber for accurate counting of white cells (WBCs) in WBC-reduced platelets: Validation and application for quality control of WBC-reduced platelets prepared by apheresis and filtration. Transfusion 1993;33(5):409-12.

104. Dzik S, Moroff G, Dumont L. A multicenter study evaluating three methods for counting residual WBCs in WBC-reduced blood components: Nageotte hemocytometry, flow cytometry, and microfluorometry. Transfusion 2000; 40(5):513-20.

105. Strobel J, Antos U, Zimmermann R, et al. Comparison of a new microscopic system for the measurement of residual leucocytes in apheresis platelets with flow cytometry and manual counting. Vox Sang 2014;107(3):233-8.

106. van der Meer PF, de Korte D. The buffy-coat method. In: Blajchman M, Cid J, Loranzo M, eds. Blood component preparation: From benchtop to bedside. Bethesda, MD: AABB Press, 2011:55-81.

107. Rowe AW, Eyster E, Kellner A. Liquid nitrogen preservation of red blood cells for transfusion. Cryobiology 1968;5(2):119-28.

108. Meryman HT, Hornblower M. A method for freezing and washing red blood cells using a high glycerol concentration. Transfusion 1972; 12:145-56.

109. Valeri CR, Zaroulis CG. Rejuvenation and freezing of outdated stored human red cells. N Engl J Med 1972;287(26):1307-13.

110. Valeri CR. Viability, function and rejuvenation of previously frozen washed red blood cells. In: Chaplin HJ, Jaffe ER, Lenfant C, Valeri CR, editors. Preservation of red blood cells. Washing-

ton, DC: National Academy of Science, 1972: 265-97.

111. Valeri CR, Ragno G, Pivacek LE, et al. A multicenter study of in vitro and in vivo values in human RBCs frozen with 40-percent (wt/vol) glycerol and stored after deglycerolization for 15 days at 4 degrees C in AS-3: Assessment of RBC processing in the ACP 215. Transfusion 2001; 41(7):933-9.

112. Lelkens CC, de Korte D, Lagerberg JW. Prolonged post-thaw shelf life of red cells frozen without prefreeze removal of excess glycerol. Vox Sang 2015;108(3):219-25.

113. Valeri CR, Pivacek LE, Cassidy GP, Ragno G. The survival, function and hemolysis of human RBCs stored at 4°C in additive solution (AS-1, AS-3 or AS-5) for 42 days and then biochemically modified, frozen, thawed, washed and stored at 4°C in sodium chloride and glucose solution for 24 hours. Transfusion 2000;40(11):1341-5.

114. Valeri CR, Feingold H, Marchionni LD. A simple method for freezing human platelets using 6 per cent dimethylsulfoxide and storage at -80 degrees C. Blood 1974;43:131-6.

115. Cid J, Escolar G, Galan A, et al. In vitro evaluation of the hemostatic effectiveness of cryopreserved platelets. Transfusion 2016;56(3):580-6.

116. Valeri CR, Ragno G, Khuri SF. Freezing human platelets with 6 percent dimethyl sulfoxide with removal of the supernatant solution before freezing and storage at -80 degrees C without posthaw processing. Transfusion 2005;45:1890-8.

117. Noorman F, van Dongen TT, Plat MJ, et al. Transfusion: -80 degrees C frozen blood products are safe and effective in military casualty care. PLoS One 2016;11(12):e0168401.

118. Slichter SJ, Dumont LJ, Cancelas JA, et al. Safety and efficacy of cryopreserved platelets in bleeding patients with thrombocytopenia. Transfusion 2018;58(9):2129-38.

119. Dumont LJ, Cancelas JA, Dumont DF, et al. A randomized controlled trial evaluating recovery and survival of 6% dimethyl sulfoxide-frozen autologous platelets in healthy volunteers. Transfusion 2013;53(1):128-37.

120. Reade MC, Marks DC, Johnson L, et al. Frozen platelets for rural Australia: The CLIP trial. Anaesth Intensive Care 2013;41(6):804-5.

121. Waters L, Cameron M, Padula MP, et al. Refrigeration, cryopreservation and pathogen inactivation: An updated perspective on platelet storage conditions. Vox Sang 2018;113(4):317-28.

122. Stolla M, Fitzpatrick L, Gettinger I, et al. In vivo viability of extended 4 degrees C-stored autologous apheresis platelets. Transfusion 2018; 58(10):2407-13.

123. Moroff G, Luban NLC. The irradiation of blood and blood components to prevent graft-versus-host disease: Technical issues and guidelines. Transfus Med Rev 1997;11(1):15-26.

124. Moroff G, Leitman SF, Luban NL. Principles of blood irradiation, dose validation, and quality control. Transfusion 1997;37(10):1084-92.

125. Serrano K, Chen D, Hansen AL, et al. The effect of timing of gamma-irradiation on hemolysis and potassium release in leukoreduced red cell concentrates stored in SAGM. Vox Sang 2014; 106(4):379-81.

126. de Korte D, Thibault L, Handke W, et al. Timing of gamma irradiation and blood donor sex influences in vitro characteristics of red blood cells. Transfusion 2018;58:917-26.

127. Strauss RG. RBC storage and avoiding hyperkalemia from transfusions to neonates and infants. Transfusion 2010;50(9):1862-5.

128. Voak D, Chapman J, Finney RD, et al. Guidelines on gamma irradiation of blood components for the prevention of transfusion-associated graft-versus-host disease. BCSH Blood Transfusion Task Force. Transfus Med 1996;6(3):261-71.

129. O'Leary MF, Szklarski P, Klein TM, Young PP. Hemolysis of red blood cells after cell washing with different automated technologies: Clinical implications in a neonatal cardiac surgery population. Transfusion 2011;51(5):955-60.

130. Tobian AA, Savage WJ, Tisch DJ, et al. Prevention of allergic transfusion reactions to platelets and red blood cells through plasma reduction. Transfusion 2011;51(8):1676-83.

131. Silliman CC, Moore EE, Johnson JL, et al. Transfusion of the injured patient: Proceed with caution. Shock 2004;21(4):291-9.

132. Cholette JM, Henrichs KF, Alfieris GM, et al. Washing red blood cells and platelets transfused in cardiac surgery reduces postoperative inflammation and number of transfusions: Results of a prospective, randomized, controlled clinical trial. Pediatr Crit Care Med 2012;13(3):290-9.

133. Cortes-Puch I, Wang D, Sun J, et al. Washing older blood units before transfusion reduces plasma iron and improves outcomes in experimental canine pneumonia. Blood 2014;123(9):1403-11.

134. Hansen A, Yi QL, Acker JP. Quality of red blood cells washed using the ACP 215 cell processor:

Assessment of optimal pre- and postwash storage times and conditions. Transfusion 2013; 53(8):1772-9.

135. Gruber M, Breu A, Frauendorf M, et al. Washing of banked blood by three different blood salvage devices. Transfusion 2013;53(5):1001-9.

136. Moroff G, Friedman A, Robkin-Kline L, et al. Reduction of the volume of stored platelet concentrates for use in neonatal patients. Transfusion 1984;24(2):144-6.

137. Pisciotto PT, Snyder EL, Napychank PA, Hopfer SM. In vitro characteristics of volume-reduced platelet concentrate stored in syringes. Transfusion 1991;31(5):404-8.

138. Aster RH. Effect of acidification in enhancing viability of platelet concentrates current status. Vox Sang 1969;17(1):23-7.

139. Seltsam A. Pathogen inactivation of cellular blood products-an additional safety layer in transfusion medicine. Front Med 2017;4:219.

140. Lin L, Conlan MG, Tessman J, et al. Amotosalen interactions with platelet and plasma components: Absence of neoantigen formation after photochemical treatment. Transfusion 2005; 45(10):1610-20.

141. Irsch J, Pinkoski L, Corash L, Lin L. INTER-CEPT plasma: Comparability with conventional fresh-frozen plasma based on coagulation function—an in vitro analysis. Vox Sang 2010; 98(1):47-55.

142. Marks DC, Faddy HM, Johnson L. Pathogen reduction technologies. ISBT Science Series 2014; 9:44-50.

143. Larrea L, Calabuig M, Roldan V, et al. The influence of riboflavin photochemistry on plasma coagulation factors. Transfus Apher Sci 2009; 41(3):199-204.

144. Rock G. A comparison of methods of pathogen inactivation of FFP. Vox Sang 2011;100(2):169-78.

145. Seltsam A, Muller TH. UVC irradiation for pathogen reduction of platelet concentrates and plasma. Transfus Med Hemother 2011;38(1): 43-54.

146. Seghatchian J, Struff WG, Reichenberg S. Main properties of the THERAFLEX MB-Plasma System for pathogen reduction. Transfus Med Hemother 2011;38(1):55-64.

147. Hellstern P, Solheim BG. The use of solvent/detergent treatment in pathogen reduction of plasma. Transfus Med Hemother 2011;38(1): 65-70.

148. Hellstern P, Haubelt H. Manufacture and composition of fresh frozen plasma and virus-inactivated therapeutic plasma preparations: Correlation between composition and therapeutic efficacy. Thromb Res 2002;107(Suppl 1):S3-8.

149. Sharma AD, Sreeram G, Erb T, Grocott HP. Solvent-detergent-treated fresh frozen plasma: A superior alternative to standard fresh frozen plasma? J Cardiothorac Vasc Anesth 2000; 14(6):712-17.

150. Octaplas package insert and label information. Hoboken, NJ: Octapharma USA Inc, 2015:1-8.

151. Espinola R, O'Callaghan S, Weir L, et al. Quarantine release errors (QREs) in blood establishments: Summary of a public workshop. Transfusion 2012;52S:269A.

152. Food and Drug Administration. Guideline for the uniform labeling of blood and blood components. (August 1985) Silver Spring, MD: CBER Office of Communication, Outreach, and Development, 1985. [Available at https://www.fda.gov/vaccines-blood-biologics/biologics-guidances/blood-guidances.]

153. ISBT 128 standard technical specifications v5.9.0. (March 2018) San Bernardino, CA: IC-CBBA, 2018:185.

154. Knels R, Ashford P, Bidet F, et al. Guidelines for the use of RFID technology in transfusion medicine. Vox Sang 2010;98(Suppl 2):1-24.

CHAPTER 7
Infectious Disease Screening

Lauren A. Crowder, MPH; Whitney R. Steele, PhD, MPH; and Susan L. Stramer, PhD

BLOOD COMPONENTS, LIKE ALL OTH-er medications in the United States, are regulated by the Food and Drug Administration (FDA). The FDA requires drug manufacturers to verify the suitability of every raw material in their products.[1] For biologic pharmaceuticals, the donor is the key ingredient whose suitability must be verified.

A sample of blood from each donation must be tested with screening tests approved by the FDA to identify donors and donated components that might harbor infectious agents. This screening process is critically important because most blood components (eg, red cells, platelets, plasma, and cryoprecipitate) are infused without other treatments to inactivate infectious agents. Thus, infectious agents in a donor's blood at the time of donation that are not detected by the screening process may be transmitted directly to recipients.

HISTORICAL OVERVIEW OF BLOOD DONOR SCREENING

Table 7-1 shows the progression over time of donor testing for infectious diseases in the United States. Initially, donors were screened only for syphilis. In the 1960s, studies showed that greater than 30% of patients who received multiple transfusions developed posttransfusion hepatitis (PTH).[2] Studies in the early 1970s found that the newly discovered hepatitis B vi-

rus (HBV) accounted for only 25% of PTH cases.[2] Both HBV and non-A, non-B (NANB) hepatitis occurred more frequently in recipients of blood from commercial (paid) blood donors than in recipients of blood from volunteer donors. By the mid-1970s, implementation of sensitive tests for hepatitis B surface antigen (HBsAg) and conversion to a volunteer donor supply resulted in a dramatic reduction in the incidence of both HBV and NANB PTH. Still, NANB PTH continued to occur in approximately 6% to 10% of recipients of multiple transfusions.[2,3]

In the absence of a specific test for the causative agent of NANB PTH, investigators searched for surrogate markers that could be used to identify donations associated with NANB hepatitis. The presence of antibody to hepatitis B core antigen (anti-HBc) and/or the presence of elevated alanine aminotransferase in blood donors was shown to be associated with an increased risk of NANB PTH.[4-7] However, concerns about the nonspecific nature of these tests led to a delay in their implementation for donor screening.

The concept of surrogate testing was revisited in the early 1980s when concerns arose about the transmission of AIDS by transfusions before the identification of its causative agent. In an effort to reduce the potential transfusion transmission of AIDS, some blood banks implemented donor testing for anti-HBc, because this antibody was highly prevalent in populations at increased risk of AIDS, and/or donor screening

Lauren A. Crowder, MPH, Epidemiologist, Scientific Affairs, American Red Cross, Rockville, Maryland; Whitney R. Steele, PhD, MPH, Director of Epidemiology, Scientific Affairs, American Red Cross, Rockville, Maryland; and Susan L. Stramer, PhD, Vice President, Scientific Affairs, American Red Cross, Gaithersburg, Maryland
The authors have disclosed no conflicts of interest.

TABLE 7-1. Changes in Licensed US Donor Screening Tests for Infectious Diseases

Year First Implemented	Screening Test	Comments
1940s-1950s	Syphilis	The syphilis test was mandated by FDA in the 1950s.
1970s	HBsAg	The first-generation test was available in 1970, and a higher-sensitivity test was required in 1973.
1985	Antibody to HIV (anti-HTLV-III)	The initial name for HIV, the virus that causes AIDS, was HTLV-III. The first test for antibody to HIV was called "anti-HTLV-III."
1986-1987	ALT and anti-HBc	ALT and anti-HBc were recommended by AABB as surrogate tests for NANB hepatitis. These tests were initially not licensed by FDA for donor screening. AABB's recommendation for donor ALT testing was dropped in 1995 after antibody testing for HCV was in place. Anti-HBc was licensed and required by FDA in 1991.
1988	Anti-HTLV-I	Although HTLV-I infection is usually asymptomatic, a small percentage of infected individuals develop leukemia, lymphoma, or a neurologic disease.
1990	Antibody to HCV, Version 1 (anti-HCV 1.0)	HCV was identified as the cause of most cases of NANB hepatitis.
1991	Anti-HBc	Anti-HBc was previously recommended by AABB as a surrogate screen for NANB hepatitis. It was required by FDA in 1991 as an additional screen for HBV.
1992	Anti-HCV 2.0	This version had improved ability to detect antibody to HCV.
1992	Anti-HIV-1/2	The new HIV antibody tests had improved ability to detect early infection and an expanded range of detection that included HIV-2 in addition to HIV-1.

Year	Test	Description
1996	HIV-1 p24 antigen test	This test was found to detect HIV-1 infection 6 days earlier than the antibody test. FDA permitted discontinuation of HIV-1 p24 antigen testing with the implementation of a licensed HIV-1 NAT.
1996	Anti-HCV 3.0	This version has improved ability vs anti-HCV 2.0 to detect antibody to HCV.
1997-1998	Anti-HTLV-I/II	The new HTLV antibody tests detected HTLV-II in addition to HTLV-I.
1999	HIV-1 and HCV NAT to detect HIV and HCV RNA	These tests were implemented initially as investigational assays and were licensed by FDA in 2002. They detect infection earlier than antibody or antigen assays and are performed using MP-NAT in pools of 6-16.
2003	West Nile virus NAT to detect WNV RNA	This test was implemented initially as an investigational assay and was licensed by FDA during 2005-2007. Testing by ID-NAT, rather than MP-NAT, at times of increased WNV activity in a region was recommended by AABB in 2004 and FDA in 2009. Updated AABB recommendations were issued in 2013.
2004	Sampling of platelet components to detect bacterial contamination	Testing was recommended by AABB in 2004. Some tests are approved by FDA as quality-control tests. Since 2011, AABB has accepted only FDA-approved tests or those validated to have equivalent sensitivity. Pathogen-reduced platelets meet the AABB requirement.
2006-2007	Antibody to *Trypanosoma cruzi*	This test was approved by FDA as a donor screen late in 2006, and widespread testing was implemented in 2007. The rarity of seroconversion in US residents led to endorsement in FDA 2010 guidance of one-time donor screening.
2007-2008	HBV NAT to detect HBV DNA	This test was initially implemented as part of automated multiplex assays that detect HIV RNA, HCV RNA, and HBV DNA simultaneously. HBV DNA screening was explicitly recommended by FDA guidance issued in October 2012. Testing is performed using MP-NAT in pools of 6-16.

(Continued)

TABLE 7-1. Changes in Licensed US Donor Screening Tests for Infectious Diseases (Continued)

Year First Implemented	Screening Test	Comments
2016	ZIKV NAT to detect ZIKV RNA	Universal ID-NAT was recommended by FDA guidance issued in August 2016 in response to the epidemic in the Americas (with immediate implementation in Puerto Rico, 4-week implementation in high-risk Southern states and New York, and 12-week implementation in all other states). Guidance released in July 2018 allows the use of MP-NAT in place of ID-NAT (in pools of 6-16), unless a region is experiencing a local outbreak in which ID-NAT must be used. Licensed pathogen inactivation may be used in place of testing.
2019	*Babesia* NAT to detect *B. microti* DNA/RNA	This NAT assay was licensed and mandated for use in 2019. Licensed pathogen inactivation may be used in place of testing. No licensed serologic assay is available.

FDA = Food and Drug Administration; HBsAg = hepatitis B surface antigen; HIV = human immunodeficiency virus; AIDS = acquired immune deficiency syndrome; HTLV = human T-cell lymphotropic virus; ALT = alanine aminotransferase; HBc = hepatitis B core antigen; NANB = non-A, non-B; HCV = hepatitis C virus; HBV = hepatitis B virus; RNA = ribonucleic acid; NAT = nucleic acid testing; MP-NAT = minipool nucleic acid testing; ID-NAT = individual donor nucleic acid testing; WNV = West Nile virus; DNA = deoxyribonucleic acid; ZIKV = Zika virus.

for inverted CD4/CD8 T-cell ratio, which is an immune abnormality found both in AIDS patients and in people during the pre-AIDS incubation period of what was subsequently identified as human immunodeficiency virus (HIV) infection.[8] However, it was initially believed that the risk of transmitting AIDS by transfusion was too low to warrant surrogate interventions.[9] After HIV was isolated and identified as the causative agent of AIDS, donor screening tests for antibody to HIV were rapidly developed and implemented in 1985.

Once the HIV antibody test became available and cases of HIV were recognized in both prior donors and transfusion recipients, it became clear that the risk of transmitting HIV via blood transfusion had been greatly underestimated.[10] The HIV experience highlighted the fact that an infectious agent associated with a lengthy asymptomatic carrier state could be present in the blood supply for years without being recognized.

In the wake of this realization, the approach to donor screening was extended beyond known agents. Current donor history evaluations include screening for, and the exclusion of, donors with an increased risk of exposure to blood-borne or sexually transmitted infections. The intention is to reduce the likelihood that the blood supply will be subject to other as-yet-unidentified agents that are potentially transmissible by blood.

Transfusion transmission of HIV persisted even after implementation of donor testing because of a delay of weeks or months between the time a person is infected with HIV and the time the screening test for HIV antibody shows positive results.[11] Blood donated during this seronegative "window period" contains infectious HIV that is not detected by the donor screening tests.

The most straightforward means of protecting the blood supply from HIV window-period donations is to exclude potential donors with an increased likelihood of exposure to HIV. The FDA initially recommended in 1983 that blood banks provide donors with informational materials listing HIV risk activities and requesting that individuals not donate if they had engaged in these behaviors. Experience from San Francisco, CA, clearly documented the efficacy of this approach.[12] In 1990, the FDA recommended asking each donor directly about each risk activity. In 1992, the FDA issued comprehensive guidance describing this questioning process.

In the years since the discovery of HIV, the risk of transfusion-transmitted disease has been progressively reduced through a variety of measures:

1. Use of donor education and screening questionnaires to exclude donors at increased risk of blood-borne/window-period infections and transfusion-transmitted diseases for which no tests are available.
2. Improving and/or adding tests to shorten the window period for specific agents by detecting earlier stages of infection and implementing new donor screening tests, when necessary.
3. Adoption of current good manufacturing practice (cGMP) regulations to ensure that unsuitable units are not collected and/or distributed.
4. Surveillance of the known and emerging transfusion-transmissible diseases.

The approach used to screen potential donors for an agent depends on whether specific risk factors are identifiable and whether donor screening tests are available. Table 7-2 lists the screening approaches used for different types of infectious agents.

DONOR SCREENING TESTS

The donor infectious disease tests required by the FDA are specified in Title 21, Part 610.40, of the *Code of Federal Regulations* (CFR).[1] In addition to the CFR, the FDA communicates changes in its recommendations by issuing guidance publications. Although FDA guidance documents do not constitute legal requirements, they define the standard of practice in the United States, and many blood collectors consider them legal imperatives. AABB also issues recommendations and requirements to the blood

TABLE 7-2. Approaches to Donor Screening

Approach	Context for Use	Example(s)
Questioning only	Infectious agents with defined risk factors and no sensitive and/or specific test	Malaria, prions
Testing only	Donor test is available, but no question to distinguish individuals at risk of infection	West Nile virus
Questioning and testing	Agents for which there are both identified risk factors and effective tests	Human immunodeficiency virus, hepatitis B and C viruses, *Babesia*
Use of blood components that test negative for specific recipients	Agents with a high prevalence in donors but for which an identifiable subset of recipients can benefit from blood components that test negative	Cytomegalovirus (universal leukocyte reduction of cellular blood components has nearly replaced the use of cytomegalovirus-seronegative blood except in selected patient populations)
Testing of blood components	Infectious agent not detectable in donor samples; detection in blood component (platelets) required	Bacteria

banking community. These are communicated either by Association Bulletins or by inclusion in AABB *Standards for Blood Banks and Transfusion Services (Standards)*. AABB recommendations and *Standards* do not have the force of law, except in California, where some sets of AABB standards have been incorporated into state law.

Since 1985, the FDA and AABB have issued a series of recommendations, regulations, and/or standards for additional screening tests in addition to the long-standing donor screens for syphilis and HBsAg. Table 7-1 summarizes the chronology of changes in donor infectious disease testing, and Table 7-3 lists the licensed donor screening tests that are performed by US blood banks.

Logistics of Testing

All infectious disease testing for blood donor qualification purposes is performed on samples collected at the time of donation and sent to the testing laboratory. In addition, most platelet components are tested for bacterial contamination typically by the component manufacturing facility.

Laboratories that perform donation sample testing mandated by the FDA must be registered with the FDA as biologics manufacturers because this "qualification of raw materials" is considered part of the blood component manufacturing process. The infectious disease tests and testing equipment used to screen donation samples must be approved (licensed or cleared) for this purpose by the FDA's Center for Biologics Evaluation and Research. The FDA website maintains lists of assays approved for donor screening.[13] The tests must be performed exactly as specified in the manufacturers' package inserts. Tests and test platforms that are approved only for diagnostic use may not be used for screening blood donors.

TABLE 7-3.   Licensed Blood Donor Screening Tests Performed in the United States

Agent	Marker Detected	Screening Test Method	Supplemental Assays*
Babesia	*Babesia* spp. DNA/RNA	TMA or PCR	Research antibody and PCR
HBV	Hepatitis B surface antigen	ChLIA or EIA	Positive HBV DNA (FDA)[†] Neutralization (FDA)
	Total (IgM and IgG) antibody to hepatitis B core antigen	ChLIA or EIA	
	HBV DNA[‡]	TMA or PCR	
HCV	IgG antibody to HCV peptides and recombinant proteins	ChLIA or EIA	Positive HCV RNA (FDA)[†] RIBA (FDA),[§] line immunoblots (not FDA licensed)
	HCV RNA[‡]	TMA or PCR	
HIV-1/2	IgM and IgG antibody to HIV-1/2	ChLIA or EIA	Positive HIV RNA (FDA)[†] HIV-1: IFA or Western blot (FDA) HIV-2: EIA (FDA)
	HIV-1 RNA[‡]	TMA or PCR	
HTLV-I/II	IgG antibody to HTLV-I/II	ChLIA or EIA	Western blot (FDA) and line immunoblots (not FDA licensed)

(Continued)

TABLE 7-3. Licensed Blood Donor Screening Tests Performed in the United States (Continued)

Agent	Marker Detected	Screening Test Method	Supplemental Assays*
Treponema pallidum	IgG or IgG + IgM antibody to *Treponema pallidum* antigens *or*	Microhemagglutination, particle agglutination, immunofluorescence, or EIA	Second FDA-cleared *T. pallidum* screening test
	Nontreponemal serologic test for syphilis (eg, rapid plasma reagin)	Macroscopic flocculation	*T. pallidum* antigen-specific immunofluorescence, agglutination assays, or EIA
Trypanosoma cruzi	IgG antibody to *T. cruzi* (one time)[?]	ChLIA or EIA	ESA (FDA)
WNV and ZIKV	WNV or ZIKV RNA¶	TMA or PCR	Repeat or alternate NAT and antibody (IgM, IgG)

*Supplemental assays with "(FDA)" are FDA-approved supplemental assays. Other supplemental assays listed are not required but may be useful for donor counseling.

†Positive results on NAT screening tests are approved by the FDA as providing confirmation for reactive HBsAg, HIV antibody, and HCV antibody serology tests. If NAT is negative, a serologic supplemental test(s) must be performed.

‡Screening for HIV, HCV, and HBV nucleic acid in the United States is performed on minipools of 6 to 16 donor samples.

§As of 2013, RIBA is not available. Revised guidance provides alternate methods of confirmation.

? *T. cruzi* antibody testing may be limited to one-time testing of each donor.

¶ZIKV RNA testing is now performed using licensed NAT assays. See WNV text for specific use of ID- and MP-NAT.

TMA = transcription-mediated amplification; PCR = polymerase chain reaction; IND = Investigational New Drug (application); HBV = hepatitis B virus; ChLIA = chemiluminescent immunoassay; EIA = enzyme immunoassay; FDA = Food and Drug Administration; NAT = nucleic acid testing; HBsAg = hepatitis B surface antigen; HIV = human immunodeficiency virus; HCV = hepatitis C virus; Ig = immunoglobulin; RIBA = recombinant immunoblot assay; HIV-1/2 = HIV types 1 and 2; IFA = immunofluorescence assay; HTLV-I/II= human T-cell lymphotropic virus, types I and II; ESA = enzyme strip assay; WNV = West Nile virus; ZIKV = Zika virus; ID-NAT = individual donation NAT; MP-NAT = minipool NAT.

Serologic Testing Process

Most serologic screening tests (assays for the detection of antibody or antigen) are enzyme immunosorbent assays (EIAs) or chemiluminescent immunoassays (ChLIAs). Typically, the screening process involves performing the required test once on each donor sample. If the screening test is nonreactive, the test result is considered negative. If a test is "initially reactive," the package insert for the test typically requires that the test be repeated in duplicate. If both repeat results are nonreactive, the final interpretation is nonreactive or negative, and the unit may be used. If one or both repeat results are reactive, the donor sample is characterized as "repeatedly reactive," and the blood unit is not permitted to be used for allogeneic transfusion. In the case of cellular therapy products, there are some circumstances in which repeatedly reactive donations may be used. (See "Considerations in Testing Donors of Human Cells, Tissues, and Cellular and Tissue-Based Products" later in this chapter.)

The infectious disease tests approved for donor screening have performance characteristics chosen to make them highly sensitive. They are designed to detect infected individuals and minimize false-negative results. However, the assays also react with samples from some individuals who are not infected (false-positive results). Because the blood donor population is preselected by questioning to be at low risk of infection, the vast majority of repeatedly reactive results in donors do not represent true infections. To determine whether a repeatedly reactive screening result represents a true infection rather than a false-positive result, additional, more specific testing should be performed on the donor sample.

The FDA requires that repeatedly reactive donor specimens be further evaluated by FDA-approved supplemental assays when such assays are available.[1] The FDA has approved supplemental assays for HBsAg; HIV type 1 (HIV-1) antibodies; hepatitis C virus (HCV) antibodies; antibodies to human T-cell lymphotropic virus, types I and II (HTLV-I/II); and antibodies to *Trypanosoma cruzi*. The original HCV antibody confirmatory test (the recombinant immunoblot assay) is no longer available, but revised FDA guidance provides an alternate HCV supplemental testing pathway.[14] Table 7-3 displays the available supplemental assays. If no licensed supplemental assay is available, the FDA requires retesting of the donor sample using another FDA-licensed, -approved, or -cleared test to provide additional information for donor counseling; unlicensed supplemental testing may also provide useful information but cannot be used to requalify a donor or donation.

A donation that is repeatedly reactive on a screening test may not be used for allogeneic transfusion, regardless of the results of further testing. Syphilis is the only disease for which negative results on supplemental tests can, in some circumstances, enable use of a screening-test-reactive unit; this applies only to donations screened using a nontreponemal assay. This is discussed in the "Syphilis" section.

Nucleic Acid Testing

Nucleic acid testing (NAT) was implemented to reduce the seronegative window periods described earlier. Screening for viral nucleic acid [ribonucleic acid (RNA) or deoxyribonucleic acid (DNA)] is somewhat different from the serologic screening process. NAT requires the extraction of nucleic acid from a donor plasma or serum sample followed by nucleic acid amplification and detection of viral genetic sequences.

The test systems that were implemented in 1999 to screen donors for HIV and HCV RNA were semiautomated and had insufficient throughput to allow individual testing of each donor sample. Testing of seroconversion panels showed little loss of sensitivity if donor plasma samples were tested in small pools [minipools (MPs)], because levels of HIV and HCV RNA are typically high in the blood of infected individuals, and NAT assays are exquisitely sensitive.

Thus, in the initially approved NAT donor screening systems, MPs of 16 to 24 donor samples were prepared and tested. Current systems use pools of 6 to 16. If a pool is negative, all donations in that pool are considered negative for HIV and HCV RNA. If a pool showed NAT reactivity, further testing to the individual samples was performed to determine which donation was responsible for the reactive test result. Donations that were nonreactive on this additional testing could be released for transfusion. Donations that were reactive at the individual-sample level were considered reactive for viral nucleic acid and could not be released for transfusion.

In recent years, fully automated NAT systems have been developed. The automated test platforms approved by the FDA for donor screening use multiplex assays that detect HIV RNA, HCV RNA, and HBV DNA in one reaction. Some directly discriminate the reactive target during the initial screen; others require separate discriminatory testing to identify which virus is present. These systems are approved for testing of individual donations and pools of 6 to 16 donor samples, depending on the platform. The availability of fully automated NAT platforms creates the possibility of performing routine screening on individual donor samples [individual donation screening (ID-NAT)] rather than testing of pools (MP-NAT). However, the predicted frequency of reactive donations identified solely by ID-NAT as compared with MP-NAT at present does not justify this practice in the United States. It has been estimated that ID-NAT screening would minimally increase detection of infected donors, whereas the associated testing cost would be significantly higher than with MP-NAT.[15] An additional concern is that donors might be deferred for false-positive results more frequently with ID-NAT screening than with pooled screening.

In contrast to serologic testing policies, repeat testing is not permitted by the FDA for an individually reactive NAT sample to determine whether the initially reactive result represents a true-positive result. If an individual (unpooled) sample is reactive by NAT for HIV, HCV, or HBV, the FDA requires that the corresponding blood component be discarded and the donor be deferred for specified periods. FDA-approved donor reentry algorithms are available (Table 7-4).[27] In countries where donor screening for HIV/HCV/HBV is routinely performed by ID-NAT, it is common practice for initially reactive specimens to be subjected to repeat testing. Practices vary regarding the management of donors and components in cases where initial testing is reactive and repeat testing is nonreactive; in many countries, such donations are discarded because these results would not rule out the presence of a low concentration of virus. Donor management for this scenario varies and may include a deferral and reentry algorithm.

In the case of West Nile virus (WNV), ID-NAT screening rather than MP-NAT screening is recommended when WNV activity is occurring in a specific geographic area. Zika virus (ZIKV) testing by investigational NAT was introduced in response to the explosive ZIKV outbreak in the Americas during 2015-2017. Initially ID-NAT was required, but recently MP-NAT has been allowed, using 6 to 16 donations per pool and with triggers for converting to ID-NAT that are similar to those used for WNV.[26]

Implications of Reactive Test Results

A repeatedly reactive result on a screening test (or individually reactive NAT result) typically results in discard of the reactive donation. Linkage of laboratory information systems to blood bank computer systems prevents labeling and/or release of components from donations with reactive test results. A reactive test result may also indicate that the donor should be prohibited from making future donations, because many infections are persistent. Furthermore, past donations may also be considered suspect because the exact onset of a donor's infection cannot be determined.

Both the FDA and AABB have issued recommendations regarding whether reactive test results affect a donor's eligibility for future donations, whether components from prior donations should be retrieved (and if so, how far back in time), and whether recipients who previously received components from that donor should be notified. These recommendations are often guided by the results of supplemental or confirmatory testing performed on the donor sample.

Because these recommendations are complex, creating checklists detailing each action to be performed after a specific reactive test result is obtained may be helpful. Staff use these checklists to document completion of each

TABLE 7-4. Donor Reentry Eligibility Requiring Donor Follow-Up Testing and Temporary Deferrals Not Requiring Donor Follow-Up, by Infectious Disease Marker

Reactive Marker or Screening Test	Eligible for Reentry: Index Donation Test Results	Required for Reentry		
		Minimum Interval	Test Results on Predonation Sample or Other Requirements	

Hepatitis B Virus (HBV): Follow-Up Predonation Testing Requirements Differ (see below)

HBsAg[16]	Unconfirmed HBsAg • HBsAg—repeat reactive (RR), neutralization negative (NEG) or not done • anti-HBc—nonreactive (NR)	56 days	Subsequent donation meets all eligibility criteria and screens NR for required tests: • HBsAg • anti-HBc (Predonation testing of a follow-up sample before subsequent donation is not required)	
HBsAg within 28 days of HBV vaccine—no risk of exposure to HBV[17]	Confirmed positive (POS) HBsAg • HBsAg—RR, neutralization POS, and anti-HBc—NR *and* • Received HBV vaccine within 28 days of index donation *and* • Vaccine was given solely as protection from possible future exposure (ie, not for specific incident of potential exposure such as a needlestick*)	56 days	Subsequent donation meets all eligibility criteria and screens NR for required tests: • HBsAg • anti-HBc (Predonation testing of a follow-up sample before subsequent donation is not required)	
Anti-HBc[18]	Anti-HBc—RR on more than one occasion	8 weeks	Follow-up sample test results: • HBsAg—NR • Anti-HBc—NR • HBV NAT†—NR	

(Continued)

TABLE 7-4. Donor Reentry Eligibility Requiring Donor Follow-Up Testing and Temporary Deferrals Not Requiring Donor Follow-Up, by Infectious Disease Marker (Continued)

Reactive Marker or Screening Test	Eligible for Reentry: Index Donation Test Results	Required for Reentry	
		Minimum Interval	Test Results on Predonation Sample or Other Requirements
HBV NAT[19]	HBV NAT—reactive *and* HBsAg—NR and anti-HBc—RR *or* HBsAg—NR and anti-HBc—NR *or* HBsAg—RR, not confirmed, and anti-HBc—NR	6 months	Follow-up sample test results: • HBsAg—NR • Anti-HBc—NR • HBV NAT[†]—NR
NOT ELIGIBLE FOR REENTRY	• HBsAg—RR, confirmed (POS) by neutralization • HBV NAT—reactive, and HBsAg—RR (confirmed using either an HBsAg neutralization test or an HBV NAT with a supplemental claim), regardless of anti-HBc results • HBV NAT—reactive using a NAT assay that does not have a supplemental indication, and HBsAg—RR but unconfirmed by neutralization, and anti-HBc—RR		

Human Immunodeficiency Virus Types 1 and 2 (HIV-1/2)[20]: Follow-Up Required

HIV-1 NAT	HIV-1 NAT—reactive Anti-HIV-1/2[‡]—NR HIV-1 p24 EIA[§]—NR	8 weeks	• HIV-1 NAT—NR • Anti-HIV-1/2—NR

Test	Time	Results	Reentry criteria
Anti-HIV-1/2	8 weeks	• Anti-HIV-1/2—RR or • Anti-HIV-2—RR • HIV-1 NAT—NR or not done • HIV-1 p24 EIA[§]—NR • HIV-1 Western blot (WB)—NEG, or immunofluorescent assay (IFA)—NEG, indeterminate, unreadable, or not done	• HIV-1 NAT—NR • Anti-HIV-1/2—NR
HIV-1 p24	8 weeks	• HIV-1 p24 EIA—RR, neutralization POS or indeterminate (nonneutralized or invalid) • HIV-1 NAT—NR or not done • Anti-HIV-1/2—NR	• HIV-1 NAT—NR • Anti-HIV-1/2—NR
NOT ELIGIBLE FOR REENTRY		• HIV-1 NAT—reactive, and anti-HIV-1/2—RR (regardless of HIV-1 WB or IFA or HIV-1 p24 EIA test results) • HIV-1 NAT—reactive, and HIV-1 p24 EIA—RR (regardless of anti-HIV-1/2 test results) • HIV-1 NAT—NR (or not done), and anti-HIV-1/2—RR, HIV-1 WB or IFA—POS (regardless of HIV-1 p24 EIA test result) • HIV-1 NAT—NR (or not done), and anti-HIV-1/2—RR (regardless of WB or IFA result), and HIV-1 p24 EIA—RR (regardless of neutralization test result)	

Hepatitis C Virus (HCV)[20]: Follow-Up Required

Test	Time	Results	Reentry criteria
HCV NAT	6 months	• HCV NAT—reactive • Anti-HCV—NR	• HCV NAT—NR • Two different licensed tests for anti-HCV—NR
Anti-HCV	6 months	• HCV NAT—NR or not done • Anti-HCV—RR	• HCV NAT—NR • Two different licensed tests for anti-HCV—NR?
NOT ELIGIBLE FOR REENTRY		• HCV NAT—reactive, and anti-HCV—RR (regardless of historical HCV RIBA result) • HCV NAT—NR (or not done), and anti-HCV—RR, and historical HCV RIBA—POS	

(Continued)

TABLE 7-4. Donor Reentry Eligibility Requiring Donor Follow-Up Testing and Temporary Deferrals Not Requiring Donor Follow-Up, by Infectious Disease Marker (Continued)

Reactive Marker or Screening Test	Eligible for Reentry: Index Donation Test Results	Required for Reentry	
		Minimum Interval	Test Results on Predonation Sample or Other Requirements
***Treponema pallidum* (Syphilis)**[21,22]**: Predonation Testing Not Required for Reentry**			
Nontreponemal	• Nontreponemal test—reactive[¶] • Treponemal test—POS	3 months[#]	• Written evidence from a physician or public health clinic of completion of known effective treatment • Subsequent donation meets all eligibility criteria
Treponemal	• Treponemal screening test—reactive • Alternate treponemal screening test—NEG	N/A	• Different FDA-cleared treponemal screening test than the screening test—NEG on index or follow-up sample
	• Treponemal screening test—reactive • Alternate treponemal screening test—POS • Nontreponemal test—NEG	3 months[#]	• Written evidence from a physician or public health clinic of completion of known effective treatment • Subsequent donation meets all eligibility criteria
	• Treponemal screening test—reactive • Alternate treponemal screening test—POS • Nontreponemal test—POS	3 months[#]	• Written evidence from a physician or public health clinic of completion of known effective treatment • Subsequent donation meets all eligibility criteria

Trypanosoma cruzi (Chagas Disease)[23]: **Follow-Up Required**

Antibodies to *T. cruzi*	Antibodies to *T. cruzi*—RR *and* • Investigational/licensed supplemental test for antibodies to *T. cruzi*—NEG *or* • *T. cruzi* RIPA (unlicensed)—NEG *or* • Not tested with an investigational or licensed supplemental test for antibodies to *T. cruzi* and not tested with the unlicensed *T. cruzi* RIPA test	6 months	• Two different** licensed screening tests for antibodies to *T. cruzi*—NR *and* • Licensed supplemental test for antibodies to *T. cruzi*—NEG
NOT ELIGIBLE FOR REENTRY	• Positive or indeterminate with an investigational or licensed supplemental test for antibodies to *T. cruzi* • Positive or indeterminate with the unlicensed *T. cruzi* RIPA test		

Human T-Cell Lymphotropic Virus, Types I and II (HTLV-I/II)[24]: **Follow-Up Required**

Anti-HTLV-I/II	Anti-HTLV-I/II—RR • Anti-HTLV-I/II investigational or licensed supplemental test—NEG or not done *or* • HTLV research-use supplemental algorithm final interpretation—NEG	6 months	• Two different** licensed screening tests for anti-HTLV-I/II—NR
NOT ELIGIBLE FOR REENTRY	• POS or indeterminate for anti-HTLV-I/II with an investigational or licensed supplemental test • POS or indeterminate final interpretation with a research-use supplemental HTLV algorithm (eg, California Department of Public Health Laboratory HTLV algorithm)		

(Continued)

TABLE 7-4. Donor Reentry Eligibility Requiring Donor Follow-Up Testing and Temporary Deferrals Not Requiring Donor Follow-Up, by Infectious Disease Marker (Continued)

Reactive Marker or Screening Test	Eligible for Reentry: Index Donation Test Results	Required for Reentry		
		Minimum Interval	Test Results on Predonation Sample or Other Requirements	

***Babesia* spp.[25]: Predonation Testing Not Required for Reentry**

Babesia	*Babesia* NAT—reactive	2 years	Subsequent donation meets all eligibility criteria and screens NR by licensed NAT	

West Nile Virus (WNV)[26]: Predonation Testing Not Required for Reentry

WNV NAT	WNV NAT—reactive	120 days	Subsequent donation meets all eligibility criteria	

Zika virus (ZIKV)[27]: Predonation Testing Not Required for Reentry

ZIKV NAT	ZIKV NAT—reactive	120 days	Subsequent donation meets all eligibility criteria	

*If possible exposure (eg, needlestick) occurred, defer donor for 3 months.

†HBV NAT with sensitivity ? 2 IU/mL at 95% detection rate using specific procedures according to the package insert (eg, replicate testing).

‡Anti-HIV-1 or -2 or -1/2.

§If performed.

? If one anti-HCV test is RR and one anti-HCV test is NR, the FDA allows reconsideration of the donor for reentry by testing a follow-up sample after one more waiting period of at least 6 months using an HCV ID-NAT and two different licensed anti-HCV screening tests. If an anti-HCV test is still RR on a second follow-up sample at any time after the original donation, the FDA recommends permanent deferral of the donor.

¶"Reactive" includes "repeatedly reactive," as defined in the package insert.

#3 months after completion of a known effective treatment for syphilis.

**Testing should include the screening assay that resulted RR on the original donation.

HBV = hepatitis B virus; HBsAg = hepatitis B surface antigen; RR = repeat reactive; NR = nonreactive; NEG = negative; POS = positive; HBc = hepatitis B core antigen; NAT = nucleic acid testing; HIV-1/2 = human immunodeficiency virus, types 1 and 2; EIA = enzyme immunoassay; WB = Western blot; IFA = immunofluorescent assay; HCV = hepatitis C virus; RIBA = recombinant immunoblot assay; RIPA = radioimmunoprecipitation assay; HTLV-I/II = human T-cell lymphotropic virus, types I and II; ZIKV = Zika virus; ID-NAT = individual donation NAT.

action as they perform it, and they should be part of standard operating procedures.

Table 7-5 lists federal regulations, FDA guidance documents, AABB standards, and AABB Association Bulletins with recommendations regarding management of blood donors with reactive test results, retrieval of other components, and notification of prior recipients. These regulations and recommendations are described briefly below.

Donor Eligibility

FDA regulations in Title 21, CFR Part 610.41 address the deferral of donors with reactive screening test results. FDA guidance documents and AABB Association Bulletins contain more detailed recommendations regarding additional testing, donor eligibility, and donor counseling for these and other tests. Donors must be notified of any test results that affect their eligibility to donate or that could have important implications for their health. Systems that prevent future collections from ineligible donors and the release of any components inadvertently collected from such individuals are required.

The FDA has issued guidance documents (referenced in Table 7-4) that define reentry pathways for donors deferred for reactivity on anti-HIV, anti-HCV, HBsAg, and anti-HBc tests; serologic tests for syphilis and *T. cruzi*; and HIV/HCV/HBV, WNV, *Babesia*, and ZIKV NAT. Most of the pathways require that the donor have negative results on specified tests after a defined waiting period. Reentry of donors must follow the FDA-defined algorithms explicitly.[28]

Retrieval of Prior Donations and Notification of Prior Recipients ("Look-Back")

The FDA and AABB offer guidance regarding the appropriate management of previously collected blood components from donors whose current donation is repeatedly reactive (or, in the case of NAT, individually reactive) on an infectious disease screening test. These recommendations address the concern that at the time of the previous donation(s), the donor could have been in the window period of an infection

even though the screening test results were negative.

For HIV and HCV tests, the algorithms for managing prior donations and recipients of prior donations are detailed in 21 CFR 610.46 and 610.47. These requirements are replicated in the Centers for Medicare and Medicaid Services regulations (Title 42, CFR Part 482.27) to ensure hospital transfusion service compliance with recipient notification requirements. For other agents, recommendations for the management of previously donated components may be found in the FDA guidance documents or AABB Association Bulletins (or both) listed in Table 7-5.

In most cases, the FDA and AABB recommend retrieval and quarantine of any remaining components from prior donations of that donor. It is essential that the retrieval of in-date components be initiated immediately after the repeatedly reactive result is obtained. This prevents transfusion of these components while confirmatory testing is performed. The FDA requires initiation of retrieval within 3 calendar days of a reactive HIV, HCV, WNV, ZIKV, or *T. cruzi* test and within 1 week of a reactive HBsAg, anti-HBc, or anti-HTLV screening test. Babesia tests also require component retrieval; however, no specific time-frame has been mandated by the FDA. If confirmatory test results on the current donation are negative, the FDA, in some circumstances, permits re-release of the prior donations. In many cases, some or all components from prior donations will have been transfused. For some infectious agents, the FDA and AABB recommend that the recipients of prior donations from confirmed-positive donors be notified within 12 weeks via their physicians of their possible exposure to the infectious agent.

Recommendations for notification of recipients of prior donations ("look-back") are usually issued by AABB, the FDA, or both, at the time a new test is implemented, but these recommendations may evolve as supplemental (confirmatory) tests become available or medical treatments are developed for the infection in question. Look-back is required by law only for HIV and HCV tests (21 CFR 610.46 and 610.47). For an HIV look-back investigation involving a deceased prior recipient, the next of kin must be notified. The CFR spells out specific

TABLE 7-5. Regulations and Standards Related to Blood Donor Testing and Actions Following Reactive Test Results*

Agent/Test	Relevant Document	Topics				
		Donor Testing and PRT	Donor Management	Product Retrieval	Recipient Notification	Donor Reentry
HIV-1/2	Title 21, CFR Part 610.40[1]	X				
	Title 21, CFR Part 610.41[1]		X			
	Title 21, CFR Part 610.46[1]			X	X	
	Title 42, CFR Part 482.27[29]			X	X	
	FDA guidance, October 2004[30]	X				
	FDA guidance, December 2017[20]	X	X	X	X	X
	AABB BB/TS Standard 5.8.5, 5.8.6[31(p34)]	X				
HIV-1 group O	FDA guidance, August 2009[32]	X	X			X
HBV	Title 21, CFR Part 610.40[1]	X				
	Title 21, CFR Part 610.41[1]		X			
	FDA guidance, October 2012[19]	X	X			X
	AABB BB/TS Standard 5.8.5, 5.8.6[31(p34)]	X				
	FDA guidance, September 2017[33]					X

Analyte	Reference					
HBsAg	FDA memorandum, December 1987[16]	X			X	
	AABB BB/TS Standard 5.8.5, 5.8.6[31(p34)]	X				
HBsAg and anti-HBc†	FDA memorandum, July 1996[34]			X		
Anti-HBc	FDA guidance, May 2010[18]	X				
	AABB BB/TS Standard 5.8.5, 5.8.6[31(p34)]	X				
HBV (vaccine)	FDA guidance, November 2011[17]	X				
HCV	Title 21, CFR Part 610.40[1]					X
	Title 21, CFR Part 610.41[1]				X	
	Title 21, CFR Part 610.47[1]		X	X		
	Title 42, CFR Part 482.27[29]		X	X		
	FDA guidance, October 2004[30]					X
	FDA guidance, December 2010[35]		X	X		
	FDA guidance, December 2017[20]	X	X	X		X
	FDA Guidance, October 2019[36]				X	
	AABB BB/TS Standard 5.8.5, 5.8.6[31(p34)]		X	X		X

(Continued)

TABLE 7-5. Regulations and Standards Related to Blood Donor Testing and Actions Following Reactive Test Results* (Continued)

Agent/Test	Relevant Document	Topics				
		Donor Testing and PRT	Donor Management	Product Retrieval	Recipient Notification	Donor Reentry
HTLV-I/II	Title 21, CFR Part 610.40[1]	X				
	Title 21, CFR Part 610.41[1]		X			
	FDA guidance, February 2020[24]	X	X	X	X	X
	AABB BB/TS Standard 5.8.5, 5.8.6[31(p34)]	X				
Syphilis	Title 21, CFR Part 610.40[1]	X				
	Title 21, CFR Part 610.41[1]		X			
	FDA guidance, September 2014[21]	X	X			X
	AABB BB/TS Standard 5.8.5, 5.8.6[31(p32)]	X				
Trypanosoma cruzi	FDA guidance, December 2017[23]	X	X	X	X	X
	FDA draft guidance, December 2017[22]					X
	AABB BB/TS Standard 5.8.5, 5.8.6[31(p34)]	X				

Agent	Document					
WNV	FDA guidance, June 2005[37]	X	X	X	X	X
	FDA guidance, November 2009[26]	X	X	X	X	
	AABB BB/TS Standard 5.8.5, 5.8.6[31(p34)]		X			
	Association Bulletin #13-02[38]		X			
ZIKV	FDA guidance, July 2018[27]	X	X	X	X	X
ZIKV (and DENV and CHIKV)	Association Bulletin #16-07[39]	X	X	X	X	X
Bacteria	FDA guidance, September 2019[40]		X			
	AABB BB/TS Standards 5.1.5.1, 5.1.5.2, 5.1.5.3[31(pp11-12)]	X	X	X‡		
	Association Bulletin #05-02[41]	X		X		
	Association Bulletin #12-04[42]		X			
	Association Bulletin #04-07[43]	X	X	X	X	
Parvovirus B19§	FDA guidance, July 2009[44]		X			
Babesia spp.	FDA guidance, May 2019[25]	X	X	X	X	X

*Recommendations in effect as of August 2018. Blood centers may be bound by additional requirements, such as specifications in Recovered Plasma contracts.

†Memorandum also includes recommendations regarding HCV and HTLV, but these recommendations have been superseded by subsequent documents.

‡Co-components of current donation.

§Plasma for further manufacture only.

HIV-1/2 = human immunodeficiency virus, types 1 and 2; CFR = Code of Federal Regulations; FDA = Food and Drug Administration; BB/TS Standards = *Standards for Blood Banks and Transfusion Services*; HBV = hepatitis B virus; HBsAg = hepatitis B surface antigen; anti-HBc = antibody to hepatitis B core antigen; HCV = hepatitis C virus; HTLV-I/II = human T-cell lymphotropic virus, types I and II; WNV = West Nile virus; ZIKV = Zika virus; DENV = dengue viruses; CHIKV = chikungunya virus.

timelines for component retrieval and recipient notification. It also specifies how far back in time (ie, to which donations) the retrieval and notification should extend. For other agents, such as WNV, ZIKV, *Babesia* spp, and *T. cruzi*, recommendations regarding retrieval and recipient notification are included in FDA guidance documents and AABB Association Bulletins. Investigational protocols for unlicensed screening assays may also include these requirements. Table 7-5 indicates which of these documents address product retrieval or recipient notification.

In the absence of published guidance, it is not always obvious whether or when it is appropriate to notify prior recipients of their possible exposure to infection. If there is no supplemental assay available or further testing performed, it is not possible to determine whether a repeatedly reactive screening test result for a donor represents a true infection. Furthermore, if there is no effective treatment for that infection, there may be no medical benefit to the recipient of being told that he or she might have been exposed. There could, however, be a public health benefit from such a notification; specifically, a recipient who is alerted of a potential exposure can be tested and, if the results are positive, take precautions to avoid further spread of the infection.

Cytomegalovirus Testing of Components for Immunocompromised Recipients

Some common infections cause relatively innocuous illnesses in immunocompetent individuals but can cause severe disease in immunocompromised patients; such is the case with cytomegalovirus (CMV).

CMV is a lipid-enveloped DNA virus in the *Herpesviridae* family. Like other herpesviruses, CMV causes lifelong infection, typically in a latent state, with the potential for reactivation. Primary CMV infection in immunologically competent individuals is mild, with symptoms ranging from none to an infectious mononucleosis-type syndrome. In immunocompromised patients, however, both primary infection and reactivated disease can be overwhelming and even fatal. CMV can be transmitted by blood transfusion, primarily through intact white cells contained in cellular blood components. Frozen/thawed plasma components do not appear to transmit CMV infection. Immunocompromised patients who are at increased risk of transfusion-transmitted disease include fetuses, low-birthweight premature infants who are born to CMV-seronegative mothers, and CMV-seronegative recipients of solid organ or allogeneic hematopoietic stem cell (HSC) transplants from seronegative donors.[45]

Most blood donors have had prior exposure to CMV, indicated by the presence of CMV antibodies. Therefore, it would not be possible to produce an adequate supply of blood if all CMV antibody-positive donations were discarded.

It is possible, however, to minimize CMV transmission to patients at risk of severe CMV disease, such as those described above. These patients should be supported with cellular blood components that have a reduced risk of transmitting CMV. These reduced-risk options include using blood components from donors who are CMV antibody negative or components that have been effectively leukocyte reduced. The literature suggests that these two methods have similar but not identical efficacy, with an estimated transmission risk by seronegative components of 1% to 2% vs a risk of 2% to 3% with leukocyte-reduced components.[45-47] Recent studies, however, found no CMV transmissions among a total of 176 carefully monitored allogeneic stem cell transplant recipients who received CMV-untested, leukocyte-reduced components.[48,49] Because many at-risk patients receive leukocyte-reduced components and are monitored closely for CMV infection, treated early with anti-CMV drugs, or both, it is difficult to measure a benefit from also providing CMV-seronegative components to these patients. There has been a transition to reduced use of CMV-seronegative blood in favor of universally leukocyte-reduced blood, particularly because there is no evidence that CMV continues to be transmitted by leukocyte-reduced components. However, there remains a small but theoretical risk of transmission from blood components collected before seroconversion or following early antibody production because such units contain the highest levels of CMV DNA[50]; CMV DNA screening or pathogen inactivation (when universally available) would likely eliminate this risk. The major risk of transmission occurs in low-birthweight infants as a result of breastfeeding from a CMV-infected mother.[51,52]

Autologous Donations

The FDA requires infectious disease testing of autologous donations that are shipped from one facility to another. If the receiving facility does not permit autologous donations to be crossed over to the general inventory, the FDA requires testing of only the first donation in each 30-day period [21 CFR 610.40(d)(3)]. The labeling of the unit must be consistent with its testing status. Units from donors with repeatedly reactive tests must be labeled with biohazard labels. Some hospitals have policies that prohibit acceptance of autologous units with positive results on some tests because there is a potential for an infectious unit to be transfused to the wrong patient.

Considerations in Testing Donors of Human Cells, Tissues, and Cellular and Tissue-Based Products

Both the questions and tests required by the FDA to screen donors of human cells, tissues, and cellular and tissue-based products (HCT/Ps) differ from those for blood donors, and the requirements vary by type of tissue. The general requirements are spelled out in 21 CFR 1271 and an August 2007 FDA guidance document and are summarized in Table 7-6.[54,55] The FDA has issued additional guidance regarding testing of HCT/Ps for syphilis[56] and WNV,[57] as well as draft guidance documents on other infectious agents, including ZIKV. An up-to-date list of FDA HCT/P guidance documents may be found on the "Tissue Guidances" page of the FDA website.[58]

The time frames for testing HCT/P donors are specified in 21 CFR 1271 and the August 2007 FDA guidance document.[54,55] In most cases, the samples for infectious disease testing must be obtained within 7 days before or after the tissue donation. Samples from donors of peripheral blood hematopoietic progenitor cells or marrow may be tested up to 30 days before donation; however, longer intervals between testing and transplantation may be associated with transmission of infectious agents.[59] Autologous tissues and reproductive tissues from recipients' sexually intimate partners may be exempt from some testing requirements.

Laboratories that test samples from HCT/P donors must be registered with the FDA and must use tests approved for testing of these donors, when such tests are available. HCT/P testing requirements and approved tests may be found on the FDA website.[60] Testing laboratories must take care to check package inserts for HCT/P testing methods; a package insert may require a different testing method for HCT/P donors than for blood donors. For example, NAT for most types of HCT/P donors must be performed on individual donor samples; MP-NAT is not permitted for most HCT/P donor categories.

In some cases, FDA regulations permit the use of HCT/P donations that are reactive on infectious disease screening tests. These exceptions are listed in 21 CFR 1271.65. The FDA has issued specific labeling, storage, and notification requirements for these tissues. Testing of HCT/P donors for antibody to *T. cruzi* is not required by the FDA (at the time of writing this chapter).

International Variations in Donor Testing

Although this chapter focuses on infectious disease screening in the United States, the general approach to donor screening is similar in other countries. However, the specific donor questions and tests vary from country to country based on the regional epidemiology of infections and tests available. For example, most countries where WNV is not endemic do not test for this agent, although they may question donors and defer them for travel to WNV-affected countries. Countries where HBV is hyperendemic cannot exclude donations from individuals who test reactive for anti-HBc, without adversely affecting the adequacy of their blood supply. The AABB Subcommittee for the Evaluation of Variances considers variance applications from facilities desiring accreditation in countries where national practices and available testing methods are different from those used in the United States. Some blood donations outside the

TABLE 7-6. FDA Testing Requirements for HCT/Ps (as of October 2018)

Tissue Type	Agent	Tests
All tissues	HIV	Antibody to HIV-1 and HIV-2* HIV-1 RNA*
	HBV	Hepatitis B surface antigen* Antibody to hepatitis B core antigen*
	HCV	Antibody to hepatitis C* HCV RNA*
	Treponema pallidum	FDA-licensed, -approved, or -cleared donor screening test
All living donors[†]	WNV	WNV RNA*
For donors of viable leukocyte-rich HCT/Ps (eg, hematopoietic progenitor cells or semen), test for the following in addition to the above:	HTLV-I/II	Antibody to HTLV-I/II*
	CMV	FDA-cleared screening test for anti-CMV (total IgG and IgM)
For donors of reproductive tissues, test for the following in addition to the above:	*Chlamydia trachomatis*	FDA-licensed, -approved, or -cleared diagnostic test
	Neisseria gonorrhea	FDA-licensed, -approved, or -cleared diagnostic test

*These tests must be FDA licensed for donor screening.
[†]Living donors must meet clinical and behavioral eligibility requirements for ZIKV exposure, but no testing is required to be considered eligible.[53]
FDA = Food and Drug Administration; HCT/Ps = human cells, tissues, and cellular and tissue-based products; HIV = human immunodeficiency virus; HBV = hepatitis B virus; HCV = hepatitis C virus; WNV = West Nile virus; HTLV = human T-cell lymphotropic virus; CMV = cytomegalovirus; Ig = immunoglobulin.

United States are tested for agents not included in routine US donor testing. Hepatitis E virus (HEV), discussed later in this chapter, is an example.

RESIDUAL INFECTIOUS RISKS OF TRANSFUSION

Despite donor screening, blood components may still transmit infections. The residual risk of transmission varies according to the incidence of the infection in the donor population and the nature of the donor screening processes in place.

Agents for Which Blood Is Tested

Transfusion transmissions of HIV, HCV, and HBV are now so rare that the rates of transmission cannot be measured by prospective clinical studies. The risk can only be estimated by modeling.

One theoretical source of risk is a virus strain that the current test kits do not detect. The Centers for Disease Control and Prevention (CDC), blood providers, and the test manufacturers conduct surveillance for such emerging strains.[61] Over time, the FDA has required that test manufacturers expand their detection capabilities to include new strains. A second potential cause of transmission is a quarantine failure (ie, a blood bank's failure to quarantine a unit that tests reactive). Quarantine errors are thought to be rare in facilities that use electronic systems to control blood component labeling and release because these systems are designed to prevent the labeling and release of any unit with incomplete testing or a reactive test result. Erroneous releases appear to occur more frequently in facilities that rely on manual records and quarantine processes; facilities using manual processes are rare.[62]

The primary cause of residual transmissions is thought to be donations from individuals in the window period of early infection, before test results are positive. Figure 7-1 displays the sequence in which different types of donor screening tests demonstrate reactivity. Over time, the window periods have been shortened by the implementation of donor screening tests that detect earlier infections. However, because no test gives a positive result immediately after an individual acquires an infection, the infectious window period remains a concern. With MP-NAT, the average duration of the window period is estimated to be 9.0 to 9.1 days for HIV and 7.4 days for HCV.[15,63] The window period for HBV is longer, currently estimated to be 18.5 to 26.5 days, the reasons for which will be discussed later in this chapter.

The likelihood that a blood donation has been obtained from a donor in the window period can be estimated mathematically using the incidence × window-period model[64]:

Residual risk of window period donation = length of window period × incidence of infections in repeat donors

The incidence of infections in repeat donors can be calculated from the observed number of donors with a negative test result on one donation but a positive result on a subsequent donation (ie, seroconverting donors), divided by the amount of time (usually in person-years) of surveillance or follow-up of the sampled population. This method is limited by considering incidence rates only in repeat donors and does not permit assessment of the likelihood that first-time donors might be in the window period. This method also does not consider NAT-converting donors.

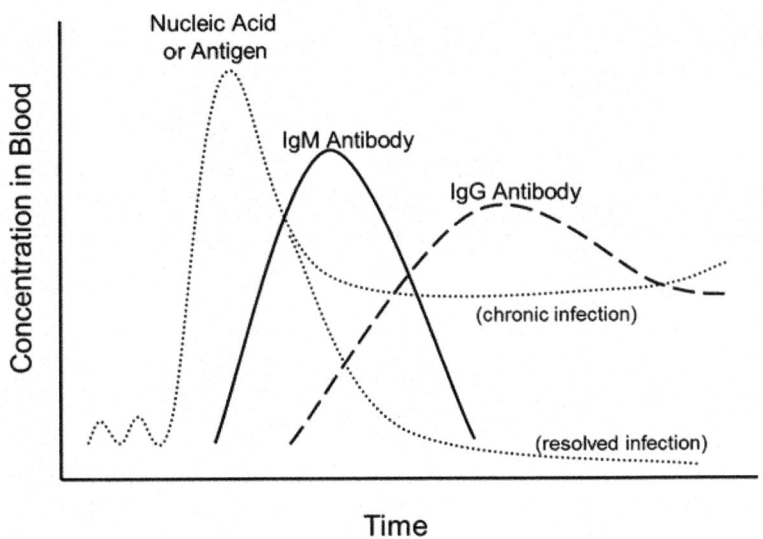

FIGURE 7-1. Time sequence of the appearance of various markers of infection.

Other methods permit measurement of new infection rates in both first-time and repeat donors using tests that differentiate new from established infections. Such tests include NAT (ie, with NAT, donor blood that contains HIV or HCV RNA or HBV DNA, but not antibodies to these infections, can be interpreted as representing a very early infection) and "sensitive/less sensitive," "detuned" antibody, or limiting antigen (LAg) avidity testing.[15,63,65,66] When these alternative methods have been used, new HIV and HCV infections were two to four times more common among first-time donors than among repeat donors.[63,65-67] However, both of these donor populations have significantly lower infection rates than the general population. The continued importance of using donor education and questioning to select donors with a low incidence of infection is explored in more detail in the HIV section below.

The current estimated risks of HIV, HCV, and HBV transmission in donors, based on window-period and incidence calculations, are shown in Table 7-7.[63,68]

Agents for Which No Donor Screening Tests Are Available

Essentially any infectious agent that can circulate in the blood of an apparently healthy person might be transmitted by transfusion. It is impossible to estimate the risk of transmission for each of the infectious agents for which donors are not tested. The infections that are most likely to be recognized as transmitted by transfusion are those that have a distinctive clinical presentation and are otherwise rare in the United States. The likelihood that an infection will be recognized as transfusion transmitted is enhanced if the infection is usually associated with a clinical or behavioral risk that the transfusion recipient lacks (eg, when malaria develops in a transfusion recipient who has not traveled to a known malaria-endemic region).

If a life-threatening agent is recognized as a potential threat to the blood supply, both AABB and the FDA typically consider whether a donor screening question could be used to exclude potentially exposed donors in the absence of a donor screening test. Donor questioning regarding travel to, and residence in, areas where an agent is endemic is currently the only means of protecting the US blood supply from malaria and variant Creutzfeldt-Jakob disease. Most infectious agents, however, do not have such clear geographic risk areas. In general, it is difficult to design donor questions that are both sensitive (ie, detect most infected individuals) and specific (ie, exclude only infected individuals).

TABLE 7-7. Estimated Risks of Transfusion-Transmitted Infection in the United States Based on the Incidence/Window-Period Model

Study Period	Agent	Incidence per 10⁵ Person-Years	Infectious Window Period (days)	Residual Risk per Donated Unit
2007-2008[63]*	HIV	3.1	9.1	1:1,467,000
2007-2008[63]*	HCV	5.1	7.4	1:1,149,000
2009-2011[68]†	HBV	1.6	26.5-18.5	1:843,000 to 1:1,208,000

*HIV and HCV risk estimates are based on MP-NAT in pools of 16.
†HBV risk estimates are based on MP-NAT in pools of 16 using the Grifols Ultrio Plus assay. The range indicated for the HBV window period reflects uncertainty regarding the minimum infectious dose of HBV (1 copy in 20 mL plasma vs 10 copies in 20 mL plasma).
HIV = human immunodeficiency virus; HCV = hepatitis C virus; HBV = hepatitis B virus; MP-NAT = minipool nucleic acid testing.

An alternative method of protecting the blood supply from infectious agents is pathogen inactivation. Heat-inactivation, solvent/detergent (SD) treatment, nanofiltration, chromatography, cold ethanol fractionation, and other approaches have been used with remarkable success to inactivate or remove residual pathogens in plasma derivatives. Pathogen inactivation systems for platelets and transfusable plasma have been available outside the United States for several years, and one manufacturer's system was FDA approved for use in the United States in December 2015 (INTERCEPT Blood System). SD-treated plasma (SD plasma) is also available for transfusion in the United States; Octaplas (Octapharma) is manufactured from pools of human source plasma (630-1520 individual donors).[69] Pathogen inactivation systems are discussed later in this chapter.

The AABB Transfusion-Transmitted Diseases Committee published an extensive review of infectious agents that are possible threats to the blood supply.[70] Potential mitigation strategies were discussed for each agent, including the documented or theoretical efficacy of pathogen inactivation processes. AABB periodically updates this information via its website, adding materials for new potential threats as they are identified.[71] The agents deemed to pose the highest threat from either a scientific or public perspective are briefly discussed in this chapter. (See the 2009 supplement to *TRANSFUSION* and updates on the AABB website for a more thorough review of these potential infectious risks.[70,71])

SCREENING FOR SPECIFIC AGENTS

Human Immunodeficiency Virus

HIV-1, a lipid-enveloped, single-stranded RNA spherical retrovirus containing two linear, positive-sense strands of RNA, was identified in 1984 as the causative agent of AIDS. Blood donation screening for antibodies to this virus was implemented in the United States in 1985. In 1992, donor screening tests were modified to include detection of antibodies to HIV-2, a closely relat-ed virus identified initially in West Africa, only rarely seen in the United States.[72]

HIV is transmitted by infected body fluids either through sexual or parenteral contact (eg, injection drug use), or vertically (from infected mothers to their infants). Although heterosexual and vertical HIV transmission predominates in some parts of the world, new HIV cases in the United States continue to be concentrated in men who have sex with men (MSM), injection drug users, and individuals with high-risk heterosexual contact (defined as contact with an individual who is HIV positive or in an identified risk group for HIV, such as MSM or injection drug users).[73]

Current donation screening for HIV includes NAT for HIV-1 RNA and serologic testing for antibodies to HIV. The antibody tests approved for donor screening detect both immunoglobulin M (IgM) and IgG antibody to both HIV-1 and HIV-2. Current-generation assays also detect antibody to HIV-1 group O, a strain of HIV-1 found primarily in Central and West Africa. With this detection claim, donor centers no longer need to exclude individuals who have resided in, received medical treatment in, or had sex partners from HIV-1 group O endemic areas.[32]

The average window period after HIV-1 infection to test detection is currently estimated to be 9.0 to 9.1 days for MP-NAT.[15,63] Based on window-period and incidence-rate calculations, the current risk in the United States of acquiring HIV from transfusion from repeat blood donors is estimated to be approximately 1 in 1.5 million units (Table 7-7). Unpublished data indicate that the residual risk has further declined to 1 in 2 million to 1 in 3 million units. However, residual risks would be two to four times higher if first-time donor risk was included in these estimates.[66] Also, it should be noted that these risks are based on the transfusion of only 1 unit, and risk increases if multiple units are transfused.

In the United States, blood donor screening questions exclude very broadly defined populations at increased risk of HIV. Given the short delay of only days between infection and detection of infection by NAT, experts have questioned whether donor interviews and exclusion of donors with increased risk remain medically necessary. The continued importance of a low-risk donor population becomes evident if different HIV incidence figures are used for the blood safety calculation. For example, HIV incidence rates as high as 1% to 8% have been observed in some high-risk populations, such as young urban MSM.[74,75] If an individual from a population with a 1% incidence of HIV donates blood, the likelihood that this individual is in the window period and that the component will transmit HIV can be calculated as follows:

Risk that the donation is in window period =
length of window period × incidence of
infection in donor population =
(9.0 days/365 days/year) ×
(1/100 person-years) = 1/4100.

This is the likelihood that a unit from this high-risk donor would harbor HIV but be missed by the current donor screening. This risk is clearly much higher than the estimated HIV transmission risk of 1 in 1.5 million for a unit of blood obtained from the current donor population. Thus, despite the short window period with current testing, inclusion of donors with a high risk of HIV would have a profoundly adverse impact on blood safety. Accordingly, questioning of donors for risk and temporarily excluding those at increased risk to minimize window-period donations continue to be critical for preserving blood safety.

Although there has been great interest in developing a more specific donor-screening algorithm based on specific behaviors instead of sexual preference that would exclude only individuals who are truly at increased risk of HIV, the FDA guidance issued in December 2015 indicated that the efficacy of a more specific algorithm had not yet been established. An April FDA guidance lists the current definitions of potential risks for HIV exposure in the United States that require donor deferral. Most of these risk categories, including MSM behavior, now require a 3-month deferral.[22]

Hepatitis B Virus

HBV is a lipid-enveloped, spherical virus in the *Hepadnaviridae* family. It is unique in that it has a partially double-stranded circular DNA genome with overlapping reading frames. Like HIV, HBV is transmitted by contact with body fluids from HBV-infected individuals. Jaundice is noted in only 25% to 40% of adult cases and in a smaller proportion of childhood cases. A large percentage of perinatally acquired cases result in chronic infection, but most HBV infections acquired in adulthood are cleared. HBV is highly prevalent in certain parts of the world, such as eastern Asia and Africa, where perinatal transmission and resultant chronic infection have amplified infection rates in the population. In the United States, the incidence of acute HBV infection has decreased by at least 80% with the implementation of routine vaccination programs. Maternal screening for HBV and newborn prophylaxis have also been effective in reducing perinatal transmission.

During HBV infection, DNA and viral envelope antigen (HBsAg) are typically detectable in circulating blood. Antibody to the core antigen is produced soon after the appearance of HBsAg, initially in the form of IgM antibody, followed by IgG. As infected individuals produce antibody to the surface antigen (anti-HBsAg), HBsAg is cleared.

The FDA requires donor screening for HBsAg, HBV DNA, and total anti-HBc (IgM and IgG antibody). Measurements of HBV incidence in donors have been complicated by the transience of HBsAg and false-positive results on the HBsAg test.[68] Published estimates of the infectious window have varied because of differences in the sensitivity of various HBV assays and lack of certainty regarding the level of virus in a blood component that is required for infectivity.[76,77] Recent publications provide window-period estimates for different potential infectious doses of virus (eg, 10 copies/20 mL of plasma vs 1 copy/20 mL of plasma). The infectious window before a positive result on the Abbott PRISM (Abbott Laboratories) HBsAg test has been estimated to be 30 to 38 days.[76] With the addition of HBV DNA testing in MPs of 16, the window period is estimated to have been reduced to 18.5 to 26.5 days (range dependent on whether the infectious dose is assumed to be 1 copy or 10 copies).[68] Using these MP-testing estimates, US HBV transfusion-transmission risk has been estimated to be between 1 in 843,000 donations and 1 in 1.2 million donations (Table 7-7).[68] Residual risks have been declining for HBV and are likely now in the 1 in 2 million to 1 in 3 million range based on unpublished data.

Donor screening for HBV DNA is of value in detecting HBV-infected donors. HBV DNA is detected during the infectious window period before HBsAg detection; however, DNA levels may be below the limits of detection of MP-NAT assays.[76,77] Later in infection, following the clearance of HBsAg, HBV NAT may detect persistent (ie, "occult") infection.[76,77] Such infections are interdicted in the United States by the donor screening test for anti-HBc, with about 1% of anti-HBc repeat-reactive donations considered to be from donors with occult HBV infection due to the presence of HBV DNA in the absence of detectable HBsAg.[68] High-sensitivity NAT is required to detect occult HBV infections because viral loads are typically low. HBV NAT can also detect acute HBV infections in individuals who have previously been vaccinated.[78,79] Such individuals may never develop detectable HBsAg, but they may have detectable DNA. The infectivity of such donations is not known because these units contain vaccine-induced antibodies to HBsAg. Routine HBV DNA screening of US blood donations detects at least some of these infections. There may come a time when HBsAg testing is deemed unnecessary due to the use of HBV NAT; the additional risk, if HBsAg were discontinued with testing only by NAT and anti-HBc, has been projected to be 1 per 4.4 million donations.[80]

Hepatitis C Virus

HCV is a small, lipid-enveloped, single-stranded RNA virus in the family *Flaviviridae*. HCV was shown to be the cause of up to 90% of cases previously called NANB transfusion-related hepatitis.[81] Most HCV infections are asymptomatic. However, HCV infection is associated with a high risk of chronicity, which can result in liver cirrhosis, hepatocellular carcinoma, and a variety of extrahepatic syndromes.

HCV is transmitted primarily through blood exposure. In the United States, about 55% of HCV infections are associated with injection drug use or receipt of transfusion before donor screening in 1992, but the risk factors for the remainder of the infections are not clear.[82] Sexual and vertical transmissions are uncommon, although coinfection with HIV increases transmission rates by these routes.

Current donor screening for HCV includes NAT for HCV RNA and serologic testing for antibodies to HCV. FDA guidance released in October 2019 recommends further testing of repeat-reactive donations by HCV NAT and, if nonreactive, by a second licensed screening test.[36] The average window period between infection and detection of infection by MP-NAT is estimated to be 7.4 days.[15] The serologic test detects only IgG antibody, a relatively late marker of infection. Therefore, there may be a significant lag (1.5 to 2 months) between detection of RNA and detection of antibody.[83] Donor questioning has limited potential to exclude individuals who may be harboring HCV infection because a large proportion of infected individuals are asymptomatic and admit to no risk factors or possible exposure. Despite this limitation, the current estimated US risk of HCV transmission by transfusion is extremely low—approximately 1 in 1.1 million (Table 7-7).[63] As already mentioned for HIV and HBV, the residual risk of HCV has been declining as well, possibly as low as the 1 in 2 million to 1 in 3 million range.

Human T-Cell Lymphotropic Virus, Types I and II

HTLV-I is a lipid-enveloped RNA retrovirus. It was the first human retrovirus identified, isolated in 1978 from a patient with cutaneous T-cell lymphoma. A closely related virus, HTLV-II, was later isolated from a patient with hairy cell leukemia. Both viruses are highly cell associated, infect lymphocytes, and cause lifelong infections, but most of these infections remain asymptomatic. Approximately 2% to 5% of HTLV-I-infected individuals develop adult T-cell leukemia/lymphoma after a lag of 20 to 30 years. A smaller percentage develop a neurologic disease called HTLV-associated myelopathy or tropical spastic paraparesis. HTLV-II disease associations remain unclear. Both infections are thought to be spread through blood, sexual contact, and breastfeeding.

HTLV-I infection is endemic in certain parts of the world, including regions of Japan, South America, the Caribbean, and Africa. In the United States, infections are found in immigrants from areas where it is endemic, injection drug users, and the sexual partners of these individuals. Approximately one-half of the HTLV infections in US blood donors are with HTLV-II.[84,85]

The only FDA-approved donor tests for HTLV infection are screening assays for IgG antibody to HTLV-I and HTLV-II. Units that are reactive on the screening assay may not be released for transfusion. Until recently, only screening assays were licensed by the FDA for HTLV-I/II antibody detection. The screening tests do not differentiate between HTLV-I and HTLV-II antibodies. A Western blot licensed in December 2014 (MP Biomedicals, version 2.4) uses recombinant and peptide antigens in addition to HTLV-I viral lysate to detect and differentiate between HTLV-I and HTLV-II antibodies. In February 2020, the FDA released guidance allowing a reentry algorithm for certain categories of donors who were previously deferred due to reactive screening results.[24]

Risk estimates for transfusion-transmitted HTLV are somewhat uncertain, given the absence of well-defined window periods for the current HTLV antibody tests. However, there is no evidence of residual HTLV transfusion-transmission risk, which is estimated at less than 1 per several million. Because HTLV is cell associated, leukocyte reduction likely reduces infectivity; in addition, infectivity is reduced with increased refrigerated red cell storage.[86,87] Like CMV, HTLV is thought to be transmitted only by white-cell-containing blood components and not by frozen/thawed plasma components.[84,85] The low frequency of HTLV transfusion transmission (even in the absence of testing) is related to the low incidence of infection in the United States, for example. Because of this, the nearly universal use of leukocyte reduction, and the poor persistence of HTLV in stored blood components, some countries (eg, the United Kingdom and the Netherlands) have transitioned or are considering transition from testing each donation to testing donors only one time, so that donors with negative results on their initial do-

nation remain qualified as HTLV-negative for all future donations.[88,89]

Hepatitis E Virus

One agent that has received recent attention globally is HEV, a small, nonenveloped, icosahedral, single-stranded RNA virus in its own family, *Hepeviridae*. HEV was first recognized in the 1980s in Afghanistan among soldiers with unexplained hepatitis. There is a single serotype but at least four genotypes with differing geographic distributions and epidemiologic patterns. Genotypes 1 and 2 are generally associated with large, waterborne (fecal-oral transmitted) outbreaks in less-developed tropical countries. Genotypes 3 and 4 appear to be animal viruses that result in zoonotic infection of humans, most often through consumption of inadequately cooked pork products. Genotype 3 is widely distributed and is present in developed countries, and genotype 4 seems to be more common in certain Asian countries.

The incubation period is 3 to 8 weeks, with resulting illness that is generally self-limited but can result in fulminant hepatitis in those who are immunosuppressed or patients with chronic liver disease. Genotypes 1 and 2 can be lethal in pregnant women and their fetuses. Transfusion transmission, mostly of genotype 3, has been well documented in Japan, France, England, the Netherlands, and Spain, with greater than 30 transfusion transmissions documented to date.[90] Recent studies suggest a wide range of seroprevalence rates of 20% to 40% in areas where HEV is endemic, but some of the variability may be attributable to the differences in performance characteristics of the tests used, and some to dietary habits. Most studies indicate a cohort effect, with prevalence rates increasing with age. Transfusion infectivity is associated with the presence of viral RNA in plasma; reported frequencies of RNA prevalence in donations have ranged from approximately 1 in 1000 to 1 in 10,000. In a large study in England, 225,000 donations were tested, and 79 (1 in 2848) were positive when tested for HEV RNA by an in-house NAT assay.[91] Tracing was possible for 43 recipients, of whom 18 (42%) showed evidence of transfusion-transmitted infection, with 10 having prolonged infection; three were immunosuppressed individuals requiring treatment to clear the virus, and another had clinical hepatitis. In contrast, in a smaller, blinded study in the United States, 7.7% of donors were anti-HEV positive and only two of approximately 19,000 were RNA positive (1:9500).[92] The main concern is the finding that highly immunosuppressed patients (such as solid-organ transplant recipients) develop chronic HEV infections with long-term clinical sequelae, although these have not been specifically linked to infection via transfusion in the United States.

As a nonenveloped agent, HEV is not susceptible to SD treatment or to current-generation pathogen inactivation technologies. Breakthrough infection following treatment has been documented, and commercial pooled lots of SD plasma (Octaplas) are screened for HEV RNA.[69,93] Asking donors about risk would not be an effective screening measure because most donors would be considered at risk due to dietary factors (eg, consumption of pork or wild game). NAT screening is the only effective protective measure. Routine NAT has been implemented in several European countries (eg, England, Ireland, and the Netherlands) and areas of Japan with documented higher HEV incidence; other countries are evaluating such testing, particularly for patients at increased risk, including solid-organ transplant and HSC recipients.

Syphilis

Syphilis is caused by the spirochete *Treponema pallidum*. Donor screening for syphilis has been performed for almost 80 years. Donors were initially screened by nontreponemal serologic tests that detect antibody to cardiolipin [eg, rapid plasma reagin (RPR)]. In recent years, tests that detect specific antibodies to *T. pallidum* have replaced RPR because these tests can be performed with automated testing instruments.

Most reactive donor test results do not represent infectious syphilis. Most reflect either biologic false-positive results or persistent antibody in previously treated individuals (the former has negative and the latter has positive treponemal-specific antibody screening tests). FDA recommendations vary depending on whether the initial screening is performed using a nontreponemal test (eg, RPR) or a treponemal-specific test. If screening is performed with a nontreponemal test, additional testing with a treponemal-specific test can be used to guide donor and component management. The FDA permits release of units from donors who have reactive nontreponemal screening test results and negative treponemal-specific results if the units are labeled with both test results.[1,21] If screening is performed using a treponemal-specific test, the FDA recommends additional testing by a second FDA-cleared treponemal test. If the second test is nonreactive, the donor can be reentered, although the component cannot be released. If the result of the second treponemal-specific test is reactive, the donor must be deferred for at least 12 months, and before reentry must have documented evidence from his or her physician or a public health laboratory of effective treatment.[79] The same is true if a nontreponemal screening test was used and if subsequent testing using a treponemal test is reactive.

The current value of donor screening for syphilis is controversial.[94-96] Although numerous cases of transfusion-transmitted syphilis were reported before World War II, no cases have been reported in the United States in over 40 years. The low transmission risk is probably related to a declining incidence of syphilis in donors as well as the limited survival of the *T. pallidum* spirochete during blood storage.[97] Syphilis rates have been increasing since 2000, particularly in the MSM population, dampening hopes for elimination of donation testing.[98]

One issue that has been considered is whether the syphilis screen improves blood safety by serving as a surrogate marker of high-risk sexual activity. However, studies have demonstrated that donor screening for syphilis does not provide incremental value in detecting other blood-borne and sexually transmitted infections, such as HIV, HBV, HCV, or HTLV.[96]

Other Bacteria

Bacterial contamination of blood components (mainly platelets) continues to cause transfusion-related morbidity and fatalities.[40,99] As defined by FDA guidance, platelets are associated with a higher risk of sepsis and related fatality than any other transfusable blood component and are a leading cause of infection from blood transfusion, with a rate of approximately 1 per 100,000 transfused apheresis platelet units.[40,100] Bacteria are detected in approximately 1 in 6000 apheresis platelet donations by routine quality-control culture, but some escape detection to cause septic transfusion reactions.[40,100,101] The source of the bacteria is most commonly the donor's skin but can also be asymptomatic bacteremia in the donor.

The level of bacteria in components just after collection is generally too low to detect or to cause symptoms in the recipient. However, bacteria can multiply during component storage, particularly in platelet components, due to storage at room temperature. Bacteria proliferate to a lesser extent in refrigerated red cells, and septic reactions occur much less commonly with these components. In rare cases, Red Blood Cell (RBC) units contaminated with bacteria capable of growth at cold temperatures during the storage period have caused life-threatening sepsis.[99,101] In 2004, to reduce the risk of septic transfusion reactions associated with platelets, AABB implemented a standard for facilities to limit and detect bacterial contamination in all platelet components. AABB recognized in 2009 the availability in some countries of pathogen inactivation methods, which can replace bacteria detection methods for platelet components.[31(p11)]

To limit blood component contamination by bacteria from donor skin, two elements of the blood collection process are critical. Before venipuncture, the donor skin must be carefully disinfected using a method with demonstrated efficacy. Most of these methods involve iodophors, chlorhexidine, or alcohol.[106] Second, diversion of the first 40 mL or more of donor blood containing the contaminated skin plug into a sample pouch and away from the platelet component further reduces the likelihood that skin contaminants will enter the component.[40,100-102] Since 2008, AABB has required that collection sets with diversion pouches be used for all platelet collections, including whole blood collections from which platelets are made.[31(p22)]

A variety of technologies are available for detection of bacteria in platelet components. AABB *Standards* requires blood centers to use a bacteria detection method that is approved by the FDA or validated to provide sensitivity equivalent to FDA-approved methods.[31(p11)] None of these methods is sensitive enough to detect bacteria immediately after collection. All methods require a waiting time for bacteria contaminants to multiply before the component is sampled.

The process most commonly used in the United States to screen apheresis platelets is a single-step, culture-based system inoculated at least 24 hours after phlebotomy. After that time, a sample is withdrawn and inoculated into one or more culture bottles. The bottles are then incubated in the culture system. Some blood centers continue to hold the platelet components during the first 12 to 24 hours of culture and release them for use only if the culture is negative at the end of that time. In all cases, the culture is continued for the shelf life of the unit. If the culture becomes positive after the component is released, the blood center attempts to retrieve it. If the component has not been transfused, resampling of the component for culture is informative because approximately two-thirds of the initially positive signals are caused by either contamination of the bottle (and not the component) or false signals from the culture system.[100,101] All positive cultures should be tested to determine the identity of the organism. If a true-positive result is related to an organism that is not a common skin contaminant but could indicate asymptomatic bacteremia, the donor should be notified and advised to seek medical consultation.[41]

All testing methods are approved for leukocyte-reduced apheresis platelets, and some are approved for testing pools of leukocyte-reduced, whole-blood-derived platelets.[103] Single-step culture testing applies to whole-blood-derived platelets and poststorage pools of whole-blood-derived platelets. Low-technology methods for screening platelets just before issue, such as visually inspecting the platelets for swirling or testing them for low glucose or pH, lack both sensitivity and specificity and do not fulfill the AABB standard for bacteria detection.[31,102] However, visual inspection of all platelets for signs of bacterial contamination should occur before transfusion regardless of the method of platelet testing. FDA-cleared point-of-issue assays can be used for detection of bacterial contamination of platelet concentrates that are pooled immediately before issue.[104,105]

Since the implementation of routine bacteria screening of apheresis platelets, the frequency of FDA-reported fatalities from contaminated apheresis platelets has declined.[99] However, approximately 50% of contaminated apheresis platelets escape detection by this early testing, presumably because bacterial concentrations remain below the limits of detection at the time of sampling; thus, septic, and even fatal, reactions occur. AABB has recommended consideration of policies to further reduce the risk of bacterially contaminated platelets, and the FDA finalized guidance in September 2019, which classified methods as either single-step strategies or parts of two-step strategies.[40,100-102] The point-of-issue assays mentioned above are cleared by the FDA as adjunct tests for apheresis platelets that have been screened by another method. In a large clinical trial, one of these assays detected 9 bacterially contaminated components among 27,620 apheresis platelet units (1 in 3069 components) that were negative by an early-storage culture-based assay.[106] There were also 142 false-positive results. At the time of writing, results for point-of-issue retesting of apheresis platelets in routine use have been presented in a single report, but without demonstrating additional yield. As of yet, point-of-issue retesting using FDA-approved tests has not been widely implemented in the United States.[107]

The culture approaches used to date in the United States provide incomplete assurance of bacteria detection. Enhancements include secondary culture at days 3 or 4, use of point-of-issue secondary testing, or primary culture using delayed-sampling, large-volume methods.[108] In addition, some of these testing options may allow extension of platelet dating to 7 days, provided that platelets are collected in devices with the appropriate 7-day labeling. Licensed pathogen inactivation methods for platelets, which impair proliferation of bacteria, have been documented by active hemovigilance in Switzerland, France, and Belgium to reduce the risk of septic transfusion reactions.[105] In such countries, pathogen inactivation has replaced bacteri-

al culture for platelets, with no documented confirmed bacterial breakthrough infections in over 2 million units of inactivated platelets transfused through 2017. Replacement of bacterial culture by pathogen inactivation has not been widely adopted in the United States due to operational issues with the approved process. The 2019 FDA guidance for industry[40] recommends interventions beyond those included in AABB *Standards*. These additional measures include: secondary testing with a point-of-issue test of previously cultured apheresis platelets or prestorage pooled platelets within 24 hours of transfusion, reculture of platelets on day 4 with a hold for at least the first 12 hours after reculture, or pathogen inactivation per device instructions for use. Enhanced primary culture methods as used in England and in Canada (ie, delayed-sampling, large-volume culture) are now also recommended by the FDA. These methods use a culture no sooner than 48 hours from the time of collection with a sample volume of 16 mL inoculated evenly into aerobic and anaerobic culture bottles. This practice allows for 7-day platelet dating and has demonstrated significant reductions in the frequency of septic transfusion reactions to rates of approximately 1 in 1.2 million transfused platelets, although one *Staphylococcus aureus* breakthrough infection and three other *S. aureus* near misses caught by visual platelet inspection before transfusion were documented. Another enhanced culture method has been proposed (minimal proportional sampling volume) involving proportional culture of a minimum of 3.8% of collected apheresis platelets vs a fixed volume of 1.1% to 2.7% (ie, 8 to 10 mL into only a single aerobic bottle), but there are no data on outcomes comparable to those from England.[104,109]

Vector-Borne Infections

Before the late 1990s, malaria was the most common vector-borne infection recognized as having the potential for transfusion transmission. Since 2002, additional vector-borne diseases have been recognized as having the potential for secondary transmission by blood transfusion. Each one has been evaluated as it emerged and has been addressed for the threat it posed to the blood supply. For some, interventions such as new blood donor screening assays were developed and implemented, while for others donor screening questions were added. Not all required immediate intervention, and surveillance continues. The extent to which these vector-transmitted infections have been perceived as threats to the US blood supply, as well as the ease of developing a reasonable intervention strategy, has often influenced what action is taken.

West Nile Virus

WNV is a lipid-enveloped RNA virus in the *Flaviviridae* family. The first WNV cases were identified in the West Nile district of Uganda in 1937. Afterward, outbreaks occurred in the Middle East, South Africa, and Europe. First detected in the United States in 1999, WNV subsequently spread throughout North America, appearing in virtually every US state in cyclical, annual epidemics every summer and autumn. Transmission primarily occurs in a bird-to-bird transmission cycle by culicine mosquitoes, and human infections occur incidentally. WNV viral loads in humans are too low to re-infect mosquitoes. Approximately 80% of human cases are asymptomatic, 20% are associated with a self-limited febrile illness, and less than 1% are associated with severe neuroinvasive disease, such as meningoencephalitis or acute flaccid paralysis.

During the summer of 2002, a model suggesting a significant risk for WNV infection in blood donors was published.[110] Concurrently, four recipients of organ allografts from a single organ donor infected by transfusion developed neuroinvasive WNV infection.[111] Transfusion transmission was documented in 23 recipients in 2002 compared with a background of 2946 cases of WNV-meningoencephalitis in the general population.[111] A multidisciplinary effort led to the implementation of WNV investigational screening assays by the following summer. Because RNA-positive units, not antibody-positive units, were considered to pose the greatest risk from this acute infection, NAT, rather than serologic testing, was required to protect the blood supply. Donor tests for WNV RNA are required for use by both the FDA and AABB.[26,30,38] In

retrospective cohort studies of blood donors with positive WNV RNA tests, 29% to 61% described symptoms before or after donation, compared to 3% to 20% of control uninfected donors, demonstrating that screening with donor history questionnaires is neither sensitive nor specific enough to prevent transfusion transmission.[112]

To maximize efficiency, donation samples are tested by MP-NAT in pools of 6 to 16 donations, as is done for HCV, HBV, and HIV. However, because circulating levels of WNV RNA are low (the highest viral load documented has been 720,000 copies/mL), a donor sample may contain a low concentration of RNA that will not be detected by MP-NAT.[113] It has been observed that MP-NAT screening for WNV RNA fails to detect 50% or more of donations from infected donors due to dilution of low levels of RNA during pooling.[38,113,114] Therefore, both the FDA and AABB recommend testing by ID-NAT, not MP-NAT, during periods of WNV activity in a particular geographic collection region.[26,38] Regional WNV activity is monitored through active communications between neighboring blood collection agencies and includes monitoring RNA-reactive donations, public health surveillance of clinical WNV cases, and animal and mosquito surveillance in the area.

Following the 23 cases of transfusion-transmitted WNV documented before the initiation of NAT screening in 2003, an additional 14 cases were reported, most related to donations having only low levels of RNA.[92] All implicated donations, except one in 2002, have been IgM negative.[113,115] Blood centers must remain vigilant to make the rapid conversion from MP- to ID-NAT needed for this seasonal strategy to be effective.

Zika Virus

ZIKV is a tropical arbovirus of the flavivirus group, closely related to dengue viruses and transmitted to humans through the same *Aedes* mosquito vector. ZIKV was first recognized in Africa in 1947, then moved through Asia and subsequently the Pacific Islands. In 2007, the first large-scale human outbreak was recognized on the island of Yap in Micronesia, with subsequent spread to French Polynesia and other Pacific Island groups in 2013, to Brazil in May 2015, and to the Caribbean in December 2015.[115,116] At the time of writing, 86 countries or areas had reported active transmission, including 48 countries or territories in the Americas, all involved in the pandemic from 2013 to 2017.[117] Most cases (~80%) of ZIKV infection are asymptomatic.[118] However, ZIKV infection causes fetal loss, congenital ZIKV-related syndromes including microcephaly, and Guillain-Barré syndrome and other neurologic complications in adults.[116,119-124]

The primary route of infection in US residents is travel to areas with active vector-borne ZIKV transmission.[125,126] At the time of writing, there were 5430 travel-associated ZIKV cases in the continental United States reported to the CDC, 52 sexually transmitted cases, and two laboratory-acquired cases.[125] In addition, a fatal, rapidly progressive infection acquired outside of the United States resulted in a secondary local transmission to a caregiver without other ZIKV risk factors.[127] During 2016 and 2017, local mosquito-borne transmission was reported in two states: Florida (226 cases) and Texas (11 cases); none in 2018. In contrast, 37,115 locally transmitted cases of ZIKV clinical disease were reported in the US territories, mostly in Puerto Rico. An additional 13 cases of Guillain-Barré syndrome associated with ZIKV infection have been reported to the CDC in the continental United States, and 51 in US territories.[125]

ZIKV RNA can be recovered from blood donors, as demonstrated in the 2013-2014 ZIKV outbreak in French Polynesia, in which 2.8% of donors tested RNA positive by NAT, and subsequently in Martinique and Puerto Rico with rates of 1.8% in blood donors.[118,128-130] At the time of writing, there have been four probable transfusion transmissions, all reported in Brazil.[131,132] These were identified when three donors reported postdonation information of dengue/ZIKV-like symptoms. None of the recipients developed ZIKV-related symptoms following transfusion. In addition to mosquito-borne transmission and transfusion transmission, sexual transmission has been documented, mostly from an infected male to his partner (male or female)[116]; female-to-male sexual transmission has also been reported in one case.[133]

The duration of ZIKV viremia is believed to be 1 to 2 weeks, consistent with other mosquito-borne viruses. Viral clearance was estimated, using diagnostic assays, to be 19 days for 95% of affected patients (95% confidence interval of 13 to 80 days in a pooled analysis of published studies).[134] ZIKV RNA has been reported to persist longer in whole blood, semen, vaginal fluid, and urine, vs serum and plasma. One report found persistence of ZIKV RNA (as opposed to infectious virus) in whole blood for 5 to 58 days after symptom onset despite RNA-negative findings in corresponding serum samples; RNA positivity for 5 to 26 days occurred in urine from these same individuals.[135] The longest persistence of ZIKV has been in semen. In one case, RNA was detected for 62 days, and in others for 92 to 93 days with the longest at 188 days, all in travelers returning from ZIKV-active or previously active areas.[136-139] ZIKV RNA duration was estimated from following 150 ZIKV patients in Puerto Rico positive by polymerase chain reaction (PCR).[140] The medians and 95th percentiles (plus 95% confidence limits) for ZIKV RNA persistence were 15 (14-17) and 41 (37-44) days in serum, 11 (9-12) and 34 (30-38) days in urine, and 42 (35-50) and 120 (100-139) days in semen.[140]

Because of concern about severe disease associations, rapid virus spread in the Americas, recovery of RNA from blood of asymptomatic donors, and reports of probable transfusion transmission, blood centers initially asked donors about travel to or residence in ZIKV-active areas using a specific question with an associated 28-day deferral.[141] Because of increased concern about the probability of autochthonous transmission and travel-related and sexual transmission, the FDA revised its guidance in August 2016 to require universal ZIKV ID-NAT or the use of approved pathogen inactivation technologies.[39,142]

Two NAT assays were used under investigational new drug (IND) applications; both were subsequently licensed in late 2017 and mid-2018. These assays have been used in the continental United States and in Puerto Rico. The donor screening NAT assays are more sensitive than FDA-cleared diagnostic assays.[143] RNA has been reported in donor plasma samples as long as 71 and 97 days after donor return from ZIKV-endemic areas.[144,145] A recent report using one assay presented data from 15 months of investigational testing of 4.3 million donations with nine confirmed-positive donors identified (of 160 initially reactive, or a positive predictive value of 5.6%), yielding 99.997% specificity.[146] Upon further investigation of the nine confirmed-positive donors, two infections were locally acquired, six were acquired while traveling to ZIKV-endemic areas, and one donor tested positive following receipt of an experimental ZIKV vaccine. RNA levels were detectible in RBCs for up to 154 days after donation and in plasma for up to 80 days after donation. The costs for identifying the eight donors infected by mosquito (assuming associated donations would be infectious) was $5.3 million/infected donor. This is true primarily because there was little vector-borne transmission in the United States during the 2015-2017 outbreak, and subsequently, cases of ZIKV infection have appeared to be declining worldwide. Whether ZIKV will return in epidemic proportions remains to be seen. There have been no local transmissions reported in the United States during 2018, and all 68 cases reported in Florida (at time of writing) have been from travelers to areas that remain ZIKV active.[125]

The FDA has approved pathogen inactivation for platelets and plasma, which has been shown to be effective for reducing relevant arbovirus titers. Published data using the FDA-approved method demonstrated more than a 6 $\log_{10}$ reduction in ZIKV infectivity in plasma and platelets, with similar reductions observed for RBCs. ZIKV is also readily inactivated in SD plasma and other plasma-derived products.[147-150]

An amended FDA guidance, published in July 2018, allows for the use of MP-NAT universally in place of ID-NAT.[27] Conversion from MP-NAT to ID-NAT is required when triggered by local vector-borne ZIKV activity in a collection region or if a donation tests NAT reactive for ZIKV, and local vector-borne transmission is possible (ie, other modes of transmission have been excluded). Pathogen inactivation for plasma and platelet collections remains an alternative to testing. In addition, the guidance requests donors to self-defer based on a ZIKV disease diagnosis; donors testing NAT reactive and/or with a clinical diagnosis are deferred for 120 days, with subsequent reinstatement allowed after that period.[27] Predonation screening of donors for possible exposure to ZIKV through travel activity is no longer recommended.

Other Arboviruses

There are other vector-transmitted infections that could be secondarily transmitted by transfusion. These agents and potential intervention strategies are reviewed in the AABB emerging infectious disease resources.[70,71] Two of these agents, dengue and chikungunya viruses (DENV and CHIKV), have received attention because donations containing viral nucleic acid were documented during epidemics outside the continental United States; however, to date no specific interventions for either agent have been introduced. Like ZIKV, the magnitude and clinical significance of transfusion transmission for these agents remains unclear.

Forty percent of the world's population lives in areas with risk for DENV, including many areas visited by US travelers. It has spread rapidly in Latin America and the Caribbean since the 1980s. DENV is endemic in Puerto Rico, the US Virgin Islands, and American Samoa, and there have been outbreaks in Hawaii, Texas, and Florida during the last 10 years.[151] DENV is caused by four related flaviviruses spread person to person by *Aedes aegypti* and *A. albopictus* (these are the same vectors that transmit ZIKV). Most infections are asymptomatic, but illness ranges from undifferentiated fever to classic breakbone fever and severe dengue (dengue hemorrhagic fever and dengue shock syndrome). An approximately 7-day viremia is a feature of both asymptomatic and symptomatic infection, and asymptomatic blood donors from Hong Kong, Singapore, Brazil, and Puerto Rico have transmitted DENV to blood recipients in seven clusters. Although the number of reports of transfusion-transmitted infections is limited compared to the high rates of vector-borne infection, the lack of systematic surveillance for transfusion-transmitted DENV makes its recognition in the face of widespread outbreaks problematic.[152] RNA-positive, asymptomatic donors have been identified in Brazil, Central America, and Puerto Rico using NAT and antigen detection tests. Rates of donor RNA positivity in Puerto Rico are comparable to those found in US donors during the most active WNV seasons.[153,154] A study in Brazil documented transfusion transmission from RNA-positive donors; however, when the medical charts of infected recipients of blood components from those donors were compared to control recipients who did not receive an RNA-positive unit, there was no measurable apparent clinical illness.[155] The pathogenesis and phenotypic expression of disease may differ after transfusion vs infection from mosquitoes, due to the absence of promoters that are present in mosquito saliva and other alterations of the virus that occur after mosquito infection.[156,157]

In the absence of sustained outbreaks of locally transmitted DENV in the continental United States, transfusion risk relates mainly to return of infected, asymptomatic or presymptomatic travelers. A 3- to 14-day incubation period precedes symptom onset. Deferral for travel to malaria-endemic areas (12 weeks for US residents) offers some protection, but a large proportion of dengue-affected areas frequently visited from the United States are malaria free, and travelers to those areas could potentially introduce the virus into the community and the blood supply. The conditions for sustained spread of DENV exist in large areas of the United States: a source of infection from travelers, a susceptible population, and competent mosquito vectors.

CHIKV is another tropical arbovirus also transmitted by *Aedes* spp. mosquitoes. It is a togavirus of the alphavirus group first recognized in Africa. It has been responsible for explosive outbreaks in the islands of the Indian Ocean, followed by spread to the Caribbean, where more than 1.7 million clinical cases were reported from the end of 2013 to the middle of 2015, including RNA positivity in blood donors.[158,159] There have been no reported cases of transmission by transfusion, but the similarity of early infection to that of dengue has resulted in significant concern. Notably, French authorities responded to the outbreak in the islands of the Indian Ocean by halting local collection of red cells (providing for the islands' needs by supplying blood from the French mainland) and by implementation of limited NAT and the use of pathogen inactivation for platelets.[159] Other precautions that have been used include strengthening requirements of postdonation information from donors, a process enhanced by the high (50%-80%) frequency of symptoms among infected subjects, along with deferrals for residence in affected areas. Chikungunya symptoms are like those of dengue, but without the impact on the circulatory system. Arthralgia is a prominent symptom and may be prolonged. Although routine tests are currently available, as combination NAT assays with DENV, they are not widely used. Rates of CHIKV RNA detection in unlinked blood donation samples reached 2.1% in Puerto Rico during the 2014 outbreak.[160] Viral titers in positive donations ranged from 10^4 to 10^9 RNA copies per mL.[158-160]

Trypanosoma cruzi

T. cruzi is the protozoan parasitic agent of Chagas disease. Chagas disease is endemic in parts of Mexico, Central America, and South America. It is transmitted to humans most commonly by an infected triatomine or reduviid bug, but human-to-human transmission is possible via blood transfusion, organ/tissue transplantation, congenitally, and from ingestion of contaminated food or beverages. The insect vector is associated with a wide variety of mammalian reservoir hosts in rural areas of countries where *T. cruzi* is endemic; human infections most commonly occur when the vector cannot find an alternative mammalian host for a blood meal. Acute infection is usually self-limited, involving localized swelling at the bite site and fever, but may be severe in immunocompromised patients. Most infections become chronic but remain asymptomatic. Decades after the initial infection, 10% to 40% of infected individuals develop late-stage manifestations, including intestinal dysfunction or cardiac disease, which can be fatal. Transfusion transmission of *T. cruzi* from the blood of chronically infected, asymptomatic donors has been recognized for decades in areas where it is endemic, although it has become uncommon with decreasing use of fresh whole blood and implementation of donor serologic screening.

The first blood donation screening EIA for antibodies to *T. cruzi*, using parasite lysate, was approved by the FDA for use in the United States in December 2006. Although not initially required by the FDA, the test was widely implemented by US blood centers during 2007. Subsequently, a second licensed screening test using ChLIA was approved using recombinant antigens for antibody capture instead of parasite lysate as used for the EIA. Initially there was no FDA-approved supplemental assay, but additional testing of reactive donations using an unlicensed radioimmunoprecipitation assay (RIPA) was helpful for guiding donor counseling. Based on the results of the latter assay, about 25% of reactive US donors appear to be truly infected.[161,162] An enzyme strip assay (ESA) using the same *T. cruzi* recombinant antigens as used in ChLIA is now approved by the FDA as a supplemental assay but yields high rates of false positivity.

Most US donations with reactive *T. cruzi* screening test results and positive supplemental results are from donors born in *T. cruzi*-endemic areas of Latin America. The minority have congenital acquired infections transmitted from a mother from a *T. cruzi*-endemic area. Only a small number of donor infections appear to have been acquired from vector exposure within the United States (autochthonous cases). In the first 2 years of universal donor screening in the United States, no donor seroconversions (ie, incident infections) were identified.[162] In December 2010, the FDA issued guidance recommending one-time testing of each US donor for *T. cruzi* antibodies.[163] A subsequent 2017 guidance maintains one-time screening of donors in the United States. For blood donors not found to be positive or indeterminate on supplemental testing, the guidance provides an algorithm for donor reentry.[23] Finally, the FDA recommends removal of the question on the Donor History Questionnaire (DHQ) about a history of Chagas disease, due to the lack of specificity of the question and the efficacy of one-time donor screening.[23,164]

Before implementation of donor screening, seven cases of transfusion-transmitted *T. cruzi*

had been identified in the United States and Canada; cases with available data were linked to platelet transfusion, and none were from a donor with recent infection. Twenty cases of transfusion transmission in the United States, Canada, and Spain have now been documented—again, all related to platelets from remotely infected donors who had formerly resided in areas where *T. cruzi* was highly endemic.[165] Since the implementation of US donor screening, confirmed-positive donors have been identified, and recipients of their prior donations have been notified and tested. Only two prior recipients of platelets from one remotely infected donor born in a Chagas-endemic country appear to have been infected by transfusion since 2007, and they were identified only through look-back procedures.[166] Despite historically reported transmission rates of 10% to 20% from whole blood from infected donors in *T. cruzi*-endemic areas, no *T. cruzi* transmissions by red cells in the United States have been documented (only one case has ever been reported).[167] The lower infectivity of red cell components compared to platelets or fresh whole blood is likely attributable to the limited survival of the parasite in refrigerated components.

Babesia

Babesia are intraerythrocytic parasites that are the causative agent of babesiosis. Well over 100 species have been described worldwide. Human *Babesia* infections are zoonotic, usually acquired through the bite of an infected tick. In the Northeastern and Midwestern United States, the most common *Babesia* species is *B. microti*. The vector is *Ixodes scapularis*, the same tick that transmits Lyme disease. In the Western United States, *Babesia* infections are less common, and a different species, *B. duncani*, predominates. The vector for *B. duncani* in the United States is likely *I. pacificus*. Reported human infections with *Babesia* are becoming more frequent, and in 2011, the CDC made babesiosis nationally notifiable, although not all states require reporting. *Babesia* infection is usually asymptomatic, even though parasites can circulate for months to years. In some individuals, however, *Babesia* infection presents as a severe malaria-like illness that can be fatal. Generally, fatalities range from 6% to 9% but may be as high as 21% in immunocompromised patients.[25,168] Immunocompromised, elderly, and asplenic patients are at increased risk of severe disease, but following a review of published transfusion-transmitted babesiosis (TTB) cases, it has become clear that any recipient is susceptible to infection and serious illness.[169] Treatment with antibiotics is very effective, most commonly including oral atovaquone with azithromycin for 7 to 10 days; more severe cases often receive red cell exchange transfusion. The key is prompt recognition and diagnosis of infection.

TTB is being identified with increasing frequency. From 1979 to 2009, 162 TTB cases were described, but there were greater than 200 through October 2018.[168,170,171] This is an underestimate because most infections are asymptomatic. In March 2018, the FDA approved two independent donor screening tests for *B. microti* (one antibody and one PCR assay), but neither remain commercially available.[25] Subsequently in January 2019, the FDA licensed a NAT assay for multiple *Babesia* spp. (*B. microti*, *B. duncani*, *B. divergens*, and *B. venatorum*) that because of enhanced sensitivity can be used without antibody testing. In May 2019, the FDA released final guidance for *Babesia* via testing for nucleic acids using licensed NAT. Through 2016, 95% of *Babesia* cases occurred in the seven states considered to be *Babesia*-endemic areas (all in the Northeast and upper Midwest).[25] However, the FDA guidance considers 14 US states and the District of Columbia to be at risk (defined as being either a *Babesia*-endemic state/district or adjacent to states where *Babesia* are highly endemic) and thus recommended for testing. The past FDA requirement that donors be asked if they have had a history of babesiosis and permanently deferred for affirmative responses can be replaced in areas of the country with testing, now that the guidance is final. Blood establishments must either test by licensed NAT in the 14 states plus DC (or other areas if added by the FDA in the future) or retain a history of the babesiosis risk question regarding prior test reactivity or a medical diagnosis. In either case (test reactivity or a medical diagnosis), the donor is deferred for at least 2 years and can donate only if the donor has not had a positive *Babesia* test in the last 2 years and the donation tests NAT negative using a licensed test. The licensed NAT assay and an additional NAT assay in use investigationally both have increased analytic sensitivity compared to the initial licensed NAT (PCR) assay.[172] Licensed pathogen inactivation technology is capable of significantly reducing *B. microti* infectivity and may be used as an alternate to a licensed NAT.[25,173]

Babesia infection is most commonly diagnosed when the intraerythrocytic parasites are seen on a blood smear; tetrads of parasites in infected red cells, referred to as a Maltese cross, are characteristic of *B. microti* (vs malaria) infection. If a patient is suspected of having acquired the infection by transfusion, donors of the patient's components can be recalled and may be tested by research assays for *Babesia* antibodies, by NAT, or both; typically, the presence of *B. microti* nucleic acids or high-titer antibody in the donor is suggestive of recent infection. Most of the donors implicated in TTB cases have been residents of *Babesia*-endemic areas, although rarely nonresidents of these areas are infected during travel to such areas and implicated in TTB cases.[25,168,170,174] The frequency of TTB from travelers is estimated at 1 per 10 million donations.[171]

The results of investigational blood donation screening describing the testing yield, the duration of donor positivity, the relationship of test-negative units to transfusion transmission, the infectivity of test-positive units, and residual risks have been reported.[171] Approximately 90,000 donations from consenting donors were tested by two investigational assays: automated immunofluorescence for antibody detection and ID-NAT by PCR to detect the parasite's DNA (these were the first two FDA-licensed assays that are no longer commercially available). Donors reactive by either test were further tested to confirm infection. The frequency of infected donors in an area where *Babesia* are highly endemic and where screening occurred was 1 per 300 donations, with 1 per 10,000 donations in the PCR-positive, antibody-negative window period. The current risk of TTB from an unscreened RBC unit in *Babesia*-endemic states is

1 per 100,000 but as high as 1 per 18,000 in areas where *Babesia* are highly endemic. Receipt of unscreened RBCs in areas where *Babesia* are highly endemic was nine times more likely to result in TTB than screened blood (screened blood was not associated with any case of TTB). DNA clearance in 95% of infected donors occurred after 1 year, but antibody clearance occurred in less than 10% during that interval.

The current versions of NAT assays (including the licensed test in use and an additional investigational test) are ultrasensitive and run on fully automated platforms. These assays detect and amplify the parasite's ribosomal RNA (rRNA), of which thousands of copies per infecting parasite are present, vs amplifying and detecting the single chromosomal DNA template; DNA will also be amplified and detected. Thus, if even one infected red cell is sampled, it likely will be detected. In addition, these assays are able to detect multiple *Babesia* species, in addition to *B. microti,* that are human pathogens. The use of these ultrasensitive rRNA NAT assays is also consistent with the recommendations of the AABB Ad Hoc Babesia Policy Working Group.[172]

Malaria

Malaria is caused by an intraerythrocytic parasite of the genus *Plasmodium.* Infection is transmitted to humans through a mosquito bite. Five species account for most human infections: *P. falciparum, P. vivax, P. malariae, P. ovale,* and *P. knowlesi.* Disease symptoms include periodic fever, rigors and chills, and hemolytic anemia.

Plasmodium parasites are present in the circulation during asymptomatic infection and are readily transmitted by blood transfusion. Recognition of infected recipients, as is true of *Babesia* infection, may be complex and requires a high index of suspicion and identification of the parasite in red cell blood smears, detection of parasite DNA by PCR, or detection by antibody tests. Transfusion transmission is common in tropical malaria-endemic areas and occurs elsewhere when infected travelers return from these areas or especially when residents of these areas with partial or incomplete immunity donate in areas where malaria is not endemic. No FDA-approved test is available to screen US blood donations for malaria infection. Screening is accomplished solely by donor questioning. Donors are excluded temporarily from donating blood after traveling to malaria-endemic areas, after residing in malaria-endemic countries, or after recovery from clinical malaria. Donor questioning has been effective at preventing transfusion-transmitted malaria (TTM) in the United States with only 11 cases reported between 2000 and 2017, eight of which were due to *P. falciparum.* Risk of TTM continues in the United States at rates of fewer than 1 per million collected blood units. Approximately 70% of TTM cases occur due to failure to appropriately defer a donor during the screening interview, most notably because the donor may not complete the DHQ correctly. In a large majority of cases, this is linked to donors with a history of residence (as opposed to short-term travel) in Africa.[175-177]

This level of transfusion safety has been achieved at a substantial cost in terms of donor loss; malaria-related questions have excluded hundreds of thousands of otherwise acceptable US donors annually. Since 2013, FDA guidance has redefined malaria-endemic areas as only those for which chemoprophylaxis is recommended.[178] With this new definition, travel to many popular tourist locations is no longer considered a malarial risk; for example, in the past, Mexico has accounted for the largest proportion of deferred donors while having risk that is exceedingly low.[179] However, the 2013 guidance adds a complex algorithm for evaluating travel by donors who have lived for more than 5 years in malaria-endemic countries, because of a concern about partial immunity causing prolonged asymptomatic parasitemia in such donors.

Outside of the United States, some countries that exclude donors after travel to malaria-endemic areas permit reentry of these donors if they test negative for malaria 4 to 6 months after completion of travel using an antibody test relying on recombinant antigens to two *Plasmodium* spp. (*P. falciparum* and *P. vivax*; other species are detected at lower rates due to cross-reactivity). This is done routinely in France, England, and Australia, with only one suspected TTM case associated with a reentered donor (in France in 2012). A review of practices in five countries where malaria is not endemic reported 11 TTM cases from 2002 to 2013 (three in France, one in England, and seven in the United States). In the absence of an approved assay, such a "test-in" reentry strategy has not been accepted by the FDA.[180]

Pathogen inactivation methods have been shown to be effective at reducing transfusion transmission in malaria-endemic areas.[181] FDA guidance in April 2020 allowed for an alternative procedure whereby platelets and/or plasma components may be collected from residents of countries where malaria is not endemic after travel to or through malaria-endemic areas. These residents may become donors without a deferral period, provided the components are pathogen reduced with an appropriate device, and the donor meets all other eligibility requirements.[178] A randomized clinical trial involved 214 patients in Africa (Kumasi, Ghana) who completed a blinded evaluation comparing the efficacy of pathogen-reduced vs untreated whole blood for prevention of TTM (107 treated and 107 untreated patients).[181] Overall, 65 nonparasitemic recipients (28 treated and 37 untreated) were exposed to parasitemic blood. The incidence of TTM was significantly lower for the patients treated with pathogen-reduced blood [1 (4%) of 28 patients] than the untreated group [8 (22%) of 37 patients].

Prions

Prions are proteinaceous infectious particles that induce disease by triggering conformational changes in their naturally occurring protein counterparts. These agents cause fatal infections of the nervous system called transmissible spongiform encephalopathies (TSEs).

Sporadic Creutzfeldt-Jakob disease (CJD) is a TSE that occurs sporadically throughout the world at an incidence rate of approximately 1 case per million population. Iatrogenic CJD has been transmitted by injection of human-derived growth hormone or implantation of products from infected central nervous system tissues, including dura mater grafts, corneal tissue, and pituitary-derived hormones. Surveillance studies in the United Kingdom and United States since the mid-1900s have shown no evidence of transmission of sporadic CJD through blood transfusion.[182,183] Nevertheless, blood donations are not accepted from donors who are perceived at increased risk for this disease or from family members of those who have died of sporadic CJD.[184]

Genetic prion disease makes up approximately 15% of all forms of human prion disease and is inherited from one or both parents through an autosomal dominant mutation of the prion protein gene.

In contrast, variant CJD (vCJD), is transmissible by blood transfusion. It is caused by the prion that causes bovine spongiform encephalopathy (BSE), also known as "mad cow disease," with human infection occurring after ingesting neural tissues from infected animals. vCJD differs from CJD in that infected individuals are younger, present with psychiatric symptoms, and have a longer course from diagnosis to death than those with sporadic CJD. Postmortem diagnosis involves unusual florid plaques in the brain. Clinical cases have occurred primarily in the United Kingdom, but cases have occurred in other areas worldwide due to the export of contaminated animal tissues. The number of cases reported has declined since the peak of the epidemic at the turn of the century. Approximately 230 cases have been seen in 12 countries, with over 95% of these occurring in the United Kingdom and Europe. Of those, four were cases of vCJD transmission by transfusion in the United Kingdom.[185] Three of these four resulted in the development of clinical vCJD; the fourth was identified at autopsy of an individual who died of underlying disease but whose spleen and one lymph node contained vCJD prions. In addition, one latent vCJD infection was identified in a patient with hemophilia in the United Kingdom who died of other causes. This patient had received UK-plasma-derived Factor VIII, including material from a donor who later developed vCJD, suggesting that vCJD might have been transmitted by clotting factor concentrates.[70,71] vCJD infection is extremely rare in the United States. The few reported cases have been in individuals who most likely acquired their infections elsewhere, and no US transfusion-transmitted cases have been reported.

Although all but a single vCJD case reported to date have occurred on the genetic background of methionine homozygosity at the condon 129 sequence of the prion protein gene, the occurrence of a single case in a methionine-valine heterozygote raises questions about a potential prolonged incubation period and suggests that vCJD deferrals will be maintained for the foreseeable future.[186]

There are no FDA-approved donor screening tests for prion infections. Recent reports indicate that some research technologies may be adaptable for prion diagnostics[187]; however, none of these technologies as of yet has adequate performance characteristics, including testing turnaround time suitable for blood donation screening. If tests became available, the issue of donor acceptance of screening for a fatal, incurable disease would be an ethical and social challenge.[188] However, the need to screen for prion-related diseases may not be necessary considering that sporadic CJD has not been demonstrated to be transmitted by transfusion and the incidence of vCJD is miniscule and continues to decline. It is thought that plasma-derivative manufacturing processes remove substantial amounts of TSE infectivity.[184] Blood donors in the United States are screened solely by questioning and are excluded if they have an increased risk of either CJD or vCJD. In April 2020 guidance, the FDA revised long-standing deferral criteria, broadening the potential donor base. The new recommendations include removing deferrals for 1) cumulative residence in Europe outside of the United Kingdom, France, and Ireland, and 2) military personnel who lived on any US military base anywhere in Europe. In addition, donors are no longer asked about receipt of human growth hormone derived from pituitary glands or for receipt of UK bovine insulin, among other changes. CJD exclusions are based on family history of the disease or on receipt of a cadaveric dura mater tissue graft. vCJD exclusions are now for residence in the United Kingdom (1980-1996) or Ireland or France (1980-2001) during times when BSE was endemic, as specified, or for receipt of a transfusion in these countries.[184] Ireland represents a new addition to the residence criteria.

Screening of Plasma Derivatives

Commercial plasma derivatives are prepared from pools of plasma derived from thousands of donors. Before the incorporation of specific pathogen inactivation processes, contamination of these large pools with viral agents was common. Today, plasma-derivative manufacturing processes incorporate methods such as prolonged heat or SD treatment to remove or inactivate most known pathogens. SD treatment inactivates lipid-enveloped agents, such as HIV, HCV, and HBV. Pathogen infectivity may also be reduced by nanofiltration, chromatography, or cold ethanol fractionation, which are used in the production of certain products. Not all infectious agents, however, are removed or inactivated by these processes.

One agent that can persist in plasma-derivative products is human parvovirus B19. This small, nonenveloped DNA virus is extremely resistant to physical inactivation. Acute infection is typically mild and self-limited; clinical manifestations include "fifth disease" (erythema infectiosum) and polyarthropathy. Acute infection is associated with transient red cell aplasia that may be clinically significant in immunodeficient individuals and those with underlying hemolytic processes. The aplasia in immunodeficient individuals can be prolonged. Intrauterine infection is associated with severe fetal anemia and hydrops fetalis. Parvovirus B19 infection is very common; most adults have antibodies to this agent, indicating previous exposure. Levels of viral DNA during acute infection may exceed 10^{12} IU/mL, decreasing over weeks to months in association with antibody production. Viral DNA, mostly at low concentrations, has been detected in approximately 1% of blood donations and in essentially all lots of pooled plasma derivatives. Transmission of parvovirus B19 by transfusion has been linked only to blood components or plasma products that contain high concentrations of viral DNA; only one transmission has been documented with a product containing less than 10^4 IU/mL.[71]

Currently, there is no FDA-approved test to screen fresh blood donations for parvovirus B19 infection, although automated assays are available outside of the United States and cleared for use by European regulatory agencies. However, plasma-derivative manufacturers require screening of incoming plasma units for the presence of high-titer parvovirus B19. This is accomplished by performing NAT on pools of samples from plasma units, with sensitivity adjusted to detect only units with a high concentration of virus. By excluding high-titer units from the plasma pools, the final titer in the plasma pool is kept below 10^4 IU/mL.

Other Agents

AABB maintains a publicly accessible electronic resource containing expert analyses of emerging infectious disease agents that have received attention as potential threats to the United States or global blood supply.[71] This digital resource contains up-to-date fact sheets on a variety of agents. Each fact sheet includes information about clinical manifestations and epidemiology of infection, evidence of transfusion transmissibility, and analyses of the potential effectiveness of various mitigation strategies (eg, donor questioning, serologic testing or NAT, or pathogen inactivation). Readers are encouraged to use this rich resource.

PATHOGEN INACTIVATION TECHNOLOGY

Donor screening reduces, but cannot eliminate, the infectious risks of blood transfusion. The efficacy of blood donor testing is limited by several factors, including the following[189]:

1. It is not logistically feasible to test donors for every infection that is conceivably transmissible by transfusion.
2. For every test, there is a lag time (ie, window period) between when a person becomes infected and when the test detects infection.
3. Every test has limited sensitivity (concentration of the target marker that can be detected by the test).
4. Developing a donor test can be a long, multiphase process that includes identification of the infectious agent, selection of the type of

test that would be effective in detecting infectious donations (eg, serology vs NAT), development of a test suitable for donor screening, performance of clinical trials of the test, and regulatory approval. During this development process, infections can be transmitted.
5. Testing cannot interdict unknown pathogens or pathogens not yet recognized or suspected to be transfusable.

Pathogen inactivation provides an attractive and proactive alternative to relying on donor questioning and testing to prevent infectious donations from reaching recipients. Pathogen inactivation processes reduce the infectivity of residual pathogens in blood components. This approach could reduce the transmission of infectious agents for which there are no donor screening tests and further reduce the residual transmission risks of known agents. Once approved and implemented, pathogen inactivation could theoretically enable discontinuation of some testing that is currently performed (eg, CMV testing and bacteria testing of platelets, ID-NAT, others), and pathogen inactivation methods have been shown to obviate the need for irradiation, potentially offsetting some of its cost.

As discussed above, pathogen inactivation methods are an essential component of the plasma-derivative manufacturing process. An SD-treated pooled plasma product has been approved for transfusion in the United States (Octaplas).[69] Because SD treatment and methylene blue/visible light treatment used on plasma damage cell membranes, these methods are not used for platelets or red cells. The pooling of plasma components for use with these technologies results in an increased risk of transmitting an agent that lacks a lipid envelope and is particularly resistant to inactivation. Hence, incoming lots of plasma intended for manufacture of plasma derivatives are prescreened to eliminate the risk of contamination by these agents, such as parvovirus B19, HEV, and hepatitis A virus (another nonenveloped hepatitis agent rarely transfusion transmitted). Such prescreening also occurs for SD plasma lots used for transfusion in the United States.

One manufacturer's pathogen inactivation process is now approved in the United States for treatment of individual units of plasma and platelets (INTERCEPT) using amotosalen (a psoralen) and ultraviolet A (UVA) light. Additional technologies are in use outside the United States. Riboflavin (vitamin B2) and UVB and UVA light are being used for plasma and platelets (Mirasol). The nucleic-acid-damaging pathogen inactivation technologies provide significant activity against all agents for which tests are performed currently: HIV, HBV, HCV, HTLV, WNV, CMV, ZIKV, *Babesia* spp, and parasites, as well as syphilis and agents causing bacterial contamination of platelets. However, pathogen inactivation methods appear to differ greatly in their capacity. Amotosalen/UV treatment also inactivates white cells to prevent transfusion-associated graft-vs-host disease, decreases formation and release of cytokines during storage, and reduces febrile nonhemolytic transfusion reactions. Amotosalen/UV treatment appears to have no effect on the rate of white-cell-induced alloantibody (eg, HLA antibody) formation.[190] Clinical trials are under way in the United States and in-ternationally on pathogen-reduced red cells using amustaline plus glutathione (INTERCEPT) and whole blood using riboflavin and UV light (Mirasol). Processes that are available or in development have been recently reviewed in detail and are summarized in Table 7-8.[191-193]

Pathogen inactivation technologies that target nucleic acids usually do so by generation of nucleic acid crosslinking, preventing pathogen replication. Platelets treated with these technologies have somewhat lower 1-hour posttransfusion corrected count increments.[193] In clinical trials, mild and moderate bleeding frequency is increased, but not severe bleeding complications; the time between transfusions and the total number of platelet transfusions have not generally been different. Pulmonary toxicity, like transfusion-related acute lung injury (TRALI), was reported in clinical trials and in animal model experiments with amotosalen/UV, but does not appear to be a material issue in general in the European Union. Previous clinical trials of one red cell inactivation method were halted because of asymptomatic immunoreactivity against the red cell neoantigens believed to be

TABLE 7-8. Pathogen Inactivation Technologies for Transfusable Blood Components

Component	Technology	Manufacturer
Plasma: commercially prepared pools	Solvent/detergent treatment	Octapharma (FDA cleared)
Plasma: individual units	Amotosalen (psoralen) + UV light	Cerus (FDA cleared)
	Riboflavin (vitamin B2) + UV light	Terumo BCT
	Methylene blue + light	Macopharma
Platelets	Amotosalen (psoralen) + UV light	Cerus (FDA cleared)
	Riboflavin (vitamin B2) + UV light	Terumo BCT
	UV light	Macopharma
Red Blood Cells/Whole Blood	Amustaline and glutathione	Cerus
	Riboflavin (vitamin B2) + UV light	Terumo BCT

FDA = Food and Drug Administration; UV = ultraviolet.

the result of treatment, and trials are being resumed with a reformulated process (amustaline plus glutathione). Preliminary reports suggest riboflavin/UV causes functional impairment in red cells stored nearest the 42-day expiration. Although there have been discussions about the potential for adverse reactions to treated components, extensive reviews of European data on pathogen-reduced platelets and plasma do not support the additional concern. Nevertheless, the FDA has required Phase IV postmarketing studies in the United States as part of the implementation of the approved system, and this is likely for other methods approved in the future.

The benefit to be gained from pathogen inactivation in the United States is primarily the mitigation of emerging pathogens and platelet-associated bacterial sepsis. Currently, the quantifiable infectious risks of transfusion in the United States are low. Therefore, it is critically important to demonstrate that inactivating treatments do not introduce new hazards to patients. Rigorous preclinical and clinical studies are required for US regulatory approval. Extensive toxicology studies have been critical because most of the pathogen inactivation agents interact with nucleic acid, raising the theoretical potential of carcinogenicity and mutagenicity. Treated components should be assessed for neoantigen formation and the impact of the inactivating process on the final product's clinical efficacy. The evaluation processes required for approval of pathogen inactivation methods in North America have been reviewed.[191-193]

Interest in pathogen inactivation remains high because it has the potential to 1) reduce sepsis-related platelet transfusion complications and eliminate the need for complex testing procedures to reduce risk related to bacterially contaminated platelets; 2) inactivate parasites such as *B. microti* and *P. falciparum;* 3) mitigate risks associated with recognized emerging pathogens such as DENV, CHIKV, and ZIKV; and 4) proactively decrease threats from unknown, emerging pathogens. Again, it should be noted that inactivation capabilities differ greatly between the various technologies, and each must be evaluated for its intended use.

SUMMARY

The current level of safety of blood components is based on two critical elements of donor screening: donor education and questioning, which is the sole method of screening for certain agents, such as malaria and prions, and donor testing. Testing must be performed carefully and in accordance with manufacturers' instructions, FDA regulations, and AABB *Standards*, and facilities must have robust systems for quarantining components of donations that test reactive and for retrieving prior donations from donors whose samples have tested positive.

Current quantifiable risks of infectious disease transmission through the US blood supply are very low; the published estimated risk of HIV transmission by transfusion in the United States is approximately 1 in 1.5 million units, the risk of HCV transmission is approximately 1 in 1.1 million units, and the risk of HBV transmission is approximately 1 in 800,000 to 1 in 1.2 million units,[63,68] and as noted, these risks are further decreasing. However, it is critical to remain vigilant for changes in rates of known agents as donor eligibility policies change, and for evidence of new infectious agents so that mitigation measures are implemented as quickly as feasible or required.[141,142,61,194] Pathogen inactivation technologies show promise in replacing or augmenting current screening strategies such as for bacteria in platelets and may be effective in providing protection against infectious agents for which no screening is currently in place.

KEY POINTS

1. Infectious disease screening of donors is accomplished by a) questioning potential donors and excluding those with an increased risk of infection, and b) testing donated blood.

2. There is a delay between the time when an individual is exposed to an infection and the time when the donor screening test for the infection yields a positive result. Blood donated during this window period can transmit infections.

3. The estimated window period with MP-NAT of donor samples is less than 10 days for HIV and HCV and less than 28 days for HBV.

4. The residual risk of transfusion-transmitted infection is a function of the length of the window period and the incidence of infection in the donor population. Maintaining a donor population that has a low incidence of infection continues to play a key role in preserving blood safety.

5. The residual risk of HIV, HCV, and HBV is very low and declining. Based on window-period and incidence calculations, the current risk of HIV transmission by transfusion in the United States is approximately 1 in 1.5 million units, the risk of HCV transmission is approximately 1 in 1.1 million units, and the risk of HBV transmission is approximately 1 in 800,000 to 1 in 1.2 million units.

6. There are no donor screening tests approved by the FDA for malaria or vCJD. Donor questioning about potential exposure is the sole means of protecting the US blood supply from these diseases.

7. AABB requires blood banks to have processes that limit and detect or inactivate bacteria in platelet components. Either pathogen inactivation or bacteria testing can satisfy this requirement; however, enhancements to the existing bacterial culture method are being considered to further reduce septic transfusion events.

8. Infections transmitted to humans by vectors are increasingly recognized as a potential source of transfusion-transmitted infection. These include WNV, *T. cruzi*, *Babesia* species, DENV, potentially CHIKV, and most recently ZIKV.

9. Pathogen inactivation may reduce the transmission of infectious agents for which there are no donor screening tests and may further reduce the residual transmission risks of known agents. Pathogen-reduced products include commercially manufactured plasma derivatives and pooled solvent/detergent-treated plasma, as well as pathogen-reduced platelet and plasma components.

10. Blood banks must have processes in place to ensure that donations with positive test results are not released for transfusion. In some circumstances, 1) prior donations from those donors must also be retrieved and quarantined, and 2) recipients of prior donations must be notified of their possible exposure to infection.

REFERENCES

1. Code of federal regulations. Title 21, CFR Parts 211 and 610. Washington DC: US Government Publishing Office, 2019 (revised annually).

2. Alter HJ, Klein HG. The hazards of blood transfusion in historical perspective. Blood 2008; 112:2617-26.

3. Seeff LB, Wright EC, Zimmerman HJ, McCollum RW. VA cooperative study of post-transfusion hepatitis, 1969-1974: Incidence and characteristics of hepatitis and responsible risk factors. Am J Med Sci 1975;270:355-62.

4. Alter HJ, Purcell RH, Holland PV, et al. Donor transaminase and recipient hepatitis. Impact on blood transfusion services. JAMA 1981;246: 630-4.

5. Aach RD, Szmuness W, Mosley JW, et al. Serum alanine aminotransferase of donors in relation to the risk of non-A, non-B hepatitis in recipients: The transfusion-transmitted viruses study. N Engl J Med 1981;304:989-94.

6. Alter HJ, Holland PV. Indirect tests to detect the non-A, non-B hepatitis carrier state. Ann Intern Med 1984;101:859-61.

7. Stevens CE, Aach RD, Hollinger FB, et al. Hepatitis B virus antibody in blood donors and the occurrence of non-A, non-B hepatitis in transfusion recipients. An analysis of the Transfusion-Transmitted Viruses Study. Ann Intern Med 1984;101:733-8.

8. Galel SA, Lifson JD, Engleman EG. Prevention of AIDS transmission through screening of the blood supply. Annu Rev Immunol 1995;13:201-27.

9. Joint statement on acquired immune deficiency syndrome (AIDS) related to transfusion. Transfusion 1983;23:87-8.

10. Busch MP, Young MJ, Samson SM, et al. Risk of human immunodeficiency virus (HIV) transmission by blood transfusions before the implementation of HIV-1 antibody screening. The Transfusion Safety Study Group. Transfusion 1991;31:4-11.

11. Ward JW, Holmberg SD, Allen JR, et al. Transmission of human immunodeficiency virus (HIV) by blood transfusions screened as negative for HIV antibody. N Engl J Med 1988;318:473-8.

12. Perkins HA, Samson SM, Busch MP. How well has self-exclusion worked? Transfusion 1988;28:601-2.

13. Food and Drug Administration. Infectious disease tests. Silver Spring, MD: CBER Office of Communication, Outreach, and Development, 2019. [Available at https://www.fda.gov/vaccines-blood-biologics/blood-donor-screening/infectious-disease-tests.]

14. Food and Drug Administration. Information for blood establishments: Unavailability of CHIRON RIBA HCV 3.0 SIA (RIBA). Silver Spring, MD: CBER Office of Communication, Outreach, and Development, 2012.

15. Busch MP, Glynn SA, Stramer SL, et al. A new strategy for estimating risks of transfusion-transmitted viral infections based on rates of detection of recently infected donors. Transfusion 2005;45:254-64.

16. Food and Drug Administration. Memorandum to all registered blood establishments: Recommendations for the management of donors and units that are initially reactive for hepatitis B surface antigen (HBsAg). Silver Spring, MD: CBER Office of Communication, Outreach, and Development, 1987.

17. Food and Drug Administration. Guidance for industry: Requalification method for reentry of donors who test hepatitis B surface antigen (HbsAg) positive following a recent vaccination against hepatitis B virus infection. Silver Spring, MD: CBER Office of Communication, Outreach, and Development, 2011.

18. Food and Drug Administration. Guidance for industry: Requalification method for reentry of blood donors deferred because of reactive test results for antibody to hepatitis B core antigen (Anti-HBc). Silver Spring, MD: CBER Office of Communication, Outreach, and Development, 2010.

19. Food and Drug Administration. Guidance for industry: Use of nucleic acid tests on pooled and individual samples from donors of whole blood and blood components, including source plasma, to reduce the risk of transmission of hepatitis B virus. Silver Spring, MD: CBER Office of Communication, Outreach, and Development, 2012.

20. Food and Drug Administration. Guidance for industry: Nucleic acid testing (NAT) for human immunodificiency virus type 1 (HIV-1) and hepatitis C virus (HCV): Testing, product disposition, and donor deferral and reentry. Silver Spring, MD: CBER Office of Communication, Outreach, and Development, 2017.

21. Food and Drug Administration. Guidance for industry: Recommendations for screening, testing and management of blood donors and blood and blood components based on screening tests for syphilis. Silver Spring, MD: CBER Office of Communication, Outreach, and Development, 2014.

22. Food and Drug Administration. Guidance for industry: Revised recommendations for reducing the risk of human immunodeficiency virus transmission by blood and blood products. (April 2020) Silver Spring, MD: CBER Office of Communication, Outreach, and Development, 2020.

23. Food and Drug Administration. Guidance for industry: Use of serological tests to reduce the risk of transmission of *Trypanosoma cruzi* infection in blood and blood components. Silver Spring, MD: CBER Office of Communication, Outreach, and Development, 2017.

24. Food and Drug Administration. Guidance for industry: Use of serological tests to reduce the risk of transfusion-transmitted human T-lymphotropic virus types I and II (HTLV-I/II). Silver Spring, MD: CBER Office of Communication, Outreach, and Development, 2020.

25. Food and Drug Administration. Guidance for industry: Recommendations for reducing the risk of transfusion-transmitted babesiosis. Silver Spring, MD: CBER Office of Communication, Outreach, and Development, 2019.

26. Food and Drug Administration. Guidance for industry: Use of nucleic acid tests to reduce the risk of transmission of West Nile virus from donors of whole blood and blood components intended for transfusion. (November 2009) Silver

Spring, MD: CBER Office of Communication, Outreach, and Development, 2009.

27. Food and Drug Administration. Guidance for industry: Revised recommendations for reducing the risk of Zika virus transmission by blood and blood components. (July 2018) Silver Spring, MD: CBER Office of Communication, Outreach, and Development, 2018. [Available at https://www.fda.gov/vaccines-blood-biologics/biologics-guidances/blood-guidances.]

28. Eder AF. Donor reentry. In: Eder AF, Goldman M, eds. Screening blood donors with the donor history questionnaire. Bethesda, MD: AABB Press, 2019:209-47.

29. Code of federal regulations. Title 42, CFR Part 482.27. Washington, DC: US Government Publishing Office, 2019 (revised annually).

30. Food and Drug Administration. Guidance for industry: Use of nucleic acid tests on pooled and individual samples from donors of whole blood components (including Source Plasma and Source Leukocytes) to adequately and appropriately reduce the risk of transmission of HIV-1 and HCV. Silver Spring, MD: CBER Office of Communication, Outreach, and Development, 2004.

31. Gammon R, ed. Standards for blood banks and transfusion services. 32nd ed. Bethesda, MD: AABB, 2020.

32. Food and Drug Administration. Guidance for industry: Recommendations for management of donors at increased risk for human immunodeficiency virus type 1 (HIV-1) group O infection. Silver Spring, MD: CBER Office of Communication, Outreach, and Development, 2009.

33. Food and Drug Administration. Guidance for industry: Requalification of donors previously deferred for a history of viral hepatitis after the 11th birthday. Silver Spring, MD: CBER Office of Communication, Outreach, and Development, 2017.

34. Food and Drug Administration. Memorandum to all registered blood and plasma establishments: Recommendations for the quarantine and disposition of units from prior collections from donors with repeatedly reactive screening tests for hepatitis B virus (HBV), hepatitis C virus (HCV), and human T-lymphotropic virus type I (HTLV-I). Silver Spring, MD: CBER Office of Communication, Outreach, and Development, 1996.

35. Food and Drug Administration. Guidance for industry: Lookback for hepatitis C virus (HCV): Product quarantine, consignee notification, fur-

ther testing, product disposition, and notification of transfusion recipients based on donor test results indicating infection with HCV. Silver Spring, MD: CBER Office of Communication, Outreach, and Development, 2010.

36. Food and Drug Administration. Guidance for industry: Further testing of donations that are reactive on a licensed donor screening test for antibodies to hepatitis c virus. Silver Spring, MD: CBER Office of Communication, Outreach, and Development, 2019.

37. Food and Drug Administration. Guidance for industry: Assessing donor suitability and blood and blood product safety in cases of known or suspected West Nile virus infection. Silver Spring, MD: CBER Office of Communication, Outreach, and Development, 2005.

38. West Nile virus nucleic acid testing - revised recommendations. Association bulletin #13-02. Bethesda, MD: AABB, 2013.

39. Updated recommendations for Zika, dengue, and chikungunya viruses. Association bulletin #16-07. Bethesda, MD: AABB, 2016.

40. Food and Drug Administration. Draft guidance for industry: Bacterial risk control strategies for blood collection establishments and transfusion services to enhance the safety and availability of platelets for transfusion. Silver Spring, MD: CBER Office of Communication, Outreach, and Development, 2019.

41. Guidance on management of blood and platelet donors with positive or abnormal results on bacterial contamination tests. Association bulletin #05-02. Bethesda, MD: AABB, 2005.

42. Recommendations to address residual risk of bacterial contamination of platelets. Association bulletin #12-04. Bethesda, MD: AABB, 2012.

43. Actions following an initial positive test for possible bacterial contamination of a platelet unit. Association bulletin #04-07. Bethesda, MD: AABB, 2004.

44. Food and Drug Administration. Guidance for industry: Nucleic acid testing (NAT) to reduce the possible risk of parvovirus B19 transmission by plasma-derived products. Silver Spring, MD: CBER Office of Communication, Outreach, and Development, 2009.

45. Blajchman MA, Goldman M, Freedman JJ, Sher GD. Proceedings of a consensus conference: Prevention of post-transfusion CMV in the era of universal leukoreduction. Transfus Med Rev 2001;15:1-20.

46. Vamvakas E. Is white blood cell reduction equivalent to antibody screening in preventing

transmission of cytomegalovirus by transfusion? A review of the literature and meta-analysis. Transfus Med Rev 2005;19:181-99.

47. Bowden RA, Slichter SJ, Sayers M, et al. A comparison of filtered leukocyte-reduced and cytomegalovirus (CMV) seronegative blood products for the prevention of transfusion-associated CMV infection after marrow transplant. Blood 1995;86:3598-603.

48. Nash T, Hoffmann S, Butch S, et al. Safety of leukoreduced, cytomegalovirus (CMV)-untested components in CMV-negative allogeneic human progenitor cell transplant recipients. Transfusion 2012;52:2270-2.

49. Hall S, Danby R, Osman H, et al. Transfusion in CMV seronegative T-depleted allogeneic stem cell transplant recipients with CMV-unselected blood components results in zero CMV transmissions in the era of universal leukocyte reduction: A U.K. dual centre experience. Transfus Med 2015;25:418 23.

50. Ziemann M, Thiele T. Transfusion-transmitted CMV infection – current knowledge and future perspectives. Transfus Med 2017;27:238-48.

51. Furui Y, Yamagishi N, Morioka I, et al. Sequence analyses of variable cytomegalovirus genes for distinction between breast milk- and transfusion-transmitted infections in very-low-birth-weight infants. Transfusion 2018;9999:1-9.

52. Josephson CD, Caliendo AM, Easley KA, et al. Blood transfusion and breast milk transmission of cytomegalovirus in very-low-birth-weight infants: A prospective cohort study. JAMA Pediatr 2014;168:1054-62.

53. Food and Drug Administration. Guidance for industry: Donor screening recommendations to reduce the risk of transmission of Zika virus by human cells, tissues, and cellular and tissue-based products. Silver Spring, MD: CBER Office of Communication, Outreach, and Development, 2018.

54. Code of federal regulations. Title 21, CFR Part 1271 21. Washington, DC: US Government Publishing Office, 2019 (revised annually).

55. Food and Drug Administration. Guidance for industry: Eligibility determination for donors of human cells, tissues, and cellular and tissue-based products (HCT/Ps). Silver Spring, MD: CBER Office of Communication, Outreach, and Development, 2007.

56. Food and Drug Administration. Guidance for industry: Use of donor screening tests to test donors of human cells, tissues and cellular and tissue-based products for infection with Trepo-

nema pallidum (syphilis). Silver Spring, MD: CBER Office of Communication, Outreach, and Development, 2015.

57. Food and Drug Administration. Guidance for industry: Use of nucleic acid tests to reduce the risk of transmission of West Nile virus from living donors of human cells, tissues, and cellular and tissue-based products (HCT/Ps). Silver Spring, MD: CBER Office of Communication, Outreach, and Development, 2016.

58. Food and Drug Administration. Tissue guidances. Silver Spring, MD: CBER Office of Communication, Outreach, and Development, 2016. [Available at https://www.fda.gov/vaccines-blood-biologics/biologics-guidances/tissue-guidances.]

59. Mezochow AK, Henry R, Blumberg EA, Kotton CN. Transfusion transmitted infections in solid organ transplantation. Am J Transplantation 2015;15:547-54.

60. Food and Drug Administration. Testing donors of human cells, tissues, and cellular and tissue-based products: Specific requirements. Silver Spring, MD: CBER Office of Communication, Outreach, and Development, 2015. [Available at https://www.fda.gov/vaccines-blood-biologics/safety-availability-biologics/testing-donors-human-cells-tissues-and-cellular-and-tissue-based-products-hctp-specific-requirements.]

61. Custer B, Stramer SL, Glynn S, et al. Transfusion-transmissible infection monitoring system: A tool to monitor changes in blood safety. Transfusion 2016;56:1499-502.

62. Anderson SA, Yang H, Gallagher LM, et al. Quantitative estimate of the risks and benefits of possible alternative blood donor deferral strategies for men who have had sex with men. Transfusion 2009;49:1102-14.

63. Zou S, Dorsey KA, Notari EP, et al. Prevalence, incidence, and residual risk of human immunodeficiency virus and hepatitis C virus infections among United States blood donors since the introduction of nucleic acid testing. Transfusion 2010;50:1495-504.

64. Schreiber GB, Busch MP, Kleinman SH, Korelitz JJ. The risk of transfusion-transmitted viral infections. The Retrovirus Epidemiology Donor Study. N Engl J Med 1996;334:1685-90.

65. Stramer SL, Glynn SA, Kleinman SH, et al. Detection of HIV-1 and HCV infections among antibody-negative blood donors by nucleic acid-amplification testing. N Engl J Med 2004;351:760-8.

66. Dodd RY, Notari EP 4th, Stramer SL. Current prevalence and incidence of infectious disease markers and estimated window-period risk in the American Red Cross blood donor population. Transfusion 2002;42:975-9.

67. Duong YT, Kassanjee R, Welte A, et al. Recalibration of the limiting antigen avidity EIA to determine mean duration of recent infection in divergent HIV-1 subtypes. PLoS One 2015;10: e0114947.

68. Stramer SL, Notari EP, Krysztof DE, Dodd RY. Hepatitis B virus testing by minipool nucleic acid testing: Does it improve blood safety? Transfusion 2013;53:2449-58.

69. Octaplas, pooled plasma (human), solvent/detergent treated solution for intravenous infusion insert (prescribing information). Hoboken, NJ: Octapharma USA.

70. Stramer SL, Hollinger FB, Katz LM, et al. Emerging infectious disease agents and their potential threat to transfusion safety. Transfusion 2009;49(Suppl 2):1S-29S.

71. Emerging infectious disease agents and their potential threat to transfusion safety. Bethesda, MD: AABB, 2017. [Available at http://www.aabb.org/tm/eid/Pages/default.aspx (accessed October 1, 2019).]

72. Stramer SL, Yu G, Herron R, et al. Two human immunodeficiency virus Type 2 cases in US blood donors including serologic, molecular, and genomic characterization of an epidemiologically unusual case. Transfusion 2016;56: 1560-8.

73. Centers for Disease Control and Prevention. HIV surveillance report, 2016. Vol. 28. Atlanta, GA: CDC, 2017. [Available at https://www.cdc.gov/hiv/library/reports/hiv-surveillance.html.]

74. Centers for Disease Control and Prevention. HIV prevalence, unrecognized infection, and HIV testing among men who have sex with men—five U.S. cities, June 2004-April 2005. MMWR Morb Mortal Wkly Rep 2005;54:597-601.

75. Truong HM, Kellogg T, Klausner JD, et al. Increases in sexually transmitted infections and sexual risk behaviour without a concurrent increase in HIV incidence among men who have sex with men in San Francisco: A suggestion of HIV serosorting? Sex Transm Infect 2006;82: 461-6.

76. Kleinman SH, Busch MP. Assessing the impact of HBV NAT on window period reduction and residual risk. J Clin Virol 2006;36(Suppl 1):S23-9.

77. Stramer SL. Pooled hepatitis B virus DNA testing by nucleic acid amplification: Implementation or not. Transfusion 2005;45:1242-6.

78. Linauts S, Saldanha J, Strong DM. PRISM hepatitis B surface antigen detection of hepatits B virus minipool nucleic acid testing yield samples. Transfusion 2008;48:1376-82.

79. Stramer SL, Wend U, Candotti D, et al. Nucleic acid testing to detect HBV infection in blood donors. N Engl J Med 2011;364:236-47.

80. Dodd RY, Nguyen ML, Krysztof DE, et al. Blood donor testing for hepatitis B virus in the United States: Is there a case for continuation of hepatitis B surface antigen detection? Transfusion 2018;58:2166-70.

81. Alter HJ. Descartes before the horse: I clone, therefore I am: The hepatitis C virus in current perspective. Ann Intern Med 1991;115:644-9.

82. Smith BD, Morgan RL, Beckett GA, et al. Recommendations for the identification of chronic hepatitis C virus infection among persons born during 1945-1965. MMWR Recomm Rep 2012;61:1-32.

83. Page-Shafer K, Pappalardo BL, Tobler LH, et al. Testing strategy to identify cases of acute hepatitis C virus (HCV) infection and to project HCV incidence rates. J Clin Microbiol 2008;46:499-506.

84. Guidelines for counseling persons infected with human T-lymphotropic virus type I (HTLV-I) and type II (HTLV-II). Centers for Disease Control and Prevention and the U.S.P.H.S. Working Group. Ann Intern Med 1993;118:448-54.

85. Vrielink H, Zaaijer HL, Reesink HW. The clinical relevance of HTLV type I and II in transfusion medicine. Transfus Med Rev 1997;11:173-9.

86. Aubron C, Nichol A, Cooper DJ, Bellomo R. Age of red blood cells and transfusion in critically ill patients. Ann Intensive Care 2013;3:2.

87. Eikelboom JW, Cook RJ, Liu Y, Heddle NM. Duration of red cell storage before transfusion and in-hospital mortality. Am Heart J 2010;159:737-43.

88. UK BTS Joint Professional Advisory Committee's (JPAC) HTLV Working Group. Options for human T-lymphotropic virus (HTLV) screening within the UK Blood Services (updated October 2015). [Available at https://www.transfusionguidelines.org/document-library/options-for-human-t-lymphotropic-virus-htlv-screening-with-the-uk-blood-services-updated-october-2015-r.]

89. Hewitt PE, Davison K, Howell DR, Taylor GP. Human T-lymphotropic virus lookback in NHS

Blood and Transplant (England) reveals the efficacy of leukoreduction. Transfusion 2013;53: 2168-75.

90. Petrik J, Lozano M, Seed CR, et al. Hepatitis E. Vox Sang 2016;110:93-130.

91. Hewitt PE, Ijaz S, Brailsford SR, et al. Hepatitis E virus in blood components: A prevalence and transmission study in southeast England. Lancet 2014;384:1766-73.

92. Stramer SL, Moritz ED, Foster GA, et al. Hepatitis E virus: Seroprevalence and frequency of viral RNA detection among US blood donors. Transfusion 2016;56:481-8.

93. Hauser L, Roque-Afonso AM, Beylouné A, et al. Hepatitis E transmission by transfusion of Intercept blood system-treated plasma. Blood 2014; 123:796-7.

94. Orton S. Syphilis and blood donors: What we know, what we do not know, and what we need to know. Transfus Med Rev 2001;15:282-91.

95. Katz LM. A test that won't die: The serologic test for syphilis. Transfusion 2009;49:617-19.

96. Zou S, Notari EP, Fang CT, et al. Current value of serologic test for syphilis as a surrogate marker for blood-borne viral infections among blood donors in the United States. Transfusion 2009; 49:655-61.

97. Orton SL, Liu H, Dodd RY, et al. Prevalence of circulating *Treponema pallidum* DNA and RNA in blood donors with confirmed-positive syphilis tests. Transfusion 2002;42:94-9.

98. Centers for Disease Control and Prevention. Sexually transmitted diseases (STDs): Syphilis statistics. Atlanta, GA: CDC, 2016. [Available at http://www.cdc. gov/std/syphilis/stats.htm.]

99. Food and Drug Administration. Fatalities reported to FDA following blood collection and transfusion: Annual summary for fiscal year 2015. Silver Spring, MD: CBER Office of Communication, Outreach, and Development, 2015.

100. Eder AF, Kennedy JM, Dy BA, et al. Limiting and detecting bacterial contamination of apheresis platelets: Inlet-line diversion and increased culture volume improve component safety. Transfusion 2009;49:1554-63.

101. Ramirez-Arcos SM, Goldman M, Blajchman MA. Bacterial infection: Bacterial contamination, testing and post-transfusion complications. 2nd ed. Philadelphia: Church Livingstone, 2007.

102. Suggested options for transfusion services and blood collectors to facilitate implementation of BB/TS Interim Standard 5.1.5.1.1. Association bulletin #10-05. Bethesda, MD: AABB, 2010.

103. Benjamin RJ, Kline L, Dy BA, et al. Bacterial contamination of whole-blood-derived platelets: The introduction of sample diversion and prestorage pooling with culture testing in the American Red Cross. Transfusion 2008;48: 2348-55.

104. McDonald C, Allen JM, Brailsford S, et al. Bacterial screening of platelet components by National Health Service Blood and Transplant, an effective risk reduction measure. Transfusion 2017;57:1122-31.

105. Benjamin RJ, Braschler T, Weingand T, Corash LM. Hemovigilance monitoring of platelet septic reactions with effective bacterial protection systems. Transfusion 2017;57:2946-57.

106. Jacobs MR, Smith D, Heaton WA, et al. Detection of bacterial contamination in prestorage culture-negative apheresis platelets on day of issue with the Pan Genera Detection test. Transfusion 2011;51:2573-82.

107. Ruby KN, Thomasson RR, Szczepiorkowski ZM, Dunbar NM. Bacterial screening of apheresis platelets with a rapid test: A 113-month single center experience. Transfusion 2018;58:1665-9.

108. Erony SM, Marshall CE, Gehrie EA, et al. The epidemiology of bacterial culture-positive and septic transfusion reactions at a large tertiary academic center: 2009 to 2016. Transfusion 2018;58:1933-9.

109. Kamel H, Townsend M, Bravo M, Vassallo RR. Improved yield of minimal proportional sample volume platelet bacterial culture. Transfusion 2017;57:2413-19.

110. Biggerstaff BJ, Petersen LR. Estimated risk of transmission of the West Nile virus through blood transfusion in the US, 2002. Transfusion 2003;43:1007-17.

111. Pealer L, Marfin A, Petersen LR. Transmission of West Nile virus through blood transfusion in the United States in 2002. N Engl J Med 2003;349: 1236-45.

112. Zou S, Foster GA, Dodd RY, et al. West Nile fever characteristics among viremic persons identified through blood donor screening. J Infect Dis 2010; 202:1354-61.

113. Dodd RY, Foster GA, Stramer SL. Keeping blood transfusion safe from West Nile virus: American Red Cross experience, 2003 to 2012. Transfus Med Rev 2015;29:153-61.

114. O'Brien SF, Scalia V, Zuber E, et al. West Nile virus in 2006 and 2007: The Canadian Blood Services' experience. Transfusion 2010;50:1118-25.

115. Groves JA, Shafi H, Nomura JH, et al. A probable case of West Nile virus transfusion transmission. Transfusion 2017;57:850-6.

116. Petersen LR, Jamieson DJ, Powers AM, Honein MA. Zika virus. N Engl J Med 2016;374:1552-63.

117. Pan American Health Organization, World Health Organization. Zika - epidemiological update. (August 25, 2017) Washington, DC: PAHO/WHO, 2017. [Available at http://www.paho.org/hq/dmdocu ments/2017/2017-aug-25-phe-epi-update-zika-virus.pdf (accessed October 1, 2019).]

118. Gallain P, Cabie A, Richard P, et al. Zika virus in asymptomatic blood donors in Martinique. Blood 2017; 129:263-6.

119. Rasmussen SA, Jamieson DJ, Honein MA, Petersen LR. Zika virus and birth defects—reviewing the evidence for causality. N Engl J Med 2016;374:1981-7.

120. Brasil P, Pereira JP Jr, Moreira ME, et al. Zika virus infection in pregnant women in Rio de Janeiro. N Engl J Med 2016;375:2321-34.

121. Franca GV, Schuler-Faccini L, Oliveira WK, et al. Congenital Zika virus syndrome in Brazil: A case series of the first 1501 livebirths with complete investigation. Lancet 2016;388:891-7.

122. Johansson MA, Mier-y-Teran-Romero L, Reefhuis J, et al. Zika and the risk of microcephaly. N Engl J Med 2016;375:1-4.

123. Garcez PP, Loiola EC, Madeiro da Costa R, et al. Zika virus impairs growth in human neurospheres and brain organoids. Science 2016;352:816-18.

124. Cao-Lormeau VM, Blake A, Mons S, et al. Guillain-Barre Syndrome outbreak associated with Zika virus infection in French Polynesia: A case-control study. Lancet 2016;387:1531-9.

125. Centers for Disease Control and Prevention. Zika virus: Statistics and maps. Atlanta, GA: CDC, 2019. [Available at http://www.cdc.gov/zika/reporting/index.html.]

126. Porse CC, Messenger S, Vugia DJ, et al. Travel-associated Zika cases and threat of local transmission during global outbreak, California, USA. Emerg Infect Dis 2018;24:1626-32.

127. Swaminathan S, Schlaberg R, Lewis J, et al. Fatal Zika virus infection with secondary nonsexual transmission. N Engl J Med 2016;375:1907-9.

128. Musso D, Nhan T, Robin E. Potential for Zika virus transmission through blood transfusion demonstrated during an outbreak in French Polynesia, November 2013 to February 2014. Euro Surveill 2014;19:20761.

129. Kuehnert MJ, Basavaraju SV, Moseley RR, et al. Screening of blood donations for Zika virus infection - Puerto Rico, April 3-June 11, 2016. MMWR Morb Mortal Wkly Rep 2016;65:627-8.

130. Benjamin RJ. Zika virus in the blood supply. Blood 2017;129:144-5.

131. Barjas-Castro ML, Angerami RN, Cunha MS, et al. Probable transfusion-transmitted Zika virus in Brazil. Transfusion 2016;56:1684-8.

132. Motta IJ, Spencer BR, Cordeiro da Silva SG, et al. Evidence for transmission of Zika virus by platelet transfusion. N Engl J Med 2016;375:1101-3.

133. Davidson A, Slavinski S, Komoto K, et al. Suspected female-to-male sexual transmission of Zika virus - New York City, 2016. MMWR Morb Mortal Wkly Rep 2016;65:716-17.

134. Lessler J, Ott CT, Carcelen AC, et al. Times to key events in Zika virus infection and implications for blood donation: A systematic review. Bull World Health Organ 2016;94:841-9.

135. Lustig Y, Mendelson E, Paran N, et al. Detection of Zika virus RNA in whole blood of imported Zika virus disease cases up to 2 months after symptom onset, Israel, December 2015 to April 2016. Euro Surveill 2016;21(26).

136. Atkinson B, Hearn P, Afrough B, et al. Detection of Zika virus in semen. Emerg Infect Dis 2016;22:940.

137. Mansuy JM, Pasquier C, Daudin M, et al. Zika virus in semen of a patient returning from a non-epidemic area. Lancet Infect Dis 2016;16:894-5.

138. Gaskell KM, Houlihan C, Nastouli E, Checkley AM. Persistent Zika virus detection in semen in a traveler returning to the United Kingdom from Brazil, 2016. Emerg Infect Dis 2017;23:137-9.

139. Medina FA, Torres G, Acevedo J, et al. Duration of the presence of infectious Zika virus in semen and serum. J Infect Dis 2019;219:31-40.

140. Paz-Bailey G, Rosenberg ES, Doyle K, et al. Persistence of Zika virus in body fluids - final report. N Engl J Med 2018;13:1234-43.

141. Food and Drug Administration. Guidance for industry: Recommendations for donor screening, deferral, and product management to reduce the risk of transfusion transmission of Zika virus. Silver Spring, MD: CBER Office of Communication, Outreach, and Development, 2016.

142. Food and Drug Administration. Guidance for industry: Revised recommendations for reducing

the risk of Zika virus transmission by blood and blood components. Silver Spring, MD: CBER Office of Communication, Outreach, and Development, 2016.

143. Stone M, Lanteri MC, Bakkour S, et al. Relative analytical sensitivity of donor nucleic acid amplification technology screening and diagnostic real-time polymerase chain reaction assays for detection of Zika virus RNA. Transfusion 2017; 57:734-47.

144. Galel SA, Williamson PC, Busch MP, et al. First Zika-positive donations in the continental United States. Transfusion 2017;57:762-9.

145. Williamson PC, Linnen JM, Kessler DA, et al. First cases of Zika virus-infected US blood donors outside states with areas of active transmission. Transfusion 2017;57:770-8.

146. Saa P, Proctor M, Foster G, et al. Investigational testing for Zika virus among U.S. blood donors. N Engl J Med 2018;378:1778-88.

147. Aubry M, Richard V, Green J, et al. Inactivation of Zika virus in plasma with amotosalen and ultraviolet A illumination. Transfusion 2016;56: 33-40.

148. Laughhunn A, Santa Maria F, Broult J, et al. Amustaline (S-303) treatment inactivates high levels of Zika virus in red blood cell components. Transfusion 2017;57:779-89.

149. Blumel J, Musso D, Teitz S, et al. Inactivation and removal of Zika virus during manufacture of plasma-derived medicinal products. Transfusion 2017; 57:790-6.

150. Kuhnel D, Muller S, Pichotta A, et al. Inactivation of Zika virus by solvent/detergent treatment of human plasma and other plasma-derived products and pasteurization of human serum albumin. Transfusion 2017;57:802-10.

151. Anez G, Rios M. Dengue in the United States of America: A worsening scenario? Biomed Res Int 2013;2013:678645.

152. Tomashek KM, Margolis HS. Dengue: A potential transfusion-transmitted disease. Transfusion 2011;51:1654-60.

153. Stramer SL, Linnen JM, Carrick JM, et al. Dengue viremia in blood donors identified by RNA and detection of dengue transfusion transmission during the 2007 dengue outbreak in Puerto Rico. Transfusion 2012;52:1657-66.

154. Matos D, Tomashek KM, Perez-Padilla J, et al. Probable and possible transfusion-transmitted dengue associated with NS1 antigen-negative but RNA confirmed-positive red blood cells. Transfusion 2016; 56:215-22.

155. Sabino EC, Loureiro P, Lopes ME, et al. Transfusion-transmitted dengue and associated clinical symptoms during the 2012 epidemic in Brazil. J Infect Dis 2016;213:694-702.

156. Matos D, Tomashek KM, Perez-Padilla J, et al. Probable and possible transfusion-transmitted dengue associated with NS1 antigen-negative but RNA confirmed-positive red blood cells. Transfusion 2016; 56:215-22.

157. Vogt MB, Lahon A, Arya RP, et al. Mosquito saliva alone has profound effects on the human immune system. PLoS Negl Trop Dis 2018;12: e0006439.

158. Chiu CY, Bres V, Yu G, et al. Genomic assays for identification of Chikungunya virus in blood donors, Puerto Rico, 2014. Emerg Infect Dis 2015;21:1409-13.

159. Brouard C, Bernillon P, Quatresous I, et al. Estimated risk of Chikungunya viremic blood donation during an epidemic on Reunion Island in the Indian Ocean, 2005 to 2007. Transfusion 2008;48:1333-41.

160. Simmons G, Bres V, Lu K, et al. High incidence of chikungunya virus and frequency of viremic blood donations during epidemic, Puerto Rico, USA, 2014. Emerg Infect Dis 2016;22:1221-8.

161. Otani MM, Vinelli E, Kirchhoff LV, et al. WHO comparative evaluation of serologic assays for Chagas disease. Transfusion 2009;49:1076-82.

162. Food and Drug Administration. Blood Products Advisory Committee, 94th meeting. Silver Spring, MD: CBER Office of Communication, Outreach, and Development, 2009. [Available at https://wayback. archive-it.org/7993/ 20170111012330/http://www.fda.gov/Advi soryCommittees/Committees MeetingMateri als/BloodVaccinesandOtherBiolo gics/Blood-ProductsAdvisoryCommittee/ucm121612. htm.]

163. Food and Drug Administration. Guidance for industry: Use of serological tests to reduce the risk of transmission of *Trypanosoma cruzi* infection in whole blood and blood components intended for transfusion. Silver Spring, MD: CBER Office of Communication, Outreach, and Development, 2010.

164. Steele WR, Hewitt EH, Kaldun AM, et al. Donors deferred for self-reported Chagas disease history: Does it reduce risk? Transfusion 2014; 54:2092-7.

165. Benjamin RJ, Stramer SL, Leiby DA, et al. *Trypanosoma cruzi* infection in North America and Spain: Evidence in support of transfusion transmission. Transfusion 2012;52:1913-21; quiz 2.

166. Kessler DA, Shi PA, Avecilla ST, Shaz BH. Results of lookback for Chagas disease since the inception of donor screening at New York Blood Center. Transfusion 2013;53:1083-7.

167. Blumental S, Lambermont M, Heijmans C, et al. First documented transmission of *Trypanosoma cruzi* infection through blood transfusion in a child with sickle-cell disease in Belgium. PLoS Negl Trop Dis 2015;9:e0003986.

168. Herwaldt BL, Linden JV, Bosserman E, et al. Transfusion-associated babesiosis in the United States: A description of cases. Ann Intern Med 2011;155:509-19.

169. Fang DC, McCullough J. Transfusion-transmitted *Babesia microti*. Transfus Med Rev 2016;30: 132-8.

170. Linden JV, Prusinski MA, Crowder LA, et al. Transfusion-transmitted and community-acquired babesiosis in New York, 2004 to 2015. Transfusion 2018;58:660-8.

171. Moritz ED, Winton CS, Tonnetti L, et al. Screening for *Babesia microti* in the U.S. blood supply. N Engl J Med 2016;375:2236-45.

172. Ward SJ, Stramer SL, Szczepiokowski ZM. Assessing the risk of *Babesia* to the United States blood supply using a risk-based decision-making approach: Report of AABB's Ad Hoc Babesia Policy Working Group (original report). Transfusion 2018;58:1916-23.

173. Tonnetti L, Laughhunn A, Thorp AM, et al. Inactivation of *Babesia microti* in red blood cells and platelet concentrates. Transfusion 2017;57: 2404-12.

174. Tonnetti L, Eder AF, Dy B, et al. Transfusion-transmitted *Babesia microti* identified through hemovigilance. Transfusion 2009;49:2557-63.

175. Mali S, Steele S, Slutsker L, Arguin PM. Malaria surveillance - United States, 2007. MMWR Surveill Summ 2009;58:1-16.

176. Mali S, Tan KR, Arguin PM. Malaria surveillance—United States, 2009. MMWR Surveill Summ 2011;60:1-15.

177. Anand A, Mace KE, Townsend RL, et al. Investigation of a case of suspected transfusion-transmitted malaria. Transfusion 2018;58:2115-21.

178. Food and Drug Administration. Guidance for industry: Revised recommendations to reduce the risk of transfusion-transmitted malaria. Silver Spring, MD: CBER Office of Communication, Outreach, and Development, 2020.

179. Spencer B, Steele W, Custer B, et al. Risk for malaria in United States donors deferred for travel

to malaria-endemic areas. Transfusion 2009;49: 2335-45.

180. O'Brien SF, Delage G, Seed CR, et al. The epidemiology of imported malaria and transfusion policy in 5 nonendemic countries. Transfus Med Rev 2015; 29:162-71.

181. Allain JP, Owusu-Ofori AK, Assennato SM, et al. Effect of *Plasmodium* inactivation in whole blood on the incidence of blood transfusion-transmitted malaria in endemic regions: The African investigation of the Mirasol System (AIMS) randomised controlled trial. Lancet 2016;387:1753-61.

182. Crowder LA, Schonberger LB, Dodd RY, Steele WR. Creutzfeldt-Jakob disease lookback study: 21 years of surveillance for transfusion transmission risk. Transfusion 2017;57:1875-8.

183. Urwin PJ, Mackenzie JM, Llewelyn CA, et al. Creutzfeldt-Jakob disease and blood transfusion: Updated results of the UK Transfusion Medicine Epidemiology Review Study. Vox Sang 2016; 110:310-16.

184. Food and Drug Administration. Guidance for industry: Recommendations to reduce the possible risk of transmission of Creutzfeldt-Jakob Disease (CJD) and variant Creutzfeldt-Jakob disease (vCJD) by blood and blood products. Silver Spring, MD: CBER Office of Communication, Outreach, and Development, 2020.

185. Seed CR, Hewitt PE, Dodd RY, et al. Creutzfeltd-Jakob disease and blood transfusion safety. Vox Sang 2018;113:220-31.

186. Mok T, Jaunmuktane Z, Joiner S, et al. Variant Creutzfeldt–Jakob disease in a patient with heterozygosity at PRNP codon 129. N Engl J Med 2017;379:292-4.

187. Bougard D, Brandel JP, Bélondrade M, et al. Detection of prions in the plasma of presymptomatic and symptomatic patients with variant Creutzfeldt-Jakob disease. Sci Transl Med 2016; 8:370ra182.

188. Cooper JK, Andrews N, Ladhani K, et al. Evaluation of a test for its suitability in the diagnosis of variant Creutzfeldt-Jakob disease. Vox Sang 2013;105:196-204.

189. Snyder E, Stramer S, Benjamin RJ. The safety of the US blood supply - time to raise the bar. N Engl J Med 2015;372:1882-5.

190. Norris PJ, Kaidarova Z, Maiorana E, et al. Ultraviolet light-based pathogen inactivation and alloimmunization after platelet transfusion: Results from a randomized trial. Transfusion 2018;58: 1210-17.

191. Webert KE, Cserti CM, Hannon J, et al. Proceedings of a Consensus Conference: Pathogen inactivation-making decisions about new technologies. Transfus Med Rev 2008;22:1-34.

192. Klein HG, Anderson D, Bernardi MJ, et al. Pathogen inactivation: Making decisions about new technologies. Report of a consensus conference. Transfusion 2007;47:2338-47.

193. Seghatchian J, Hervig T, Putter JS. Effect of pathogen inactivation on the storage lesion in red cells and platelet concentrates. Transfus Apher Sci 2011;45:75-84.

194. Food and Drug Administration. Guidance for industry: Recommendations for assessment of blood donor eligibility, donor deferral and blood product management in response to Ebola virus. Silver Spring, MD: CBER Office of Communication, Outreach, and Development, 2017.

CHAPTER 8

Molecular Biology and Immunology in Transfusion Medicine

Sean R. Stowell, MD, PhD, and James D. Gorham, MD, PhD

THIS CHAPTER REVIEWS FUNDAMEN-
tal principles and approaches for analyzing
nucleic acids and proteins, particularly antibodies, and introduces basic concepts in humoral (antibody-mediated) immunity.

In the practice of transfusion medicine, analyses of nucleic acids and antibodies are extensively employed to 1) detect infectious pathogens in donated components; 2) predict the
phenotypic expression of antigens on the surface of cells (red cells, platelets, and neutrophils); 3) detect and identify red cell and platelet
antibodies; 4) determine HLA type; and 5)
perform relationship testing. Although the last is
somewhat outside transfusion medicine practice, it is a component of AABB's standards and
accreditation programs.

Entire textbooks explain molecular biology
and immunology. This chapter focuses on topics
immediately relevant to the practice of transfusion testing. Moreover, within immunology, the
primary focus is humoral immunity, which is
more relevant to most of the practice of transfusion medicine than is cellular immunity. Finally,
because many assays exist, specific assay protocols are not provided here.

ANALYSIS OF DNA

The practical application of nucleic acid analysis
in transfusion medicine lies in two principal areas: 1) the detection of infectious pathogens and
2) the genotyping of blood donors and recipients. The human genome is made up of DNA,
organized into chromosomes, which are present
in the cell nucleus. Whereas most cells in the
human body are nucleated, red cells and platelets lack nuclei and therefore DNA. The genotype of an individual is his or her genetic make-
up, encoded in the DNA; in practical transfusion
medicine, the term "genotype" is commonly
used to refer to the specific allele present at a
single gene locus. Bacteria, fungi, protozoa, and
many viruses also use DNA to encode their genomes. Some viral pathogens use RNA instead.
Either DNA or RNA encodes all known genetic
material relevant to transfusion medicine, with

Sean R. Stowell, MD, PhD, Director of Apheresis, Emory University Hospital, and Medical Director of the Blood
Bank and Transfusion Services, Emory University Orthopedic and Spine Hospital, Emory University School of
Medicine, Atlanta, Georgia; and James D. Gorham, MD, PhD, Professor of Pathology, Chief, Division of Labora-
tory Medicine, and Medical Director of the Blood Bank and Transfusion Medicine Services, University of Virginia
Health System, Charlottesville, Virginia
The authors have disclosed no conflicts of interest.

the notable exception of prions, which appear to lack nucleic acids.

Basic Chemistry and Structure of Nucleic Acids

A brief overview of this topic is presented here, while more details are available elsewhere.[1] DNA is a nucleic acid polymer containing chains of nucleotides. Nucleotides are composed of three moieties: 1) a pentose sugar (five carbon atoms); 2) a phosphate group linked to carbon 5 (C5); and 3) a base group attached to carbon 1 (C1) [Fig 8-1 (A)].

There are four different nucleotides in DNA—adenine (A), guanine (G), cytosine (C), and thymine (T)—which differ from one another in the chemical structure of the C1 base group. Polymers of DNA consist of repeats of covalently bound sugars and phosphates that form the outside backbone of the double helical strand of DNA. DNA strands are described as having a "5′ end" and a "3′ end," terms that re-

fer to the end with a free phosphate attached to C5 and the opposite end with a free hydroxyl group attached to carbon 3 (C3), respectively [Fig 8-1 (B)].

The human genome consists of double-stranded DNA (dsDNA). The bases within one strand of DNA form noncovalent hydrogen bonds with complementary bases on the other strand. Specifically, T always pairs with A, using two hydrogen bonds, and G always pairs with C, using three hydrogen bonds. When two strands have complementary sequences, they can "hybridize" via hydrogen bonding between complementary base pairs to form a dsDNA molecule [Fig 8-1 (C)]. The two complementary strands align such that the 5′ and 3′ ends have opposite orientations and form a double helix in which the phosphodiester backbone is on the outside of the helix and the hydrogen-bond-paired bases are on the inside. DNA molecules vary from each other based on the sequence of

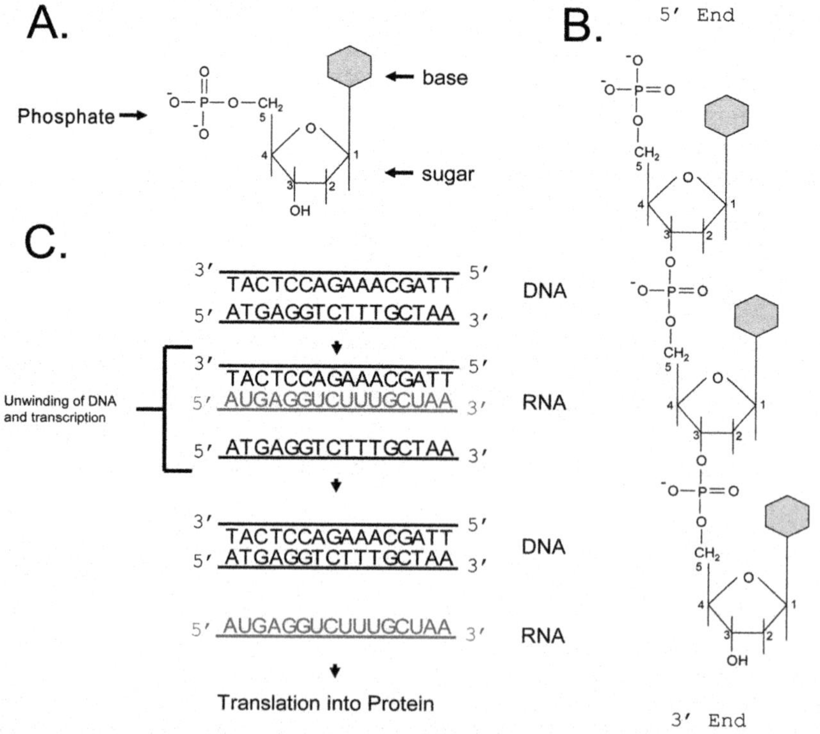

FIGURE 8-1. Chemical structure of nucleic acids and DNA.

nucleotides, determined by the bases incorporated into the polymer.

When genes are expressed, the DNA encoding a given gene is used as a template to produce RNA, which is further processed to form a messenger RNA (mRNA) that is then exported from the nucleus to the cytoplasm and used as a guide to produce proteins, the workhorses of most cellular activity. The structure of RNA is similar to that of DNA, with some differences: 1) ribonucleotides have an additional hydroxyl group on carbon 2; 2) uracil (U) is used in place of thymine (T); and 3) RNA is typically single stranded.

Several classes of RNA exist in human cells; the class that is used as a blueprint for protein synthesis is mRNA. When a gene is expressed, it is used as a template to generate a copy of itself in mRNA form, a process termed "transcription." The transcription machinery unwinds the DNA double helix, synthesizes a new mRNA strand of complementary sequence, and reanneals the DNA in its wake [Fig 8-1 (C)]. Thus, the mRNA represents a copy of the gene sequence present in the DNA. mRNA is always synthesized in the "5′ to 3′ direction," and thus for a given gene, only one of the two DNA strands is transcribed into mRNA. After synthesis in the nucleus, mRNA is processed and exported to the cytoplasm, where ribosomes use it as a template to synthesize a new protein molecule, a process called "translation."

Isolation of Nucleic Acid

The first step in most DNA and RNA analyses is the isolation of nucleic acids. Because essentially all nucleated cells of an individual contain identical genomic DNA (gDNA), gDNA can be isolated from any readily obtainable cellular source, such as peripheral blood leukocytes or buccal swabs (epithelial cells). However, mRNAs differ between cell types, because their differential expression patterns are important in defining the phenotypes of these cells. The implication of this is that for mRNA analysis, the choice of source cells is critical. Kits are readily available from multiple manufacturers for the simple and rapid isolation of high-quality cellular DNA or mRNA, or of nucleic acids from plasma.

The Polymerase Chain Reaction

Nucleic acid detection and analysis were revolutionized by the invention of the polymerase chain reaction (PCR) in the 1980s. PCR was the first amplification-based technique for generating many copies of nucleic acid fragments for direct analysis.[2] A PCR requires: 1) a DNA sample to be analyzed (the "target" or "template"); 2) gene-specific primers of around 20 nucleotides in length; 3) a thermostable DNA polymerase enzyme that recognizes primer bound to target DNA and sequentially adds the complementary nucleotide building blocks to extend the length of the primed DNA strand; 4) the four nucleotides (ATCG); and 5) the proper buffer. PCR involves repeat cycles of heating/cooling ("thermocycling"), allowing exponential DNA amplification of the fragment of interest, carried out in a thermocycler that rapidly changes temperature with accuracy and precision. A single cycle involves 1) heating to denature the template dsDNA to allow strand separation, 2) cooling to allow annealing of primer to complementary regions on the template DNA, and 3) extension and synthesis of DNA on the primer strand. Typically, 20 to 40 cycles are performed in total, depending on the abundance of the template and the required sensitivity of the assay.

Figure 8-2 shows an example, beginning with a single copy of a dsDNA template. The dsDNA is denatured by heating to near boiling (~95 C), disrupting the hydrogen bonds between complementary bases, thereby separating the two strands. The temperature is then lowered to allow gene-specific primers in the reaction mix to anneal to their complementary targets. One primer is designed to anneal "upstream" (aka "just 5′") to the region of interest, whereas the other is designed to anneal "downstream" (aka "just 3′") to this region. The temperature is then raised to 72 C, the temperature at which the thermostable polymerase functions optimally, and the primers are extended along the length of the DNA through incorporation of complementary nucleotides. Thus, at the end of extension, there are two copies of the DNA. The process of denaturing, annealing, and extension then repeats itself. Each subsequent

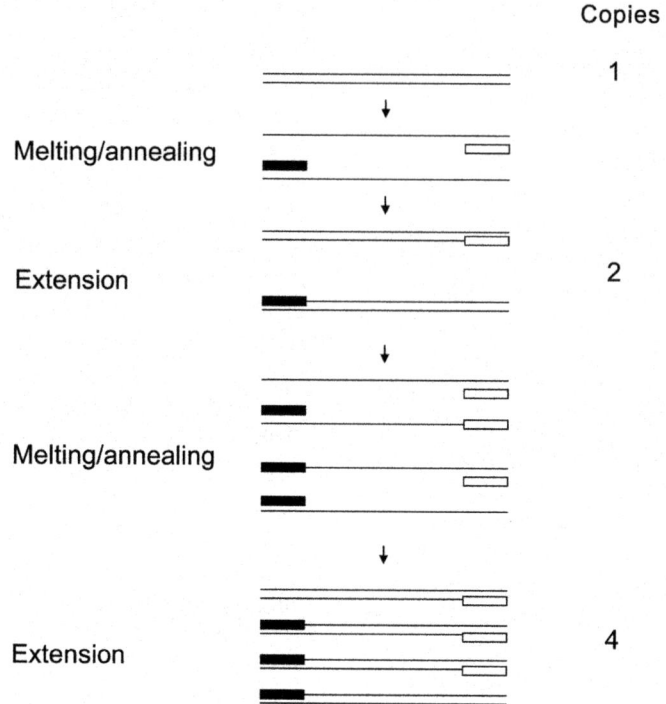

FIGURE 8-2. Overview of the polymerase chain reaction.

cycle yields a doubling in DNA copy number. PCR results in an exponential expansion of a selected DNA "amplicon," defined as the sequence bound by the two chosen primers.

PCR Considerations

Although PCR is a robust method of detecting nucleic acids, technical considerations can affect PCR and other amplification-based techniques.

Specimen Processing and Template Degradation

DNA is stable and can usually withstand variations in storage temperature and handling before being processed for genomic analysis. Exceptions include samples in which the target DNA is present in low quantity, such as fetal typing from maternal plasma and viral testing. By contrast, RNA is far less stable, as it is susceptible both to spontaneous autodegradation and to catalytic degradation mediated by abundant thermostable RNAse enzymes found in many biologic specimens.

Inhibitors

Because PCR amplification depends on the enzymatic activity of DNA polymerase, PCR can be inhibited by substances that negatively affect the activity. Heparin can inhibit PCR, and hemoglobin or lactoferrin released from erythrocytes or leukocytes also inhibits this process.[3] Most analytic systems minimize risk of interference by an inhibitor, but deviations from established protocols may introduce unintended inhibitory substances. To detect the presence of inhibitors, controls include amplifying ubiquitous target sequences (conserved regions of gDNA) and/or spiking the specimen with a positive control.

Primer Design

Although inferior performance of primers is typically not a concern for commercially available tests, understanding primer design is important in assay troubleshooting and in developing PCR-based assays for new targets. Although the ideal primer hybridizes to a target found in only one location in the entire genome, given the complexity of gDNA, primer annealing to unintended targets can occur, resulting in both the potential to amplify unintended targets and the ongoing consumption of primers. In addition, primers can anneal to each other to form a short amplicon, in a so-called primer-dimer formation.[4]

Contamination

One of the greatest strengths of PCR is its ability to amplify very small amounts of genetic material. In theory, single-copy sensitivity can be achieved. In practice, about 10 copies of target DNA are the lower limit of detection, depending on the sensitivity of the assay readout. The sensitivity makes PCR susceptible to false-positive results due to contamination either from other specimens being analyzed or, more commonly, from amplicons generated in previous PCR runs. Beginning with just 10 molecules of DNA, 30 rounds of PCR amplification yields >10^{10} amplicons. Thus, as little as 0.0000001% of a previous reaction inadvertently introduced into a pipette, picked up from a laboratory surface, or from the thermocycler can lead to a false-positive result in a subsequent reaction.

To minimize contamination, PCR laboratories routinely process samples in one geographic direction. DNA extraction is located away from testing, and PCR reactions are assembled in one room (or in a positive pressure hood) and amplified in a second room; any downstream analysis is performed in a third room. There should be no retrograde flow, and no materials or instruments used in the amplification or analysis (post-PCR) rooms should ever make their way into the DNA extraction and PCR setup (pre-PCR) room. Filtered pipette tips are routinely used to minimize carryover contamination and sample aerosols. Recent developments in which PCR extraction is avoided altogether and the PCR process uses an entirely closed system[5] may soon obviate the need for geographic directional flow in clinical laboratories.

Another effective method to avoid contamination involves the addition of deoxyuridine triphosphate (dUTP) before PCR amplification. Polymerases incorporate dUTP in place of deoxythymidine triphosphate (dTTP). The enzyme uracil-DNA glycosylase (UNG) is also added to specifically cleave DNA containing uracil[6]; thus, UNG in PCR reactions destroys contaminating amplicons from previous amplifications but not native DNA in the specimen. The initial PCR denaturation step inactivates the heat-labile UNG.

Finally, it is standard practice to include a water control, for which water, rather than a DNA sample, is used as the input sample. The water control (no-DNA control) reaction should yield no detectable signal above background. Signal in the water control indicates probable contamination of a reagent or instrument and invalidates the test run.

Reverse Transcriptase PCR

Messenger RNA is unsuitable as a template for PCR. When analysis of mRNA is desired, an additional step is employed to generate a single-stranded complementary DNA (cDNA), using mRNA as the template. The enzyme reverse transcriptase (RT) synthesizes cDNA from an RNA template (in the 5′ to 3′ direction), requiring the annealing of a primer to initiate transcription. The cDNA is then a suitable substrate for PCR.

Transcription-Mediated Amplification and Sequence-Based Amplification

There are additional non-PCR amplification techniques; among these, transcription-mediated amplification (TMA) and nucleic acid sequence-based amplification (NASBA) are further described (Fig 8-3).[7,8]

TMA plays a large role in nucleic acid testing (NAT) for human immunodeficiency virus (HIV), hepatitis C virus (HCV), and West Nile virus, for which viral RNA is the target. The reaction contains two primers, RT, DNA polymerase, RNAse H, and a sequence-specific RNA polymerase called T7 polymerase. A sequence-specific downstream primer hybridizes to the 3′ end of the target RNA, and RT synthesizes a

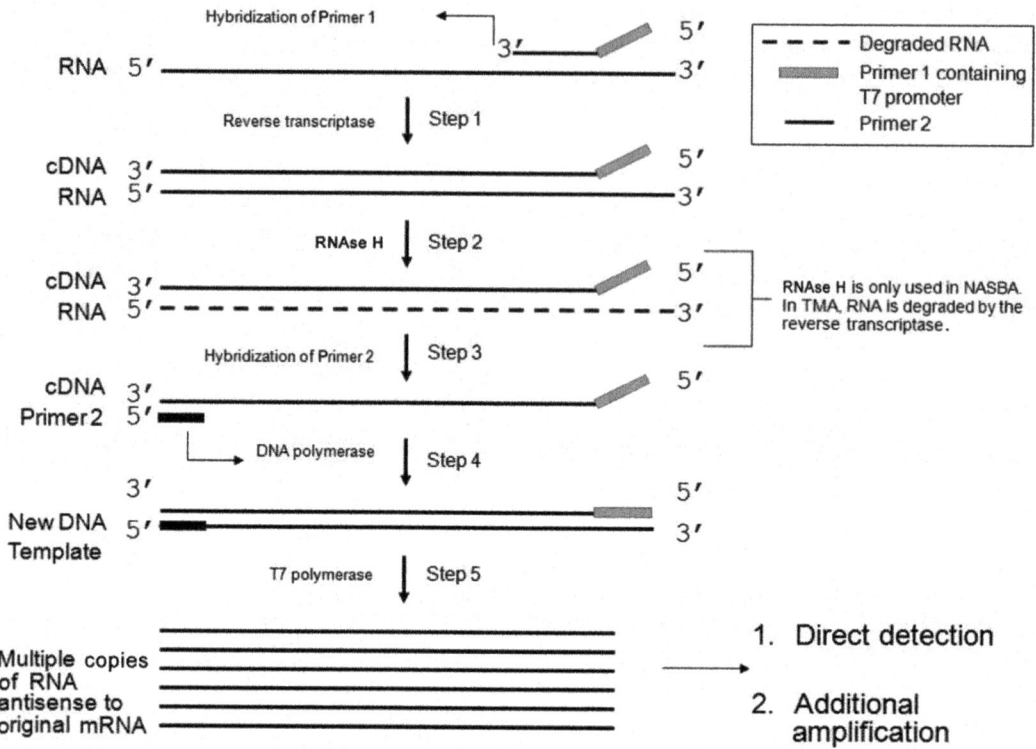

FIGURE 8-3. Overview of transcription-mediated amplification and nucleic acid sequence-based amplification. RNA = ribonucleic acid; cDNA = complementary deoxyribonucleic acid; mRNA = messenger RNA; RNAse = ribonuclease.

cDNA copy (Fig 8-3, step 1). Primer 1 contains a sequence at its 3′ end that hybridizes to the target RNA and a specific sequence at its 5′ end that serves as a promoter for the T7 polymerase. The RNA template is degraded either by RT itself (TMA assay) or by RNAse H (NASBA assay) (step 2). A second primer (primer 2) then binds to the newly synthesized cDNA (step 3) and utilizes DNA polymerase to synthesize a dsDNA molecule (step 4). This molecule now has a T7 promoter at one end (from primer 1), and thus T7 polymerase drives transcription of new RNA (step 5). The numerous RNA transcripts synthesized from a single DNA template can reenter the amplification cycle, with primer 2 initiating reverse transcription, followed by RNA degradation and subsequent synthesis of DNA using primer 1 and DNA polymerase. This leads to additional amplification, with ongoing cycles of transcription and template synthesis. One ad-

vantage of NASBA over PCR is that repeat nucleic acid denaturation is unnecessary; amplification of RNA is isothermal and thus does not require a thermocycler.

Detection of Amplification Products

Traditionally, amplicons were detected through separation by gel electrophoresis, followed by visualization of fragment length using a fluorescent DNA intercalating agent such as ethidium bromide. Because gel electrophoresis is time-consuming and not readily automated, more advanced techniques for detecting amplicons have become routine in the clinical laboratory.

Real-Time PCR

Real-time PCR employs one or more "probes" that fluoresce only when the target amplicon is present. A probe is a short oligomer of DNA that hybridizes to a specific cDNA sequence located within the amplicon. For real-time PCR approaches, the thermocycler used also incorporates a built-in fluorescence spectrophotometer, allowing for the detection of amplification products with each cycle. Real-time PCR is highly sensitive and quantitative and (through the use of multiple reporter dyes with distinct fluorescence spectra) permits the detection of multiple targets in a single reaction tube (multiplex amplification). In addition, because detection allows analysis without opening the reaction tube, the risk of laboratory contamination with amplicons (and subsequent false-positive results) is greatly minimized.

Several approaches can be used to detect fluorescence resulting from amplicon production. The TaqMan system (Applied Biosystems) employs a probe built with a fluorescent chemical tag (a "fluorochrome") at one end and a fluorescence quencher tag at the other [Fig 8-4 (A)]. Tethered to the probe, the two tags are close enough that the quencher effectively blocks the fluorescent signal. During amplicon synthesis, DNA polymerase, moving along the template strand, encounters the hybridized probe. DNA polymerase also has a nuclease activity, which causes probe degradation. The fluorochrome is now liberated from the probe and, no longer in proximity to the quencher, begins to fluoresce. Because fluorochrome liberation occurs only when 1) the probe hybridizes to its target and 2) DNA polymerase degrades the bound probe, fluorescence generation is a highly specific function of amplicon generation.

A second approach uses a molecular "beacon" that, like the TaqMan probe, has a fluorochrome tag at one end and a quencher tag at the other. The beacon probe is built such that the target sequence is flanked by complementary sequences. Unbound probe forms a hairpin loop, thus closely juxtaposing the fluorochrome with the quencher. As the amplicon is generated, the beacon hybridizes to its target, and the hairpin loop unfolds; the quencher is now sufficiently distant from the fluorochrome that fluorescence is generated [Fig 8-4 (B)].

A third approach uses two probes, each of which has a distinct tag tethered to it. Fluorescence does not occur unless the two tags are near to one other. If the amplicon is present, the probes anneal so that the two tags are in close proximity, and fluorescence ensues [Fig 8-4 (C)].

A fourth method (not shown) uses a dye called SYBR green (Thermo Fisher Scientific), which fluoresces only when bound to dsDNA. Unlike the above approaches, SYBR green is not sequence-specific but detects all dsDNA in the reaction tube. It is thus less specific than approaches that use sequence-specific probes and is more prone to false-positive results. Fortunately, authentic amplicons typically can be distinguished from aberrant products by making use of a "melting curve" analysis, which assesses the temperature profile at which the amplicon denatures ("melts"). Because the melting curve is a function of amplicon size and of GC content, and the size and sequence of the correct amplicon is known, the melting curve is useful to confirm the identity of the amplicon.

These fluorescent-probe techniques are applicable not only to real-time PCR, but also to other amplification technologies, such as TMA (above).

DNA Arrays

Evaluation at the DNA level of differences in the genes encoding protein blood groups is becoming much more commonly employed in the practice of transfusion medicine.[9] The vast majority of blood group antigens are the result of small differences in membrane proteins, often a single amino acid residue, that are encoded by single nucleotide polymorphisms (SNPs) at the level of gDNA.

Methods for detecting blood group SNPs primarily use PCR amplification followed by analysis by DNA-array technologies. After the region of interest in a blood group gene is amplified by PCR, specific products are detected by primers (or probes) designed such that hybridization and signal output depends on the presence of one allele but not the other. Multiplex PCR and DNA-array systems can determine the genotypes of blood group antigens in individual specimens and offer high throughput and automated readout.[10-12]

A.

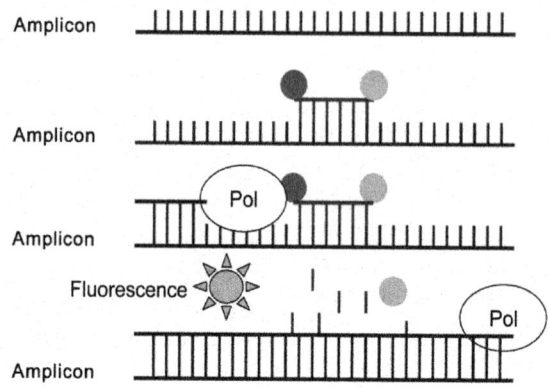

B.

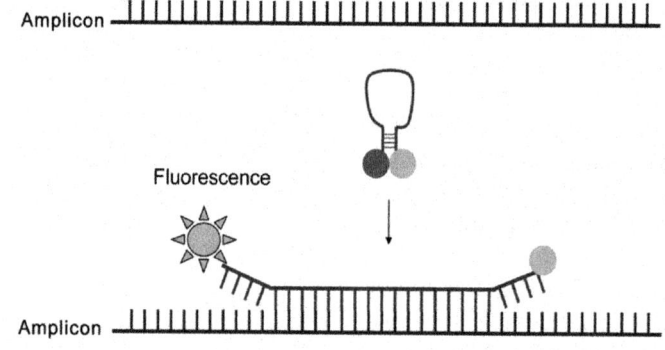

C.

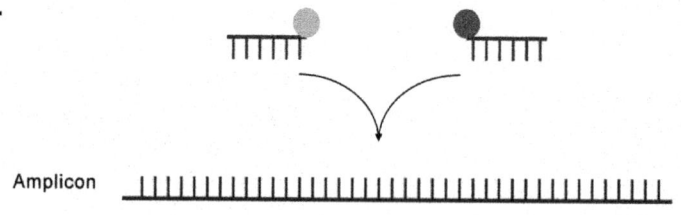

FIGURE 8-4. Methods of detection by sequence-specific probes during real-time polymerase chain reaction. Pol = polymerase enzyme.

Genotyping to predict red cell antigens can be more efficient than traditional serologic typing.[13-16] In the case of the patient who has had multiple transfusions, where it may not be possible to distinguish the patient's own red cells from transfused red cells, genotyping patient DNA can reliably predict the patient's red cell phenotype.[17] When serologic reagents inadequately characterize certain antigens (eg, partial D), genotyping can provide detailed information[18] and is helpful in identifying which patients with a weak D identified using serologic testing would benefit from Rh Immune Globulin (RhIG) immunoprophylaxis.[19] Genotyping can also be helpful when assessing alloantigens that may not be detected serologically, such as those of the DO (Dombrock) system, some forms of weak D (eg, DEL), and Fy^{X}[20]; identifying these antigens is particularly helpful when investigating patients manifesting hemolytic transfusion reactions in the absence of detectable alloantibodies.[21] Genotyping to predict multiple blood group antigens is especially useful in sickle cell disease (SCD) patients and other disease states in which frequent transfusion is expected and antigen-matching to prevent alloimmunization is an important component of long-term care.[22-25]

Genotyping platforms currently approved by the Food and Drug Administration (FDA) focus on known single nucleotide and other common polymorphisms, including those that regulate antigen expression [eg, GATA mutation impacting FY (Duffy) expression],[21] and allow the identification in parallel of multiple polymorphisms, greatly facilitating the selection of appropriate Red Blood Cell (RBC) units for transfusion for patients with multiple antibodies.[25,26] However, some haplotypes, such as *RHCE*ce* alleles that express Rhce variants may be inferred based on results generated on current platforms, although confirmatory studies are typically required. Some blood group antigens arise from complex genetic interactions or from alleles not fully represented on FDA-approved platforms. Genotyping platforms do not clarify complex antigen determinants such as *ABO, GLOB, RHD, RHCE, GYPA,* and *GYPB.*[17] Despite prophylactic matching, alloimmunization toward Rh variants continues to be a significant challenge in transfusion practice. The reliable determination of *RhD* and

RhCE allele sequences is particularly important, and genotyping platforms are often incapable of resolving the underlying allelic composition.[27] Because current FDA platforms require inclusion of specific targets a priori, a new (hitherto unknown) polymorphism in a coding region that alters protein structure, or in a noncoding region (such as the gene promoter) that regulates expression, would not be detected. As the relationship between genetic polymorphisms and antigen expression continues to be refined, the prediction of antigen expression will continue to improve.

Next-Generation Sequencing

The entire human genome was sequenced by traditional sequencing methods in 2001 at a cost of nearly 13 billion US dollars. Defining the sequence of the human genome was expected to dramatically change approaches to genetic analysis of clinical disease and to biomedical research, but the high cost and excessively long turnaround time of whole genome sequencing by traditional methods prohibited its use in routine clinical practice. However, over the last decade or so, more robust sequencing technologies have emerged, collectively referred to as next-generation sequencing (NGS), allowing the realization of the practical potential of DNA sequencing.[28]

Whereas early sequencing approaches addressed one stretch of DNA at a time, NGS involves sequencing massive amounts of distinct stretches of DNA in parallel. Although different NGS approaches use a variety of platforms and technologies, all involve sequencing individual sections of target DNA multiple times as "reads." A bioinformatic algorithm incorporates overlapping reads with a prior sequencing database to determine the location of a relevant read within a reference genome. NGS aligns reads in silico to produce the genetic signature of a given individual. Although the fidelity of a single NGS read is less robust than older sequencing approaches, an increased read number greatly enhances statistical confidence. The ability of NGS to simultaneously sequence multiple stretches of DNA has dramatically reduced the time and cost of sequencing an entire genome, with costs approaching 1000 US dollars per genome.[28]

Despite significant advantages over traditional sequencing technologies, NGS has limitations. First, although the cost of acquiring the raw sequence has dropped dramatically,[28] the bioinformatics infrastructure required to store and process the very large dataset is substantial and can be cost prohibitive. These costs may be partially offset by mining extant sequence data previously acquired for other clinical indications. Indeed, some groups have begun to develop promising bioinformatic methods interrogating NGS data for blood group characterization, with high accuracy.[29-32] Second, due to relatively short reads, NGS is often limited in its ability to distinguish highly similar genetic sequences, such as the paralogs *RHD* and *RHCE*, which are 93% identical.[33] However, recent paralog-specific NGS approaches can successfully detect variations in *RHD* and *RHCE*.[34] Although such strategies are still at an investigative stage, they illustrate the potential impact of genomic approaches on the practice of transfusion medicine. For example, coupling robust paralog-specific NGS approaches in donors and recipients with targeted efforts to increase minority blood donor participation holds significant promise in reducing the deleterious consequences of RhD and RhCE alloimmunization in patients with SCD.[35]

ANALYSIS OF PROTEIN

Much laboratory testing in transfusion medicine involves the detection and identification of antibodies in patients' plasma. In the following sections, the principles of the more common laboratory assays used to detect antibodies are described. Less routinely used technologies that are nevertheless important to understand are also presented.

Fluid-Phase Assays (Agglutination-Based Methods)

Depending on antibody isotype, immunoglobulins contain two (IgG) to 10 (IgM) antigen-binding sites per molecule. Each antibody can bind more than one target molecule, allowing antibodies to crosslink antigens present in multiple copies on red cells. A standard serologic method for detecting antibody-antigen interactions, agglutination, is used extensively in transfusion medicine.

The antigen copy number and density vary depending on the blood group. Agglutination is used for serologic crossmatching (donor red cells incubated with recipient plasma or serum), screening for unexpected antibodies (reagent red cells of known blood group antigen composition incubated with recipient plasma or serum), and blood group antigen phenotyping of the donor or recipient (test red cells incubated with monoclonal antibodies or reagent-quality antisera of known specificity).

Agglutination can be detected by several methods. With manual tube testing, agglutination is visually detected by the adhesion of red cells to one another in the postcentrifuge pellet. Agglutination in microtiter plates is visualized by the spread pattern of red cells in individual wells. Gel-based testing is used widely; after agglutination is allowed to take place, the reaction mixture is centrifuged through a gel matrix, typically composed of dextran-acrylamide. Unagglutinated red cells pass through the gel, while the larger, agglutinated complexes are retained at the top of, or within, the matrix. Advantages of gel-based testing over tube testing include standardization of reaction strength, sensitivity, and streamlined throughput, because of both the use of automated platforms and the opportunity to eliminate some wash steps.[36]

Although agglutination reaction tests are sensitive and easy to perform, the formation of agglutinates depends on the proper stoichiometric ratio of antibody to antigen. The "zone of equivalence" refers to the ratio of antigen to antibody that permits ready agglutination. Each arm of the antibody binds to a different particle, and a network (lattice) of linked particles results in agglutination [Fig 8-5 (B)].

A false-negative result is generated if the stoichiometric ratio is outside the zone of equivalence at either extreme. A prozone effect can occur with an unusually high antibody concentration, diminishing the likelihood of an antibody binding to two separate particles or red

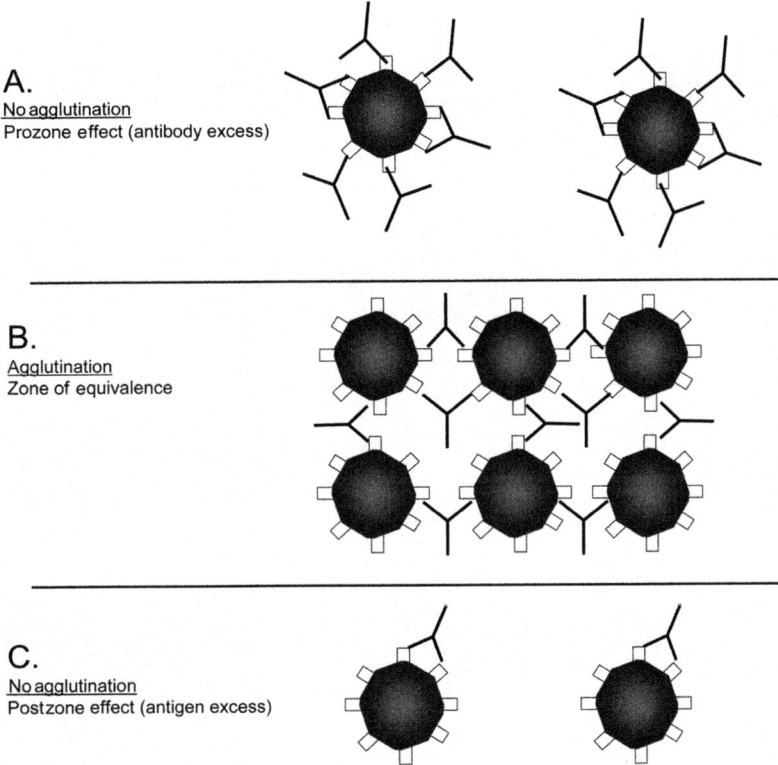

A.
<u>No agglutination</u>
Prozone effect (antibody excess)

B.
<u>Agglutination</u>
Zone of equivalence

C.
<u>No agglutination</u>
Postzone effect (antigen excess)

FIGURE 8-5. Effects of relative concentrations of antigen and antibody on the outcome of agglutination reactions.

cells [Fig 8-5 (A)]. Although unusual in classical red cell serology, prozone has been observed when titers of red cell antibodies are very high and can cause discrepant reverse ABO typing.[37] Diluting the serum being tested, or using diluents containing EDTA, decreases the likelihood of prozone.[38] False-negative agglutination reactions can also be the result of a postzone effect, which occurs when there is excess antigen [Fig 8-5 (C)] and each antibody binds to multiple epitopes on the same particle, thereby preventing crosslinking and agglutination.

Solid-Phase Assays

In solid-phase assays, a specific antigen or antibody is immobilized on a solid matrix, typically made of plastic. A solution containing the protein of interest is placed into a well; the polystyrene (or other plastic employed) directly absorbs protein from solution and irreversibly binds protein to the plastic. The well is washed, the analyte is added and incubated with the protein-coated solid phase, and its adherence is measured. Several combinations of adherence and detection approaches have been described.

Solid-Phase Assays for Phenotyping Red Cells

Antibodies specific for a known blood group antigen are coated onto round-bottom microtiter plates [Fig 8-6 (A)]. Red cells to be analyzed are added to the wells and allowed to adhere; then the plate is centrifuged. If no binding occurs (negative reaction), the red cells cluster together as a "button" at the well bottom. In contrast, specific binding results in dispersion of the red cells over the surface of the entire well (positive reaction), which indicates the presence of the antigen on the red cells.

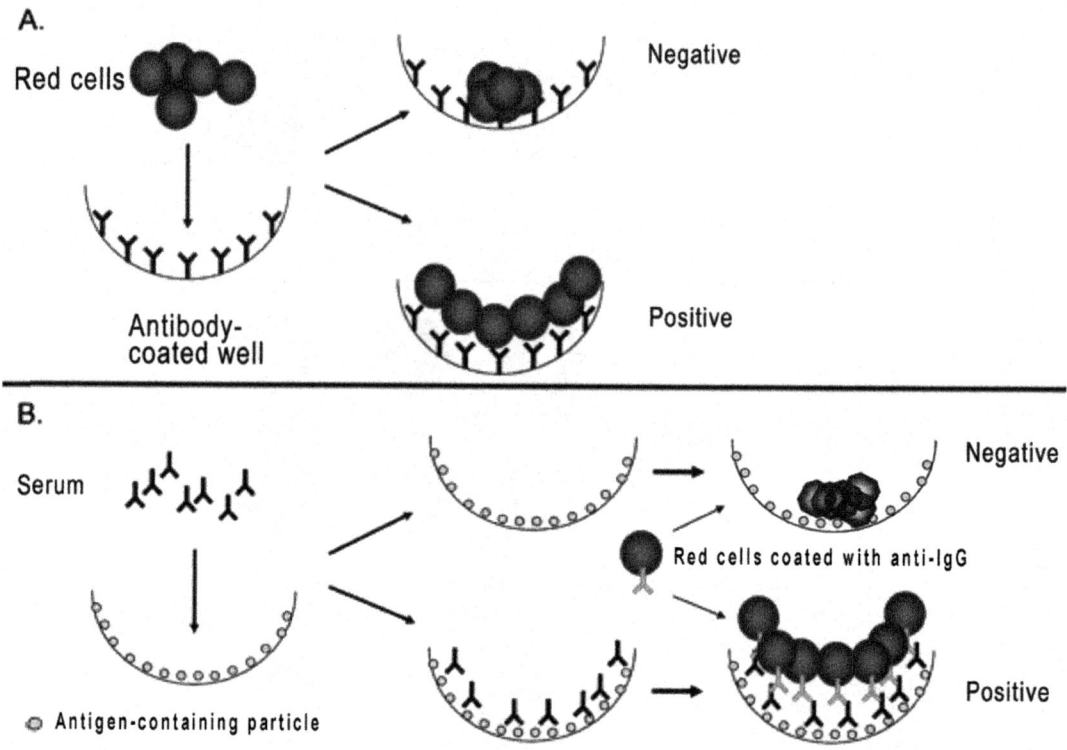

FIGURE 8-6. Schematic of (A) phenotyping red cells and (B) detecting antibodies by solid-phase assay.

Solid-Phase Assays for Detecting Antibodies to Red Cell Antigens

Antigen-coated particles, typically red cells (or red cell fragments), are coated onto microtiter plate wells [Fig 8-6 (B)]. Patient serum is then added, followed by incubation and washing. If the patient serum contains antigen-specific antibodies, they will bind to the red cells. Indicator red cells (coated with antihuman IgG) are then added. A positive reaction is demonstrated by diffuse adherence of the indicator red cells to the well, whereas a negative reaction is demonstrated by clustering of indicator cells in a button.

Solid-Phase Assays for Platelet Testing

Using the approaches described above, solid-phase red cell adherence (SPRCA) technology has been adapted to detect antigens on platelets,

such as HPA-1a, as well as to detect antibodies against platelet antigens.[39]

Enzyme-Linked Immunosorbent Assay

Enzyme-linked immunosorbent assay (ELISA, aka "enzyme immunoassay") can detect either antibodies or antigens. To generate a signal, a secondary antibody is used that is tethered to an enzyme, that modifies an added enzyme-specific substrate to generate either color (chromogenic reaction) or photons (chemiluminescent reaction). The use of secondary antibodies and enzymatic signal generation renders ELISAs capable of robust signal amplification; ELISAs are therefore much more sensitive than fluid-phase agglutination or SPRCA assays.

ELISAs typically use purified or recombinant antigens or antibodies, depending on the analyte to be detected. However, intact red cells can be used to screen for red cell antibodies, and this is referred to as the enzyme-linked antiglobulin test.[40]

Detection of Antibodies by the Indirect ELISA. To detect antibodies against a specific antigen, the antigen is coated onto microtiter plate wells [Fig 8-7 (A)]. The test sample is then added, incubated, and washed. Antigen-specific antibodies bound to the antigen-coated well are then detected by incubating with an antibody (eg, anti-IgG) that serves as a reporter, as it is engineered to be tethered to an enzyme such as alkaline phosphatase or horseradish peroxidase. After further washing, enzyme substrate is added and enzymatically converted to a detectable color. A spectrophotometer is used to measure light absorbance at the wavelength specific for that enzyme/substrate. Color intensity is positively related to the amount of antibody bound to the antigen. Quantification is possible through use of a standard curve. Sometimes samples need to be diluted to ensure that they yield absorbance values in the linear range of the assay. Detection of antigens carried on multipass transmembrane proteins can be difficult in ELISAs, because epitopes may not retain antigenic conformation when deposited onto a solid surface such as a microtiter well.

Detection of Antigens by Sandwich ELISA. The sandwich ELISA is used to detect and quantify a specific soluble antigen. For this assay, two different antibodies [typically monoclonal antibodies (MoAbs)] are used, each of which binds separate epitopes on the same target antigen without cross-interference. Microtiter plate wells are first coated with one MoAb (the "capture" antibody) [Fig 8-7 (B)]. The sample is then added, and antigen in solution binds to the capture antibody. Next, the plate is

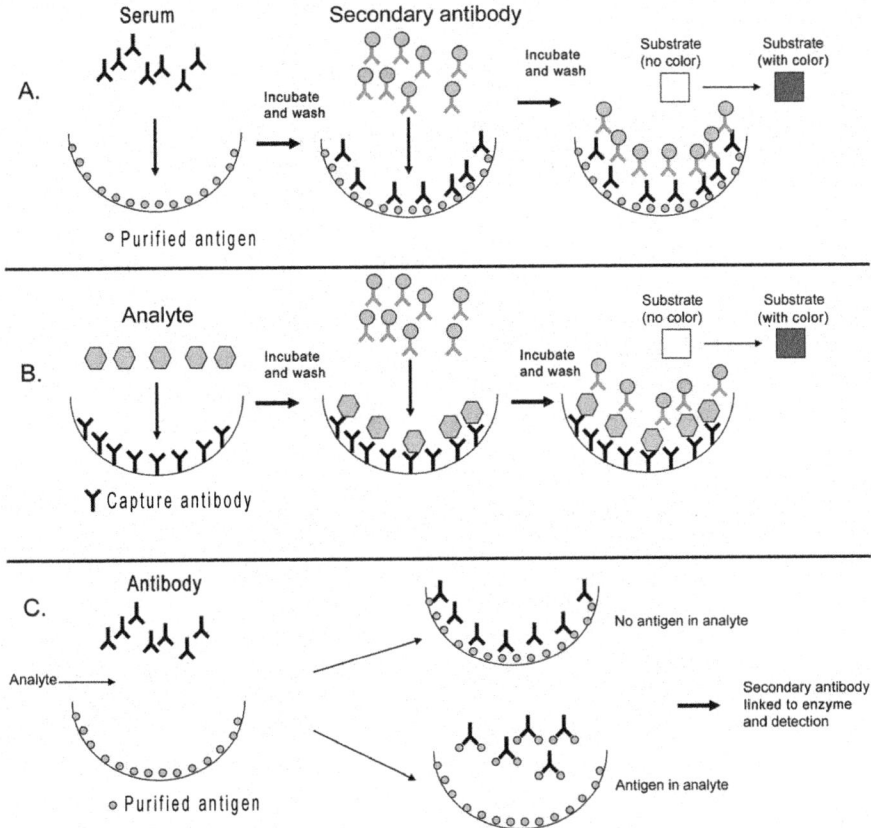

FIGURE 8-7. (A) indirect enzyme-linked immunosorbent assay (ELISA), (B) sandwich ELISA, and (C) competitive ELISA.

washed and incubated with a second MoAb linked to a reporter enzyme. Because it is specific for the target antigen, the reporter antibody binds to the well only if antigen is already bound via the capture antibody. After additional washing, enzyme substrate is added, and it is converted to a detectable color if antibody with enzyme has been bound.

Detection of Antigens by Competitive ELISA. Competitive ELISA begins similarly to indirect ELISA, using wells in which target antigen is already bound. The test sample is preincubated with solution-phase antibody, and this mixture is added to the well [Fig 8-7 (C)]. If no antigen is in the specimen, then reagent antibodies bind unimpeded to the solid-phase antigen. If antigen is present in the specimen, the antigen binds to reagent antibodies, preventing them from binding to the solid-phase antigen. As the amount of soluble antigen in the specimen increases, the amount of reagent antibody free to bind to the solid-phase antigen decreases. Thus, the signal is *inversely* related to the amount of soluble antigen in the specimen.

Competitive ELISA is also used for antibody detection. In this case, the test sample is added to an antigen-coated well along with a labeled antigen-specific reagent antibody. Patient antibody and labeled reagent antibody compete with each other for antigen-binding sites in the well. Again, a higher signal is generated if the antibody level in the sample is low or absent. Although more difficult to optimize than sandwich ELISAs, competitive ELISAs do not require two separate antibodies against different epitopes on the target antigen.

Technical Problems with ELISAs. ELISAs are usually straightforward and robust. False-negative signals can result from enzymatic inhibitors in the sample, and false-positive signals from nonspecific enzymatic activity; however, the use of proper controls and thorough washing typically prevents these problems. Falsely low signals can occur if the amount of antigen exceeds the amount of antibody present, a phenomenon termed the "hook effect." Similar to the prozone effect (see "Fluid-Phase Assays" section above), excess antigen can cause the signal to decrease in some sandwich ELISAs in which the antigen and detection antibody are added simultaneously. The hook effect can be readily overcome by diluting the antigen. Finally, patients exposed to mice or to mouse-based biologic drugs may develop human anti-mouse antibodies (HAMAs) that crosslink the capture antibody and/or detection antibody in sandwich ELISAs, resulting in very high signals.

Protein Assays Encountered Less Commonly in Transfusion Medicine

A number of other technological approaches can be used in the analysis of proteins. For a variety of reasons, these approaches have not been widely adopted in blood banking and transfusion medicine, although some reference laboratories use such technologies as laboratory-developed tests (LDTs).

Protein Microarrays

Microarray technology dramatically increases the number of substrates that can be simultaneously assayed by solid-phase methods. When numerous different proteins are placed (spotted) on a small chip, a single specimen can be assayed for binding activity to multiple analytes simultaneously. For example, a microarray chip spotted with different blood group antigens can be used to assess a single patient specimen for several alloantibodies simultaneously. Like ELISAs, protein microarrays require that the structural conformation required for antibody recognition be maintained. The practical application of protein microarrays to blood bank serology has yet to be realized.

Western Blotting

Although highly sensitive, ELISAs are prone to false-positive results if the antigen used to coat the well is not pure (eg, cell lysates of viruses grown in tissue culture), leading to cross-reactivity with other components in the antigen preparation. In Western blot (WB) assays, the antigen mixture is first separated by high-resolution protein electrophoresis, using polyacrylamide gels. The separated proteins are then transferred to a membrane to serve as the solid phase for probing with an antibody-containing patient sample. Using molecular-weight size markers in an adjacent lane, one can determine the molecular weight of the antigens recognized by the antibodies. Alternatively, antigens can be separated on the basis of other physical properties, such as charge.

Because of the low likelihood of a cross-reactive antigen sharing the same physical characteristics as the intended analyte, WB provides more specificity than ELISAs. WB can be used to confirm positive serologic screening assays of transfusion-transmitted infectious agents, such as HIV or HCV, although NAT testing has become the approach of choice in confirmation of infection by these viruses.

Flow Cytometry

Flow cytometry revolutionized the analysis of cell populations. The basic principle is that fluorescent-tag-labeled antibodies against cell-surface molecules are incubated with a target population of cells; these "stained" cells are then passed through a flow cytometer. As they travel, cells are exposed to lasers that excite the fluorescent tags, causing emission of photons of very specific wavelengths that can be detected by sensors in the flow cytometer. Fluorescence is assessed on a cell-by-cell basis, allowing for the visualization and quantification of minor populations of cells within a complex mixture.[41] Although use in transfusion practice is limited, some laboratories use flow cytometry to quantify RhD-positive fetal red cells in a sample of maternal blood in order to determine appropriate dosing of RhIG to prevent sensitization to the RhD antigen in RhD-negative pregnant females.[42]

Suspension Array Technology

Suspension array technology (SAT) combines the specificity of solid-state antibody/antigen interaction (ELISA) with the sensitivity and high throughput of optical detection by flow cytometry.[43] Through selection of fluorescent dyes during the manufacturing process, populations of microspheres (beads) are generated with distinct fluorescent properties and used as solid supports for the initial binding of specific receptors (capture antigens or antibodies). By pairing beads of specific fluorescent optical properties with specific receptors, it is possible to prepare arrays of microspheres capable of detecting multiple analytes at the same time.

For sample analysis, a suspension of beads covalently tethered with receptors is first incubated with the solution of interest (eg, plasma) to bind the target analyte (antigen or antibody). Next, the bead-receptor-analyte suspension is incubated with a secondary MoAb. The secondary (reporter) MoAb is labeled with its own fluorochrome, rather than with an enzyme (as done in ELISA). Detection is rendered by sending bead suspensions through a flow cytometer, which detects individual beads (as opposed to individual cells). Software in the flow cytometer can recognize the specific capture antibody on each individual bead based on the unique fluorescent signature of the bead and can determine the quantity of analyte bound based on the fluorescent intensity of the secondary MoAb. Multiple specific analytes can be measured simultaneously. The system allows for high throughput using very small quantities of sample.

An example of SAT applicable to transfusion medicine is the use of the Luminex system (Luminex) in the detection and identification of HLA-specific alloantibodies for screening platelet donors and for workup of platelet refractoriness.[44] This system is also used for blood group genotyping.

BASIC IMMUNOLOGY

The process by which the immune system generates antibodies against foreign antigens (yet maintains tolerance to self-antigens) is complicated and elegant, with multiple cellular players and intricate regulation. Of necessity, this section is primarily limited to antibody structure, function, and role in transfusion complications.

Antibody Structure

At its simplest, an antibody is a tetramer composed of two identical heavy chains and two identical light chains (Fig 8-8). Each heavy chain and light chain contains a variable region, which is the part of the molecule that varies between antibodies and binds antigen, and a constant region. Two light-chain families (kappa and lamb-

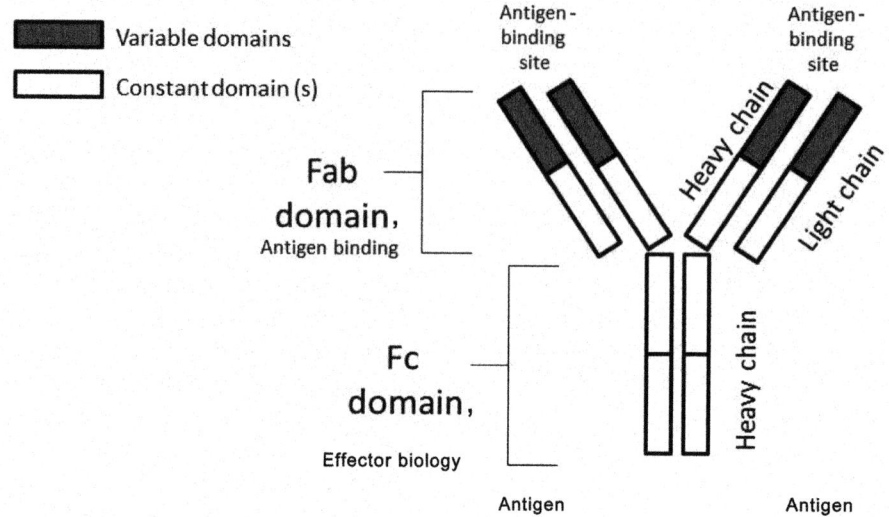

FIGURE 8-8. General structure of a monomeric immunoglobulin.

da) are found in humans. A given antibody has either two kappa light chains or two lambda light chains.

Immunoglobulins treated with the enzyme papain can be digested into two functional fragments. The "Fab" fragment consists of the heavy- and light-chain variable regions, the light-chain constant regions, and one heavy-chain constant region domain. The Fab fragment binds antigen but does not activate effector mechanisms. In contrast, the Fc fragment, consisting only of heavy-chain constant regions, activates effector mechanisms, allowing destruction of the antibody target. Fc constant regions differ between antibody molecules based on antibody isotype and subclass.

There are five different antibody isotypes (IgM, IgG, IgE, IgA, IgD), determined by the constant region of the heavy chain. Antibodies of different isotypes differ both in the number of antigen-binding sites per molecule and in the potency of their effector functions [Fig 8-9 (A)]. The "affinity" of an antibody for its antigen reflects the binding ability of a single binding site, whereas the "avidity" refers to the total binding strength conferred by the combined effects of multiple binding sites. Thus, although the indi-

vidual binding sites of IgM are of relatively low affinity, IgM demonstrates high antigen avidity because it has 10 antigen-binding sites. In IgM, the five immunoglobulin molecules are held together by an additional protein (the J chain) and by extensive disulfide binding. Treatment with dithiothreitol (DTT) can destroy IgM binding because it cleaves (reduces) disulfide bonds; DTT treatment is used in the clinical laboratory to distinguish IgM antibodies from IgG antibodies. IgM potently activates complement by changing its three-dimensional structure after antigen-binding. In general, IgM (and some IgG) can cause hemolysis during transfusion reactions and in autoimmune hemolytic anemia. Importantly, unlike IgG, IgM does not cross the placenta and is therefore not involved in hemolytic disease of the fetus and newborn.

Whereas IgM is generated early in the antigen-specific immune response, IgG antibodies are important in mature humoral immune effector functions, and are divided into four subclasses: IgG1, IgG2, IgG3, and IgG4. Each subclass has a different constant region and a different capacity to activate complement and/or interact with Fc receptors on phagocytes [Fig 8-9 (B)]. IgG1 and IgG3 are the most potent,

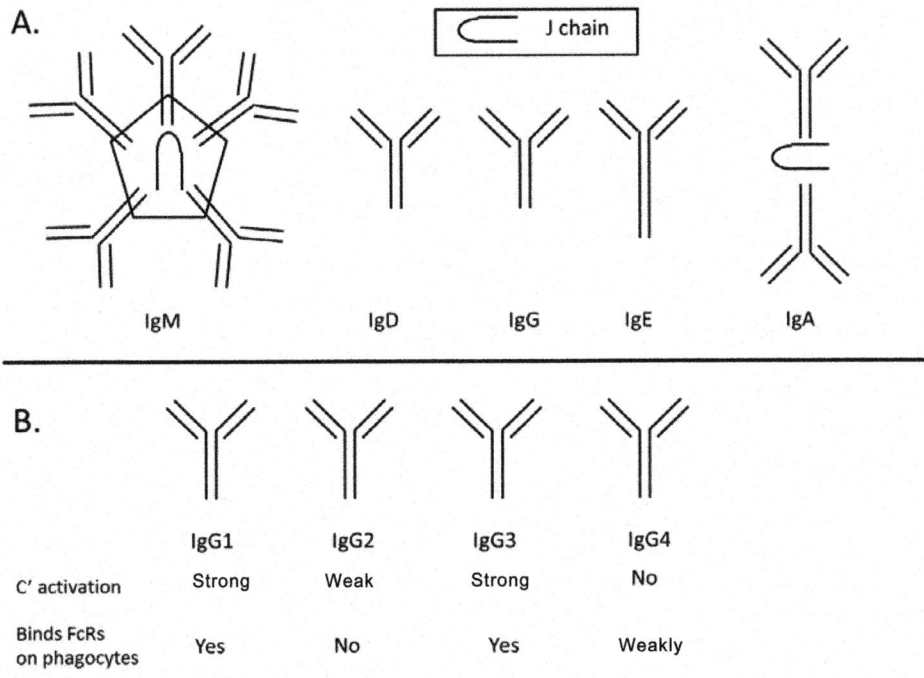

FIGURE 8-9. Immune globulin (Ig) isotypes (A), IgG subclasses, and their relative activation of complement and binding to Fc-gamma receptors (FcγRs) (B).

whereas IgG2 only weakly activates complement, and IgG4 largely lacks effector activity. Consistent with these observations, patients with only IgG4 subclass red cell antibodies typically do not exhibit hemolysis. In contrast, IgG1, IgG2, and IgG3 red cell antibodies can all induce hemolysis.

IgA is the primary antibody isotype secreted at mucosal surfaces; therefore, it is largely responsible for neutralizing pathogens encountered in the gastrointestinal, genitourinary, and respiratory tracts. Although IgA exists in either monomeric or dimeric forms (Fig 8-9 shows a dimer), in serum it is often monomeric. IgA is further divided into IgA1 and IgA2 subclasses (not shown). Dimeric IgA is composed of monomers connected by the J chain (the same J chain found in IgM). Only rarely is immunoglobulin-mediated hemolysis due to IgA. Antiglobulin (Coombs) reagents do not detect IgA, and the potential presence of IgA red cell antibodies

should be considered when analyzing a patient with both hemolysis and a negative direct antiglobulin test result.

IgE antibodies bind to Fc receptors on mast cells, inducing histamine release upon antigen encounter, and are the predominant cause of allergic and anaphylactic responses (Type I hypersensitivity). IgD primarily remains membrane bound on the B-cell surface, with only minimal levels in serum, but its functions remain unclear.

Antibody screens use reagents that recognize IgG, the primary isotype produced following red-cell-induced alloimmunization. In contrast, naturally occurring antibodies against carbohydrate blood group antigens, such as A and B, are typically, but not exclusively, IgM. The pentameric structure of IgM allows it to directly agglutinate alloreactive A and B red cells and represents the underlying principle of the forward and reverse typing reaction. However, it should be noted that IgM directed against other antigens may be present but not cause agglutination, possibly due to lower target antigen levels, and therefore can be missed using current assay systems. Similarly, IgA antibodies, which have been shown to cause autoimmune hemolytic anemia,[45] are not directly detected using standard clinical assays. Some anti-IgG reagents also fail to detect all IgG subtypes, leading to the possibility that some IgG alloantibodies in certain patients may be missed.[46] What drives distinct alloantibody isotypes to blood group antigens remains largely unknown. Red-cell-induced alloantibody formation and class switching is thought to require CD4 T-cell help,[47] although recent studies suggest that CD4 T cells may not be required for all red-cell-induced IgG alloantibodies.[48] Naturally occurring antibodies can occur in the absence of any exogenous stimulus,[49] suggesting that environmental exposure and immunologic mechanisms distinct from RBC-transfusion-induced alloimmunization likely drive A and B antibody formation and may be responsible for the persistence of IgM antibodies against these antigens.

Antibody Receptors (FcγRs) in Target Clearance

The Fc regions of antigen-bound IgGs are recognized by the gamma family of Fc receptors (FcγRs) found on the surface of cells. At least four FcγRs have been described, each with different properties that can have opposite functions. FcγR2a and FcγR3 promote phagocytosis of targets. Because of the relatively low affinity of these receptors, monomeric IgG does not engage FcγR2a or FcγR3; these receptors are preferentially engaged when an antigenic target is bound by multiple IgGs simultaneously. In contrast, FcγR2b is an inhibitory receptor that prevents phagocytosis. FcγR1 has an unusually high affinity for IgG and binds monomeric IgG such that FcγR1 binds IgG whether or not it is complexed with a target; the function of this activity is currently unclear.

FcγR biology is complex, as 1) a given IgG-bound cell or particle may simultaneously activate multiple (potentially antagonistic) receptors, and 2) each IgG subclass (IgG1, IgG2, IgG3, IgG4) has a different affinity for the vari-ous FcγRs [Fig 8-9 (B)]. A mixture of IgGs may bind a particle or cell bearing a foreign antigen. The net effect on phagocytosis depends on the relative binding of different IgG subclasses and their interactions with different FcγRs. Thus, direct binding of Fc domains to FcγRs promotes red cell clearance in many but not all cases.

Complement in Target Cell Opsonization and Destruction

Fc regions of IgG antibodies can also activate complement. The complement system consists of a cascade of proteases that, once activated, amplifies the initial signal, leading to the production of a large number of effector molecules. Although there are several pathways to complement activation, this discussion focuses on the "classical pathway" initiated by Fc regions.

IgM is highly efficient in activating complement. However, to avoid indiscriminate activation, IgM must undergo a conformational shift, which occurs only after binding antigen, thereby exposing complement-binding sites in the heavy-chain constant region. This interaction is so potent that, in theory, a single antigen-bound IgM is sufficient to lyse a target.

In contrast, complement activation by IgG does not involve a conformational change. Rather, complement activation requires clustered binding to the same target by multiple IgG molecules. This ensures against indiscriminate complement activation by unbound circulating IgG.

Once activated, the complement system initiates at least two distinct mechanisms of target destruction. The first involves decoration of the target by complement components labeling it for destruction; this process is known as "opsonization." Early in activation, a portion of one complement component (termed "C3") covalently attaches (by cleavage of a thioester bond, generating a highly labile carbonyl group that reacts with free amines or hydroxyl groups on the cell surface) to the surface of the antigen. Multiple copies of C3b can be recognized by specific receptors on phagocytic cells. Upon encountering a C3b-coated molecule, a phagocyte ingests and destroys it. However, C3b can also rapidly degrade to C3dg, which is not recognized by phagocytes, thus bypassing phagocytosis. C3dg is recognized by B-cell complement receptors and therefore may affect alloantibody development.

In the second mechanism, activation of C3 promotes the assembly of the membrane attack complex (MAC). The MAC consists of complement proteins (C5b-C9) arranged into a structure resembling a hollow tube that is inserted into the membrane of the target cell. This creates a channel between the inside of a target cell and its external environment, typically resulting in osmotic lysis of the target.

Outcomes of Complement Activation

The effector mechanisms induced by antibody binding have different effects on bacteria, viruses, particles, and various human tissues. In general, once an IgG antibody binds to a red cell, the target cell may undergo FcγR-mediated phagocytosis (Fig 8-10). If the antibody initiates the complement cascade, C3b deposition on the red cell surface contributes to opsonization, leading to phagocytosis mediated by the C3b receptors CR1, CR3, CR4, and CRIg. Finally, if

complement activation is complete, MAC insertion causes red cell lysis.

The relative contribution of each pathway varies based on the relative amounts of antibody isotype and subclass, and on the properties of the antigen (eg, antigen density and/or linkage to cytoskeleton), which likely converge to dictate the overall outcome of an incompatible RBC transfusion.[50-52] The sections below describe what is known about these processes with regard to red cell destruction and the clinical manifestations of hemolysis.

Extravascular Hemolysis

Extravascular hemolysis refers to the consumption of antibody- and/or C3b-bound red cells by phagocytes in the reticuloendothelial system (RES), found predominantly in the spleen and liver. The term "extravascular" is used because the red cells are destroyed outside of their normal compartment, the intravascular space. In contrast, "intravascular" hemolysis (see below) occurs rapidly during or following transfusion and is often associated with an acute hemolytic transfusion reaction (AHTR). Unlike AHTRs, de-

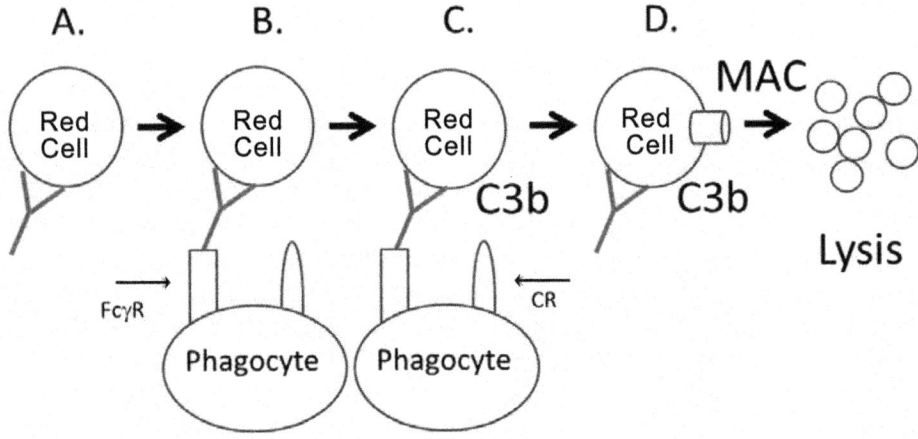

FIGURE 8-10. Mechanisms of red cell destruction by antibody binding. Upon binding (A), an immune globulin G (IgG) represents a ligand for Fc-gamma receptors (FcγRs) on phagocytes (B). If the red cell avoids FcγR-mediated phagocytosis, opsonization may be increased by activation of complement with deposition of C3b (C). If the combined opsonization of FcγR binding and C3b is not sufficient to mediate clearance, completion of the complement cascade may lead to insertion of the membrane attack complex (MAC) into the red cell surface, resulting in lysis (D). These processes likely occur simultaneously, with the outcome representing the aggregate effect of competing pathways.
CR = complement receptor.

layed hemolytic transfusion reactions (DHTRs) demonstrate delayed kinetics because the antibodies implicated are often absent or of low titer initially, requiring some time to develop and increase in titer before the onset of significant red cell destruction. This results in manifestations of delayed hemolysis, which is often, but not exclusively, extravascular in nature.

Extravascular hemolysis is markedly different from intravascular hemolysis, in which red cell contents are directly released into the circulating blood. The term "hemolysis" in this context can cause confusion for health-care providers not accustomed to transfusion medicine terminology; hemolysis is often thought of as just described—the rupture of red cells within the circulation. In contrast, in extravascular hemolysis, the red cells are destroyed by phagocytes, typically within the lysosomes. This is a very important distinction because phagocytes in the RES consume a substantial number of senescent, autologous red cells each day in the normal process of red cell turnover. Thus, consumption of red cells by this pathway follows a process that evolved specifically to break down and recycle red cell contents (hemoglobin and iron) in a manner that avoids tissue damage.

This does not mean, however, that extravascular removal of antibody-coated red cells is biologically equivalent to clearance of normal, senescent red cells. On the contrary, DHTRs can cause substantial morbidity (and occasional mortality).

It is not clear why some red cell antibodies preferentially promote opsonization and phagocytosis instead of osmotic lysis by the MAC. The antibody type and the topology and copy number of the target antigen on the red cells are important. In addition, although complement may be activated, the aggregate opsonization of red cells by C3b and antibody may result in phagocytosis before MAC-induced lysis occurs. Consistent with these explanations, extravascular hemolysis is typically induced by IgG red cell antibodies, whereas intravascular hemolysis is typically induced by IgM red cell antibodies. IgM can be much more efficient at activating complement and promoting MAC formation.

Intravascular Hemolysis

In some cases of incompatible transfusion, the MAC rapidly assembles and lyses the red cells before C3b and/or IgG opsonization can induce phagocytosis. Because these red cells lyse while still circulating, this process is termed "intravascular hemolysis." In addition, because antibody-mediated intravascular hemolysis occurs at a brisker pace than extravascular hemolysis, the clinical signs and symptoms may be more quickly noticed.

As discussed, AHTRs are typically caused by IgM antibodies, which efficiently activate complement, leading to rapid formation of the MAC. Although an IgM-specific Fc receptor has been described (FcμR), its role in promoting the clearance of IgM-coated red cells in the setting of incompatible RBC transfusion is not known. Complement activation by IgM red cell antibodies can result in opsonization by C3b, leading to some receptor-mediated phagocytosis. Overall, however, IgM antibodies are thought to predominantly induce intravascular hemolysis.

Intravascular hemolysis, unlike the removal of senescent red cells through extravascular mechanisms, does not occur at any appreciable level under normal conditions. The release of red cell contents directly into the circulation can be highly toxic, with free hemoglobin inducing perhaps the greatest insult. Although much free hemoglobin is scavenged by the circulating molecule haptoglobin, this system can be easily overwhelmed. AHTRs often result in tea-colored urine (hemoglobinuria) and can induce renal dysfunction, which likely reflects heme-induced cell injury that results from a confluence of compromised mitochondrial function, altered oxidative stress, perturbed metabolism, and increased inflammation.[53] Moreover, the signs and symptoms of AHTRs can be dramatic and include disseminated intravascular coagulation, shock, and death. This type of reaction most often occurs as a result of a clerical error with ABO-incompatible transfusion. To prevent such an occurrence, transfusion service practices have evolved multiple redundant checkpoints to prevent AHTRs from ABO incompatibility.

Hyperhemolysis and Antibody-Negative DHTRs

Occasionally, patients who experience AHTRs or DHTRs may also hemolyze their own (non-transfused) red cells, a process often referred to as hyperhemolysis. Although hyperhemolysis has been recognized, in particular, in patients with SCD, it is sometimes observed in other clinical settings. As hyperhemolysis results in the loss of the patient's own red cells, sometimes with no detectable autoantibody, it may be antibody-independent. Several studies indicate a role for complement; case series suggest that patients experiencing hyperhemolysis may benefit from eculizumab, an antibody that inhibits complement activation beyond C5.[54,55]

In addition to hyperhemolysis, some patients experience accelerated clearance of transfused red cells, but without any detectable alloantibody, a process referred to as antibody-negative DHTR (AN-DHTR). AN-DHTRs can be fatal and can be accompanied by hyperhemolysis, but the underlying mechanism(s) remain unknown. Awareness of this phenomenon is critical, as traditional approaches designed to identify red cell incompatibility focus entirely on the presence of an alloantibody, and therefore fail to directly detect AN-DHTR. Monitoring of hemoglobin A values immediately following transfusion and at the time of suspected AN-DHTR can be especially helpful when evaluating such cases.[56] Given the mortality rate associated with these reactions, a greater understanding of the underlying biology is needed in order to discover and implement effective treatment options for AN-DHTRs, with or without accompanying hyperhemolysis.[57,58]

Nonhemolytic Red Cell Antibodies

Given the redundant pathways leading to the destruction of antibody-coated red cells, it makes sense that transfusions of crossmatch-incompatible red cells can produce hemolysis. Curiously, many red cell antibodies are actually not hemolytic. For some blood group antigens, hemolysis is only very rarely observed following incompatible transfusion (eg, JMH or CH/RG antigens). Moreover, approximately 1% of healthy blood donors have positive direct antiglobulin test results (indicating that IgG autoantibodies are bound to their own red cells), yet there is no evidence of hemolysis. For antigens known to be frequently responsible for antibody-mediated hemolysis (in the RH, KEL, JK, FY, and MNS systems), hemolysis is variable. Indeed, in patients who mistakenly received ABO-incompatible RBC units, clinically significant hemolysis occurs in only 50% of cases even for this robustly hemolytic antigen/antibody combination.

Several explanations may account for the lack of hemolysis during incompatible transfusions. For antigens rarely implicated in hemolysis, antigen cell surface density or topography may not be conducive to initiating the hemolytic pathway. For antigens variably involved in hemolysis, the antibody response (thermal range, titer, affinity, isotype, or IgG subclass) may play roles. Distinct antibodies of the same antigenic specificity may have different capacities for activating complement. This is the rationale for including the anti-C3 component in the antiglobulin (Coombs) reagent: it provides information on whether an antibody can activate (fix) complement. Recent studies also suggest that engagement of some antigens by antibodies may result in the selective loss of the antigen from the cell surface, thereby rendering the cells inert to additional alloantibody-mediated hemolysis.[59,60]

IgG blood group antibodies are typically polyclonal responses, and a number of early studies demonstrated that clinically significant red cell IgG responses are primarily IgG1 and IgG3 isotypes, with IgG2 and IgG4 isotypes much less frequently observed[61-63]; indeed, some clinically insignificant blood group antibodies (eg, antibodies to CH/RG antigens) show a converse relationship, exhibiting a higher frequency of IgG4.[61] In this regard, it is notable that one anti-human globulin MoAb in common use in pretransfusion testing fails to detect IgG4 isotypes, as well as some IgG3 allelic variants present in specific populations.[46] The studies establishing that clinically significant antibodies are often IgG1 and IgG3, and clinically insignificant antibodies are IgG2 and IgG4, are now decades old. Using new exquisitely specific reagents could potentially establish, for each blood group antigen, the relationship between IgG isotype and clinical significance.

Different genetic polymorphisms and/or deficiencies may regulate hemolysis vs red cell clearance on a patient-by-patient basis, including perturbations in complement, complement-regulatory proteins, and allelic polymorphisms in FcγRs. Furthermore, the status of the reticulo-endothelial system of a given patient may dictate the extent to which antibody-coated cells are efficiently removed. The monocyte monolayer assay (MMA) provides the only available method aimed at determining the potential clinical significance of a given red cell alloantibody. Although useful, the MMA does not address important additional recipient factors, such as alterations in complement within a potential recipient. Recent data suggest that some cases of immune-mediated platelet refractoriness may occur independent of alloantibodies, facilitated instead by CD8 T cells,[64] and that regulation of clearance may have alloantibody-independent mechanisms.

It is fair to state that there is only a rudimentary understanding of the underlying basis for the development and manifestation of immune red cell destruction.[65] Because the testing approach for the presence of alloantibodies is not an activity assay, the historical significance of a particular alloantibody is used as an indicator of its clinical relevance. From a practical standpoint, crossmatch-incompatible RBC units may be issued for transfusion if the offending entity is in the category of a "clinically insignificant antibody," especially if the antigen is of very high frequency and antigen-negative blood is difficult or impossible to obtain. The transfusion service must be prepared to address appropriate concerns from health-care providers managing these patients. Although an antibody deemed "clinically significant" may not actually produce hemolysis in all patients, there is no practical method of predicting hemolysis in a given recipient in the acute setting. RBC transfusion strategies can include units that are antigen-matched to the patient for common clinically significant blood group antigens. RBC units that are crossmatch incompatible should not be issued for clinically significant antibodies, except as a lifesaving intervention. If compatible RBC units are unavailable, the potential for hemolysis may be less deleterious than the patient's severe anemia; in such cases, immunosuppression can be considered. Close and frequent communication between a given patient's clinical care team and the transfusion medicine physician should take place, so as to determine optimal approaches to managing patients in these unfortunate circumstances.

New Approaches to Understanding the Mechanistic Basis for Alloantibody Development

Although research characterizing the structural basis of blood group antigens and the regulation of their expression has been extensive, the factors responsible for alloantibody formation following red cell exposure have remained obscure. In solid organ transplantation, a plethora of animal models described, defined, and refined the roles of major histocompatibility antigens and immune mechanisms in transplant rejection; by contrast, analogous animal models for transfusion-induced alloimmunization were, for many years, not available.

Recent advances in the development of relevant animal models are providing important insights into factors responsible for the development of alloantibodies in the setting of blood transfusion. Studies using these systems, coupled with compelling corollary studies in patients, are beginning to clarify the mechanisms responsible for this fundamental process in transfusion medicine.[47,66-71] Historically, a given blood group antigen becomes defined as clinically relevant only after a patient generates an immune response to it and suffers a hemolytic event. Understanding the process of red cell alloimmunization using these newly available research tools opens up possibilities for the prevention of alloantibody development.

Summary of Immunologic Responses to Red Cells

In aggregate, when an antibody binds a red cell, multiple pathways are activated that can lead to cell destruction. Complement activation promotes phagocytosis through the opsonizing properties of C3b and through direct red cell lysis via assembly of the MAC. The presence of IgG Fc domains promotes red cell phagocytosis by binding FcγRs on the phagocyte surface. The relative contributions of these different pathways vary depending on the nature of the target antigen and the properties of the cognate antibodies. The activation of immune pathways and the toxicity associated with red cell hemolysis can lead to negative clinical consequences far beyond simple loss of efficacy of the transfused red cells. Indeed, substantial toxicity can occur, leading to morbidity and, in some cases, mortality. The reader is referred to a more in-depth reference if additional mechanistic details on immunobiology and the immune response are desired.[72]

KEY POINTS

1. Hybridization-based methods can be used to detect genes, gene products, and polymorphisms. However, hybridization methods are less sensitive than amplification-based methods.
2. Amplification-based nucleic acid detection methods (PCR, TMA, NASBA) are highly sensitive but susceptible to false-positive or false-negative results caused by contamination (eg, amplicons) or inhibitors, respectively.
3. Analysis of protein expression detects the actual gene product(s), whereas nucleic acid testing predicts protein expression.
4. Protein analysis is less sensitive than NAT because no amplification is involved, but it is also less susceptible to contamination and inhibition.
5. Methods of detecting protein suffer from non-amplification-based artifacts (HAMA, prozone effects, hook effects) that can lead to erroneous results.
6. Different methods of detecting antigens and antibodies can result in variability in test performance.
7. IgMs and IgGs cause destruction of red cells by multiple mechanisms, based largely on the antigen recognized and the antibody structure.
8. IgG antibodies that cause red cell destruction induce extravascular hemolysis by promoting phagocyte consumption of red cells (through Fc receptors and/or complement-based opsonization). Such destruction typically presents as a DHTR.
9. IgM antibodies (and in some rare cases IgG) that cause red cell destruction typically induce intravascular hemolysis through complement activation, resulting in insertion of the membrane attack complex. Such destruction typically presents as an acute hemolytic transfusion reaction.
10. Antibody-independent DHTRs can occur; careful evaluation of a patient's clinical status and response to transfusion are necessary to diagnose and provide supportive treatment in a timely manner.
11. Not all antibodies to red cell antigens result in destruction of red cells. Incompatibility is best avoided whenever possible, but if compatible blood is unavailable, incompatible RBC units can be used when the antibodies are known to be clinically insignificant. Transfusion of incompatible blood should be considered on a case-by-case basis and with extensive communication with the clinicians requesting the blood components.

REFERENCES

1. Alberts B, Johnson A, Lewis J, et al. Molecular biology of the cell. 6th ed. New York: Garland Science, 2014.
2. Mullis KB, Faloona FA. Specific synthesis of DNA in vitro via a polymerase-catalyzed chain reaction. Methods Enzymol 1987;155:335-50.
3. Al-Soud WA, Radstrom P. Purification and characterization of PCR-inhibitory components in blood cells. J Clin Microbiol 2001;39(2):485-93.
4. Rychlik W. Selection of primers for polymerase chain reaction. Mol Biotechnol 1995;3(2):129-34.

5. Wagner FF, Flegel WA, Bittner R, Döscher A. Molecular typing for blood group antigens within 40 min by direct polymerase chain reaction from plasma or serum. Br J Haematol 2017; 176(5):814-21.

6. Pang J, Modlin J, Yolken R. Use of modified nucleotides and uracil-DNA glycosylase (UNG) for the control of contamination in the PCR-based amplification of RNA. Mol Cell Probes 1992; 6(3):251-6.

7. Compton J. Nucleic acid sequence-based amplification. Nature 1991;350(6313):91-2.

8. Kwoh DY, Davis GR, Whitfield KM, et al. Transcription-based amplification system and detection of amplified human immunodeficiency virus type 1 with a bead-based sandwich hybridization format. Proc Natl Acad Sci U S A 1989; 86(4):1173-7.

9. Elkins MB, Davenport RD, O'Malley BA, Bluth MH. Molecular pathology in transfusion medicine. Clin Lab Med 2013;33(4):805-16.

10. Denomme GA, Van Oene M. High-throughput multiplex single-nucleotide polymorphism analysis for red cell and platelet antigen genotypes. Transfusion 2005;45(5):660-6.

11. Bugert P, McBride S, Smith G, et al. Microarray-based genotyping for blood groups: Comparison of gene array and 5'-nuclease assay techniques with human platelet antigen as a model. Transfusion 2005;45(5):654.

12. Hashmi G, Shariff T, Seul M, et al. A flexible array format for large-scale, rapid blood group DNA typing. Transfusion 2005;45(5):680.

13. van der Schoot CE, de Haas M, Engelfriet CP, et al. Genotyping for red blood cell polymorphisms. Vox Sang 2009;96(2):167-79.

14. Flegel WA, Castilho L, Delaney M, et al. Molecular immunohaematology round table discussions at the AABB Annual Meeting, Denver 2013. Blood Transfus 2015;13(3):514-20.

15. Flegel WA, Johnson ST, Keller MA, et al. Molecular immunohaematology round table discussions at the AABB Annual Meeting, Boston 2012. Blood Transfus 2014;12(2):280-6.

16. Flegel WA, Chen Q, Castilho L, et al. Molecular immunohaematology round table discussions at the AABB Annual Meeting, Orlando 2016. Blood Transfus 2018;16(5):447-56.

17. Denomme GA. Molecular basis of blood group expression. Transfus Apher Sci 2011;44(1):53-63.

18. Denomme GA, Dake LR, Vilensky D, et al. Rh discrepancies caused by variable reactivity of partial and weak D types with different serologic techniques. Transfusion 2008;48(3):473-8.

19. Sandler SG, Flegel WA, Westhoff CM, et al. It's time to phase in RHD genotyping for patients with a serologic weak D phenotype. College of American Pathologists Transfusion Medicine Resource Committee Work Group. Transfusion 2015;55(3):680-9.

20. Baumgarten R, van Gelder W, van Wintershoven J, et al. Recurrent acute hemolytic transfusion reactions by antibodies against Doa antigens, not detected by cross-matching. Transfusion 2006;46(2):244-9.

21. Fasano RM, Sullivan HC, Bray RA, et al. Genotyping applications for transplantation and transfusion management: The Emory experience. Arch Pathol Lab Med 2017;141(3):329-40.

22. Svensson AM, Delaney M. Considerations of red blood cell molecular testing in transfusion medicine. Expert Rev Mol Diagn 2015;15(11):1455-64.

23. Wheeler MM, Johnsen JM. The role of genomics in transfusion medicine. Curr Opin Hematol 2018;25(6):509-15.

24. Chou ST, Westhoff CM. The role of molecular immunohematology in sickle cell disease. Transfus Apher Sci 2011;44(1):73.

25. Wilkinson K, Harris S, Gaur P, et al. Molecular blood typing augments serologic testing and allows for enhanced matching of red blood cells for transfusion in patients with sickle cell disease. Transfusion 2012;52(2):381-8.

26. Klapper E, Zhang Y, Figueroa P, et al. Toward extended phenotype matching: A new operational paradigm for the transfusion service. Transfusion 2010;50(3):536-46.

27. Chou ST, Jackson T, Vege S, et al. High prevalence of red blood cell alloimmunization in sickle cell disease despite transfusion from Rh-matched minority donors. Blood 2013;122(6):1062-71.

28. Metzker ML. Sequencing technologies - the next generation. Nat Rev Genet 2010;11(1):31-46.

29. Lane WJ, Westhoff CM, Uy JM, et al. Comprehensive red blood cell and platelet antigen prediction from whole genome sequencing: Proof of principle. Transfusion 2016;56(3):743-54.

30. Lane WJ, Westhoff CM, Gleadall NS, et al. Automated typing of red blood cell and platelet antigens: A whole-genome sequencing study. Lancet Haematol 2018;5(6):e241-e51.

31. Fichou Y, Audrézet MP, Guéguen P, et al. Next-generation sequencing is a credible strategy for

blood group genotyping. Br J Haematol 2014; 167(4):554-62.

32. McBean RS, Hyland CA, Flower RL. Approaches to determination of a full profile of blood group genotypes: Single nucleotide variant mapping and massively parallel sequencing. Comput Struct Biotechnol J 2014;11(19):147-51.

33. Okuda H, Suganuma H, Kamesaki T, et al. The analysis of nucleotide substitutions, gaps, and recombination events between RHD and RHCE genes through complete sequencing. Biochem Biophys Res Commun 2000;274(3):670-83.

34. Wheeler MM, Lannert KW, Huston H, et al. Genomic characterization of the RH locus detects complex and novel structural variation in multiethnic cohorts. Genet Med 2019;21:477-86.

35. Chou ST, Evans P, Vege S, et al. RH genotype matching for transfusion support in sickle cell disease. Blood 2018;132(11):1198-207.

36. Harmening DM, Walker PS. Alternative technologies and automation in routine blood bank testing. In: Harmening DM, ed. Modern blood banking and transfusion practices. 5th ed. Philadelphia: FA Davis, 2005:293-302.

37. Judd WJ, Steiner EA, O'Donnell DB, Oberman HA. Discrepancies in reverse ABO typing due to prozone. How safe is the immediate-spin crossmatch? Transfusion 1988;28(4):334-8.

38. Salama A, Mueller-Eckhardt C. Elimination of the prozone effect in the antiglobulin reaction by a simple modification. Vox Sang 1982; 42(3):157-9.

39. Procter JL, Vigue F, Alegre E, et al. Rapid screening of platelet donors for PlA1 (HPA-1a) alloantigen using a solid-phase microplate immunoassay. Immunohematology 1998;14(4):141-5.

40. Leikola J, Perkins HA. Enzyme-linked antiglobulin test: An accurate and simple method to quantify red cell antibodies. Transfusion 1980; 20(2):138-44.

41. Arndt PA, Garratty G. A critical review of published methods for analysis of red cell antigen-antibody reactions by flow cytometry, and approaches for resolving problems with red cell agglutination. Transfus Med Rev 2010;24(3):172-94.

42. Dziegiel MH, Nielsen LK, Berkowicz A. Detecting fetomaternal hemorrhage by flow cytometry. Curr Opin Hematol 2006;13(6):490-5.

43. Nolan JP, Sklar LA. Suspension array technology: Evolution of the flat-array paradigm. Trends Biotechnol 2002;20(1):9-12.

44. Kopko PM, Warner P, Kresie L, Pancoska C. Methods for the selection of platelet products for alloimmune-refractory patients. Transfusion 2015;55(2):235-44.

45. Chadebech P, Michel M, Janvier D, et al. IgA-mediated human autoimmune hemolytic anemia as a result of hemagglutination in the spleen, but independent of complement activation and FcalphaRI. Blood 2010;116(20):4141-7.

46. Howie HL, Delaney M, Wang X, et al. Serological blind spots for variants of human IgG3 and IgG4 by a commonly used anti-immunoglobulin reagent. Transfusion 2016;56(12):2953-62.

47. Calabro S, Gallman A, Gowthaman U, et al. Bridging channel dendritic cells induce immunity to transfused red blood cells. J Exp Med 2016;213(6):887-96.

48. Mener A, Patel SR, Arthur CM, et al. Complement serves as a switch between CD4+ T cell-independent and -dependent RBC antibody responses. JCI Insight 2018;3(22).

49. Haury M, Sundblad A, Grandien A, et al. The repertoire of serum IgM in normal mice is largely independent of external antigenic contact. Eur J Immunol 1997;27(6):1557-63.

50. Stowell SR, Winkler AM, Maier CL, et al. Initiation and regulation of complement during hemolytic transfusion reactions. Clin Dev Immunol 2012;2012:307093.

51. Liepkalns JS, Hod EA, Stowell SR, et al. Biphasic clearance of incompatible red blood cells through a novel mechanism requiring neither complement nor Fcgamma receptors in a murine model. Transfusion 2012;52(12):2631-45.

52. Girard-Pierce KR, Stowell SR, Smith NH, et al. A novel role for C3 in antibody-induced red blood cell clearance and antigen modulation. Blood 2013;122(10):1793-801.

53. Tracz MJ, Alam J, Nath KA. Physiology and pathophysiology of heme: Implications for kidney disease. J Am Soc Nephrol 2007;18(2):414-20.

54. Dumas G, Habibi A, Onimus T, et al. Eculizumab salvage therapy for delayed hemolysis transfusion reaction in sickle cell disease patients. Blood 2016;127(8):1062-4.

55. Chonat S, Quarmyne MO, Bennett CM, et al. Contribution of alternative complement pathway to delayed hemolytic transfusion reaction in sickle cell disease. Haematologica 2018; 103:e483-5.

56. Mekontso Dessap A, Pirenne F, Razazi K, et al. A diagnostic nomogram for delayed hemolytic transfusion reaction in sickle cell disease. Am J Hematol 2016;91(12):1181-4.

57. Habibi A, Mekontso-Dessap A, Guillaud C, et al. Delayed hemolytic transfusion reaction in adult sickle-cell disease: Presentations, outcomes, and treatments of 99 referral center episodes. Am J Hematol 2016;91(10):989-94.

58. Vidler JB, Gardner K, Amenyah K, et al. Delayed haemolytic transfusion reaction in adults with sickle cell disease: A 5-year experience. Br J Haematol 2015;169(5):746-53.

59. Stowell SR, Liepkalns JS, Hendrickson JE, et al. Antigen modulation confers protection to red blood cells from antibody through Fcgamma receptor ligation. J Immunol 2013;191(10):5013-25.

60. Sullivan HC, Gerner-Smidt C, Nooka AK, et al. Daratumumab (anti-CD38) induces loss of CD38 on red blood cells. Blood 2017;129(22):3033-7.

61. Devey ME, Voak D. A critical study of the IgG subclasses of Rh anti-D antibodies formed in pregnancy and in immunized volunteers. Immunology 1974;27(6):1073-9.

62. Szymanski IO, Huff SR, Delsignore R. An autoanalyzer test to determine immunoglobulin class and IgG subclass of blood group antibodies. Transfusion 1982;22(2):90-5.

63. Michaelsen TE, Kornstad L. IgG subclass distribution of anti-Rh, anti-Kell and anti-Duffy antibodies measured by sensitive haemagglutination assays. Clin Exp Immunol 1987;67(3):637-45.

64. Arthur CM, Patel SR, Sullivan HC, et al. CD8+ T cells mediate antibody-independent platelet clearance in mice. Blood 2016;127(14):1823-7.

65. Flegel WA. Pathogenesis and mechanisms of antibody-mediated hemolysis. Transfusion 2015;55(Suppl 2):S47-58.

66. Yazdanbakhsh K, Ware RE, Noizat-Pirenne F. Red blood cell alloimmunization in sickle cell disease: Pathophysiology, risk factors, and transfusion management. Blood 2012;120(3):528-37.

67. Stowell SR, Henry KL, Smith NH, et al. Alloantibodies to a paternally derived RBC KEL antigen lead to hemolytic disease of the fetus/newborn in a murine model. Blood 2013;122(8):1494-504.

68. Patel SR, Cadwell CM, Medford A, Zimring JC. Transfusion of minor histocompatibility antigen-mismatched platelets induces rejection of bone marrow transplants in mice. J Clin Invest 2009;119(9):2787-94.

69. Bao W, Yu J, Heck S, Yazdanbakhsh K. Regulatory T-cell status in red cell alloimmunized responder and nonresponder mice. Blood 2009;113(22):5624-7.

70. Evers D, van der Bom JG, Tijmensen J, et al. Absence of the spleen and the occurrence of primary red cell alloimmunization in humans. Haematologica 2017;102(8):e289-e92.

71. Elayeb R, Tamagne M, Pinheiro M, et al. Anti-CD20 antibody prevents red blood cell alloimmunization in a mouse model. J Immunol 2017;199(11):3771-80.

72. Murphy K, Weaver C. Janeway's immunobiology. 9th ed. New York: Garland Science, 2016.

CHAPTER 9
Blood Group Genetics

Margaret A. Keller, PhD, and Sandy Wortman, MT(ASCP)^{CM}SBB

THE SCIENCE OF **GENETICS** IS THE study of heredity—that is, the mechanisms by which particular characteristics are passed from parents to offspring.[1] A **genome** refers to all of the genetic information of a cell, and **genomics** is the study of the entire genome of an organism.[2] This chapter describes the genetics of blood groups. The term "blood group" can be applied to any detectable, variable characteristic of a component of the blood. But in this chapter, the term applies primarily to antigens on the surface of the red cell membrane that are defined serologically by an antibody. Platelet and white cell antigens are discussed in Chapter 15.

That blood groups are inherited characteristics was first shown by von Dungern and Hirszfeld in 1910, 10 years after Landsteiner's discovery of the ABO blood group.[3] Blood groups became an ideal tool for geneticists because they could be identified by specific antibodies in simple hemagglutination tests and, once identified, their inheritance could easily be followed in family studies. Red cell antigens were (and still are) valuable as **markers** (detectable characteristics to recognize a gene's presence and allelic forms) in genetic and anthropologic studies.[4,5]

Differences in antigen expression on the red cells from different people can be used to provide safe blood transfusion. Therefore, an understanding of the principles of human genetics (including the patterns of inheritance and the language or terminology in use) is an important aspect of immunohematology and transfusion medicine. This chapter outlines the fundamental principles of genetics as they apply to blood group antigens and relates them to examples relevant to transfusion medicine. This requires the use of numerous genetic terms; each term, when first used or when fully described, will be in **bold** type and usually is closely followed by a definition.

Molecular genetics is the study of genes at the nucleic acid level for a variety of clinical and research purposes.[1,6] Molecular genetic research has provided an understanding of the genes and their associated regulatory elements that control the expression of blood groups. With the links between genetic variation and antigen status came the ability to predict blood group types using DNA-based molecular methods.[7] The use of molecular immunohematologic testing is becoming commonplace in clinical scenarios that challenge transfusion medicine practitioners. Whereas transfusion medicine has been "personalized" since the advent of compatibility testing, the integration of genomics into the field is elevating transfusion medicine to the status of genome-informed precision medicine.

Margaret A. Keller, PhD, Senior Director, National Molecular and Genomics Laboratories, American Red Cross, and Adjunct Associate Professor, Thomas Jefferson University, Philadelphia, Pennsylvania; and Sandy Wortman, MT(ASCP)^{CM}SBB, Reference and Transfusion Laboratory Services Director, Carter BloodCare, Bedford, Texas
The authors have disclosed no conflicts of interest.

GENOMIC ORGANIZATION AND GENE REGULATION

Many excellent texts offer greater insight into classical genetics[8] and genomics.[2] The fundamental principles of genetics and genomics outlined in this chapter are intended to serve as a review of the inheritance and expression of blood group antigens and for background on the mechanism of molecular methods that are commonly used to predict antigen phenotypes.

Genes

A **gene** is a functional unit of heredity. It is a segment of deoxyribonucleic acid (DNA) within a chromosome that codes for a molecule that has a function. Many but not all genes encode polypeptide chains. A gene is the basic unit of inheritance of any **trait** (defined as a genetically determined characteristic or condition), including blood group antigens, that is passed from parents to offspring. A **locus** is a fixed position on a chromosome, such as a gene or genetic marker. A locus may be occupied by one of several alternative forms of the gene, called **alleles**. For example, the gene that encodes the protein carrying the Jk^a antigen is an alternative form (allele) of the one that encodes the Jk^b antigen. The terms "gene" and "allele" can be used interchangeably. *JK*01* and *JK*02* are the allele names of the *SLC14A1* gene encoding the polymorphic common antigens Jk^a and Jk^b, respectively. (See the section on terminology for more information.) A group of alleles that tend to be inherited together are referred to as a **haplotype**. *RHD* and *RHCE* alleles in the *RH* locus are an example of a haplotype.

Chromosomes

Chromosomes contain the genetic material (DNA) necessary to maintain the life of the cell and the organism. A human **somatic cell** (any nonreproductive cell) contains 46 chromosomes made up of 23 pairs; each pair has one paternally- and one maternally-derived chromosome. In humans, 22 of the pairs are **homologous chromosomes** (a pair of chromosomes in which paternally- and maternally-derived chromosomes

carry equivalent genes) and are referred to as the **autosomes** (any chromosome that is not a sex chromosome). The remaining pair is nonhomologous and consists of the **sex chromosomes**; they determine an individual's gender. Males carry X and Y chromosomes, whereas females carry two X chromosomes. The **karyotype** represents the chromosome complement of a person; this is written as "46,XY" and "46,XX" for a normal male and female, respectively. The hereditary information carried by the chromosomes is passed from a parent cell to a daughter cell during somatic cell division (**mitosis**; see "Mitosis" section below), and from parents to offspring (children) by the **gametes** or germ cells produced by **meiosis** during reproduction (see "Meiosis" section below).

Cytogenetics is the study of chromosomes. Chromosome structures can be studied during mitosis when they can be visualized by various staining and imaging techniques. Each chromosome has two sections, or **arms**, that are joined at a central constricted region called the **centromere** (Fig 9-1). All chromosomes have some common morphologic features but differ in other characteristics, including size, location of the centromere, DNA content, and staining properties.

Staining techniques provide a means to distinguish individual chromosomes. Selected dyes do not stain chromosomes uniformly, and the different banding patterns can be used to distinguish each human chromosome and detect gross rearrangements. Giemsa stains well the chromosomal regions that are rich in adenine (A) and thymine (T), also known as **heterochromatic regions**. **Euchromatic regions** that are rich in guanine (G) and cytosine (C) stain poorly. This results in a chromosomal banding pattern that can be used to identify and characterize chromosomes. The so-called **G-bands** are numbered from the centromere outward. Using chromosome 1 as an example, the region closest to the centromere on the short or long arm is numbered 1p1 or 1q1, respectively. With greater resolution, there is further distinction into subbands (eg, 1p11 and 1p12) that, in turn, can be subdivided (eg, 1p11.1 and 1p11.2). Genes can be individually mapped to a specific band location (Fig 9-2). Other stains can be used to

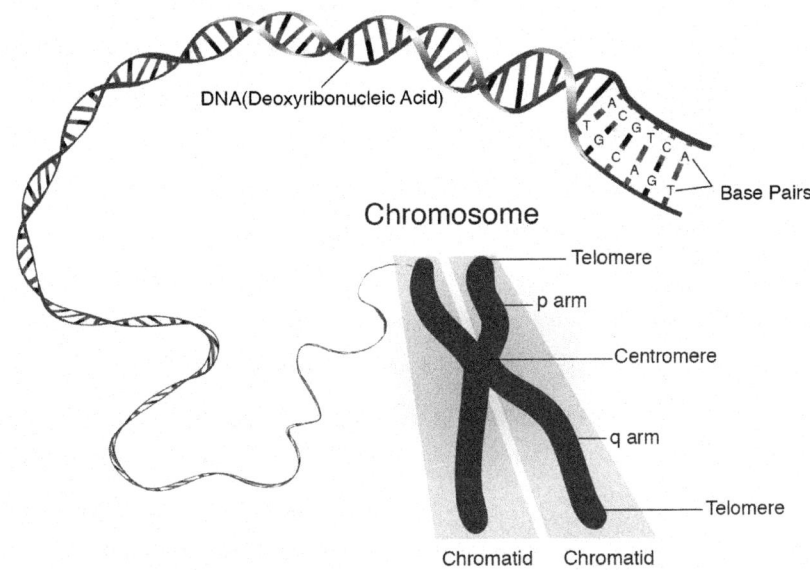

FIGURE 9-1. Chromosomes are made up of one linear double-stranded DNA molecule, packaged in an organized fashion. Each chromosome has a centromere, or constricted region, with the regions on either side referred to as "arms": the short arm, or **p arm**, on the top, and the long arm, or **q arm**, on the bottom. The chromosomes differ in their overall size, the location of the centromere, and their DNA content. [Image courtesy of National Human Genome Research Institute (genome.gov).]

study chromosomes; fluorescent in-situ hybridization (FISH) uses fluorescent dyes to identify specific regions and detect gross structural abnormalities and trisomies. The chromosomal locations of the genes encoding the 39 red cell systems[9-13] are listed in Table 9-1, and Fig 9-2 illustrates some of these.

Cell Division

As a cell divides, the chromosomes replicate, and each daughter cell receives a full complement of genetic material. In somatic cells, this occurs through **mitosis**; in reproductive cells, a similar process called **meiosis** takes place. A feature common to both types of cell division is that, before the start of the process, each chromosome replicates to form two identical daughter **chromatids** attached to each other through the centromere (Fig 9-1).

Mitosis

Somatic cells divide for growth and repair by **mitosis** (Fig 9-3). Through this process, a single cell gives rise to two daughter cells with identical sets of chromosomes. The daughter cells, like the parent cell, are **diploid (2N)**; that is, they contain 46 chromosomes in 23 pairs and have all the genetic information of the parent cell.

Meiosis

Meiosis occurs only in germ cells that are intended to become gametes (sperm and egg cells). Somatic cells are diploid (2N), whereas gametes are **haploid** [having half the chromosomal complement of somatic cells (1N)]. **Meiosis** is a process of cell division and replication that leads to the formation of haploid gametes. During meiosis, diploid cells undergo DNA replication, followed by two cycles of cell division

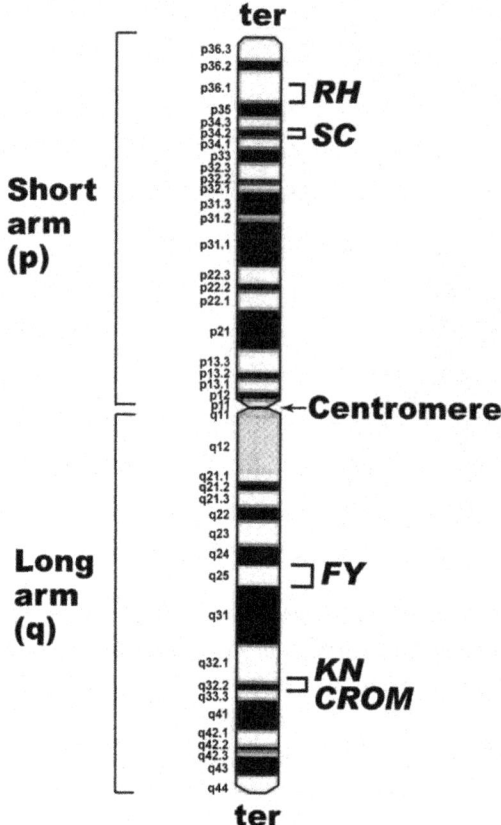

FIGURE 9-2. The morphology and banding pattern of a Giemsa-stained human chromosome 1. The locations of the genes controlling the expression of antigens for the RH, SC, FY, KN, and CROM blood group systems are shown. (Table 9-1 lists the ISBT symbols for the blood groups.)

to produce four haploid gametes (Fig 9-4). Sperm and egg cells fuse at fertilization such that the gametes, each carrying a haploid (1N) set of chromosomes come together to form a zygote with 46 chromosomes. Eggs fertilized by X-bearing sperm become females (XX) while those fertilized by Y-bearing sperm become males (XY).

Meiosis ensures genetic diversity through two mechanisms: **independent assortment** and **crossing over**. Through independent assortment, each daughter cell randomly receives either maternally or paternally derived homologous chromosomes. Crossing over involves ex-

change of genetic material between homologous chromosome pairs. Such shuffling of genetic material ensures diversity and produces genetically unique gametes that fuse to produce a unique zygote.

X Chromosome Inactivation (Lyonization)

Based on the inheritance of the sex chromosomes, females have two copies and males have only one copy of genes carried by the X chromosome. Because most genes carried by the X chromosome do not have a homolog on the Y chromosome, there is a potential imbalance in the dosage of the gene products between males and females. Dosage compensation involves **X chromosome inactivation** (also called lyonization), a process through which most of the genes on one of the two X chromosomes in each female somatic cell are inactivated at a very early stage of embryonic development.[23] It is a matter of chance whether the maternal or paternal X chromosome is inactivated in any one cell, but once inactivation has occurred, all descendants of that cell will have the same inactive X chromosome. Some genes carried by the X chromosome escape inactivation; the first gene found to escape inactivation was *XG*, the gene encoding the antigens of the XG blood group system. Like *XG*, most of the genes that escape inactivation are located on the extreme tip of the short arm of the X chromosome, but several are clustered in regions on the short and long arms of the chromosome.[24(pp359-370),25]

The *XK* gene, which encodes the XK blood group system, is the only other gene carried by the X chromosome known to encode a red cell antigen. Changes or deletions in *XK* result in McLeod phenotype red cells that lack Kx antigen and have reduced expression of KEL antigens.[26,27] The *XK* gene, unlike *XG*, is subject to X chromosome inactivation, with the result that a female who is a **carrier** (a person who carries one gene for a recessive trait and one normal gene) of a gene that is responsible for the McLeod phenotype can have a dual population of Kx– (McLeod phenotype) and Kx+ (non-McLeod phenotype) red cells. Flow cytometry, using selected KEL antibodies, shows the weaken-

TABLE 9-1. Blood Group Systems

ISBT System Symbol / Name (Number)	Gene Name: ISBT (HGNC)*	Chromosome Location	Gene Product (Component Name) [CD number]	Associated Blood Group Antigens [Null phenotype]
ABO (001)	*ABO* (*ABO*)	9q34.2	Glycosyltransferase, carbohydrate	A; B; A,B; A1 [Group O]
MNS (002)	*MNS* (*GYPA* *GYPB*)	4q31.21	Glycophorin A (GPA) [CD235a] Glycophorin B (GPB) [CD235b]	M, N, S, s, U, He, Mi^a, Vw, M^c, and 40 more [En(a−); U−; M^{k}M^k]
P1PK (003)	*P1* (*A4GALT*)	22q13.2	Galactosyltransferase, carbohydrate	P1, P^k, NOR
RH / Rh (004)	*RH* (*RHD* *RHCE*)	1p36.11	RhD [CD240D] RhCE [CD240CE]	D, G C, E, c, e, V, VS, and 47 more [Rh$_{null}$]
LU / Lutheran (005)	*LU* (*BCAM*)	19q13.32	Lutheran glycoprotein, B-cell adhesion molecule [CD239]	Lu^a, Lu^b, Lu3, Lu4, Au^a, Au^b, and 19 more [Recessive Lu(a−b−)]
KEL / Kell (006)	*KEL* (*KEL*)	7q34	Kell glycoprotein [CD238]	K, k, Kp^a, Kp^b, Ku, K11, Js^a, Js^b, and 28 more [K$_0$ or K$_{null}$]
LE / Lewis (007)	*LE* (*FUT3*)	19p13.3	Fucosyltransferase, carbohydrate (adsorbed from plasma)	Le^a, Le^b, Le^{ab}, Le^{bh}, Ale^b, Ble^b [Le(a−b−)]
FY / Duffy (008)	*FY* (*ACKR1*)	1q23.2	FY glycoprotein [CD234]	Fy^a, Fy^b, Fy3, Fy5, Fy6 [Fy(a−b−)]
JK / Kidd (009)	*JK (SLC14A1)*	18q12.3	Human urea transporter (HUT), Kidd glycoprotein	Jk^a, Jk^b, Jk3 [Jk(a−b−)]
DI / Diego (010)	*DI* (*SLC4A1*)	17q21.31	Band 3, anion exchanger 1 [CD233]	Di^a, Di^b, Wr^a, Wr^b, Wd^a, Rb^a, and 16 more

(Continued)

TABLE 9-1. Blood Group Systems (Continued)

ISBT System Symbol / Name (Number)	Gene Name: ISBT (HGNC)*	Chromosome Location	Gene Product (Component Name) [CD number]	Associated Blood Group Antigens [Null phenotype]
YT / Yt (011)	YT (ACHE)	7q22.1	Acetylcholinesterase	Yt^a, Yt^b, YTEG, YTLI, YTOT
XG / Xg (012)	XG (XG)	Xp22.33 Yp11.2	Xg^a glycoprotein CD99 (MIC2 product)	Xg^a, CD99
SC / Scianna (013)	SC (ERMAP)	1p34.2	Erythroid membrane-associated protein (ERMAP)	Sc1, Sc2, Sc3, Rd, and 3 more [Sc:−1,−2,−3]
DO / Dombrock (014)	DO (ART4)	12p12.3	Do glycoprotein, ART 4 [CD297]	Do^a, Do^b, Gy^a, Hy, Jo^a, and 5 more [Gy(a−)]
CO / Colton (015)	CO (AQP1)	7p14.3	Aquaporin 1 (AQP1)	Co^a, Co^b, Co3, Co4 [Co(a−b−)]
LW / Landsteiner-Wiener (016)	LW (ICAM4)	19p13.2	LW glycoprotein, intracellular adhesion molecule 4 (ICAM4) [CD242]	LW^a, LW^{ab}, LW^b [LW(a−b−)]
CH/RG / Chido/Rodgers (017)	CH/RG (C4A, C4B)	6p21.32	Complement component: C4A, C4B	Ch1, Ch2, Rg1, and 6 more [Ch−Rg−]
H (018)	H (FUT1)	19q13.33	Fucosyltransferase, carbohydrate [CD173]	H [Bombay (O$_h$)]
XK / Kx (019)	XK (XK)	Xp21.1	XK glycoprotein	Kx [McLeod phenotype]
GE / Gerbich (020)	GE (GYPC)	2q14.3	Glycophorin C (GPC) [CD236] Glycophorin D (GPD)	Ge2, Ge3, Ge4, and 8 more [Leach phenotype]
CROM / Cromer (021)	CROM (CD55)	1q32.2	DAF [CD55]	Cr^a, Tc^a, Tc^b, Tc^c, Dr^a, Es^a, IFC, and 13 more [Inab phenotype]
KN / Knops (022)	KN (CR1)	1q32.2	CR1 [CD35]	Kn^a, Kn^b, McC^a, Sl^a, Yk^a, and 4 more

TABLE 9-1. Blood Group Systems (Continued)

ISBT System Symbol / Name (Number)	Gene Name: ISBT (HGNC)*	Chromosome Location	Gene Product (Component Name) [CD number]	Associated Blood Group Antigens [Null phenotype]
IN / Indian (023)	IN (CD44)	11p13	Hermes antigen [CD44]	In^a, In^b, and 4 more
OK / Ok (024)	OK (BSG)	19p13.3	Neurothelin, basigin [CD147]	Ok^a, OKGV, OKGM
RAPH / Raph (025)	RAPH (CD151)	11p15.5	CD151	MER2 [Raph–]
JMH / John Milton Hagen (026)	JMH (SEMA7A)	15q24.1	Semaphorin 7A [CD108]	JMH and 5 more [JMH–]
I (027)	GCNT2 (IGNT)	6p24.2	Glucosaminyltransferase, carbohydrate	I [I– or i adult]
GLOB / Globoside (028)	GLOB (B3GALNT1)	3q26.1	Transferase, carbohydrate (Gb$_4$, globoside)	P, PX2 [P–]
GIL / Gill (029)	GIL (AQP3)	9p13.3	Aquaporin 3 (AQP3)	GIL [GIL–]
RHAG / Rh-associated glycoprotein (030)	RHAG	6p21.3	Rh-associated glycoprotein [CD241]	Duclos, Ol^a, DSLK
FORS[14] (031)	FORS (GBGT1)	9q34.2	Globoside 3-α-N-acetylgalactosaminyltransferase 1	FORS1
JR[15,16] (032)	JR (ABCG2)	4q22.1	Jr glycoprotein, ATP-binding cassette, subfamily G, member 2 (ABCG2) [CD338]	Jr^a [Jr(a–)]
LAN[17] (033)	LAN (ABCB6)	2q36	Lan glycoprotein, ATP-binding cassette, subfamily B, member 6 (ABCB6)	Lan [Lan–]

(Continued)

TABLE 9-1. Blood Group Systems (Continued)

ISBT System Symbol / Name (Number)	Gene Name: ISBT (HGNC)*	Chromosome Location	Gene Product (Component Name) [CD number]	Associated Blood Group Antigens [Null phenotype]
VEL / Vel[18-20] (034)	VEL (SMIM1)	1p36	Small integral membrane protein 1 (SMIM1)	Vel [Vel–]
CD59[21] (035)	CD59	11p13.33	CD59	CD59.1 [CD59:–1]
AUG / Augustine[22] (036)	ENT1 (SLC29A1)	6p21.1	Equilibrative nucleoside transporter 1 (ENT1)	AUG1, At^a (AUG2), and 2 more [AUG:–1,–2]
KANNO (037)	PRNP	20p13	Prion protein (PRNP)	KANNO1
SID / Sid (038)	B4GALNT2	17q21.32	Beta-1,4-N-acetylgalac-tosaminyltransferase 2	Sd^a (SID1)
CTL2[†] (039)	SLC44A2	19p13.2	Solute carrier family 44, member 2	CTL2.1 (global), CTL2.2 (Rif)

*If the genetic information is obtained by blood group typing, the gene name is the italicized form of the blood group system ISBT name. For example, SLC14A1 (HGNC terminology) would be written as JK*A and JK*B or JK*01 and JK*02 (ISBT terminology).
[†]As the manual went to press, the ISBT Working Party meeting to approve CTL as blood group 039 was delayed. See ISBT website for updates.
ISBT = International Society of Blood Transfusion; HGNC = Human Gene Nomenclature Committee; ATP = adenosine triphosphate.

ing of KEL antigens on red cells of the McLeod phenotype and demonstrates two red cell populations in carrier females. This mixed-cell population reflects the randomness in whether the maternal or paternal X chromosome is inactivated in any single somatic cell lineage.

GENETIC VARIATION

A **polymorphism** refers to the occurrence in the population of genomes with allelic variation (two or more alleles at one locus), each with appreciable (>1%) frequency. Some blood group systems (RH and MNS, for example) are highly polymorphic and have many more alleles at a given locus than other systems, such as FY and CO.[9] An allele that is polymorphic in one population is not necessarily polymorphic in all populations; for example, the FY allele associated with silencing of Fy^b in red cells (FY*02N.01) is polymorphic in populations of African ancestry, with a prevalence of >70%, but this allele is not typically found in other populations. A gene polymorphism may represent an evolutionary advantage for a population, and a polymorphic population is likely to adapt to evolutionary change more rapidly than if the population had genetic uniformity. It is not yet understood what, if any, evolutionary advantages were derived from the extensive polymorphism displayed by red cell antigens, but many publica-

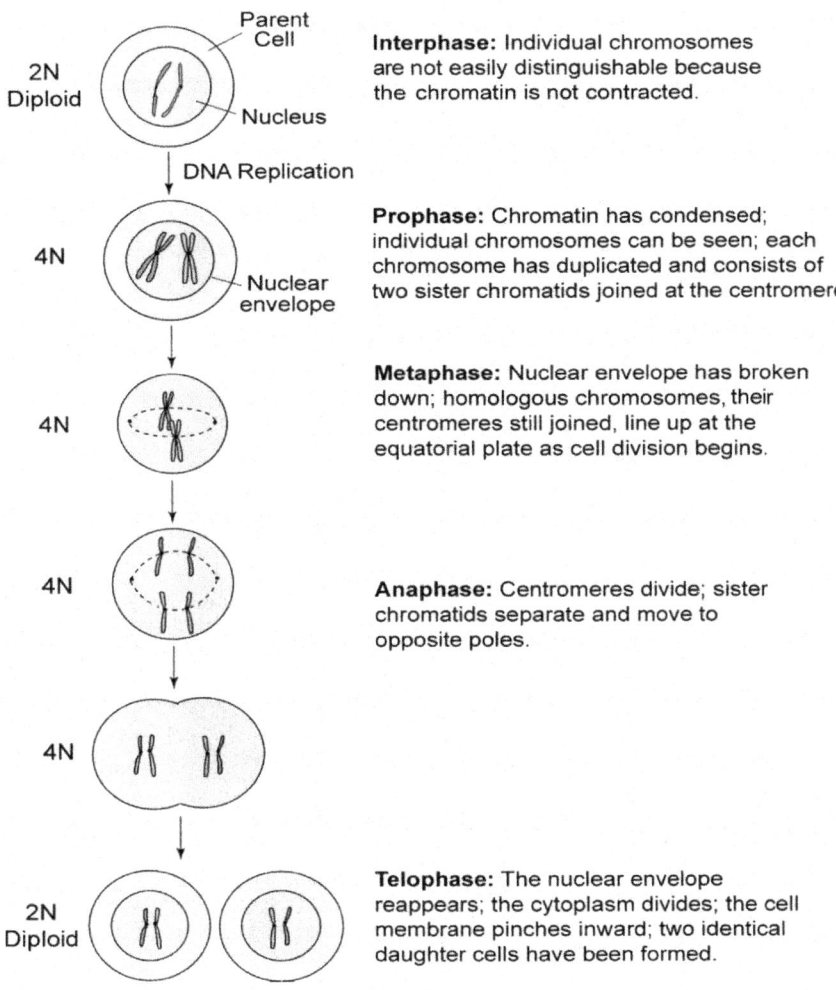

FIGURE 9-3. Diagram showing mitosis.

tions associate resistance to, or susceptibility for, particular diseases with particular blood types.[28]

Mutations can be inherited (germline) or acquired. Germline mutations are present in every cell and will be passed on to offspring. Acquired or **de-novo** mutations can occur spontaneously or be brought about by agents such as radiation (eg, ultraviolet rays or x-rays) or chemicals. A mutation may occur within a gene or in the intergenic regions. It may be **silent**—that is, have no effect on the encoded protein—or it may alter the gene product and potentially cause an observable effect in the phenotype. The mutation rate of expressed genes resulting in a *new*

phenotype has been estimated to be $<10^{-5}$ (<1 in 100,000) in humans.

There are three types of genetic variation: single base-pair substitutions, also known as **single nucleotide variants** (SNVs); insertions or deletions (**in/dels**) of a single stretch of DNA, ranging from two to several hundred base pairs; and **structural variants**, which involve larger stretches of DNA and include deletions, insertions, inversions, duplications, and copy number variants. All three types of genetic variation are seen in the genes that encode red cell antigen phenotypes. SNVs have given rise to most of the diversity in the human genome.[29-31] Accordingly,

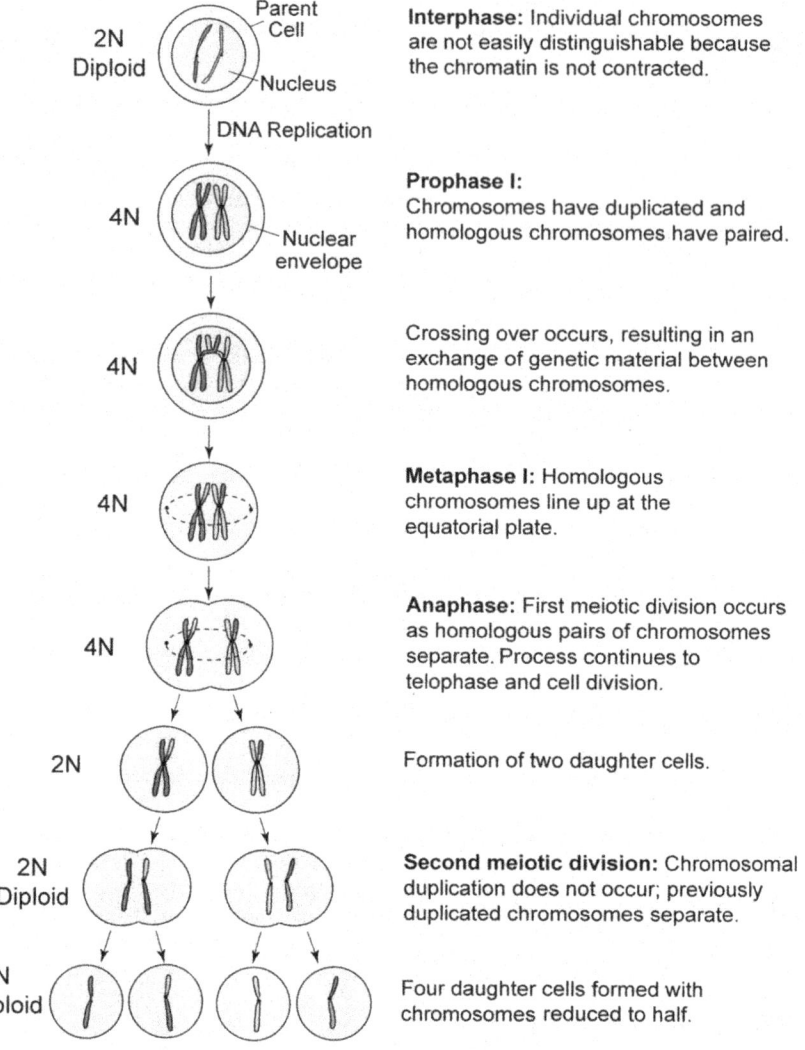

2N
Diploid

Parent
Cell

Nucleus

DNA Replication

4N

Nuclear
envelope

4N

4N

4N

2N

2N
Diploid

N
Haploid

Interphase: Individual chromosomes are not easily distinguishable because the chromatin is not contracted.

Prophase I: Chromosomes have duplicated and homologous chromosomes have paired.

Crossing over occurs, resulting in an exchange of genetic material between homologous chromosomes.

Metaphase I: Homologous chromosomes line up at the equatorial plate.

Anaphase: First meiotic division occurs as homologous pairs of chromosomes separate. Process continues to telophase and cell division.

Formation of two daughter cells.

Second meiotic division: Chromosomal duplication does not occur; previously duplicated chromosomes separate.

Four daughter cells formed with chromosomes reduced to half.

FIGURE 9-4. Diagram showing meiosis.

the majority of polymorphic blood group antigens are the result of SNVs.[7,32,33] SNVs located in gene-coding regions can be **synonymous**, meaning that they encode the same amino acid as the reference sequence; or **nonsynonymous**, meaning they result in substitution of a different amino acid; or **nonsense**, meaning they encode a stop codon. Because of the triplet nature of codons encoding amino acids, in/dels can result in frameshifts if the number of nucleotides inserted or deleted is not divisible by three; frameshifts often cause premature termi-

nation of a polypeptide, often resulting in a nonfunctional protein product. **Genotyping** or DNA-based assays designed to determine the sequence at the location of an SNV can be used to predict a red cell phenotype. This is discussed in more detail in the "Blood Group Genomics" section. In the context of an allele that encodes a protein that carries red cell antigens, any genetically induced change in the antigen must be recognized by a specific antibody before an allele can be said to encode an antigen.

Alleles

A gene at a given locus on a chromosome may exist in more than one form; that is, it may be allelic. Each person has two alleles for a trait, one that is maternally derived and another that is paternally derived. At the simplest level, and for the purpose of explaining the concept, the ABO gene locus can be considered to have three alleles: *A*, *B*, and *O* (although genotyping has revealed many variant alleles). With three alleles, there are six possible genotypes (*A/A*, *A/O*, *A/B*, *B/B*, *B/O*, and *O/O*). Depending on the parental contribution, a person could inherit any combination of two of the alleles and express the corresponding antigens on their red cells. For example, inheritance of *A/A* and *A/O* would result in group A red cells, *A/B* would result in group AB red cells, *B/B* and *B/O* would result in group B red cells, and *O/O* would result in group O red cells.

When identical alleles for a given locus are present on both chromosomes, the person is said to be **homozygous** for the particular allele. A person who is **hemizygous** for an allele has only a single copy of an allele instead of the customary two copies; an example is the deletion of one *RHD* in a D+ phenotype. When different (ie, not identical) alleles are present at a particular locus, the person is said to be **heterozygous**. For example, a person who is homozygous at the *KEL* locus for the allele encoding the k antigen (*KEL*02*) will have K–k+ red cells. A person who is heterozygous for *KEL*01* and *KEL*02* (*KEL*01/02* genotype), would have red cells that are K+k+.

Antigens that are encoded by alleles at the same locus are said to be **antithetical** (meaning opposite); thus, K and k are a pair of antithetical antigens. It is incorrect to refer to red cells that are, for example, K–k+ or Kp(a–b+) as being homozygous for the k or Kp^b antigen; rather, it should be said that the cells have a double dose of the antigen and that they are from a person who is homozygous for the allele. Genes are allelic, whereas some antigens are antithetical.

The quantity of antigen expressed (antigen density) is influenced by whether a person is heterozygous or homozygous for an allele; the antigen density is generally greater when a person is homozygous. In some blood group systems, this difference in antigen density is manifested by antibodies giving stronger reactions with cells that have a double dose of the antigen. Red cells with the Jk(a+b–) phenotype, encoded by a *JK*A/A* genotype, have a double dose of the Jk^a antigen and often are more strongly reactive with anti-Jk^a than those that are Jk(a+b+) and have a single dose of the antigen. Similarly, M+N– red cells tend to be more strongly reactive with anti-M than are M+N+ red cells. Antibodies that are weakly reactive may not be detected if they are tested with red cells expressing a single dose of the antigen. This observable difference in strength of reaction, based on homozygosity or heterozygosity for an allele, is termed the "**dosage effect.**" (See Table 9-2.)

Genotype and Phenotype

The **genotype** of a person is the complement of genes inherited from his or her parents; the term is frequently also used to refer to the set of alleles at a single gene locus. The **phenotype** is the observable expression of the genes inherited by a person and reflects the biologic activity of the gene(s). Thus, the presence or absence of

TABLE 9-2. Example of How Genotyping Can Be Used to Determine Zygosity and Antigen Dose

Allelic State	Genotype*	Phenotype	Jk^a Dose	Jk^b Dose
Homozygous	JK*01/JK*01	Jk(a+b–)	Double dose	N/A
Heterozygous	JK*01/JK*02	Jk(a+b+)	Single dose	Single dose
Hemizygous	*JK*01/JK*01N.01* (null)	Jk(a+b–)	Single dose	N/A

*JK*01 encodes Jk^a, and *JK*02* encodes Jk^b. *JK*01N.01* is silenced for Jk^a expression.
N/A = not applicable.

antigens on the red cells, as determined by serologic testing, represents the phenotype; the presence or absence of antigens on the red cells predicted by DNA-based testing represents the genotype. Sometimes the genotype can be predicted from the phenotype; for example, when a person's red cells are reactive with anti-Jk^a and anti-Jk^b, which is a Jk(a+b+) phenotype, a *JK*A/JK*B* genotype can be inferred. Frequently, the phenotype provides only a partial indication of the genotype; for example, red cells that are group B reflect the presence of a *B* gene, but the genotype may be *ABO*B/B* or *ABO*B/O*. For decades, family studies were often used to infer a person's genotype, but now that most antigens and phenotypes can be defined at the DNA level, family studies to determine genotype can be mostly replaced by DNA analysis. (See "Blood Group Genomics" section below.)

INHERITANCE OF GENETIC TRAITS

A genetic trait is the observed expression of one or more genes. The inheritance of a trait (and red cell antigens) is determined by whether the gene responsible is located on an autosome or on the X chromosome (sex-linked) and whether the trait is dominant or recessive.

Pedigrees

A family study follows the inheritance of a genetic characteristic—for example, an allele encoding the expression of a red cell antigen—as it is transmitted through a kinship. A diagram that depicts the relationship of family members and shows which family members express (are **affected**), or do not express, the trait under study is termed a **pedigree**. A review of a pedigree should reveal the pattern or type of inheritance for the trait, or antigen, of interest. The person who first caused the family to be investigated is considered the index case and is often referred to as the **proband** or **propositus/proposita** (male singular form or gender unknown/female singular form); propositi is the plural form regardless of gender. Details of the conventions

and symbols used for the construction of pedigrees are provided in Figs 9-5 and 9-6.

Autosomal Dominant Inheritance

An antigen (or any trait) that is inherited in an **autosomal dominant** manner is always expressed when the relevant allele is present, regardless of whether a person is homozygous or heterozygous for the allele. The antigen appears in every generation and occurs with equal frequency in both males and females. A person who carries an autosomal dominant trait transmits it, on average, to half of his or her children. The pedigree in Fig 9-7 demonstrates autosomal dominant inheritance and shows that the *B* allele is dominant over *O*.

Autosomal Codominant Inheritance

Blood group antigens that appear to be autosomal dominant may be encoded by alleles that are inherited in a **codominant** manner—that is, when two different alleles are present (the heterozygous condition), the products of both

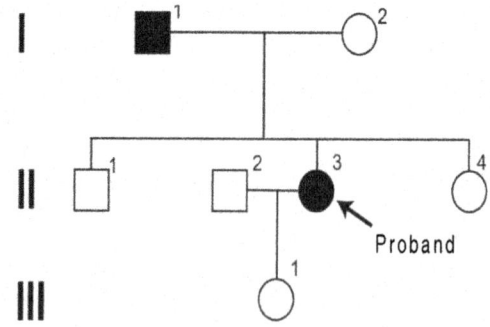

FIGURE 9-5. An example of a pedigree. Males are denoted by squares and females by circles, and each different generation in a pedigree is identified by Roman numerals. Persons in each generation are identified by Arabic numbers; the numbering is sequential from left to right, with the eldest child for each family unit being placed on the left of any series of siblings. Closed symbols represent family members affected by the trait, whereas open symbols are unaffected members.

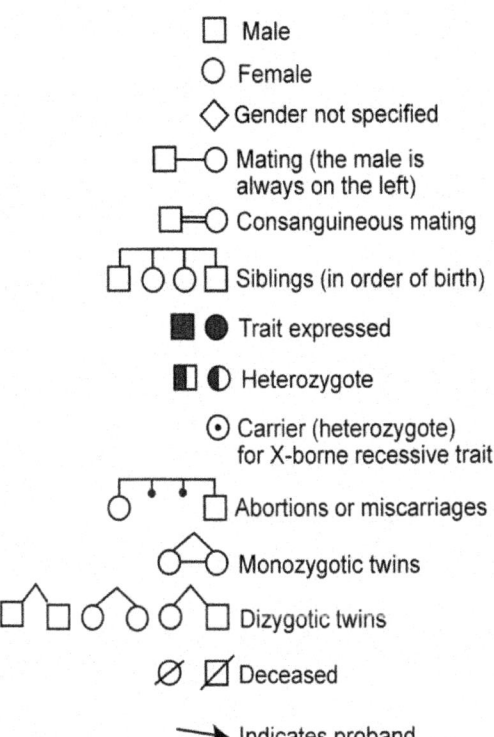

FIGURE 9-6. Symbols, and their significance, used in the construction of pedigrees.

alleles are expressed. Thus, when red cells have the S+s+ phenotype, the presence of one allele encoding S and another allele encoding s [or an *S/s* (*GYPB*S/s*) genotype] can be inferred.

Autosomal Recessive Inheritance

A trait with **autosomal recessive** inheritance is expressed only in a person who is homozygous for the allele and has inherited the recessive allele from both parents. When a person inherits a single copy of a recessive allele in combination with a silent or deleted (null) allele—that is, a nonfunctioning allele or one that encodes a product that cannot be detected—the recessive trait is expressed and the person appears to be homozygous. It is difficult or impossible to distinguish such a combination from homozygosity for the recessive allele through serologic testing, but DNA-based testing can usually make this distinction.

A mating between two heterozygous carriers results in one chance in four that the children will be homozygous for the trait. The parents of a child who is homozygous for a recessive trait are obligate carriers of the trait. If the frequency of the recessive allele is low, the condition is rare and usually found only among

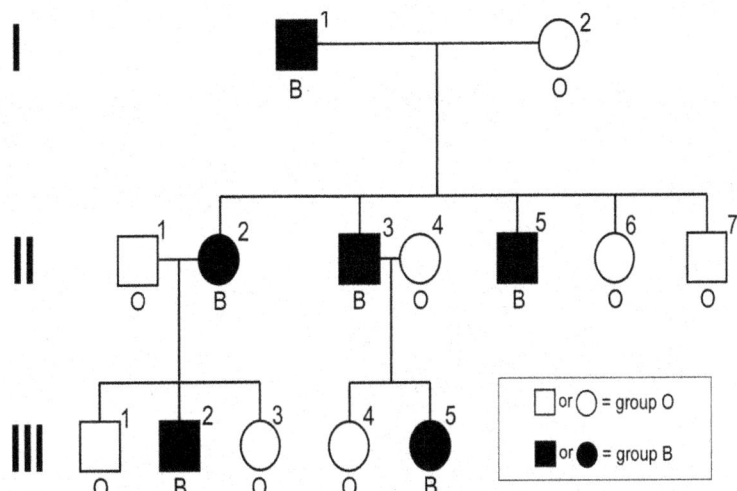

FIGURE 9-7. Autosomal dominant inheritance of the ABO alleles. Based on the ABO groups of his children, I-1 would be expected to have a *B/O* rather than a *B/B* genotype (showing that the B allele is dominant over *O*) because two of his children (II-6 and II-7) are group O and must have inherited an O allele from their father (I-1) in addition to the O allele inherited from their mother (I-2). Similarly, II-2 and II-3 are *B/O*, based on the ABO type of their children, showing the dominance of *B* over *O*.

siblings (brothers and sisters) of the person and not in other relatives. The condition is not found in preceding or successive generations unless **consanguineous** mating (ie, between blood relatives) occurs. When a recessive allele is very rare, the parents of an affected person are most likely consanguineous because a rare allele is more likely to occur in blood relatives than in unrelated persons in a random population. When a recessive trait is one that is common, consanguinity is not a prerequisite for homozygosity; for example, the O allele of the ABO system, although recessive, is not rare, and persons who are homozygous for O are easily found in the random population.

In blood group genetics, a recessive trait almost always involves homozygosity for a **silenced** allele that encodes no product such that the red cells express a **null** phenotype [eg, the Lu(a–b–) or Rh_null or O phenotypes]. The family in Fig 9-8 demonstrates the codominant inheri-

tance of antithetical antigens Lu^a and Lu^b as well as autosomal recessive inheritance of a null *LU* gene, which in the homozygous state results in the Lu(a–b–) phenotype. The proband, II-3, who received multiple transfusions, developed anti-Lu3 (an antibody to a high-prevalence Lutheran antigen) in his plasma. Because his Lu(a–b–) phenotype is the result of recessive inheritance, his siblings are potential donors, with a probability of one in four that the offspring of the mating between I-1 and I-2 would have the Lu(a–b–) phenotype. However, in this case, only the proband had red cells with the Lu(a–b–) phenotype.

Sex-Linked Inheritance

A **sex-linked** trait is one that is encoded by a gene located on the X or Y chromosome. The Y chromosome carries few functional genes, and discussion of sex-linked inheritance generally is

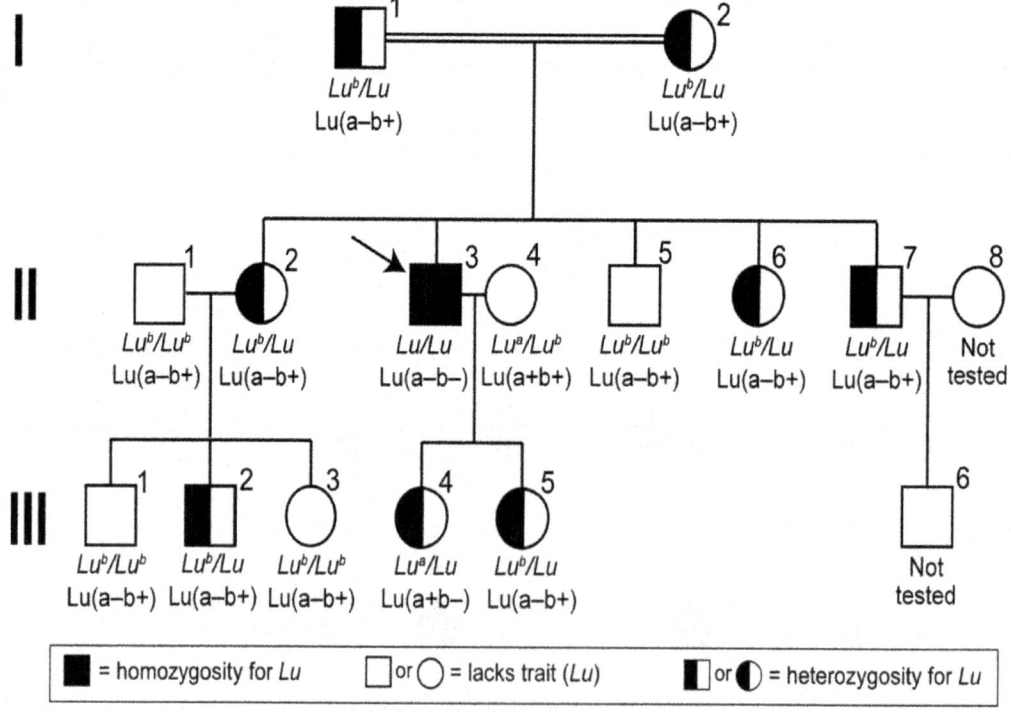

FIGURE 9-8. Autosomal recessive inheritance. The offspring of II-3, the Lu(a–b–) proband, and II-4, his Lu(a+b+) wife, demonstrate that *Lu* (depicting a Lutheran null allele, or *LU*02N*) is recessive to *Lu^a* (*LU*A*) and *Lu^b* (*LU*B*) and that the presence of the silenced Lutheran allele is masked by the product of *Lu^a* (*LU*A*) or *Lu^b* (*LU*B*) at the phenotype level.

synonymous with inheritance of genes carried by the X chromosome. In females (who have two X chromosomes), the inheritance of genes carried by the X chromosome, like the inheritance of genes carried on the autosomes, can be dominant or recessive. Males, in contrast, have one X chromosome (always maternally derived) and one Y chromosome (always paternally derived) and are hemizygous for genes on the X or Y chromosome because only one chromosome (and thus one copy of a gene) is present. Most genes carried by the X chromosome do not have a **homolog** (a similar sequence of DNA) on the Y chromosome. As a consequence, inheritance of an X-linked dominant trait is the same in males and females. However, an X-linked recessive trait is expressed by all males who carry the gene for the trait. There is no male-to-male transmission of either dominant or recessive X-linked traits; that is, X-linked traits are not transmitted from father to son.

Sex-Linked Dominant Inheritance

Sex-linked dominant inheritance describes a trait encoded by a gene on a sex chromosome showing dominant inheritance. For X-linked genes, the trait is expressed by males and by females heterozygous or homozygous for the gene. A male passes his single X chromosome to all of his daughters and all daughters will express the condition or trait. When a female is heterozygous for an allele that encodes a dominant trait, each of her children, whether male or female, has a 50% chance of inheriting the trait. When a female is homozygous for an X-linked trait with dominant inheritance, the encoded trait is expressed by all her children. (See Fig 9-9.)

The Xg^a antigen (XG blood group system) is encoded by an allele on the X chromosome and is inherited in a sex-linked dominant manner. The first indication that the Xg^a antigen was X-linked came from the observation that the

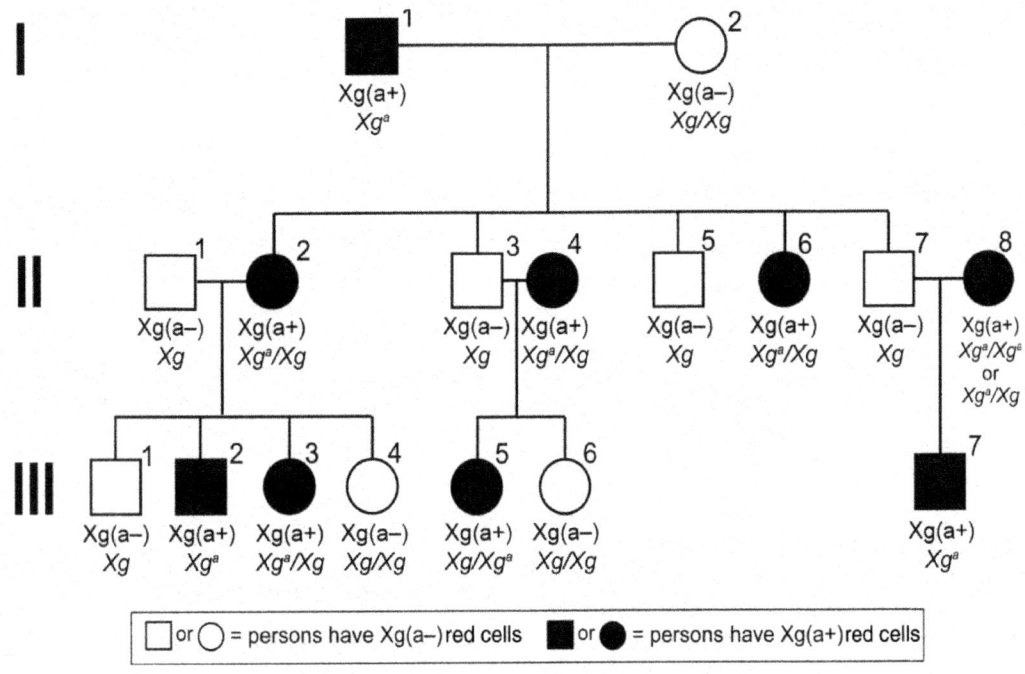

FIGURE 9-9. Sex-linked dominant inheritance. The Xg^a antigen is encoded by an allele on the tip of the short arm of the X chromosome. This family demonstrates the sex-linked dominant inheritance of the Xg^a antigen.

prevalence of the Xg(a–) and Xg(a+) phenotypes differed noticeably between males and females, with the Xgª antigen having a prevalence of 89% in females and only 66% in males.[9] Recently, differential expression of Xgª was found to be linked to disruption of GATA-binding motif in the *XG* gene.[34]

Figure 9-9 shows the inheritance of the Xgª antigen in a three-generation family. In generation I, the father (I-1) is Xg(a+) and has transmitted *Xgª* to all his daughters but to none of his sons. His eldest daughter (II-2), for example, must be heterozygous for *Xgª/Xg*; she received the allele encoding the Xgª antigen from her Xg(a+) father and a silent allele, *Xg*, from her Xg(a–) mother. II-2 has transmitted *Xgª* to half her children, regardless of whether they are sons or daughters.

Sex-Linked Recessive Inheritance

Sex-linked recessive inheritance describes a trait encoded by a sex chromosome that is not expressed in carriers of a single copy, such as in heterozygous females. A male inherits the trait from his mother, who is usually a carrier (or homozygous for the trait). An affected male transmits the trait to all of his daughters, who in turn transmit the trait to approximately half of their sons. Therefore, the prevalence of the expression of an X-linked recessive trait is much higher in males than in females. A carrier female who mates with a male lacking the trait transmits the trait to one-half of her daughters (who will also be carriers) and to one-half of her sons (who will be affected). If mating is between an affected male and a female who lacks the trait, all of the sons will lack the trait and all of the daughters will be carriers. If an X-linked recessive trait is rare in the population, the trait is expressed almost exclusively in males.

The *XK* gene encodes the Kx protein and demonstrates X-linked recessive inheritance. Mutations in or deletions that include *XK* result in red cells with the **McLeod phenotype**, in which red cells lack Kx and have reduced expression of KEL antigens. **McLeod syndrome** is associated with late-onset clinical or subclinical myopathy, neurodegeneration, and central nervous system manifestations, as well as with ac-anthocytosis and, frequently, compensated hemolytic anemia. More than 30 different *XK* gene mutations associated with a McLeod phenotype have been found. Different *XK* mutations appear to have different clinical effects and may account for the variability in the prognosis.[35] Sequencing of *XK* to determine the specific type of mutation in individuals with McLeod phenotypes has clinical prognostic value. McLeod syndrome is an X-linked recessive condition and, as demonstrated by the family in Fig 9-10, is found only in males.

The Principles of Independent Segregation and Independent Assortment

The passing of a trait from one generation to the next follows certain patterns or principles. The principle of independent segregation refers to the separation of homologous chromosomes and their random distribution to the gametes during meiosis. Only one member of an allelic pair is passed on to the next generation, and each gamete has an equal probability of receiving either member of a parental homologous allelic pair; these chromosomes are randomly united at fertilization and thus segregate independently from one generation to the next. The family in Fig 9-11 demonstrates the independent segregation of the ABO alleles on chromosome 9.

The principle of **independent assortment** states that alleles determining various traits are inherited independently from each other. In other words, the inheritance of one allele (eg, a *B* allele, on chromosome 9) does not influence the inheritance of another allele (eg, an *M* allele, on chromosome 4). This is demonstrated by the family in Fig 9-11.

STRUCTURAL VARIATION

Linkage and Crossing Over

Linkage is the physical association between two genes that are located on the same chromosome and are inherited together. Examples include *RHD* and *RHCE* encoding the antigens of the RH system, which are both on chromosome

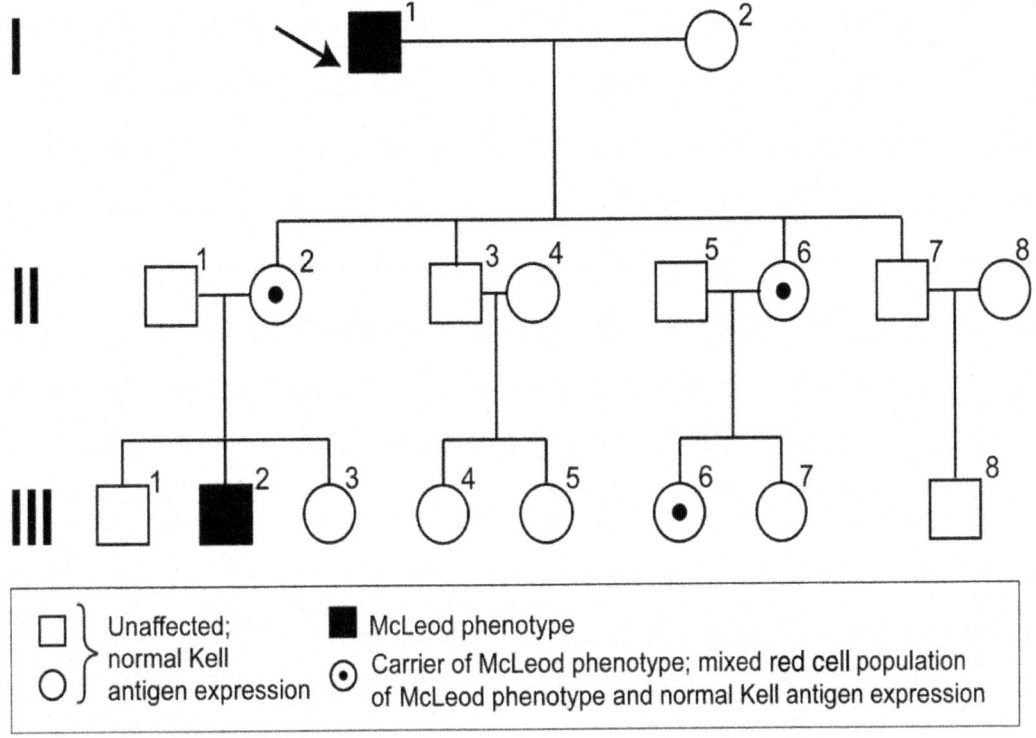

Unaffected; normal Kell antigen expression

■ McLeod phenotype

⊙ Carrier of McLeod phenotype; mixed red cell population of McLeod phenotype and normal Kell antigen expression

FIGURE 9-10. Sex-linked recessive inheritance. This family demonstrates that a sex-linked trait that is recessive in females will be expressed by any male who inherits the trait. Homozygosity for such a trait is required for it to be expressed in females. The trait skips one generation and is carried through females.

1 and represent linked loci that do not assort independently.

Crossing over is the exchange of genetic material between homologous chromosome pairs (Fig 9-4). In this process, a segment from one chromatid (and any associated genes) changes places with the corresponding part of the other chromatid (and its associated genes); the segments are rejoined, and some genes will have switched chromosomes. Thus, crossing over is a means to shuffle genetic material. Because crossing over can result in new gene combinations on the chromosomes involved, it is also referred to as **recombination**, and the rearranged chromosomes can be referred to as **recombinants**. Crossing over and recombination, using chromosome 1 as an example, are explained in Fig 9-12.

Two gene loci carried by the same chromosome that are not closely linked are referred to as being **syntenic**. For example, the loci for *RH* and *FY*, both located on chromosome 1, are syntenic because the distance between them (*RH* on the short arm and *FY* on the long arm) is great enough for them to undergo crossing over and to assort independently.

The frequency of crossing over involving two genes on the same chromosome is a measure of the distance [measured in centimorgans (cM)] between them; the greater the distance between two loci, the greater the probability that crossing over (and recombination) will occur. In contrast, genes located very close together (linked) tend to be transmitted together with no recombination. The degree of crossing over between two genes can be calculated by analyzing pedigrees of families informative for the genes of

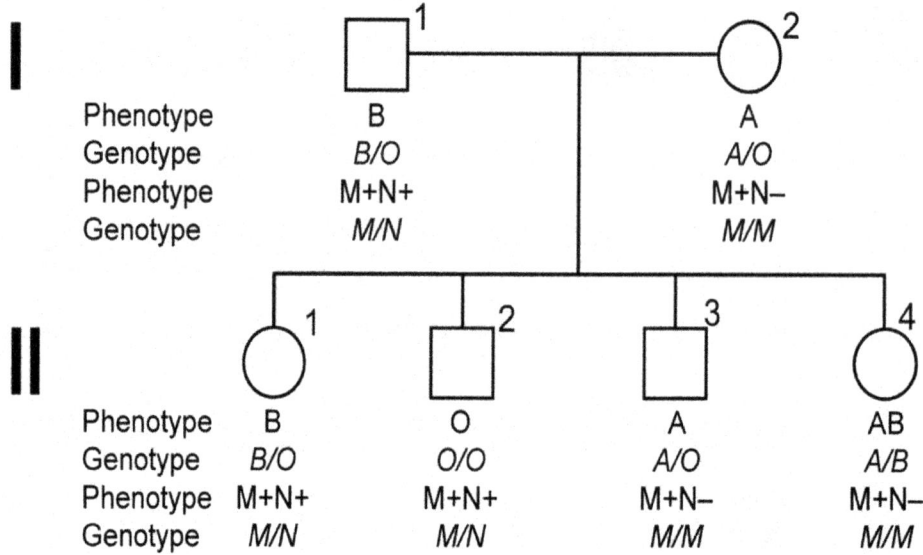

FIGURE 9-11. Independent segregation and independent assortment are illustrated by the inheritance of blood group alleles in one family. Parental ABO alleles were randomly transmitted (independent segregation), and each child has inherited a different combination. The family also illustrates that the alleles encoding antigens of the ABO and MNS blood group systems are inherited independently from each other.

interest and observing the extent of recombination. The traditional method of linkage analysis requires the use of LOD (logarithm of the odds) scores.[36] Linkage analysis was the basis through which chromosomes were mapped and the relative position and distance between genes established. Linkage between Lutheran (*LU*) and ABH secretion (*SE* or *FUT2*) was the first recognized example of autosomal linkage in humans and is explained in Fig 9-13.

Although crossing over occurs readily between distant genes, rare examples of recombination have been documented for genes that are very closely linked or adjacent on a chromosome. Such genes include those encoding the MN (*GYPA*) and Ss (*GYPB*) antigens on chromosome 4 and are reviewed by Daniels.[24(pp96-142)]

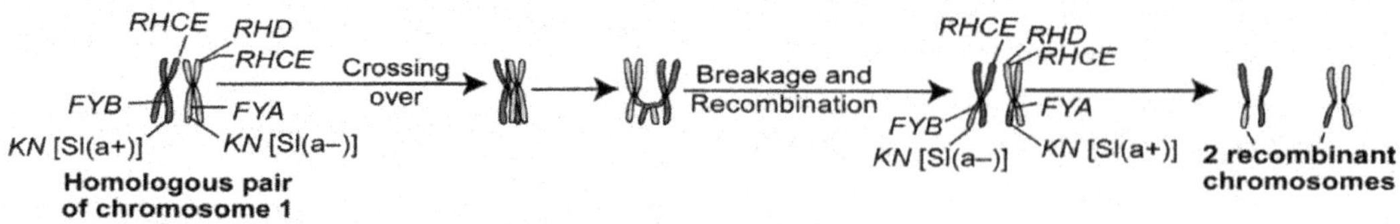

FIGURE 9-12. Crossing over and recombination. In the diagram, chromosome 1 is used as an example. The very closely linked RH genes, *RHD* and *RHCE*, are located near the tip of the short arm of chromosome 1. The loci for *FY* and *KN* are on the long arm of the chromosome and are not linked. During meiosis, crossing over occurs between this homologous chromosome pair, and portions of chromosome break and become rejoined to the partner chromosome. Crossing over of the long arm of chromosome 1 results in recombination between the loci for *FY* and *KN* such that the gene encoding Fy[b] antigen is now traveling with a gene that encodes the Sl(a−) phenotype of the KN system.

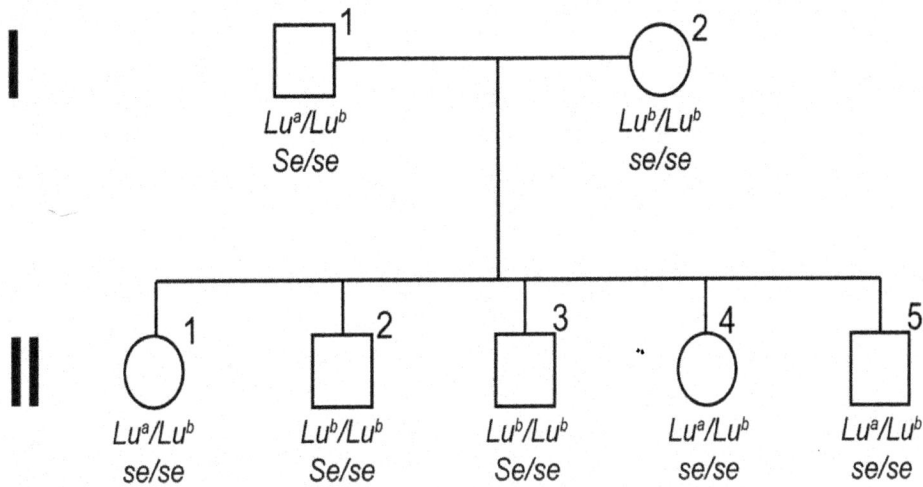

FIGURE 9-13. Linkage between *LU* and *SE* (*FUT2*). I-2 is homozygous for *Lu*^{b} (*LU*B*) and *se* and must transmit these alleles to all her offspring. I-1 is doubly heterozygous [*Lu*^{a}/*Lu*^{b} (*LU*A/B*) and *Se/se*]. He has transmitted *Lu*^{b} (*LU*B*) with *Se*, and *Lu*^{a} (*LU*A*) with *se*, showing linkage between *LU* and *Se* (*FUT2*). Several such informative families would need to be analyzed to statistically confirm linkage.

Linkage Disequilibrium

As mentioned earlier, genes at closely linked loci tend to be inherited together and constitute a **haplotype** (a combination of alleles at two or more closely linked loci on the same chromosome). The alleles encoding the MNS antigens are inherited as four haplotypes: *MS*, *Ms*, *NS*, or *Ns* [in the International Society of Blood Transfusion (ISBT) allele terminology, these haplotypes would be written as *GYPA*M-GYPB*S*, *GYPA*M-GYPB*s*, *GYPA*N-GYPB*S*, or *GYPA*N-GYPB*s*, respectively). Because linked genes do not assort independently, the antigens encoded by each of these haplotypes have a different prevalence in the population than would be expected by random assortment. If *M* and *S* were not linked, the expected prevalence for M+ and S+ in the population would be 17% (from frequency calculations), whereas the actual or observed prevalence (obtained from testing and analyzing families) of the *MS* haplotype is 24%.[24(pp96-142)] This constitutes **linkage disequilibrium**, which is the tendency of specific combinations of alleles at two or more linked loci to be inherited together more frequently than would be expected by chance.

CHIMERISM

The observation that a sample gives mixed-field agglutination is not an unusual one in transfusion medicine. Often this is the result of artificially induced chimerism through the transfusion of donor red cells or the result of a hematopoietic stem cell transplant. On rare occasions, the observation of mixed-field agglutination identifies a true **chimera**, that is, a person with a dual population of cells derived from more than one zygote. Indeed, the first example of a human chimera was a female blood donor discovered through mixed-field agglutination during antigen typing. Most human chimeras can be classified as either twin chimeras or tetragametic (dispermic) chimeras. Chimerism is not a hereditary condition.[37]

Twin chimerism occurs through the formation of placental blood vessel anastomoses, which results in the mixing of blood between two fetuses. This vascular bridge allows hematopoietic stem cells to migrate to the marrow of the opposite twin. Each twin may have two distinct populations of cells (red cells and leukocytes), that of his or her true genetic type and that of the twin. The percentage of the two cell lines in each twin tends to vary; the major cell line is not necessarily the autologous cell line, and the proportions of the two cell lines may change throughout life. Chimeric twins have immune tolerance; they do not make antibody against the A or B antigens that are absent from their own red cells but are present on the cells of the engrafted twin. This tolerance extends beyond red cells to negative mixed-lymphocyte cultures and the mutual acceptance of skin grafts.

In twin chimeras, the dual cell population is strictly confined to blood cells. Tetragametic or dispermic chimeras present chimerism in all tissues and are more frequently identified because of infertility than because of mixed populations of red cells. The mechanism(s) leading to the development of tetragametic chimeras are unknown, but they arise through the fertilization of two maternal nuclei by two sperm, followed by fusion of the two zygotes and development into one person containing two cell lineages.

More commonly, chimeras occur through medical intervention and arise from the transfer of actively dividing cells, such as through hematopoietic cell transplantation.[37] However, chimerism may be more prevalent than once thought, based on the discovery of people with dual red cell populations when performing DNA analysis to predict red cell phenotypes, and chimerism has been the cause of disputed maternity.[38,39]

GENE POSITION EFFECTS

Alleles that are carried on the same chromosome are referred to as being in **cis** position, whereas those on opposite chromosomes of a homologous pair are in **trans** position. Alleles that are in *cis* and linked are always inherited together on the same chromosome, whereas genes in *trans* segregate independently.

Historically, the RH blood group system was used to explain the meaning of *cis* and *trans*. For example, the *DCe/DcE* genotype was described as having *C* and *e* alleles in *cis* in the *DCe* haplotype, with *c* and *E* alleles in *cis* in the partner *DcE* haplotype, whereas *C* and *E* and also *c* and *e* are in opposing haplotypes and are in *trans*. In this alignment, *C* and *e*, for exam-

ple, are always inherited together, but *C* and *E* are not. The preceding explanation, which implies that one gene encodes C and c antigens while another linked gene encodes E and e antigens, was based on the Fisher-Race theory of three genes at the *RH* locus. In contrast, genomic analysis indicates that only one gene (*RHCE*), with four alleles (*RHCE*Ce*, *RHCE*cE*, *RHCE*ce*, and *RHCE*CE*), encodes one protein that carries the CcEe antigens. Thus, for Rh, *DCe* is an example of a haplotype, and the *RHD* allele is in *cis* to the *RHCE*Ce* allele.

The expression of red cell antigens may be modified or affected by gene or protein interactions that manifest primarily as reduced antigen expression. One example in which the haplotype on one chromosome affects the expression of the haplotype on the paired chromosome is commonly referred to as the **position effect** and can be observed with Rh antigen expression. When a *Ce* haplotype (note the absence of *RHD*) is in *trans* to a D-antigen-encoding haplotype, the expression of D is dramatically reduced and a weak D phenotype can result. When the same D-encoding haplotype is inherited with either *ce* or *cE*, D antigen is normally expressed. The cause of this reduced antigen expression is not known, but it may involve differences in gene expression levels or altered assembly of proteins in the membrane. In the presence of the KEL system antigen Kp^a, expression of other KEL system antigens encoded by the same allele is suppressed to varying degrees (*cis*-modifier effect). This is best observed in persons who have a silenced *KEL* gene (K_0) in *trans*. The amino acid change that results in the expression of Kp^a adversely affects trafficking of the Kell glycoprotein to the red cell surface, so that the quantity of Kp^a carrying Kell glycoprotein that reaches the red cell surface is greatly reduced.

GENETIC MODIFIERS OF BLOOD GROUP ANTIGEN EXPRESSION

A genetic modifier is a gene or locus that affects the expression of another gene or genes. Genetic modifiers can be **unlinked** or inherited independently from the genes they modify. For example, *KLF1*, located on chromosome 19p13.3-p13.12, encodes erythroid Krüppel-like factor (EKLF), which is a transcription factor essential for expression of genes critical to terminal differentiation of red cells. Singleton et al[40] first discovered that heterozygosity for nucleotide variants in *KLF1* is responsible for the dominant Lu(a–b–) phenotype,[9] which is also known as the ***In(Lu)* phenotype**. This heterozygosity is characterized by reduced expression of antigens in the Lutheran system, P1, In^b, and AnWj antigens. X-linked forms of the *In(Lu)* phenotype have been associated with mutations in the transcription factor GATA1, encoded by the X-borne *GATA-1* gene, known to be essential for erythroid and megakaryocyte differentiation.[41] Typing of red cells for one or more of these other antigens can help differentiate the *In(Lu)* phenotype from Lu(a–b–). Sequencing of the relevant genes also can be used to make the distinction.

Another example of an unlinked modifier of a blood group system is the regulator type (as opposed to the amorph type) of Rh$_{null}$. Family studies have been employed to locate silencing mutations in *RHAG*, a gene located on chromosome 6 that encodes the Rh-associated glycoprotein RhAG. Red cell membrane expression of RhAG is required for Rh antigen expression. *RHAG* has also been found to carry variants associated with the Rh$_{mod}$ phenotype.[9]

Several red cell antigens require the interaction of the products of two or more independent genes for their expression. Amino acids 75 to 99 of GPA, the glycoprotein that carries the M and N antigens, must be present in the red cell membrane for expression of Wr^b, an antigen in the Diego blood group system carried on band 3. An absence of RhD and RhCE protein (Rh$_{null}$) results in red cells that lack LW antigens and have reduced or no expression of U, S, and s antigens encoded by GPB, again demonstrating the interaction in the membrane of the products of two or more independent blood group genes.

The sequential interaction of gene products from several loci is required for the expression of ABO, H, LE, and I antigens on red cells and in secretions. These antigens are carbohydrate determinants carried on glycoproteins or glycolipids. The genes responsible for carbohydrate-based antigens do not encode membrane proteins but instead encode a glycosyltransferase that catalyzes the sequential transfer of the appropriate immunodominant monosaccharide. The carbohydrate antigens are carried on oligosaccharide chains that are assembled by the stepwise addition of monosaccharides. Each monosaccharide structure is transferred by a separate glycosyltransferase, such that two genes are required for a disaccharide, three for a trisaccharide, and so on. If the enzyme encoded by one locus is inactive due to a genetic variant, this can prevent or modify the expression of the other gene products. The product encoded by the *H* gene is the biosynthetic precursor for A and B antigen production. Thus, if the *H* gene is silenced, A or B antigens cannot be produced. Genetic variation in *ABO*A* and *ABO*B* alleles can result in expression of a glycosyltransferase that is less functional or inactive. Details on the biosynthesis of the ABO, H, LE, and I antigens may be found in Chapter 10.

POPULATION GENETICS

Population genetics is the study of the distribution patterns of genes and of the factors that maintain or change gene (or allele) frequencies. A basic understanding of population genetics, probability, and the application of simple algebraic calculations is important in transfusion medicine, where the knowledge can be applied to clinical situations such as predicting the likelihood of finding compatible blood for a patient who has made antibody(ies) to red cell antigens. It may be helpful to define three commonly used words so that their appropriate use is understood. **Frequency** is used to describe prevalence at the genetic level—that is, the occurrence of an allele (gene) in a population. **Prevalence** is used to describe the occurrence of a permanent inherited characteristic at the phenotypic level—for example, a blood group antigen—in any given population. **Incidence** is used when describing the rate of occurrence in a population of a condition that changes over time, such as a disease.

Phenotype Prevalence

The prevalence of a blood group antigen or phenotype can be determined by testing red cells from a large random sample of people of the same race or ethnicity with a specific antibody and calculating the percentage of positive and negative reactions. The larger the cohort being tested, the more statistically significant is the result. For antithetical antigens, the sum of the percentages for the prevalence of the phenotypes should equal 100%. For example, in the FY blood group system, the prevalence in a random population of African ancestry for the Fy(a+b−), Fy(a−b+), Fy(a+b+), and Fy(a−b−) phenotypes is 9%, 22%, 1%, and 68%, respectively; together, these percentages total 100%. If the red cells from 1000 donors of European ancestry are tested with anti-c, and 800 of the samples are positive and 200 are negative for the Rh antigen c, the prevalence of the c+ phenotype is 80% and that of the c− phenotype is 20%. Thus, in this donor population, approximately 20% of ABO-compatible units of blood, or 1 in 5, should be compatible with serum/plasma from a patient who has made anti-c.

Calculations for Antigen-Negative Phenotypes

When blood is provided for a patient with antibodies directed at one or more red cell antigens, a simple calculation can be used to estimate the number of units that need to be tested to find the desired antigen combination. To calculate the prevalence of the combined antigen-negative phenotype, the prevalence of each of the individual antigens are multiplied together if the antigens are inherited independently of each other. This approach is not valid when the antigens are encoded by alleles that are closely linked and are inherited as haplotypes (M, N, S, s) or reside on the same carrier protein (C, c, E, e). If a patient with antibodies to K, S, and Jk^a antigens requires 3 units of blood, for example, prevalence of the antigen-negative phenotype and the number of units that need to be tested to find it can be calculated as follows:

- The prevalence of donors of European ancestry who are: K− = 91%; S− = 48%; Jk(a−) = 24%.
- The percentage of such donors negative for each antigen is expressed as a decimal and multiplied: 0.91 (K−) × 0.48 (S−) × 0.24 [Jk(a−)] = 0.1048.
- 0.1048 expressed as a % = 0.1048 × 100% = 10.48%.
- 10.48% expressed as occurrence = 10.48/100 = approximately 1/10.
- Thus, approximately 1 in 10 ABO-compatible Red Blood Cell (RBC) units are expected to be K−, S−, Jk(a−).
- The patient in question requires 3 units, so on average, 30 units would need to be tested. This can be calculated as follows:
  0.1 of X = 3.
  X = 3/0.1.
  X = 30 units.

The prevalence of a particular antigen (or phenotype) can vary with race,[5] and the prevalence for a combined antigen-negative phenotype calculation should be selected on the basis of the predominant race found in the donor population.

Allele (Gene) Frequency

The allele frequency is the proportion of one allele relative to all alleles at a particular gene locus in a given population at a given time. This frequency can be calculated from the prevalence of each phenotype observed in a population. The sum of allele frequencies at any given locus must equal 100% (or 1 in an algebraic calculation) in the population sample tested. The genotype frequency is the number of individuals with a given genotype divided by the total number of individuals sampled in a population.

The Hardy-Weinberg Equilibrium

Gene frequencies tend to remain constant from generation to generation in any relatively large population unless they are influenced by factors such as selection, mutation, migration, or nonrandom mating, any of which would have to be significant to have a discernible effect. According to the principles proposed by the British mathematician Hardy and the German physician Weinberg, gene frequencies reach equilibrium. This equilibrium can be expressed in algebraic terms by the Hardy-Weinberg formula or equation:

$$p^2 + 2pq + q^2 = 1$$

If two alleles, classically referred to as A and a, have gene frequencies of p and q, the homozygotes and heterozygotes are present in the population in the following proportions:

$$AA = p^2; \, Aa = 2pq; \, aa = q^2$$

In such a two-allele system, if the gene frequency for one allele, say p, is known, q can be calculated by $p + q = 1$.

The Hardy-Weinberg equation permits the estimation of genotype frequencies from the phenotype prevalence in a sampled population and, reciprocally, allows the determination of genotype frequency and phenotype prevalence from the gene frequency. The equation has a number of applications in blood group genetics, and its use is demonstrated below.

In a population of European ancestry, the frequencies of the two alleles encoding the antithetical antigens K (*KEL*01*) or k (*KEL*02*) can be determined as follows:

Frequency of the *KEL*01* allele = p

Frequency of the *KEL*02* allele = q

Frequency of the *KEL*01* genotype = p^2

Frequency of the *KEL*01/KEL*02* genotype = 2pq

Frequency of the *KEL*02/KEL*02* genotype = q^2

The K antigen is expressed on the red cells of 9% of people of European ancestry; therefore:

$p^2 + 2pq$ = the frequency of people who carry *KEL*01* and are K+

Thus, $p^2 + 2pq = 0.09$

$q^2 = 1 - (p^2 + 2pq)$ = the frequency of people who carry *KEL*02/02* and are K–

$q^2 = 1 - 0.09$

$q = \sqrt{0.91}$

$q = 0.95$ = the frequency of *KEL*02*

Because the sum of the frequencies of both alleles must equal 1.00:

$p + q = 1$

$p = 1 - q$

$p = 1 - 0.95$

$p = 0.05$ = the frequency of *KEL*01*

Having calculated the allele frequencies for *KEL*01* and *KEL*02*, it is possible to calculate the percentage of k+ (both K+k+ and K–k+) and K+ (both K+k– and K+k+) people:

Prevalence of k+ $\quad = 2pq + q^2$
$\quad\quad = 2(0.05 \times 0.95) + (0.95)^2$
$\quad\quad = 0.9975 \times 100$
$\quad\quad$ = a calculated prevalence of 99.75% (the observed prevalence of the k+ phenotype is 99.8%)

Prevalence of K+ $\quad = 2pq + p^2$
$\quad\quad = 2(0.05 \times 0.95) + (0.05)^2$
$\quad\quad = 0.0975$
$\quad\quad = 0.0975 \times 100$ = a calculated prevalence for K+ of 9.75% (the observed prevalence of the K+ phenotype is 9%)

The Hardy-Weinberg equation also can be applied to calculate the frequencies of the three possible genotypes *KEL*01/KEL*01*, *KEL*01/KEL*02*, and *KEL*02/KEL*02* from the gene frequencies *KEL*01* (p) = 0.05 and *KEL*02* (q) = 0.95:

$p^2 + 2pq + q^2 = 1$

Frequency of *KEL*01/KEL*01* = $p^2 = 0.0025$

Frequency of *KEL*01/KEL*02* = $2pq = 0.095$

Frequency of *KEL*02/KEL*02* = $q^2 = 0.9025$

If antibodies are available to test for the products of the alleles of interest (in this example, anti-K and anti-k), the allele frequencies also can be obtained by direct counting as demonstrated in Table 9-3. The allele frequencies obtained by direct testing are the **observed frequencies** for the population being sampled, whereas those obtained by gene frequency calculations (above) are the **expected frequencies**. The various calculations above, when applied to a two-allele situation, are relatively simple; the calculations for three or more alleles are much more complex and beyond the scope of this chapter.

For a given population, if the prevalence of one genetic trait, such as a red cell antigen, is known, the Hardy-Weinberg equation can be applied to calculate allele and genotype frequencies. The Hardy-Weinberg equilibrium principle is valid when the population is sufficiently large that chance alone cannot alter an allele frequency and when the mating is random. A selective advantage or disadvantage of a particular trait and other influencing factors, such as mutation or migration in or out of the population, are assumed to be absent when the Hardy-Weinberg equilibrium principle is applied. When all of these conditions are met, the gene pool is said to be in equilibrium and allele frequencies do not change from one generation to the next. If the conditions are not met, changes in allele frequencies may occur over a few generations and

may explain many of the differences in allele frequencies between populations.

RELATIONSHIP TESTING

Polymorphisms are inherited characteristics or genetic markers that can distinguish between people. The blood groups with the greatest number of alleles (greatest polymorphism) have the highest power of discrimination. Blood is a rich source of inherited characteristics that can be detected, including red cell, HLA, and platelet antigens. Red cell and HLA antigens are easily identifiable, are polymorphic, and follow Mendelian laws of inheritance. The greater the level of genetic variation in a system, the less chance there is of finding two people who are identical. The extensive polymorphism of the HLA system alone allows the exclusion of >90% of falsely accused men in cases of disputed paternity. However, serologic methods of identity testing were surpassed and replaced by DNA-based assays[42] (referred to as DNA fingerprinting or DNA profiling) that were pioneered by Jeffreys and colleagues.[43,44] Tandemly repeated sequences of DNA of varying lengths occur predominantly in the noncoding genomic DNA, and they are classified into groups depending on the size of the repeat region. The extensive vari-

TABLE 9-3. Allele Frequencies of *K (KEL*01)* and *k (KEL*02)* Calculated Using Direct Counting (assuming the absence of null alleles)

Phenotype	No. of Persons	No. of Alleles	K (*KEL*01*)	k (*KEL*02*)
K+k−	2	4	4	0
K+k+	88	176	88	88
K−k+	910	1820	0	1820
Totals	1000	2000	92	1908
Allele frequency			0.046	0.954

A random sample of 1000 people tested for K and k antigens has a total of 2000 alleles at the *KEL* locus because each person inherits two alleles, one from each parent. Therefore, the two persons with a K+k− phenotype (each with two alleles) contribute a total of four alleles. To this are added 88 *K (KEL*01)* alleles from the K+k+ group, for a total of 92 *K (KEL*01)* alleles, or an allele frequency of 0.046 (92 ÷ 2000). The frequency of the *k (KEL*02)* allele is 0.954 (1908 ÷ 2000).

ation of these tandemly repeated sequences between individuals makes it unlikely for the same number of repeats to be shared by two individuals, even if these individuals are related. Minisatellite [also referred to as variable number of tandem repeats (VNTR)] loci have tandem-repeat units of 9 to 80 base pairs, whereas microsatellite [also referred to as short tandem repeat (STR)] loci consist of two to five base-pair tandem repeats.[45]

Commonly used assays for VNTR and STR sequences involve the electrophoretic separation of DNA fragments according to size. DNA profiling involves amplification of selected, informative VNTR and STR loci using locus-specific oligonucleotide primers, and subsequently measuring the size of the **polymerase chain reaction (PCR)** products. Hundreds of STR loci have been mapped throughout the human genome, and many have been applied to identity testing. Analysis of different STR loci (usually at least 12) is used to generate a person's DNA profile that is virtually guaranteed to be unique to that person (or to two identical twins). DNA fingerprinting is a powerful tool not only for identity testing and population genetics but also for monitoring chimerism after marrow transplantation.[46] STR analysis also has been used to monitor patients for graft-vs-host disease after organ transplantation, particularly after a liver transplant.[47] With the advent of **next-generation sequencing (NGS)**, SNV panels are being developed for use in genetic identification.[48]

In a case of disputed paternity, if an alleged father cannot be excluded from paternity, the probability of his paternity can be calculated. The calculation compares the probability that the alleged father transmitted the paternal obligatory genes with the probability that any other randomly selected man from the same racial or ethnic group transmitted the genes. The result is expressed as a likelihood ratio (paternity index) or as a percentage. AABB has developed standards and guidance documents for laboratories that perform relationship testing.[49]

BLOOD GROUP GENE MAPPING

Gene mapping is the process through which a gene locus is assigned to a location on a chromosome. The initial mapping of blood group genes was accomplished by testing many families for selected red cell antigens. Pedigrees were analyzed for evidence of recombination between the genes of interest to rule out or establish linkage of a blood group with another marker having a known chromosomal location.

The gene encoding the antigens of the FY blood group system was the first to be assigned to a chromosome, by showing that the gene is linked to an inherited deformity of chromosome 1.[50] Subsequently, recombinant DNA methods were used to establish the physical locations of genes. The Human Genome Project,[51] completed in 2003, resulted in construction of a physical gene map indicating the position of gene loci, and the distance between loci is expressed by the number of base pairs of DNA. The 1000 Genomes Project,[52] completed in 2015, created the largest public catalogue of human genetic variation.

Currently, 39 blood group systems are recognized by the ISBT.[10] The genes for all of them have been cloned and assigned to their respective chromosomes (Table 9-1). For the more recently mapped blood group antigen genes, a variety of methods was used, including peptide sequencing, massively parallel sequencing, and bioinformatics approaches. Mapping of the VEL blood group system was performed by two different groups. Storry et al used SNV mapping of 20 Vel-negative individuals in Sweden, which identified a region on chromosome 1 that tracked with the Vel-negative phenotype.[18] Sanger sequencing of several candidate genes expressed in red cells identified a 17-base-pair deletion in *SMIM1* in the Vel-negative individuals. Details on procedures for gene mapping are beyond the scope of this chapter, but reviews are available.[12]

GENE, PROTEIN, AND BLOOD GROUP TERMINOLOGY

Gene and protein nomenclature is dictated by the Human Genome Organization (HUGO) Gene Nomenclature Committee.[53] HUGO approves both abbreviated gene symbols and longer descriptive names. Gene symbols are written in italics (eg, *KEL*). Genes may have one or more aliases, such as *ACKR1*, which encodes the FY system antigens, with aliases *DARC*, *CD234*, and *FY*, which is the ISBT gene name. A Locus Reference Genomic (LRG) record, including curated genomic, transcript, and protein reference sequences, is being developed for the blood group antigen genes.[54] Coordinates of nucleotides within the coding region of a gene are numbered starting with the A of the translational start codon ATG. Thus, the location of the SNV in the *FY* gene that determines the Fy^a or Fy^b antigen expression is expressed *FY* c.125, such that a heterozygote can be written *FY* c.125A/G, with the nucleotide found in the reference sequence (in this case A) written first. Coordinates of polypeptides are numbered starting with the first amino acid of the mature protein. Thus, the location of the amino acid determinant of the Fy^a or Fy^b antigen is expressed FY p.Asp42Gly, with the amino acid found in the reference protein (in this case Asp) written first.

Blood group antigens were originally named using an alphabetical (eg, A/B, C/c) notation, or they were named after the proband whose red cells carried the antigen or who made the first known antibody (eg, Duclos). A symbol with a superscript letter (eg, Lu^a, Lu^b; Jk^a, Jk^b) was used, and a numerical terminology (eg, Fy3, Jk3, Rh32) was introduced. In blood group systems, antigens are named using more than one scheme (eg, the KEL blood group system: K, k, Js^a, Js^b, K11, K17, TOU).

In 1980, the ISBT established its Working Party on Terminology for Red Cell Surface Antigens.[10] The working party was charged to develop a uniform nomenclature that would be "both eye and machine readable" and "in keeping with the genetic basis of blood groups." A **blood group system** consists of one or more antigens under the control of a single gene locus or of two or more homologous genes. Thus,

each blood group system is genetically independent from every other blood group system and represents a single gene or a cluster of two or more homologous genes.

The failure of an antibody to be reactive with red cells of a particular null phenotype is not sufficient for assignment of the corresponding antigen to a system. Some null phenotypes are the result of inhibitor or modifying genes that may suppress the expression of antigens from more than one system [eg, the Rh$_{null}$ phenotype lacks not only Rh antigens but also LW system antigens, Fy5 antigen (FY system), and sometimes U antigen (MNS system)]. Similarly, a blood group antigen must be shown to be inherited through family studies, or the expression of the antigen must be demonstrated to be associated with a variation in the nucleotide sequence of the gene controlling the system, to be assigned antigen status by the ISBT terminology working party. A blood group antigen must be defined serologically by an antibody; a genetic variant that is detectable only by DNA analysis and for which there is no corresponding antibody cannot be called a blood group antigen.

The working party established a terminology consisting of uppercase letters and Arabic numerals to represent blood group systems and antigens.[10,55] Each system can be identified by a set of numbers (eg, ABO system = 001; RH system = 004). Similarly, each antigen in the system is assigned a number (eg, A antigen = 001; B antigen = 002; D antigen = 001). Thus, 001001 identifies the A antigen and 004001 identifies the D antigen. Alternatively, the sinistral zeros may be omitted so that the A antigen becomes 1.1 and the D antigen becomes 4.1. Each system also has an alphabetical abbreviation (Table 9-1 gives the abbreviated system names, which are often analogous to the gene names); thus, KEL is the ISBT symbol for the Kell system, the Rh ISBT system symbol is RH, and an alternative name for the D antigen is RH1. This alphanumeric terminology, which was designed primarily for computer use, is not ideal for everyday communication. To achieve uniformity, a recommended list of user-friendly alternative names was compiled.[56]

The ISBT working party meets periodically to assign names and numbers to newly discovered antigens. The working party is also charged to develop, maintain, and monitor a terminology for blood group genes and their alleles; this is reflected by its current name, the Red Cell Immunogenetics and Blood Group Terminology Working Party.[10] The terminology takes into account the guidelines for human gene nomenclature published by HUGO, which is responsible for naming genes based on the International System for Human Gene Nomenclature.[57] For antigen terminology criteria; tables listing the systems, antigens, and phenotypes; and information regarding the current status of gene and allele terminology, see the ISBT Red Cell Immunogenetics and Blood Group Terminology web resources.[10] An example of ISBT terminology as it applies to blood group names, alleles, phenotypes, and antigens is shown in Table 9-4. Clinical significance of alloantibodies to specific antigens varies widely.[58]

BLOOD GROUP GENOMICS

As discussed in earlier sections of this chapter, the antigens expressed on red cells are the products of genes and can be detected directly by hemagglutination techniques (as long as relevant antisera are available). Their detection is an important aspect of the practice of transfusion medicine because an antigen can, if it is introduced into the circulation of an individual who lacks that antigen, elicit an immune response.

It is the antibody from such an immune response that causes problems in clinical practice, such as patient/donor blood transfusion incompatibility or maternal-fetal incompatibility, and it is the reason why antigen-negative blood is required for safe transfusion in these patients. Hemagglutination is simple, quick, and relatively inexpensive. When carried out correctly, it has a specificity and sensitivity that is appropriate for most testing. However, hemagglutination has limitations; for example, it is difficult and often impossible to obtain an accurate phenotype for a recent transfusion recipient or to type red cells that are coated with immunoglobulin G (IgG), and some typing reagents are in short supply or not available. Because the genes encoding the 39 known blood group systems have been cloned and sequenced and the genetic bases of most blood group antigens and phenotypes are known, several of the more recent blood group antigen gene discoveries involved the use of genomic approaches, such as SNV analysis for JR,[15] and NGS of Vel-negative individuals.[19] Additionally, targeted exome sequencing has been employed to resolve problematic serologic cases.[59]

DNA-based methods (genotyping) are increasingly being used as an indirect method to predict a blood group phenotype. This approach has introduced blood group genomics, often referred to as molecular immunohematology, into the practice of transfusion medicine. Prediction of a blood group antigen by testing DNA is simple and reliable for the majority of antigens because most result from SNVs that are inherited in a straightforward Mendelian manner. For example, the **antithetical** antigens S and s arise from *GYPB* alleles that differ by one nucleotide,

TABLE 9-4. Examples of ISBT Terminology in Blood Group Systems

Blood Group Name		First Antigen in the System		Phenotype of Example Antigen		Allele Encoding Example Antigen	Antibody to Example Antigen
Traditional	ISBT Symbol	Traditional	ISBT Terminology	Traditional	ISBT Terminology		
Rh	RH	D	RH1	D+	RH:1	*RHD*01*	Anti-D
Kell	KEL	K	KEL1	K+	KEL:1	*KEL*01.01*	Anti-K
Duffy	FY	Fy^a	FY1, or 008001, or 8.1	Fy(a+)	FY:1	*FY*01* or *FY*A*	Anti-Fy^a

143T for S and 143C for s, and the resulting proteins differ by one amino acid, methionine at amino acid residue p.48 for S and threonine for s (designated c.143T>C p.Met48Thr).

Detailed serologic and genetic studies, including whole genome sequencing, have shown that there are far more alleles than phenotypes, and this is especially relevant clinically for ABO and Rh. Hundreds of alleles encoding the glycosyltransferases responsible for the four ABO types have been identified, and a single nucleotide variant in an *A* or *B* allele can result in an inactive transferase and a group O phenotype (see Chapter 10). Testing for the common Rh antigens D, C/c, and E/e is uncomplicated for most populations, but antigen expression is more complex in some ethnic groups. There are >500 *RHD* alleles, including those encoding weak D or partial D phenotypes, and >150 *RHCE* alleles, including those encoding altered, or novel, hybrid Rh proteins, some of which result in weakened antigen expression (see Chapter 11). RH genotyping, particularly in minority populations, requires sampling of multiple regions of the gene(s) and algorithms for interpretation.

Molecular Methods for Predicting Blood Group Antigen Phenotypes

Genomic DNA for molecular genotyping can be isolated from any nucleated cell source. Peripheral blood mononuclear cells (MNC) are by far the most common specimen type used for predicting a red cell phenotype. If a patient has a low MNC count that hampers DNA isolation from peripheral blood, buccal swabs are an alternate source; this source is also useful for comparison in marrow transplant recipients if antibody formation suggests a loss of engraftment. Complementary DNA (cDNA) can be made from messenger RNA (mRNA) from red cells for investigation of splicing or for cloning of distinct transcripts to determine if the multiple DNA variants identified in a blood group antigen gene are in *cis* or *trans*.

Most DNA-based assays involve amplification of a target gene sequence through PCR, followed by one of a variety of downstream analyses. (See also Chapter 8.) Genotyping methods can be grouped by their level of resolution at the nucleotide level. Any PCR-based testing method can result in a false-negative prediction due to failure to detect an allele resulting from the presence of variation in the gene that inhibits amplification or detection of the variant being interrogated. This is a phenomenon called **allele dropout**.

Low-resolution molecular methods typically interrogate an SNV or other genetic variant in a DNA sample. This includes **sequence-specific primer PCR (SSP-PCR)**, also known as allele-specific PCR, where each DNA sample is amplified using two sets of primers, each of which amplifies only one allele, when the alleles differ by a single nucleotide. Another low-resolution method follows PCR amplification with digestion of the resulting PCR product using a restriction enzyme [**PCR-RFLP (restriction fragment length polymorphism)**]. Both of these methods typically use agarose gel electrophoresis to separate the DNA fragments by size, and imaging to visualize the fragments. These methods are considered low throughput and are not easily automated. **Real-time PCR** uses fluorescent probes with quantitative or qualitative readout. This method is less labor-intensive and can be automated, yet each reaction typically interrogates only one SNV. Bead-based or slide-based DNA arrays or single-base primer extension followed by **matrix-assisted laser desorption/ionization time-of-flight (MALDI-TOF)** mass spectrometry allows for higher throughput genotyping involving a multiplex PCR reaction with multiple gene targets amplified simultaneously and the ability to test multiple samples (typically 48, 96, or 384) simultaneously. These approaches allow for the determination of numerous antigens in a single assay.

Medium-resolution molecular methods include SNV genotyping panels that simultaneously interrogate multiple variants in a single gene. For blood group antigen genotyping, array-based and mass-spectrometry-based assays are used to interrogate many variants in a single gene (eg, *RHD*) to obtain a more accurate prediction, including weak and partial antigens as well as low- and high-prevalence antigens. It is important to note that both low- and medium-resolution genotyping approaches can result in false-positive antigen predictions, because they would typically not detect a null mutation that would silence expression of an antigen.

High-resolution molecular methods involve interrogating, at the very least, the coding region of a gene or genes, thus obtaining the nucleotide sequence that can be used to predict the amino acid sequence and splice sites. A commonly used high-resolution method is Sanger sequencing, which can be performed using DNA fragments generated by gene-specific PCR of genomic DNA or cDNA. When cDNA is used as template, splice variants can be detected. **Massively parallel sequencing** (MPS), which includes NGS, is a high-resolution method that can be used to sequence the whole genome, the whole exome (covering all protein-coding regions), or a set of selected or targeted genomic regions (such as the genes critical for blood group antigen expression). MPS is being employed in research and clinical settings, where it has the potential to revolutionize and personalize diagnostics, prognostics, and selection of optimal therapies, including blood components.[60] High-resolution approaches are more accurate than low- and medium-resolution approaches but often involve a more complex analysis process and interpretation. These approaches can also identify **variants of unknown significance** (VUS) that can complicate a clinical interpretation.

Molecular immunohematology laboratories use methods that are similar to those used for HLA typing, that is, low-resolution typing of one or a few SNVs as well as high-resolution sequencing of entire gene regions. High-resolution methods are often used to investigate new alleles and resolve discordant findings comparing serologic and molecular results. The application of these methods has been reviewed by several groups.[61-64]

Public databases of blood group antigen variation are critical to the sharing of information for both research and clinical purposes. Besides the blood group allele tables managed by the ISBT working party that include phenotype information, when available, there are other resources, either specific to blood group antigens[65-67] or more general,[68] that are useful catalogues of human variation. These resources

further the understanding of the impact of genetic variation on antigen expression as well as the frequency of such variation.

Clinical Application of the Prediction of Blood Groups by Molecular Testing

A major use of DNA-based molecular testing is to predict the red cell phenotype of a fetus or of a transfusion recipient, or when red cells are coated with IgG. Additional applications include the resolution of discrepancies in the ABO and RH systems and identification of the genetic basis of unusual serologic results. Molecular DNA analysis also provides information to aid in distinguishing alloantibodies from autoantibodies. This section gives an overview of some of the major applications of molecular testing that are currently employed in patient and donor testing. These and additional clinical applications are summarized in Table 9-5.

Molecular Testing to Predict the Red Cell Phenotype

Recent Recipients of Transfusion. In patients receiving chronic or massive transfusions, the presence of donor red cells makes typing by hemagglutination inaccurate. Time-consuming and cumbersome cell separation methods that are often unsuccessful in isolating the patient's reticulocytes for typing can be avoided when DNA typing is used. PCR-based assays primarily use DNA extracted from MNCs isolated from a sample of peripheral blood. Interference from donor-derived DNA is avoided by targeting and amplifying a region of the gene that is common to all alleles so that the minute quantity of donor DNA is not detected. This approach makes possible reliable blood group determination with DNA prepared from a blood sample collected after transfusion. DNA isolated from a buccal swab or saliva is also suitable for testing. In transfusion-dependent patients who produce alloantibodies, an extended antigen profile is important to determine additional blood group antigens to which the patient can become sensitized.

In the past, when a patient with autoimmune hemolytic anemia received transfusion

TABLE 9-5. Applications of Molecular Testing to Predict Red Cell Antigens in Patients and Donors

To predict a patient's red cell phenotype:

- After a recent transfusion
    - Aid in antibody identification and RBC unit selection
    - Select red cells for adsorption

- When antibody typing reagent is not available (eg, anti-Do^a, -Do^b, -Js^a, -V, -VS)

- Distinguish an alloantibody from an autoantibody (eg, anti-e, anti-Kp^b)

- Help identify alloantibody when a patient's type is antigen-positive and a variant phenotype is possible (eg, anti-D in a D-positive patient, anti-e in an e-positive patient)

- When the patient's red cells are coated with immunoglobulin (DAT+)
    - When direct-agglutinating antibodies are not available
    - When the antigen is sensitive to the IgG removal treatment (eg, antigens in the Kell system are denatured by EDTA-glycine-acid elution)
    - When testing requires the indirect antiglobulin test and IgG removal techniques are not effective at removing cell-bound immunoglobulin
    - When antisera are weakly reactive and reaction is difficult to interpret (eg, anti-Do^a, anti-Do^b, anti-Fy^b)

- Obtain a patient's phenotype before or after administration of monoclonal antibody therapeutic drugs (eg, anti-CD38, anti-CD47, daratumumab) that cause interferences with serologic testing methods

- After allogeneic stem cell transplantation [If an antibody problem arises, test stored DNA samples (or buccal swab) from the patient and the donor(s) to guide selection of units for transfusion]

- To detect weakly expressed antigens (eg, Fy^b with the Fy^x phenotype)

- Identify genetic basis of unusual serologic results, especially Rh variants

- Resolve blood group discrepancies (eg, A, B, and Rh)

- Aid in the resolution of complex serologic investigations, especially those involving high-prevalence antigens when reagents are not available

- Identify if a fetus is at risk for HDFN (mother with anti-D; father homozygous or heterozygous for *RHD*)

To predict a donor's red cell phenotype:

- Screen for antigen-negative donors

- When antibody is weak or not available (eg, anti-Do^a, -Do^b; -Js^a, -Js^b; -V/VS)

- Mass screening to increase antigen-negative inventory

- Find donors whose red cells lack a high-prevalence antigen

- Identify donors with RH variant alleles that express partial Rh antigens (for Rh allele-matching to patients)

- Resolve blood group discrepancies (eg, A, B, and Rh)

- Resolve antigen-typing discrepancies caused by alleles encoding weak or partial antigens

- Type donors for reagent red cells for antibody screening cells and antibody identification panels (eg, Do^a, Do^b, Js^a, V, VS)

- Determine zygosity of donors on antibody detection/identification reagent panels, especially D, S, Fy^a, and Fy^b

RBCs = Red Blood Cells; DAT = direct antiglobulin test; HDFN = hemolytic disease of the fetus and newborn.

before the patient's red cell phenotype for minor antigens was established, time- and resource-consuming differential allogeneic adsorptions were required to determine the presence or absence of alloantibodies underlying the autoantibody. Establishing the patient's most probable phenotype through molecular testing makes it possible to match the antigen profile of the adsorbing red cells to that of the patient, thereby reducing the number of cell types required for adsorption. This approach also allows matching of the antigen profile of the donor to that of the patient for the most clinically significant, common antigens (eg, Rh; Jk^a, Jk^b, S, s) when transfusion is required. Transfusion of units that are antigen-matched for clinically significant blood group antigens prevents delayed transfusion reactions and avoids additional alloimmunization.

When Red Cells Are Coated with IgG. In patients with or without autoimmune hemolytic anemia, the presence of immunoglobulin bound to the red cells [positive result on direct antiglobulin testing (DAT)] often makes antigen typing results by serologic methods invalid. Certain methods, such as treatment of the red cells with chloroquine diphosphate or EDTA-glycine acid (EGA), may be employed to remove the red-cell-bound IgG. These methods are not always successful or accurate[69]; the antigen of interest may be denatured by the treatment (eg, EGA destroys antigens of the Kell blood group system), and direct agglutinating antibodies for the antigen of interest may not be available. Molecular testing allows determination of an extended antigen profile to select antigen-negative RBC units for transfusion that match the antigen profile.

When Red Cells Are Coated with Therapeutic Drugs. As a result of the increasing success of treating patients with monoclonal antibody (MoAb) therapeutic drugs (eg, anti-CD38, anti-CD47), there has been an increase in interfering substance detection, causing several serology methods to become invalid. For example, anti-CD38 is broadly reactive when performing antibody detection with an indirect antiglobulin test (IAT), due to the expression of CD38 on the red cell, and anti-CD47 presents with a broader reactivity range than anti-CD38 due to its large

amounts of CD47 expression on the red cell. Also, in some cases a patient who is sensitized may cause an initial positive DAT that may be negative upon subsequent testing. The detection of MoAbs is dependent on when the last dose was received in relation to pretransfusion testing, on the patient disease, and on serologic method used.[70]

Many laboratories use thiol-treated red cells to test the patient's serum/plasma after anti-CD38 administration; however, they are unable to rule out antibodies to the KEL, LU, KN, LW, and YT blood group system antigens. Currently, several anti-CD47 clones are in clinical trial. The interference due to HU5F9-G4 can be avoided using a monoclonal anti-IgG that is nonreactive with IgG4 or by allogeneic platelet or red cell adsorption.[71] The development of methods to negate interference by different clones of anti-CD47 is under way as the trial continues.

Molecular testing may help with mitigating the MoAb interferences with serologic testing by obtaining a baseline genotype before the patient begins drug therapy. Molecular testing may also be used to predict a patient's phenotype after drug therapy is already started if whole blood or buffy coat is used for DNA extraction. The patient's extended phenotype can be used to predict the potential antibodies that the patient might make. Phenotype-similar red cells can be provided for transfusion while the patient is receiving MoAb drug treatments.[72]

DNA-Based Assays to Distinguish Alloantibody from Autoantibody

When an antibody specificity is found in a patient whose red cells express the corresponding antigen, it is essential to know whether the antibody is an allo- or autoantibody, and molecular testing is helpful for transfusion management. If molecular testing predicts the red cells to be antigen positive, further investigation of the blood group antigen coding regions by a higher-resolution molecular method such as Sanger sequencing should be considered, because the sample may have an amino acid change from the reference sequence in the protein carrying the antigen. Amino acid changes can result in new epitopes or altered (weakened or partial) expression of the conventional antigen.

This is especially relevant in patients with sickle cell disease (SCD) or thalassemia who require long-term transfusion support and are at risk of alloimmunization that is often complicated by the presence of antibodies. In patients of African ancestry who have SCD, partial expression of common Rh antigens (D, C, c, and e) is prevalent. Such patients frequently present with a combination of anti-D, -C, and -e, and yet their red cells type serologically as D+, C+, and/or e+. Although such patients may make alloantibodies to these antigens, autoantibody production with Rh-related specificity is common, and distinguishing between the two is critical for safe transfusion practice to avoid hemolytic transfusion reactions (and conserve rare blood).[73,74] Delayed hemolytic transfusion reactions, in particular, places patients with SCD at risk for life-threatening anemia, pain crisis, acute chest syndrome, and/or acute renal failure. Patients may also experience hyperhemolysis, in which hemoglobin levels decline below pretransfusion levels as a result of bystander hemolysis of the patients' own antigen-negative red cells. RH genotyping has revealed that many of these patients have variant RHD and/or RHCE alleles that encode amino acid changes in Rh proteins, resulting in altered or partial antigens. For details on RHD and RHCE alleles that encode partial antigens, refer to Chapter 11.

Reports of autoantibodies to Jk[a] and Jk[b] are not uncommon. With the discovery of variant JK alleles that encode partial Jk[a] and Jk[b] antigens, it is probable that some previously identified autoantibodies were alloantibodies. (The JK system is discussed in Chapter 12.) DNA analysis for JK variants is helpful to clarify the situation. As in some other blood group systems, JK system genetic diversity is higher in populations of African ancestry.

Molecular Testing in Prenatal Practice

DNA-based testing has affected prenatal practice in the areas that are discussed below. Hemagglutination, including antibody titers, gives only an indirect indication of the risk and severity of hemolytic disease of the fetus and newborn (HDFN). Antigen prediction by molecular methods can be used to identify the fetus who is not at risk of HDFN (ie, who is predicted to be antigen negative) so that the mother need not be aggressively monitored. Testing of fetal DNA should be considered when a mother's serum contains an IgG alloantibody that has been associated with HDFN and the father's status for the corresponding antigen is heterozygous or indeterminable, or he is not available for testing. For more detail on perinatal issues, including HDFN, see Chapter 23.

Molecular Testing to Identify a Fetus at Risk for HDFN. The first application of a DNA-based method for the prediction of blood group phenotype occurred in the prenatal setting and was reported by Bennett et al,[75] who tested fetal DNA for the presence of RHD. Because of the clinical significance of anti-D, RHD is probably the most frequent target gene for fetal testing, but molecular testing can be used to predict the antigen type of the fetus for any antigen if the genetic basis is known. When the implicated IgG antibody in the maternal circulation is not anti-D, it is prudent, when possible, to also test the fetal DNA for RHD to preempt unnecessary requests for D– blood for intrauterine transfusion; this is particularly relevant to avoid the use of rare rr′ or rr″ blood when anti-c or anti-e is the implicated antibody.

PCR analyses for the prediction of fetal D phenotype are based on detecting the presence or absence of specific portions of RHD. In populations of European ancestry, the genetic basis of the D– phenotype is usually associated with deletion of the entire RHD, but several other molecular bases have been described. In populations of Asian ancestry, 15% to 30% of D– people have an intact but inactive RHD, while others with red cells that are nonreactive with anti-D have the Del phenotype. Approximately a quarter of D– people of African ancestry have an inactive RHD gene (RHDΨ), which does not encode the D antigen, and many others have a hybrid RHD-CE-D gene (eg, the r′[s] phenotype). (For details on the RH system, see Chapter 11.) Predicting the D type by molecular methods requires probing for multiple nucleotide changes. The choice of assays depends on the patient's ethnicity and the degree of discrimination desired.[76] Establishing the fetal *KEL* genotype is also of great clinical value in determining whether a fetus is at risk for severe anemia, because the strength of the mother's K antibody often does not correlate with the severity of the infant's anemia. The same is true for anti-Ge3.[77]

The risk of HDFN can be predicted by determining whether the fetus carries the antigen that corresponds to the mother's antibody. If the father demonstrates heterozygous expression of the antigen or if antigen expression is indeterminable, testing of fetal DNA should be considered. If the fetus is predicted not to carry an antigen against the mother's antibody, the invasive and expensive monitoring of the mother may not be necessary.

Amniocytes, harvested from amniotic fluid, are the most common source of fetal DNA. Chorionic villus sampling and cordocentesis are not favored because of their more invasive nature and associated risk to the fetus. A noninvasive sample source is the cell-free fetal DNA that is present in maternal plasma as early as 5 weeks of gestation; the amount of DNA increases with gestational age, and reliable results in DNA-based assays are obtained starting at about 15 weeks of gestation (sometimes earlier, depending on the gene of interest).[78] Because fetal DNA is generally composed of shorter fragments, the testing capability may be limited compared to cellular DNA.[79] However, these assays are particularly successful for D typing because the D– phenotype in the majority of samples is due to the absence of the *RHD* gene.

Testing for the presence or absence of a gene is less demanding than testing for a single gene polymorphism or SNV to predict, for example, the K/k antigen status. Cell-free fetal DNA from the maternal plasma is routinely used in some European countries[80,81] to test for the presence of a fetal *RHD* gene to eliminate the unnecessary administration of antepartum Rh Immune Globulin (RhIG) to the ~ 40% of D– women who are carrying a D– fetus.[82] In a multiethnic population, accuracy of noninvasive fetal *RHD* genotyping requires distinguishing normal *RHD* from hybrid or inactive alleles.[76]

RHD Genotyping to Determine D Antigen Status in Pregnant Women. Serologic typing for D cannot easily distinguish women whose red cells lack some epitopes of D (partial D) and are at risk for D immunization, from those with a weak D phenotype who are not at risk for D immunization. Red cells with partial D may type as D+, some by direct tests and others by indirect tests. These women might benefit from receiving RhIG prophylaxis if they carry a D+ fetus. *RHD* genotyping can distinguish D variants to guide RhIG prophylaxis and blood transfusion recommendations.[64] *RHD* genotyping is recommended in females of childbearing potential, to avoid treatment of females with weak D types 1, 2, or 3 who have little or no risk of RhD alloimmunization, as well as to identify women with other D variants, including women of African ancestry, in whom partial D is common and who may benefit from Rh immunoprophylaxis.[83,84]

Molecular Testing of Paternal Samples. The father's red cells should be tested for the antigen corresponding to the antibody in the maternal plasma. If the red cells are negative, the fetus is not at risk. If the father is positive for the antigen, **zygosity** testing can be performed. Zygosity describes the number and similarity of two alleles; whereas homozygous or heterozygous individuals carry two copies, in scenarios where there is copy number variation, individuals can be hemizygous, or only carry a single gene copy.

Zygosity testing of paternal samples is most often performed when testing for possible HDFN due to anti-D or anti-K. If the paternal red cells are K+ and the mother has anti-K, they can be tested serologically for expression of the allelic k antigen. However, many centers do not have a licensed reagent available, such that genetic counselors often request DNA testing of the father to predict K antigen status. If the paternal red cells are K–, the maternal anti-K is most likely the result of immunization through transfusion, or pregnancy by another partner.

When molecular methods are used to determine paternal *RHD* zygosity, several different genetic events cause a D– phenotype, and multiple assays are often used to accurately determine *RHD* zygosity, especially in non-European ethnic groups. If the father is homozygous (carries two functional *RHD* alleles), all of his children will be D+, and any pregnancy in his partner needs to be monitored. If the father is heterozygous, the fetus has a 50% chance of being at risk. Determining the D type of the fetus can prevent unnecessary monitoring of the pregnancy and use of immune-modulating agents.

Using Molecular Methods to Screen for Antigen-Negative Blood Donors

DNA-based typing to predict donor antigen profiles in the search for antigen-negative units is routine for most blood centers, especially when suitable antibodies are not available. Because red cell typing for DO antigens is notoriously difficult, one of the most frequent approaches is to type for Do[a] and Do[b]. Many other antibody specificities are unavailable for mass donor screening. These specificities include anti-Hy, -Jo[a], -Js[a], -Js[b], -C[W], -V, and -VS.

Red cell genotyping panels are used by many blood donor centers to screen for multiple minor antigens in a single assay format and have been used for mass screening of blood donors.[85] Several platforms licensed by the Food and Drug Administration (FDA) are now available. The results can be used for the labeling of donor units for extended antigen profiles. This practice not only increases the antigen-negative inventory by expanding combinations of the minor antigens and some high-prevalence antigens, but also allows provision of donor components that are molecularly matched to the patient's type. Licensed genotyping tests that predict ABO and RhD are not available for the labeling of donor units.

Using Molecular Methods to Resolve Serologic Typing Discrepancies

It is not uncommon in either the donor center or hospital blood bank setting to have a discrepancy between two serologic typings of a donor or patient. The discrepancy may involve the current vs a historical type, or two typings on a current sample. In the latter scenario, the discrepancy may involve the use of two different methods (eg, solid-phase vs tube testing) or two different reagents (eg, monoclonal vs polyclonal antisera). Molecular methods can be employed as part of discrepancy investigations. Such methods are typically focused on ruling out variant antigens that are known to be associated with variability in antigen typing. Examples of discrepancies that have been resolved using molecular methods are listed in Table 9-6. A detailed discussion of causes of both ABO and RhD typing discrepancies is beyond the scope of this chapter; several publications describe approaches to handling such findings.[86-88]

Molecular Testing to Confirm the D Type of Donors

Donor centers must serologically test donors for weak D to avoid labeling a product as D− that might result in anti-D in response to transfused RBCs. Some donor red cells with very weak D expression (weak D type 2, and especially those with the Del phenotype) are not typed as D+ using current methods and are labeled as D−. The prevalence of weak D red cells not detected by serologic reagents is approximately 0.1% (but may vary depending on the test method and population). Although the clinical significance has not been established, donor red cells with weak D expression have been associated with alloimmunization. *RHD* genotyping could be used to confirm blood donors who type D−,[89] but a high-throughput and cost-effective platform is not yet available.

Molecular Testing to Match Red Cell Donors to Rh-Alloimmunized Patients Carrying Rh Variants

Rh variant antigen expression is common in individuals of African ancestry.[90,91] Antibodies to variant Rh antigens, including anti-hr[B] and anti-hr[S], have been associated with insufficient decrease in sickle hemoglobin (HbS) after exchange transfusion in patients with SCD, as well as with transfusion reactions and/or monocyte monolayer assay incompatibility. In some cases, patients have benefited from transfusion with RBC units matched to their RH alleles. RH allele-matching describes the process of selecting blood donors based on the *RHCE* and *RHD* alleles of the patient, using a tiered system.[92] This approach has yet to be implemented on a large scale but has been modeled.[93,94]

TABLE 9-6. Examples of Serologic Discrepancies Resolved Using Molecular Methods

Blood Group System	Discrepancy	Molecular Method	Findings
RH	Sample typed D− previously, currently types weak D+	*RHD* array and *RHD* cDNA analysis	*RHD* array detected no variants cDNA analysis identified *RHD* c.19T (p.7W) associated with weak D type 18
RH	Sample typed C+ previously, currently types C−	RBC panel, *RHCE* and *RHD* arrays	*RHCE* array identified *RHCE*ceTI*; *RHD* array identified *RHD*DIV*; this haplotype is associated with anti-C reactivity
FY	Sample typed Fy(b−) previously; now types Fy(b+w) with one antisera, Fy(b−) with another, and Fy(b+) with a third	RBC panel	*FY*01/FY*02W.01* Fy(a+b+w)
JK	Sample typed Jk(a+) previously, now types Jk(a−)	SSP-PCR for *JK* c.130G/A	*JK*01W.01/JK*02* (Jka+ʷb+)

SSP-PCR = sequence-specific primer polymerase chain reaction.

ABO Genotyping of Solid-Organ Donors

Due to insufficient ABO-compatible donors for kidney transplantation, ABO-incompatible transplantations have become routine. A recent meta-analysis showed good, albeit inferior, outcomes of such transplantations.[95] Transplantation of other ABO-incompatible solid organs is on the rise.[96] Living-donor registries that use buccal swabs (instead of peripheral blood) for initial DNA testing can use ABO genotyping strategies to predict the blood type. ABO genotyping is also useful for predicting the blood type of recently deceased individuals of unknown ABO type who received massive transfusion.

Discrepancies between Serologic (Phenotype) and Molecular (Genotype) Testing

Differences between serologic and DNA testing results do occur and should be investigated. Often, these discrepancies lead to interesting discoveries such as the presence of a novel allele or genetic variant, particularly when people of diverse ethnicities are tested. Causes of discrepancies include recent transfusions, stem cell transplantation, and natural chimerism. Stem cell transplantation and natural chimerism also may cause differences between the results of testing DNA from somatic cells and results of testing DNA extracted from peripheral MNCs. Thus, when using molecular methods, it is important to obtain an accurate medical history. Many genetic events can cause apparent discrepant results between hemagglutination and molecular test results (Table 9-7). Weak antigen expression may not be detected by hemagglutination, and the genotype may not always predict the phenotype.[7,9] Table 9-8 lists some important considerations when resolving discrepancies between serologic and molecular testing.

Challenges in Using SNV Genotyping to Predict Red Cell Phenotypes

Molecular testing interrogates a single SNV or a few SNVs associated with antigen expression and cannot sample every nucleotide in the gene.

TABLE 9-7. Examples of Some Molecular Events Where Analysis of Gene and Phenotype May Not Agree

Molecular Event	Mechanism	Example(s)
Alternative splicing	Nt change in splice site: partial/ complete skipping of exon	S–s–; Gy(a–)
Premature stop codon	Deletion of nt(s) → frameshift	Fy(a–b–); D–; c–E–; Rh_{null}; Gy(a–); GE:–2,–3,–4; K_0; McLeod
	Insertion of nt(s) → frameshift	D–; Co(a–b–)
	Nt change	Fy(a–b–); r′; Gy(a–); K_0; McLeod
Amino acid variant	Missense nucleotide variant	D–; Rh_{null}; K_0; McLeod
Reduced amount of protein	Missense nucleotide variant	Fy^x; Co(a–b–)
Hybrid genes	Crossing over	GP.Vw; GP.Hil; GP.TSEN
	Gene conversion	GP.Mur; GP.Hop; D––
Interacting protein	Absence of RhAG	Rh_{null}
	Absence of Kx	Weak expression of KEL antigens
Modifying gene	*KLF1* mutations	*In(Lu)* phenotype

Nt = nucleotide.

Although a gene may be detected by DNA testing, there are times when the gene product is not expressed on the red cells, because of a mutation that silences the gene or reduces expression levels, and it is not detected by routine hemagglutination testing. Such changes result in discrepancies in the typing of patients and donors. Homozygosity (or compound heterozygosity) for a silenced gene results in a null phenotype, and most null phenotypes have more than one genetic basis.[9]

With donor typing, the presence of a grossly normal gene whose product is not expressed on the red cell surface results in the donor being falsely typed as antigen positive. Although this situation means loss of an antigen-negative donor, it does not jeopardize the safety of blood transfusion. However, if a grossly normal gene is detected in a patient but the gene is not expressed, the patient remains at risk for the corresponding antibody if he or she receives a transfusion of antigen-positive blood.

To avoid misinterpretation, routine assays must include appropriate tests to detect variants that silence gene expression if prevalent in the population tested. Silenced alleles can be specific to a particular ethnic group. For example, in the FY blood group system, an SNV (c.–67T>C) within the promoter region (GATA box) of *FY* prevents transcription of *FY*A* and/or *FY*B* in red cells but not in other tissues. Although silencing of *FY*A* is rare, silencing of *FY*B* is frequent in persons of African ancestry where homozygosity for the –67T>C SNV in *FY*B* results in the Fy(a–b–) phenotype, which has a prevalence of 60% or higher. To ensure accuracy, testing for the GATA box variant must be included in typing for FY in persons of African ancestry.

When an assay is used to predict the presence or absence of D antigen, particularly in populations of African ancestry, it is essential to include a test for the complete but inactive *RHD* gene *RHDΨ*. If an assay is designed to predict S and s antigen expression in persons of African ancestry, it should include interrogation of a

TABLE 9-8. Common Methods for Resolving Discrepancies between Serologic (Phenotype) and Molecular (Genotype) Testing

- Some common factors that can lead to discordant results:
  - The number of epitopes present on the red cell at testing
  - The use of human, polyclonal, or monoclonal reagents on historical typing
  - Process errors during testing
  - Clerical errors during computer entry

- Review of serologic and molecular results entry to verify no clerical errors:
  - Data entry errors
  - Sample labeled with the incorrect patient/donor information
  - Sample tubes switched during testing and/or DNA extraction

- Clerical error detected:
  - Invalidate the test result(s); order and result the corrected interpretation
  - Obtain a new properly labeled sample with the correct patient/donor information
  - Repeat sample testing and/or DNA extraction if a switched sample tube(s) is suspected

- Repeat serologic testing:
  - If the sample is available, repeat serologic testing on the current sample
  - Repeat testing of the current sample with a different source of serologic reagent(s)
  - If the sample is not available for repeat testing, try to obtain another sample from the patient/donor for additional testing upon subsequent donation or next encounter

- Repeat molecular testing:
  - If the sample is available, repeat molecular testing on the current sample and indicate if a new DNA extraction was used for repeat sample testing
  - Repeat testing of the current sample with a different molecular platform, if available
  - Sample may need to be sent to an outside laboratory for further testing (eg, sequencing)

- Determination of final results:
  - If the repeat testing resolved the discrepancy, no further action is required
  - If repeat testing does not resolve the discrepancy, notify management team, including CLIA laboratory director or designee for further instructions

C>T SNV at nucleotide c.230 in *GYP*B* exon 5 or an SNV in intron 5 (+5g>t) because both SNVs prevent expression of S antigen and result in expression of U^{VAR}.

Other common causes of discrepancies include the presence in the sample of an altered *FY*B* allele that encodes an amino acid variant causing the Fy^X phenotype with greatly reduced expression of Fy^b antigen. The red cells type as Fy(b−) with most serologic reagents. The prevalence of the allele encoding the Fy^X phenotype in people of European ancestry is as high as 2%, and the allele has been found in persons of African ancestry also. Silencing mutations associated with the loss of JK antigen expression occur more often in people of Asian ancestry, whereas nucleotide variants encoding amino acid variant that weaken JK expression occur in people of African ancestry.

SUMMARY

Blood group genetics has become an essential component of the practice of transfusion medicine. The field of molecular immunohematology has provided a greater understanding of genetic blood group variants, including the complexity of Rh variants and the associated partial Rh antigens. Molecular methods used to predict blood group antigen expression vary in their throughput capabilities and resolution. Genotyping assays that can predict many antigens in multiple samples simultaneously are being used routinely by blood centers to identify red cell donors lacking antigens of clinical significance. The use of these red cell panels in chronic transfusion recipients, especially those with hemoglobinopathies, is growing. Increasingly, *RHD* genotyping is being used to resolve discrepancies and assess candidacy for RhIG. Blood group genomics, including the use of massively parallel sequencing, is poised to provide even richer information about patient and donor red cell phenotypes that has the potential to make transfusion medicine even more personalized.

KEY POINTS

1. Genetics is the study of heredity; that is, the mechanisms by which a trait, such as expression of a blood group antigen, is passed from parents to offspring.

2. A gene is a segment of DNA and is the basic unit of inheritance; it occupies a specific location on a chromosome (the gene locus).

3. Alleles are alternative forms of a gene (eg, alleles *JK*A* and *JK*B* are different forms of *SLC14A1* that encode the Jk^a and Jk^b antigens, respectively).

4. A human somatic cell is diploid, containing 46 chromosomes in 23 pairs: 22 pairs are autosomes, and the remaining pair are the sex chromosomes, with males carrying X and Y, and females, two X chromosomes.

5. Somatic cells divide by mitosis, where the chromosomes replicate and are divided into two new diploid cells that have all the genetic information of the parent cell.

6. Germ cells divide by meiosis, where after chromosomal replication and two divisions, four haploid gametes are formed, each having half the chromosomal complement of the parent somatic cell.

7. The term "genotype" traditionally refers to the complement of genes inherited by each person from his or her parents; the term is also used to refer to the set of alleles at a single gene locus. Whereas the genotype of a person is his or her genetic constitution, the phenotype is the observable expression of the genes and reflects the biologic activity of the gene(s). Thus, the presence or absence of antigens on the red cells, as determined by serologic testing, represents the phenotype.

8. When identical alleles for a given locus are present on both chromosomes, a person is homozygous; when nonidentical alleles are present at a particular locus, the person is heterozygous; and a person carrying only one allele copy is hemizygous.

9. The expression of blood group antigens on the red cell may be modified or affected by gene interactions. This can involve structural interactions (eg, *RHAG* gene mutations associated with Rh$_{null}$ phenotype) or transcriptional interactions [eg, *KLF1* mutations associated with *In(Lu)* phenotype].

10. There are multiple types of genetic variation, including single nucleotide, insertion/deletion, and structural variants. SNVs can result in changes to amino acids, cause premature stop codons, and alter messenger RNA splicing, all of which can alter blood group antigen expression.

11. A blood group system consists of one or more antigens under the control of a single gene locus (eg, *KEL* encodes the Kell blood group antigens) or of two or more homologous genes (eg, *RHD* and *RHCE* encode the Rh blood group antigens). Thus, each blood group system is genetically independent. Currently, 39 blood group systems are recognized.

12. The genes encoding the blood group systems have been identified, and the genetic bases of most antigens and phenotypes are known.

13. DNA-based assays of varying resolution and throughput are being used by molecular immunohematology laboratories to predict antigen status in both donors and patients.

14. DNA-based assays can be used to predict the red cell phenotype to assess alloimmunization risk, predict antigen status when serologic reagents are unavailable or unreliable, identify antigen-negative donors, resolve typing discrepancies, and identify variant antigens.

15. Genomic approaches, including massively parallel sequencing, can predict an individual's red cell phenotype with a single test and has the potential to revolutionize transfusion medicine.

REFERENCES

1. Brown TA. Introduction to genetics: A molecular approach. London, UK: Garland Science, 2011.
2. Lesk A. Introduction to genomics. 3rd ed. New York: Oxford University Press, 2017.
3. Reid ME, Shine I. The discovery and significance of the blood groups. Cambridge, MA: SBB Books, 2012.
4. Schurr TG. The peopling of the New World: Perspectives from molecular anthropology. Annu Rev Anthropol 2004;33:551-83.
5. Pierron D, Heiske M, Razafindrazaka H, et al. Strong selection during the last millennium for African ancestry in the admixed population of Madagascar. Nat Commun 2018;9(1):932.
6. Clark DP, Russell LD. Molecular biology: Made simple and fun. St. Louis, MO: Cache River Press, 2010.
7. Reid ME, Denomme GA. DNA-based methods in the immunohematology reference laboratory. Transfus Apher Sci 2011;44:65-7.
8. Nussbaum RL, McInnes RR, Willard HF. Thompson & Thompson genetics in medicine. 8th ed. Philadelphia: Elsevier/Saunders, 2016.
9. Reid ME, Lomas-Francis C, Olsson ML. The blood group antigen factsbook. 3rd ed. San Diego, CA: Academic Press, 2012.
10. International Society of Blood Transfusion. Red Cell Immunogenetics and Blood Group Terminology (working group). Blood group terminology. Amsterdam, the Netherlands: ISBT, 2019. [Available at http://www.isbtweb.org/working-parties/red-cell-immunogenetics-and-blood-group-terminology/ (accessed October 4, 2019).]
11. An international system for human cytogenetic nomenclature (1978) ISCN (1978). Report of the Standing Committee on Human Cytogenetic Nomenclature. Cytogenet Cell Genet 1978; 21:309-404.
12. Lewis M, Zelinski T. Linkage relationships and gene mapping of human blood group loci. In: Cartron J-P, Rouger P, eds. Molecular basis of major human blood group antigens. New York: Plenum Press, 1995:445-75.
13. Lögdberg L, Reid ME, Zelinski T. Human blood group genes 2010: Chromosomal locations and cloning strategies revisited. Transfus Med Rev 2011;25:36-46.
14. Svensson L, Hult AK, Stamps R, et al. Forssman expression on human erythrocytes: Biochemical and genetic evidence of a new histo-blood group system. Blood 2013;121:1459-68.
15. Zelinski T, Coghlan G, Liu XQ, et al. ABCG2 null alleles define the Jr(a–) blood group phenotype. Nat Genet 2012;44:131-2.
16. Saison C, Helias V, Ballif BA, et al. Null alleles of ABCG2 encoding the breast cancer resistance protein define the new blood group system Junior. Nat Genet 2012;44:174-7.
17. Helias V, Saison C, Ballif BA, et al. ABCB6 is dispensable for erythropoiesis and specifies the new blood group system Langereis. Nat Genet 2012;44:170-3.
18. Storry JR, Jöud M, Christophersen MK, et al. Homozygosity for a null allele of SMIM1 defines the Vel-negative blood group phenotype. Nat Genet 2013;45:537-41.
19. Cvejic A, Haer-Wigman L, Stephens JC, et al. SMIM1 underlies the Vel blood group and influences red cell traits. Nat Genet 2013;45:542-5.
20. Ballif BA, Helias V, Peyrard T, et al. Disruption of SMIM1 causes the Vel– blood type. EMBO Mol Med 2013;5:751-61.
21. Anliker, M, von Zabern I, Höchsmann B, et al. A new blood group antigen is defined by anti-CD59, detected in a CD59 deficient patient. Transfusion 2014;54:1817-22.
22. Daniels G, Ballif BA, Helias V, et al. Lack of the nucleoside transporter ENT1 results in the Augustine-null blood type and ectopic mineralization. Blood 2015;125:3651-4.
23. Lyon MF. X-chromosome inactivation. Curr Biol 1999;9:R235-R237.
24. Daniels G. Human blood groups. 3rd ed. Oxford, UK: Blackwell Science, 2013.
25. Clemson CM, Hall LL, Byron M, et al. The X chromosome is organized into a gene-rich outer rim and an internal core containing silenced

nongenic sequences. Proc Natl Acad Sci U S A 2006;103:7688-93.

26. Redman CM, Reid ME. The McLeod syndrome: An example of the value of integrating clinical and molecular studies. Transfusion 2002;42:284-6.

27. Russo DCW, Lee S, Reid ME, Redman CM. Point mutations causing the McLeod phenotype. Transfusion 2002;42:287-93.

28. Garratty G. Blood groups and disease: A historical perspective. Transfus Med Rev 2000;14:291-301.

29. Thorisson GA, Stein LD. The SNP consortium website: Past, present and future. Nucleic Acids Res 2003;31:124-7.

30. Blumenfeld OO, Patnaik SK. Allelic genes of blood group antigens: A source of human mutations and cSNPs documented in the Blood Group Antigen Gene Mutation Database. Hum Mutat 2004;23:8-16.

31. US Department of Energy and National Institutes of Health. Human Genome Project. Washington, DC: US Department of Energy Genome Programs, Office of Biological and Environmental Research, 2010. [Available at http://web.ornl.gov/sci/techresources/Human_Genome/index.shtml.]

32. Reid ME. Molecular basis for blood groups and function of carrier proteins. In: Silberstein LE, ed. Molecular and functional aspects of blood group antigens. Bethesda, MD: AABB, 1995:75-125.

33. Storry JR, Olsson ML. Genetic basis of blood group diversity. Br J Haematol 2004;126:759-71.

34. Möller M, Lee YQ, Vidovic K, et al. Disruption of a GATA1-binding motif upstream of XG/PBDX abolishes Xg(a) expression and resolves the Xg blood group system. Blood 2018;132(3):334-8.

35. Roulis E, Hyland C, Flower R, et al. Molecular basis and clinical overview of McLeod syndrome compared with other neuroacanthocytosis syndromes: A review. JAMA Neurol 2018;75:1554-62.

36. Rice JP, Saccone NL, Corbett J. The lod score method (review). Adv Genet 2001;42:99-113.

37. Bluth MH, Reid ME, Manny N. Chimerism in the immunohematology laboratory in the molecular biology era. Transfus Med Rev 2007;21:134-46.

38. Yu N, Kruskall MS, Yunis JJ, et al. Disputed maternity leading to identification of tetragametic chimerism. N Engl J Med 2002;346(20):1545-52.

39. Cho D, Lee JS, Yazer MH, et al. Chimerism and mosaicism are important causes of ABO phenotype and genotype discrepancies. Immunohematology 2006;22:183-7.

40. Singleton BK, Burton NM, Green C, et al. Mutations in EKLF/KLF1 form the molecular basis of the rare blood group In(Lu) phenotype. Blood 2008;112:2081-8.

41. Singleton BK, Roxby D, Stirling J, et al. A novel GATA-1 mutation (Ter414Arg) in a family with the rare X-linked blood group Lu(a–b–) phenotype (abstract). Blood 2009;114:783.

42. Pena SDJ, Chakraborty R. Paternity testing in the DNA era. Trends Genet 1994;10:204-9.

43. Jeffreys AJ, Wilson V, Thein SL. Hypervariable 'minisatellite' regions in human DNA. Nature 1985;314:67-73.

44. Jeffreys AJ, Wilson V, Thein SL. Individual-specific 'fingerprints' of human DNA. Nature 1985;316:76-9.

45. Butler JM, Reeder DJ. Short tandem repeat DNA internet database. NIST standard reference database SRD 130. Gaithersburg, MD: National Institute of Standards and Technology, 2017. [Available at http://www.cstl.nist.gov/div831/strbase/index.htm (accessed March 20, 2017).]

46. Clark JR, Scott SD, Jack AL, et al. Monitoring of chimerism following allogeneic haematopoietic stem cell transplantation (HSCT): Technical recommendations for the use of short tandem repeat (STR) based techniques, on behalf of the United Kingdom National External Quality Assessment Service for Leucocyte Immunophenotyping Chimerism Working Group. Br J Haematol 2015;168(1):26-37.

47. Domiati-Saad R, Klintmalm GB, Netto G, et al. Acute graft versus host disease after liver transplantation: Patterns of lymphocyte chimerism. Am J Transplant 2005;5:2968-73.

48. Alvarez-Cubero MJ, Saiz M, Martínez-García B, et al. Next generation sequencing: An application in forensic sciences? Ann Hum Biol 2017;44(7):581-92.

49. Maha GC, ed. Standards for relationship testing laboratories. 14th ed. Bethesda, MD: AABB, 2020.

50. Donahue RP, Bias WB, Renwick JH, McKusick VA. Probable assignment of the Duffy blood group locus to chromosome 1 in man. Proc Natl Acad Sci U S A 1968;61(3):949-55.

51. National Human Genome Research Institute. The Human Genome Project. Bethesda, MD: National Institutes of Health, 2019. [Available at

https://www.genome.gov/human-genome-project.]

52. International Genome Sample Resource. Genome browsers: 1000 Genomes data in Ensembl. Hinxton, UK: European Bioinformat ics Institute, 2018. [Available at http://www.internationalgenome.org/1000-genomes-browsers/ (accessed October 4, 2019).]

53. Yates B, Braschi B, Gray K, et al. Gene names.org: The HGNC and VGNC resources in 2017. Nucleic Acids Res 2017;45(D1):D619-25.

54. MacArthur JA, Morales J, Tully RE, et al. Locus Reference Genomic: Reference sequences for the reporting of clinically relevant sequence variants. Nucleic Acids Res 2014;42(Database issue):D873-8.

55. Daniels GL, Anstee DJ, Cartron J-P, et al. Blood group terminology 1995. ISBT Working Party on Terminology for Red Cell Surface Antigens. Vox Sang 1995;69:265-79.

56. Garratty G, Dzik WH, Issitt PD, et al. Terminology for blood group antigens and genes: Historical origins and guidelines in the new millennium. Transfusion 2000;40:477-89.

57. HGNC guidelines. Cambridge, UK: HUGO Gene Nomenclature Committee, 2002. [Available at https://www.genenames.org/about/guidelines/ (accessed October 4, 2019).]

58. Reid ME, Lomas-Francis C. Blood group antigens and antibodies: A guide to clinical relevance and technical tips. New York: SBB Books, 2007.

59. Schoeman EM, Roulis EV, Liew YW, et al. Targeted exome sequencing defines novel and rare variants in complex blood group serology cases for a red blood cell reference laboratory setting. Transfusion 2018;58(2):284-93.

60. Yohe S, Thyagarajan B. Review of clinical next-generation sequencing. Arch Pathol Lab Med 2017;141(11):1544-57.

61. Avent ND. Large scale blood group genotyping. Transfus Clin Biol 2007;14:10-15.

62. Monteiro F, Tavares G, Ferreira M, et al. Technologies involved in molecular blood group genotyping. ISBT Sci Ser 2011;6:1-6.

63. Gassner C, Meyer S, Frey BM, et al. Matrix-assisted laser desorption/ionization, time of flight mass spectrometry-based blood group genotyping – the alternative approach. Transfus Med Rev 2013;27:2-9.

64. Keller MA. The role of red cell genotyping in transfusion medicine. Immunohematology 2015;31(2):49-52.

65. The Human RhesusBase. Version 2.4. [Available at http://www.rhesusbase.info/ (accessed October 4, 2019).]

66. Möller M, Jöud M, Storry JR, Olsson ML. Erythrogene: A database for in-depth analysis of the extensive variation in 36 blood group systems in the 1000 Genomes Project. Blood Adv 2016; 1(3):240-9.

67. Lane WJ, Westhoff CM, Gleadall NS, et al. Automated typing of red blood cell and platelet antigens: A whole-genome sequencing study. Lancet Haematol 2018;5(6):e241-e251. [Available at https://bloodantigens.com/cgi-bin/a/a.fpl (accessed October 4, 2019).]

68. Single Nucleotide Polymorphism Database (dbSNP). Bethesda, MD: National Center for Biotechnology Information, US National Library of Medicine, 2019. [Available at https://www.ncbi.nlm.nih.gov/projects/SNP/ (accessed October 4, 2019).]

69. Horn T, Hamilton J, Kosanke J, et al. Assessment of common red blood cell pretreatments to yield an accurate serologic antigen phenotype compared with genotype-predicted phenotype. Immunohematology 2017;33(4):147-51.

70. Dizon MF. The challenges of daratumumab in transfusion medicine. Lab Med 2017;48(1):6-9.

71. Liu J, Wang L, Zhao F, et al. Pre-clinical development of a humanized anti-CD47 antibody with anti-cancer therapeutic potential. PLoS One 2015;10(9):e0137345.

72. Mitigating the anti-CD38 interference with serologic testing. Association bulletin #16-02. Bethesda, MD: AABB, 2016. [Available at http://www.aabb.org/programs/publications/bulletins/Documents/ab16-02.pdf (accessed October 4, 2019).]

73. Chou ST, Westhoff CM. The role of molecular immunohematology in sickle cell disease. Transfus Apher Sci 2011;44:73-9.

74. Noizatt-Pirenne F, Tournamille C. Relevance of RH variants in transfusion of sickle cell patients. Transfus Clin Biol 2011;18:527-35.

75. Pate LL, Myers J, Palma J, et al. Anti-Ge3 causes late-onset hemolytic disease of the newborn: The fourth case in three Hispanic families. Transfusion 2013;53:2152-7.

76. Hyland CA, Millard GM, O'Brien H, et al. Non-invasive fetal RHD genotyping for RhD negative women stratified into RHD gene deletion or variant groups: Comparative accuracy using two blood collection tube types. Pathology 2017; 49(7):757-64.

77. Daniels G, Finning K, Martin P, Soothill P. Fetal blood group genotyping from DNA from maternal plasma: An important advance in the management and prevention of haemolytic disease of the fetus and newborn. Vox Sang 2004;87: 225-32.

78. Clausen FB, Christiansen M, Steffensen R, et al. Report of the first nationally implemented clinical routine screening for fetal RHD in D– pregnant women to ascertain the requirement for antenatal RhD prophylaxis. Transfusion 2012; 52:752-8.

79. Li Y, Zimmermann B, Rusterholz C, et al. Size separation of circulatory DNA in maternal plasma permits ready detection of fetal DNA polymorphisms. Clin Chem 2004;50(6):1002-11.

80. Haimila K, Sulin K, Kuosmanen M, et al. Targeted antenatal anti-D prophylaxis program for RhD-negative pregnant women - outcome of the first two years of a national program in Finland. Acta Obstet Gynecol Scand 2017;96(10):1228-33.

81. de Haas M, Thurik FF, van der Ploeg CP, et al. Sensitivity of fetal RHD screening for safe guidance of targeted anti-D immunoglobulin prophylaxis: Prospective cohort study of a nationwide programme in the Netherlands. BMJ 2016;355: i5789.

82. Clausen FB. Lessons learned from the implementation of non-invasive fetal RHD screening. Expert Rev Mol Diagn 2018;18(5):423-31.

83. Sandler S, Flegel W, Westhoff CM, et al. It's time to phase in RHD genotyping for patients with a serologic weak D phenotype. Transfusion 2015:55:680-9.

84. Johnson ST, Katz L, Queenan JT, et al for the Interorganizational Work Group on *RHD* Genotyping. Joint statement on phasing-in *RHD* genotyping for pregnant women and other females of childbearing potential with a serologic weak D phenotype. Bethesda, MD: AABB. [Available at http://www.aabb.org/advocacy/statements/Pages/statement150722.aspx (accessed October 4, 2019).]

85. Denomme GA, Schanen MJ. Mass-scale donor red cell genotyping using real-time array technology (review). Immunohematology 2015; 31(2):69-74.

86. Luo X, Keller MA, James I, et al. Strategies to identify candidates for D variant genotyping. Blood Transfus 2018;16(3):293-301.

87. Meny GM. Recognizing and resolving ABO discrepancies. Immunohematology 2017;33(2):76-81.

88. Vege S. Resolution of discordances between serology and DNA. In: Vege S, Gannett M, Delaney M. Introduction to moleclar immunohematology. Bethesda, MD: AABB Press, 2020:91-114.

89. Wagner FF. RHD PCR of D-negative blood donors. Transfus Med Hemother 2013;40:172-81.

90. Pham B-N, Peyrard T, Tourret S, et al. Anti-HrB and anti-hrB revisited. Transfusion 2009;49: 2400-5.

91. Reid ME, Hipsky CH, Velliquette RW, et al. Molecular background of RH in Bastiaan, the RH:-31,-34 index case, and two novel RHD alleles. Immunohematology 2012;28:97-103.

92. Keller MA, Horn T, Crowley J, et al. Genotype compatibility tables for matching patients and donors for RH variants. Transfusion 2013; 53(2S):174A.

93. Gaspardi AC, Sippert EA, De Macedo MD, et al. Clinically relevant RHD-CE genotypes in patients with sickle cell disease and in African Brazilian donors. Blood Transfus 2016;14(5):449-54.

94. Chou ST, Evans P, Vege S, et al. *RH* genotype matching for transfusion support in sickle cell disease. Blood 2018;132(11):1198-207.

95. de Weerd AE, Betjes MGH. ABO-incompatible kidney transplant outcomes: A meta-analysis. Clin J Am Soc Nephrol 2018;13(8):1234-43.

96. Dean CL, Sullivan HC, Stowell SR, et al. Current state of transfusion practices for ABO-incompatible pediatric heart transplant patients in the United States and Canada. Transfusion 2018;58(9):2243-9.

CHAPTER 10

ABO and Other Carbohydrate Blood Group Systems

Martin L. Olsson, MD, PhD, and Julia S. Westman, PhD

THE 19 BLOOD GROUP ANTIGENS IN the ABO, P1PK, LE (Lewis), H, I, GLOB (Globoside), FORS, and SID blood group systems are defined by immunodominant carbohydrate epitopes on glycoproteins and glycolipids. The synthesis of these antigens requires the action of a series of enzymes known as glycosyltransferases [Fig 10-1 (A)]. These enzymes reside mainly in the Golgi apparatus and are responsible for adding specific sugars, in a particular sequence and steric or anomeric linkage (α-linked or β-linked), to growing oligosaccharide chains on glycolipids and/or glycoproteins.[1,2] Most, but not all, carbohydrate blood group antigens are located at the ends of these chains. Because of their wide tissue distribution, the carbohydrate-based systems are often referred to as histo-blood groups.[3]

Previously, the dogma was that each glycosyltransferase typically uses one specific donor substrate molecule and one specific acceptor substrate molecule, but many examples of broader, more "promiscuous" use of acceptor substrates have come to light, including those involving carbohydrate-based blood groups. Transcriptional regulation together with the specificity of these enzymes for both their nucleotide sugar donor substrates [eg, uridine diphosphate (UDP)-galactose] and acceptor substrates

(eg, type 1 chain vs type 2 chain) are responsible for the tissue-specific distribution of many blood group antigens.[4,5] Studies have shown that these blood groups have roles in development, cell adhesion, malignancy, and infectious disease, although many of the exact mechanisms underlying these roles are still unknown.[4,6,7]

THE ABO SYSTEM (001)

The ABO system was originally described by Karl Landsteiner in 1900 and remains the most important blood group system in transfusion medicine.[7] In blood, ABO antigens are found in substantial amounts on red cells and also to a lesser extent on platelets. In individuals who have the "secretor" phenotype, antigens are present in body fluids as well. ABO antigens are also expressed on many other tissues, including those of the endothelium, kidney, heart, bowel, pancreas, and lung.[5] This is the reason why these antigens also constitute a relative barrier against ABO-incompatible organ transplantation.[8]

Transfusion of ABO-incompatible blood can be associated with acute intravascular hemolysis and renal failure, and can be fatal.[9,10] Similarly, transplanted ABO-incompatible solid organs can

Martin L. Olsson, MD, PhD, Professor of Transfusion Medicine, Department of Laboratory Medicine, Vice Dean, Faculty of Medicine, Lund University, and Medical Director, Nordic Reference Laboratory for Genetic Blood Group Typing, Office of Medical Services, Region Skåne, Lund, Sweden; and Julia S. Westman, PhD, Postdoctoral Fellow, Sanford Burnham Prebys Medical Discovery Institute, Center for Nanomedicine, University of California—Santa Barbara, Santa Barbara, California
The authors have disclosed no conflicts of interest.

10

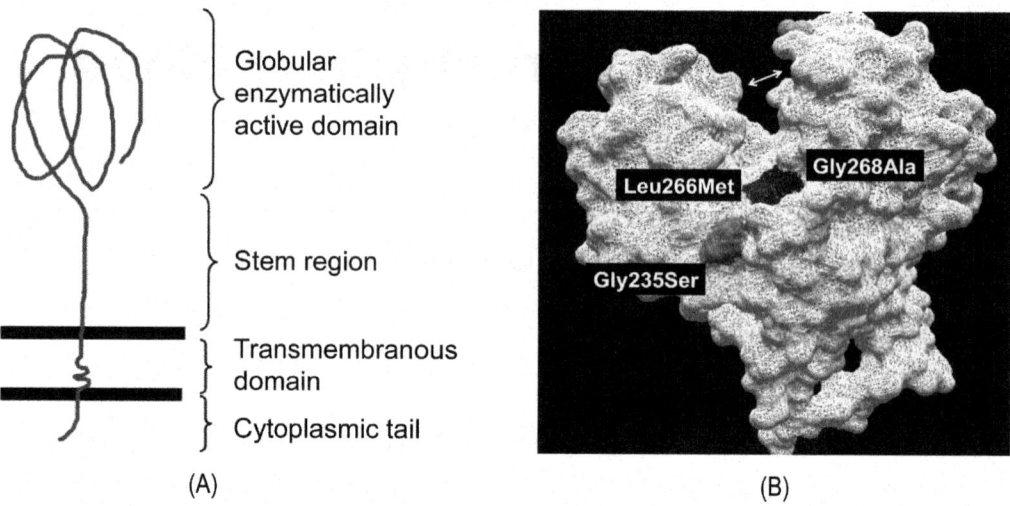

FIGURE 10-1. Model of a glycosyltransferase anchored in the Golgi membrane (A), and three-dimensional surface model of the human ABO glycosyltransferase (B). The arrow at the top shows the catalytic cleft, and the dark surfaces highlighted with black labels correspond to the amino acid positions that determine A vs B specificity.

undergo hyperacute humoral rejection if the patient has not been pretreated to remove naturally occurring anti-A and/or anti-B from plasma. Because of the serious clinical consequences associated with ABO incompatibilities, ABO typing and ABO compatibility testing remain the foundation of safe pretransfusion testing and a crucial part of a pretransplantation workup.

The ABO system contains four major ABO groups: A, B, O, and AB. The four phenotypes are determined by the presence or absence of two antigens (A and B) on red cells. (See Table 10-1.) The ABO system is also characterized by the presence or absence of naturally occurring antibodies, termed isohemagglutinins, directed against the missing A and B antigens. As shown in Table 10-1, an inverse relationship exists between the presence of A and/or B antigens on red cells and the presence of anti-A, anti-B, or both, in sera, a phenomenon often referred to as Landsteiner's rule. For example, group O individuals, who lack A and B antigens on red cells, possess both anti-A and anti-B. It is believed that the immunizing sources for such naturally occurring antibodies are gut and environmental bacteria, such as the *Enterobacteriaceae*, which

have been shown to possess ABO-like structures on their lipopolysaccharide coats.[11,12]

Biochemistry

The A and B antigens are defined by three-sugar terminal epitopes on glycolipids and glycoproteins.[7] As shown in Fig 10-2, the H antigen is characterized by a terminal $\alpha 1,2$ fucose, which is the immediate and required biosynthetic precursor for expression of either the A or B antigen. The presence of this fucose is required for the A and B glycosyltransferases to be able to use the oligosaccharide chain as their acceptor substrate. In group A individuals, an *N*-acetylgalactosamine is added in an $\alpha 1$-3 linkage to the subterminal galactose of the H antigen to form the A antigen. In group B individuals, an $\alpha 1,3$ galactose is added to the same subterminal galactose to form the B antigen. In group AB individuals, both A and B structures are synthesized. In group O individuals, neither A nor B antigens are synthesized as a result of alterations in the *ABO* genes.[7,13] Consequently, group O individuals express only H antigen. A and B antigens are also absent in the very rare Bombay phenotype

TABLE 10-1. Routine ABO Grouping

Reaction of Red Cells with Antisera (Red Cell Grouping)		Reaction of Serum/Plasma with Reagent Red Cells (Serum Grouping)			Interpre-tation	Prevalence (%) in US Population	
Anti-A	Anti-B	A₁ Cells	B Cells	O Cells	ABO Group	European Ethnicity	African Ethnicity
0	0	+	+	0	O	45	49
+	0	0	+	0	A	40	27
0	+	+	0	0	B	11	20
+	+	0	0	0	AB	4	4
0	0	+	+	+	Bombay*	Rare	Rare

*H-negative phenotype (see section on H antigen).

+ = agglutination; 0 = no agglutination.

because of the absence of the H-antigen precursor (see "The H System" below).

As terminal epitopes, the A and B antigens can be displayed on a number of oligosaccharide scaffolds that differ in their size, composition, linkages, and tissue distribution. On red cells, ABH antigens are present mainly as the N-linked portions of glycoproteins and as glycosphingolipids, but also to a lesser degree as an O-linked part of certain glycoproteins (Fig 10-3). ABH antigens are subclassified by the carbohydrate sequence immediately next to the ABH-defining sugars. In humans, ABH is expressed predominantly on four different oligosaccharide peripheral core structures (see Table 10-2). On human red cells, the majority of endogenous ABH antigen synthesized is present on type 2 chain structures. In addition, ABH-active type 1 chain structures can be adsorbed onto the red cell, especially in secretor individuals.[14]

The ability to synthesize and use different carbohydrate chains is genetically determined. In addition to the four main ABO groups mentioned above, subgroup phenotypes of A and B can be identified based on the quantity of A or B antigen expression and which types of carbohydrate chains contain the A or B antigen (see section on ABO subgroups). For example, the A phenotype can be subdivided into a number of subgroups, with A₁ and A₂ being the most common and second most common A subgroup, respectively. The A₁ phenotype, compared to A₂, has approximately five times the number of A antigens on red cells as a result of a more active A transferase.[13] There are also antigen differences between the two. For instance, the A₁ transferase is more prone to make type 3 (repetitive A) and type 4 (globo-A) A antigens than the A₂ transferase.[15,16] In addition to the above, ABH antigens expressed on type 1 chain substrates can form additional Leᵇ-associated antigens depending on secretor and LE status.[13,17] (See the H and LE system sections.)

ABO in Development and Aging

ABO antigens can be detected on red cells of embryos as early as 5 to 6 weeks of gestation.[17] The quantity of ABO antigens on umbilical cord red cells is less than that for adults, as a result of the immaturity of type 2 chain precursors on cord red cells.[18] (See section on the I blood group system below.) With increasing age, precursor chains become increasingly branched, thereby allowing more A and B antigen to be expressed.[19] Adult levels of ABO expression are generally present by age 2 to 4 years.[17,18]

Anti-A and anti-B are not present at birth or, if present, they are of maternal origin. Endogenous synthesis of anti-A and anti-B can develop

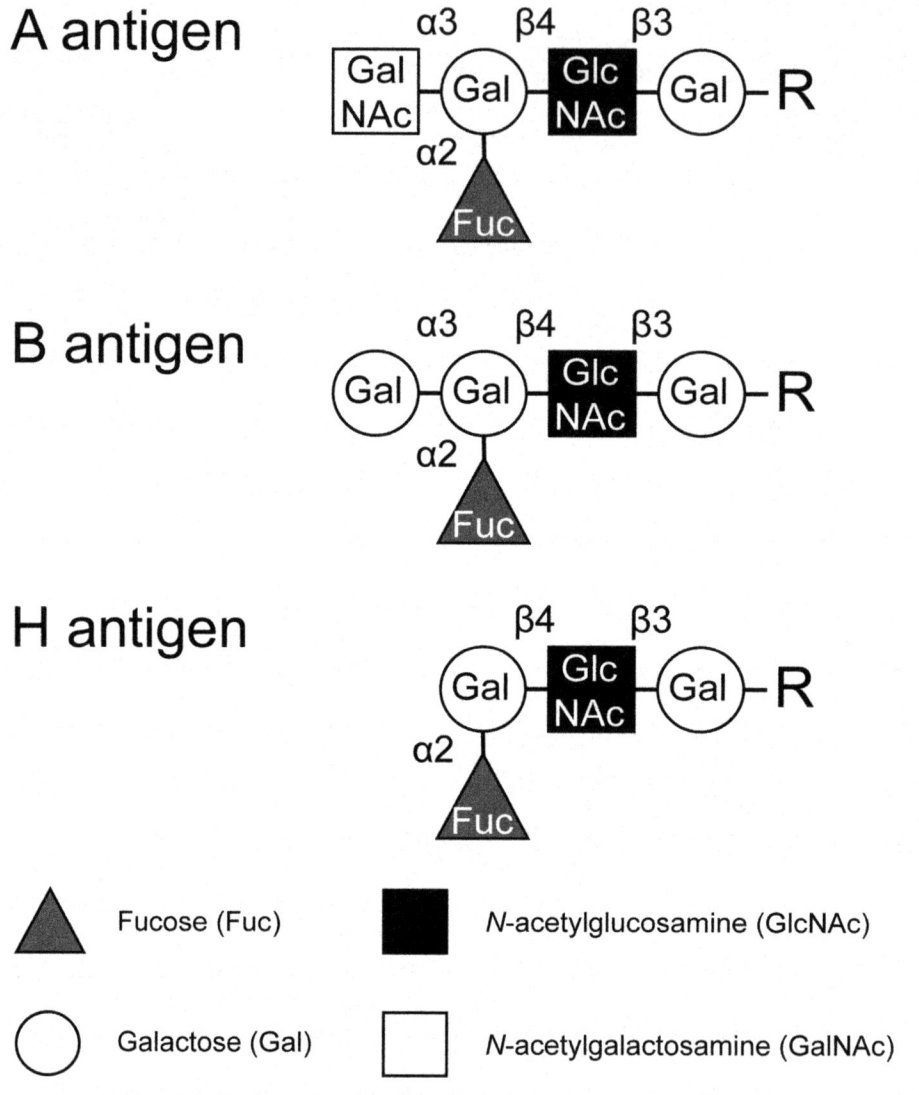

FIGURE 10-2. Schematic representation of the ABH antigens. Standard symbols for glycan annotation are used. Type 2 ABH antigens, the most common type on red cells, are shown. (See also Table 10-2.) R = upstream carbohydrate sequence.

as early as age 3 to 6 months, with nearly all children displaying the appropriate isohemagglutinins in their sera at 1 year of age.[17,20] Titers of anti-A and anti-B continue to increase during early childhood and achieve adult levels within 5 to 10 years.

Among healthy adults, ABO titers can naturally vary from 4 to 2048 or higher.[17,20,21] High-

titer ABO antibodies can be present in group O multiparous women and in patients taking certain bacteria-based nutritional supplements.[7,12,17] Although early reports indicated a decline in isohemagglutinin titers in the elderly, subsequent studies have disputed these findings.[20] In industrialized countries, isohemagglutinin titers have generally decreased, and some studies suggest

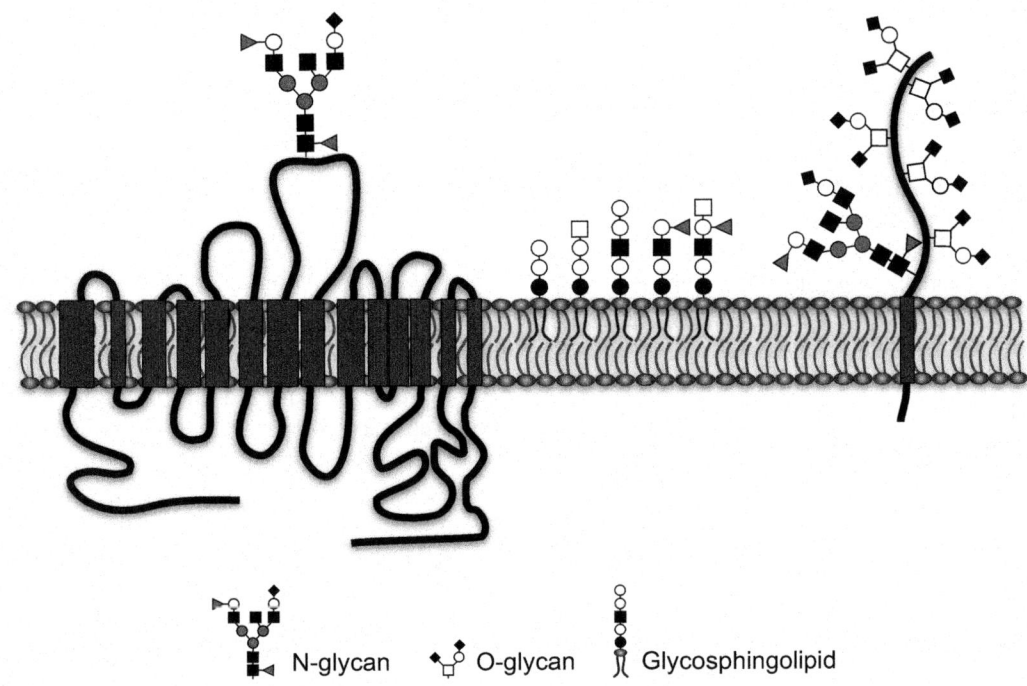

FIGURE 10-3. Schematic representation of the red cell membrane with selected carbohydrate-carrying blood group molecules representing different kinds of glycans.

TABLE 10-2. The Most Important Peripheral Core Chain Variants of A Antigen in Humans

Antigen	Oligosaccharide Sequence*
A epitope	GalNAcα1-3(Fucα1-2)Galβ1-R
A type 1	GalNAcα1-3(Fucα1-2)Galβ**1-3**GlcNAcβ1-3-R
A type 2†	GalNAcα1-3(Fucα1-2)Galβ**1-4**GlcNAcβ1-3-R
A type 3 (repetitive A)	GalNAcα1-3(Fucα1-2)Galβ**1-3**GalNAcα1-3(Fucα1-2)Galβ**1-4**GlcNAcβ1-3-R
A type 4 (globo-A)	GalNAcα1-3(Fucα1-2)Galβ**1-3**GalNAcβ1-3Galα1-4Galβ1-4Glc-Cer

*Underlined sequences denote the critical differences between type 1, 2, and 4 chains. Linkages and anomery (α- or β-linked) of the galactose in these A antigen variants are shown in bold. Bracketed sequences denote the repetitive sequence characteristic of type 3 chain A antigen. Note: There is also an alternative type 3 chain that is denoted the O-linked mucin type, which has the characteristic Galβ**1-3**GalNAc binding but not the repetitive A sequence.

†By far the predominant type on human red cells.

Cer = ceramide; Fuc = fucose; Gal = galactose; GalNAc = *N*-acetylgalactosamine; Glc = glucose; GlcNAc = *N*-acetylglucosamine; R = upstream carbohydrate sequence.

that increasing consumption of processed foods is a factor.[21]

Genetics

The *ABO* gene is located on chromosome 9q34 and consists of seven coding exons spread over ~19 kb.[7] The largest portion of the open reading frame is located in exons 6 and 7. The gene is transcriptionally regulated by several mechanisms, including promoter methylation, antisense RNA, tissue-specific transcription-factor-binding motifs, and a minisatellite enhancer region ~4 kb upstream of exon 1.[7] In addition, recent studies have shown the importance of an erythrospecific GATA-binding motif in intron 1[22] and the possibility that micro-RNAs may be involved by binding to the 3' end of the sequence.[23] ABO expression is also regulated by the *H(FUT1/FUT2)* genes, which are responsible for the synthesis of H antigen, the precursor of A and B antigens. The *H* genes are in turn tightly regulated in a tissue-specific manner through transcription factors and promoters. In the total absence of H, no A or B antigen can be expressed regardless of *ABO* genotype. This results in the Bombay or O_h phenotype.[7,13]

Following the purification of A glycosyltransferase from lung tissue[24] and the subsequent cloning of the *ABO* gene,[25] a series of studies has identified the molecular basis for A, B, O, cisAB, and weak ABO subgroups.[7,13,26] Although hundreds of *ABO* alleles have been found and characterized, the vast majority of individuals have alleles giving rise to A_1, A_2, B, or O expression. The A^1 and *B* consensus alleles are written as *ABO*A1.01* and *ABO*B.01*, respectively, in the blood group allele terminology developed by the International Society of Blood Transfusion (ISBT) (see Table 9-4 in Chapter 9 for examples of ISBT terminology applied to blood groups). These alleles are codominantly expressed, and their coding regions differ by only seven nucleotides, of which four alter amino acids in the resulting glycosyltransferases.[7,25,26] Three amino acid substitutions (A vs B; p.Gly235Ser, p.Leu266Met, and p.Gly268Ala) are important in determining whether the glycosyltransferase uses UDP-*N*-acetylgalactosamine or UDP-galactose donor substrate to synthesize A or B anti-

gens, respectively [Fig 10-1 (B)].[7,13] The rare cisAB phenotype has a chimeric enzyme with a mix of A- and B-specific amino acids at or nearby those amino acid positions.[26] A plethora of mutations associated with weak A and B subgroups has been described. As an example, group A_2 (the second most common A subgroup after A_1) is commonly the result of a nucleotide deletion (c.1061delC) resulting in a frameshift and an enzyme with an additional 21 amino acids at the C-terminus of the molecule.[7,26] Most of the weak A or B subgroups described below and in Table 10-3 depend on single nonsynonymous changes compared to A or B consensus, resulting in the substitution of a conserved amino acid that is important for the activity, specificity, or localization of the enzyme.

An *O* allele encodes a gene product without enzymatic function or no protein at all. The blood group O phenotype, therefore, is an autosomal recessive trait representing inheritance of two nonfunctional *ABO* genes. Overall, more than 100 *O* alleles have been identified.[7,26] The two most common *O* alleles are *ABO*O.01.01* (formerly known as *O^1* or *OO1*) and *ABO*O.01.02* (known as *$O^{1variant}$* or *OO2*). These alleles contain the same nucleotide deletion, c.261delG, which leads to a frameshift and premature truncation of the protein that lacks the enzymatically active domain. A principally different but infrequent *O* allele is *ABO*O.02* (originally described as *O^2* but later also called *OO3*), representing a group of nondeletional *O* alleles that contains a nonsynonymous polymorphism (c.802G>A) encoding amino acid 268 (p.Gly268Arg), which is otherwise a critical residue for donor substrate binding. These alleles were also found to be involved in cases of suspected A subgroups.[27,28] A subsequent study found that alleles with this alteration were responsible for 25% of all serologic ABO typing discrepancies caused by reverse-grouping problems in healthy donors, despite the frequency of this type of *O* allele being 1% to 3% in people of European ancestry but less common or virtually absent in other populations.[29,30] It was speculated that the weak anti-A observed in plasma could reflect weak residual glycosyltransferase activity. However, a later study was unable to demonstrate A antigen or enzyme activity in

TABLE 10-3. Serologic Reactions Observed in Selected A and B Subgroups

Red Cell Phenotype	Red Cell Reactions with Antisera or Lectins				Serum Reactions with Reagent Red Cells			Saliva (secretors)
	Anti-A	Anti-B	Anti-A,B	Anti-H	A₁ Cells	B Cells	O Cells	
A₁	4+	0	4+	0	0	4+	0	A, H
A₂	4+	0	4+	2+	0/2+ *	4+	0	A, H
A₃	3+^{mf†}	0	3+^{mf†}	3+	0/2+ *	4+	0	A, H
Aₓ	0/±	0	1-2+	4+	0/2+ *	4+	0	H
A_el	0 ‡	0	0	4+	0/2+ *	4+	0	H
A_m	0/±	0	0/±	4+	0	4+	0	A, H
B	0	4+	4+	0	4+	0	0	B, H
B₃	0	3+^{mf†}	3+^{mf†}	4+	4+	0	0	B, H
B_weak	0	±/2+	±/2+	4+	4+	0	0	H
B_el	0	0	0	4+	4+	0	0	H
B_m	0	0/±	0/±	4+	4+	0	0	B, H

*The occurrence of anti-A1 is variable in these phenotypes.

†This reaction can be read as 2+ or 3+ mixed field but typically looks like one or a few large agglutinates among a large number of free cells.

‡Positive adsorption/elution test with anti-A.

1+ to 4+ = agglutination of increasing strength; ± = weak agglutination; mf = mixed-field agglutination; 0 = no agglutination.

group O donors with the *ABO*O.02* allele but confirmed that the anti-A titers appear to be lower.[31] The clinical significance, if any, is unclear and the units are labeled group O.

ABO Subgroups

ABO subgroups are phenotypes that differ in the amount of A and B antigen carried on red cells and present in secretions (for individuals who have the secretor phenotype). Clinically, the two most common subgroups encountered are A₁ and A₂. A₁ represents the majority of group A donors (~80% among people of European ancestry) and, as previously mentioned, is characterized by approximately five times more A antigen epitopes per red cell compared to A₂, which is the second most common subgroup (20%). It is difficult to estimate the absolute number of A antigen sites per red cell. Some investigators have suggested approximately 1 million for A₁ and 220,000 for A₂,[32] but others have suggested two to three times as many.[33] Both A₁ and A₂ subgroups are strongly agglutinated by reagent anti-A in routine direct testing. A₁ can be distinguished from A₂ by the lectin *Dolichos biflorus*, which agglutinates A₁ red cells but is diluted to a level that should not agglutinate A₂ red cells. Because the A₂ phenotype reflects the inefficient conversion of H-to-A antigen, A₂ red cells have increased reactivity with anti-H lectin *Ulex europaeus*. Enzyme studies comparing A₁ and A₂ glycosyltransferase activity show that the A₁ enzyme is 5 to 10 times more active than the A₂ enzyme, resulting in quantitative and qualitative differences in A antigen expression.[7,13] The latter includes the synthesis of type 3 and type 4 chain A antigens on A_1 red cells that are either not present or expressed at much lower levels on A_2 and other weaker A subgroups.[13,15,16]

In addition to A_2, several weaker A subgroups have been described (eg, A_3, A_x, A_m, and A_{el}). Similarly, multiple weak B subgroups have been described (eg, B_3, B_x, B_m, and B_{el}). The weak A and B subgroups are infrequently encountered and are usually recognized by apparent discrepancies between red cell (forward) and serum or plasma (reverse) grouping. Most weak A and B subgroups were originally described before the advent of monoclonal typing reagents, and the hemagglutination patterns reported were based on reactivity with human polyclonal anti-A, anti-B, and anti-A,B reagents. Weak A subgroups are frequently nonreactive with human polyclonal anti-A (see Table 10-3) and can show variable reactivity with human polyclonal anti-A1 and anti-A,B and murine monoclonal antibodies (not shown).[13,15,26] The degree of reactivity with commercial murine monoclonal reagents is clone dependent, and clones may be used together as monoclonal blends as an anti-A,B reagent to allow for the agglutination of A_x red cells. This is a requirement of the European In-Vitro Diagnostic Directive (IVDD), although not required in the United States. Because of the reciprocal relationship between H and synthesis of A and B antigens, most weak A and B subgroups have H expression similar to group O cells.[7] In clinical practice, it is seldom necessary to identify a patient's specific A or B subgroup except where identifying a group A_2 kidney donor allows for transplantation of the kidney to a group O or B recipient. To avoid unnecessary use of group O Red Blood Cell (RBC) units, however, it can be worthwhile to define the ABO blood group carefully in chronic transfusion recipients. Great care should be exercised to understand the underlying reason for any ABO discrepancy in a blood donor. For instance, a chimera should be differentiated from an A_3 subgroup, even if both may exhibit a mixed-field agglutination pattern.

When performed, classification of weak A subgroups is typically based on the following:

1. Degree of red cell agglutination by monoclonal (and possibly polyclonal) anti-A and anti-A1 (in the case of the latter, *Dolichos biflorus* lectin can also be used).
2. Degree of red cell agglutination by human polyclonal and some monoclonal anti-A,B.
3. Degree of H antigen expression (reactivity with monoclonal anti-H and/or *Ulex europaeus* lectin).
4. Presence or absence of anti-A1 in serum (Method 2-9).
5. Presence of A and H in saliva (an analysis now seldom performed).
6. Adsorption and elution studies with polyclonal anti-A.
7. Family (pedigree) studies.
8. Molecular testing (genotyping).

In the case of suspected weak B subgroups, the investigation is similar to the above but anti-B replaces anti-A (and anti-A1). Presence of B and H can be investigated in saliva.

Presently, many reference laboratories also use genetic typing of the *ABO* gene as a complement to establish the underlying reason for an ABO discrepancy.[34] In addition to various genotyping methods available, Sanger sequencing of the *ABO* gene or next-generation sequencing may be used. Furthermore, some ABO subgroups exhibit characteristic patterns when tested by flow cytometry with selected monoclonal ABO reagents.[35] This method is very useful for differentiating a low-grade chimera from a weak subgroup, or the inherited A_3 subgroup from a mixed-field pattern after transfusion. It should be noted that some of the above-mentioned methods to characterize ABO subgroups have not yet obtained regulatory approval and that this varies depending on the geographic region.

B(A), A(B), and cisAB Phenotypes

The B(A) phenotype is an autosomal dominant phenotype characterized by weak A expression on group B red cells.[17,36] Serologically, red cells from B(A)-phenotype individuals are strongly reactive with anti-B and weakly reactive with certain monoclonal anti-A (<2+), and they may possess a strong anti-A that is reactive with both

A_1 and A_2 red cells in their sera. B(A) red cells can show varying reactivity with monoclonal anti-A reagents. Testing the sample with a panel of polyclonal and monoclonal anti-A may resolve the discrepancy, but genetic testing is the most accurate. Absence of the B-characteristic c.703G>A polymorphism (p.Gly235Ser) in a *B* allele will make it a *B(A)* allele, but also other genetic alterations in *B* alleles will result in this phenotype.[26] The basis of the phenotype is that the B-like glycosyltransferase in these individuals has an increased capacity to use UDP-*N*-acetylgalactosamine in addition to UDP-galactose, resulting in detectable A antigen synthesis.

An A(B) phenotype has also been described, using monoclonal anti-B. The A(B) phenotype was associated with elevated H antigen and plasma H-transferase activity.[17] It has been hypothesized that the increased H precursor on these cells may permit the synthesis of some B antigen by the A glycosyltransferase.

The cisAB phenotype can occur when an individual has inherited an *ABO* gene encoding an ABO glycosyltransferase that can use both A- and B-specific nucleotide sugars in a more equal way than in the B(A) or A(B) phenotypes.[37] If a *cisAB* allele is inherited together in *trans* with an *O* allele, an unusual phenotype with weak expression of both A and B is observed (eg, A_2B_3). Anti-B is often present in serum. There are different variants of *cisAB*, but the most common one (*ABO*cisAB.01*) is relatively prevalent in some parts of East Asia, and consequently in individuals with origin from these regions. In this variant, an A^1 allele exhibits the presence of a B-specific polymorphism, c.803G>C (p.Gly268Ala), which alters the enzyme's specificity for donor substrate.

Acquired B Phenotype

The acquired B phenotype phenomenon is a transient serologic discrepancy in group A individuals that causes red cell grouping discrepancies.[38] Acquired B should be suspected when a patient or donor who has historically typed as group A now presents with weak B expression on forward red cell typing. Serologically, the acquired B phenotype shows strong agglutination with anti-A, typically shows weak agglutination (2+ or less) with certain monoclonal and most polyclonal anti-B, and contains a strong anti-B in serum. Despite reactivity of the patient's red cells with anti-B, the patient's serum is not reactive with autologous red cells.

Acquired B is the result of deacetylation of the A antigen's *N*-acetylgalactosamine, yielding a B-like galactosamine sugar.[39,40] In patients' samples, acquired B is often present in the setting of infection by gastrointestinal bacteria. Many enteric bacteria possess a deacetylase enzyme capable of converting A antigen to a B-like analog.[40] Identification of the acquired B phenotype can also be influenced by reagent pH and specific monoclonal anti-B typing reagents.[38] In the past, anti-B reagents containing the ES-4 clone were associated with an increased detection of acquired B.

To resolve a patient's true red cell type and confirm the presence of acquired B, red cells should be retyped using a different monoclonal anti-B or acidified (pH 6.0) human anti-B. Acidified human anti-B does not react with acquired B antigen. *ABO* genotyping can also be useful. Monoclonal anti-B, which recognizes acquired B, should not be used in clinical practice.

Antibodies to ABO Blood Group System Antigens

Anti-A and Anti-B

Immunoglobulin M (IgM) is the predominant isotype found in group A and group B individuals, although small quantities of IgG antibody can be detected. In group O serum, IgG is a major isotype of anti-A and anti-B. As a consequence, the incidence of ABO hemolytic disease of the fetus and newborn (ABO-associated HDFN) is higher among the offspring of group O mothers than of mothers with other blood types, because IgG can cross the placenta but IgM cannot. However, ABO-associated HDFN is less of a clinical problem than RhD-associated HDFN.

Both IgM and IgG anti-A and anti-B preferentially agglutinate red cells at room temperature (20 to 24 C) or cooler, and both can efficiently activate complement at 37 C. The complement-mediated lytic capability of these antibodies becomes apparent if serum testing includes an incubation phase at 37 C. Hemolysis caused by ABO antibodies should be suspected when either the supernatant serum is pink to red or the cell button is smaller or absent. Hemolysis is interpreted as a positive result. The use of plasma for testing or of reagent red cells suspended in solutions that contain EDTA prevents complement activation and hemolysis.

Anti-A,B

Sera from group O individuals contain an antibody specificity known as "anti-A,B" because it is reactive with both A and B red cells. Such anti-A and anti-B reactivity cannot be separated by differential adsorption, suggesting that the antibody recognizes a common epitope shared by the A and B antigens.[7,41] This is the reason why ISBT has acknowledged A,B as the third antigen of the ABO system. Saliva containing secreted A or B substance can inhibit the activity of anti-A,B against both A and B red cells.

Anti-A1

Anti-A1 is present as an alloantibody in the serum of 1% to 8% of A_2 individuals and 22% to 35% of A_2B individuals, and is sometimes present in the sera of individuals with other weak A subgroups. Group O serum contains a mixture of anti-A and anti-A1.[40] Because of the presence of the antibody, ISBT has recognized the A1 antigen as the fourth antigen in the ABO system. Anti-A1 can cause ABO discrepancies during routine testing and lead to incompatible crossmatches with A_1 and A_1B red cells. Anti-A1 is usually of IgM isotype, reacting best at room temperature or below, and is usually considered clinically insignificant. Anti-A1 is considered clinically significant if reactivity is observed at 37 C.[40] Group A_2 patients with an anti-A1 that is reactive at 37 C should receive group A_2 or O red cells for transfusion; group A_2B patients should receive group A_2, A_2B, B, or O red cells.

Routine Testing for ABO

Donor blood samples are routinely typed for ABO at the time of donation and on receipt of red cell units in the hospital transfusion service (confirmatory typing). The latter is not always practiced outside the United States. Recipient samples are typed before transfusion. ABO grouping requires both antigen typing of red cells for A and B antigen (red cell grouping or forward type) and screening of serum or plasma for the presence of anti-A and anti-B isohemagglutinins (serum/plasma grouping or reverse type). Both red cell and serum/plasma grouping are required for donors and patients because each grouping serves as a control for the other. Reverse or serum grouping is not required in two circumstances: 1) for confirmation testing of labeled, previously typed donor red cells and 2) in infants younger than 4 months of age. As previously discussed, isohemagglutinins are not present at birth and develop only after 3 to 6 months of age.

Commercially available anti-A and anti-B for red cell typing are extremely potent and agglutinate most antigen-positive red cells directly, even without centrifugation. Most monoclonal typing reagents have been formulated to detect many weak ABO subgroups. (See manufacturers' inserts for specific reagent characteristics.) Additional reagents (anti-A1 and anti-A,B) and special techniques to detect weak ABO subgroups are not necessary for routine testing but are helpful for resolving ABO typing discrepancies.

In contrast to commercial ABO typing reagents, human anti-A and anti-B in the sera of patients and donors can be relatively weak, requiring incubation and centrifugation. Tests for serum grouping, therefore, should be performed using a method that adequately detects human anti-A and anti-B. Several methods are available for determining ABO group, including slide, tube, microplate, and column agglutination (gel) techniques.

ABO Discrepancies

Table 10-1 shows the results and interpretations of routine red cell and serum tests for ABO. A discrepancy exists when the results of red cell tests do not agree with those of serum tests, usually due to unexpected negative or positive results in either the forward or reverse typing. (See Table 10-3.) ABO discrepancies may arise from intrinsic problems with either red cells or serum or from technical errors in performing the test. (See Table 10-4 and section on resolving ABO discrepancies.)

When a discrepancy is encountered, the discrepant results must be recorded, but interpretation of the ABO group must be delayed until the discrepancy has been resolved. If the specimen is from a donor unit, the unit must be quarantined and cannot be released for transfusion. When an ABO discrepancy is identified in a patient, it may be necessary to transfuse group O red cells pending an investigation. It is important to obtain a sufficient pretransfusion blood sample from the patient to complete any additional studies that may be required.

Red Cell Testing Problems

ABO testing of red cells may give unexpected results for many reasons, including the following:

1. Weak ABO expression that results from inheritance of a weak ABO subgroup. Some patients with leukemia and other malignancies, as well as during pregnancy, can also show weakened ABO expression.[13,35,42]
2. Mixed-field agglutination with circulating red cells of more than one ABO group following out-of-group red cell transfusion or hematopoietic progenitor cell (HPC) transplantation (eg, group O to group A). Mixed-field agglutination is also present in some ABO subgroups (eg, A_3), blood group chimerism in fraternal twins, and rare cases of mosaicism arising from dispermy.
3. Neutralization of anti-A and anti-B typing reagents by high concentrations of A or B blood group substance in serum, resulting in unexpected negative reactions with serum- or plasma-suspended red cells.
4. Spontaneous agglutination or autoagglutination of serum or plasma-suspended red cells caused by heavy coating of red cells by potent autoagglutinins.
5. Nonspecific aggregation of serum- or plasma-suspended red cells caused by abnormal concentrations of serum proteins or infused macromolecular solutions.

6. False-positive reactions that are caused by a pH-dependent autoantibody, a reagent-dependent antibody (eg, EDTA or paraben), or rouleaux.
7. Anomalous red cell grouping resulting from acquired B, B(A), cisAB, or A(B) phenotypes.
8. Polyagglutination (eg, T activation) resulting from inherited or acquired abnormalities of the red cell membrane, with exposure of "cryptic autoantigens."[40] Because all human sera contain naturally occurring antibodies to such cryptic antigens, those abnormal red cells are agglutinated also by ABO-compatible human sera. Monoclonal anti-A and anti-B reagents do not detect polyagglutination.

Problems with Serum or Plasma Testing

Problems may arise during ABO testing of serum or plasma, including the following:

1. Small fibrin clots in plasma or incompletely clotted serum that can be mistaken for red cell agglutinates.
2. Lack of detectable isoagglutinins in infants younger than 4 to 6 months. Children do not develop isoagglutinins until 3 to 6 months of age. ABO antibodies present at birth are passively acquired from the mother. Children between 6 months and 1 year of age may also have lower levels of anti-A/-B.
3. Unexpected absence of ABO agglutinins caused by a weak A or B subgroup. (See Table 10-3.)
4. Unexpected absence of anti-B in children receiving long-term parenteral and enteral nutrition and who are in a sterile environment, free of bacteria.[43]
5. Unexpected absence of anti-A agglutinins in patients receiving equine-derived immunoglobulins.[44]
6. ABO-incompatible HPC transplantation with induction of tolerance. For example, a group A patient receiving a group O marrow transplant will have circulating group O red cells but will produce only anti-B in serum.[45]

TABLE 10-4. Possible Causes of ABO Typing Discrepancies

Category	Causes
Weak/missing red cell reactivity	ABO subgroup
	Leukemia/malignancy
	Transfusion
	Pregnancy
	Intrauterine fetal transfusion
	Transplantation
	Excessive soluble blood group substance
Extra red cell reactivity	Autoagglutinins/excess protein coating red cells
	Unwashed red cells: plasma proteins
	Unwashed red cells: antibody in patient's serum to reagent constituent
	Transplantation
	Acquired B antigen or other polyagglutinable conditions
	cisAB or B(A) phenomenon
	Out-of-group transfusion
Mixed-field red cell reactivity	ABO subgroup
	Recent transfusion
	Transplantation
	Fetomaternal hemorrhage
	Twin or dispermic (tetragametic) chimerism
Weak/missing serum reactivity	Age related (<4-6 months old or elderly)
	ABO subgroup
	Hypogammaglobulinemia
	Transplantation
	Excessive anti-A or anti-B (prozone effect)
	Hemodilution, eg, by excessive infusion of intravenous fluids
Extra serum reactivity	Cold autoantibody
	Cold-reactive alloantibody
	Serum antibody to reagent constituent
	Excess serum protein
	Transfusion of plasma components
	Transplantation
	Infusion of intravenous immune globulin

(See Chapter 27 for more information on ABO-mismatched transplantation.)

7. Severe hypogammaglobulinemia secondary to inherited immunodeficiency or disease therapy. Hypogammaglobulinemia with dilution of isoagglutinins can also occur after several courses of plasma exchange with albumin replacement.

8. Cold alloantibodies (eg, anti-M) or autoantibodies (eg, anti-I) reactive with corresponding antigen-positive reverse-grouping cells.

9. Antibodies directed against constituents in the diluents used to preserve reagent A_1 and B red cells.[40]

10. Nonspecific aggregation or agglutination caused by high-molecular-weight plasma expanders, rouleaux, high serum-protein concentrations, or altered serum-protein ratios.

11. Recent transfusion of out-of-group plasma-containing components (eg, a group A patient provided with platelets from a group O donor, causing unexpected passively acquired anti-A in the patient's plasma).

12. Recent infusion of intravenous immunoglobulin, which can contain ABO isoagglutinins.

13. Anti-CD47, a monoclonal antibody therapy in US clinical trials, will give positive reactions with all test red cells, as they possess the CD47 protein.

14. The test method, which may impact the ability to detect anti-A/-B. Column agglutination testing may show weaker reactivity than test tube methods.

Technical Errors

Technical problems with a sample or during testing can also lead to problems in ABO grouping, including:

1. Specimen mix-up.
2. Too-heavy or too-light red cell suspensions.
3. Failure to add reagents.
4. Missed observation of hemolysis.
5. Failure to follow the manufacturer's instructions.

6. Under- or overcentrifugation of tests.
7. Incubating forward- or reverse-typing reactions at a suboptimal temperature.
8. Incorrect interpretation or recording of test results.

Resolving ABO Discrepancies

The first step in resolving an apparent serologic testing discrepancy should be to repeat the test with the same sample to exclude the possibility of a technical error during testing. Additional studies may include testing a new sample to avoid mix-up; testing washed red cells; testing for unexpected red cell alloantibodies; and reviewing the patient's medical record for conditions, medications, or recent transfusions that may have contributed to the conflicting test results (Method 2-4). Samples with apparent weak or missing ABO antigens and/or antibodies may require tests using methods that enhance antigen-antibody binding, including incubating red cells at 4 C (Method 2-5), using enzyme-treated red cells (Method 2-6), and conducting adsorption and elution studies (Method 2-7), as well as flow cytometry and molecular testing when warranted. In some instances, it may be necessary to test for the secretion of ABH antigens in saliva (Method 2-8). Patients with suspected B(A), acquired B, or A(B) phenotypes should be retested using different monoclonal and human polyclonal reagents.

ABO discrepancies caused by unexpected serum reactions are not uncommon. Commonly encountered causes of serum-grouping discrepancies include cold autoantibodies, rouleaux, cold-reacting alloantibodies (eg, anti-M), and weak A subgroups with an anti-A1. In addition, the presence of certain nondeletional *O* alleles (*ABO*O.02*) is a common reason for lower anti-A titers in group O individuals, as discussed above.[29,46] To resolve an ABO discrepancy caused by an anti-A1 in a group A individual, red cells should be tested with *Dolichos biflorus* lectin, which agglutinates group A_1 but not A_2 and weaker A subgroups. The presence of an anti-A1 should be confirmed by testing serum against A_1, A_2, and O red cells (Method 2-9). Reverse-grouping problems resulting from either a cold alloantibody (Method 2-10) or autoantibody can be identified with a room-temperature antibody detection test and an autocontrol at room temperature. Techniques to identify ABO antibodies in the presence of cold autoantibodies include testing at 37 C without centrifugation (Method 2-11) and cold autoadsorption (Method 4-5). Serum or plasma properties can induce rouleaux formation that resembles agglutination with A_1 and B red cells. Saline replacement or saline dilution (Method 3-7) can be used to distinguish rouleaux from agglutination and identify ABO antibodies. Incubating or diluting the agglutination reaction with a citrate solution has a similar effect.

Cold autoantibodies can cause autoagglutination of red cells and unexpected reactions during red cell typing. Red cells heavily coated with autoantibodies can spontaneously agglutinate and cause false-positive reactions in tests with anti-A and anti-B. Usually, false-positive reactions caused by cold autoantibodies can be eliminated by washing red cells with warm saline (Method 2-17). Autoagglutination caused by IgM can also be inhibited or dispersed by incubating red cells in the presence of either dithiothreitol (Method 3-16) or 2-aminoethylisothiouronium bromide. These reagents reduce the disulfide bonds on IgM molecules, decreasing their polyvalency and ability to agglutinate red cells directly.

THE H SYSTEM (018)

H antigen is expressed on red cells from all individuals except those of the rare Bombay phenotype. Because H antigen serves as the precursor to both A and B antigens, the amount of H antigen on red cells depends on an individual's ABO type. H antigen is highly expressed on group O red cells because group O individuals lack a functional ABO glycosyltransferase. In group A and B individuals, the amount of H antigen is considerably less because H is converted to the A and B antigens, respectively. The amount of H antigen on red cells, based on agglutination with the anti-H lectin *Ulex europaeus*, differs between the ABO phenotypes as follows: $O>A_2>B>A_2B>A_1>A_1B$. H antigen is present on HPCs, red cells, megakaryocytes, and other tis-

sues.[5,47,48] H antigen has been implicated in cell adhesion, normal hematopoietic differentiation, and several malignancies.[6,7,49]

Biochemistry and Genetics

H antigen is defined by the terminal disaccharide fucose(α1,2)galactose. Two different fucosyltransferase (Fuc-T) enzymes are capable of synthesizing H antigen: α2Fuc-T1 (encoded by *FUT1*, also known as the *H* gene) and α2Fuc-T2 (encoded by *FUT2*, the secretor gene). The *FUT1* enzyme preferentially fucosylates type 2 chain oligosaccharides on red cell glycoproteins and glycolipids to form H type 2. In contrast, the *FUT2* enzyme prefers type 1 chain precursors to form H type 1 antigens in secretions (Fig 10-4).[13] Secretion of type 1 chain ABH antigens in saliva and other fluids requires a functional *FUT2* (secretor) gene. *FUT2* is not expressed in red cells but is expressed in salivary glands, gastrointestinal tissues, and genitourinary tissues.[13] Type 1 chain ABH antigens present on red cells are passively adsorbed from circulating glycolipid antigens present in plasma.[40] (See "The LE System.") Several inactivating and weakening gene variants have been described in both the *FUT1* and *FUT2* genes.[26] Many of the variants are geographically and ethnically restricted. For instance, approximately 20% of people of European ancestry are nonsecretors, and this is mainly due to homozygosity for the common *FUT2*01N.02* allele with c.428G>A, which leads to a premature stop codon (p.Trp143Stop) and a nonfunctional enzyme.

Null Phenotypes

Bombay (O_h) Phenotype

Originally described in Bombay, India, the O_h or Bombay phenotype is a rare, autosomal recessive phenotype characterized by the absence of H, A, and B antigens on red cells and in secretions. Genetically, O_h individuals are homozygous (or compound heterozygous) for nonfunctional *FUT1* and *FUT2* genes, resulting in a complete absence of H type 1 and H type 2 chain, and consequently also loss of A and B independent of *ABO* genotype. The original Bombay phenotype is actually due to the

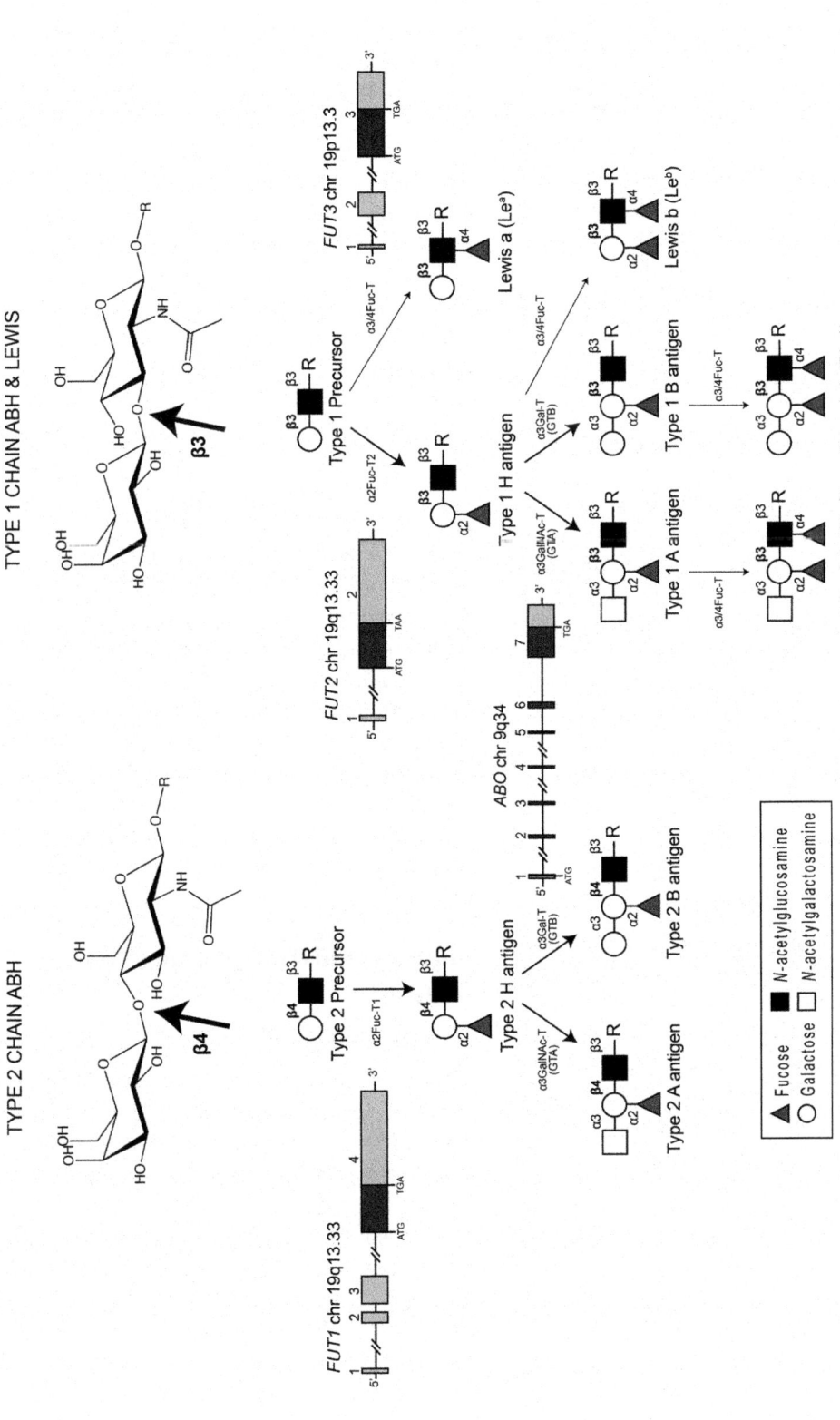

FIGURE 10-4. Type 1 and type 2 precursor chains are shown in the two figures at the top, and the difference (β3 vs β4 linkage) is highlighted with arrows. The genes and enzymes involved in the elongation of precursor to type 1 ABH and LE antigens, as well as type 2 ABH antigens, and a representation of their glycan structures are shown in the lower section of the figure. ATG and TGA in the gene symbols represent the start and stop codons, respectively. Fuc-T = fucosyltransferase; Gal-T = galactosyltransferase; GalNAc-T = *N*-acetylgalactosaminyltransferase; R = upstream carbohydrate sequence.

FUT1*01N.09 allele with a critical missense mutation (c.725T>G, p.Leu242Arg), while the entire *FUT2* gene is deleted. O_h red cells type as H negative with anti-H lectin *Ulex europaeus*, monoclonal anti-H, and human polyclonal anti-H from other O_h individuals. Because these individuals lack a functional *FUT2* (secretor) gene necessary for Le^b synthesis, O_h individuals also type as Le(b–). (See "The LE System.") Genotyping studies have described a wide range of inactivating mutations in both the *FUT1* and *FUT2* genes in O_h individuals.[13,26] The O_h phenotype is also present in leukocyte adhesion deficiency 2 (LAD2) because of mutations in the GDP-fucose transporter gene.[50]

Because they lack all ABH antigens, O_h individuals possess isoagglutinins to A, B, and H. (See Table 10-1.) In routine ABO typing, these individuals initially type as group O. The O_h phenotype becomes apparent during antibody screening tests with group O red cells, which are rich in H antigen. The anti-H present in O_h individuals strongly agglutinates all group O red cells and sometimes demonstrates in-vitro hemolysis. The O_h phenotype can be confirmed by demonstrating an absence of H antigen on red cells and the presence of a strong anti-H in serum that is reactive with group O red cells but not with O_h red cells from other individuals.

Para-Bombay Phenotype

Individuals with the para-Bombay phenotype can be secretors whose red cells are apparently deficient of H antigen.[7,13] Genetically, these individuals are homozygous for a nonfunctional *FUT1* gene, but they have inherited at least one functional *FUT2* (secretor) gene. The red cells from these H-deficient secretors lack serologically detectable H antigen but can carry small amounts of H, A, and/or B antigen because, unlike persons with classic Bombay phenotype, para-Bombay persons express type 1 chain ABH antigens in their secretions and plasma (Method 2-8).[40] Type 1 chain A and/or B antigens in plasma are then passively adsorbed onto red cells, resulting in weak A or B antigen expression. Red cells from para-Bombay individuals are designated "A_h," "B_h," and "AB_h." Para-Bombay can also occur in group O individuals, as evidenced by trace type 1 chain H on their red cells and in their secretions.

In laboratory testing, red cells from para-Bombay individuals may (or may not) have weak reactions with anti-A and anti-B reagents. In some cases, A and B antigens may be detected only after adsorption and elution. A_h and B_h para-Bombay red cells are nonreactive with anti-H lectin, monoclonal anti-H, and human anti-H from O_h individuals. The sera of para-Bombay individuals contain anti-H, anti-HI, or both and, depending on their ABO type, anti-A and anti-B.[17,40] The anti-H is typically weaker and less clinically significant in para-Bombay than Bombay individuals.

The para-Bombay phenotype can also occur in nonsecretors (ie, without a functional *FUT2* gene). In these rare cases, both *FUT1* alleles carry mutations that diminish, but do not abolish, the enzyme activity. Therefore, these individuals express small amounts of H type 2 antigen on red cells but lack H type 1 in secretions (and on red cells). If *A* or *B* alleles are inherited at the *ABO* locus, the phenotypes can be described as A_h and B_h, respectively. In principle, it is also possible to have a weak *FUT1*-encoded enzyme in combination with a fully functional *FUT2*-encoded enzyme. The resulting phenotype is para-Bombay.

Antibodies to H Blood Group System Antigens

Alloanti-H (Bombay and Para-Bombay)

The anti-H found in Bombay (O_h) individuals is clinically significant and associated with acute hemolytic transfusion reactions. These antibodies are predominantly of IgM isotype and exhibit a broad thermal range (4 to 37 C) with all red cells except O_h red cells. As with anti-A and anti-B, alloanti-H is capable of activating complement and causing red cell hemolysis intravascularly. The anti-H found in para-Bombay individuals may show lower titers and be less prone to cause direct lysis in vitro but is potentially significant, especially in nonsecretors.

Autoanti-H and Autoanti-HI

Autoantibodies to H and HI antigens can be encountered in healthy individuals. When present, these autoantibodies are most common in A_1 individuals, who have low levels of H antigen on their red cells. Autoanti-H and autoanti-HI are usually of IgM isotype and are reactive at room temperature.

Transfusion Practice

Alloanti-H is highly clinically significant and is capable of fixing complement and causing hemolytic transfusion reactions. As a result, patients with alloanti-H caused by the Bombay phenotype should be provided with H-negative (O_h) red cells for transfusion. The same is typically not necessary for para-Bombay secretor patients, but evaluation of the clinical significance and thermal range of the anti-H in the individual para-Bombay case is worthwhile, particularly in nonsecretors.

In contrast, autoantibodies against H and HI are generally clinically insignificant. In most patients, transfused group-specific or group O red cells should have normal in-vivo survival. Rarely, autoanti-HI can result in decreased red cell survival and hemolytic transfusion reactions after transfusion of group O red cells.[17,40] Hemolysis may follow transfusion of group O red cells to a group A_1, B, or A_1B patient with an unusually potent high-titer anti-HI that is reactive at 37 C.[40] In such patients, transfusion of group-specific (A_1, B, or AB) red cells is advised.

THE LE SYSTEM (007)

The LE blood group system consists of two main antigens, Le^a (LE1) and Le^b (LE2), and three common phenotypes, Le(a+b−), Le(a−b+), and Le(a−b−). Four additional LE antigens represent composite reactivity between Le^a, Le^b, and ABO antigens: Le^{ab} (LE3), Le^{bH} (LE4), ALe^b (LE5), and BLe^b (LE6).[26,50] In addition to being present on red cells, LE antigens are widely expressed on platelets, endothelial cells, and kidney, as well as on genitourinary and gastrointestinal epithelium.

LE antigens are not synthesized by the erythroid cells but are passively adsorbed onto red cell membranes from a pool of soluble LE glycolipid present in plasma.[50] The gastrointestinal tract, which is rich in LE-active glycolipid and glycoprotein, is thought to be the primary source of LE glycolipid in plasma. Because LE antigens are passively adsorbed onto red cell membranes, they can be eluted from red cells after transfusion or by increases in plasma volume and increased circulating lipoproteins, which also adsorb LE glycolipid. For example, LE antigen is often decreased on red cells during pregnancy, and some women transiently type as Le(a−b−), which is attributed to an increase in circulating plasma volume and a fourfold increase in lipoprotein.[40] The levels of LE antigens also decrease on stored red cells; therefore, LE phenotyping should be done sooner than later to avoid false-negative results. Le^b expression and immunoreactivity are also influenced by ABH type as a result of the synthesis of structures carrying both LE and ABH activity (Fig 10-4).[5,13,48]

Biochemistry and Synthesis

LE antigen synthesis depends on the interaction of fucosyltransferases encoded by two distinct genes (Fig 10-4): *FUT3* (the *LE* gene) and *FUT2* (the secretor gene).[50,51] Unlike the enzyme encoded by *FUT1*, which is relatively specific for type 2 chain substrates, the enzymes encoded by *FUT2* and *FUT3* preferentially fucosylate type 1 chain substrates. The *FUT2* gene therefore controls addition of a terminal $\alpha1,2$ fucose to type 1 chain precursors to form H type 1 antigen. *FUT3*, the *LE* gene, encodes an $\alpha1,3/4$-fucosyltransferase that transfers a fucose, in an $\alpha1$-4 linkage, to the penultimate *N*-acetylglucosamine of type 1 chain precursor (also known as Lewis c) to form Le^a antigen. The LE enzyme can also add a second fucose to H type 1 antigen to form Le^b antigen. Note that Le^b cannot be formed from Le^a because the presence of a subterminal fucose on Le^a sterically inhibits binding by the secretor enzyme.[4]

In individuals with both LE and secretor enzymes, H type 1 chain is favored over Le^a synthesis. As a result, most of the LE antigen synthesized is Le^b [Le(a–b+) phenotype]. In group A_1 and B individuals, Le^b and H type 1 chain can be further modified by ABO glycosyltransferases to form LE5 and LE6, type 1 antigens that express a combination of Le^b activity and A or B, respectively.[5,51] In group A_1 individuals, the majority of LE antigen in plasma is actually ALe^b.[52]

Genetics and LE Phenotypes

The three LE phenotypes commonly encountered represent the presence or absence of LE and secretor enzymes (see Table 10-5). Le(a+b–) individuals have inherited at least one functional FUT3 gene (traditionally denoted Le) but are homozygous for nonfunctional FUT2 alleles (denoted se/se). As a result, such individuals synthesize and secrete Le^a antigen but lack Le^b and type 1 chain ABH antigens.

The Le(a–b+) phenotype reflects inheritance of both functional FUT3 (Le) and FUT2 (Se) alleles, leading to the synthesis of Le^a, Le^b, and type 1 chain ABH. Because most type 1 chain precursor is converted to Le^b in those individuals, they appear to type as Le(a–). An Le(a+b+) phenotype is transiently observed in infants be-cause secretor activity increases with developmental age. An Le(a+b+) phenotype is also present in 10% to 40% of individuals of Asian ancestry (eg, 16% of Japanese individuals) as a result of inheritance of a very common weak secretor gene in East Asian populations (FUT2*01W.02, previously Se^w).[26,30] In the absence of a functional FUT3 gene (le/le), neither Le^a nor Le^b can be synthesized, leading to the Le(a–b–), or LE null, phenotype. Type 1 chain ABH antigens may still be synthesized and secreted in individuals who have inherited at least one functional FUT2 allele (Method 2-8). The Le(a–b–) phenotype is significantly more common in persons of African ancestry. Although rare, an Le(a–b–) phenotype is also present in patients with LAD2 due to defects in fucose transport.[50] This leads to lack of sialyl-Lewis X (sLe^x), which is normally involved in leukocyte extravasation.

Several inactivating mutations have been identified in both the FUT3 (LE) and FUT2 (secretor) genes.[26] Many of the mutations are geographically and ethnically restricted, with many populations displaying a few predominant alleles.

TABLE 10-5. Adult Phenotypes and Prevalence Rates in the LE System

Red Cell Reactions			Prevalence (%)		Genotype*		
Anti-Le^a	Anti-Le^b	Phenotype	European Ancestry	African Ancestry	LE	Secretor	Saliva†
+	0	Le(a+b–)	22	23	Le	se/se	Le^a
0	+	Le(a–b+)	72	55	Le	Se	Le^a, Le^b, ABH
0	0	Le(a–b–)	6	22	le/le le/le	se/se Se	Type 1 precursor Type 1 ABH
+	+	Le(a+b+)‡	Rare	Rare	Le	Se^w	Le^a, Le^b

*Probable genotype at the LE (FUT3) and secretor (FUT2) loci.

†Type 1 chain antigens present in saliva and other secretions.

‡Le(a+b+) is present in 10-40% of people of East Asian ancestry and is also transiently observed in infants.

Le = at least one FUT3 gene encoding functional LE enzyme (represents the genotypes Le/Le or Le/le); le/le = homozygous for FUT3 gene encoding an inactive enzyme; Se = at least one FUT2 gene encoding active secretor enzyme (represents the genotypes Se/Se or Se/se); se/se = homozygous for FUT2 gene encoding an inactive enzyme; Se^w = FUT2 gene encoding weak secretor enzyme.

LE Expression in Children

Table 10-5 shows the distribution of LE types in adults. In contrast, most newborns type as Le(a–b–). Approximately 50% of newborns subsequently type as Le(a+) after ficin or papain treatment. The prevalence of Le^b antigen, however, is low in newborns compared to adults because of developmental delays in secretor (*FUT2*-encoded fucosyltransferase) activity. An Le(a+b+) phenotype can be transiently present in children as the level of secretor activity approaches adult levels. A valid LE phenotype is not developed until age 5 or 6.[17]

Antibodies to LE Blood Group System Antigens

Antibodies against LE antigens are generally of IgM isotype and occur naturally. Clinically, LE antibodies are most often encountered in the sera of Le(a–b–) individuals and may contain a mixture of anti-Le^a, anti-Le^b, and anti-Le^{ab}, an antibody capable of recognizing both Le(a+) and Le(b+) red cells. Because small amounts of Le^a are synthesized in the Le(a–b+) phenotype, Le(a–b+) individuals do not make anti-Le^a. Anti-Le^b is present infrequently in the Le(a+b–) phenotype. A transient Le(a–b–) phenotype, accompanied by LE antibodies, is commonly observed during pregnancy. Finally, anti-Le^b can demonstrate ABO specificity (anti-Le^{bH}, anti-ALe^b, and anti-BLe^b), and is preferentially reactive with Le(b+) red cells of a specific ABO group.[40,48] Anti-Le^{bH}, the most common specificity, is more strongly reactive with Le(b+) group O and A$_2$ red cells than with group A$_1$ and B red cells, which have low H antigen levels. Anti-Le^{bL} is strongly reactive with all Le(b+) red cells, regardless of ABO group.

Most examples of LE antibodies are saline agglutinins that are reactive at room temperature. Unlike ABO, the agglutination is relatively fragile and easily dispersed, requiring gentle resuspension after centrifugation. Agglutination is sometimes observed after 37 C incubation, but the reaction is typically weaker than that at room temperature. On occasion, LE antibodies can be detected in the antihuman globulin (AHG) phase. Such detection may reflect either IgG or bound complement (if polyspecific AHG reagent is used). LE antibodies can sometimes cause hemolysis in vitro, especially when fresh serum and enzyme-treated red cells are used.

Transfusion Practice

In general, LE antibodies are not considered clinically significant. Red cells that are compatible in tests at 37 C, regardless of LE phenotype, are expected to have normal in-vivo survival. It is not necessary to transfuse antigen-negative red cells in most patients. Unlike ABO antigens, LE antigens are extrinsic glycolipid antigens that are readily eluted and shed from transfused red cells within a few days of transfusion.[50] Furthermore, LE antigens in transfused plasma can neutralize LE antibodies in the recipient. For these reasons, hemolysis in vivo is very rare following transfusion of either Le(a+) or Le(b+) red cells, but exceptions occur.[53]

LE antibodies are not a cause of HDFN.[17] LE antibodies are predominantly of IgM isotype and do not cross the placenta. In addition, LE antigens are poorly expressed on neonatal red cells, with many newborns typing as Le(a–b–). However, anti-Le^a has surprisingly been associated with stillbirth.[54]

I AND i ANTIGENS OF THE I BLOOD GROUP SYSTEM (027) AND i BLOOD GROUP COLLECTION

The I and i antigens are ubiquitous, structurally related antigens present on all cell membranes. The I antigen is the only antigen in the I blood group system, while i antigen is still genetically unsolved and remains in the Ii blood group collection. The minimum epitope common to both antigens is a repeating lactosamine (Galβ1-4GlcNAc) or type 2 chain precursor. The minimum i antigen epitope is a linear, nonbranched structure containing at least two successive lactosamine motifs.[18] The I antigen is a polyvalent, branched glycan derived from the i antigen (Fig 10-5). Both i and I serve as substrates and scaffolds for the synthesis of ABH, LE^x [Galβ1-4(Fucα1-3)GlcNAc], and other type 2 chain antigens.[4,5,18] On red cells, i and I antigens are

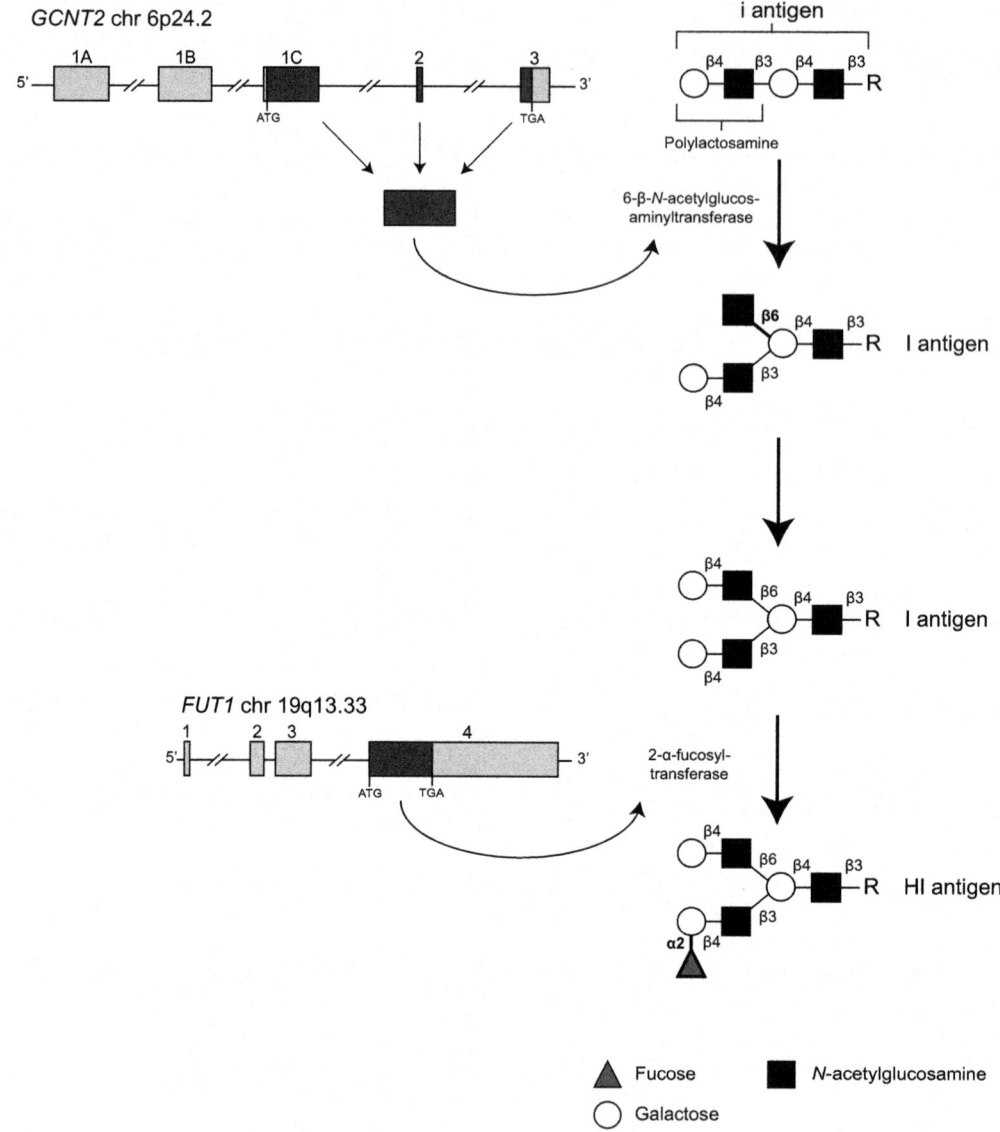

FIGURE 10-5. *GCNT2* and its erythroid transcript that gives rise to the enzyme synthesizing the I antigen from i antigen. Further elongation by *FUT1*-encoded fucosyltransferase results in the HI antigen. The linkages created by each enzyme are highlighted in bold. ATG and TGA represent the start and stop codons of the gene, respectively.
R = upstream carbohydrate sequence.

present on N-linked glycoproteins and glycosphingolipids.

Phenotypes

Two phenotypes are recognized according to the presence or absence of I antigen: I and i (I−).

The i phenotype is characteristic of neonatal red cells as well as other maturing erythroid cells, whereas I+ is the common phenotype for mature red cells as seen in an adult's peripheral circulation. With increasing age, there is a gradual increase in I antigen accompanied by a reciprocal decrease in i antigen as glycan chains are branched; most children develop an adult I+ phenotype by age 2.[18] An increase in i antigen can occur in people with chronic hemolytic disorders and is a sign of stressed erythropoiesis.[55]

Certain genetic disorders are associated with an increase in i antigen.[18] The i_{adult} phenotype (I−i+) is a rare autosomal recessive phenotype caused by mutations in the *GCNT2* (previously known as the *I* or *IGnT* gene). In patients of Asian ancestry, the i_{adult} phenotype can be associated with congenital cataract. Increased i antigen levels are also present in people with Diamond-Blackfan anemia and congenital dyserythropoietic anemia type II (also known as hereditary erythroblastic multinuclearity with positive acidified serum lysis test, or HEMPAS).

Genetics

The *GCNT2* gene encodes a β1-6-*N*-acetylglucosaminyltransferase that converts the linear i antigen into the branched I antigen.[18,26] The gene resides on chromosome 6p24 and contains five exons, including three tissue-specific exons (exons 1A, 1B, and 1C). As a result, three different messenger RNA (mRNA) transcripts are synthesized, depending on which exon 1 is used.

In the i_{adult} phenotype without cataracts, there are mutations in exon 1C, which is specific for I antigen synthesis in red cells. As a consequence, I antigen is missing on red cells but is still synthesized in other tissues that use either exon 1A or exon 1B. In the i_{adult} phenotype with cataracts, there is a loss of I antigen synthesis in all tissues, caused by either gene deletion or mutations in exons 2 and 3.

Antibodies to I and i Antigens of the I Blood Group System and i Blood Group Collection

Anti-I

Anti-I is common in the serum of healthy individuals and is typically autoreactive. Anti-I is usually of IgM isotype and is strongly reactive at 4 C with titers of <64. Samples with higher titers may also be detectable at room temperature. Anti-I is identified by strong reactions with adult red cells but weak or no agglutination with cord red cells (see Table 10-6). Anti-I can be enhanced by 4 C incubation, the presence of albumin, or use of enzyme-treated red cells. An alloanti-I can be seen in the i_{adult} phenotype.

Some examples of anti-I can demonstrate complex reactivity and are more strongly reactive with red cells of specific ABO, P_1, or LE phenotypes. Many of those antibodies appear to recognize branched oligosaccharides that have been further modified to express additional blood group antigens. Anti-HI is commonly present in the serum of A_1 individuals. Anti-HI is more strongly reactive with group O and group A_2 red cells, which are rich in H antigen, than with group A_1 red cells. Anti-HI is suspected

TABLE 10-6. Comparative Typical Serologic Behavior of Antibodies to I/i Blood Group System Antigens with Saline Red Cell Suspensions

Temperature	Cell Type	Anti-I	Anti-i
4 C	I adult	4+	0-1+
	i cord	0-2+	3+
	i adult	0-1+	4+
22 C	I adult	2+	0
	i cord	0	2-3+
	i adult	0	3+

when serum from a group A individual directly agglutinates all group O red cells but is compatible with most group A donor blood tested. Other examples of complex reactivity include anti-IA, -IP1, -IBH, and -ILe^{bH}.[40]

Anti-i

Autoanti-i is a relatively uncommon cold agglutinin in sera from healthy individuals. Like anti-I, anti-i is primarily of IgM isotype but is weakly reactive at 4 to 10 C. Anti-i is most strongly reactive with cord and i_{adult} red cells and more weakly reactive with I+ adult red cells (Table 10-6). Patients with infectious mononucleosis often have transient but potent anti-i. As with anti-I, complex reactivity can sometimes occur.

Cold Agglutinin Syndrome

Autoanti-I and autoanti-i are pathologically significant in cold agglutinin syndrome (CAS) and mixed-type autoimmune hemolytic anemia. In those disorders, autoanti-I (or anti-i) behaves as a complement-binding antibody with a high titer and wide thermal range. Primary CAS occurs with lymphoproliferative disorders (eg, Waldenström macroglobulinemia, lymphoma, and chronic lymphocytic leukemia). A potent autoanti-I can also occur in the setting of infection. *Mycoplasma pneumoniae* infections are a common cause of autoanti-I and can be accompanied by a transient intravascular hemolysis and subsequent hemoglobinuria. (See Chapter 14 for additional information on CAS.)

The specificity of the autoantibody in CAS may not be apparent when undiluted samples are tested. Titration and thermal amplitude studies may be required to discern the specificity of the autoantibodies and their potential clinical significance. Table 10-6 illustrates the serologic behavior of anti-I and anti-i at 4 C and 22 C. (See Chapters 13 and 14 and Method 4-7 for additional information regarding titration and thermal amplitude studies.)

Transfusion Practice

Autoanti-I can interfere with ABO typing, antibody detection, and compatibility testing. In laboratory testing, these antibodies can be reactive in the AHG phase of testing, particularly when polyspecific AHG is used. Such reactions rarely indicate antibody activity at 37 C but are the consequence of antibody binding, followed by complement binding, at low temperatures. Usually, avoiding room-temperature testing and using anti-IgG-specific AHG prevents detection of nuisance cold autoantibodies. For stronger antibody samples, autoantibody can be removed from serum by cold autoadsorption techniques (see Method 4-5). Cold autoadsorbed serum can also be used for ABO testing.

P1PK (003) AND GLOB (028) BLOOD GROUP SYSTEMS

The first antigen of (what was previously known as) the P blood group system was discovered by Landsteiner and Levine in 1927 in a series of experiments that also led to the discovery of M and N antigens. Because this was actually what is now called the P1 antigen (and because the P antigen belongs to another system, GLOB), it was decided in 2010 to change the name of this system to P1PK. Several related glycosphingolipid antigens belong to the P1PK system (P1, P^k, NOR) and the GLOB system (P, PX2).[26,56] In 2018, the GLOB collection was made obsolete, and the LKE antigen moved to the 901 series of antigens.[57] P^k, P, PX2, and LKE are high-prevalence antigens expressed on the red cells of nearly all individuals except in rare null phenotypes, which lack P, PX2, and LKE antigens (P^k phenotype) or P, P^k, and LKE antigens (p phenotype) (see Table 10-7), although PX2 is particularly strongly expressed on red cells of p phenotype.[58] Red cells are particularly rich in P antigen (also known as globoside), which is the most abundant neutral red cell glycolipid.[59,60] P^k and P antigens are also widely expressed on nonerythroid cells, including lymphocytes, platelets, kidney, lung, heart, endothelium, placenta, and synovium cells.[61,62] In contrast, P1 antigen seems to be mainly expressed on red cells.[61]

TABLE 10-7. Phenotypes and Prevalences in the P1PK and GLOB Group Systems

Red Cell Reactions with Antisera						Prevalence (%)		
Anti-P1	Anti-P	Anti-P^k	Anti-PP1P^k	Antibodies in Serum	Pheno-type	European Ancestry	African Ancestry	Asian Ancestry
+	+	0/+	+	None	P$_1$	79	94	20
0	+	0/±	+	Anti-P1*	P$_2$	21	6	80
0	0[†]	0	0	Anti-PP1P^k (Tj^a)	p	Rare	Rare	Rare
+	0	+	+	Anti-P, -PX2	P$_1$^{k}	Rare	Rare	Rare
0	0	+	+	Anti-P, -P1, -PX2	P$_2$^{k}	Rare	Rare	Rare

*An anti-P1 is detected in approximately 25% of P$_2$ individuals.
[†]Usually negative. Some examples of anti-P may be weakly positive as a result of cross-reactivity of anti-P with PX2 on p red cells.

Phenotypes

More than 99.9% of donors have the P$_1$ (P1+) or P$_2$ (P1–) phenotypes. (See Table 10-7.) Both phenotypes express P^k and P antigens and differ only in the expression of P1 antigen. Three rare, autosomal recessive phenotypes have been identified (p, P$_1$^{k}, P$_2$^{k}), as well as some rare weak variants.[63,64] In analogy with the ABO system, the rare p and P^k phenotypes are associated with the presence of naturally occurring antibodies against missing antigens (anti-P1, anti-P, anti-P^k, and anti-PX2).

Biochemistry

The synthesis of the P^k, P, and P1 antigens proceeds through the stepwise addition of sugars to lactosylceramide, a ceramide dihexose (CDH) (Fig 10-6 and Table 10-8). The first step in this process is the synthesis of the P^k antigen, the precursor of all globo-series glycosphingolipids. To make the P^k antigen, α1,4-galactosyltransferase (encoded by *A4GALT*) adds a terminal galactose, in an α1-4 linkage, to CDH. The P^k antigen can then serve as a substrate for β1,3-*N*-acetylgalactosaminyltransferase (encoded by *B3GALNT1*), which adds a β1-3-linked *N*-acetylgalactosamine to the terminal galactose of P^k (Gb3) to form P antigen (Gb4). In some cells, including red cells, the P antigen is further elongated to form additional, globo-family antigens, such as Luke (LKE), type 4 chain ABH antigens (globo-H, -A, and -B), and NOR. NOR+ is a rare polyagglutinable red cell phenotype and the result of unusual globo-family antigens characterized by the addition of an α1-4 galactose to the terminus of P and related long-chain globo-glycolipids (Table 10-8).[65]

Unlike P^k and P antigens, the P1 antigen is not a globo-series glycosphingolipid but a member of the neolacto family (type 2 chain glycosphingolipids). In P$_1$ individuals, *A4GALT* adds an α1-4 galactose to the terminus of paragloboside. Whether P1 antigen is present on red cell glycoproteins or not has remained unclear.[66,67] However, the P1 determinant is found on glycoproteins in other species, and paragloboside is also the precursor of H antigen, which together with A and B determinants are mostly found on N-linked glycans.[68,69] A recent study shows that, in fact, the P1 epitope is present on glycopro-

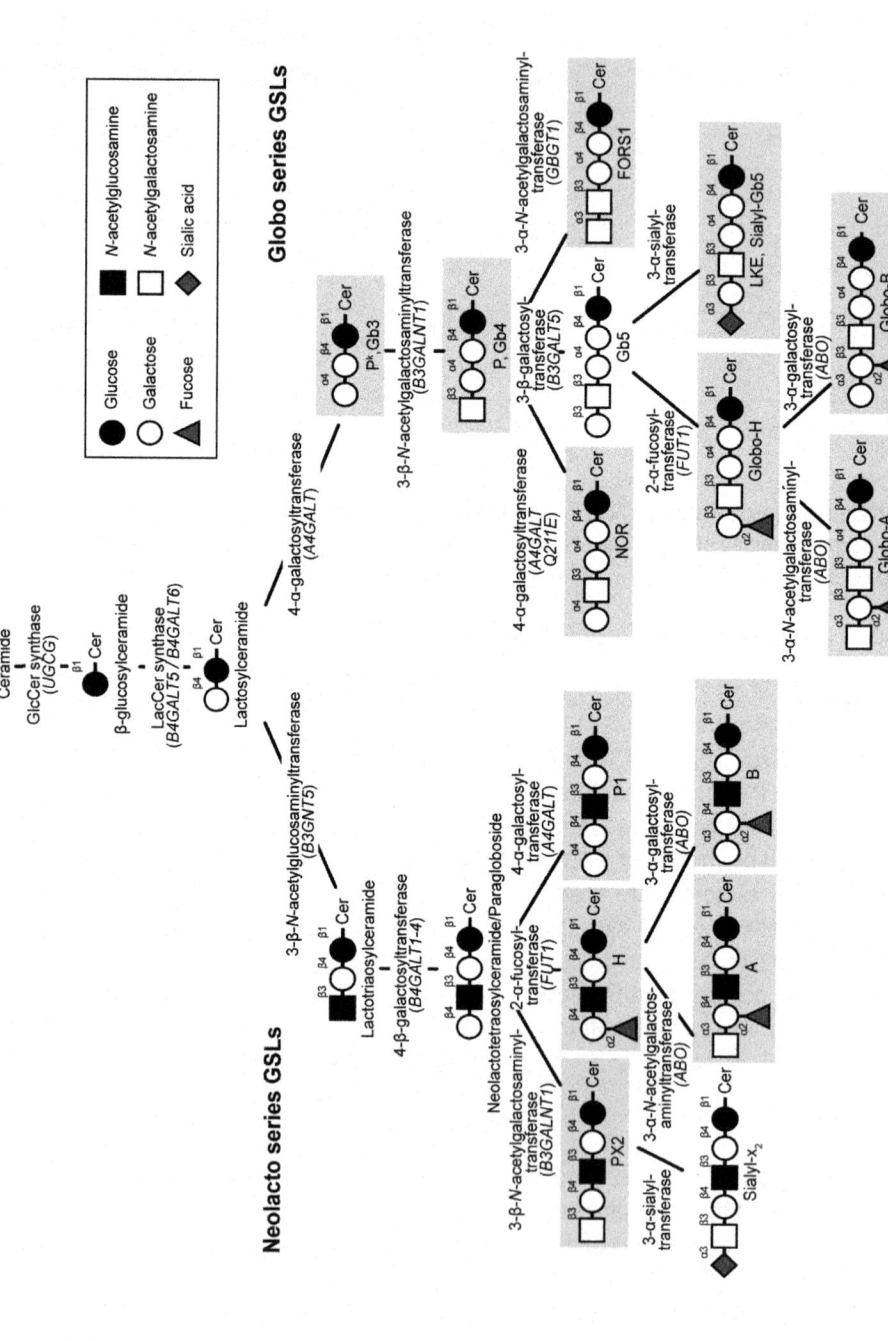

FIGURE 10-6. Synthetic pathways of glycosphingolipids in the neolacto and globo series. Structures acknowledged as blood group antigens are highlighted with a grey box. Glycosyltransferases synthesizing all glycosphingolipids depicted are included, as are the underlying genes (italicized and in brackets), if known. The ABH antigens are presented on type 2 chains in the neolacto series and as type 4 chains in the globo series. GlcCer = glucosylceramide; GSLs = glycosphingolipids; LacCer = lactosylceramide.

TABLE 10-8. Structures of Blood-Group-Carrying Molecules in the P1PK and GLOB Systems, and Related Glycosphingolipids

Family*	Name	Oligosaccharide Structure
	CDH	Galβ1-4Glcβ1-1Cer
Globo (Gb)	Gb3, Pᵏ	Galα1-4Galβ1-4Glcβ1-1Cer
	Gb4, P	GalNAcβ1-3Galα1-4Galβ1-4Glcβ1-1Cer
	Gb5	Galβ1-3GalNAcβ1-3Galα1-4Galβ1-4Glcβ1-1Cer
	NOR1	Galα1-4GalNAcβ1-3Galα1-4Galβ1-4Glcβ1-1Cer
	FORS1	GalNAcα1-3GalNAcβ1-3Galα1-4Galβ1-4Glcβ1-1Cer
	Globo-H	Fucα1-2Galβ1-3GalNAcβ1-3Galα1-4Galβ1-4Glcβ1-1Cer
	LKE	NeuAcα2-3Galβ1-3GalNAcβ1-3Galα1-4Galβ1-4Glcβ1-1Cer
	NOR2	Galα1-4GalNAcβ1-3Galα1-4GalNAcβ1-3Galα1-4Galβ1-4Glcβ1-1Cer
Neolacto (nLc)	Lc₃	GlcNAcβ1-3Galβ1-4Glcβ1-1Cer
	nLc₄, PG	Galβ1-4GlcNAcβ1-3Galβ1-4Glcβ1-1Cer
	P1	Galα1-4Galβ1-4GlcNAcβ1-3Galβ1-4Glcβ1-1Cer
	SPG	Neu5Acα2-3Galβ1-4GlcNAcβ1-3Galβ1-4Glcβ1-1Cer
	PX2 (x₂)	GalNAcβ1-3Galβ1-4GlcNAcβ1-3Galβ1-4Glcβ1-1Cer
	Sialyl-x₂	Neu5Acα2-3GalNAcβ1-3Galβ1-4GlcNAcβ1-3Galβ1-4Glcβ1-1Cer

*Glycosphingolipid family. Note: Neolacto are type 2 chain glycosphingolipids.
CDH = ceramide dihexose or lactosylceramide; Cer = ceramide; Gal = galactose; GalNAc = *N*-acetylgalactosamine; Glc = glucose, GlcNAc = *N*-acetylglucosamine; Neu5Ac = *N*-acetylneuraminic acid (sialic acid); PG = paragloboside; SPG = sialylparagloboside.

teins on human red cells.[70] The weak P-like activity on p red cells is conferred by x₂ (renamed PX2 in 2010), a related type 2 chain glycolipid. *B3GALNT1* is capable of synthesizing PX2, and this explains why PX2 is lacking on red cells of the Pᵏ phenotype.[58]

Genetics

Several inactivating mutations have been identified in both *A4GALT* and *B3GALNT1*.[26,71,72] The p phenotype is the consequence of mutations in the protein-coding sequence of *A4GALT* but can also be due to deletions in noncoding upstream exons.[73] In the absence of *A4GALT*-encoded activity, there is a loss of all globo-family and P1 antigens. These individuals have a compensatory increase in type 2 chain glycolipid synthesis, as evidenced by increased paragloboside, sialoparagloboside, and PX2.[58] Mutations in *B3GAL-NT1* give rise to the Pᵏ phenotype, which is characterized by a loss of P, LKE, and PX2 antigens and by increased Pᵏ expression.[74] The mechanism underlying the P₁ vs P₂ phenotypes has long been an enigma. Interestingly, individuals with weak P1 expression are heterozygous for P^1P^2 alleles and have fewer transcripts of $A4GALT$ as compared to homozygotes for P^1.[63] A recent study identified a transcription-factor binding site encompassing the intronic P^1/P^2-associated single nucleotide polymorphism (SNP) rs5751348 in $A4GALT$, where binding of the hematopoietic transcription factor runt-related transcription factor 1 (RUNX1) was absent on P^2 alleles.[75] In addition, another study showed binding of the transcription factor early growth response 1 (EGR1) to P^1 alleles on a motif including rs5751348.[76] To further complicate the P_1/P_2 story, haploinsufficiency for Krüppel-like factor 1 (KLF1), as seen in the In(Lu) phenotype, is connected to lowered P1 antigen expression, suggesting KLF1 involvement in $A4GALT$ regulation and P1 antigen expression.[77]

Antibodies to Antigens of the P1PK and GLOB Blood Group Systems

Anti-P1

Anti-P1 is present in the sera of one-quarter to two-thirds of P_2 donors.[40] Anti-P1 is a naturally occurring antibody of IgM isotype and is often detected as a weak, room-temperature agglutinin. In rare cases, anti-P1 is reactive at 37 C or shows in-vitro hemolysis. Because anti-P1 is nearly always IgM, anti-P1 does not cross the placenta and has not been reported to cause HDFN. Anti-P1 has only rarely been reported to cause in-vivo hemolysis. Anti-P1 titers are often elevated in patients with hydatid cyst disease or fascioliasis (liver fluke) and in bird handlers. It is believed that P1-like substance in bird excrement can stimulate anti-P1 levels. Some people with anti-P1 also have I blood group specificity (anti-IP1).[40]

P1 expression varies in strength among individuals according to genotype[63] and has been reported to decrease during in-vitro storage.[40] As a consequence, anti-P1 may not be reactive with all P1+ red cells tested. Anti-P1 can be enhanced by incubation at low temperatures (eg, 4 C) or by testing serum against enzyme-treated red cells. Anti-P1 reactivity can be inhibited in the presence of hydatid cyst fluid or P1 substance derived from pigeon eggs. Inhibiting anti-P1 activity may be helpful when testing sera containing multiple antibodies.

Alloanti-PP1P^k and Alloanti-P

Anti-PP1P^k (historically known as anti-Tj^a) is a separable mixture of anti-P, anti-P1, and anti-P^k in the sera of p individuals. Alloanti-P (and also the recently described anti-PX2[58]) is present in the sera of P_1^k and P_2^k individuals, occurs naturally, and is predominantly of IgM isotype or a mixture of IgM and IgG. (See Table 10-7.) The antibodies are potent hemolysins and are associated with hemolytic transfusion reactions and, occasionally, HDFN. There is an association between anti-PP1P^k and early, recurrent spontaneous abortions. The placenta, which is of fetal origin, is rich in P^k and P antigen and is a target for maternal cytotoxic IgG antibodies.[78]

Autoanti-P (Donath-Landsteiner)

An autoantibody with P specificity is present in patients with paroxysmal cold hemoglobinuria (PCH), a clinical syndrome that most commonly occurs in children following viral infection. In PCH, autoanti-P is an IgG biphasic hemolysin capable of binding red cells at colder temperatures, followed by intravascular hemolysis at body temperature. This characteristic can be demonstrated in vitro in the Donath-Landsteiner test (see Chapter 14 and Method 4-11).

Transfusion Practice

Alloanti-PP1P^k and alloanti-P are clinically significant antibodies associated with acute hemolytic transfusion reactions and spontaneous abortion. For transfusion, rare individuals of p and P^k phenotypes should be provided with antigen-negative, crossmatch-compatible red cells of the p and P^k phenotypes, respectively. Because P^k individuals have both anti-P and anti-PX2 in their sera, the provision of red cell units of p phenotype should be avoided even if they are P negative. The p phenotype exhibits the highest expression of PX2 of all phenotypes.[58] However, the clinical significance of anti-PX2 is not known, and p units could be considered if P^k blood is not available.

In general, anti-P1 is a clinically insignificant, room-temperature agglutinin. Patients with anti-P1, which is reactive only at room temperature or below, can safely receive P1+ red cells for transfusion, which results in normal red cell survival. It is not necessary to provide antigen-negative units to these patients. Very rarely, anti-P1 can cause decreased red cell survival and hemolytic transfusion reactions.

Anti-P1 that is capable of fixing complement at 37 C and is strongly reactive in the AHG phase of testing is considered potentially clinically significant. In such rare instances, units selected for transfusion should be nonreactive at 37 C and in an indirect antiglobulin test with either polyspecific AHG or anti-C3.[40]

THE FORS BLOOD GROUP SYSTEM (031)

Another addition to the carbohydrate blood group systems came in 2012, when the FORS system was acknowledged by ISBT. This system harbors a single low-prevalence antigen, FORS1, a glycosphingolipid synthesized by addition of *N*-acetylgalactosamine in an α1-3 linkage to the P antigen (Fig 10-6). Because this antigen bears a certain resemblance to the A antigen, which terminates with the same α1-3-linked sugar residue, some polyclonal anti-A reagents may react with FORS1-positive red cells of group O. Thus, the FORS1-positive phenotype was originally reported in 1987 as a new ABO subgroup, A_{pae}, found in three English families.[79] These red cells reacted weakly with some anti-A but were strongly positive with *Helix pomatia* lectin and negative with *Dolichos biflorus*. When *ABO* genotyping showed homozygosity for common *O* alleles, it was revealed that the reactive antigen was not A but FORS1.[80] The responsible gene is *GBGT1*, which encodes Forssman synthase, a glycosyltransferase able to create this specific linkage in many mammals. This gene had previously been considered a pseudogene in humans but was shown to be reactivated by c.887G>A (p.Arg296Gln) in FORS1-positive individuals.[80] Interestingly, most people have naturally occurring anti-FORS1 in plasma. These antibodies may cause hemolysis in vitro, but their clinical relevance is not yet known. A summary of the FORS blood group system with more information was recently published.[81]

THE SID BLOOD GROUP SYSTEM (038)

In 2019, a new carbohydrate blood group system including the Sd[a] antigen was acknowledged and designated SID (see Chapter 12).

KEY POINTS

1. The antigens of the ABO, H, LE, I, P1PK, GLOB, FORS, and SID blood group systems are defined by carbohydrate epitopes on glycoproteins and glycosphingolipids. They are synthesized by a group of Golgi-residing enzymes called glycosyltransferases and are considered histo-blood-group antigens because of their broad tissue distribution.

2. The ABO system contains four major ABO groups: A, B, O, and AB. The four phenotypes result from the combination of *ABO* alleles inherited, and are determined by the presence or absence of A and B glycosyltransferase, which synthesize A and B antigens, respectively, on red cells. An inverse reciprocal relationship exists between the presence of A and B antigens on red cells and the presence of anti-A, anti-B, or both, in sera.

3. ABO grouping requires both antigen typing of red cells for A and B antigen (red cell grouping or forward type) and typing of serum or plasma for the presence of anti-A and anti-B isoagglutinins (serum grouping or reverse type). ABO discrepancies occur when forward and reverse typing do not agree, and can be resolved with additional testing with methods to enhance missing reactivity or eliminate spurious reactivity and, if available, the use of *ABO* and *FUT1/FUT2* genotyping or gene sequencing.

4. H antigen is ubiquitously expressed on all red cells, except in the rare Bombay (O_h) phenotype, in which both H-synthesizing fucosyltransferases encoded by the *FUT1* and *FUT2* genes are inactive or absent.

5. H antigen is the precursor to both A and B antigens; thus, the amount of H antigen on red cells depends on the person's ABO group. H antigen is highly expressed on group O red cells because group O persons lack a functional *ABO* gene. In group A_1 and B persons, the amount of H antigen is considerably less because H is converted to the A and B antigens, respectively.

6. LE antigens are not synthesized by red cells but are passively adsorbed onto red cell membranes from soluble LE glycolipids present in plasma.

7. The three common LE phenotypes indicate the presence or absence of functional glycosyltransferases encoded by the *FUT3* (LE) and *FUT2* (secretor) genes.

8. As young children age, there is a gradual increase in I antigen accompanied by a reciprocal decrease in i antigen. Most children develop an adult I+ phenotype by age 2.

9. Autoanti-I and autoanti-i are pathologically significant in cold agglutinin syndrome and mixed-type autoimmune hemolytic anemia.

10. More than 99.9% of donors have the P_1 (P1+) or P_2 (P1–) phenotype. Both phenotypes synthesize P^k and P antigens and differ mainly in the expression of the P1 antigen. Other rare phenotypes (P_1^k, P_2^k, and p) exist, in which naturally occurring antibodies against P^k and P can give rise to hemolytic transfusion reactions and recurrent spontaneous abortions.

REFERENCES

1. Paulson JC, Colley KJ. Glycosyltransferases. Structure, localization, and control of cell type-specific glycosylation. J Biol Chem 1989;264 (30):17615-18.

2. Hansen SF, Bettler E, Rinnan A, et al. Exploring genomes for glycosyltransferases. Mol Biosyst 2010;6(10):1773-81.

3. Clausen H, Hakomori S. ABH and related histo-blood group antigens; Immunochemical differences in carrier isotypes and their distribution. Vox Sang 1989;56(1):1-20.

4. Lowe JB, Marth JD. A genetic approach to mammalian glycan function. Annu Rev Biochem 2003;72:643-91.

5. Marionneau S, Cailleau-Thomas A, Rocher J, et al. ABH and Lewis histo-blood group antigens, a model for the meaning of oligosaccharide diversity in the face of a changing world. Biochimie 2001;83(7):565-73.

6. Anstee DJ. The relationship between blood groups and disease. Blood 2010;115(23):4635-43.

7. Storry JR, Olsson ML. The ABO blood group system revisited: A review and update. Immunohematology 2009;25(2):48-59.

8. Rydberg L. ABO-incompatibility in solid organ transplantation. Transfus Med 2001;11(4):325-42.

9. Sazama K. Reports of 355 transfusion-associated deaths: 1976 through 1985. Transfusion 1990; 30(7):583-90.

10. Linden JV, Wagner K, Voytovich AE, Sheehan J. Transfusion errors in New York State: An analysis of 10 years' experience. Transfusion 2000; 40(10):1207-13.

11. Springer GF. Blood-group and Forssman antigenic determinants shared between microbes and mammalian cells. Prog Allergy 1971;15:9-77.

12. Daniel-Johnson J, Leitman S, Klein H, et al. Probiotic-associated high-titer anti-B in a group A platelet donor as a cause of severe hemolytic transfusion reactions. Transfusion 2009;49(9): 1845-9.

13. Daniels G. Human blood groups. 3rd ed. Oxford: Wiley-Blackwell, 2013.

14. Henry S, Oriol R, Samuelsson B. Lewis histo-blood group system and associated secretory phenotypes. Vox Sang 1995;69(3):166-82.

15. Clausen H, Levery SB, Nudelman E, et al. Repetitive A epitope (type 3 chain A) defined by blood group A1-specific monoclonal antibody TH-1: Chemical basis of qualitative A1 and A2 distinction. Proc Natl Acad Sci U S A 1985; 82(4):1199-203.

16. Svensson L, Rydberg L, de Mattos LC, Henry SM. Blood group A(1) and A(2) revisited: An im-

munochemical analysis. Vox Sang 2009;96(1):56-61.

17. Klein HG, Anstee DJ. ABO, H, LE, P1PK, GLOB, I and FORS blood group systems. In: Mollison's blood transfusion in clinical medicine. 12th ed. Oxford: Wiley-Blackwell, 2014:118-66.

18. Cooling L. Polylactosamines, there's more than meets the "Ii": A review of the I system. Immunohematology 2010;26(4):133-55.

19. Twu YC, Hsieh CY, Lin M, et al. Phosphorylation status of transcription factor C/EBPalpha determines cell-surface poly-LacNAc branching (I antigen) formation in erythropoiesis and granulopoiesis. Blood 2010;115(12):2491-9.

20. Auf der Maur C, Hodel M, Nydegger UE, Rieben R. Age dependency of ABO histo-blood group antibodies: Reexamination of an old dogma. Transfusion 1993;33(11):915-18.

21. Mazda T, Yabe R, NaThalang O, et al. Differences in ABO antibody levels among blood donors: A comparison between past and present Japanese, Laotian, and Thai populations. Immunohematology 2007;23(1):38-41.

22. Sano R, Nakajima T, Takahashi K, et al. Expression of ABO blood-group genes is dependent upon an erythroid cell-specific regulatory element that is deleted in persons with the B(m) phenotype. Blood 2012;119(22):5301-10.

23. Kronstein-Wiedemann R, Nowakowska P, Milanov P, et al. miRNA regulation of blood group ABO genes (abstract). Blood 2015;126:158.

24. Clausen H, White T, Takio K, et al. Isolation to homogeneity and partial characterization of a histo-blood group A defined Fuc alpha 1—2Gal alpha1—3-N-acetylgalactosaminyltransferase from human lung tissue. J Biol Chem 1990;265(2):1139-45.

25. Yamamoto F, Clausen H, White T, et al. Molecular genetic basis of the histo-blood group ABO system. Nature 1990;345(6272):229-33.

26. Reid ME, Lomas-Francis C, Olsson ML. The blood group antigen factsbook. 3rd ed. London: Academic Press, 2012.

27. Hosseini-Maaf B, Irshaid NM, Hellberg Å, et al. New and unusual O alleles at the ABO locus are implicated in unexpected blood group phenotypes. Transfusion 2005;45(1):70-81.

28. Seltsam A, Das Gupta C, Wagner FF, Blasczyk R. Nondeletional ABO*O alleles express weak blood group A phenotypes. Transfusion 2005;45(3):359-65.

29. Wagner FF, Blasczyk R, Seltsam A. Nondeletional ABO*O alleles frequently cause blood donor typing problems. Transfusion 2005;45(8):1331-4.

30. Möller M, Jöud M, Storry JR, Olsson ML. Erythrogene: A database for in-depth analysis of the extensive variation in 36 blood group systems in the 1000 Genomes Project. Blood Adv 2016;1(3):240-9.

31. Yazer MH, Hult AK, Hellberg Å, et al. Investigation into A antigen expression on O2 heterozygous group O-labeled red blood cell units. Transfusion 2008;48(8):1650-7.

32. Cartron JP. [Quantitative and thermodynamic study of weak A erythrocyte phenotypes]. Rev Fr Transfus Immunohematol 1976;19(1):35-54.

33. Berneman ZN, Van Bockstaele DR, Uyttenbroeck WM, et al. Flow-cytometric analysis of erythrocytic blood group A antigen density profile. Vox Sang 1991;61(4):265-74.

34. Hosseini-Maaf B, Hellberg Å, Chester MA, Olsson ML. An extensive PCR-ASP strategy for clinical ABO blood group genotyping that avoids potential errors caused by null, subgroup and hybrid alleles. Transfusion 2007;47(11):2110-25.

35. Hult AK, Olsson ML. Many genetically defined ABO subgroups exhibit characteristic flow cytometric patterns. Transfusion 2010;50(2):308-23.

36. Beck ML, Yates AD, Hardman J, Kowalski MA. Identification of a subset of group B donors reactive with monoclonal anti-A reagent. Am J Clin Pathol 1989;92(5):625-9.

37. Yazer MH, Olsson ML, Palcic MM. The cis-AB blood group phenotype: Fundamental lessons in glycobiology. Transfus Med Rev 2006;20(3):207-17.

38. Garratty G, Arndt P, Co A, et al. Fatal hemolytic transfusion reaction resulting from ABO mistyping of a patient with acquired B antigen detectable only by some monoclonal anti-B reagents. Transfusion 1996;36(4):351-7.

39. Okubo Y, Seno T, Tanaka M, et al. Conversion of group A red cells by deacetylation to ones that react with monoclonal antibodies specific for the acquired B phenotype. Transfusion 1994;34(5):456-7.

40. Issitt PD, Anstee DJ. Applied blood group serology. 4th ed. Miami, FL: Montgomery Scientific Publications, 1998.

41. Obukhova P, Korchagina E, Henry S, Bovin N. Natural anti-A and anti-B of the ABO system: Allo- and autoantibodies have different epitope specificity. Transfusion 2012;52(4):860-9.

42. Olsson ML, Irshaid NM, Hosseini-Maaf B, et al. Genomic analysis of clinical samples with serologic ABO blood grouping discrepancies: Identification of 15 novel A and B subgroup alleles. Blood 2001;98(5):1585-93.

43. Cooling LW, Sitwala K, Dake LR, et al. ABO typing discrepancies in children requiring long-term nutritional support: It is the gut after all! Transfusion 2007;47(Suppl 1):10A.

44. Shastry S, Bhat SS, Singh K. A rare case of missing antibody due to anti-snake venom. Transfusion 2009;49(12):2777-8.

45. Hult AK, Dykes JH, Storry JR, Olsson ML. A and B antigen levels acquired by group O donor-derived erythrocytes following ABO-non-identical transfusion or minor ABO-incompatible haematopoietic stem cell transplantation. Transfus Med 2017;27(3):181-91.

46. Yazer MH, Hosseini-Maaf B, Olsson ML. Blood grouping discrepancies between ABO genotype and phenotype caused by O alleles. Curr Opin Hematol 2008;15(6):618-24.

47. Mölne J, Björquist P, Andersson K, et al. Blood group ABO antigen expression in human embryonic stem cells and in differentiated hepatocyte- and cardiomyocyte-like cells. Transplantation 2008;86(10):1407-13.

48. Larson G, Svensson L, Hynsjo L, et al. Typing for the human Lewis blood group system by quantitative fluorescence-activated flow cytometry: Large differences in antigen presentation on erythrocytes between A_1, A_2, B, O phenotypes. Vox Sang 1999;77(4):227-36.

49. Hosoi E, Hirose M, Hamano S. Expression levels of H-type alpha(1,2)-fucosyltransferase gene and histo-blood group ABO gene corresponding to hematopoietic cell differentiation. Transfusion 2003;43(1):65-71.

50. Combs MR. Lewis blood group system review. Immunohematology 2009;25(3):112-18.

51. Cooling L. Carbohydrate blood group antigens and collections. In: Cooling L, Davenport R, Schwartz J. eds. Transfusion medicine: Key concepts in a changing world. Bethesda, MD: AABB Press, 2020 (in press).

52. Lindström K, Breimer ME, Jovall PA, et al. Nonacid glycosphingolipid expression in plasma of an A1 Le(a-b+) secretor human individual: Identification of an ALeb heptaglycosylceramide as major blood group component. J Biochem 1992; 111(3):337-45.

53. Höglund P, Rosengren-Lindquist R, Wikman AT. A severe haemolytic transfusion reaction caused by anti-Le(a) active at 37 degrees C. Blood Transfus 2013;11(3):456-9.

54. Fan J, Lee BK, Wikman AT, et al. Associations of Rhesus and non-Rhesus maternal red blood cell alloimmunization with stillbirth and preterm birth. Int J Epidemiol 2014;43(4):1123-31.

55. Navenot JM, Muller JY, Blanchard D. Expression of blood group i antigen and fetal hemoglobin in paroxysmal nocturnal hemoglobinuria. Transfusion 1997;37(3):291-7.

56. Storry JR, Castilho L, Chen Q, et al. International Society of Blood Transfusion Working Party on Red Cell Immunogenetics and Terminology: Report of the Seoul and London meetings. ISBT Sci Ser 2016;11(2):118-22.

57. Storry JR, Clausen FB, Castilho L, et al. International Society of Blood Transfusion Working Party on Red Cell Immunogenetics and Blood Group Terminology: Report of the Dubai, Copenhagen and Toronto meetings. Vox Sang 2019;114(1):95-102.

58. Westman JS, Benktander J, Storry JR, et al. Identification of the molecular and genetic basis of PX2, a glycosphingolipid blood group antigen lacking on globoside-deficient erythrocytes. J Biol Chem 2015;290(30):18505-18.

59. Fletcher KS, Bremer EG, Schwarting GA. P blood group regulation of glycosphingolipid levels in human erythrocytes. J Biol Chem 1979; 254(22):11196-8.

60. Suzuki A, Kundu SK, Marcus DM. An improved technique for separation of neutral glycosphingolipids by high-performance liquid chromatography. J Lipid Res 1980;21(4):473-7.

61. Cooling L, Downs T. Immunohematology. In: McPherson RA, Pincus MR, eds. Henry's clinical diagnosis and management by laboratory methods. Philadelphia: Saunders, 2007:618-68.

62. Dunstan RA. Status of major red cell blood group antigens on neutrophils, lymphocytes and monocytes. Br J Haematol 1986;62(2):301-9.

63. Thuresson B, Westman JS, Olsson ML. Identification of a novel *A4GALT* exon reveals the genetic basis of the P_1/P_2 histo-blood groups. Blood 2011;117(2):678-87.

64. Cooling L, Dake LR, Haverty D, et al. A hemolytic anti-LKE associated with a rare LKE-negative, "weak P" red blood cell phenotype: Alloanti-LKE and alloanti-P recognize galactosylgloboside and monosialogalactosylgloboside (LKE) antigens. Transfusion 2015;55(1):115-28.

65. Duk M, Singh S, Reinhold VN, et al. Structures of unique globoside elongation products present

in erythrocytes with a rare NOR phenotype. Glycobiology 2007;17(3):304-12.

66. Haselberger CG, Schenkel-Brunner H. Evidence for erythrocyte membrane glycoproteins being carriers of blood-group P1 determinants. FEBS Lett 1982;149(1):126-8.

67. Yang Z, Bergström J, Karlsson KA. Glycoproteins with Galα 4Gal are absent from human erythrocyte membranes, indicating that glycolipids are the sole carriers of blood group P activities. J Biol Chem 1994;269(20):14620-4.

68. Khoo KH, Nieto A, Morris HR, Dell A. Structural characterization of the N-glycans from Echinococcus granulosus hydatid cyst membrane and protoscoleces. Mol Biochem Parasitol 1997; 86(2):237-48.

69. Suzuki N, Yamamoto K. Molecular cloning of pigeon UDP-galactose:β-D-galactoside α1,4-galactosyltransferase and UDP-galactose:β-D-galactoside β1,4-galactosyltransferase, two novel enzymes catalyzing the formation of Galα1-4Galβ1-4Galβ1-4GlcNAc sequence. J Biol Chem 2010;285(8):5178-87.

70. Stenfelt L, Westman JS, Hellberg Å, Olsson ML. The P1 histo-blood group antigen is present on human red blood cell glycoproteins. Transfusion 2019;59(3):1108-17.

71. Hellberg Å, Ringressi A, Yahalom V, et al. Genetic heterogeneity at the glycosyltransferase loci underlying the GLOB blood group system and collection. Br J Haematol 2004;125(4):528-36.

72. Ricci Hagman J, Hult AK, Westman JS, et al. Multiple miscarriages in two sisters of Thai origin with the rare P^k phenotype caused by a novel nonsense mutation at the *B3GALNT1* locus. Transfus Med 2019;29(3):202-8.

73. Westman JS, Hellberg Å, Peyrard T, et al. Large deletions involving the regulatory upstream regions of *A4GALT* give rise to principally novel P1PK-null alleles. Transfusion 2014;54(7):1831-5.

74. Hellberg Å, Poole J, Olsson ML. Molecular basis of the globoside-deficient P^k blood group phenotype. Identification of four inactivating mutations in the UDP-*N*-acetylgalactosamine: globotriaosylceramide 3-β-*N*-acetylgalactosaminyltransferase gene. J Biol Chem 2002;277: 29455-9.

75. Westman JS, Stenfelt L, Vidovic K, et al. Allele-selective RUNX1 binding regulates P1 blood group status by transcriptional control of *A4GALT*. Blood 2018;131(14):1611-16.

76. Yeh CC, Chang CJ, Twu YC, et al. The differential expression of the blood group *P^1-A4GALT* and *P^2-A4GALT* alleles is stimulated by the transcription factor early growth response 1. Transfusion 2018;58(4):1054-64.

77. Eernstman JV, Heshusius S, Philipsen M, et al. KLF1 regulates P1 expression through transcriptional control of *A4GALT* (abstract). Vox Sang 2017;112(S1):25.

78. Lindström K, van dem Borne AE, Breimer ME, et al. Glycosphingolipid expression in spontaneously aborted fetuses and placenta from blood group p women. Evidence for placenta being the primary target for anti-Tj^a-antibodies. Glycoconj J 1992;9(6):325-9.

79. Stamps R, Sokol RJ, Leach M, et al. A new variant of blood group A: Apae. Transfusion 1987; 27(4):315-18.

80. Svensson L, Hult AK, Stamps R, et al. Forssman expression on human erythrocytes: Biochemical and genetic evidence of a new histo-blood group system. Blood 2013;121(8):1459-68.

81. Hult AK, Olsson ML. The FORS awakens: Review of a blood group system reborn. Immunohematology 2017;33(2):64-72.

CHAPTER 11

The Rh System

Thierry Peyrard, PharmD, PhD, EurSpLM, and Franz F. Wagner, MD

T HE RH SYSTEM IS COMPOSED OF two genes, each encoding a polypeptide, that together are responsible for the expression of 55 antigens (Table 11-1). The blood group system name is Rh, and the international symbol is RH. The attention to red cell alloimmunization relative to this system stems from the D antigen, which is the most immunogenic of all minor blood group antigens. The transfusion of D-positive Red Blood Cells (RBCs) to D-negative individuals results in an immunization rate of 80% to 90% in healthy volunteers,[1] and 20% to 50% in patients.[2-4]

Anti-D remains a major cause of severe hemolytic disease of the fetus and newborn (HDFN). A true success story in transfusion medicine therapy in the mid-1960s, the development of Rh Immune Globulin (RhIG) prophylaxis, arose partly from the observation that ABO incompatibility between a mother and fetus had a partial protective effect against immunization to D.[5] The administration of immunoglobulin G (IgG) anti-D obtained from human plasma was effective in the prevention of HDFN.[6] With the use of RhIG, alloimmunization to D in pregnancy has been reduced to occur in about 1 in 4000 live births.[7] Once a woman has become anti-D immunized, RhIG does not prevent strengthening of the anti-D during pregnancy. The high anti-D immunization risk, the impact of alloimmunization in D-negative females

of childbearing potential, and the significant risk of harm to a D-positive fetus make D antigen-matching a routine practice in transfusion medicine.

HISTORICAL PERSPECTIVE

The clinical impact of the D antigen dates to 1939, when Levine and Stetson made the key observation that the serum of a pregnant woman agglutinated some 80% of ABO-compatible samples. The authors proposed that "products of the disintegrating fetus" and an adverse transfusion reaction in the mother to a blood transfusion from her husband were related to the hemagglutinin found in her serum.[8] Landsteiner and Wiener used an antiserum from guinea pigs immunized with red cells from Rhesus macaques to distinguish "Rh-positive" and "Rh-negative" red cells. The fact that this serum probably represented an anti-LW (LW antigen is increased in D-positive red cells) and the failure of Levine to name their antigen triggered a fierce debate about who really discovered Rh. A good historical account of the confusion of the D antigen with the LW system has been described by Rosenfield.[9]

"Rh-positive" and "Rh-negative" refer to the D antigen status of red cells. The D and ABO antigens are the principal antigens matched for

Thierry Peyrard, PharmD, PhD, EurSpLM, Head of Department, National Immunohematology Reference Laboratory, and Assistant Director, Medical and Scientific Director, National Institute of Blood Transfusion, Paris, France; and Franz F. Wagner, MD, Priv-Doz, Head of Laboratory, Red Cross Blood Service NSTOB, Springe, Germany, and Medical Director, ambulatory health-care center Clementinenkrankenhaus, Springe, Germany

T. Peyrard has disclosed no conflicts of interest. F. Wagner receives royalties from patents on the molecular structure of Rh.

TABLE 11-1. Rh Antigens by Common Name, ISBT Terminology, and Prevalence

Antigen	ISBT Terminology Number	ISBT Terminology Symbol	Prevalence	Comment
D	004.001	RH1	Common	85%/92% Whites/Blacks
C	004.002	RH2	Common	68%/27% Whites/Blacks
E	004.003	RH3	Common	29%/22% Whites/Blacks
c	004.004	RH4	Common	80%/96% Whites/Blacks
e	004.005	RH5	98%	
ce or f	004.006	RH6	Common	65%/92% Whites/Blacks
Ce or rh_i	004.007	RH7	Common	68%/27% Whites/Blacks
C^w	004.008	RH8	2%	Whites
C^x	004.009	RH9	~2%	Finns
V	004.010	RH10	30%	Blacks
E^w	004.011	RH11	Low	
G	004.012	RH12*	Common	84%/92% Whites/Blacks
…	…	RH13-RH16	…	Obsolete
Hr_0	004.017	RH17[†]	High	
Hr or Hr^S	004.018	RH18[‡]	High	Hr^S– in Blacks
hr^S	004.019	RH19[§]	98%	hr^S– in Blacks
VS	004.020	RH20	Low	32% Blacks
C^G	004.021	RH21	Common	68% Whites
CE	004.022	RH22	Low	<1%
D^w	004.023	RH23[◊]	Low	on DVa
…	…	RH24/RH25	…	Obsolete
c-like	004.026	RH26	High	
cE	004.027	RH27	Common	28%/22% Whites/Blacks
hr^H	004.028	RH28	Low	
total Rh	004.029	RH29[¶]	High	100% except Rh_{null}

TABLE 11-1. Rh Antigens by Common Name, ISBT Terminology, and Prevalence (Continued)

Antigen	ISBT Terminology		Prevalence	Comment
	Number	**Symbol**		
Go^a	004.030	RH30$^\diamond$	Low	Blacks
hr^B	004.031	RH31§	98%	hr^B– in Blacks
Rh32	004.032	RH32$^\#$	Low	Blacks, on DBT
Ro^{Har}, DHAR	004.033	RH33	Low	<1%, Germans
Hr^B	004.034	RH34**	High	Hr^B– in Blacks
Rh35	004.035	RH35	Low	
Be^a	004.036	RH36	Low	
Evans	004.037	RH37	Low	on D/CE hybrids
...	...	RH38	...	Obsolete
C-like	004.039	RH39	High	
Tar	004.040	RH40	Low	on DVII
Ce-like	004.041	RH41	High	70% Whites
Ce^S	004.042	RH42	Low	2% Blacks
Crawford	004.043	RH43	Low	0.1% Blacks
Nou	004.044	RH44	High	
Riv	004.045	RH45	Low	
Sec	004.046	RH46	High	Sec– in Blacks
Dav	004.047	RH47	High	
JAL	004.048	RH48	Low	
STEM	004.049	RH49††	Low	6% Blacks
FPTT	004.050	RH50	Low	on DFR, R$_0^{Har}$
MAR	004.051	RH51	High	Finns
BARC	004.052	RH52$^\diamond$	Low	on DVI
JAHK	004.053	RH53	Low	

(Continued)

TABLE 11-1. Rh Antigens by Common Name, ISBT Terminology, and Prevalence (Continued)

Antigen	ISBT Terminology Number	ISBT Terminology Symbol	Prevalence	Comment
DAK	004.054	RH54$^{\Diamond}$	Low	Blacks (on DIII^a, DOL, R^N)
LORC	004.055	RH55	Low	
CENR	004.056	RH56	Low	
CEST	004.057	RH57	High	Antithetical to JAL, CEST– in Blacks
CELO	004.058	RH58	High	Antithetical to RH43, CELO– in Blacks
CEAG	004.059	RH59	High	CEAG– in Blacks
PARG	004.060	RH60	Low	
CEVF	004.061	RH61	High	CEFV– in Blacks
CEWA	004.062	RH62*	High	

*Present on red cells expressing C or D antigen.
†Antibody made by individuals with D-deletion phenotypes D––, Dc–, and DC^w–.
‡Antibody made by individuals with altered e and/or D phenotypes prevalent in groups of African ancestry.
§Absent from red cells with DcE/DcE (R$_2$R$_2$) phenotype or variant e found in groups of African ancestry.
$^{\Diamond}$Low-prevalence antigen associated with the partial D indicated.
¶Antibody made by individuals with Rh$_{null}$ red cells.
#Low-prevalence antigen expressed by red cells with R^N or the partial DBT antigen.[1]
**Antibody made by individuals with altered C, e, and/or D phenotypes prevalent in groups of African ancestry.
††Associated with 65% of hr^S– Hr^S– and 30% of hr^B– Hr^B– red cells.

transfusion. Along with the D antigen, four Rh antigens—antithetical C/c and E/e, named by Fisher using the next available letters of the alphabet—are responsible for the majority of clinically significant Rh antibodies. In sickle cell patients, antibodies to high-prevalence Rh antigens such as Hr^S and Hr^B may be a major obstacle to transfusion support.[10]

Rh proteins, unlike most membrane proteins, are neither glycosylated nor phosphorylated.[11,12] The use of immunoprecipitation followed by sodium dodecylsulfate polyacrylamide gel electrophoresis led to the discovery that Rh proteins have a molecular weight of 30,000 to 32,000 kDa.[13,14] N-terminal amino acid sequencing of Rh was accomplished in the late 1980s.[15] The findings led to the cloning of the RHCE gene in 1990[16] and of the RHD gene in 1992.[17,18] The genetic basis of four different RHCE alleles was identified in 1993[19] and confirmed in 1994.[20]

TERMINOLOGY

Early Rh nomenclature reflects the differences in opinion concerning the number of genes that encode DCEce antigens. The Fisher-Race terminology was based on the premise that three closely linked genes, *C/c*, *E/e*, and *D*, were responsible. In contrast, the Wiener nomenclature (Rh-Hr) was based on the belief that a single gene encoded several blood group factors. However, the Rh system is composed of two genes, as first proposed by Tippett.[21]

The Fisher-Race DCE terminology is often preferred for written communication, but a modified version of Wiener's nomenclature makes it possible to identify the Rh antigens present on one chromosome using a single term, that is, using a haplotype (Table 11-2). In the modified Wiener's nomenclature, "R" indicates that D is present, and a number or letter indicates the C/c and E/e antigens: R_1 for Ce, R_2 for cE, R_0 for ce, and R_z for CE. The lowercase "r" indicates haplotypes lacking D, with the C/c and E/e antigens indicated using symbols: r′ for Ce, r″ for cE, and r^y for CE (Table 11-2).

The International Society of Blood Transfusion (ISBT) Working Party on Red Cell Immunogenetics and Blood Group Terminology adopted six-digit numbers to indicate red cell antigens. The first three numbers represent the system, and the remaining three digits refer to the antigenic specificity; the Rh system was assigned number 004, with RH as the international symbol. The Rh system has recorded 62 antigens, with 7 antigens deemed obsolete. The true antigenic variability is even higher, as epitopes missing in partial D and some RhCE antigens are not given separate antigen numbers. (See Table 9-4 in Chapter 9 for examples of ISBT terminology for blood group antigens, alleles, and phenotypes.)

RH LOCUS

Chromosomal Structure

The Rh antigens are located on two proteins, RhD and RhCE, encoded by two genes, *RHD* and *RHCE*, closely linked near the 3′ end of chromosome 1p36.11. *RHD* and *RHCE* are oriented in a tail-to-tail arrangement: telomere – 5′-*RHD*-3′ – 3′-*RHCE*-5′ – centromere. A blood group irrelevant gene, *TMEM50A*, is located between *RHD* and *RHCE* and partially overlaps the

TABLE 11-2. Prevalence of the Principal Rh Haplotypes

Fisher-Race Haplotype	Modified Wiener Haplotype	Prevalence (%)		
		White	Black	Asian
Rh positive				
DCe	R_1	42	17	70
DcE	R_2	14	11	21
Dce	R_0	4	44	3
DCE	R_z	<0.01	<0.01	1
Rh negative				
ce	r	37	26	3
Ce	r′	2	2	2
cE	r″	1	<0.01	<0.01
CE	r^y	<0.01	<0.01	<0.01

3' end of *RHCE*. In addition, another gene, *RSRP1*, completely overlaps *RHD* but has opposite orientation [Fig 11-1 (A)]. *RHD* likely arose from *RHCE* in a duplication event.[22] Both genes have 10 exons, and overall they share 97% sequence identity in the coding region.

Segmental nucleotide exchanges are common between *RHD* and *RHCE* and, conversely, and are thought to be facilitated by the opposite orientation of *RHD* and *RHCE*.[23] One gene acts as a donor template during replication but remains unchanged in the process (so-called gene conversion mechanism). The donated region can be one nucleotide or span several base pairs (bp), single exons, or multiple exons, typically leading to *RHD-CE-D* or *RHCE-D-CE* hybrid alleles.

Gene Products (Rh Proteins)

RHD encodes the D antigen, and *RHCE* encodes the CcEe antigens in four combinations (ce, cE, Ce, or CE). Both genes encode 417 amino acids. The two polypeptides encoded by *RHD* vs *RHCE* differ by 32 to 35 amino acids, depending on whether RhD is compared to RhC or Rhc. The last decade has witnessed the development of an abundance of information on the genetic diversity of the *RH* locus, and antigen variants identified by DNA-based testing have far exceeded the number identified by serology. More than 500 *RHD* and 150 *RHCE* alleles with an impact on the Rh phenotype have been documented. A directory of *RHD* alleles is maintained by the RhesusBase database,[24] and on the ISBT website, where the Working Party on Red Cell Immunogenetics and Blood Group Terminology maintains, names, and catalogs new alleles.[25]

Most D-negative (Rh-negative) phenotypes are the result of complete deletion of the *RHD* gene, likely through a nonsister chromatid exchange involving regions termed the "Rhesus boxes," which flank *RHD* [Fig 11-1 (B)].[23] The result is a "hybrid Rhesus box" that may be used for direct detection of the *RHD* deleted allele. The absence of the whole *RHD* gene encoding the RhD protein explains why exposure of D-negative individuals to D-positive red cells results in a robust immune response. Indeed, RhD

differs from the next most similar protein, RhCE, in several amino acids, allowing for many possible T-cell stimulating peptides and exposing many immunogenic epitopes.

RHCE is found in all but rare D-- individuals (the dashes represent missing C/c and E/e antigens) and encodes both C/c and E/e antigens on a single protein (Ce, cE, ce, or CE). The E and e antigens differ by one amino acid: a proline or alanine at position 226 (p.Pro226Ala), located on the fourth extracellular loop of the protein. Most C-positive haplotypes derive from the c-positive haplotypes by a gene conversion leading to an *RHD*-like segment surrounding exon 2 in *RHCE*; this mechanism explains both the large number of amino acid differences between C and c (p.Trp16Cys, p.Leu60Ile, p.Asn68Ser, p.Ser103Pro) and the molecular basis of the G antigen (p.Ser130), expressed both by RhD and C from RhCE.

The five principal antigens are responsible for the majority of Rh incompatibilities, although the Rh system as a whole is more complex (Table 11-1). New antigens may result from single nucleotide polymorphisms (SNPs) or major gene rearrangements. For example, the genetic exchanges between *RHD* and *RHCE* can create hybrid proteins that express an RhD protein with a portion of RhCE, or vice versa.

RHD GENOTYPE

Inheritance studies of the five principal Rh antigens have been used to determine Rh haplotypes (Table 11-3) and to predict *RHD* zygosity: in many populations, the D-negative haplotype is associated with ce, while the D-positive haplotypes carry C or E. However, alternate haplotypes like Ce and Dce exist and prevent a meaningful prediction in some populations (eg, the frequencies of R_0R_0 vs R_0r are nearly identical in persons of African ancestry). Moreover, the use of inferred haplotype frequencies in multiethnic societies makes prediction of *RHD* zygosity uncertain. The strength of anti-D hemagglutination cannot reliably show a difference between a single or a double dose of the D antigen: less D antigen is expressed when the C antigen is present, a phenomenon called the "Ceppellini

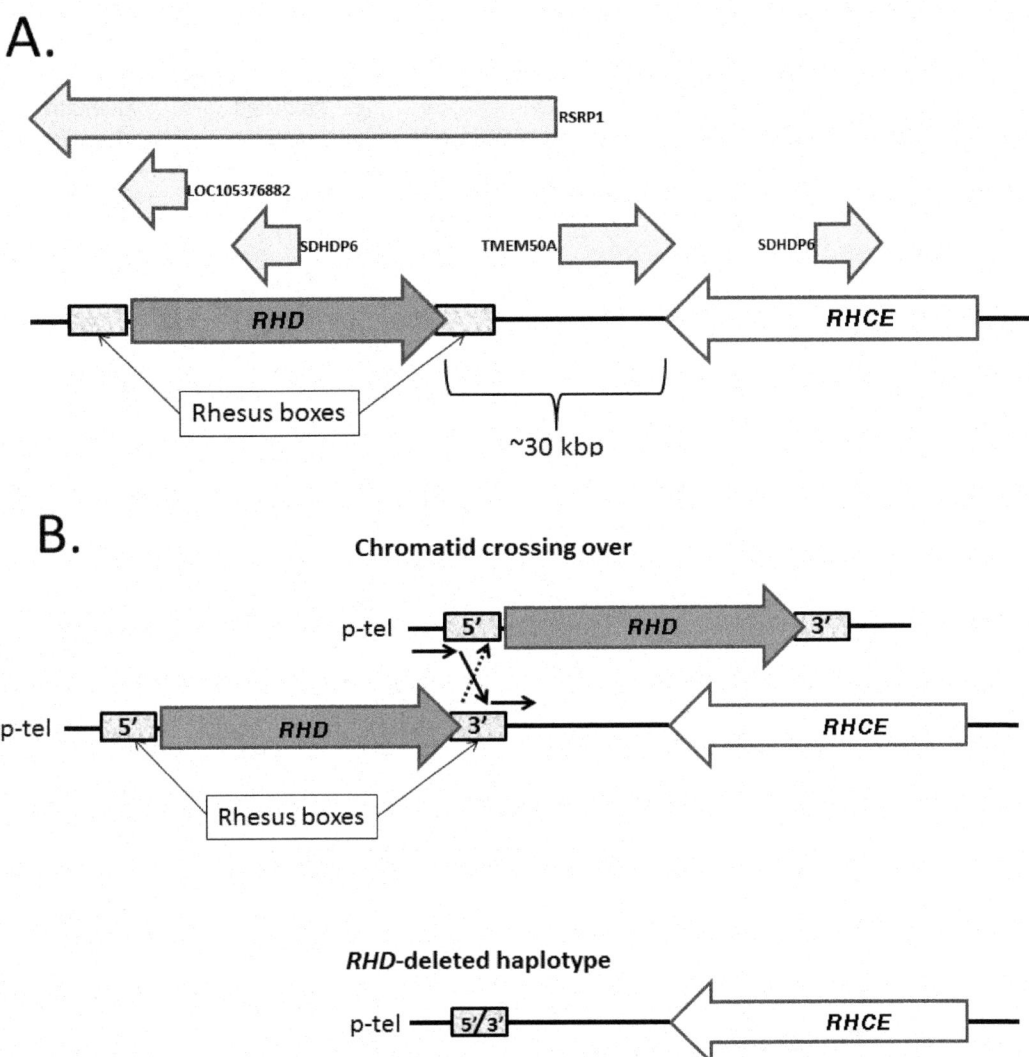

FIGURE 11-1. The *RH* locus. (A) Organization of *RHD* and *RHCE* in the short arm (p) region of chromosome 1p36.11. The two genes are each approximately 55,000 base pairs (bp) in size and are separated by approximately 30,000 bp (~30 kpb). *RHD* is flanked by two long homologous regions (Rhesus boxes) of approximately 9000 bp. The orientation of the *RH* locus is: p-telomere (p-tel) – *RHD* – *RHCE*. Other genes are in the region but are irrelevant to the expression of Rh. (B) The origin of the *RHD*-deleted haplotype. During meiosis, a chromatid crossing-over misalignment occurs between the upstream Rhesus box (5′) of one chromatid and downstream Rhesus box (3′) of another (upper figure). An *RHD*-deleted haplotype (lower figure) results from the resolution of the chromatid exchange (solid arrows), with the formation of a hybrid Rhesus box (5′/3′). The alternate haplotype, two *RHD* in tandem (hatch arrow), has not been observed.

TABLE 11-3. Results of Tests with Five Principal Rh Antisera with Phenotype and Predicted RH Genotype

Antisera							
Anti-D	Anti-C	Anti-E	Anti-c	Anti-e	Phenotype	Predicted Genotype*	Alternative Genotype
Rh positive[†]							
+	+	0	+	+	D, C, c, e	*R1 r*	*R1 R0*
						DCe/ce	*DCe/Dce*
							R0 r'
							Dce/Ce
+	+	0	0	+	D, C, e	*R1 R1*	*R1 r'*
						DCe/DCe	*DCe/Ce*
+	+	+	+	+	D, C, c, E, e	*R1 R2*	*R1 r''*
						DCe/DcE	*DCe/cE*
							R2 r'
							DcE/Ce
							Rz r
							DCE/ce
							R0 Rz
							Dce/DCE
+	0	0	+	+	D, c, e	*R0 r*	*R0 R0*
						Dce/ce	*Dce/Dce*
+	0	+	+	+	D, c, E, e	*R2 r*	*R2 R0*
						DcE/ce	*DcE/Dce*
							R0 r''
							Dce/cE
+	0	+	+	0	D, c, E	*R2 R2*	*R2 r''*
						DcE/DcE	*DcE/cE*
+	+	+	0	+	D, C, E, e	*R1 Rz*	*Rz r'*
						DCe/DCE	*DCE/Ce*
+	+	+	+	0	D, C, c, E	*R2 Rz*	*Rz r''*
						DcE/DCE	*DCE/cE*
+	+	+	0	0	D, C, E	*Rz Rz*	*Rz r^y*
						DCE/DCE	*DCE/CE*

TABLE 11-3. Results of Tests with Five Principal Rh Antisera with Phenotype and Predicted RH Genotype (Continued)

Antisera							
Anti-D	Anti-C	Anti-E	Anti-c	Anti-e	Phenotype	Predicted Genotype*	Alternative Genotype
Rh negative‡							
0	0	0	+	+	c, e	*r r*	
						ce/ce	
0	+	0	+	+	C, c, e	*r′ r*	
						Ce/ce	
0	0	+	+	+	c, E, e	*r″ r*	
						cE/ce	
0	+	+	+	+	C, c, E, e	*r′ r″*	
						Ce/cE	

*Each genotype is shown in both Wiener and Fisher-Race nomenclature.

†Rare genotypes (*R0 r^y*, *R1 r^y*, and *R2 r^y*) not shown (prevalence of <0.01%).

‡Rare genotypes (*rr^y*, *r′r^y*, *r″r^y*, and *r^yr^y*) not shown (prevalence of <0.01%).

effect."[26] This effect is seen both in *cis* [less D antigen is expressed in DCe/DCe (R_1R_1) individuals than in DcE/DcE (R_2R_2) individuals] and in *trans* [less D antigen is expressed in DCe/Ce (R_1r?) individuals than in DCe/ce (R_1r) individuals]. *RHD* homozygous (*RHD/RHD*) DCe/DCe (R_1R_1) red cells express about as much D antigen as hemizygous (*RHD/–*) DcE/ce (R_2r) red cells. For this reason, it is important to choose red cells with the same Rh phenotype when performing serial anti-D titrations in the antenatal setting because significantly different titers can be obtained if the red cells differ in their underlying zygosity. *RHD* zygosity (see below) can be determined by DNA-based testing. However, depending on the population, in addition to the *RHD* deletion, many different nonfunctional *RHD* alleles have to be detected.[27,28]

ANTIGENS

Manufactured licensed reagents are available to detect the expression of the principal Rh antigens—D, C, c, E, and e (Table 11-3). D antigen phenotyping is routinely performed on donors

and patients. Testing for the common CcEe antigens is performed primarily during antibody investigations or to provide antigen-matched blood for certain chronic transfusion recipients, such as patients with sickle cell disease (SCD) and thalassemia, to minimize alloimmunization.[29] In many European countries, CcEe typing of donors is standard, allowing for widespread use of CcEe-matched transfusion strategies (eg, in women of childbearing potential).

D Antigen

Tests with partial D red cells revealed that monoclonal anti-D reagents bind to numerous different epitopes. The main epitopes are designated epD1 to epD9. Each epitope has additional subdivisions (eg, epD6.1), leading to at least 30 different D epitopes. Most D epitopes are highly conformational and consist of more than simple linear amino acid residues.

D-Positive (Rh-Positive) Phenotypes

Most individuals with a D-positive red cell phenotype express a conventional RhD protein. However, >500 *RHD* alleles have been reported that encode amino acid changes. These alleles can cause numerous variations in the expression of D antigen, and red cells with some form of altered D expression are encountered in routine transfusion practice. An estimated 1% of individuals of European ancestry carry only *RHD* alleles that encode altered D antigens, and the incidence in individuals of African ancestry is much higher (up to 30% in some populations[30]). Altered D is organized into four groups: weak D, partial D (including category D), Del, and nonfunctional *RHD*.[31]

Weak D Types. Traditionally, the weak D phenotype was defined as red cells with a reduced amount of D antigen that required an indirect antiglobulin test (IAT) for detection (formerly called D[u]). However, the number of samples identified as having weak D expression depends on the typing reagent and method used, which have changed over the years. The vast majority of such samples carry *RHD* alleles that encode for proteins with amino acid changes predicted to be located within the intracellular or transmembrane region of the protein, rather than on the exofacial domain of the RhD protein.[32] (See Fig 11-2.) Wagner and Flegel (et al)[32] proposed a system to classify altered D red cells on the basis of their nucleotide substitutions (reviewed in Flegel and Denomme[35]). Not included in the definition is whether a person with a weak D type can or cannot make alloanti-D.

Generally, intracellular and transmembraneous amino acid changes are thought to affect the insertion of the polypeptide into the membrane and thus result in a reduced number of D-antigen sites on the red cells. More than 150 weak D types are distinguished.[24] Other mechanisms leading to diminished D antigen expression without major antigenic changes are mutations interfering with splicing[36] and deletions[37] or duplications[38] of *RHD* exons. In persons of European ancestry, the most common is weak D type 1, which has a valine-to-glycine amino acid substitution at position 270 (p.Val270Gly). Types 1, 2, and 3 represent

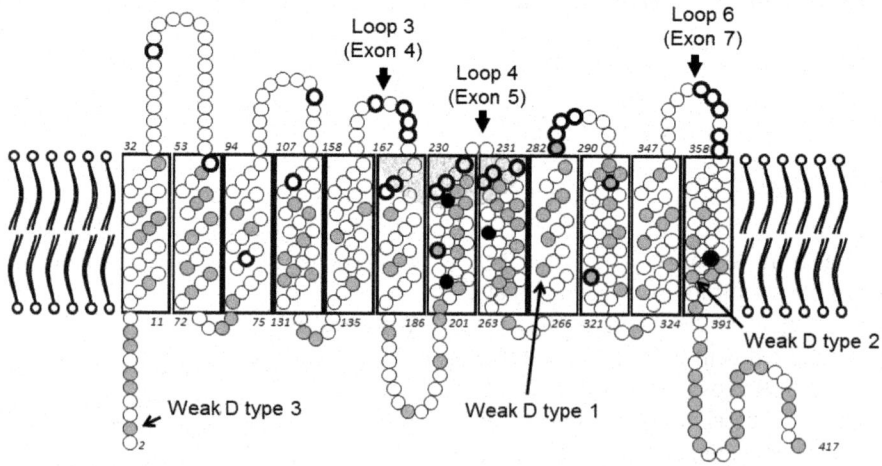

FIGURE 11-2. Structural models of weak D (according to RhesusBase[24]) and partial D (according to the ISBT listing of normal and partial D[25]). The locations of amino acid changes in alleles with single amino acid substitutions are indicated by gray disks for weak D and black rings for partial D. Black disks indicate alleles with unknown phenotype, normal D phenotype, or disputed partial D phenotype. The position of exofacial loops 3, 4, and 6 (encoded by *RHD* exons 4, 5, and 7) that harbor exofacial differences between RhD and RhCE are indicated by thick arrows. Weak D types 1, 2, and 3 (position indicated by thin arrows) are found in approximately 90% of people of European ancestry with weak D phenotypes. Partial D types are encoded by single amino acid changes that are generally present on the exterior (erythrocyte surface) of the cell. (Adapted from Flegel[33] and Wagner.[34])

approximately 90% of the weak D types.[32] Weak D types can be further weakened when C is present in *trans* to a weak D type (Ceppellini effect); for example, r′ in *trans* with weak D type 2 (R_2r').[39]

Partial D Types. Individuals with partial D type express D antigen on their red cells but may form alloanti-D. Initially, partial D types were grouped into different "category D" types (category II to VII) based on the mutual reactivity with their respective alloanti-D.[40] Nowadays, mostly monoclonal anti-D is used to investigate D epitope expression, and the molecular heterogeneity has been even greater than anticipated. Several molecular mechanisms underlie this phenotype.

First, many partial D types initially recognized as D categories were due to *RHD-CE-D* hybrid alleles that code for RhD proteins lacking RhD-specificity amino acids in certain protein parts. The phenotype is determined mainly by the origin of exons 4, 5, and 7 that encode for RhD-specific exofacial protein segments (see Fig 11-3). DFR-like phenotypes were caused by *RHCE*-like exon 4 [category D Va (DVa) by

RHCE exon 5, DIVb by *RHCE* exon 7, DVI by *RHCE* exons 4 and 5, and DBT by *RHCE* exons 5 and 7]. The novel sequences of the hybrid protein resulting from regions of RhD joined to RhCE also explain the expression of new low-frequency antigens (FPTT in DFR, D^w in DVa, BARC in DVI).

Second, amino acid substitutions in exofacial RhD protein segments have minor impact and may lead to phenotypes difficult to discriminate from standard or weak D, like DNB and DHMi. In rare cases, in-frame deletions or insertions of a single amino acid have a similar impact.

Third, often, several amino acid substitutions are dispersed along the protein, as in DIIIa, DIVa, and DAR. Such partial D are especially frequent in individuals of African ancestry. In contrast to weak D types, partial D changes are predicted to be located on the exterior membrane surface[33] or, alternatively, can be internal but alter extracellular epitopes.

The use of a panel of monoclonal antibodies to assign a D variant to a specific partial type may not be reliable.[41] Many partial D phenotypes

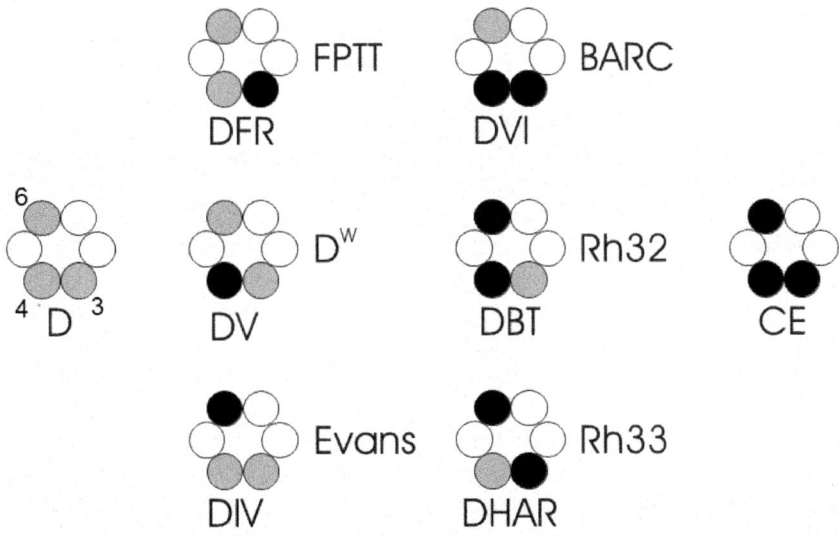

FIGURE 11-3. Schematic model of RhD as viewed from the red cell surface. RhD-like loops are indicated by gray disks, and RhCE-like loops by black disks. Loops 1, 2, and 5 show no constant differences between RhD and all RhCE proteins (loop 2 of RhD is similar to RhCe but differs from Rhce). The antigenic character of hybrid proteins depends largely on the replacement of RhD-like loops by RhCE-like loops. Each possible combination is associated with a distinct partial D phenotype and the presence of a low-prevalence antigen.

have reduced D antigen expression, making a serologic characterization difficult, and evidence of the partial D character may be difficult to assess unless an alloanti-D is observed and fully proven as an alloantibody by ad-hoc methods.

Del Types. Red cells that express extremely low levels of D antigen that cannot be detected by routine serologic methods (including IAT) are designated as "D-elution," or Del, types, because their D antigens can be detected by adsorption/elution studies only. Del cells are found in 10% to 30% of seemingly D-negative populations of Asian ancestry and are less common in individuals of European ancestry (0.027%). In Asia, the predominating allele is *RHD(1227G>A)*,[42] but the allelic background is more heterogeneous in Europeans.[28] The major mechanisms leading to Del phenotypes are mutations at splice sites and missense mutations. The discrimination of Del from D negative may be difficult, because adsorption/elution tests have a substantial rate of false positives and false negatives, and some alleles with seemingly inactivating mutations [eg, *RHD(97dupT)* with a frameshift in exon 1] may express a Del phenotype.

Nonfunctional *RHD* Alleles. *RHD* genes that do not encode a full-length polypeptide are nonfunctional and have been given the ISBT allele designation *RHD*01N* (with "N" indicating "null") to indicate that they are not expressed.[25] In D-negative individuals of African ancestry, a nonfunctional allele is prevalent, which especially contains a 37-bp insertion and results in a premature stop codon rendering the gene nonfunctional. It has been designated *RHDΨ*.[27] In addition, hybrid alleles lacking *RHCE*, like exons 4 to 7, and alleles with inactivating mutations may be the molecular basis of such alleles.

D Epitopes on RhCE. Expression of D epitopes by the protein product of the *RHCE* gene, in the absence of *RHD*, further complicates serologic determination of D status. Several RhCE proteins have D-specific amino acids and epitopes that are reactive with some monoclonal anti-D. These are more often found in a specific population. Examples include DHAR (Rhce'Har'), also named R_0^{Har}, which is found in individuals of European ancestry, and Crawford (*ceCF*),

found in individuals of African ancestry. These two examples are notable because the red cells show strong reactivity with some monoclonal anti-D reagents but are nonreactive with others, and are thus a source of D typing discrepancies (Table 11-4). Other changes in the RhCE polypeptide may mimic a D epitope. They are encoded by alleles designated by the amino acid changes as *ceRT* and *ceSL*.[43,44] The red cells are more or less reactive with some, but not all, monoclonal anti-D. A new *RHCE* allele expressing D epitopes, *RHCE*ceRG*, was recently described in a patient of European ancestry, showing a strong reactivity with several anti-D clones (MS26, HM10, ESD1, and HM16).[45] Most important, individuals with DHAR, Crawford, and *RHCE*ceRG* lack the expression of a conventional RhD protein and can be sensitized to D if no functional *RHD* gene is present in *trans*.[45-47]

Elevated D. Several rare deletion phenotypes, designated as D--, Dc-, and DC^w-, have an enhanced expression of D antigen and no or weak or altered C/c and E/e antigens.[48] These variants are the converse of partial D and result from the replacement of portions of *RHCE* by *RHD*. The additional *RHD* sequences in *RHCE* result in the additional expression of (hybrid) D antigen along with a normal *RHD* often in *trans*, which explains the enhanced D expression and reduced or missing C/c and E/e antigens.

D-Negative (Rh-Negative) Phenotype

The D-negative phenotype is more common in people of European ancestry (15-17%), is less common in people of African ancestry (approximately 8% in African-Americans), and is rare in people of Asian ancestry (<0.1%).[49] The D-negative phenotype has arisen multiple times in human history, as evidenced by the different nonfunctional alleles responsible for the lack of D expression in various ethnic groups.

Worldwide, the D-negative phenotype most frequently results from a deletion of the entire *RHD* gene.[50] In people of European ancestry, other alleles are rare and usually associated with uncommon haplotypes [r' (Ce) or r" (cE)].[28] In people of African ancestry, *RHDΨ* and a hybrid allele derived from *RHD*DIIIa* included in the so-called *(C)ce^s type 1* haplotype are almost as

TABLE 11-4. Reactivity of FDA-Licensed Anti-D Reagents with Some D-Variant Red Cells

Reagent	IgM Monoclonal	IgG	DVI IS/AHG*	DBT IS/AHG*	DHAR (Whites) IS/AHG*	Crawford (Blacks) IS/AHG*	ceRT	ceSL
Gammaclone	GAMA401	F8D8 monoclonal	Neg/Pos	Pos	Pos	Pos/Neg†		
Immucor Series 4	MS201	MS26 monoclonal	Neg/Pos	Pos	Pos	Neg/Neg	Weakly pos	Neg
Immucor Series 5	Th28	MS26 monoclonal	Neg/Pos	Pos	Pos	Neg/Neg	Weakly pos	Weakly pos
Ortho BioClone	MAD2	Polyclonal	Neg/Pos	Neg/Pos	Neg/Neg	Neg/Neg		
Ortho Gel (ID-MTS)	MS201		Neg	Pos	Pos	Neg	Weakly pos	Neg
Biotest RH1	BS226		Neg		Pos	Neg		
Biotest RH1 Blend	BS221	BS232 H4111B7	Neg/Pos		Pos†	Neg		
Alba Bioscience alpha	LDM1		Neg		Pos	Neg		
Alba Bioscience beta	LDM3		Neg		Pos	Neg		
Alba Bioscience delta	LDM1 ESD1-M		Neg		Pos	Neg		
ALBAclone blend	LDM3	ESD1	Neg/Pos	Neg/Pos	Pos	Pos/Neg†	Weakly pos‡	
Polyclonal		Polyclonal	Neg/Pos	Neg/Pos	Neg/Neg	Neg/Neg	Weakly pos‡	Neg

*Result following slash denotes anti-D test result by the indirect antiglobulin test (IAT).

†Test result is positive in the direct agglutination phase and will be negative in the IAT phase.

‡Enzyme-treated cells.

FDA = Food and Drug Administration; IgM = immunoglobulin M; IS = immediate spin; AHG = antihuman globulin; pos = positive; neg = negative.

common.[27] In people of East Asian ancestry, large hybrid alleles of the *Ce* haplotype are another frequent mechanism. In people of Asian ancestry, 10% to 30% of those who serologically type as D negative are actually Del.[42]

Testing for D

Monoclonal antibody production technology introduced in the 1980s freed manufacturers from reliance on human source material to manufacture anti-D reagents. These antibodies are specific for a single D epitope and do not detect all D-positive red cells. By the 1990s it became apparent that monoclonal antibodies could be used in a "blended" fashion to avoid deeming a pregnant woman or transfusion recipient D-positive if she or he expressed the category DVI variant. It had been known for many years that category DVI types could make anti-D and cause significant HDFN.[50,51] Reagents for D phenotyping were selected to circumvent this problem. The immediate-spin (IS) phase uses an IgM monoclonal anti-D that fails to react with red cells with partial DVI. This antibody is blended with a monoclonal or polyclonal IgG that requires an antiglobulin test (IAT) for the detection of D. In this way, typing partial DVI as D positive could be avoided in pregnancy and transfusion by performing only the IS phase of testing. Cord blood is tested in both the IS phase and the IAT phase to assign a D-positive status to most D variants.

Since their development, blended anti-D reagents from various manufacturers have used different monoclonal anti-D. Most Food and Drug Administration (FDA)-approved anti-D reagents combine a monoclonal IgM, which causes direct agglutination at room temperature, with a monoclonal or polyclonal IgG that is reactive by IAT, for the determination of weak expression of D. Anti-D for column agglutination testing may contain only monoclonal IgM or a blend of IgM and IgG. FDA-licensed reagents contain unique IgM clones, and these may exhibit different reactivity with red cells that have certain weak D, partial D, or D-like epitopes, including DHAR and Crawford (Table 11-4).

Typing Donors for D

The goal of D typing of donors, including the identification of units with weak D or partial D types, is to prevent anti-D immunization of transfusion recipients. The AABB *Standards for Blood Banks and Transfusion Services* (*Standards*) requires donor blood to be tested using a method that is designed to detect weak expression of D. There is no requirement that the typing should be done using an IAT, and some automated systems use enzymes to enhance detection of weak D. If the test results are positive, the unit is labeled "Rh positive."[52(p31)] Most weak- or partial-D-antigen units are detected, but infrequently some very weak D red cells or unusual partial D types are not detected; Del red cells will be nonreactive with anti-D. Red cells with weak D antigen are less immunogenic than normal D-positive red cells, but even Del donor units may stimulate anti-D.[53-57] Once shipped to an institution, a unit labeled "Rh negative" must be confirmed D negative by testing an integrally attached segment before transfusion, but testing by IAT is not required. Units labeled "Rh positive" do not require a confirmatory test.[52(p35)]

Typing Patients for D

When the D type of a patient is determined, a weak D test is not recommended except to assess the red cells of a newborn to determine maternal risk for D immunization. Today, monoclonal IgM reagents type many samples as D-positive by IS that would have previously been detected only by IAT.

DVI is one of the most common partial D types found in people of European ancestry, and anti-D produced by women with partial DVI has resulted in fatal HDFN.[51] Current FDA-licensed monoclonal IgM reagents are selected to be nonreactive with red cells with partial DVI in direct tests (Table 11-4). Therefore, performing only the direct test on red cells from female children and women of childbearing potential avoids the risk of sensitization by classifying females with DVI as D-negative for transfusion and RhIG prophylaxis. However, the results of positive rosetting tests (to detect fetomaternal hemorrhage) must be carefully evaluated; maternal weak D types that are reactive only in the

IAT phase have a false-positive rosette result.

D Typing Discrepancies

D typing discrepancies should always be investigated and resolved. (See "Resolving D Typing Discrepancies.") D-negative blood is an appropriate option for female patients needing immediate transfusion, but a thorough clerical and serologic investigation should be performed. *RHD* genotyping is also useful to resolve D typing discrepancies.[58] (See "Clinical Considerations.")

Because donor centers use test methods to detect weak D phenotypes, and generally hospitals do not, a donor who is correctly classified as D-positive may be classified as D-negative as a transfusion recipient. This discrepancy should not be considered problematic but, rather, should be communicated to the patient and health-care staff and be noted in the patient's medical record.

Clinical Considerations

The long history of providing recipients who have weak D phenotype cells with D-positive RBCs has suggested that some weak D phenotypes are unlikely to make anti-D. In 2015, a work group evaluated the scientific literature on anti-D alloimmunization among individuals whose red cells have a weak D phenotype and concluded that weak D types 1, 2, and 3 can be safely treated as D-positive in pregnancy.[59] The recommendations have been adopted by AABB, the College of American Pathologists, the American College of Obstetricians and Gynecologists, and the Armed Services Blood Program. *RHD* genotyping can be performed with reasonable cost recovery that is in line with the costs associated with unnecessary administration of RhIG.[60] Thus, implementing the committee recommendations can help to avoid exposing pregnant women to RhIG unnecessarily. Recent data suggest that anti-D immunization in weak D type 4.0 and 4.1 is very rare, too, but opinions on the transfusion strategy in these genotypes remain controversial.[61-63] Other weak D types such as 11 and 15 have been reported to make anti-D,[64] and information on risk for alloanti-D for other weak D types is not yet available.

Unfortunately, licensed anti-D reagents cannot distinguish individuals with partial D from those expressing a normal D antigen. Many partial D red cells such as DIIIa or DAR, two of the most common partial D types in people of African ancestry, type strongly D positive in the IS phase and, in the absence of *RHD* genotyping, are recognized as a D variant only after the patients produce anti-D.

Policies regarding D typing procedures and selection of blood components for transfusion should be based on the patient population, risk of immunization to D, and supply of D-negative blood. Policies should address procedures when an unexpected D phenotype is encountered. Although it is important to prevent D immunization in females of childbearing potential to avoid HDFN, for other patients the complications of anti-D are less serious, and the decision to transfuse D-positive or D-negative blood should take into consideration the D-negative blood supply.[65]

As previously stated, not all D-negative patients make anti-D when they are exposed to D-positive red cells. The incidence in D-negative hospitalized patients receiving D-positive blood components is variable but approximates 30%.[2-4] AABB *Standards* requires that transfusion services have policies that address the administration of D-positive red cells to D-negative patients and the use of RhIG, which is a human blood product that is not entirely without risk.[52(pp38,47)]

G Antigen

The G antigen is found on red cells possessing C or D and maps to the shared exon 2 and the 103 serine residue on RhD, RhCe, and RhCE proteins. Antibodies to G appear as anti-D plus anti-C that cannot be separated. However, the antibody can be adsorbed by either D–C+ or D+C– red cells. The presence of anti-G can explain why a D-negative person who received D–C+ blood, or a D-negative woman who delivered a D–C+ child, can subsequently appear to have made anti-D. Anti-D, -C, and -G can usually be distinguished by adsorption and elution studies.[66] The analyses are not often necessary in the pretransfusion setting. However, it is important to provide RhIG prophylaxis to pregnant women who have anti-G only and are at risk for anti-D.

C/c and E/e Antigens

The *RHCE* alleles encode the principal C/c and E/e antigens. More than 150 different *RHCE* alleles are known, and many are associated with altered or weak expression of the principal antigens and, in some cases, loss of high-prevalence antigens.[25] Partial C and many partial e antigens are well recognized, with the majority reported among individuals of African ancestry.

Altered or Variant C and e Antigens

Nucleotide changes in *RHCE* result in quantitative and qualitative changes in C/c or E/e antigen expression; altered or partial C and e antigens are encountered most frequently. In persons of European ancestry, altered C is associated with amino acid changes on the first extracellular loop of RhCe and the expression of C^W (Gln41Arg) or C^X (Ala36Thr) antigens. In people of African ancestry, variability of *RHCE* is much greater than in those of European ancestry, and altered or partial C and e antigens are frequent.

Altered or partial C is associated with changes that result in the expression of the novel antigens JAHK (p.Ser122Leu) and JAL (p.Arg114Trp), but partial C expression most often results from the inheritance of an *RHD*DIIIa-CE(4-7)-D* hybrid, and less often of an *RHD-CE(4-7)-D* hybrid.[48] These two hybrids are located in the *RHD* gene but do not encode the D antigen; rather, they encode a C reactivity on a hybrid background that differs from the normal background (Fig 11-4). The allele has an incidence of approximately 20% in people of African ancestry. It is inherited with an *RHCE* allele, designated as *RHCE*ce^S* (capital S), that encodes partial e antigen and a V–VS+ phenotype.[67] The expressed product of the hybrid *RHD*DIIIa-CE(4-7)-D* linked to *RHCE*ce^S* is referred to as the (C)ce^S type 1 or r'^S haplotype. Red cells with the r'^S haplotype express a partial C and lack the high-prevalence antigen Hr^B but type as moderately to strongly C positive with monoclonal reagents. Anti-C is not uncommon

among people of African ancestry receiving C+ blood, and anti-Hr^B immunization may become an obstacle to transfusion support.

Transfusion recipients who express partial e antigens frequently appear to make antibodies with e-like specificity, such as anti-hr^B or anti-hr^S. The red cells may lack the high-prevalence Hr^B or Hr^S antigens.[10,68,69] Partial e expression is associated with several *RHCE*ce* alleles.[10] These alleles are found primarily in people of African ancestry; some examples are shown in Fig 11-4. The molecular variability suggests that anti-hr^B/anti-Hr^B and anti-hr^S/anti-Hr^S may not represent a single entity; in fact, red cells designated as hr^B–/Hr^B– or hr^S–/Hr^S– by serologic testing may not be compatible with anti-hr^B/-Hr^B or -hr^S/-Hr^S produced by patients with other *RHCE* alleles.[70,71]

An additional complication is that altered *RHCE*ce* is often inherited with a partial D (eg, DIII, DAU, or DAR).[72] As discussed above, patients with partial-D red cells are at risk of producing anti-D.

CE, Ce, cE, and ce Compound Antigens

Compound antigens define epitopes that depend on conformational changes resulting from amino acids associated with both C/c and E/e. These antigens were referred to previously as *cis* products to indicate that the antigens were expressed from the same haplotype; that is, on a single Rhce polypeptide protein. These antigens are shown in Table 11-5 and include ce (f), Ce (rh_i), CE (Rh22), and cE (Rh27).

Clinical Considerations

It has long been recognized that alloimmunization represents a significant problem in patients with SCD because 25% to 30% or more of those who are chronic transfusion recipients develop red cell antibodies in the absence of minor blood group antigen-matching.[73] To address the problem, many treatment programs determine the pretransfusion red cell phenotype in patients with SCD and transfuse RBCs that are C, E, and K antigen matched (ie, antigen negative if the patient lacks the antigen), because these antigens are considered to be the most immunogenic. In addition, some programs attempt to supply

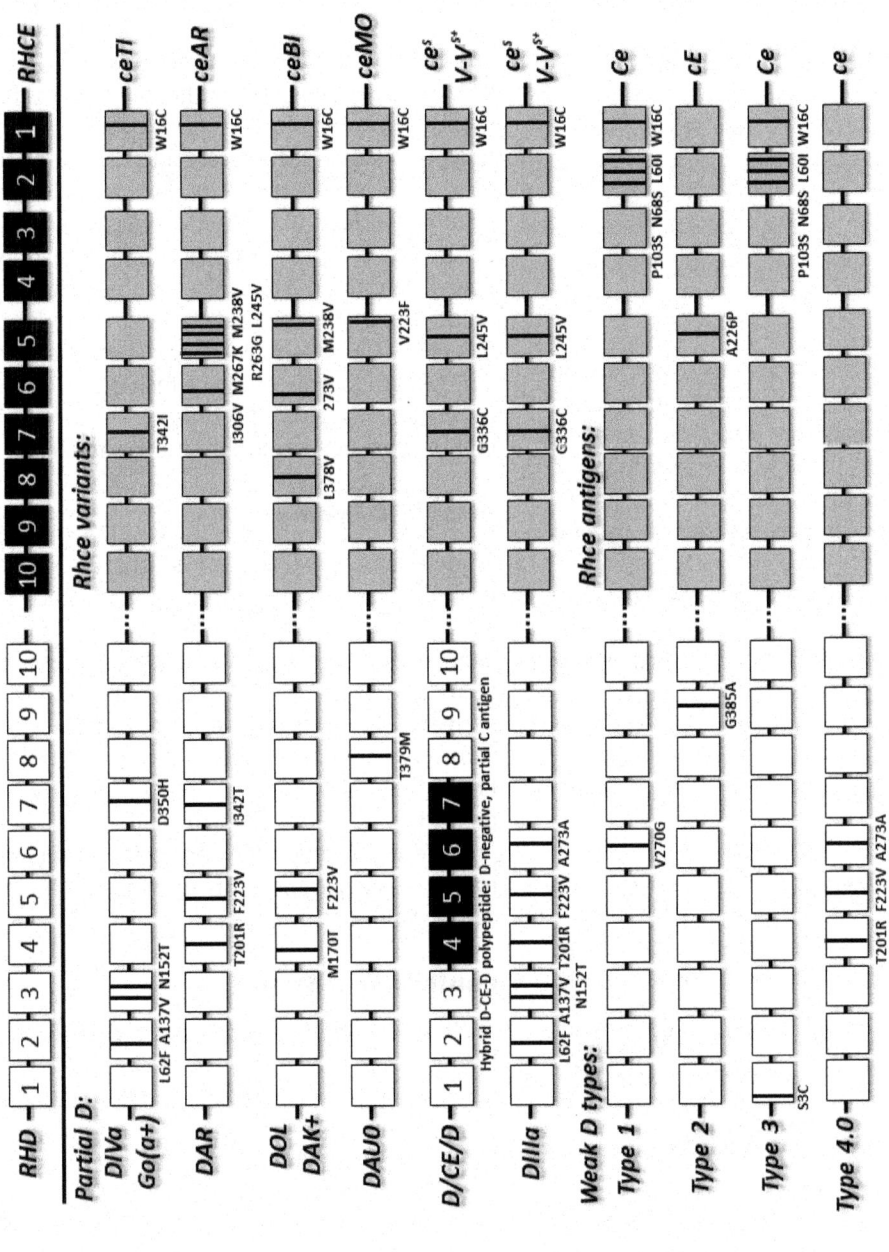

FIGURE 11-4. *RHD* and *RHCE* genes. The 10 exons of *RHD* and *RHCE* are depicted as white and gray boxes, respectively. Also shown are examples of *RHD* encoding partial D and weak D types, and of *RHCE* alleles with nucleotide polymorphisms often found in *cis* with the *RHD* alleles shown. The expression of the *RHCE* alleles with nucleotide polymorphisms can result in alloimmunization to conventional Rh proteins, which complicates transfusions in patients with sickle cell disease.

TABLE 11-5. Compound Rh Antigens on Rh Proteins

Compound Antigen Designation	Rh Protein	Present on Red Cells with These Haplotypes
ce or f	Rhce	Dce (R_0) or ce (r)
Ce or rh_i, Rh7	RhCe	DCe (R_1) or Ce (r')
cE or Rh27	RhcE	DcE (R_2) or cE (r")
CE or Rh22	RhCE	DCE (R_z) or CE (r^y)

RBCs from donors of African ancestry whenever possible. Determining the donor and patient genotypes may improve matching. Antigen-matching reduces alloimmunization significantly, although there is not complete international consensus on antigen-matching for all patients with SCD.[74,75]

Despite matching for D, C/c, and E/e, some patients become sensitized because they express Rh variants.[76] It is not possible to predict who will become alloimmunized, and prophylactic antigen-matching of blood for these patients is not feasible because of the low prevalence of antigen-negative blood.

RH GENOTYPING

RH genotyping is a powerful adjunct to serologic testing for the typing of transfusion recipients, *RHD* zygosity determination, fetal *RHD* typing, confirmation of D status, and identification of antigen-matched blood for patients with SCD.

Typing Transfusion Recipients

In patients receiving chronic or massive transfusions, the presence of donor red cells in the peripheral blood makes red cell phenotyping by agglutination inaccurate. Genotyping overcomes this limitation because blood grouping can be determined with DNA prepared from a blood sample, even if the sample was collected after transfusion.[77]

RHD Zygosity Testing

RHD zygosity can be determined by two approaches: assaying *RHD* dosage or confirming the presence of a hybrid Rhesus box.[24,78] In prenatal practice, paternal *RHD* zygosity testing is important to predict fetal D status when the mother has anti-D. The management of HDFN can vary depending on whether the father is homozygous or hemizygous *RHD* positive. Care must be taken in the interpretation of testing results using either approach. For *RHD* dosage, testing of at least two target exons is needed to accurately determine zygosity, and nucleotide polymorphisms in hybrid Rhesus boxes can confound the analysis, especially in ethnic minorities.[78,79] The presence of the nonfunctional *RHDΨ* pseudogene should be included in zygosity analysis as a routine practice because it is common among persons of African ancestry.[27]

Fetal *RHD* Typing

To determine the D-antigen status of a fetus, fetal DNA can be isolated from cells obtained by amniocentesis or chorionic villus sampling. An alternative, noninvasive approach is to test the maternal plasma, which contains cell-free, fetal-derived DNA beyond 5 weeks' gestation.[80,81] As is the case now in several countries, determination of fetal *RHD* status using this noninvasive procedure will likely become routine in clinical practice to eliminate the unnecessary administration of antepartum RhIG to women who are carrying a D-negative fetus.[80]

Confirming D Status

RHD genotyping is useful to distinguish partial D from weak D or to resolve serologic D typing discrepancies. Although patients with an uncertain D status can be treated as D-negative for transfusion and RhIG administration, this approach may be unsatisfactory for females of childbearing potential who face unnecessary RhIG injections, and it puts a strain on the limited D-negative blood supply. It is also important to confirm the D status in weak D patients with a c– or e– phenotype, to know whether they do or do not need to be provided with rare blood for transfusion. *RHD* genotyping in pregnancy allows informed decisions to be made on the administration of antenatal RhIG. (See "D Typing Discrepancies" and "Clinical Considerations" in the "Testing for D" section above.)

For donors, D typing discrepancies must be resolved because errors in determining D status may be reportable to the FDA and result in the recall of blood components. D-negative, first-time donors are screened for *RHD* to detect red cells with very weak D in some centers.[82]

RH Genotyping for Patients with SCD

Currently, extensive RH genotyping is time-consuming and is used primarily for patients with complex Rh antibody reactivity and to find compatible donors in the American Rare Donor Program for patients with antibodies to high-prevalence Rh antigens.[69] The availability of high-throughput RH genotyping platforms enables donors to be identified by genotyping. However, RH genotype-matching for patients with SCD who have rare Rh variant types may not be possible for chronic prophylactic transfusions.[83] Patients with SCD who cannot be supported with crossmatch-compatible transfusions may be candidates for stem cell transplantation.[84]

RH_{NULL} SYNDROME AND THE RHAG (030) BLOOD GROUP SYSTEM

In the red cell membrane, the two Rh proteins RhD and RhCE are organized as trimeric "Rh complexes" with a third protein, RhAG, which shares 38% of its identity with RhD/RhCE, has the same membrane topology, and is encoded by a single gene on chromosome 6. Amino acid substitutions in the RhAG protein lead to the three antigens of the RHAG blood group system, recognized as the 30th system by the ISBT in 2008: Duclos (RHAG1), Ol^a (RHAG2), and DSLK (RHAG3).[85] Of note, RHAG4 has been declared recently obsolete.

Although the RhD/RhCE presence in the Rh complex is believed to be stochastic, RhAG is a critical component, and lack of functional RhAG prevents Rh antigen expression. Furthermore,

RhAG variants may lead to reduced expression of all Rh proteins[86] or of RhD only.[87]

Red cells lacking all Rh antigens are designated as Rh$_{null}$. In the "amorph" type, both *RHD* and *RHCE* are inactive, usually due to the commonly observed deletion of *RHD* in D-negative people combined with molecular alterations in *RHCE*. In the more frequent "regulatory" type, molecular alterations in *RHAG* prevent Rh antigen expression.

Rh$_{null}$ red cells are stomatocytic and associated with mild anemia, suggesting that the Rh proteins have an important structural role in the erythrocyte membrane. The Rh complex is associated with the membrane skeleton through CD47 protein 4.2, ankyrin, band 3, Duffy, and glycophorin B and C interactions.[88,89] Absence of RhCE, as in D– –, leads to diminished CD44 and CD47 expression,[90] whereas absence of RhD diminishes LW expression.

ANTIBODIES TO RH BLOOD GROUP SYSTEM ANTIGENS

Most Rh antibodies are IgG but may have an IgM component. Typically, Rh antibodies do not activate complement, although rare exceptions have been reported. As a result, in a transfusion reaction involving Rh antibodies, hemolysis is primarily extravascular rather than intravascular.

Rh antibodies have the potential to cause clinically significant HDFN. Anti-c may cause severe HDFN, but anti-C, -E, and -e do not commonly cause HDFN, and when they do, it is usually mild to moderate. For antibody investigations, Rh antibodies are enhanced by enzyme treatment of red cells, and most are optimally reactive at 37 C.

Concomitant Rh Antibodies

Some Rh antibodies are often found together. For example, a DCe/DCe (R$_1$R$_1$) patient with anti-E most certainly has been exposed to the c antigen as well. Anti-c may be present in addition to anti-E, but the anti-c may be weak and undetectable at the time of testing. When seemingly compatible E-negative blood is transfused, it is most likely to be c-positive and may elicit an immediate or delayed transfusion reaction. Therefore, some experts advocate for avoiding the transfusion of c-positive blood in this situation. In contrast, testing for anti-E in serum containing anti-c is not warranted because the patient has probably been exposed to c without being exposed to E. In addition, the vast majority of c-negative donor blood is E-negative. (See Table 11-3.) In many European countries, consideration of the full Rh phenotype (C, E, c, e) is standard practice once the patient is immunized to one Rh antigen.

Antibodies to High-Prevalence Rh Antigens

Alloantibodies to high-prevalence Rh antigens include anti-Rh29, made by some Rh_{null} individuals who lack Rh antigens, and others (anti-Hr^B, -Hr^S, -Sec, etc) that are most often encountered in transfusion recipients with SCD.

TECHNICAL CONSIDERATIONS FOR RH TYPING

High-Protein Reagents and Controls

Some Rh reagents for use in slide, rapid tube, or microplate tests contain high concentrations of protein (20-24%) and other macromolecular additives. These reagents are prepared from pools of human sera and give reliable results; however, high protein levels and macromolecular additives may cause false-positive reactions. (See "Causes of False-Positive and False-Negative Rh Typing Results" below.) These reagents must be used according to the manufacturers' instructions and with the appropriate controls. False-positive results could cause a D-negative patient to receive D-positive blood and become immunized. If red cells exhibit aggregation in the control test, the results of the test are not valid.

Low-Protein Reagents and Controls

Most Rh antisera in routine use are low-protein reagents formulated predominantly with IgM monoclonal antibodies. Spontaneous agglutination causing a false-positive result can occur, although this happens much less frequently than with high-protein reagents. A negative result from a test that was performed concurrently with a similar reagent serves as a control. For example, for ABO and Rh typing, the absence of agglutination by anti-A or anti-B serves as a negative control for spontaneous hemagglutination. For red cells that show agglutination with all reagents (eg, group AB or D+), a control performed as described by the reagent manufacturer is required (with the exception of donor retyping).

In most cases, a suitable control is a suspension of the patient's red cells with autologous serum or 6% to 10% albumin. Indirect antiglobulin testing is not valid for red cells with a positive direct antiglobulin test (DAT) result unless a method is used to remove the IgG antibody. Antigen-positive and -negative controls should be tested, and the positive control cells should have a single dose of the antigen or be known to demonstrate weak reactivity.

Rh Testing Considerations in HDFN

Red cells from an infant with HDFN are coated with immunoglobulin, and a low-protein reagent is usually necessary to test these cells. Occasionally, red cells with a strongly positive DAT result may be so heavily coated that they are not agglutinated by a reagent with the same specificity as the bound antibody. This "blocking" phenomenon probably results from steric hindrance, or the epitope targeted by the monoclonal antiserum is occupied by maternal anti-D, causing a false-negative result. Heat elution of the antibody performed at 45 C permits red cell typing, but elution must be performed with appropriate controls to check for antigen denaturation. Detection of the antibody in an eluate confirms the presence of the antigen on the red cells, and *RHD* genotyping can be used for confirmation of D typing.

Causes of False-Positive and False-Negative Rh Typing Results

False-positive typing results can be caused by any of the following:

1. Immunoglobulin-coating of the cells as a result of warm or cold autoagglutinins. The

red cells should be washed several times and retested with low-protein reagents by direct methods. If an IAT is required, IgG coating the red cells can be removed by treating the cells with glycine/EDTA (Method 2-21) or chloroquine (Method 2-20) and retesting.

2. Induction of rouleaux by serum factors that can be eliminated by thoroughly washing the red cells and retesting.
3. Use of the wrong reagent.
4. Contamination with reagent from another vial.
5. Nonspecific aggregation of the red cells due to some component of the reagent other than the antibody (ie, a preservative, antibiotic, or dye).
6. Testing of polyagglutinable red cells agglutinated with reagents that contain human serum.
7. Reactivity of the antiserum with a rare RhCE variant.

False-negative typing results can be caused by any of the following:

1. Failure to add the reagent. It is good practice to add typing reagent to all test tubes or wells before adding the red cells.
2. Use of the wrong reagent.
3. A red cell suspension that is too heavy for a tube test or too weak for a slide test.
4. Failure to detect a weak D reaction with direct testing (immediate centrifugation).
5. Nonreactivity of a reagent with a weak or partial form of the antigen.
6. Aggressive resuspension of the red cell button, dispersing the agglutination.
7. Contamination, improper storage, or outdating of the reagent.
8. Red cells with a strongly positive DAT result and antigen sites blocked because of a large amount of bound antibody (most common in severe HDFN caused by anti-D).

Resolving D Typing Discrepancies

To investigate D typing discrepancies, errors in sample identification or of a clerical nature should be eliminated by obtaining and testing a new sample. Beyond clerical errors, multiple variables contribute to D typing discrepancies. These variables include the use of different methods (eg, slide, tube, microplate, gel, and automated analyzers using enzyme-treated red cells), the phase of testing (DAT or IAT), different IgM clones in manufacturers' reagents, and the large number of *RHD* gene variations that affect the level of expression and epitopes of the D antigen.

It is important to know the characteristics of the D typing reagent used and to always consult and follow the manufacturer's instructions during D typing. The FDA has drafted recommendations that require manufacturers to specify the reactivity of their reagents with partial DIV, DV, and DVI red cells.[91]

The IgM anti-D in all of the tube reagents currently licensed by the FDA is reactive by direct testing (initial spin) with DIV and DV red cells but has been selected to be nonreactive with partial DVI red cells in direct testing. Limited studies have been performed to characterize the reactivity of anti-D reagents with other partial D and weak D red cells. These studies have shown that the anti-D reagents cannot reliably predict whether a D variant is a weak or partial D antigen.[92,93] Table 11-4 shows the reactivity of important D variant red cells that have predictable patterns among the different anti-D reagents. In general, females of childbearing potential with partial D should be considered to be D positive when they are blood donors, but D negative when they are transfusion recipients and with regard to antenatal prophylaxis with anti-D immunoglobulin.

KEY POINTS

1. The Rh system is highly immunogenic, complex, and polymorphic. Currently, 55 Rh antigens have been characterized, although the five principal antigens—D, C, E, c, and e—are responsible for the majority of clinically significant antibodies.

2. "Rh positive" and "Rh negative" refer to the presence or absence, respectively, of the D antigen.

3. Contemporary Rh terminology distinguishes between antigens (such as D and C), genes (such as *RHD* and *RHCE*), alleles (such as *RHCE*ce* and *RHCE*Ce*), and proteins (such as RhD and RhCE).

4. Most D-negative (Rh-negative) phenotypes result from complete deletion of the *RHD* gene. Exposure of D-negative individuals to RhD often results in the development of anti-D.

5. *RHCE* encodes both C/c and E/e antigens on a single protein. C and c differ by four amino acids, whereas E and e differ by one amino acid.

6. Routine donor and patient Rh typing procedures test only for D. Testing for other common Rh antigens is used to resolve or confirm antibody identification and, for many SCD transfusion programs or for other patients receiving chronic transfusions, to match patients and donors for D, C, and E.

7. Weak D phenotypes are defined as having a reduced amount of D antigen and may require an IAT for detection. Weak D usually results from amino acid changes that impair the insertion of the protein in the membrane. Many different mutations cause weak expression of D.

8. *RHD* genotyping can identify those pregnant females and blood transfusion recipients with a serologic weak D phenotype who can be managed safely as D positive.

9. Most anti-D reagents approved by the FDA combine a monoclonal IgM (that is reactive at room temperature for routine testing) and a monoclonal or polyclonal IgG (that is reactive by IAT for the determination of weak D). Anti-D for column agglutination testing may contain only IgM. These reagents may show different reactivity with red cells that have weak D, partial D, or D-like epitopes.

10. When determining the D type of a patient, an IAT for weak expression of D is not recommended except when testing the red cells of an infant born to a mother at risk of D immunization. D-negative donors must be tested by a method that detects weak D.

11. Most Rh antibodies are IgG, although some may have an IgM component. With rare exceptions, Rh antibodies do not activate complement and, thus, cause primarily extravascular rather than intravascular hemolysis. Antibodies almost always result from red cell immunization through pregnancy or transfusion.

REFERENCES

1. Klein HG, Anstee DJ. The Rh blood group system (including LW and RHAG). In: Mollison's blood transfusion in clinical medicine. 12th ed. Hoboken, NJ: Wiley-Blackwell, 2014:167-213.

2. Selleng K, Jenichen G, Denker K, et al. Emergency transfusion of patients with unknown blood type with blood group O Rhesus D positive red blood cell concentrates: A prospective, single-centre, observational study. Lancet Haematol 2017;4:e218-24.

3. Flommersfeld S, Mand C, Kühne CA, et al. Unmatched type O RhD+ red blood cells in multiple injured patients. Transfus Med Hemother 2018;45(3):158-61.

4. Frohn C, Dumbgen L, Brand J-M, et al. Probability of anti-D development in D– patients receiving D+ RBCs. Transfusion 2003;43:893-8.

5. Mollison PL, Hughes-Jones NC, Lindsay M, Wessely J. Suppression of primary RH immunization by passively-administered antibody: Experiments in volunteers. Vox Sang 1969;16:421-39.

6. Freda V, Gorman J, Pollack W. Rh factor: Prevention of isoimmunization and clinical trials in mothers. Science 1966;151:828-30.

7. Zwingerman R, Jain V, Hannon J, et al. Alloimmune red blood cell antibodies: Prevalence and pathogenicity in a Canadian prenatal population. J Obstet Gynaecol Can 2015;37:784-90.

8. Levine P, Stetson RE. An unusual case of intragroup agglutination. JAMA 1939;113:126-7.

9. Rosenfield R. Who discovered Rh? A personal glimpse of the Levine-Wiener argument. Transfusion 1989;29:355-7.

10. Noizat-Pirenne F, Lee K, Pennec PY, et al. Rare RHCE phenotypes in black individuals of Afro-Caribbean origin: Identification and transfusion safety. Blood 2002;100:4223-31.

11. Green FA. Phospholipid requirement for Rh antigenic activity. J Biol Chem 1968;243:5519.

12. Gahmberg CG. Molecular characterization of the human red cell Rho(D) antigen. EMBO J 1983;2:223-7.

13. Bloy C, Blanchard D, Lambin P, et al. Human monoclonal antibody against Rh(D) antigen: Partial characterization of the Rh(D) polypeptide from human erythrocytes. Blood 1987;69:1491-7.

14. Moore S, Woodrow CF, McClelland DB. Isolation of membrane components associated with human red cell antigens Rh(D), (c), (E) and Fy. Nature 1982;295:529-31.

15. Saboori AM, Smith BL, Agre P. Polymorphism in the Mr 32,000 Rh protein purified from Rh(D)-positive and -negative erythrocytes. Proc Natl Acad Sci U S A 1988;85:4042-5.

16. Cherif-Zahar B, Bloy C, Le Van Kim C, et al. Molecular cloning and protein structure of a human blood group Rh polypeptide. Proc Natl Acad Sci U S A 1990;87:6243-7.

17. Le Van Kim C, Mouro I, Cherif-Zahar B, et al. Molecular cloning and primary structure of the human blood group RhD polypeptide. Proc Natl Acad Sci U S A 1992;89:10925-9.

18. Arce MA, Thompson ES, Wagner S, et al. Molecular cloning of RhD cDNA derived from a gene present in RhD-positive, but not RhD-negative individuals. Blood 1993;82:651-5.

19. Mouro I, Colin Y, Chérif-Zahar B, et al. Molecular genetic basis of the human Rhesus blood group system. Nat Genet 1993;5(1):62-5.

20. Simsek S, de Jong CAM, Cuijpers HTM, et al. Sequence analysis of cDNA derived from reticulocyte mRNAs coding for Rh polypeptides and demonstration of E/e and C/c polymorphism. Vox Sang 1994;67:203-9.

21. Tippett P. A speculative model for the Rh blood groups. Ann Hum Genet 1986;50(Pt 3):241-7.

22. Wagner FF, Flegel WA. RHCE represents the ancestral RH position, while RHD is the duplicated gene. Blood 2002;99:2272-3.

23. Wagner FF, Flegel WA. RHD gene deletion occurred in the Rhesus box. Blood 2000;95:3662-8.

24. Wagner FF, Flegel WA. The human RhesusBase. Version 2.3. [Available at http://www.rhesusbase.info (accessed August 8, 2018).]

25. International Society of Blood Transfusion Working Group on Red Cell Immunogenetics and Blood Group Terminology. Blood group terminology: Blood group allele tables. Amsterdam: ISBT, 2019. [Available at http://www.isbtweb.org/working-parties/red-cell-immunogenetics-and-blood-group-terminology/ (accessed October 8, 2019).]

26. Ceppellini R, Dunn LC, Turri M. An interaction between alleles at the RH locus in man which weakens the reactivity of the Rh(0) Factor (D). Proc Natl Acad Sci U S A 1955;41:283-8.

27. Singleton BK, Green CA, Avent ND, et al. The presence of an RHD pseudogene containing a 37 base pair duplication and a nonsense mutation in Africans with the Rh D-negative blood group phenotype. Blood 2000;95:12-18.

28. Wagner FF, Frohmajer A, Flegel WA. RHD positive haplotypes in D negative Europeans. BMC Genet 2001;2:10.

29. Compernolle V, Chou ST, Tanael S, et al. International Collaboration for Transfusion Medicine Guidelines. Red blood cell specifications for patients with hemoglobinopathies: A systematic review and guideline. Transfusion 2018;58(6):1555-66.

30. Granier T, Beley S, Chiaroni J, et al. A comprehensive survey of both RHD and RHCE allele frequencies in sub-Saharan Africa. Transfusion 2013;53(Suppl 2):3009-17.

31. Flegel WA. Molecular genetics and clinical applications for RH. Transfus Apher Sci 2011;44(1):81-91.

32. Wagner FF, Gassner C, Muller TH, et al. Molecular basis of weak D phenotypes. Blood 1999;93:385-93.

33. Flegel WA. Molecular genetics of RH and its clinical application. Transfus Clin Biol 2006;13:4-12.

34. Wagner FF. Molecular genetics: The two Rhesus genes and their Rhesus boxes (presentation). Ulm, Germany: DRK Blutspendedienst Baden-Württemberg-Hessen, 2004. [Available at http://www.uni-ulm.de/~wflegel/RH/SympDGTI2004/4WagnerDGTI2004MA.pdf (accessed October 8, 2019).]

35. Flegel WA, Denomme GA. Allo- and autoanti-D in weak D types and in partial D. Transfusion 2012;52:2067-9.

36. Ogasawara K, Sasaki K, Isa K, et al. Weak D alleles in Japanese: A c.960G>A silent mutation in exon 7 of the RHD gene that affects D expression. Vox Sang 2016;110(2):179-84.

37. Fichou Y, Chen JM, Le Maréchal C, et al. Weak D caused by a founder deletion in the RHD gene. Transfusion 2012;52(11):2348-55.

38. Fichou Y, Parchure D, Gogri H, et al. Molecular basis of weak D expression in the Indian population and report of a novel, predominant variant RHD allele.Transfusion 2018;58(6):1540-9.

39. Wagner FF, Frohmajer A, Ladewig B, et al. Weak D alleles express distinct phenotypes. Blood 2000;95:2699-708.

40. Tippett P, Sanger R. Observations on subdivisions of the Rh antigen D. Vox Sang 1962;7:9-13.

41. Denomme GA, Dake LR, Vilensky D, et al. Rh discrepancies caused by variable reactivity of partial and weak D types with different serologic techniques. Transfusion 2008;48:473-8.

42. Shao CP, Maas JH, Su YQ, et al. Molecular background of Rh D-positive, D-negative, D(el) and weak D phenotypes in Chinese. Vox Sang 2002; 83:156-61.

43. Wagner FF, Ladewig B, Flegel WA. The RHCE allele ceRT: D epitope 6 expression does not require D-specific amino acids. Transfusion 2003; 43:1248-54.

44. Chen Q, Hustinx H, Flegel WA. The RHCE allele ceSL: The second example for D antigen expression without D-specific amino acids. Transfusion 2006;46:766-72.

45. Vrignaud V, Ramelet S, Gien D, et al. A novel RHCE allele expressing RHD epitopes responsible for a false-positive D typing and post-transfusion anti-D alloimmunization in a patient of Western European descent (abstract). Transfusion 2018;58(Suppl S2):44A.

46. Beckers EA, Porcelijn L, Ligthart P, et al. The Ro^HAR antigenic complex is associated with a limited number of D epitopes and alloanti-D production: A study of three unrelated persons and their families. Transfusion 1996;36:104-8.

47. Westhoff CM. Review: The Rh blood group D antigen: Dominant, diverse, and difficult. Immunohematol 2005;21:155-63.

48. Daniels G. Human blood groups. 2nd ed. Cambridge, MA: Blackwell Science, 2002.

49. Race RR, Sanger R. Blood groups in man. 6th ed. Oxford: Blackwell, 1975.

50. Colin Y, Cherif-Zahar B, Le Van Kim C, et al. Genetic basis of the RhD-positive and RhD-negative blood group polymorphism as determined by Southern analysis. Blood 1991;78: 2747-52.

51. Lacey PA, Caskey CR, Werner DJ, Moulds JJ. Fatal hemolytic disease of a newborn due to anti-D in an Rh-positive Du variant mother. Transfusion 1983;23:91-4.

52. Gammon R, ed. Standards for blood banks and transfusion services. 32nd ed. Bethesda, MD: AABB, 2020.

53. Schmidt PJ, Morrison EC, Shohl J. The antigenicity of the Rh_o (D^u) blood factor. Blood 1962; 20:196-202.

54. Wagner T, Kormoczi GF, Buchta C, et al. Anti-D immunization by D_EL red blood cells. Transfusion 2005;45:520-6.

55. Yasuda H, Ohto H, Sakuma S, Ishikawa Y. Secondary anti-D immunization by D_el red blood cells. Transfusion 2005;45:1581-4.

56. Flegel WA, Khull SR, Wagner FF. Primary anti-D immunization by weak D type 2 RBCs. Transfusion 2000;40:428-34.

57. Mota M, Fonseca NL, Rodrigues A, et al. Anti-D alloimmunization by weak D type 1 red blood cells with a very low antigen density. Vox Sang 2005;88:130-5.

58. Flegel WA, Denomme GA, Yazer MH. On the complexity of D antigen typing: A handy decision tree in the age of molecular blood group diagnostics. J Obstet Gynaecol Can 2007;29:746-52.

59. Sandler SG, Flegel WA, Westhoff CM, et al. It's time to phase in RHD genotyping for patients with a serologic weak D phenotype. College of American Pathologists Transfusion Medicine Resource Committee Work Group. Transfusion 2015;55:680-9.

60. Kacker S, Vassallo R, Keller MA, et al. Financial implications of RHD genotyping of pregnant women with a serologic weak D phenotype. Transfusion 2015;55:2095-103.

61. Ouchari M, Srivastava K, Romdhane H, et al. Transfusion strategy for weak D Type 4.0 based on RHD alleles and RH haplotypes in Tunisia. Transfusion 2018;58(2):306-12.

62. Flegel WA, Peyrard T, Chiaroni J, et al. A proposal for a rational transfusion strategy in patients of European and North African descent with weak D type 4.0 and 4.1 phenotypes. Blood Transfus 2019;17(2):89-90.

63. Westhoff CM, Nance S, Lomas-Francis C, et al. Experience with RHD*weak D type 4.0 in the USA. Blood Transfus 2019;17(2):91-3.

64. Flegel WA. Homing in on D antigen immunogenicity. Transfusion 2005;45:466-8.

65. Schonewille H, van de Watering LM, Brand A. Additional red blood cell alloantibodies after blood transfusions in a nonhematologic alloimmunized patient cohort: Is it time to take pre-

cautionary measures? Transfusion 2006;46:630-5.

66. Issitt PD, Anstee DJ. Applied blood group serology. 4th ed. Durham, NC: Montgomery Scientific Publications, 1998.

67. Daniels GL, Faas BH, Green CA, et al. The VS and V blood group polymorphisms in Africans: A serologic and molecular analysis. Transfusion 1998;38:951-8.

68. Reid ME, Storry JR, Issitt PD, et al. Rh haplotypes that make e but not hr^B usually make VS. Vox Sang 1997;72:41-4.

69. Vege S, Westhoff CM. Molecular characterization of GYPB and RH in donors in the American Rare Donor Program. Immunohematol 2006; 22:143-7.

70. Pham BN, Peyrard T, Tourret S, et al. Anti-HrB and anti-hrb revisited. Transfusion 2009;49: 2400-5.

71. Pham BN, Peyrard T, Juszczak G, et al. Analysis of RhCE variants among 806 individuals in France: Considerations for transfusion safety, with emphasis on patients with sickle cell disease. Transfusion 2011;51:1249-60.

72. Westhoff CM, Vege S, Halter-Hipsky C, et al. DIIIa and DIII Type 5 are encoded by the same allele and are associated with altered RHCE*ce alleles: Clinical implications. Transfusion 2010; 50:1303-11.

73. Vichinsky EP, Earles A, Johnson RA, et al. Alloimmunization in sickle cell anemia and transfusion of racially unmatched blood. N Engl J Med 1990;322:1617-21.

74. Ness PM. To match or not to match: The question for chronically transfused patients with sickle cell anemia. Transfusion 1994;34:558-60.

75. Vichinsky EP, Luban NL, Wright E, et al. Prospective RBC phenotype matching in a stroke prevention trial in sickle cell anemia: A multicenter transfusion trial. Transfusion 2001;41: 1086-92.

76. Chou ST, Jackson T, Vege S, et al. High prevalence of red blood cell alloimmunization in sickle cell disease despite transfusion from Rh-matched minority donors. Blood 2013;122: 1062-71.

77. Reid ME, Rios M, Powell VI, et al. DNA from blood samples can be used to genotype patients who have recently received a transfusion. Transfusion 2000;40:48-53.

78. Pirelli KJ, Pietz BC, Johnson ST, et al. Molecular determination of RHD zygosity: Predicting risk of hemolytic disease of the fetus and newborn related to anti-D. Prenat Diagn 2010;12-13: 1207-12.

79. Matheson KA, Denomme GA. Novel 3' rhesus box sequences confound RHD zygosity assignment. Transfusion 2002;42:645-50.

80. Lo YM, Corbetta N, Chamberlain PF, et al. Presence of fetal DNA in maternal plasma and serum. Lancet 1997;350:485-7.

81. Van der Schoot CE, Soussan AA, Koelewijn J, et al. Non-invasive antenatal RHD typing. Transfus Clin Biol 2006;13:53-7.

82. Wagner FF. *RHD* PCR of D-negative blood donors. Transfus Med Hemother 2013;40:172-81.

83. Chou St, Westhoff CM. The role of molecular immunohematology in sickle cell disease. Transfus Apher Sci 2011;44:73-9.

84. Fasano RM, Monaco A, Meier ER, et al. RH genotyping in a sickle cell disease patient contributing to hematopoietic stem cell transplantation donor selection and management. Blood 2010; 116:2836-8.

85. Tilley L, Green C, Poole J, et al. A new blood group system, RHAG: Three antigens resulting from amino acid substitutions in the Rh-associated glycoprotein. Vox Sang 2010;98:151-9.

86. Cherif-Zahar B, Raynal V, Gane P, et al. Candidate gene acting as a suppressor of the RH locus in most cases of Rh-deficiency. Nat Genet 1996; 12(2):168-73.

87. Mu S, Cui Y, Wang W, et al. A RHAG point mutation selectively disrupts Rh antigen expression. Transfus Med 2019;29(2):121-7.

88. Dahl KN, Parthasarathy R, Westhoff CM, et al. Protein 4.2 is critical to CD47-membrane skeleton attachment in human red cells. Blood 2004; 103:1131-6.

89. Nicolas V, Le Van Kim C, Gane P, et al. RhRhAG/ankyrin-R, a new interaction site between the membrane bilayer and the red cell skeleton, is impaired by Rh(null)-associated mutation. J Biol Chem 2003;278:25526-33.

90. Flatt JF, Musa RH, Ayob Y, et al. Study of the D-- phenotype reveals erythrocyte membrane alterations in the absence of RHCE. Br J Haematol 2012;158(2):262-73.

91. Food and Drug Administration. Draft guidance: Recommended methods for blood grouping reagents evaluation. (March 1992) Silver Spring, MD: CBER Office of Communication, Outreach, and Development, 1992. [Available at https://www.fda.gov/downloads/Biologics BloodVaccines/GuidanceComplianceRegulato ryInformation/Guidances/Blood/UCM080926. pdf.]

92. Judd WJ, Moulds M, Schlanser G. Reactivity of FDA-approved anti-D reagents with partial D red blood cells. Immunohematol 2005;21:146-8.

93. Denomme GA, Dake LR, Vilensky D, et al. Rh discrepancies caused by variable reactivity of partial and weak D types with different serologic techniques. Transfusion 2008;48:473-8.

CHAPTER 12

Other Blood Group Systems and Antigens

Cami Melland, MLS(ASCP)[CM]SBB, and Sandra Nance, MS, MT(ASCP)SBB

THIS CHAPTER DESCRIBES 31 OF the 39 blood group systems recognized by the International Society of Blood Transfusion (ISBT). A blood group system is defined by one or more antigens controlled at a single gene locus, or by two or more very closely linked homologous genes with little or no observable recombination between them.[1,2] The blood group systems are listed in ISBT order in Table 12-1. The full ISBT classification can be found on the ISBT website (http://www.isbtweb. org/working-parties/red-cell-immunogenetics-and-blood-group-terminology/), and Appendix 6 lists all antigens assigned to systems. ISBT abbreviations (symbols) for blood group systems—for example, JK instead of Kidd—will be used in this chapter. See Table 9-4 in Chapter 9 for examples of ISBT terminology applied to blood group system antigens, alleles, and phenotypes. Many more references to blood group systems and antigens than can be provided here are available in various textbooks and reviews.[3-5]

The other groups of antigens described at the end of this chapter are not yet assigned to a system. Those that are serologically, biochemically, or genetically related to a blood group system but do not meet all the criteria are grouped into "collections." Others are classified together in the low- or high-prevalence groups from most major populations and make up the 700 and 901 series, respectively.[1] Several references relating to these antigens and their corresponding antibodies are available for guidance.[3-5]

Blood group antigens may be glycoproteins, polypeptides, or glycolipids. The structure of blood group antigens provides information about function, which can be helpful not only for antibody identification but also for assessing the potential immunogenicity of an antigen and for applications related to the emerging interest in immunotherapy. (See Tables 12-1 and 12-2.) However, the most important aspect of blood group antigens in transfusion medicine is whether their corresponding antibodies are clinically significant and therefore have the potential to cause hemolytic transfusion reactions (HTRs) and hemolytic disease of the fetus and newborn (HDFN). Identifying antibodies to these antigens and determining their clinical significance or lack thereof can determine the clinical course of action for a patient who has produced these antibodies. Emerging drug regimens that interfere with blood bank testing (eg, anti-CD38 therapy) and autoantibodies add to the difficulty in not only determining alloantibody specificity but also finding compatible blood.[7] Fortunately, advances in molecular red cell genotyping have helped predict the patient phenotype for some of the antigens discussed in this chapter.[7,8]

Cami Melland, MLS(ASCP)[CM]SBB, Immunohematology Reference Lab Manager, Vitalant Mountain Division, Denver, Colorado; and Sandra Nance, MS, MT(ASCP)SBB, Senior Director, National Laboratories, American Red Cross, Senior Director, American Rare Donor Program, and Adjunct Assistant Professor, University of Pennsylvania, Philadelphia, Pennsylvania
The authors have disclosed no conflicts of interest.

TABLE 12-1. Clinical Significance of Antibodies to Blood Group Antigens

ISBT No.	System Symbol	No. of Antigens	Hemolytic Transfusion Reaction (HTR), Acute (AHTR) or Delayed (DHTR)	Hemolytic Disease of the Fetus and Newborn (HDFN)
001	ABO	4	See Chapters 10 and 22.	See Chapters 10 and 23.
002	MNS	49	Rare examples of anti-M and -N active at 37 C cause AHTRs and DHTRs; anti-S, -s, -U, and some other antibodies may cause AHTRs and DHTRs.	Anti-S, -s, -U, and some other antibodies cause severe HDFN; anti-M rarely causes severe HDFN.
003	P1PK	3	Only very rare examples active at 37 C cause AHTRs and DHTRs.	No.
004	RH	55	RH system antibodies can cause severe AHTRs and DHTRs. (See Chapters 11 and 22.)	Anti-D can cause severe HDFN. (See Chapter 23.)
005	LU	25	Anti-Lu^a and -Lu^b have caused mild DHTRs; anti-Lu8 has caused AHTRs.	No.
006	KEL	36	KEL antibodies can cause severe AHTRs and DHTRs.	KEL antibodies can cause HDFN; anti-K has caused severe HDFN.
007	LE	6	Anti-Le^a and -Le^b are not generally considered to be clinically significant.	No.
008	FY	5	Anti-Fy^a, -Fy^b, and -Fy3 cause AHTRs and DHTRs; anti-Fy5 causes DHTRs.	Anti-Fy^a and -Fy^b have caused HDFN.
009	JK	3	All JK antibodies may cause HTRs. Anti-Jk^a is a common cause of DHTRs; anti-Jk^a and -Jk3 also cause AHTRs.	Anti-Jk^a does not usually cause HDFN.
010	DI	22	One anti-Di^a caused a DHTR, but there is little evidence; anti-Di^b has rarely caused mild DHTRs; and anti-Wr^a causes HTRs.	Anti-Di^a, -Di^b (rarely), and -Wr^a, plus some others, have caused severe HDFN.
011	YT	5	Anti-Yt^a has very rarely caused HTRs.	No.
012	XG	2	No.	No.
013	SC	7	No.	SC antibodies have caused HDFN.

No.	Symbol	No. of antigens	HTR	HDFN
014	DO	10	Anti-Do^a and -Do^b cause AHTRs and DHTRs.	No.
015	CO	4	Anti-Co^a causes AHTRs and DHTRs; anti-Co^b and -Co3 have caused mild HTRs.	Anti-Co^a has caused severe HDFN; anti-Co^b and -Co3 have caused mild HDFN.
016	LW	3	No.	No.
017	CH/RG	9	No.	No.
018	H	1	Anti-H in Bombay phenotype can cause severe intravascular HTRs; anti-H in para-Bombay is not usually clinically significant. (See Chapter 10.)	Anti-H in Bombay phenotype has the potential to cause severe HDFN.
019	XK	1	Anti-Kx and -Km in McLeod syndrome have caused severe HTRs.	Antibodies reported only in males.
020	GE	11	Anti-Ge3 has caused mild to moderate HTRs.	Three examples of anti-Ge3 have caused HDFN.
021	CROM	20	No.	No.
022	KN	9	No.	No.
023	IN	6	There is one example of anti-In^b causing an HTR. Anti-AnWj has caused severe HTRs.	No.
024	OK	3	Anti-Ok^a is very rare and no cases of HTR have been reported.	No.
025	RAPH	1	No.	No.
026	JMH	6	One example of anti-JMH has been reported to have caused an AHTR.	No.
027	I	1	Anti-I in adult i phenotype has caused increased destruction of transfused I+ red cells.	No.
028	GLOB	2	Globoside antibodies have caused intravascular HTRs.	Anti-PP1P^k has been associated with a high rate of spontaneous abortion.
029	GIL	1	No.	No.

(Continued)

TABLE 12-1. Clinical Significance of Antibodies to Blood Group Antigens (Continued)

ISBT No.	System Symbol	No. of Antigens	Hemolytic Transfusion Reaction (HTR), Acute (AHTR) or Delayed (DHTR)	Hemolytic Disease of the Fetus and Newborn (HDFN)
030	RHAG	3	No.	RHAG4 has caused one case of HDFN.
031	FORS	1	No.	No.
032	JR	1	Mild DHTRs and one case of AHTR have been reported to be caused by anti-Jr^a.	Two examples of anti-Jr^a have caused severe HDFN.
033	LAN	1	Mild to severe HTR due to anti-Lan has been reported.	Cases of mild HDFN have been reported.
034	VEL	1	Severe AHTR and mild to severe DHTR due to anti-Vel have been reported.	Cases of severe HDFN have been reported.
035	CD59	1	Not reported.	Not reported.
036	AUG	4	AHTR due to anti-At^a has been reported.	Cases of severe HDFN by anti-At^a and anti-ATML have been reported.
037	KANNO	1	Not reported.	Not reported.
038	SID	1	Not reported.	Not reported.
039*	CTL2	2	Not reported.	Not reported.

*As the manual went to press, the ISBT Working Party meeting to approve CTL as blood group 039 was delayed. See ISBT website for updates.

ISBT = International Society of Blood Transfusion.

TABLE 12-2. Blood Group Function[6]

Group	Function
	Receptors and Adhesion
FY	Proinflammatory chemokine receptor and *Plasmodium vivax* and *knowlesi* receptor
KN/CROM	Receptor to remove complement-coated immune complexes
MNS	*Plasmodium falciparum* receptor and association with the anion transporter band 3
IN (CD44)	Adhesion of leukocytes to endothelial and stromal cells, stimulating T- and B-cell activation
LU/LW	Ig superfamily adhesion moleculars, receptors, and signal transducers
OK (CD147)	Receptor for cyclophilin A; facilitation of dermoblasts to increase matrix metalloproteinases for healing and/or development
CH/RG	Complement activation; null types associated with lupus
	Transporters and Channels
DI	Anion exchange; maintenance of the red cell shape/structure
JK	Urea transport
CO	Water channel
	Enzymatic Reactivity
YT	Acetylcholinesterase essential in neurotransmission

Ig = immunoglobulin; ATP = adenosine triphosphate.

THE MNS SYSTEM (002)

MNS is a complex blood group system consisting of 49 antigens on two glycoproteins. Much of its complexity arises from recombination between closely linked homologous genes. Although there are many antigens in the MNS system, the most well known are M, N, S, and s. The M and N antigens are located on glycophorin A (GPA, CD235A), and the S and s antigens are located on glycophorin B (GPB, CD235B).

Both GPA and GPB cross the membrane once and have an external N-terminal domain and a C-terminal cytosolic domain. The extracellular domains of both molecules have many sialic-acid-rich O-glycans. GPA is N-glycosylated at asparagine-45 (position 26 in the mature protein), whereas GPB is not N-glycosylated. The long cytosolic tail of GPA interacts with the cy-

toskeleton. GPA is abundant, with about 10^6 copies per red cell, whereas GPB has only about 200,000 copies per cell. GPA forms an association in the membrane with band 3 (DI blood group system), and both GPA and GPB appear to be part of the band 3/Rh ankyrin macrocomplex (Fig 12-1).[9] The relatively few copies of GPB on the red cell surface could be linked to the somewhat low incidence of identification of antibodies to S and s antigens.[10]

GYPA and *GYPB*, the genes encoding GPA and GPB, are located on chromosome 4q31.21 and include seven and five exons, respectively. Most genetic recombination between *GYPA* and *GYPB* genes occurs in a 2-kb stretch from exons 2 to 4, resulting in many polymorphisms and diversity of antigen expression within this system (Fig 12-2).[9] A third gene in this GPA gene family, *GYPE*, probably produces a third glycoprotein, glycophorin E, but this plays little or no

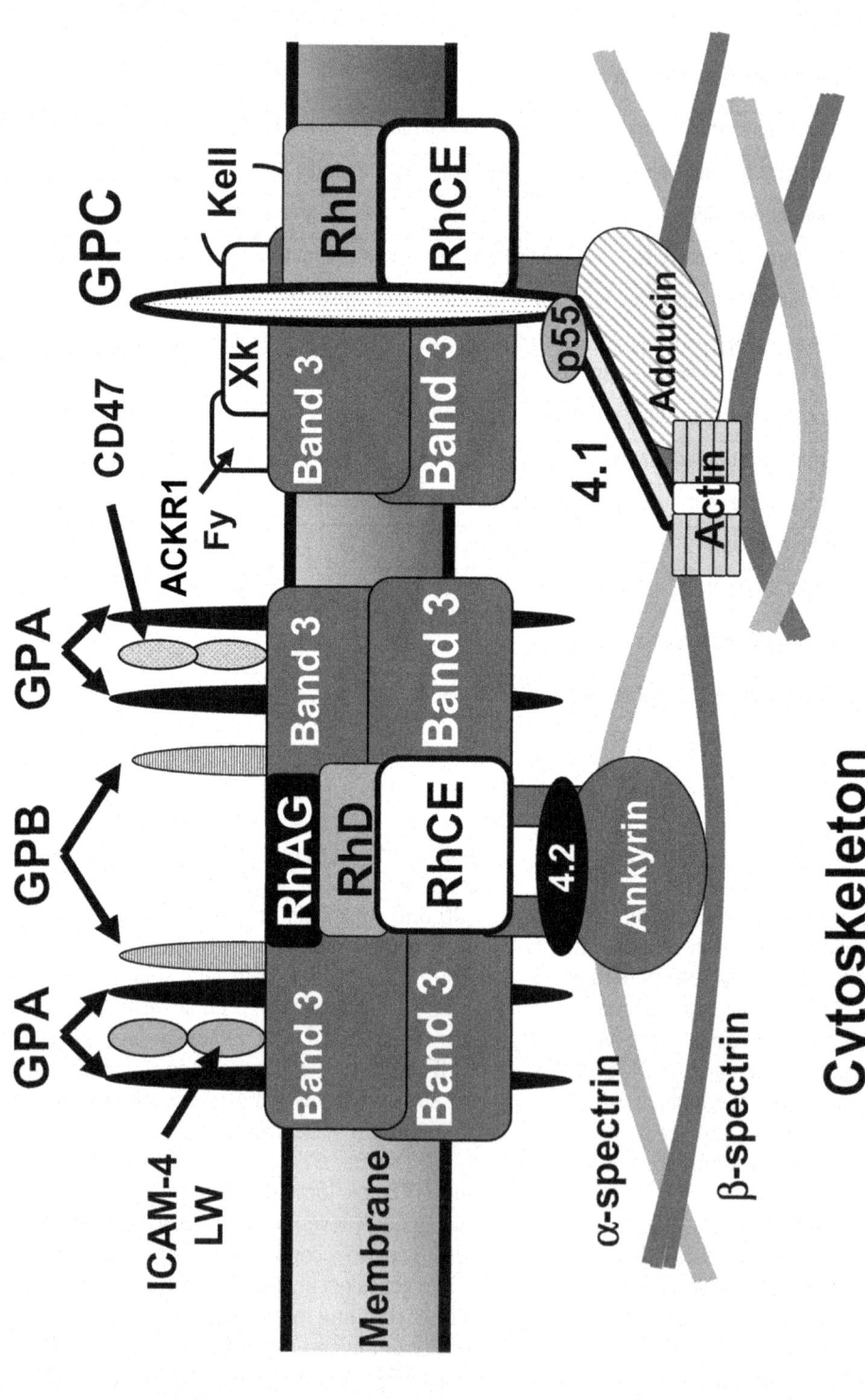

FIGURE 12-1. Model of two proposed membrane complexes containing band 3 and Rh proteins: 1) containing tetramers of band 3 and heterotrimers of RhD, RhCE, and RhAG, and linked to the spectrin matrix of the cytoskeleton through band 3, protein 4.2, and ankyrin; and 2) containing band 3, RhD, and RhCE, and linked to the spectrin/ actin junction through glycophorin C (GPC), p55, and protein 4.1, and through band 3 and adducin.

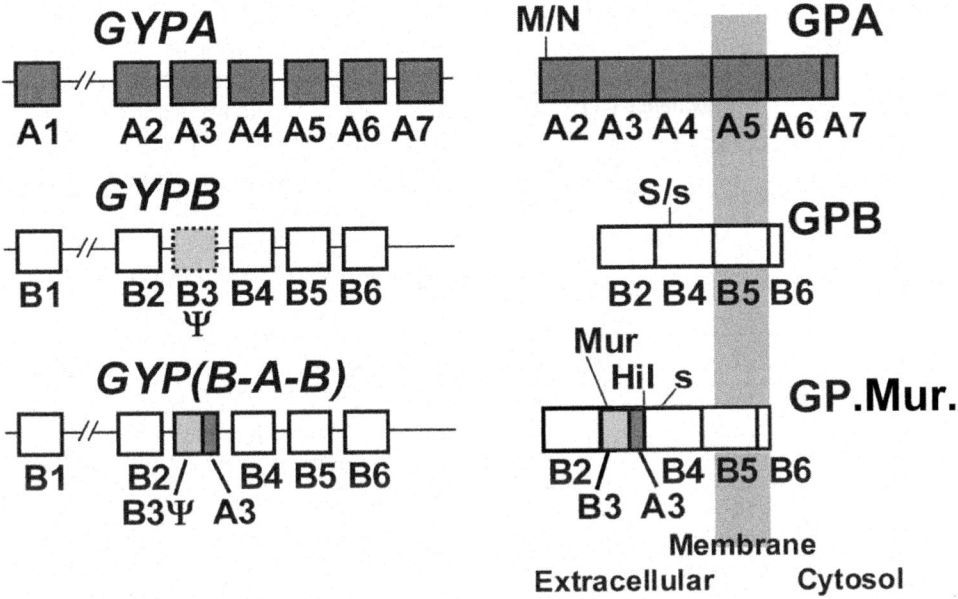

FIGURE 12-2. *GYPA*, *GYPB*, and the hybrid *GYP(B–A–B)* gene responsible for GP.Mur, and a representation of the proteins they encode, showing the regions of proteins encoded by the various exons. ψ = pseudoexon not represented in the mRNA or the encoded protein.

part in MNS antigen expression and is not detectable by routine methods.

GPA is restricted to blood cells of erythroid origin and is often used as an erythroid marker. A GPA-like molecule has been detected on renal endothelium. Both GPA and GPB are exploited by the malaria parasite *Plasmodium falciparum* as receptors for binding to red cells and may be critical to the invasion process.[11] As a result of this phenomenon, individuals from ethnic groups in areas where *P. falciparum* is endemic are more likely to be negative for the S and s antigens than other populations. This fact can be helpful information during the course of antibody identification.

M (MNS1), N (MNS2), S (MNS3), and s (MNS4)

M and N are antithetical antigens and polymorphic in all populations tested (see Table 12-3 for phenotype frequencies). M and N are located at the N-terminus, or free-amine group (-NH₂), at the end of GPA in M+ and/or N+ red cells. M+ GPA has serine and glycine at the first and fifth positions of the mature protein. The first and fifth proteins are also known as positions 20 and 25 because *GYPA* creates 19 amino acids that are removed when the GPA protein binds to the red cell membrane and becomes a mature protein. The N+ GPA has leucine and glutamic acid at those positions. The amino-terminal 26 amino acids of the GPB mature protein are usually identical to those of the N form of GPA, including the cleaved amino acids 1 to 19. Thus, in almost all people of European ancestry and most people of other ethnicities, GPB expresses 'N.' However, because GPB is much less abundant than GPA, most anti-N reagents do not detect the 'N' antigen on GPB.

S and s are another pair of polymorphic antithetical antigens of the MNS system, carried on GPB. Family studies show linkage between *M/N* and *S/s*. S+ GPB has methionine at the 29th position of the mature protein, whereas s+ GPB has threonine.

The N-terminal region of GPA is cleaved from intact red cells by trypsin, whereas that of GPB is not. Consequently, M and N antigens on GPA are trypsin sensitive, and S, s, and 'N' on GPB are trypsin resistant. In contrast, with α-chymotrypsin treatment of red cells, M and N

TABLE 12-3. Prevalence of Some Phenotypes of the MNS System

Phenotype	Prevalence (%)	
	Whites	African Americans
M+ N−	30	25
M+ N+	49	49
M− N+	21	26
S+ s−	10	6
S+ s+	42	24
S− s+	48	68
S− s−	0	2

activity is only partially reduced, whereas S, s, and 'N' expression is completely destroyed. M, N, S, s, and 'N' are all destroyed by treatment of the red cells with papain, ficin, bromelin, or pronase, although this effect with S and s may be variable.

S–s–U– Phenotype

The red cells of about 2% of Americans of African ancestry and a higher proportion of Africans are S–s– and lack the high-prevalence antigen U (MNS5). The S–s–U– phenotype often results from homozygosity for a deletion of the coding region of *GYPB*, but other, more complex molecular phenomena involving hybrid genes may also give rise to an S–s– phenotype with expression of a variant U antigen (U+^{VAR}). U is generally resistant to denaturation by proteases—papain, ficin, trypsin, and α-chymotrypsin. However, anti-U is not reactive with papain-treated red cells in rare cases.

Antibodies to M, N, S, s, and U Antigens and Their Clinical Significance

Anti-M is a relatively common antibody, whereas anti-N is less common. Most anti-M and -N

are not active at 37 C, are not clinically significant, and can generally be ignored in transfusion practice. If room-temperature incubation is eliminated from compatibility testing and screening for antibodies, these antibodies are often not detected. When M or N antibodies active at 37 C are encountered, antigen-negative red cells or those that are compatible by an indirect antiglobulin test (IAT) should be provided. Very occasionally, anti-M has been implicated as the cause of acute and delayed HTRs, and anti-M has very rarely been responsible for severe HDFN.[12] Anti-N is not generally associated with HTR or HDFN. A few cases of warm autoimmune hemolytic anemia (AIHA) caused by auto-anti-N have been described, one of which had a fatal outcome. However, in the absence of hemolysis, the specificity of an autoantibody is generally not significant. (See Chapter 14 for more information on autoantibodies with alloantibody specificity.)

Anti-S and -s are usually IgG antibodies that are active at 37 C. They have been implicated in HTRs and have caused severe and fatal HDFN. Autoanti-S has caused AIHA. If immunized, individuals with S–s–U– red cells may produce anti-U. Anti-U has been responsible for severe and fatal HTRs and HDFN. Autoanti-U has been implicated in AIHA. Because U– types are rare and are most often encountered in people of African ancestry, it can be helpful to screen those donors for S and s. If S–s– is determined serologically, it is helpful to submit samples for molecular testing to detect U+^{VAR}, which is difficult to determine serologically due to the unreliability of antisera.

Other MNS System Antigens and Antibodies

The other MNS system antigens are of either high or low prevalence in most populations. The similarity of sequence between certain regions of *GYPA* and *GYPB* may occasionally lead to *GYPA* pairing with *GYPB* during meiosis. If recombination then occurs, either by crossing over or by gene conversion, a hybrid gene can be formed consisting partly of *GYPA* and partly of *GYPB*. A large variety of these rare hybrid genes exist, and they give rise to low-prevalence antigens and, in the homozygous state, to phenotypes that lack high-prevalence antigens.[9] One well-known example of an antigen created by this recombination is the Mi(a+) phenotype created by the hybrid gene that is responsible for the GP.Mur (previously Mi.III) phenotype. The hybrid gene is mostly *GYPB*, but a small region of *GYPB* encompassing the 3′ end of the pseudo-exon and the 5′ end of the adjacent intron has been replaced by the equivalent region from *GYPA*. This means that the defective splice site in *GYPB* is now replaced by the functional splice site from *GYPA*, and the new, composite exon is expressed in the messenger RNA (mRNA) and represented in the protein.[13] This provides an unusual amino acid sequence that is immunogenic and represents the antigens Mur and Mi^a. Another recombination example is the amino acid sequence that results from the junction of exons B3 and A3, which gives rise to Hil and MINY (Fig 12-2).

Mur antigen is rare in people of European and African ancestry but has a prevalence of about 7% in people of Chinese ancestry and 10% in people of Thai ancestry. Anti-Mur has the potential to cause severe HTRs and HDFN. In Hong Kong and Taiwan, anti-Mur is the most common blood group antibody after anti-A and -B. In Southeast Asia, it is important that red cells for antibody detection include a Mur+ sample.[14]

Antibodies with the generic name anti-En^a may be made by very rare individuals who lack all or part of GPA; these antibodies have caused severe HTRs and HDFN. There are some extremely rare individuals who lack both GPA and GPB as a result of being homozygous for the M^k silencing allele. The red cells of these individuals type M–, N–, S–, s–, U–, and En(a–).[15] An antibody made by an individual with this phenotype did cause severe HDFN requiring intrauterine transfusion with blood donated by family members. Three types of anti-En^a have been recognized serologically (anti-En^{a}FS, -En^{a}FR, and -En^{a}TS), based on reactivity with ficin- and trypsin-treated red cells.

THE LU SYSTEM (005)

LU (Lutheran) is a polymorphic system consisting of 25 antigens, the majority of which are highly prevalent in all populations tested. There are four antithetical pairs—Lu^a/Lu^b, Lu6/Lu9, Lu8/Lu14, and Au^a/Au^b—of which Lu^a, Lu9, and Lu14 are of low prevalence.[16] Au^a and Au^b have a prevalence of around 80% and 50%, respectively, in people of European ancestry. Of most relevance in transfusion medicine, Lu^a (LU1) has a prevalence of about 8% in people of European or African ancestry but is rare elsewhere; its antithetical antigen, Lu^b (LU2), is common everywhere.

LU antigens are destroyed by treatment of the red cells with trypsin or α-chymotrypsin, whereas papain and ficin have little effect. Most LU antibodies are not reactive with red cells treated with the sulfhydryl reagents 2-aminoethylisothiouronium bromide (AET) or dithiothreitol (DTT), which reduce the disulfide bonds of the immunoglobulin superfamily (IgSF) domains (Method 3-18).

The LU antigens are located on a pair of glycoproteins that differ by the length of their cytoplasmic domains as a result of alternative RNA splicing. They are encoded by the *BCAM* allele located on chromosome 19q13.2, and the molecule is called CD239. The proteins span the membrane once and have five extracellular IgSF domains. The function of IgSF proteins is thought to be associated with mediation of cell-to-cell adhesion for cell recognition and innate and adaptive immune responses, and they possess structural features shared with immunoglobulins.[17] The isoform or protein with the longer cytoplasmic domain interacts with spectrin of the red cell membrane skeleton. The location of the LU antigens on the IgSF domains is shown in Fig 12-3. The LU glycoproteins are adhesion molecules that bind isoforms of laminin that contain α-5 chains. Laminin is a glycoprotein of the extracellular matrix, and LU-laminin interactions may play a role in the migration of mature erythroid cells from the marrow to the peripheral blood at the latest stages of erythropoiesis. Upregulation of LU glycoproteins on red

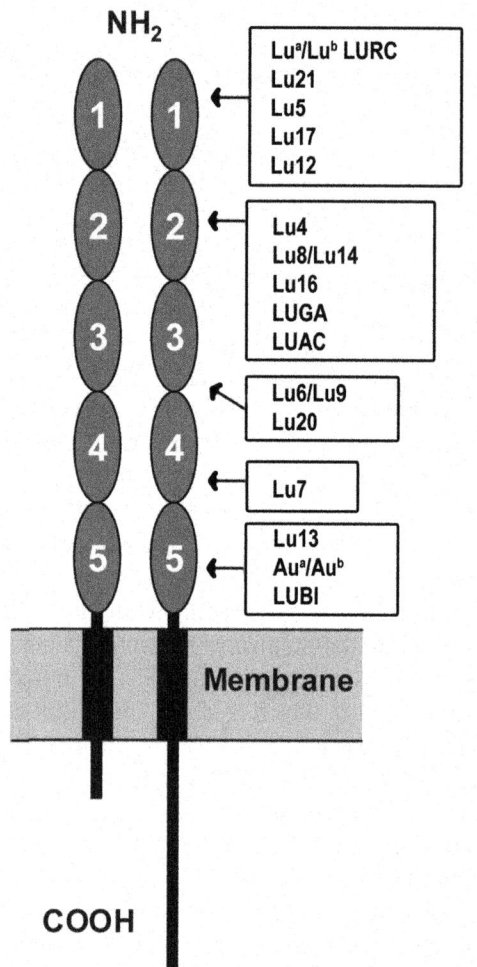

FIGURE 12-3. Diagram of the two isoforms of the LU glycoprotein, showing the five extracellular immunoglobulin superfamily domains and the location of the LU antigens on these domains, the single membrane-spanning domain, and the cytoplasmic domains.

cells of patients with sickle cell disease could play a part in adhesion of these cells to the vascular endothelium and the resultant crises of vascular occlusion.[18]

Rare LU Phenotypes

The extremely rare Lu_{null} phenotype arises due to homozygous inheritance of the inactive *LU* gene.[19] Red cells from these individuals lack expression of LU antigens, may produce anti-Lu3,

reacting with all red cells except those from Lu(a–b–) individuals. The In(Lu) phenotype is another rare group with extremely weak expression of LU antigens detectable only by adsorption/elution or predicted by molecular techniques. *In(Lu)* is the result of mutations in the erythroid transcription factor gene *KLF1*. Mutations in *KLF1* also affect other blood group genes and cause weakened expression of several other antigens, including P1, In^b, and AnWj and can be associated with hematologic abnormalities.[20,21] This is a rare, dominant suppressor of LU antigens. The In(Lu) phenotype has a prevalence of around 0.03%. In one family, hemizygosity for a mutation in the X-linked gene for the major erythroid transcription factor GATA-1 resulted in a Lu(a–b–) phenotype with an X-linked mode of inheritance.[20]

Clinical Significance of Antibodies to LU Blood Group System Antigens

LU antibodies are most often IgG and demonstrate reactivity best by IAT; they have generally been implicated only in mild delayed HTRs. Anti-Lu^a may be "naturally occurring" or immune, and it is often IgM but may also be IgG and IgA. These antibodies are usually reactive by direct agglutination of Lu(a+) red cells but often also reactive by an IAT. Anti-Lu^b may show a "mixed-field"-like agglutination. Lu(a–b–) people may form anti-Lu3, which appears to be anti-Lu^a plus anti-Lu^b.

THE KEL (006) AND XK (019) SYSTEMS

The antigen often referred to as "Kell," but correctly named "K" or "KEL1," is the original antigen of the KEL system and the first blood group antigen to be identified following the discovery of the antiglobulin test in 1946. Its antithetical antigen, k or KEL2, was identified 3 years later. The KEL system consists of 36 antigens numbered from KEL1 to KEL39, of which three are obsolete.[22] The KEL system includes seven pairs (K/k, Js^a/Js^b, K11/K17, K14/K24, VLAN/VONG, KYO/KYOR, and KHUL/KEAL) and one triplet (Kp^a/Kp^b/Kp^c) of KEL antithetical antigens. Initially, most antigens joined the KEL system through genetic associations observed in family studies. These associations have now been confirmed by DNA sequencing of the *KEL* gene.

The KEL Glycoprotein and the *KEL* Gene

The KEL antigens are located on a red cell membrane glycoprotein (CD238). KEL is a type II membrane glycoprotein; it spans the membrane once and has a short N-terminal domain in the cytosol and a large C-terminal domain outside the membrane.[23,24]

The extracellular domain has 15 cysteine residues and is extensively folded by disulfide bonding, although crystallographic studies are required to determine the molecule's three-dimensional structure. KEL system antigens depend on the conformation of the glycoprotein and are sensitive to disulfide-bond-reducing agents, such as 0.2M DTT and AET (Fig 12-4).

The KEL glycoprotein is linked through a single disulfide bond to the Xk protein (Fig 12-4), an integral membrane protein that expresses the Kx blood group antigen (XK1). Absence of Xk protein from the red cell results in reduced expression of the KEL glycoprotein and weakened KEL antigens (McLeod phenotype, see below).

The *KEL* gene is located on chromosome 7q33. It is organized into 19 exons: exon 1 encodes the probable translation-initiating methionine; exon 2, the cytosolic domain; exon 3, the membrane-spanning domain; and exons 4 through 19, the large extracellular domain.

KEL Antigens

The K antigen has a prevalence of about 9% in people of European ancestry, about 2% in people of African ancestry, and is rare in East Asia (Table 12-4). The k antigen is highly prevalent in all populations. K and k result from a single nucleotide polymorphism (SNP) in exon 6, which encodes Met193 in K and Thr193 in k.

Kp[a] (KEL3) is found in about 2% of people of European ancestry and is not present in people of African or Japanese ancestry (Table 12-4); Kp[b] (KEL4) has high prevalence in all populations. Kp[c] (KEL21), an antigen with very low preva-

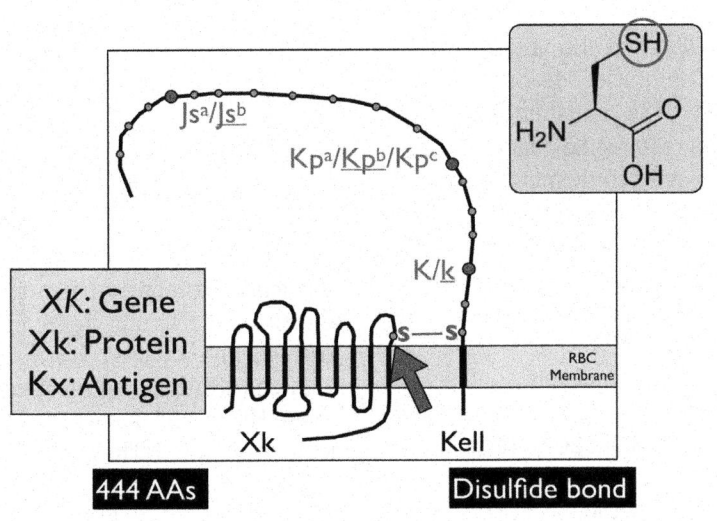

FIGURE 12-4. Diagram of the KEL and XK proteins, whose cysteine residues are linked by disulfide bonds. The remaining 14 cysteine residues on the KEL protein link with one another with more disulfide bonds. This configuration makes the KEL system antigens sensitive to dithiothreitol (DTT), which destroys disulfide bonds.

TABLE 12-4. Prevalence of Some KEL Phenotypes

Phenotype	Prevalence (%)*	
	Whites	African Americans
K– k+	91.0	98
K+ k+	8.8	2
K+ k–	0.2	Rare
Kp(a–b+)	97.7	100
Kp(a+b+)	2.3	Rare
Kp(a+b–)	Rare	0
Js(a–b+)	100.0	80
Js(a+b+)	Rare	19
Js(a+b–)	0	1

*K, Kp^a, and Js^a are extremely rare in populations of Asian ancestry.

lence, is the product of another allele at the same locus as *Kp^a* and *Kp^b*, and the antigen results from different single nucleotide substitutions within codon 281. The mutation associated with Kp^a expression reduces the quantity of KEL glycoprotein in the red cell membranes, giving rise to a slight reduction in expression of KEL antigens in *Kp^a/Kp^a* homozygotes but a more obvious weakening of KEL antigens in individuals who are heterozygous for *Kp^a* and the null allele *K^0*.

Js^a (KEL6) is almost completely confined to people of African ancestry. The prevalence of Js^a in African Americans is about 20% (Table 12-4). Js^b (KEL7) is highly prevalent in all populations, and Js(a+b–) has not been found in persons of non-African ancestry.

The expression of antigen is based largely on the inheritance of two alleles. The inheritance of one normal *KEL* allele generally results in the expression of the k, Js^b, and Kp^b antigens on red cells (Fig 12-5). If the second allele inherited by an individual carries an SNP producing the K antigen, instead of the k antigen for example, the person will express the K antigen in addition to the k antigen.[25]

The remaining five antithetical antigen pairs (K11/K17, K14/K24, VLAN/VONG, KYO/KYOR, KHUL/KEAL); the low-prevalence antigens Ul^a and K23; and the high-prevalence antigens K12, K13, K18, K19, K22, TOU, RAZ, KALT, KTIM, KUCI, KANT, KASH, KELP, and KETI all result from single amino acid substitutions in the KEL glycoprotein.

KEL antigens are resistant to papain, ficin, trypsin, and α-chymotrypsin but are destroyed by a mixture of trypsin and α-chymotrypsin. They are also destroyed by 0.2M DTT and AET and by EDTA-glycine.

Clinical Significance of Antibodies to KEL Blood Group System Antigens

KEL system antibodies are usually IgG, and predominantly IgG1. They should be considered potentially clinically significant from the perspective of causing severe HDFN and HTRs. Patients with KEL system antibodies should receive antigen-negative blood whenever possible.

Anti-K is the most common immune red cell antibody outside the ABO and RH systems; one-third of all non-Rh red cell immune antibodies investigated are anti-K. An antiglobulin test is usually the method of choice for detecting anti-K, although occasional samples may agglutinate red cells directly. Most anti-K appears to be induced by blood transfusion. Anti-K can cause severe HDFN, and in some countries, it is the practice for girls and women of childbearing potential to receive only K– red cells. Antibodies to K, k, Kp^a, Kp^b, Js^a, Js^b, Ku, Ul^a, K11, K19, K22, and KEAL are all reported to have caused severe HDFN and many have been implicated in acute or delayed HTRs.

The pathogenesis of HDFN caused by anti-K differs from that resulting from anti-D. Anti-K HDFN is associated with lower concentrations of amniotic fluid bilirubin than anti-D HDFN of comparable severity. Postnatal hyperbilirubinemia is not prominent in infants with anemia caused by anti-K. There is also an unexpected

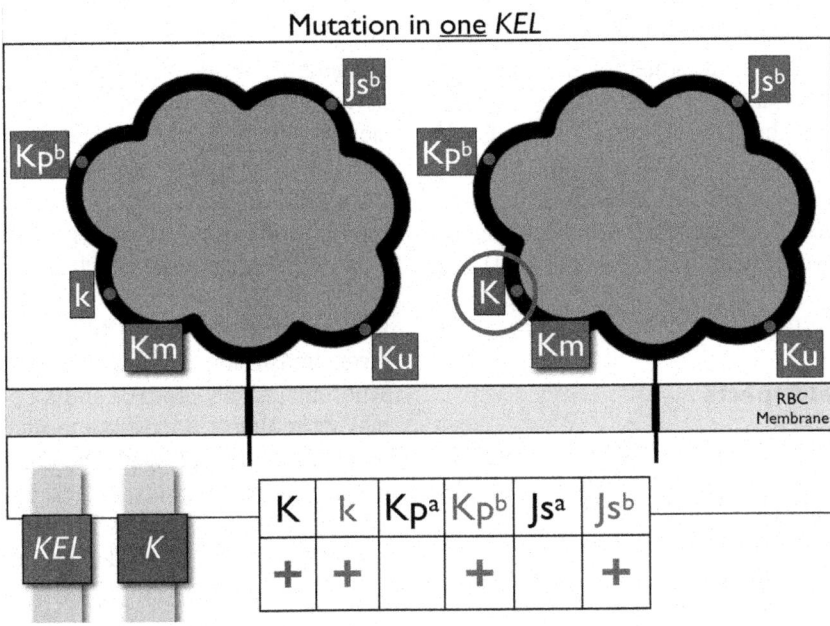

FIGURE 12-5. Diagram of a KEL protein resulting from inheritance of one mutated allele *K*, which expresses the K antigen. If the second allele inherited is the normal *KEL* allele, the individual will also express the k, Kp^b, and Js^b antigens.

low reticulocyte count in the presence of profound anemia and erythroblastosis in HDFN caused by anti-K compared with anti-D. These symptoms suggest that anti-K HDFN is associated with a lower degree of hemolysis and that fetal anemia in anti-K HDFN results predominantly from a suppression of erythropoiesis.[25] The KEL glycoprotein appears on erythroid progenitors at a much earlier stage of erythropoiesis than do RH system antigens. Consequently, anti-K probably facilitates phagocytosis of K+ erythroid progenitors at an early stage of development by macrophages in the fetal liver, before the erythroid cells produce hemoglobin.

Antibodies mimicking KEL system specificities have been responsible for severe AIHA. Presence of the autoantibody is often associated with apparent depression of all KEL antigens. Although most examples of anti-K are stimulated by pregnancy or transfusion, a few cases of apparently non-red-cell immune anti-K have been described. In some cases, the antibodies were found in healthy, male blood donors who had

not received transfusion; in another, microbial infection was implicated as an immunizing agent.[26]

KEL Null (K$_0$) and K$_{mod}$ Phenotypes

Like most blood group systems, KEL has a null phenotype (K$_0$), in which no KEL antigens are expressed and the KEL glycoprotein cannot be detected in the membrane. Immunized K$_0$ individuals may produce anti-Ku (anti-KEL5), an antibody reactive with all cells except those of the K$_0$ phenotype. Homozygosity for a variety of nonsense, missense, and splice-site mutations has been associated with K$_0$ phenotype.[27]

K$_{mod}$ red cells have only very weak expression of KEL antigens, and individuals with this phenotype are homozygous (or doubly heterozygous) for missense mutations, resulting in single-amino-acid substitutions within the KEL glycoprotein. Some K$_{mod}$ individuals make an antibody that resembles anti-Ku but differs in being nonreactive with K$_{mod}$ red cells. Other phenotypes in which KEL antigens have substantially depressed expression result from Kp^a/K_0 heterozygosity, absence of Xk protein, and absence of the GE system antigens Ge2 and Ge3, which are located on the glycophorins C and D (GPC, GPD). The reason for this phenotypic association between KEL and GE is not well defined, although there is biochemical evidence to show that KEL glycoprotein, Xk, GPC, and GPD are all located within the 4.1R membrane protein complex (Fig 12-1).[28,29]

Functional Aspects

The KEL protein has structural and sequence homology with a family of zinc-dependent endopeptidases that process a variety of peptide hormones. Although the physiologic function of the KEL glycoprotein is not known, it is enzymatically active and can cleave the biologically inactive peptide big-endothelin-3 to create the biologically active vasoconstrictor endothelin-3. Consequently, KEL might play a role in regulating vascular tone, but there is no direct evidence for this.[30] No obvious pathogenesis is associated with the K_0 phenotype.

In addition to erythroid cells, KEL antigens may be present on myeloid progenitor cells, and KEL glycoprotein has been detected in testis and lymphoid tissues, and with Xk protein in skeletal muscle.

Kx Antigen (XK1), McLeod Syndrome, and McLeod Phenotype

Kx is the only antigen of the XK blood group system. It is located on a polytopic protein that spans the red cell membrane 10 times and is linked to the Kell glycoprotein by a single disulfide bond (Fig 12-4). Xk protein is encoded by the XK gene on chromosome Xp21.1. The function of the Xk-Kell complex is not known, but Xk has structural resemblance to a family of neurotransmitter transporters.

McLeod syndrome is a very rare X-linked condition that develops almost exclusively in males and is associated with acanthocytosis and a variety of late-onset muscular, neurologic, and psychiatric symptoms.[31] It results from hemizygosity for inactivating mutations and deletions of the XK gene.[32] McLeod syndrome is associated with the McLeod phenotype, in which Kell antigens are expressed weakly, and Km (KEL20) as well as Kx are absent. When given transfusion, people with the McLeod phenotype without chronic granulomatous disease (CGD) produce anti-Km only, which is compatible with both McLeod and K_0 phenotype red cells.

Deletion of part of the X chromosome that includes XK may also include CYBB, absence of which is responsible for X-linked CGD. When given transfusion, CGD patients with McLeod syndrome usually produce anti-Kx plus anti-Km, making it almost impossible to find compatible donors, because the would-be donors are most often patients themselves. It is recommended that transfusion for males with CGD and McLeod syndrome be avoided when possible.

THE FY SYSTEM (008)

The FY (Duffy) system includes five antigens that reside on the FY glycoprotein, which is also known as the atypical chemokine receptor 1 (ACKR1, previously known as DARC). The ACKR1 gene consists of two exons, with exon 1 encoding only the first seven amino acids of the FY glycoprotein.[33] ACKR1 is on chromosome 1q21-q22.

Fy^a (FY1) and Fy^b (FY2)

The antigens Fy^a and Fy^b differ by a single amino acid change in the N-terminus of the FY glycoprotein (Gly42 and Asp42, respectively; see Fig 12-6). They are polymorphic in people of European ancestry, giving rise to three phenotypes: Fy(a+b−), Fy(a+b+), and Fy(a−b+) (Table 12-5). In Asia, Fy^a is a high-prevalence antigen, and the phenotype Fy(a−b+) is rarely encountered. In individuals of African ancestry, the Fy(a−b−) phenotype is most common, caused by homozygosity for a silenced FY*B allele (FY*02N.01). Fy^a and Fy^b are very sensitive to most proteolytic enzymes, including bromelin, α-chymotrypsin, ficin, papain, and pronase, but are not destroyed by trypsin.

The FY*02N.01 allele in people of African ancestry encodes the Fy^b antigen but is silenced

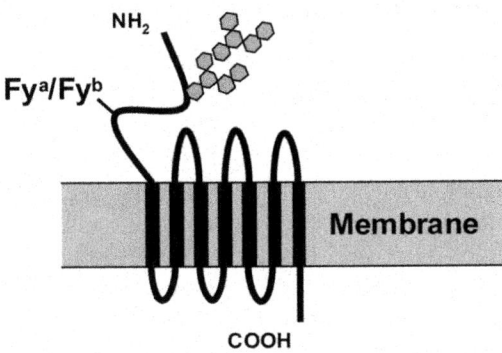

NH₂

Fyª/Fyᵇ

Membrane

COOH

FIGURE 12-6. Diagram of the FY glycoprotein (previously DARC but renamed ACKR1), with a glycosylated external N-terminal domain, seven membrane-spanning domains, and a cytoplasmic C-terminus. The position of the Fyª/Fyᵇ polymorphism is shown.

by a mutation in the promoter region, 67T>C.[34] This mutation disrupts the binding site for the erythroid-specific GATA-1 transcription factor and prevents expression of the gene in erythroid tissue. FY glycoprotein is present on many cells throughout the body; thus, Fy(a–b–) people of African ancestry lack the FY glycoprotein on their red cells only. This explains why they do not make anti-Fyᵇ and only rarely make anti-Fy3 or anti-Fy5 (see below). The GATA-1 binding-site mutation in people of African ancestry has been found only in FY genes encoding Fyᵇ; however, the same mutation has been detected in *FY*A* alleles in people of Papua New Guinea and Brazil.

A weak form of Fyᵇ antigen known as Fyˣ occurs rarely. The allele, *FY*02W.01*, encodes an amino acid substitution, Arg89Cys, in the cytosolic domain of the glycoprotein. Fyᵇ antigen may be undetected by some sources of anti-Fyᵇ (and is usually noted in the manufacturer's insert). This weak Fyᵇ antigen can be detected by adsorption/elution or predicted by molecular methods.

Fy3, Fy5, and Fy6

Very rarely people of non-African ancestry with Fy(a–b–) red cells are homozygous for inactivating mutations in *ACKR1*. These individuals make no FY glycoprotein at all and were identified through the presence in their sera of anti-Fy3, an antibody that is reactive with all red cells except those of the Fy(a–b–) phenotype. Fy6, like Fyª and Fyᵇ, is sensitive to protease treatment, whereas Fy3 and Fy5 are resistant. Fy5 is absent not only from cells of the Fy(a–b–) phenotype but also from cells of the Rh_null phenotype. The FY glycoprotein may belong to the junctional membrane protein complex, which also contains Rh proteins (Fig 12-1).[35]

Clinical Significance of Antibodies to FY Blood Group System Antigens

Anti-Fyª is a relatively common antibody; anti-Fyᵇ is about 20 times less common. IgG subclass IgG1 usually predominates, and naturally occurring examples are very rare. Anti-Fyª and anti-Fyᵇ may cause acute or delayed HTRs. Although generally mild, some have proven fatal. These antibodies have also been responsible for mild to

TABLE 12-5. FY Phenotypes and Genotypes in Selected Populations

	Genotype		Frequency (%)		
Phenotype	**Whites or Asians**	**African Americans**	**Whites**	**African Americans**	**Japanese**
Fy(a+b–)	Fyª/Fyª	Fyª/Fyª or Fyª/Fy	20	10	81
Fy(a+b+)	Fyª/Fyᵇ	Fyª/Fyᵇ	48	3	15
Fy(a–b+)	Fyᵇ/Fyᵇ	Fyᵇ/Fyᵇ or Fyᵇ/Fy	32	20	4
Fy(a–b–)	Fy/Fy	Fy/Fy	0	67	0

severe HDFN. Anti-Fy3 has been responsible for acute and delayed HTRs, and anti-Fy5, for delayed HTRs. Anti-Fy5 has been found only in individuals of African ancestry who have received multiple transfusions. Anti-Fy6 is defined by a monoclonal antibody only and reacts with all red cells except Fy(a–b–) cells. It reacts with an epitope on the N-terminus of the FY glycoprotein regardless of Fy^a/Fy^b phenotype. Anti-Fy4 is obsolete.

Functional Aspects of the FY Glycoprotein

The FY glycoprotein is a red cell receptor for a variety of chemokines, including interleukin-8, monocyte chemotactic protein-1, and melanoma growth stimulatory activity.[36] It traverses the membrane seven times, with a 63-amino-acid extracellular N-terminal domain that contains two potential N-glycosylation sites and a cytoplasmic C-terminal domain (Fig 12-6). This arrangement is characteristic of the G-protein-coupled superfamily of receptors that includes chemokine receptors.

The function of ACKR1 on red cells is not known. It has been suggested that it might act as a clearance receptor for inflammatory mediators and that red cells function as a "sink," or as scavengers, for the removal of unwanted chemokines. If so, this function must be of limited importance because FY antigens are absent on the red cells of most individuals of African ancestry. It has been suggested that ACKR1 on red cells reduces angiogenesis and, consequently, the progression of prostate cancer by clearing angiogenic chemokines from the tumor microenvironment. This potential effect of erythroid ACKR1 could provide an explanation for the substantially higher levels of prostate cancer in men of African ancestry compared with those of European ancestry.[37]

ACKR1 is present in many organs, where it is expressed on endothelial cells lining postcapillary venules. FY glycoprotein on vascular endothelium may be involved in the inhibition of cancer-cell metastasis and induction of cellular senescence.[38] ACKR1 may also facilitate movement of chemokines across the endothelium.

The FY Glycoprotein and Malaria

The FY glycoprotein is a receptor for merozoites of *Plasmodium vivax*, the parasite responsible for a form of malaria that is widely distributed in Africa and Asia but is less severe than malaria resulting from *P. falciparum* infection. Red cells with the Fy(a–b–) phenotype are resistant to invasion by *P. vivax* merozoites. Consequently, the *FY*02N.01* allele confers a selective advantage in geographic areas where *P. vivax* is endemic; this advantage probably balances out any potential disadvantage resulting from the absence of the chemokine receptor on red cells.

THE JK SYSTEM (009)

The JK (Kidd) system consists of three antigens located on the urea transporter glycoprotein with 10 membrane-spanning domains, cytoplasmic N- and C-termini, and one extracellular N-glycosylation site (Fig 12-7).[22,31] The *JK* gene (*SLC14A1*) is located on chromosome 18q11-

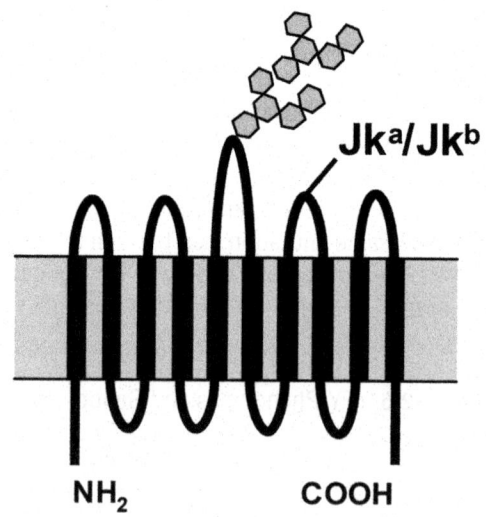

FIGURE 12-7. Diagram of the JK glycoprotein, a urea transporter, with cytoplasmic N- and C-terminal domains, 10 membrane-spanning domains, and an N-glycan on the third extracellular loop. The position of the Jk^a/Jk^b polymorphism is shown on the fourth external loop.

q12 and contains 11 exons, of which 4 through 11 encode the mature protein.

Jkᵃ (JK1) and Jkᵇ (JK2)

Jkᵃ and Jkᵇ are the products of antithetical alleles and represent Asp280 and Asn280 in the fourth external loop of the JK glycoprotein (Fig 12-7). They have similar prevalence in populations of European and Asian ancestry, but Jkᵃ is more common than Jkᵇ in people of African ancestry (Table 12-6). The antigens are resistant to proteolytic enzymes, such as papain and ficin.

Jk(a–b–) and Jk:–3

The null phenotype, Jk(a–b–) or Jk:–3, usually results from homozygosity for a silent gene at the *JK* locus. Although very rare in most populations, the null phenotype is relatively more common in people of Polynesian ancestry, with a prevalence of around 1 in 400 but as high as 1.4% in those of Niuean ancestry. The Polynesian null allele (*JK*02N.01*) contains a splice-site mutation in intron 5 that results in the absence of the protein from the membrane. In people of Finnish ancestry, where Jk(a–b–) is less rare than in other populations of European ancestry, the allele responsible (*JK*02N.06*) encodes a Ser291Pro substitution. Immunized individuals with no JK glycoprotein may produce anti-Jk3, an antibody that is reactive with all red cells except those of the Jk(a–b–) phenotype. An extremely rare form of Jk(a–b–) phenotype found in people of Japanese ancestry results from heterozygosity for a dominant inhibitor

gene, named *In(Jk)* in analogy with the *In(Lu)* dominant inhibitor of LU and other antigens. Very weak expression of Jkᵃ and/or Jkᵇ can be detected on In(Jk) red cells by adsorption/elution tests.

Clinical Significance of Antibodies to JK Blood Group System Antigens

Anti-Jkᵃ and -Jkᵇ are usually IgG1 and IgG3, but some are partly IgG2, IgG4, or IgM. Anti-Jkᵃ and -Jkᵇ are often found with other antibodies and about 50% bind complement. The Jkᵃ antigen compared to other blood group antigens is quite immunogenic, surpassed only by the K and D antigens.[10]

Although anti-Jkᵃ is immunogenic, the titer of not only anti-Jkᵃ but also anti-Jkᵇ often decreases to below the level of detection. Some agglutinate antigen-positive cells directly, but the reactions are usually weak. Generally, an antiglobulin test is required, and use of enzyme-treated cells may be necessary to detect weaker antibodies. These characteristics make JK antibodies dangerous. For example, if a patient has anti-Jkᵃ and later moves to a different hospital without the patient antibody history, the antibody may not show in testing. If anti-Jkᵃ is not identified, transfusion of Jk(a+) red cells may occur, causing a potential HTR.

JK antibodies may cause severe acute or delayed HTRs. They are a very common cause of delayed HTRs, probably because they may not be detected in pretransfusion testing due to their tendency to decrease to low or undetectable levels in plasma. Despite their hemolytic potential, JK antibodies only very rarely cause severe HDFN.[39] JK antibodies have been implicated in acute renal transplant rejection, suggesting that JK antigens can behave as histocompatibility antigens.[40]

The JK Glycoprotein in Urea Transportation

The JK antigens are located on the red cell urea transporter, SLC14A1 (also known as HUT11 or UT-B1). When red cells approach the renal medulla, which contains a high concentration of urea, the urea transporter permits rapid uptake

TABLE 12-6. JK Phenotypes in Three Populations

	Prevalence (%)		
Phenotype	Whites	African Americans	Asians
Jk(a+b–)	26	52	23
Jk(a+b+)	50	40	50
Jk(a–b+)	24	8	27

of urea and prevents the cells from shrinking in the hypertonic environment. As the red cells leave the renal medulla, urea is transported rapidly out of the cells, preventing the cells from swelling and carrying urea away from the kidney. SLC14A1 has been detected on endothelial cells of the vasa recta, the vascular supply of the renal medulla, but it is not present in renal tubules.

Normal red cells are rapidly lysed by 2M urea because urea transported into the cells makes them hypertonic and they burst as a result of the osmotic influx of water. Because of the absence of the urea transporter, Jk(a–b–) cells are not hemolyzed by 2M urea, and this can be used as a method for screening for Jk(a–b–) donors.[41]

The Jk(a–b–) phenotype is not associated with any clinical defect, although two unrelated Jk(a–b–) individuals had a mild urine-concentrating defect.[42]

THE DI SYSTEM (010)

Band 3, the Red Cell Anion Exchanger

The 22 antigens of the DI (Diego) system are located on band 3, the common name for the red cell anion exchanger or solute carrier family 4A1 (SLC4A1). Band 3 is a major red cell membrane glycoprotein with ~10^6 copies per red cell and contributes to red cell structural integrity. Band 3 has a transmembrane domain that traverses the membrane 14 times, with an N-glycan on the fourth extracellular loop. Band 3 also has a long, cytoplasmic N-terminal domain that interacts with the membrane skeleton proteins ankyrin, 4.1R, and protein 4.2 and functions as a binding site for hemoglobin (Figs 12-1 and 12-8). The short cytoplasmic C-terminal domain binds carbonic anhydrase II. Carbonic anhydrase II is an enzyme involved in CO_2 exchange on the red cell membrane.[43]

Band 3 in red cells has at least two major functions: the rapid exchange of HCO_3^- and Cl^- ions, which are important in CO_2 transport, and attachment of the red cell membrane to the cytoskeleton.[44] Tetramers of band 3 form the core of the band 3/Rh ankyrin macrocomplex of

red cell membrane proteins, which could function as a gas channel for O_2 and CO_2. Band 3 is also a component of the junctional complex that links the red cell membrane to the membrane skeleton via GPC and protein 4.1 (Fig 12-1). SLC4A1 encodes band 3. It is located on chromosome 17q21.31 and consists of 20 exons.

Di^a (DI1) and Di^b (DI2); Anti-Di^a and -Di^b

Di^a, the original DI antigen, is very rare in people of European or African ancestry but has a prevalence of 5% in people of Chinese or Japanese ancestry and an even higher prevalence in the indigenous peoples of North and South America, reaching 54% in the Kainganges Indians of Brazil. Di^b is a high-prevalence antigen in almost all populations. Di^a and Di^b represent an amino acid substitution in the seventh

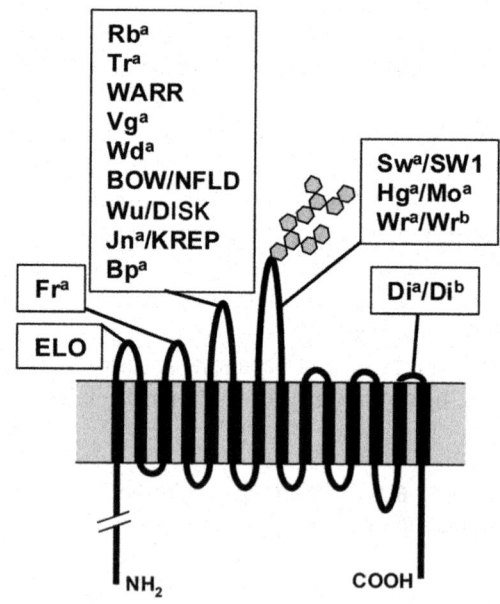

FIGURE 12-8. Diagram of band 3, the DI glycoprotein and anion exchanger, with cytoplasmic N and C-terminal domains, 14 membrane-spanning domains, and an N-glycan on the fourth extracellular loop (although the precise conformation is still controversial). The locations of the 22 antigens of the DI system on the extracellular loops are shown.

extracellular loop of band 3: Leu854 and Pro854, respectively.

Anti-Di^a and -Di^b are usually IgG1 plus IgG3, which can induce hemolysis. The antibodies typically require an antiglobulin test for detection. Anti-Di^a, which is present in ~3.6% of multiple-transfusion recipients in Brazil, can cause severe HDFN. Anti-Di^b has rarely been responsible for serious HDFN. Generally, neither anti-Di^a nor anti-Di^b cause HTRs; one example of anti-Di^a causing a delayed reaction has been reported, and anti-Di^b rarely causes mild delayed reactions.[22]

Wr^a (DI3) and Wr^b (DI4); Anti-Wr^a and -Wr^b

The low-prevalence antigen Wr^a and its antithetical antigen of extremely high prevalence, Wr^b, represent an amino acid substitution in the fourth loop of band 3: Lys658 and Glu658, respectively. Wr^b expression depends on the presence of GPA. Despite the presence of Glu658 on band 3, Wr^b is not expressed in the rare phenotypes associated with a complete absence of the MN glycoprotein GPA or of the part of GPA that is close to insertion into the red cell membrane. This provides strong evidence for an interaction between band 3 and GPA within the red cell membrane. Band 3 has been associated with clearance of senescent and oxidatively stressed red cells.[44]

Anti-Wr^a is a relatively common antibody and can be naturally occurring. It is usually detected by an antiglobulin test but sometimes by direct agglutination of red cells. Wr^a antibodies are mostly IgG1 but sometimes IgM or IgM plus IgG. Anti-Wr^a has been responsible for severe HDFN and HTRs. Alloanti-Wr^b is rare and little is known about its clinical significance, but auto-anti-Wr^b is a relatively common autoantibody and may be implicated in AIHA.

Other DI Antigens

Over the years, many antigens of very low prevalence have been shown to represent amino acid substitutions in band 3 and have joined the DI system: Wd^a, Rb^a, WARR, ELO, Wu, Bp^a, Mo^a, Hg^a, Vg^a, Sw^a, BOW, NFLD, Jn^a, KREP, Tr^a, Fr^a, and SW1. Anti-DISK detects a high-prevalence antigen that is antithetical to Wu and has caused severe HDFN. Anti-ELO and anti-BOW have also caused severe HDFN.

Antigens of the DI system are not destroyed by proteolytic enzymes, such as papain, ficin, or trypsin; however, the antigens carried on the third extracellular loop (Rb^a, Tr^a, WARR, Vg^a, Wd^a, BOW, NFLD, Wu, DISK, Jn^a, KREP, and Bp^a) are sensitive to α-chymotrypsin.

THE YT SYSTEM (011)

The YT system consists of five antigens encoded by the *ACHE* gene on the long arm of chromosome 7. Yt^a (YT1; His353) and Yt^b (YT2; Asn353) are antithetical antigens on acetylcholinesterase. High-prevalence antigen YT3, or YTEG, is the result of the nucleotide change 266G>A in exon 2 with the predicted amino acid change Gly89Glu. Acetylcholine-esterase (AChE), an enzyme that is important in neurotransmission, has an unknown function in red cells. Yt^b has a prevalence of about 8% in people of European ancestry but is more common in people from the eastern Mediterranean; Yt^a has relatively high prevalence in all populations. Yt^a is not affected by trypsin but is destroyed by α-chymotrypsin treatment of the red cells. The Yt^a antigen is variably sensitive to papain and ficin. Yt^a and Yt^b are sensitive to the disulfide-bond-reducing agents AET and DTT.

Three high-prevalence antigens—YTEG (YT3), YTLI (YT4), and YTOT (YT5)—were added to this system in 2018 with the help of soluble recombinant proteins. All three originated from homozygous mutations in exon 2 resulting in amino acid changes in AChE.[45]

YT antibodies are usually IgG and require an IAT for detection. They are not generally considered to be clinically significant, although anti-Yt^a may cause accelerated destruction of Yt(a+) transfused red cells and has been implicated in acute and delayed HTRs.[46] Rare blood may be required for a patient with anti-Yt^a. Often a monocyte monolayer assay is used to determine whether the anti-Yt^a is predicted to cause overt destruction of transfused antigen-positive red cells.

THE XG SYSTEM (012)

The two antigens of the XG blood group system, Xg^a (XG1) and CD99 (XG2), are encoded by homologous genes. The *XG* gene lies partly within the X chromosome pseudoautosomal region (Xp22.32), a section at the tip of the short arm that pairs with the Y chromosome. *XG* is one of few genes not inactivated by lyonization, which is the random inactivation of one of two X alleles in females.[47] The *CD99* gene is homologous to *XG* and is located on both X and Y chromosomes (Yp11), with pairing occurring at meiosis. Xg^a is polymorphic and has a prevalence of about 66% in males and 89% in females. Both CD99 and Xg^a expression are controlled by a common regulator gene, *XG*. *XG* transcription is impacted by allele *rs311103C*, which disrupts a GATA binding site on the *XG* gene, ultimately resulting in an Xg(a−) phenotype.[48] Although Xg^a antibodies occasionally agglutinate red cells directly, they are generally IgG and are reactive by an IAT. They are not reactive with red cells treated with proteolytic enzymes. Anti-Xg^a is not clinically significant. CD99 antibodies in common use are mostly monoclonal and of mouse origin; a few human alloanti-CD99 occur, although little is known about their characteristics.

THE SC SYSTEM (013)

The SC (Scianna) system consists of seven antigens on erythrocyte membrane-associated protein (ERMAP), a member of the IgSF that has one IgSF domain.[49] Sc1 (Gly57) and Sc2 (Arg57) are antithetical antigens of high and low prevalence, respectively. Rd (SC4) is of low prevalence; Sc3, STAR, SCER, and SCAN are of high prevalence. Anti-Sc3 is produced by individuals with the very rare SC$_{null}$ phenotype and are predicted to have red cell membrane integrity issues.

Antibodies to SC antigens are rare and few have been implicated in an HTR, but several have been implicated in mild to severe HDFN. Evidence is limited due to the scarcity of the antibodies. Although directly agglutinating SC1 antibodies are known, SC antibodies are generally reactive by an IAT. Treatment of red cells by proteolytic enzymes has little effect, but disulfide-bond-reducing agents (AET and DTT) substantially reduce reactivity.

Emerging progress in the use of monoclonal antibodies to treat disease is increasing interest in the function of various antigens. ERMAP is known to inhibit T-cell function by decreasing cell proliferation and cytokine secretion. This understanding has led to proposals to employ soluble ERMAP to help regulate the immune system for individuals with autoimmune disease.[50]

THE DO SYSTEM (014)

The DO (Dombrock) system consists of 10 antigens: the polymorphic antithetical antigens Do^a (DO1; Asn265) and Do^b (DO2; Asp265) and the high-prevalence antigens Gy^a, Hy, Jo^a, DOYA, DOMR, DOLG, DOLC, and DODE.[51] Do^a and Do^b have a prevalence of 66% and 82%, respectively, in populations of European ancestry (Table 12-7). The prevalence of Do^a is somewhat lower in populations of African ancestry and substantially lower in people of East Asian ancestry. Anti-Gy^a is the antibody that is characteristically produced by immunized individuals with the DO$_{null}$ [Gy(a−)] phenotype that results from various inactivating mutations. Two uncommon phenotypes are present in individuals of African ancestry: Hy−, Jo(a−) (Gly108Val); and Hy+^{w}, Jo(a−) (Thr117Ile). These are usually associated with weak expression of Do^b and Do^a, respectively (Table 12-7). The DO glycoprotein (ART4; CD297) is an adenosine diphosphate ribosyltransferase encoded by *ART4*, located on chromosome 12p13-p12, although its function on red cells is not known.

DO antigens are resistant to papain and ficin treatment of red cells but are sensitive to trypsin, α-chymotrypsin, and pronase. They are also sensitive to the disulfide-bond-reducing agents AET and DTT.

The Do^a and Do^b antigens are poor immunogens and therefore are uncommon antibodies. When formed, the antibodies are weak or variably reactive, usually IgG, and reactive by an IAT. The antibodies are usually found in the sera

TABLE 12-7. Phenotypes of the DO System and Their Approximate Prevalence

Phenotype	Do^a	Do^b	Gy^a	Hy	Jo^a	Prevalence (%)	
						Whites	**African Americans**
Do(a+b−)	+	−	+	+	+	18	11
Do(a+b+)	+	+	+	+	+	49	44
Do(a−b+)	−	+	+	+	+	33	45
Gy(a−)	−	−	−	−	−	Rare	0
Hy−	−	+^{w}	+^{w}	−	−	0	Rare
Jo(a−)	+^{w}	−/+^{w}	+	+^{w}	−	0	Rare
DOYA−	−	−	+^{w}	+^{w}	+^{w}	Rare	Rare
DOMR−	−	+	−	+^{w}	+^{w}	Rare	Rare
DOLG−	+	−	+^{w}	+	+	Rare	Rare

+^{w} = weakened expression of antigen.

of individuals with other alloantibodies.[52] Screening for DO-compatible donors, therefore, is best performed by molecular genotyping.

Anti-Do^a and -Do^b have been responsible for acute and delayed HTRs. Anti-Hy, anti-Gy^a, and anti-Jo^a have been reported to cause moderate transfusion reactions but are not always clinically significant. DO antibodies have not been reported to cause HDFN, although some neonates have been born with a positive direct antiglobulin test (DAT) result.

THE CO SYSTEM (015)

The CO (Colton) system consists of 4 antigens. Co^a (CO1; Ala45) is a high-prevalence antigen; Co^b (CO2; Val45), its antithetical antigen, has a prevalence of about 8% in people of European ancestry but is less common in other ethnic groups; Co:−3 is the rare CO$_{null}$ phenotype; and Co4 is a high-prevalence antigen originally thought to be Co3.[53] Anti-Co3 is reactive with all red cells except those of the extremely rare Co(a−b−) phenotype that results from various inactivating mutations. Co4 (Gln47) is a high-prevalence antigen whose presence is required for the expression of Co^a because of the proximity of the polymorphism.[54] The CO antigens are located on the red cell's water transporter, aquaporin-1, encoded by *AQP1* on chromosome 7p14 (Fig 12-9). CO antibodies are usually IgG and reactive by an IAT, although agglutinating IgM anti-Co^a has been found. CO antibodies have been implicated in severe HDFN and HTRs. CO antigens are resistant to proteolytic enzymes.

THE LW SYSTEM (016)

The LW (Landsteiner-Wiener) system consists of three antigens. LW^a (LW5) and LW^b (LW7; Gln100Arg) are antithetical antigens of high and low prevalence, respectively.[55] Anti-LW^{ab} is reactive with all red cells except those of the ex-

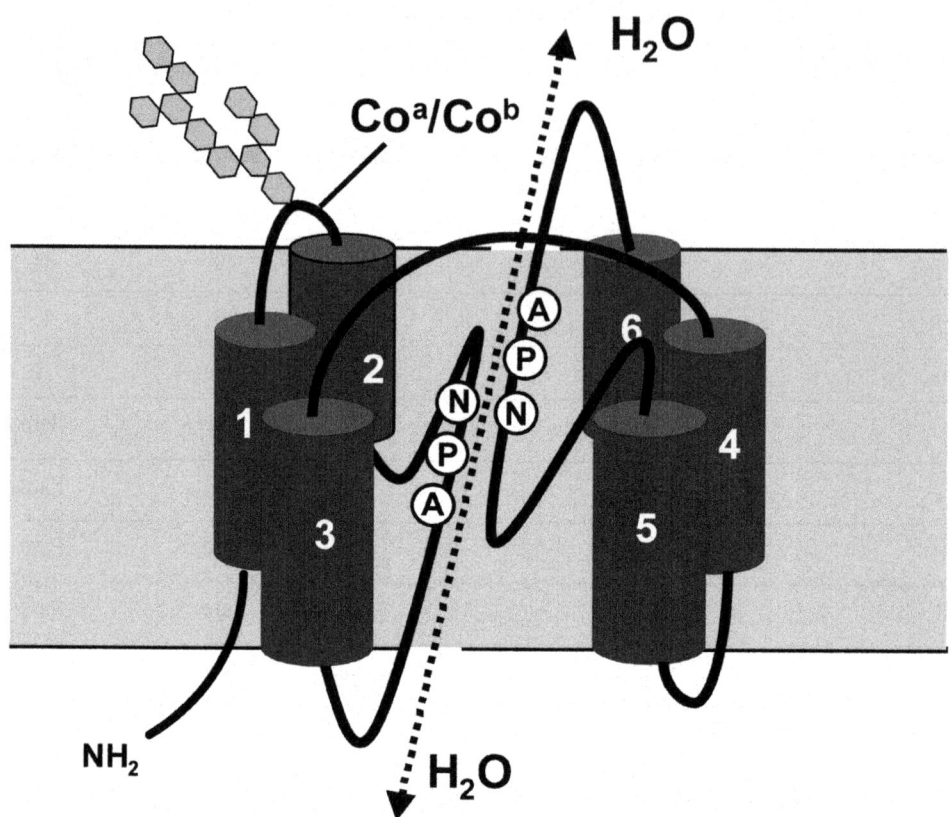

FIGURE 12-9. A model of aquaporin-1, showing the six membrane-spanning domains as cylinders. The first extracellular loop is glycosylated and contains the Co^a/Co^b polymorphism. The third extracellular loop and first intracellular loop contain alanine (A), proline (P), asparagine (N) motifs and form a channel in the membrane through which water molecules pass.

tremely rare LW_{null} phenotype and Rh_{null} cells, which are also LW(a–b–). LW antigens are expressed more strongly on D+ than D– red cells and more strongly on umbilical cord red cells, even D– red cells, than on those of adults, making D– cord red cells valuable in identification studies for anti-LW. LW antigens are unaffected by treatment of the red cells with papain, ficin, trypsin, or α-chymotrypsin but are destroyed by pronase. Disulfide-bond-reducing agents (AET and DTT) either destroy or greatly reduce LW^a or LW^{ab} (LW6) on red cells.

The LW glycoprotein is intercellular adhesion molecule-4 (ICAM-4), an IgSF adhesion molecule encoded by *ICAM4* on chromosome 19p13.2. ICAM-4 binds integrins on macrophages and erythroblasts, and it is probably involved in the stabilization of erythroblastic islands in the marrow during the later stages of erythropoiesis.[54] ICAM-4 is also part of the band 3/Rh ankyrin macrocomplex (Fig 12-1) of red cell surface antigens and might maintain close contact between the red cell surface and the vascular endothelium. Upregulation of ICAM-4 on red cells of patients with sickle cell disease has been implicated in the adhesion of these cells to the vascular endothelium and the resultant crises of vascular occlusion.[56]

Most LW antibodies are reactive by an IAT. They do not require exposure to the LW antigen, are not generally considered to be clinically significant, and have not been implicated in HTRs or HDFN. Acquired and often temporary LW-negative phenotypes sometimes occur with production of anti-LW^a or anti-LW^{ab}. This phenomenon is usually associated with pregnancy or hematologic malignancy. The transient antibodies seem like alloantibodies because they present when the patient's antigen is undetectable. If the patient recovers and the red cells are tested later, the LW antigens are again expressed.

THE CH/RG SYSTEM (017)

The nine antigens of the CH/RG (Chido/Rodgers) system, although considered blood group antigens, are not produced by erythroid cells. They are located on a fragment of the fourth component of complement (C4d) that attaches to the red cells from the plasma. Ch1 to Ch6, Rg1, and Rg2 each have a prevalence >90%; WH has a prevalence of about 15%. A complex relationship exists between the nine determinants and SNPs in *C4A* and *C4B*, the genes encoding the C4α chains. The expression of CH/RG on red cells is destroyed by treatment of the cells with proteolytic enzymes, such as papain or ficin.

No CH/RG antibodies are known to have caused HTRs or HDFN, and antigen-negative blood is not required for transfusion. However, rare cases of anaphylactic reactions and decreased red cell survival caused by these antibodies have been described.[57] CH/RG antibodies are generally IgG. Detection of these antibodies with native red cells usually requires an IAT, but they directly agglutinate red cells coated artificially with C4d. Binding of CH/RG antibodies to red cells is readily inhibited by plasma from CH/RG-positive individuals; this is a useful aid to identification of these antibodies (Method 3-17).

THE GE SYSTEM (020)

The GE (Gerbich) system consists of six high-prevalence antigens—Ge2, Ge3, Ge4, GEPL, GEAT, and GETI—and five antigens with very low prevalence: Wb, Ls^a, An^a, Dh^a, and GEIS. These antigens are located on GPC, GPD, or both. These two glycoproteins are produced by the same gene, *GYPC*, located on chromosome

2q14-q21, by initiation of translation at two different sites on the mRNA. GPD lacks the N-terminal 21 amino acids of GPC. GPC and GPD are part of the junctional complex of membrane proteins.[58] Their C-terminal cytoplasmic domains interact with the membrane skeleton through 4.1R, p55, and adducin and serve as an important link between the membrane and its skeleton.

GPC is exploited as a receptor by some strains of the malaria parasite *P. falciparum*. There are three types of "GE-negative" phenotypes (Table 12-8). Ge:−2,−3,−4 is the true null, in which both GPC and GPD are absent from the red cells, and the cells are elliptocytic. In the other phenotypes, Ge:−2,3,4 and Ge:−2, −3,4, GPD is absent and an abnormal form of GPC is present. Ge2, Ge3, and Ge4 are destroyed by trypsin treatment of red cells. Although Ge2 and Ge4 are also sensitive to papain treatment, Ge3 is resistant. Consequently, papain-treated red cells can be used for distinguishing anti-Ge2 from anti-Ge3 in the absence of red cells of the very rare Ge:−2,3,4 phenotype.

GE antibodies may be IgM and directly agglutinating, but most are IgG and require an IAT for detection. Anti-Ge2 is not generally considered to be clinically significant, but anti-Ge3 has caused mild to moderate HTRs. Anti-Ge3 has caused HDFN that tends to manifest 2 to 4 weeks after birth, and with severe neonatal anemia associated with suppression of erythropoiesis. Ge:−2,−3 blood is rare and difficult to obtain. Monocyte monolayer assays may be of value in determining potential clinical significance. Some autoantibodies with specificities

TABLE 12-8. Phenotypes Lacking High-Prevalence GE Antigens and the Antibodies That May Be Produced

Phenotype	Antibodies
Ge:−2,3,4 (Yus type)	Anti-Ge2
Ge:−2,−3,4 (Gerbich type)	Anti-Ge2 or -Ge3
Ge:−2,−3,−4 (Leach type)	Anti-Ge2, -Ge3, or -Ge4

resembling anti-Ge2 or -Ge3 have been responsible for AIHA.

THE CROM SYSTEM (021)

The 20 CROM (Cromer) antigens are located on the complement-regulatory glycoprotein called decay-accelerating factor (DAF or CD55).[59] They include the antithetical antigens Tc^a/Tc^b/ Tc^c and WES^a/WES^b. Tc^a and WES^b have high prevalence, and Tc^b, Tc^c, and WES^a have low prevalence, although both Tc^b and WES^a are present in approximately 0.5% of people of African ancestry, and WES^a is present in 0.6% of people of Finnish ancestry. The other antigens have high prevalence: Cr^a, Dr^a, Es, IFC, UMC, GUTI, SERF, ZENA, CROV, CRAM, CROZ, CRUE, CRAG, and CROK.

Anti-IFC is the antibody made by individuals with the very rare CROM$_{null}$ phenotype (Inab phenotype), and it is reactive with all red cells other than those of the Inab phenotype. CROM antigens are readily destroyed by α-chymotrypsin treatment of red cells but not by papain, ficin, or trypsin treatment. The disulfide-bond-reducing agents AET and DTT reduce antigen expression only slightly.

CD55 helps protect the red cells from lysis resulting from autologous complement by inhibiting the action of C3-convertases. Inab-phenotype red cells do not undergo undue hemolysis, however, because of the activity of another complement-regulatory glycoprotein, CD59. Because CD55 and CD59 are both linked to the red cell membrane by a glycosyl-phosphatidylinositol (GPI) anchor, pathologic levels of hemolysis occur in paroxysmal nocturnal hemoglobinuria, which is associated with a clonal defect in GPI biosynthesis and the absence of both CD55 and CD59 in affected red cells. CD55 has recently been identified as a receptor for *P. falciparum*.[60]

CROM antibodies are not usually considered to be clinically significant because there is little evidence that any have caused an HTR, and the evidence from functional cellular assays is equivocal. CROM antibodies have not been implicated in HDFN, and they are probably sequestered by high levels of CD55 in the placenta. CROM

antibodies are usually IgG and require an IAT for detection. They may be inhibited by serum or concentrated urine from antigen-positive individuals.

THE KN SYSTEM (022)

The 10 antigens of the KN (Knops) system are located on the complement-regulatory glycoprotein called complement receptor 1 (CR1 or CD35).[61] All are polymorphic, although Kn^a, McC^a, Sl1 (Sl^a), Sl3, and Yk^a have relatively high prevalence (Table 12-9).

The Helgeson phenotype, an apparent KN$_{null}$ phenotype, has very low levels of red cell CR1 and very weak expression of KN system antigens. KN system antigens are generally resistant to papain and ficin, although this may depend on the antibodies used, and are destroyed by trypsin or α-chymotrypsin treatment. They are also weakened or destroyed by AET and DTT.

CR1 is a receptor for *P. falciparum* and appears to be involved in the rosetting of red cells that is associated with severe malaria. The McC^b

TABLE 12-9. Approximate Prevalence of KN Antigens in Two Populations

Antigen		Prevalence (%)	
		Whites	African Americans
Kn^a	KN1	99	100
Kn^b	KN2	6	0
McC^a	KN3	98	94
Sl1 (Sl^a)	KN4	98	60
Yk^a	KN5	92	98
McC^b	KN6	0	45
Sl2	KN7	0	80
Sl3	KN8	100	100
KCAM	KN9	98	20
KDAS	KN10	23	87

and Sl2 alleles, present almost exclusively in individuals of African ancestry, may confer a degree of protection from the parasite. This might explain the very strong difference in the prevalence of some antigens, especially Sl1, McC[b], Sl2, and KCAM, among populations of European and African ancestry (Table 12-9).

KN system antibodies are not clinically significant and can be ignored when selecting blood for transfusion. They are usually challenging to work with, often making it difficult to distinguish antigen-negative cells from those with weak expression. Recombinant CR1 reagents or recombinant blood group antigens may be useful as inhibiting reagents to help in identification of these antibodies. They are generally IgG and reactive only by an IAT.

THE IN SYSTEM (023)

The low-prevalence antigen In[a] and its antithetical antigen In[b] plus four other high-prevalence antigens (INFI, INJA, INRA, and INSL) are located on CD44, the predominant cell surface receptor for the glycosaminoglycan hyaluronan, a component of the extracellular matrix.[62] AnWj (901009), an antigen with very high prevalence, may also be located on or associated with CD44, but the evidence is incomplete. IN antigens have reduced expression on red cells with the In(Lu) phenotype, and AnWj is virtually undetectable on In(Lu) cells. In[a] and In[b] are sensitive to treatment of red cells with proteolytic enzymes—papain, ficin, trypsin, α-chymotrypsin—and are also destroyed by the disulfide-bond-reducing agents AET and DTT. AnWj, however, is resistant to all these enzymes but shows variable outcomes with reducing agents.

Anti-In[a] and -In[b] often agglutinate red cells directly, but the reaction is usually enhanced by an IAT. IN antibodies are not generally considered to be clinically significant, although there is one report of anti-In[b] causing an HTR. Anti-AnWj, however, has caused severe HTRs, and In(Lu) red cells should be selected for transfusion. In(b−) and In(Lu) are rare blood types, and use of a monocyte monolayer assay may be of value in determining the potential clinical significance of the corresponding antibodies.

THE OK SYSTEM (024)

The OK system consists of three antigens: Ok[a], OKGV, and OKVM. All three antigens have very high prevalence and are located on the IgSF molecule CD147, or basigin, which has two IgSF domains. Ok[a] is resistant to proteolytic enzymes and disulfide-bond-reducing agents. Very few alloanti-Ok[a] antibodies and a single example each of anti-OKGV and -OKVM are known; all are reactive by an IAT.[63] In-vivo survival tests and cellular functional assays with one anti-Ok[a] have suggested that it could be clinically significant, but no clinical information exists. Basigin is another important receptor for *P. falciparum* invasion.[64]

THE RAPH SYSTEM (025)

The RAPH system consists of one antigen. MER2 (RAPH1), which is located on the tetraspanin CD151, was initially defined by mouse monoclonal antibodies that recognized a quantitative polymorphism, and about 8% of the population has undetectable levels of MER2 on their mature red cells. Alloanti-MER2 was found in three Israeli Jews originating from India who had a RAPH-null phenotype resulting from a single nucleotide deletion that led to a premature stop codon. These three individuals were CD151-deficient and had end-stage renal failure, sensorineural deafness, and pretibial epidermolysis bullosa, suggesting that CD151 is essential for the proper assembly of basement membranes in kidney, inner ear, and skin.[65,66] MER2− individuals with anti-MER2 but only single amino acid substitutions in CD151 do not have these symptoms.

MER2 antigen is resistant to treatment of red cells with papain but is destroyed by trypsin, α-chymotrypsin, and pronase and by AET and DTT. MER2 antibodies react in an IAT. There is no evidence that anti-MER2 is clinically significant.

THE JMH SYSTEM (026)

The JMH (John Milton Hagen) system consists of six antigens with very high prevalence—

JMH, JMHK, JMHL, JMHG, JMHN, and JMHQ—on the semaphorin glycoprotein CD108 (Sema7A). Anti-JMH is typically produced by individuals with an acquired loss of CD108. This most often occurs in elderly patients and is associated with a weakly positive DAT result. The absence of the other JMH antigens results from different missense mutations in *SEMA7A*.[67] JMH antigens are destroyed by proteolytic enzymes and disulfide-bond-reducing agents. They are not detected on cord red cells. Sema7A has also been shown to be a receptor for *P. falciparum*.[11]

JMH antibodies are usually reactive in an IAT but they are often not detected unless the laboratory uses an anti-IgG reagent that contains anti-IgG4. This lack of detection is usually not problematic, as they are not generally considered to be clinically significant, although one example was implicated in an acute HTR.

THE GIL SYSTEM (029)

The GIL (Gill) system consists of one very high-prevalence antigen, GIL, located on aquaporin 3 (AQP3). GIL is a member of the aquaporin superfamily of water and glycerol channels (like the CO blood group system).[68] AQP3 enhances the permeability of the red cell membrane by glycerol and water.

GIL antigen is resistant to proteolytic enzymes and disulfide-bond-reducing agents. GIL antibodies are reactive by an IAT. Anti-GIL has not been implicated in HTRs or HDFN, although monocyte monolayer assays have suggested a potential to cause accelerated destruction of GIL+ red cells.

THE RHAG SYSTEM (030)

The three antigens of the RHAG system (Olª, Duclos, DSLK) are located on the Rh-associated glycoprotein (RhAG), which is described in more detail in Chapter 11.[69] RhAG is closely associated with the Rh protein in the membrane as part of the band 3/Rh ankyrin macrocomplex (Fig 12-1). Olª is very rare, and homozygosity for the allele encoding Olª is associated with an Rh_{mod} phenotype. Duclos and DSLK have high

prevalence, and absence of these antigens is associated with an aberrant U (MNS5) antigen.

THE JR SYSTEM (032)

The high-prevalence antigen Jrª is currently the only antigen in the JR blood group system, following the independent findings of two groups demonstrating that the Jr(a–) phenotype was the result of inactivating nucleotide changes in *ABCG2*.[70,71] The gene encodes ABCG2, a multipass membrane-protein family member of the adenosine triphosphate (ATP)-binding cassette transporters that is broadly distributed throughout the body. Jrª has long been associated with drug resistance in cancer and resistance to xenobiotics, and it might be important for porphyrin homeostasis.[71]

The Jr(a–) phenotype is present predominantly in people of Japanese ancestry. Jrª antigen is resistant to proteolytic enzymes and disulfide-bond-reducing agents. Anti-Jrª is reactive by an IAT and has caused HTRs. It is not usually implicated in HDFN, although two fatal cases have been reported. ABCG2 transporter expression is stronger on cord cells than adult cells, which may lead to early anti-Jrª binding to fetal cells.[72]

THE LAN SYSTEM (033)

The LAN system consists of one antigen, Lan. Lan is a high-prevalence antigen that became a new blood group system following the discovery that it was carried on *ABCB6*. The antigen is an ATP-binding cassette transporter molecule on the erythrocyte membrane.[73] Unlike Jrª, Lan is not associated with any single geographic or ethnic group, and this is mirrored by the diversity of mutant alleles in the Lan– individuals studied. *ABCB6* is associated with porphyrin transport and was thought to have an important role in heme synthesis; however, the existence of *ABCB6*-deleted individuals indicates that there may be compensation by other transporters in the absence of *ABCB6*.

The Lan antigen is expressed variably on red cells in different individuals but is resistant to proteolytic enzymes and disulfide-bond-reducing agents. Anti-Lan is reactive by an IAT and has been implicated in HTRs but not generally in HDFN. Lan– blood is rare and use of a monocyte monolayer assay may be of value in determining potential clinical significance.

THE VEL SYSTEM (034)

Vel is a high-prevalence blood group antigen that has been assigned its own system. It has been shown to depend on the presence of small integral protein 1 (SMIM1), a protein of unknown function newly discovered on the erythrocyte surface.[74-76] Absence of Vel antigen in the majority of Vel– individuals, regardless of ethnic background, is caused by a 17-base-pair deletion in *SMIM1*, which results in the absence of the protein at the cell membrane.

Vel antigen expression is generally weak on cord red cells and differs substantially from one individual to another. Patterns of expression are a consequence both of zygosity for the 17-bp deletion and of polymorphism in the transcription regulatory region in intron 2. Serologic expression is not affected by protease treatment, although sensitivity to reducing agents such as 0.2M DTT is variable. Anti-Vel is often a mixture of IgG and IgM, readily activates complement, and has been implicated in mild to severe HTRs, although HDFN is rare.

THE CD59 SYSTEM (035)

An antibody to a high-prevalence antigen detected in the plasma of a CD59-deficient child recipient of transfusion was shown to be specific for CD59.[77] The antibody was readily inhibited with soluble protein. Sequence analysis of samples from the family revealed that the parents (first-degree cousins) were heterozygous and the child homozygous for a silencing mutation in *CD59*. The antibody was IgG, and although the child's red cells had been weakly DAT-positive following transfusion, incompatible blood was well tolerated. Thus, CD59 has been ratified as

a blood group system, and the antigen to which the antibody was directed was named CD59.1.[2]

CD59 deficiency causes chronic inflammatory demyelinating neuropathy resulting in muscular weakness, lesions in the central nervous system, and hemolytic episodes. This deficiency has been reported in over 10 children suffering from severe illness. Several of these patients had received transfusion, but only one made anti-CD59.[78]

THE AUG SYSTEM (036)

The AUG (Augustine) system consists of four antigens on the erythrocyte protein called equilibrative nucleoside transporter 1 (ENT1). The At(a–) phenotype in individuals of African ancestry is defined by an amino acid polymorphism on the ENT1 protein, and At(a–) members of a rare family affected by bone malformation lacked the protein because of an inactivating mutation in the ENT1 gene (*SLC29A1*).[79] Based on the evidence, the blood group system AUG was created. The antigen defined by the antibody produced by the null phenotype was named AUG1, and the antigen defined by the amino acid Glu391 (At^a) was named AUG2.

Anti-At^a is an antibody to a high-prevalence antigen, reactive by IAT. It has been implicated in an acute HTR and severe HDFN. At(a–) donor units are extremely rare in the United States, and use of a monocyte monolayer assay may be of value in determining potential clinical significance.

The low-prevalence antigen AUG3 (named ATML) and the high-prevalence antigen AUG4 (named ATAM) were added to the AUG blood group at the 2018 ISBT working party meeting. ATML is caused by a variant in *SLC29A1*, encoding p.Thr387Pro in the fifth extracellular loop of the ENT1 protein. Anti-ATML has caused severe HDFN. Anti-ATAM was found in 1995 in a pregnant woman of European ancestry who had received a transfusion. ATAM is caused by a homozygous missense mutation in *SLC29A1* encoding p.Asn81Ser.[45,80]

THE KANNO SYSTEM (037)

Anti-KANNO, described as a broadly reactive alloantibody, was reported in some Japanese pregnant women.[81] A genome-wide association study was performed on four KANNO-negative individuals and normal KANNO individuals. By using whole-exome sequencing, the genome variation was found and confirmed. The KANNO antigen was located on red-cell-specific membrane protein by monoclonal antibody-specific immobilization of erythrocyte antigens assay.[82] The KANNO polymorphism was located on the prion protein gene on chromosome 20p13 locus.

THE SID SYSTEM (038)

Sd^a was described in 1967 as an antigen of somewhat high prevalence with a positivity rate of about 90%.[83,84] Some of the antigen characteristics noted through the years include the loss of Sd^a reactivity in pregnancy, possible interference with binding of *Escherichia coli* in the intestines, inhibition of the entrance of malaria parasites into red cells, and exhibition by the antibody of unique refractile agglutinates in tube testing. Sd^a is a carbohydrate antigen on red cells synthesized by enzyme β(1,4)N-acetylgalactosaminyltransferase. The strength of Sd^a on red cells is highly variable from one individual to another, and Sd^a is not detected on cord red cells. Anti-Sd^a agglutination of red cells has a characteristic mixed-field appearance with free red cells when viewed microscopically. Anti-Sd^a is inhibited by urine from Sd(a+) individuals (Method 3-19) and by guinea pig urine. In 2019, Sd^a was connected to variants of *B4GALNT2* gene, and a new blood group system was established.[85] Because Sd^a is present in other tissues, it is likely that only a fraction of the 10% of the population who do not have detectable Sd^a on their red cells are actually Sd(a–), and would produce anti-Sd^a.

THE CTL2 SYSTEM (039)

The CTL2 system was named as a system in 2019 and is made up of two antigens, CTL2.1 and Rif. There have been no reports of transfusion reaction or HDFN.[86] [As the manual went to press, the ISBT Working Party meeting to approve CTL as blood group 039 was delayed. See ISBT website for updates.]

ANTIGENS THAT DO NOT YET BELONG TO A BLOOD GROUP SYSTEM

Blood Group Collections

Although many antigens are categorized to one of the 39 known blood group systems, five blood groups remain uncharacterized: 205 [Cost (symbol: COST)], 207 [Ii (symbol: I)], 208 [Er (symbol: ER)], 210, and 213 (symbol: MN CHO). Within these collections are 14 antigens, mostly with high or low prevalence. Some blood group collections contain two or more antigens that are related serologically, biochemically, or genetically to a blood group system but do not fit the criteria for system status.[1]

The COST collection contains Cs^a and Cs^b, antithetical antigens with relatively high and low prevalence, respectively. These antigens are serologically related to those of the KN system but do not appear to be located on CR1. COST antibodies are not clinically significant. The 207 collection is named Ii and has one antigen, i. This appears with variable prevalence in serologic testing, depending on the method of testing. Er^a and Er^b are antithetical antigens in the ER collection with very high and low prevalence, respectively. Anti-Er3 is produced by individuals with Er(a–b–) red cells. There is no evidence that Er antibodies are clinically significant. The 210 collection contains Le^c and Le^d, both lower-prevalence antigens. MN CHO contains carbohydrate antigens associated with MNS system antigens that are not encoded by *GYPA* or *GYPB*. These antigens have been shown to result from altered glycosylation of the *O*-linked sugars on GPA and GPB.

The 201, 202, 203, 204, 206, 209, 211, and 212 collections have been made obsolete, as they have been assigned to a system.

High-Prevalence Antigens (901 Series)

The 901 series of the ISBT classification contains six antigens (Table 12-10): all high prevalence. All are inherited, although none is eligible to join a system. All antigens are resistant to papain, trypsin, α-chymotrypsin, and DTT/AET treatment of the red cells, and all except AnWj are well-expressed on cord cells.

The first in the series is 901008, with the symbol Emm. Little is known about the Emm antigen. Seven examples of anti-Emm have been described, and of those, six have occurred as naturally occurring antibodies, all in males who have not received transfusion. The clinical significance is unknown.

Anton is next (901009), with the symbol AnWj. AnWj is a high-prevalence antigen that serves as the receptor for *Haemophilus influenza* on red cells. Alloanti-AnWj has been reported in few individuals and may cause severe HTRs, although no cases are known of HDFN.[87] Auto-

TABLE 12-10. Antigens of the ISBT 901 Series (High Prevalence)

Antigen	Number	Clinical Significance
Emm	901008	No evidence of clinical significance
AnWj	901009	Severe AHTRs
PEL	901014	No evidence of clinical significance
ABTI	901015	No evidence of clinical significance
MAM	901016	Severe HDFN
LKE	901017	No evidence of clinical significance

ISBT = International Society of Blood Transfusion; AHTR = acute hemolytic transfusion reaction; HDFN = hemolytic disease of the fetus and newborn.

anti-AnWj is more common and is associated with a transiently AnWj– phenotype. The antigen may be carried on CD44. AnWj is absent on cord red cells and is severely suppressed in red cells of the In(Lu) phenotype.

PEL is numbered as 901014. The PEL– phenotype and has been found in only two families, and two examples of anti-PEL have been described. A related antibody, anti-MTP, was nonreactive with PEL– red cells, but anti-PEL was weakly reactive with red cells of the antibody makers.

The high-prevalence antigen ABTI, number 901015, is serologically related to Vel. However, it has been excluded from SMIM1 by sequencing analysis and thus has returned to the 901 series. Like Vel, ABTI expression differs substantially, and it is generally expressed only weakly on cord red cells. ABTI is resistant to treatment of red cells with proteolytic enzymes or disulfide-bond-reducing agents. Anti-ABTI has not caused HDFN, and clinical data are limited.

For MAM (901016), there is good evidence that the antibodies are clinically significant. Severe HDFN and, in one case, neonatal thrombocytopenia have been reported to be caused by anti-MAM.

LKE is the last antigen in this series and is numbered 901017. Anti-LKE is rare, usually IgM, and is generally not known to cause HTRs or HDFN. One case of a clinically significant anti-LKE has been reported.[88]

Low-Prevalence Antigens (700 Series)

Seventeen antigens of very low prevalence in all of the populations tested constitute the 700 series of the ISBT classification: By, Chr[a], Bi, Bx[a], To[a], Pt[a], Re[a], Je[a], Li[a], Milne, RASM, JFV, Kg, JONES, HJK, HOFM, and REIT. All are inherited and do not fit any criteria for joining or forming a system.

Antibodies to low-prevalence antigens do not present transfusion problems because compatible blood is readily available; however, these antibodies remain undetected if a serologic crossmatch including antiglobulin phase is not employed. Antibodies to JFV, Kg, JONES, HJK, and REIT have all caused HDFN.

HLA Antigens on Red Cells

"Bg" is the name given to HLA Class I antigens expressed on mature red cells. Bg^a represents HLA-B7; Bg^b, HLA-B17 (B57 or B58); and Bg^c, HLA-A28 (A68 or A69, which cross-reacts with HLA-A2). Many individuals, however, do not express Bg antigens on their red cells, despite having the corresponding HLA antigens on their lymphocytes.

There are a few reports of Bg antibodies causing HTRs.[87] These antibodies are sometimes present as contaminants in reagents.[89] HLA antigens on red cells are not destroyed by papain, ficin, pronase, trypsin, α-chymotrypsin, AET, or DTT. They can be decreased or removed from red cells with chloroquine (Method 2-20) or acid glycine/EDTA (Method 2-21).

ERYTHROID PHENOTYPES CAUSED BY MUTATIONS IN TRANSCRIPTION FACTOR GENES

Mutations in genes encoding erythroid transcription factors are emerging as important modifiers of blood group antigen expression. As described in the LU system section above, heterozygosity for different mutations in *KLF1* has been identified in individuals with the In(Lu) phenotype. In these individuals, expression of antigens carried on CD44 (In^a/In^b) and the AnWj and P1 antigens is weak.[90] However, *KLF1* mutations have also been shown to affect other genes, notably the β-globin gene, resulting in the hereditary persistence of fetal hemoglobin syndrome.[91] Affected individuals have elevated hemoglobin F levels, some >30%, and demonstrate an In(Lu) phenotype. Furthermore, discrete mutations in *KLF1* appear to give rise to different phenotypes; for example, the change of Glu325Lys does not result in the In(Lu) phenotype but is associated with severe congenital dyserythropoietic anemia. These red cells demonstrate weakened expression of the antigens in the CO (AQP1), CROM (DAF), and LW (ICAM-4) blood group systems.[92]

Although mentioned above in the LU system section, it is worth repeating that a mutation in *GATA-1* resulted in the X-linked Lu(a–b–) phenotype in one family.[93] It is likely that additional mutations in these and other erythroid-specific transcription factors will be identified as the causes of altered blood group antigen expression.

KEY POINTS

1. Of 363 recognized antigen specificities, 326 belong to one of 39 blood group systems representing either a single gene or two or more closely linked homologous genes. Some groups of antigens that are not eligible to join a system are classified together as collections. Antigens not classified in a system or collection have either low or high prevalence and make up the 700 and 901 series, respectively.

2. M and N are antithetical, polymorphic antigens. M, N, S, s, and 'N' are generally thought to be destroyed by treatment of the red cells with papain, ficin, bromelin, or pronase, although this effect with S and s is variable. M and N, but not S, s, or 'N', are destroyed by trypsin treatment.

3. Anti-M is relatively common, while anti-N is uncommon. Most anti-M and -N are reactive only at room temperature and are not clinically significant. When M or N antibodies active at 37 C are encountered, antigen-negative or crossmatch-compatible red cells should be provided. Anti-S, -s, and -U are generally IgG antibodies that are active at 37 C. They have been implicated in HTRs and severe and fatal HDFN.

4. Because anti-K can cause severe HDFN and HTRs, patients with anti-K should receive K– blood whenever possible. Anti-K is the most common immune red cell antibody not in the ABO and RH systems.

5. The FY glycoprotein consists of five antigens. Fy^a and Fy^b present in four phenotypes: Fy(a+b–), Fy(a+b+), Fy(a–b+), and Fy(a-b-). Fy3, Fy5, and Fy6 are high-prevalence antigens. Fy^a and Fy^b

are sensitive to most proteolytic enzymes. In people of African ancestry, a silent allele, *FY*02N.01*, is often present. These individuals do not express Fy^b on their red cells but are not at risk for anti-Fy^b because expression in tissues is not silenced. They may be at risk for anti-Fy3/-Fy5. Individuals who are homozygous for *FY*02N.01* have the red cell phenotype Fy(a–b–). Anti-Fy^a (common) and anti-Fy^b (uncommon) are generally detected by an IAT and may cause acute or delayed HTRs that are usually mild, although some have been fatal.

6. The polymorphic antigens Jk^a and Jk^b in the JK system are resistant to proteolytic enzymes, such as papain and ficin. Anti-Jk^a and -Jk^b are not common, are generally present in antibody mixtures, and are often difficult to detect. An IAT is usually required, and use of enzyme-treated cells may be necessary to detect weaker antibodies. These antibodies have been reported to be associated with evanescence, and historical antibody identification is important to carry forward in provision of antigen-negative units. JK antibodies may cause severe acute HTRs and are a common cause of delayed HTRs.

7. The 22 antigens of the DI system are located on band 3, the red cell anion exchanger. Anti-Di^a and -Wr^a can cause severe HDFN. Anti-Wr^a can also cause HTRs.

REFERENCES

1. Daniels GL, Fletcher A, Garratty G, et al. Blood group terminology 2004: From the International Society of Blood Transfusion committee on terminology for red cell surface antigens. Vox Sang 2004;87:304-16.
2. Storry JR, Castilho L, Chen Q, et al. International Society of Blood Transfusion Working Party on Red Cell Immunogenetics and Terminology: Report of the Seoul and London meetings. ISBT Sci Ser 2016;11:118-22.
3. Poole J, Daniels G. Blood group antibodies and their significance in transfusion medicine. Transfus Med Rev 2007;21:58-71.
4. Reid ME, Lomas-Francis C, Olsson ML. The blood group antigen factsbook. 3rd ed. London: Academic Press, 2012.
5. Daniels G. Human blood groups. 3rd ed. Oxford: Wiley-Blackwell, 2013.
6. Daniels G. Blood group diversity and its impact on transfusion medicine. Transfusion science education course. Emeryville, CA: Grifols, 2018.
7. Anani W, Marchan M, Bensing K, et al. Practical approaches and costs for provisioning safe transfusions during anti-CD38 therapy. Transfusion 2017;57(6):1470-9.
8. Lux SE 4th. Anatomy of the red cell membrane skeleton: Unanswered questions. Blood 2016;127:187-99.
9. Blumenfeld OO, Huang CH. Molecular genetics of the glycophorin gene family, the antigens for MNSs blood groups: Multiple gene rearrangements and modulation of splice site usage result

in extensive diversification. Hum Mutat 1995;6:199-209.
10. Stack G, Tormey CA, Estimating the immunogenicity of blood group antigens: A modified calculation that corrects for transfusion exposures. Br J Haematol 2016;175:154-60.
11. Satchwell TJ. Erythrocyte invasion receptors for *Plasmodium falciparum*: New and old. Transfus Med 2016;26:77-88.
12. Wikman A, Edner A, Gryfelt G, et al. Fetal hemolytic anemia and intrauterine death caused by anti-M immunization. Transfusion 2007;47:911-17.
13. Huang CH, Blumenfeld OO. Molecular genetics of human erythrocyte MiIII and MiVI glycophorins: Use of a pseudoexon in construction of two delta-alpha-delta hybrid genes resulting in antigenic diversification. J Biol Chem 1991;266:7248-55.
14. Heathcote DJ, Carroll TE, Flower RL. Sixty years of antibodies to MNS system hybrid glycophorins: What have we learned? Transfus Med Rev 2011;25:111-24.
15. Al-Jada NA. A Jordanian family with three sisters apparently homozygous for M^K and evidence for clinical significance of antibodies produced by M^{K}M^K individuals. Transfusion 2017;57(2):376-8.
16. Crew VK, Green C, Daniels G. Molecular bases of the antigens of the Lutheran blood group system. Transfusion 2003;43:1729-37.
17. Eng-Hui Y, Rosche T, Almo S, Fiser A. Functional clustering of immunoglobulin superfamily proteins with protein-protein interaction infor-

mation calibrated Hidden Markov model sequence profiles. J Mol Biol 2014;426(4):945-61.

18. Eyler CE, Telen MJ. The Lutheran glycoprotein: A multifunctional adhesion receptor. Transfusion 2006;46:668-77.

19. Karamatic Crew V, Mallinson G, Green C, et al. Different inactivating mutations in the LU genes of three individuals with the Lutheran-null phenotype. Transfusion 2007;47:492-8.

20. Singleton BK, Burton NM, Green C, et al. Mutations in EKLF/KLF1 form the molecular basis of the rare blood group In(Lu) phenotype. Blood 2008;112:2081-8.

21. Keller J, Vege S, Horn T, et al. Novel mutations in KLF1 encoding the In(Lu) phenotype reflect a diversity of clinical presentations. Transfusion 2018;58(1):196-9.

22. Westhoff CM, Reid ME. Review: The Kell, Duffy, and Kidd blood group systems. Immunohematology 2004;20:37-49.

23. Lee S, Zambas ED, Marsh WL, Redman CM. Molecular cloning and primary structure of Kell blood group protein. Proc Natl Acad Sci U S A 1991;88:6353-7.

24. Chaffin J. Kell kills (video). Blood Bank Guy, February 2014. [Available at https://www.bbguy.org/education/videos/kellkills/ (accessed October 10, 2019).]

25. Daniels G, Hadley A, Green CA. Causes of fetal anemia in hemolytic disease due to anti-K. Transfusion 2003;43:115-16.

26. Marsh WL, Nichols ME, Oyen R, Thayer RS, et al. Naturally occurring anti-Kell stimulated by E. coli enterocolitis in a 20-day-old child. Transfusion 1978;18:149-54.

27. Denomme GA. Kell and Kx blood group systems. Immunohematology 2015;31:14-19.

28. Salomao M, Zhang X, Yang Y, et al. Protein 4.1R-dependent multiprotein complex: New insights into the structural organization of the red blood cell membrane. Proc Natl Acad Sci U S A 2008;105:8026-31.

29. Azouzi S, Collec E, Mohandas N, et al. The human Kell blood group binds the erythroid 4.1R protein: New insights into the 4.1R-dependent red cell membrane complex. Br J Haematol 2015;171:862-71.

30. Lee S, Debnath AK, Redman CM. Active amino acids of the Kell blood group protein and model of the ectodomain based on the structure of neutral endopeptidase 24.11. Blood 2003; 102:3028-34.

31. Gassner C, Brönnimann C, Merki Y, et al. Stepwise partitioning of Xp21: A profiling method for XK deletions causative of the McLeod syndrome. Transfusion 2017;57(9):2125-35.

32. Danek A, Rubio JP, Rampoldi L, et al. McLeod neuroacanthocytosis: Genotype and phenotype. Ann Neurol 2001;50:755-64.

33. Meny GM. The Duffy blood group system: A review. Immunohematology 2010;26:51-6.

34. Tournamille C, Colin Y, Cartron JP, Le Van Kim C. Disruption of a GATA motif in the Duffy gene promoter abolishes erythroid gene expression in Duffy-negative individuals. Nat Genet 1995;10: 224-8.

35. Mohandas N, Gallagher PG. Red cell membrane: Past, present, and future. Blood 2008; 112:3939-48.

36. Horuk R, Chitnis CE, Darbonne WC, et al. A receptor for the malarial parasite *Plasmodium vivax*: The erythrocyte chemokine receptor. Science 1993;261:1182-4.

37. Shen H, Schuster R, Stringer KF, et al. The Duffy antigen/receptor for chemokines (DARC) regulates prostate tumor growth. FASEB J 2006; 20:59-64.

38. Xu L, Ashkenazi A, Chaudhuri A. Duffy antigen/receptor for chemokines (DARC) attenuates angiogenesis by causing senescence in endothelial cells. Angiogenesis 2007;10:307-18.

39. Lawicki S, Coberly E, Lee L, et al. Jk3 alloantibodies during pregnancy-blood bank management and hemolytic disease of the fetus and newborn risk. Transfusion 2018;58;1157-62.

40. Holt S, Donaldson H, Hazlehurst G, et al. Acute transplant rejection induced by blood transfusion reaction to the Kidd blood group system. Nephrol Dial Transplant 2004;19:2403-6.

41. Heaton DC, McLoughlin K. Jk(a-b-) red blood cells resist urea lysis. Transfusion 1982;22:70-1.

42. Sands JM, Gargus JJ, Frohlich O, et al. Urinary concentrating ability in patients with Jk(a-b-) blood type who lack carrier-mediated urea transport. J Am Soc Nephrol 1992;2:1689-96.

43. Everaert N, Willemsen H, Hulikova A, et al. The importance of carbonic anhydrase II in red blood cells during exposure of chicken embryos to CO2. Respir Physiol Neurobiol 2010;172(3): 154-61.

44. Lutz H. Naturally occurring anti-band 3 antibodies in clearance of senescent and oxidatively stressed human red blood cells. Transfus Med Hemother 2012;39(5):321-7.

45. Storry J, Banch Clausen F, Castilho L, et al. International Society of Blood Transfusion Work-

ing Party on Red Cell Immunogenetics and Blood Group Terminology: Report of the Dubai, Copenhagen and Toronto meetings. Vox Sang 2019;114(1):95-102.

46. Byrne KM, Byrne PC. Review: Other blood group systems—Diego,Yt, Xg, Scianna, Dombrock, Colton, Landsteiner-Wiener, and Indian. Immunohematology 2004;20:50-8.

47. Johnson NC. XG: The forgotten blood group system. Immunohematology 2011;27:68-71.

48. Möller M, Lee Y, Vidovic K, et al. Disruption of the GATA1-binding motif upstream of XG/PBDX abolishes Xgª expression and resolves the Xg blood group system. Blood 2018;132:334-8.

49. Velliquette RW. Review: The Scianna blood group system. Immunohematology 2005;21:70-6.

50. Zang X, Ghosh K. BTNL9 and ERMAP as novel inhibitors of the immune system for immunotherapies. United States patent application publication. New York, NY: Albert Einstein College of Medicine, 2018.

51. Reid ME. Complexities of the Dombrock blood group system revealed. Transfusion 2005;45:92S-99S.

52. Gubin AN, Njoroge JM, Wojda U, et al. Identification of the Dombrock blood group glycoprotein as a polymorphic member of the ADP-ribosyltransferase gene family. Blood 2000;96:2621-7.

53. Halverson GR, Peyrard T. A review of the Colton blood group system. Immunohematology 2010;26:22-6.

54. Daniels G. Functions of red cell surface proteins. Vox Sang 2007;93:331-40.

55. Grandstaff Moulds MK. The LW blood group system: A review. Immunohematology 2011;27:136-42.

56. Zennadi R, Moeller BJ, Whalen EJ, et al. Epinephrine-induced activation of LW-mediated sickle cell adhesion and vaso-occlusion in vivo. Blood 2007;110:2708-17.

57. Mougey R. A review of the Chido/Rodgers blood group. Immunohematology 2010;26(1):30-8.

58. Walker PS, Reid ME. The Gerbich blood group system: A review. Immunohematology 2010;26:60-5.

59. Storry JR, Reid ME, Yazer MH. The Cromer blood group system: A review. Immunohematology 2010;26:109-18.

60. Egan ES, Jiang RH, Moechtar MA, et al. Malaria. A forward genetic screen identifies erythrocyte CD55 as essential for *Plasmodium falciparum* invasion. Science 2015;348:711-14.

61. Moulds JM. The Knops blood-group system: A review. Immunohematology 2010;26:2-7.

62. Xu Q. The Indian blood group system. Immunohematology 2011;27:89-93.

63. Smart EA, Storry JR. The OK blood group system: A review. Immunohematology 2010;26:124-6.

64. Crosnier C, Bustamante LY, Bartholdson SJ, et al. Basigin is a receptor essential for erythrocyte invasion by *Plasmodium falciparum*. Nature 2011;480:534-7.

65. Karamatic Crew V, Burton N, Kagan A, et al. CD151, the first member of the tetraspanin (TM4) superfamily detected on erythrocytes, is essential for the correct assembly of human basement membranes in kidney and skin. Blood 2004;104:2217-23.

66. Hayes M. Raph blood group system. Immunohematology 2014;30:6-10.

67. Seltsam A, Strigens S, Levene C, et al. The molecular diversity of Sema7A, the semaphorin that carries the JMH blood group antigens. Transfusion 2007;47:133-46.

68. Roudier N, Ripoche P, Gane P, et al. AQP3 deficiency in humans and the molecular basis of a novel blood group system, GIL. J Biol Chem 2002;277:45854-9.

69. Chou ST, Westhoff CM. The Rh and RhAG blood group systems. Immunohematology 2010;26:178-86.

70. Zelinski T, Coghlan G, Liu XQ, Reid ME. ABCG2 null alleles define the Jr(a-) blood group phenotype. Nat Genet 2012;44:131-2.

71. Robey RW, To KK, Polgar O, et al. ABCG2: A perspective. Adv Drug Deliv Rev 2009;61:3-13.

72. Fujita S, Kashiwagi H, Tomimatsu T, et al. Expression levels of ABCG2 on cord red blood cells and study of fetal anemia associated with anti-Jr(a). Transfusion 2016;56:1171-81.

73. Helias V, Saison C, Ballif BA, et al. ABCB6 is dispensable for erythropoiesis and specifies the new blood group system Langereis. Nat Genet 2012;44:170-3.

74. Storry JR, Joud M, Christophersen MK, et al. Homozygosity for a null allele of SMIM1 defines the Vel-negative blood group phenotype. Nat Genet 2013;45:537-41.

75. Ballif BA, Helias V, Peyrard T, et al. Disruption of SMIM1 causes the Vel- blood type. EMBO Mol Med 2013;5:751-61.

76. Cvejic A, Haer-Wigman L, Stephens JC, et al. SMIM1 underlies the Vel blood group and influences red blood cell traits. Nat Genet 2013;45:542-5.

77. Anliker M, von Zabern I, Hochsmann B, et al. A new blood group antigen is defined by anti-CD59, detected in a CD59-deficient patient. Transfusion 2014;54:1817-22.

78. Weinstock C, Anliker M, von Zabern I. An update on the CD59 blood group system. Immunohematology 2019;35:7-8.

79. Daniels G, Ballif BA, Helias V, et al. Lack of the nucleoside transporter ENT1 results in the Augustine-null blood type and ectopic mineralization. Blood 2015;125:3651-4.

80. Daniels G. An update on the Augustine blood group system. Immunohematology 2019;35:1-2.

81. Kawabata K, Uchikawa M, Ohio H, et al. Anti-KANNO: A novel alloantibody against a red cell antigen of high frequency. Transfus Med Rev 2014:28:23-8.

82. Omae Y, Ito S, Takeuchi M, et al. Integrative genome analysis identified the KANNO blood group antigen as prion protein. Transfusion 2019;59;2429-35.

83. Macvie SJ, Morton JA, Pickels MM. The reactions and inheritance of a new blood group antigen Sd^a. Vox Sang 1967;13:485-92.

84. Benton PH, Howell P, Ikin EW. Anti-Sd^a, a new blood group antibody. Vox Sang 1967;13:493-501.

85. Stenfelt l, Hellberg A, Moller M, et al. Missense mutations in the C-terminal portion of the *B4GALNT2*-encoded glycosyltransferase underlying the Sd(a-) phenotype. Biochem Biophys Rep 2019;19:100659.

86. Peyrard T, Vrignaud C, Mikdar M, et al. IGT4: Alloantibodies directed to the SLC4412/CTL2 transporter define two new red cell antigens and a novel human blood group system (abstract). Transfusion 2019;59(Suppl):18A.

87. Zhaodong X, Duffett L, Tokessy M, et al. Anti-AnWj causing hemolytic transfusion reactions in a patient with aplastic anemia. Transfusion 2012;52:1476-81.

88. Cooling L, Dake LR, Haverty D, et al. A hemolytic anti-LKE associated with a rare LKE-negative, "weak P" red blood cell phenotype: Alloanti-LKE and alloanti-P recognize galactosylgloboside and monosialogalactosylgloboside (LKE) antigens. Transfusion 2015;55(1):115-28.

89. Nance ST. Do HLA antibodies cause hemolytic transfusion reactions or decreased RBC survival? Transfusion 2003;43:687-90.

90. Anti-Fy^a and Anti-Fy^b (package insert). Rev 02/2013. Peachtree Corners, GA: Immucor, 2013.

91. Borg J, Papadopoulos P, Georgitsi M, et al. Haploinsufficiency for the erythroid transcription factor KLF1 causes hereditary persistence of fetal hemoglobin. Nat Genet 2010;42:801-5.

92. Arnaud L, Saison C, Helias V, et al. A dominant mutation in the gene encoding the erythroid transcription factor KLF1 causes a congenital dyserythropoietic anemia. Am J Hum Genet 2010;87:721-7.

93. Singleton BK, Roxby DJ, Stirling JW, et al. A novel GATA1 mutation (Stop414Arg) in a family with the rare X-linked blood group Lu(a-b-) phenotype and mild macrothrombocytic thrombocytopenia. Br J Haematol 2013;161:139-42.

CHAPTER 13

Identification of Antibodies to Red Cell Antigens

Lay See Er, MSTM, SBB(ASCP)^{CM}, CQA(ASQ), and Debra J. Bailey, MT(ASCP)SBB

NATURALLY OCCURRING ANTI-A and anti-B are the only red cell antibodies commonly found in human serum or plasma. All other antibodies are called "unexpected red cell antibodies." This chapter discusses methods for identifying unexpected red cell antibodies once pretransfusion testing (see Chapter 17) indicates an unexpected antibody is present.

There are two types of unexpected red cell antibodies: alloantibodies and autoantibodies. When an individual produces an antibody to an antigen that he or she lacks, the antibody is called an alloantibody. When an individual produces an antibody to an antigen that he or she possesses, the antibody is called an autoantibody. Therefore, by definition, alloantibodies react only with allogeneic red cells that express the corresponding antigens—not with the antibody producer's red cells. Conversely, autoantibodies are reactive with the red cells of the antibody producer. In fact, autoantibodies usually are reactive with most reagent red cells as well as with autologous red cells because they typically target an antigen commonly expressed on all red cells except those of rare phenotypes.

Immunization to red cell antigens may result from pregnancy, transfusion, transplantation, needle sharing, or injections of immunogenic material. The incidence of alloimmunization is extremely variable depending on the patient population being studied. In chronic transfusion recipient populations, such as those with sickle cell anemia or thalassemia, as many as 14% to 50% of individuals are reported to be alloimmunized, whereas in the general population, alloimmunization is estimated to be 0.5% to 1.5%.[1-4]

In some instances, no specific immunizing event due to red cell exposure can be identified. Non-red-cell-stimulated or "naturally occurring" antibodies have presumably resulted from exposure to environmental, bacterial, or viral antigens that are similar to blood group antigens. Antibodies detected in serologic tests may also be passively acquired from injected immunoglobulin, donor plasma, passenger lymphocytes in transplanted organs, or hematopoietic progenitor cells (HPCs) or, in the case of neonates, may be of maternal origin.

After an antibody has been detected, its type (auto and/or allo)—and in the case of alloantibody, its specificity—should be determined and its clinical significance assessed. A clinically significant red cell antibody is defined as an antibody that is associated with hemolytic disease of the fetus and newborn (HDFN), hemolytic transfusion reactions, or a notable decrease in transfused red cell survival. Determining the specificity of the antibody is the most commonly used way of predicting its possible clinical significance. Yet, the degree of clinical significance varies among antibodies with the same specificity;

Lay See Er, MSTM, SBB(ASCP)^{CM}, CQA(ASQ), Manager, Immunohematology Reference Laboratory, Bloodworks Northwest, Seattle, Washington; and Debra J. Bailey, MT(ASCP)SBB, Lead Technologist, Immunohematology Reference Laboratory, American Red Cross Blood Services, Detroit, Michigan
The authors have disclosed no conflicts of interest.

some cause destruction of incompatible red cells within hours or even minutes, whereas others decrease red cell survival by only a few days, and still others do not shorten red cell survival discernibly. Some antibodies are known to cause HDFN, whereas others may cause a positive direct antiglobulin test (DAT) result in the fetus without clinical evidence of HDFN.

BASIC CONCEPTS IN RED CELL ANTIGEN EXPRESSION

Antibody identification is dependent on the reactivity of the serum or plasma with red cells of known antigen expression. A basic understanding of variables in antigen expression is critical to interpreting reactivity in identification studies.

Zygosity and Dosage

The reaction strength of some antibodies may vary because of dosage, meaning that antibodies are more strongly reactive (or only reactive) with red cells that possess a "double-dose" expression of the antigen. *Dosage* describes the expression of an antigen on red cells, while *zygosity* describes the degree of similarity of alleles (alternative forms of the same gene) present at a given locus. Double-dose antigen expression occurs when an individual is homozygous for the gene for a given allele that encodes the antigen. Red cells from individuals who are heterozygous for the gene would be expected to express a single-dose of the corresponding antigen(s). Red cells with a single-dose expression of an antigen would typically have fewer antigen sites than those that express a double dose and, therefore, may be weakly reactive or nonreactive with a weak example of the corresponding antibody. Alloantibodies vary in their tendency to demonstrate dosage (see "Alleles" in Chapter 9). Many antibodies to antigens in the RH, FY (Duffy), MNS, and JK (Kidd) blood group systems demonstrate dosage. (See Table 9-4 in Chapter 9 for examples of International Society of Blood Transfusion terminology applied to blood group systems.)

Variation in Adults and Neonates

Some antigens (eg, I, P1, Le[a], and Sd[a]) show variable expression on red cells from different adults. The antigenic differences can be demonstrated serologically; however, the variability from one antigen-positive adult to another is unrelated to zygosity. Some antigens are expressed differently on cord/neonate red cells compared to adult red cells. Antigen expression on cord/neonate red cells may be absent, weaker, or stronger as compared to adult red cells. (Table 13-1 provides some examples.)

Changes with Storage

Blood group antibodies may be more weakly reactive with stored red cells than with fresh red cells. Some antigens (eg, Fy[a], Fy[b], M, P1, Kn[a], McC[a], and Bg) deteriorate more rapidly than others during storage, and the rate varies among red cells from different individuals.[4] Because red cells from donors are often fresher than commercial reagent red cells, some antibodies have stronger reactions with donor red cells than with reagent red cells. Similarly, storage of red cells in a freezer may cause antigens to deteriorate, thus producing misleading antibody identification results.

The pH or other characteristics of the storage medium can affect the rate of antigen deterioration.[4,6] For example, Fy[a] and Fy[b] antigens may weaken when the red cells are stored in a medium with low pH and low ionic strength. Thus, certain antibodies may demonstrate differences

TABLE 13-1. Antigen Expression on Cord Red Cells*

Expression	Antigens
Negative	Le[a], Le[b], Sd[a], Ch, Rg, and AnWj
Weak	I, H, P1, Lu[a], Lu[b], Yt[a], Vel, Bg, KN, and DO antigens, Yk[a], Cs[a], and Fy3
Strong	i, LW[a], and LW[b]

*Modified with permission from Reid et al.[5]

in reactivity with red cells from different manufacturers if the suspending media are different.

The age and nature of the specimen must be considered when red cells are typed. Antigens on red cells from clotted samples tend to deteriorate more quickly than antigens on red cells from donor units that are collected in citrate anticoagulants, such as acid-citrate-dextrose or citrate-phosphate-dextrose. Red cells in donor units collected in approved anticoagulants retain their antigens throughout the standard shelf life of the blood component. Samples with EDTA up to 14 days old are suitable for antigen typing.[7] However, the manufacturer's instructions pertaining to sample suitability for antigen typing should always be consulted when commercial typing reagents are used.

INITIAL ANTIBODY IDENTIFICATION CONSIDERATIONS

Specimen Requirements

Serum and plasma are interchangeable for antibody testing unless complement is required for antibody detection. In such rare cases, only serum provides complement. Throughout this chapter, serum can be considered interchangeable with plasma unless the text indicates otherwise. The use of serum or plasma may also be dictated by the test method or the manufacturer's instructions for the reagents employed.

Depending on the test methods used and the hematocrit of the patient, a 5-mL to 10-mL aliquot of whole blood usually contains enough serum or plasma for identifying simple antibody specificities; more whole blood (ie, 10 mL to 20 mL) may be required for complex studies. When autologous red cells are tested, the use of samples anticoagulated with EDTA avoids problems associated with the in-vitro uptake of complement components by red cells, which may occur when clotted samples are used.

Reagents and Test Methods

Antibody Detection Red Cells

Group O red cells suitable for pretransfusion antibody screening are commercially available and most frequently offered as sets of either two or three (sometimes four) samples of reagent single-donor red cells. All reagent red cell sets licensed by the US Food and Drug Administration (FDA) for this purpose must contain red cell samples that collectively express the following antigens: D, C, E, c, e, M, N, S, s, P1, Le^a, Le^b, K, k, Fy^a, Fy^b, Jk^a, and Jk^b. Three-red-cell-sample antibody-detection sets often offer red cells from donors presumed homozygous for the respective genes with double-dose expression for the following common antigens: D, C, E, c, e, k, M, N, S, s, Fy^a, Fy^b, Jk^a, and Jk^b. As mentioned above, antibodies to antigens of the RH, MNS, FY, and JK blood group systems most commonly demonstrate dosage. Each laboratory should decide whether to use two or three reagent single-donor red cell samples for antibody detection testing. When antibody detection is automated, the instrument platform may dictate the reagent red cell configuration. In the United States, pooled red cells for antibody detection are obtained from two different donors and may be used only when testing donor samples. Reagent red cells should be refrigerated when not in use and should be in date when used for antibody detection tests.

Antibody Identification Red Cell Panels

Identification of antibodies to red cell antigens detected in pretransfusion antibody screening requires testing the serum/plasma against a panel of red cell samples (typically 8-16) with known antigenic composition. Usually, the red cell samples are obtained from commercial suppliers, but institutions may assemble their own panels using red cells from local sources. Except in special circumstances, panel cells are group O, thereby allowing serum/plasma of any ABO group to be tested.

Each reagent red cell sample in the panel is from a different donor. The reagent red cells are selected so a distinctive pattern of positive and negative reactions will result when the reactivity of all the panel cells is considered. To be functional, a reagent red cell panel must make it possible to identify with confidence those clinically significant alloantibodies that are most commonly encountered, such as anti-D, -E, -K, and -Fy^a. The phenotypes of the reagent red cells should be distributed so that single common alloantibody specificities can be clearly identified and most others can be excluded. Ideally, patterns of reactivity for most examples of single alloantibodies should not overlap with any other (eg, all of the K+ red cells should not be the only ones that are also E+). Reagent red cells with double-dose antigen expression are included to detect common antibodies that frequently show dosage. Commercial panels are accompanied by a common antigen profile sheet that lists the phenotypes of the red cells. Table 13-2 provides an example of a common antigen profile sheet for a hypothetical antibody identification panel. It is essential to use the correct panel antigen profile sheet when interpreting results because the combination of red cell samples is different for each lot of panel cells. Commercial reagent red cells for tube testing are diluted to a 2% to 5% suspension in a preservative solution that can be used directly from the bottle. Washing the red cells before use is usually unnecessary unless the preservative solution is suspected of interfering with antibody identification.

Panel cells beyond their expiration date should not be used as the sole resource for antibody identification. Most laboratories use in-date reagent red cells for initial antibody identification and, if necessary, use expired reagent red cells to exclude or confirm uncommon specificities. Any laboratory that uses expired reagent red cells should establish a policy and validate any procedures associated with this practice.[8(p21)]

Test Methods

All techniques for antibody detection and identification in general use today are based on the principle of hemagglutination (tube or column agglutination systems) or red cell adherence (solid phase). AABB *Standards for Blood Banks and Transfusion Services (Standards)* requires that "methods of testing shall be those that demonstrate clinically significant antibodies" and "include incubation at 37 C preceding an antiglobulin test."[9(p36)] All methods meet this standard, but each method offers different advantages. Tube testing offers flexibility to test at different phases and the option to use a variety of additive solutions (and thus obtain varying degrees of sensitivity). It also requires little specialized equipment. Column agglutination and solid-phase technology offer stable and possibly less subjective endpoints, workflow standardization, and the ability to be incorporated into semiautomated or automated systems. They provide a sensitive detection system for most blood group antibodies. Column agglutination, solid-phase methods, and very sensitive tube tests have also been shown to enhance serologic reactivity that may not be clinically significant in the selection of units for transfusion, including the reactivity of warm autoantibodies. The different methods offer laboratories choice in selecting a primary antibody detection and identification method that, with its sensitivity, specificity, automation capabilities (if desired), and cost, is suitable for the patient population served, the laboratory size, and its staff expertise/experience.

Published studies have compared the various methods for detection of wanted and unwanted red cell alloantibodies as well as the potential effect of using red cell membranes vs intact red cells.[10-16] Laboratories should be familiar with the unique reactivity characteristics of their selected method. They frequently will choose to have one or more additional methods available and develop testing algorithms that involve the different methods to aid in the investigation and resolution of results that are not easily apparent with their primary method.

Additive Solutions

Although the test method may consist solely of serum or plasma and red cells (either reagent red cells as provided by the manufacturer or saline-suspended red cells), as in Method 3-2, most serologists use some type of additive solution when tube methods are used to decrease incubation time and/or increase sensitivity. Several different additive solutions are available,

TABLE 13-2. Example of a Reagent Red Cell Panel for Antibody Identification

Cell	RH								MNS				KEL				P1	LE		FY		JK		Others	Cell	Results 37 C IAT
	D	C	E	c	e	f	C^w	V	M	N	S	s	K	k	Kp^a	Js^a	P1	Le^a	Le^b	Fy^a	Fy^b	Jk^a	Jk^b			
1	+	+	0	0	+	0	0	0	+	0	0	+	0	+	0	0	–	0	+	+	+	0	+	Bg(a+)	1	
2	+	+	0	0	+	0	+	0	+	+	+	0	0	+	0	0	–	0	0	0	0	+	0		2	
3	+	0	+	+	0	0	0	0	0	+	0	+	0	+	0	0	0	+	0	0	+	+	+		3	
4	0	+	0	+	+	+	0	0	+	0	+	+	0	+	0	0	–	0	+	+	0	+	0		4	
5	0	0	+	+	+	+	0	0	0	+	+	+	0	+	0	0	–	0	+	0	+	0	+		5	
6	0	0	0	+	+	+	0	0	+	0	+	0	+	+	0	0	–	0	+	+	0	0	+		6	
7	0	0	0	+	+	+	0	0	+	+	0	+	0	+	0	0	+	0	+	0	+	+	0		7	
8	+	0	0	0	+	+	0	+	0	+	+	0	0	+	0	0	0	0	0	0	0	0	+		8	
9	0	0	0	+	+	+	0	0	+	0	0	+	+	+	0	0	+	+	0	+	+	+	+		9	
10	0	0	0	+	+	+	0	0	+	0	0	+	+	+	+	0	+	0	0	0	+	+	+	Yt(b+)	10	
11	+	+	0	0	+	0	0	0	+	+	0	+	0	+	0	0	+	0	+	0	+	0	+		11	
AC																									AC	

+ indicates presence of antigen; 0 indicates absence of antigen; AC = autocontrol; IAT = indirect antiglobulin test.

including low-ionic-strength saline (LISS), poly-ethylene glycol (PEG), and 22% bovine albumin. Additional enhancement techniques may be used for complex studies. Some enhancement techniques are discussed in more detail later in this chapter. Specifics regarding the mechanism of action for 22% bovine albumin, LISS, and PEG can be found in the methods describing their use (Methods 3-3, 3-4, and 3-5). Non-tube methods typically prescribe the use of an additive solution, most often LISS, for the same reasons they are used in tube methods.

Antiglobulin Reagents

Most antibody detection and identification studies include an indirect antiglobulin test (IAT) phase. Either antihuman globulin (AHG) specific only for human immunoglobulin G (IgG) or a polyspecific reagent that contains anti-IgG and anticomplement may be used. A polyspecific reagent may detect—or may detect more readily—antibodies that bind complement, because a single IgG molecule can deposit multiple complement molecules. Therefore, presence of a low-level IgG antibody may be visualized by its complement activation. To detect complement binding, serum rather than plasma must be used: the anticoagulant in plasma binds calcium, making it unavailable for complement activation. Complement binding may be advantageous in some rare instances, such as the detection of certain JK system antibodies. Because of the sensitivity of current test methods, most serologists prefer IgG-specific AHG reagents for routine use. This avoids unwanted reactivity resulting from in-vitro complement binding by cold-reactive antibodies.[17]

Antiglobulin reagents may be derived from monoclonal or polyclonal source material. Polyclonal reagents, by nature, contain antibodies from many B-cell clones, and collectively their reactivity is directed at many epitopes of the target antigen. Monoclonal reagents have selective reactivity with only specific epitopes. Reagents made from different clones may have subtle reactivity differences: some monoclonal-based reagents are blended to cover a wider range of epitope specificities. The anticomplement reagents licensed in the United States are

monoclonal. Anti-IgG can be either polyclonal or monoclonal. Some US-licensed monoclonal anti-IgG does not detect antibodies of IgG4 subclass. This has little clinical significance, as red cell antibodies of pure IgG4 subclass are rare, and they are not associated with increased red cell destruction because monocytes do not have receptors for the Fc portion of IgG4 molecules. The property of an anti-IgG reagent not to react with IgG4 subclass antibodies may be a testing advantage in some cases. It has been described to be a valuable tool for excluding common clinically significant alloantibodies of IgG1, IgG2, and IgG3 subclasses in patients who either have made a pure IgG4 alloantibody (eg, anti-JMH) or have a passively acquired IgG4 antibody due to a biologic therapy (ie, anti-CD47, Hu5F9-G4).[18-20] However, a recent report has described lack of reactivity of this monoclonal anti-IgG also with several IgG3 isoallotypes (genetic variations within an IgG subclass).[21] These reactivity patterns could lead to missing a clinically significant IgG3 red cell antibody if it is predominantly of an isoallotype not detected by the reagent. Differences in anti-IgG reactivity can also be a source of variation in detection of antibody reactivity between laboratories testing the same sample. It is important to reference the manufacturer's instructions for unique performance characteristics of each reagent.

BASIC ANTIBODY IDENTIFICATION

Patient History

Before antibody identification testing begins, the patient's medical history should be considered, if such information can be obtained. Multiple aspects of the patient's medical history may influence antibody identification test selection as well as interpretation.

Prior Red Cell Exposure

Exposure to foreign red cells through blood transfusion or pregnancy is the usual cause of red cell immunization. It is uncommon for patients who have never had a transfusion or been pregnant to produce clinically significant alloantibodies, although naturally occurring antibodies may be present. Women are more likely to have alloantibodies than men because of exposure to foreign (ie, fetal) red cells during pregnancy. Infants <6 months usually do not produce alloantibodies, but newborns may have passive antibody of maternal origin.

If the patient has received transfusion, it is critical to know when the most recent transfusion was given. If transfusion was given during the past 3 months, primary immunization to red cell antigens may be a risk, and the presence of circulating donor red cells affects testing. Mixed-field results caused by the donor red cells in antigen typing tests interfere with interpretation of an autologous phenotype. In situations where warm autoantibodies are present in a sample, autologous adsorption techniques would not be used because alloantibodies could be adsorbed onto transfused donor red cells.

Diagnosis and Disease

Certain diseases have been associated with red cell antibodies; depending on the methods used, such antibodies may be detectable in antibody detection and identification tests. Cold agglutinin syndrome, Raynaud phenomenon, and infections with *Mycoplasma pneumoniae* are often associated with anti-I. Infectious mononucleosis is sometimes associated with anti-i. Patients with paroxysmal cold hemoglobinuria, which is associated with syphilis in adults and viral infections in children, may demonstrate autoantibodies with anti-P specificity confirmed by the Donath-Landsteiner test. Warm autoantibodies often accompany diagnoses such as warm autoimmune hemolytic anemia, systemic lupus erythematosus, multiple myeloma, chronic lymphocytic leukemia, or lymphoma. Patients who have received solid-organ or HPC transplants may demonstrate passive antibodies that originate from donor passenger lymphocytes.

Medications and Biologic Therapies

Certain drugs are known to cause antibody identification problems. (See Chapter 14 for a discussion of drug-related mechanisms and drugs that are associated with serologic problems.) Administration of intravenous immune globulin (IVIG) and Rh Immune Globulin (RhIG) can interfere with antibody screening tests. Some lots of IVIG have been reported to contain unexpected antibodies, including anti-A and anti-B. Intravenous RhIG, which is sometimes used to treat immune thrombocytopenia, could explain the presence of anti-D in an Rh-positive patient.

Monoclonal antibodies developed as immunotherapeutic agents may also interfere with serologic results. Anti-CD38 treatment [daratumumab (Darzalex; Janssen Biotech)] for multiple myeloma and other B-cell malignancies has been used for a number of years and is known to cause positive reactions in serologic tests employing the antiglobulin phase when the infused monoclonal IgG anti-CD38 binds to the small amount of CD38 present on all normal red cells, including reagent red cells of antibody detection and identification tests.[22-24] Anti-CD38 can also, although less often, be the cause of a weakly positive DAT in the treated patient. Clinical trials of an anti-CD47 [humanized monoclonal antibody Hu5F9-G4 (Forty Seven, Inc, in collaboration with Merck KGaA and Genentech)] alone or with other immunotherapeutic agents and at least one additional source of monoclonal anti-CD38 [Isatuximab (ImmunoGen and Sanofi-Aventis)] are under way and have also been reported to interfere with pretransfusion testing.[18-20,25-27] Development of other novel immunotherapies might cause similar serologic interferences depending on their target antigen. Communication from the health-care team identifying patients being treated with a monoclonal immunotherapy can streamline pretransfusion testing.

Elements of Basic Antibody Identification

Autologous Control and DAT

The autologous control (autocontrol), in which serum or plasma and autologous red cells are tested under the same conditions as reagent red cells, is an important part of antibody identification and should be performed when the test method allows. The autocontrol is not the same as or equivalent to a DAT (Method 3-14). Incubation and the presence of additive solutions may cause reactivity in the autocontrol that is an in-vitro phenomenon only. If the autocontrol is positive in the antiglobulin phase, a DAT should be performed. If the DAT result is negative, antibodies to an additive solution constituent or autoantibodies that are reactive only in the presence of the additive solution should be considered. Warm autoantibodies and cold autoantibodies, such as anti-I, -IH, or -Pr, may be reactive in an IAT when certain enhancement techniques are used; therefore, testing should be repeated in another medium. If the DAT result is positive, it must be interpreted with careful attention to the transfusion history. Autoantibodies or drugs could explain a positive DAT result; however, if the patient has an alloantibody and recently received blood that expressed the corresponding antigen, the positive DAT result may be caused by coating of the donor red cells with alloantibody. This situation can be associated with a clinically significant delayed transfusion reaction. More information about interpreting a positive DAT result can be found in Chapter 14.

Initial Identification Panel

For initial antibody identification, it is common to use a complete commercial reagent red cell panel with the same methods and test phases as in the antibody detection test or crossmatch. The gel-column and solid-phase methods involve a single reading of the test at the IAT phase. Tube-testing protocols have greater flexibility for reading at different test phases (eg, immediate spin, room temperature, 37 C, and IAT), but many serologists also use a single IAT reading because this test detects the overwhelming majority of clinically significant alloantibodies.

Some serologists using tube methods may choose to include an immediate centrifugation reading, a room-temperature incubation that is read before an additive solution is included, or both during initial antibody identification. Such an approach may enhance the detection of certain antibodies (eg, anti-M, -N, -P1, -I, -Le^a, or -Le^b) and may help explain reactions detected in other phases. These steps are frequently omitted in initial antibody identification studies because

most antibodies that are reactive only at lower temperatures have little or no clinical significance.

Readings for direct agglutination taken after 37 C incubation in tube testing are influenced by the additive solution used. Tests employing PEG enhancement cannot be centrifuged and read because the reagent causes nonspecific aggregation of all red cells. LISS, albumin, and saline (no enhancement) tests do not have this restriction. A 37 C reading can detect some antibodies (eg, potent anti-D, -E, or -K) that may cause direct agglutination of red cells. Other antibodies (eg, anti-Le^a or -Jk^a) may occasionally be detected by the lysis of antigen-positive red cells during the 37 C incubation if serum is tested. Omitting centrifugation and the reading at 37 C should lessen the detection of unwanted positive reactions caused by clinically insignificant autoantibodies and alloantibodies. However, in some instances, potentially clinically significant antibodies are detected only by their 37 C reactivity. In 87,480 samples, 103 examples of such antibodies were identified (63 anti-E; 27 -K; 5 -Jk^a; 4 -D; 3 -cE; and 1 -C).[28] If the 37 C reading is desired in a specific antibody study, an alternative strategy is to set up duplicate tests. One test is read after the 37 C incubation, and the other test is read only at the IAT phase.

Abbreviated Identification Panel

If a patient has antibodies that were identified previously, the known antibodies should be considered when selecting reagent red cells to test. For example, if the patient has known anti-e, it will not be helpful to test the patient's serum with a complete commercial reagent red cell panel in which 9 of 10 red cell samples are e-positive. Testing a selected panel of e-negative red cells is a better approach to find any newly formed antibodies. It is not necessary to test e-positive red cells to reconfirm the previously identified anti-e because e-negative donor units will be selected for transfusion regardless of the reactivity.

If the patient's red cell phenotype is known, reagent red cells may be selected to detect only those alloantibodies that the patient would potentially form. For example, if the patient's Rh phenotype is C–E+c+e–, red cells selected to exclude anti-E and anti-c should not be necessary or can be limited to a single selected cell sample because the patient is not expected to form alloantibodies to these antigens. Exceptions include patients with weak or altered (partial) Rh antigens, which are usually found in populations of African ancestry and patients whose Rh phenotype was predicted by DNA testing rather than serology and who could be carrying a silenced or altered allele. This approach can minimize the amount of testing required.

Autologous Red Cell Phenotype

Determining the phenotype of an individual's autologous red cells by serology or genotyping is an important part of antibody identification because the antibody maker's red cells are expected to lack antigens to which they make alloantibodies. This information can guide the antibody identification process.

Obtaining an autologous red cell phenotype may not always be simple. Recent transfusions or immunoglobulins coating the patient's red cells make obtaining a valid phenotype difficult. Misleading results may occur unless techniques are used to circumvent these issues.[29] Many of these special phenotyping techniques, such as separation of autologous cells or removal of bound immunoglobulin, are described later in this chapter under "Selected Procedures." Red cell genotyping is now commonly performed to obtain phenotype information. This approach avoids interference from circulating donor red cells or immunoglobulin-coated patient red cells. Molecular testing relies on the extraction of DNA from white cells. Because of nearly universal leukocyte reduction, the short life span of white cells in vivo, and, importantly, the assay design, the presence of transfused white cells from donors, if present, is not a limiting factor in determining the patient's red cell genotype. There are situations, however, where the genotype of a person may not predict the red cell phenotype. Mutations that inactivate gene expression or rare new alleles may not be identified by the specific assay performed. In addition, the genotype obtained from DNA isolated from leukocytes and hematopoietic cells may differ from that of other tissues in people with a history of transplantation.[30]

Interpretation of Results

Antibody detection results are interpreted as positive or negative according to the presence or absence of reactivity (ie, agglutination, hemolysis in serum tests, or red cell effacement in solid-phase tests). Interpretation of antibody identification results can be a very complex process combining technique, knowledge, and intuitive skills. Identification panels generally include both positive and negative results, sometimes at different phases of testing; each positive result should ultimately be explained. The following sections describe a systematic process for antibody identification interpretation.

General Assessment of Positive and Negative Reactions

Both positive and negative reactions are equally important in antibody identification, and they may be initially assessed to provide a general idea of the specificity(ies) present in the sample. (See Method 1-9 for grading agglutination in hemagglutination assays.) The phase and strength of positive reactions may be compared to the antigen patterns of the panel red cells to help suggest specificity. Negative reactions support the specificity suggested by the positive reactions. A single common alloantibody usually produces a clear pattern with antigen-positive and antigen-negative reagent red cells. In Table 13-2, if a sample is reactive only with red cell samples 3 and 5 of the reagent red cell panel, anti-E is very likely present. Both reactive red cells express the antigen, and all cells lacking the antigen are nonreactive. This general assessment is only the first part of the interpretation process. The rest of the process as described below must be completed even when a specificity looks apparent at this stage. Exclusion of antibodies must be performed to ensure proper identification of all antibodies potentially present.

Antibody Exclusion and Initial Specificity Assessment

A widely used first approach to the interpretation of panel results is to exclude specificities on the basis of nonreactivity of the patient's sample with red cells that express the antigen. Such a system is sometimes referred to as a "cross-out," "rule-out," or "exclusion" method. Once all panel results have been recorded, the antigen profile on the panel worksheet of the first nonreactive red cell is examined. If an antigen is *present* on the panel red cell and the patient sample was *not reactive* with it, the presence of the corresponding antibody may tentatively be excluded.

Many laboratory scientists actually cross out such antigens from the list at the top of the antigen profile sheet using a mark on the specificity to facilitate the process. Laboratories that have rule-out policies that consider whether the rule-out was done on a single or double dose of the antigen may use different notations to distinguish between the two—eg, "/" and "X" respectively. After all of the antigens for a red cell sample have been crossed out, the same process is performed with the other nonreactive red cells for the panel; additional specificities are then excluded. After the last nonreactive red cell is examined, only those antigens not "crossed out" are left for further evaluation as the specificity(ies) responsible for the reactivity.

Some laboratory scientists prefer a similar but two-phased cross-out approach. In this approach, phase one is to cross out the antigens on each red-cell-sample (panel-donor) *row* using the same or similar notation as described above for each nonreactive panel cell. Table 13-3 illustrates what an antibody identification panel might look like with phase one rule-outs complete. The second phase of this approach is to apply the laboratory's exclusion policy or criteria to the rule-outs and denote the final composite rule-out on the top row of the panel to summarize the specificities excluded. Table 13-4 depicts an antibody identification panel with phase-two rule-outs complete. In this example, final composite cross-out (and thus antibody exclusion) was indicated with an "X" on the top-row antigen list after meeting the hypothetical

laboratory's criteria of two examples of double-dose common antigens or two examples of antigens whose expression is not a result of zygosity (eg, P1, Le^a, Le^b) that were nonreactive with the patient's plasma. It should be noted that some specificities were not crossed out at the top despite being crossed out on one or more rows. Anti-E was not crossed out on the top row because although two panel red cells (#3 and #5) were E+ and nonreactive with the patient's plasma, only one was a double-dose expression (#3), and therefore anti-E did not meet this laboratory's criteria for final exclusion. There are many acceptable variations of exclusion policies; the one chosen for this example is just one alternative.

Exclusion of clinically significant alloantibodies should involve, at a minimum, those to the following antigens: D, C, E, c, e, K, Fy^a, Fy^b, Jk^a, Jk^b, S, and s. Antibodies to Le^a, Le^b, M, N, P1, and other antigens specific to certain patient populations may also be added to this list. Laboratories should have a policy for their antibody exclusion. The policy should list alloantibodies requiring exclusion as well as, based on the chosen test method and available resources, whether the exclusion is to be performed using single- or double-dose antigen-positive red cells and if more than one example of the antigen is needed. Ideally, antibody exclusion is performed on a nonreactive double-dose antigen-positive red cell sample. As antibody investigations become more complex, double-dose exclusion may become more difficult. The laboratory policy should also include any exceptions to the exclusion criteria.

The ethnicity of the donor serving as a panel cell source affects antibody exclusions. Panel red cells may appear to be double dose based on phenotype. Yet, for blood group systems having a very common silencing allele, the panel cells may carry only a single dose of the antithetical antigen. Most common is the Fy(a+b−) phenotype on the red cells of a donor of African ancestry. Because of the high frequency of the *FY*02N.01* allele with silenced Fy^b red cell expression in this population, these Fy(a+b−) cells often have only one dose of Fy^a antigen. If the Fy(a+b−) sample is also D+C−E−, V+, or Js(a+), the donor is likely of African ancestry. Exclusion

TABLE 13-3. Example of Antibody Exclusion Using the Two-Phase Cross-Out Approach: Phase One—Exclude for Each Negative Result on the Row*

Cell	RH					MNS				KEL		P1	LE		FY		JK		Cell	Results Tube PEG IAT	Results IAT CC
	D	C	E	c	e	M	N	S	s	K	k	P1	Le^a	Le^b	Fy^a	Fy^b	Jk^a	Jk^b			
1	+	+	0	0	+	+	0	0	+	0	+	+	0	+	+	+	0	+	1	2+	
2	+	0	0	0	+	0	+	0	0	0	+	+	0	0	0	0	0	0	2	0	✓
3	+	0	+	0	0	0	+	+	+	0	0	0	+	0	0	+	+	0	3	0	✓
4	0	+	0	+	+	+	0	+	+	0	+	+	0	+	+	0	+	0	4	3+	
5	0	0	0	0	+	0	+	0	+	0	+	+	0	0	0	0	0	+	5	0	✓
6	0	0	0	+	+	+	0	+	0	+	+	+	0	+	+	0	0	+	6	3+	
7	0	0	0	0	+	0	+	0	+	0	+	0	0	0	0	0	0	0	7	0	✓
8	+	0	0	0	+	0	+	0	+	0	+	0	0	0	0	0	0	0	8	0	✓
9	0	0	0	+	+	+	+	+	+	+	+	0	+	0	+	0	+	+	9	3+	
10	0	0	0	0	+	0	+	0	+	0	0	0	0	0	0	0	+	0	10	0	✓
11	0	0	0	0	+	0	+	0	+	0	0	0	0	0	0	0	0	0	11	0	✓
AC																			AC	0	✓

*Example laboratory policy applied to this table: exclude on each row with an "X" if reagent red cells express a single dose of the antigen or antigen expression is not a result of zygosity and patient's plasma is nonreactive. Note the D antigen on row 8 is excluded conservatively with a "/" indicating it is a single dose of the antigen, but the phenotype on this cell cannot exclude the possibility of a *Dce/Dce* red cell genotype which would express a double dose of D. + indicates presence of antigen; 0 indicates absence of antigen; AC = autocontrol; PEG = polyethylene glycol; IAT = indirect antiglobulin test; CC = control cells; ✓ indicates an acceptable antihuman globulin control cell result following a negative IAT.

TABLE 13-4. Example of Antibody Exclusion Using the Two-Phase Cross-Out Approach: Phase Two—Composite Cross Out*

Cell	D	C	E	c	e	M	N	S	s	K	k	P1	Le^a	Le^b	Fy^a	Fy^b	Jk^a	Jk^b	Cell	Tube PEG IAT	IAT CC
																				Results	Results
1	+	+	0	0	+	+	0	0	+	0	+	+	0	+	+	+	0	+	1	2+	
2	+	0	0	+	+	0	+	0	+	0	0	+	0	0	0	0	0	0	2	0	✓
3	+	0	0	+	0	0	+	+	0	0	0	0	0	0	0	0	+	+	3	0	✓
4	0	+	0	+	+	+	0	0	+	0	+	+	0	+	+	0	+	0	4	3+	
5	0	0	0	0	+	0	+	+	0	0	0	+	0	0	0	0	0	0	5	0	✓
6	0	0	0	+	+	+	0	+	0	+	0	+	0	+	+	0	0	+	6	3+	
7	0	0	0	+	0	0	+	0	+	0	0	0	0	0	0	0	0	0	7	0	✓
8	+	0	0	0	0	0	+	0	+	0	0	+	0	0	0	0	0	0	8	0	✓
9	0	0	0	+	+	+	+	+	+	+	0	0	+	0	+	0	+	+	9	3+	
10	0	0	0	0	0	0	+	0	0	0	+		0	0	0	0	+	+	10	0	✓
11	0	0	0	0	0	+	0	0	0	0	+		0	0	0	0	0	+	11	0	✓
AC																			AC	0	✓

*In this example, final composite cross-out (and thus antibody exclusion) was indicated with an "X" on the top row listing the antigens after meeting the hypothetical laboratory's criteria of two examples of a double dose of common antigens or two examples of antigens whose expression is not a result of zygosity (eg, P1, Le^a, Le^b) that were nonreactive with the patient's plasma. Final composite cross-out for these test results will vary with differing laboratory exclusion policies or criteria.

+ indicates presence of antigen; 0 indicates absence of antigen; AC = autocontrol; PEG = polyethylene glycol; IAT = indirect antiglobulin test; CC = control cells; ✓ indicates an acceptable antihuman globulin control cell result following a negative test.

of anti-Fy^a on such a panel red cell would probably represent only a single-dose exclusion.

For any method of crossing out, final exclusion should be done only after ensuring the laboratory's policies for eliminating the presence of antibodies are met. In most cases, this process leaves one or more antibodies that have not been excluded. The red cells that are reactive are then evaluated. If there is an antigen pattern that matches the test reactivity exactly for an antigen not excluded, this most likely identifies the specificity of the antibody. Additional testing may be needed to eliminate remaining specificities that were not excluded and confirm the suspected specificity. This process of selecting red cells for exclusion and confirmation is described in the next section. When additional testing is not needed after the initial identification panel because an initial specificity can be assigned and all other specificities can be excluded, the probability of an accurate identification can be directly assessed (see below).

Selected Red Cells for Exclusion and Confirmation

Selected red cells, chosen for the specific antigens they carry or lack, are used to confirm or rule out the presence of antibodies. For example, if a pattern of reactive red cells fits anti-Jk^a exactly, but anti-K and anti-S were not excluded, the serum should be tested with selected red cells. Ideally, red cells with the following phenotypes should be chosen: Jk(a–), K+, S–; Jk(a–), K–, S+; and Jk(a+), K–, S–. The reaction pattern with these red cells should both confirm the presence of anti-Jk^a and include or exclude anti-K and anti-S. Whenever possible, selected red cells should have a strong expression of the antigen being tested (ie, from donors presumed homozygous for the appropriate gene or red cells with double-dose expression). Such red cells help ensure that nonreactivity with the selected red cell sample indicates the absence of the antibody and not that the antibody was too weak to be reactive with a selected red cell that had a weak expression of the antigen. It must be remembered that confirmation of double-dose expression of an antigen can be accomplished only by demonstrating homozygosity of the corresponding allele through genotyping. As explained above, ethnicity influences the apparent zygosity of the *FY*A* allele. Testing at this stage of the investigation can also reveal errors in the presumptive identification when the expected positive and negative results in confirmatory testing are not obtained.

Probability of Accurate Identification

Accurate identification of antibody specificity greatly depends, first, on the antibody having a sufficient titer (ie, quantity of circulating antibody) to provide reliably positive reactions. Secondly, antigen strength on test cells must be adequate to provide a consistent target antigen. It is difficult to know exactly when both of these criteria are met. Test protocols are designed to enhance clinically significant reactivity and diminish false negatives due to poor antibody affinity, if applicable, and good laboratory practices attempt to minimize antigen deterioration while optimizing proper staff testing techniques. Assuming these variables are controlled to the greatest degree possible, it is still necessary to ensure that an observed pattern of reactions is not the result of chance alone. Conclusive antibody identification requires the sample to be tested against a sufficient number of reagent red cell samples that lack—and express—the antigen that corresponds with the antibody's apparent specificity. A standard approach (which is based on Fisher's exact method) has been to require that three antigen-positive red cell samples are reactive and that three antigen-negative red cell samples are not reactive for each specificity identified.[31] When that approach is not possible, a more liberal approach (which is derived from calculations by Harris and Hochman[32]) allows the minimum requirement for a probability (p) value of 0.05 to be met with two reactive and three nonreactive red cell samples or with one reactive and seven nonreactive red cell samples (or the reciprocal of either combination). In some cases, the use of two reactive and two nonreactive red cell samples is also an acceptable approach for antibody confirmation.[8(p25),33] Additional details on calculating probability may be found in the suggested readings list at the end of this chapter.

Consistency of Antibody Identified with Autologous Red Cell Phenotype

The patient's autologous red cell phenotype is used to support the presumptive antibody identification: the red cells should lack the corresponding antigen. The phenotype as determined by serology or genotyping may also indicate the need for further investigation. For example, if an individual appears to have anti-Fy[a], his or her red cells should type Fy(a–). However, if the autologous red cells type as Fy(a+) (and have a negative DAT result), the identification of an anti-Fy[a] is in conflict with the phenotype, and additional testing should be performed. A serologically derived antigen-positive typing should be reconfirmed by testing with more than one antibody source when possible. If genotyping predicted the antigen-positive status, this discrepancy may indicate that the patient's red cells do not actually express the antigen because of a gene-silencing mutation not targeted by the assay. Alternatively, the patient might have an altered or partial antigen because of an additional gene polymorphism. It is important to remember that the antibody in the sample could be, in fact, an alloantibody.

COMPLEX ANTIBODY IDENTIFICATION

Not all antibody identifications are straightforward. The interpretation process described above does not always lead directly to an answer, and additional testing and/or consultation with an immunohematology reference laboratory (IRL) may be required. The autologous control that is tested with initial antibody identification studies provides a starting point for complex antibody problem resolution. If the test method does not allow for testing of an autocontrol, the DAT result can be used to plan additional testing. Figure 13-1 shows some approaches to identifying antibodies in a variety of situations when the autocontrol is negative, and Fig 13-2 shows some approaches to identifying antibodies when the autocontrol is positive. Common types of antibody investigations mentioned in Figs 13-1 and 13-2 as well as others are further described below.

Multiple Antibodies

When a sample contains two or more alloantibodies, it may be difficult to interpret the results of testing performed with a single panel of reagent red cells. The presence of multiple antibodies may be suggested by a variety of test results, such as the following:

1. *The observed pattern of reactive and nonreactive red cells does not fit a single antibody.* When the exclusion approach fails to indicate a specific pattern, it is helpful to determine whether the pattern matches two combined specificities. For example, if the reactive red cells on the panel in Table 13-2 are numbers 3, 5, 6, 9, and 10, none of the specificities remaining after crossing out fits a pattern exactly. However, if both E and K are considered together, a pattern is discerned, with reagent cells 3 and 5 showing reactivity because of anti-E, and reagent cells 6, 9, and 10 because of anti-K. If the reaction pattern does not fit two combined specificities, the possibility that more than two antibodies are present must be considered. The more antibodies a sample contains, the more complex identification and exclusion become, but the basic process remains the same.

2. *Reactivity occurs at different test phases.* When tube tests are performed and reactivity occurs at several phases, each phase should be analyzed separately. The pattern at room temperature may indicate a different specificity from the pattern at the IAT phase. It is also helpful to look for variations in the strength of the reactions at each phase of testing. Table 13-5 provides information about the characteristic reactivity of many antibodies.

3. *Unexpected reactions occur when attempts are made to confirm the specificity of a suspected single antibody.* If a sample suspected to contain anti-e is reactive with some

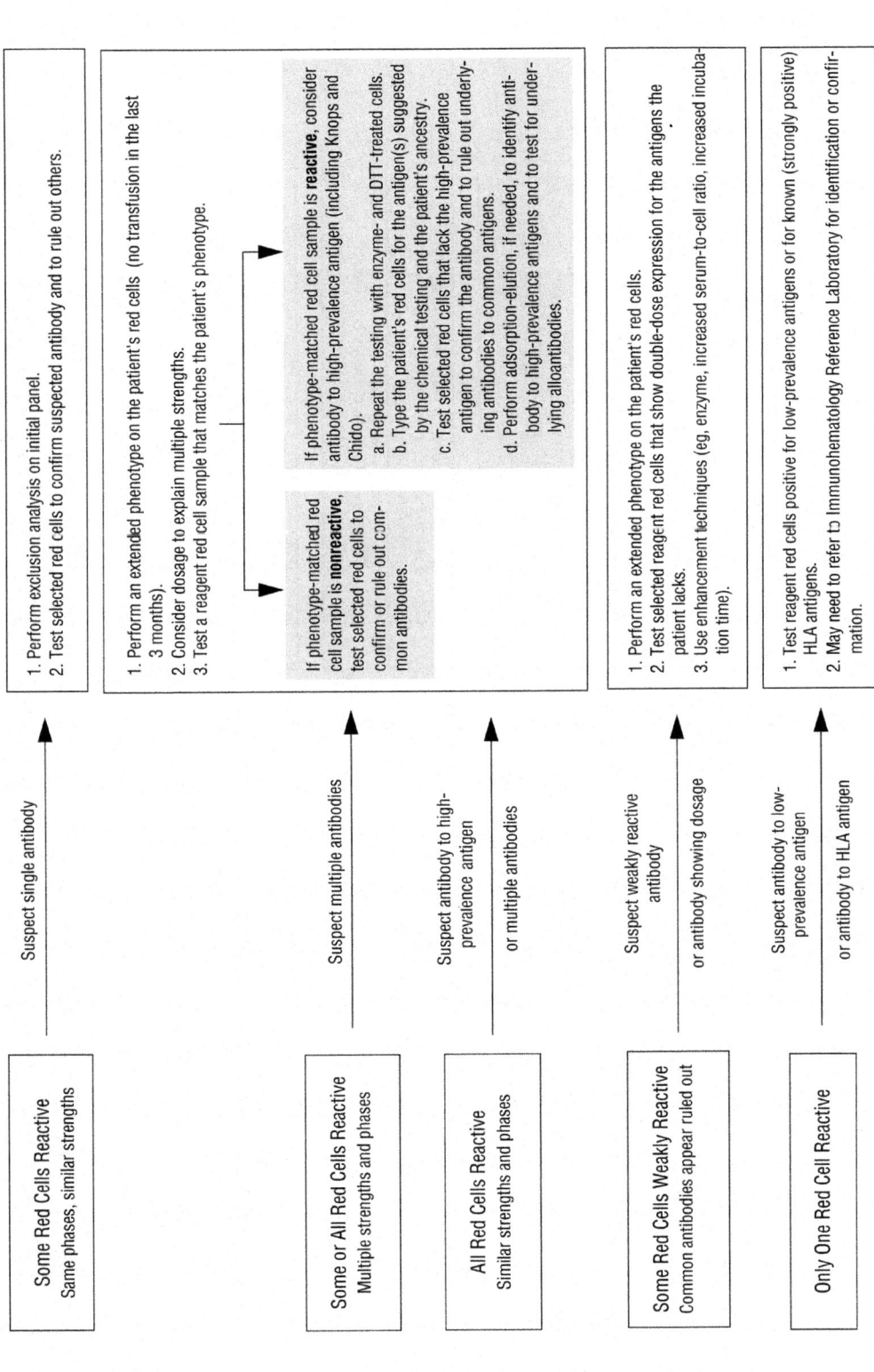

FIGURE 13-1. Antibody identification with negative autocontrol.
DTT = dithiothreitol.

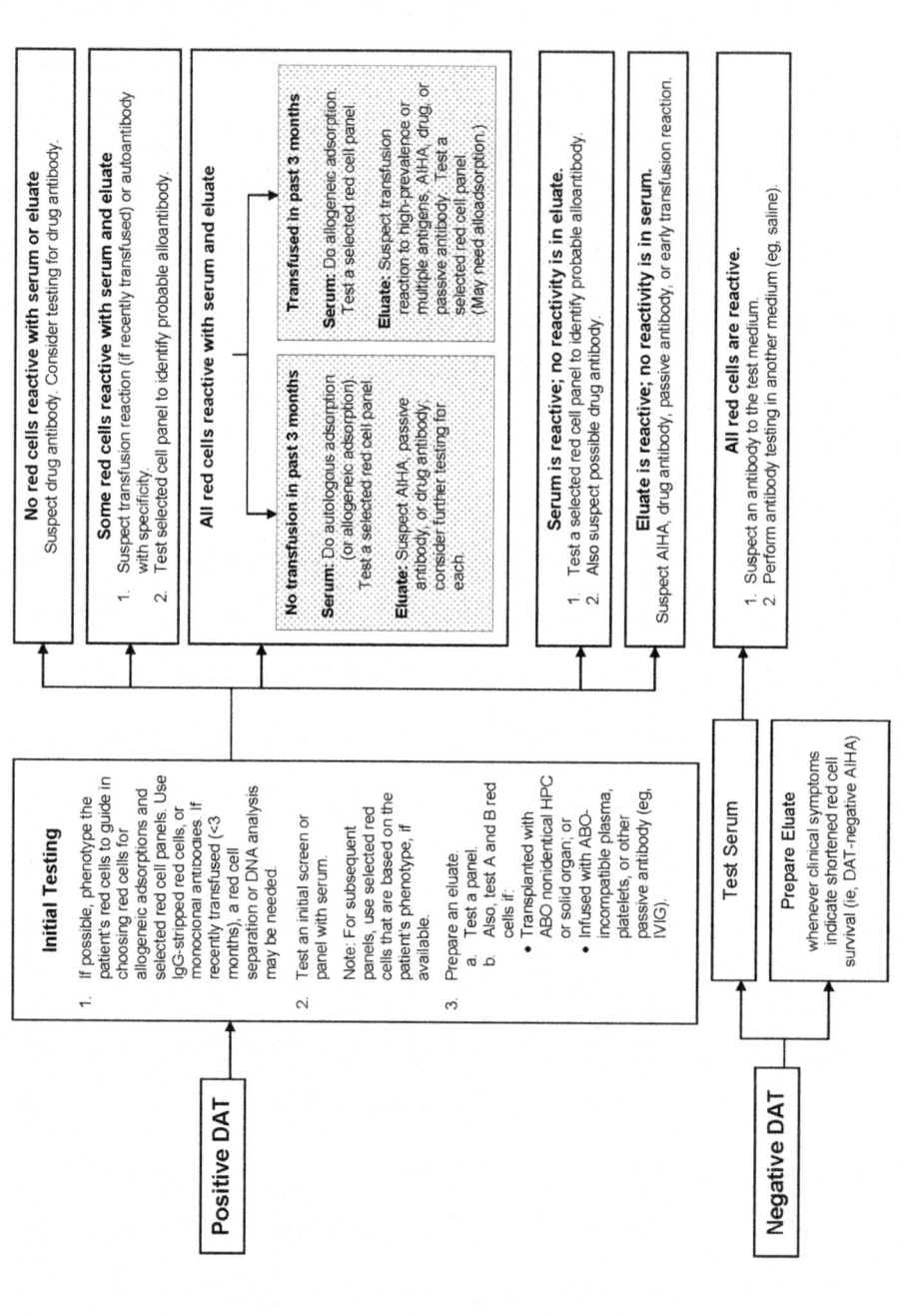

FIGURE 13-2. Antibody identification with positive autocontrol.

HPC = hematopoietic progenitor cell; IVIG = intravenous immune globulin; DAT = direct antiglobulin test; AIHA = autoimmune hemolytic anemia.

TABLE 13-5. Serologic Reactivity of Some Common Blood Group Antibodies

Antibody	Immuno-globulin Class	Reactivity				Papain/ Ficin	DTT (200 mM)	Associated with	
		4 C	22 C	37 C	IAT			HDFN	HTR
Anti-M	IgG>IgM	Most	Most		Rare	Sensitive	Resistant	Rare	Rare
Anti-N	IgM>IgG	Most	Most		Rare	Sensitive	Resistant	No	Rare
Anti-S	IgG>IgM		Most		Most	Variable	Resistant	Yes	Yes
Anti-s	IgG>IgM				Most	Variable	Resistant	Yes	Yes
Anti-U	IgG				Most	Resistant	Resistant	Yes	Yes
Anti-P1	IgM (IgG rare)	Most	Most			Resistant	Resistant	No	Rare
Anti-D	IgG>IgM (IgA rare)		Some	Some	Most	Resistant	Resistant	Yes	Yes
Anti-C	IgG>IgM		Some	Some	Most	Resistant	Resistant	Yes	Yes
Anti-E	IgG>IgM		Some	Some	Most	Resistant	Resistant	Yes	Yes
Anti-c	IgG>IgM		Some	Some	Most	Resistant	Resistant	Yes	Yes
Anti-e	IgG>IgM		Some	Some	Most	Resistant	Resistant	Yes	Yes
Anti-Lu[a]	IgM>IgG		Most		Most	Resistant or weakened	Variable	No	Mild
Anti-Lu[b]	IgG>IgM		Some		Most	Resistant or weakened	Variable	No	Mild
Anti-K	IgG>IgM		Some		Most	Resistant	Sensitive	Yes	Yes
Anti-k	IgG>IgM				Most	Resistant	Sensitive	Yes	Yes
Anti-Kp[a]	IgG				Most	Resistant	Sensitive	Yes	Yes
Anti-Kp[b]	IgG>IgM				Most	Resistant	Sensitive	Yes	Yes
Anti-Js[a]	IgG>IgM				Most	Resistant	Sensitive	Yes	Yes
Anti-Js[b]	IgG				Most	Resistant	Sensitive	Yes	Yes
Anti-Le[a]	IgM>IgG	Most	Most	Most	Most	Resistant	Resistant	No	Rare

(Continued)

TABLE 13-5. Serologic Reactivity of Some Common Blood Group Antibodies (Continued)

Antibody	Immuno-globulin Class	Reactivity				Papain/ Ficin	DTT (200 mM)	Associated with	
		4 C	22 C	37 C	IAT			HDFN	HTR
Anti-Le^b	IgM>IgG	Most	Most	Most	Most	Resistant	Resistant	No	No
Anti-Fy^a	IgG>IgM				Most	Sensitive	Resistant	Yes	Yes
Anti-Fy^b	IgG>IgM				Most	Sensitive	Resistant	Yes	Yes
Anti-Jk^a	IgG>IgM				Most	Resistant	Resistant	Rare	Yes
Anti-Jk^b	IgG>IgM				Most	Resistant	Resistant	Rare	Yes
Anti-Di^a	IgG				Most	Resistant	Resistant	Yes	Rare
Anti-Di^b	IgG				Most	Resistant	Resistant	Yes	Rare
Anti-Yt^a	IgG				Most	Variable	Sensitive or weak-ened	No	Rare
Anti-Yt^b	IgG				Most	Variable	Sensitive or weak-ened	No	No
Anti-Xg^a	IgG>IgM		Some		Most	Sensitive	Resistant	No	No
Anti-Sc1	IgG				Most	Resistant	Variable	No	No
Anti-Sc2	IgG				Most	Resistant	Variable	No	No
Anti-Do^a	IgG				Most	Resistant	Variable	No	Yes
Anti-Do^b	IgG				Most	Resistant	Variable	No	Yes
Anti-Co^a	IgG>IgM				Most	Resistant	Resistant	Yes	Yes
Anti-Co^b	IgG				Most	Resistant	Resistant	Yes	Yes

DTT = dithiothreitol; HDFN = hemolytic disease of the fetus and newborn; HTR = hemolytic transfusion reaction; IAT = indirect antiglobulin test; Ig = immunoglobulin.

e-negative red cells, another antibody may be present or the suspected antibody may not be anti-e at all. Testing a panel of selected e-negative red cells may help identify an additional specificity.

4. *A phenotypically similar red cell is nonreactive.* When all or nearly all panel red cells are reactive, the easiest way to recognize multiple antibodies is to test a phenotypically similar red cell. A phenotypically similar red cell

is one that lacks the same common antigens as the patient's red cells. Lack of reactivity with this type of red cell indicates that the alloantibodies are directed at common antigens lacking from the test red cell. A selected red cell panel can then be tested to identify or exclude the common antibodies to the red cell antigens that the patient lacks. (See the discussion on selected red cells earlier in this chapter.)

Reactivity without Apparent Specificity

Zygosity (ie, copy number), variation in antigen expression, and other factors may contribute to difficulty in interpreting results of antibody identification tests. If the reactivity of the serum is very weak and/or the pattern of reactivity and the cross-out process have excluded all likely specificities, alternative approaches should be used. Some helpful techniques and considerations include those described below.

Alternate Test Method

Depending on the method originally used, it may be necessary either to enhance antibody reactivity by using a more sensitive method (eg, PEG, enzymes, increased incubation time, or increased serum-to-cell ratio; see Methods 3-5 and 3-8 through 3-13) or to decrease the sensitivity of the method to avoid the detection of unwanted and clinically insignificant reactivity. Methods to inactivate certain antigens on the reagent red cells may also be helpful. Enzyme treatment renders red cells negative for such antigens as Fy^a and Fy^b. (See Table 13-5.) Observation of the effect a reagent red cell treatment has on the unknown serum reactivity can provide clues about its possible specificity. Adsorption or elution methods to separate antibodies (Methods 3-20, 4-1, and 4-2) may also be useful because selective adsorption can isolate unknown reactivity, and elution of unknown reactivity from adsorbing red cells can concentrate the antibody.

Optimal Phase or Temperature for Antibody Was Not Tested

If weak or questionable positive results are obtained at the IAT phase, it may be helpful to perform tube tests with readings at immediate spin, room temperature, or 37 C if these phases were not included in the original testing. This may allow an antibody that optimally reacts as a direct agglutinin at 37 C or below to be more clearly visualized.

Potential Phenotype Exclusions

When serum reactivity has no apparent specificity, a useful approach is to type the patient's red cells by serology or genotyping for common red cell antigens, and eliminate from initial consideration specificities that correspond to antigens on the patient's autologous red cells. This combined with other techniques allows the investigation to be focused on specificities more likely to be present. Phenotyping may not be possible if the patient has received transfusion recently or has had a positive DAT result.

Presence of Antigens in Common

Instead of excluding antibodies to antigens on nonreactive red cells, close observation may identify antigens that the reactive red cells have in common. For example, if all of the red cells reactive at room temperature are P1+ but the anti-P1 pattern is not complete, the antibody could be anti-P1 that is not reactive with red cells with a weaker expression of the antigen. (Such red cells are occasionally designated on the panel sheet as "+w.") In this case, it might be helpful to use a method that enhances anti-P1, such as testing after incubation at lower temperatures.

If all of the reactive red cells are Jk(b+) but not all Jk(b+) red cells are reactive [especially (Jka+Jkb+) cells], the reactive red cells might be Jk(a–b+) with a double-dose expression of the antigen. In this case, tube-based enhancement techniques, such as enzymes or PEG, or a different test method, such as solid phase, might help demonstrate reactivity with all of the Jk(b+) red cells. Typing the patient's red cells to confirm that they lack the corresponding antigen is also helpful.

If strongly positive results are obtained, the exclusion method should be used with nonreactive cells to eliminate specificities from initial consideration. The strongly reactive reagent cells may be examined for any antigen in common.

Finally, the presence of some antigens in common may suppress the expression of other antigens. This suppression can cause weak antibodies to be missed or certain red cells to be unexpectedly nonreactive when a suspected antibody fails to show reactivity with all antigen-positive red cells. For example, In(Lu) is known to suppress the expression of LU antigens, P1, In[b], and AnWj. Similarly, Kp[a] is known to weaken the expression of KEL antigens. (See Chapter 12 for a more detailed discussion.)

Inherent Variability

Nebulous reaction patterns that do not appear to fit any particular specificity are characteristic of certain antibodies, such as anti-Bg[a], -Kn[a], -McC[a], -Sl[a], -Yk[a], -Cs[a], and -JMH. Antigens corresponding to these antibodies vary markedly in their expression on red cells from different individuals. For example, the expression of Knops blood group antigens shows marked differences between individuals as a result of variations in the CR1 copy numbers on the red cells.[34]

Unlisted Antigens

A sample may react with an antigen that is not routinely listed on the antigen profile supplied by the reagent manufacturer—Do[a], Do[b], and Yt[b] are some examples. Even though serum studies yield clearly reactive and nonreactive test results, such antibodies may not be recognized. In these circumstances, it is useful to review additional phenotype information supplied with the reagent panel or consult the manufacturer. If only one cell is unexpectedly reactive, this reaction is most likely caused by an antibody to a low-prevalence antigen. These antibodies are discussed in more detail later in this chapter.

ABO Group of Red Cells Tested

The sample may be reactive with many or all of the group O reagent red cells but not with red cells of the same ABO group as the autologous red cells. Such a reaction pattern occurs most frequently with anti-H, anti-IH, or anti-Le[bH]. Group O and A_2 red cells have more H antigen than A_1 and A_1B red cells, which express very little H. (See Chapter 10 for more information.) Thus, sera containing anti-H or anti-IH are strongly reactive with group O reagent red cells, whereas autologous A_1 or A_1B red cells or donor red cells used for crossmatching may be weakly reactive or nonreactive. Anti-Le[bH] is strongly reactive with group O, Le(b+) red cells but weakly reactive or nonreactive with Le(b+) red cells from A_1 or A_1B individuals.

Unexpected Reagent Red Cell Problems

Rarely, a pattern of reactive and nonreactive red cells cannot be interpreted because the typing result for a reagent red cell is incorrect or the reagent red cell has a positive DAT result. If the red cell sample is from a commercial source, the manufacturer should be notified immediately of the discrepancy.

Warm Autoantibodies

The presence of warm-reactive autoantibodies in a patient's serum creates a special challenge because the antibody is reactive with virtually all red cells tested. The majority of warm autoantibodies are IgG; IgM warm autoantibodies are unusual, but they have caused severe (often fatal) autoimmune hemolytic anemia.[35] If a patient with warm autoantibodies requires a transfusion, it is important to detect any underlying clinically significant alloantibodies. Solid-phase and gel-column methods frequently greatly enhance warm autoantibodies. PEG, enzymes, and, to a lesser extent, LISS also may enhance these autoantibodies. It is often helpful to omit the additive solutions when testing sera that contain warm autoantibodies. If such tests are nonreactive, common alloantibody specificities can be excluded and the same procedure can be used for compatibility testing without the need for adsorptions. If such tests remain reactive, adsorptions are typically required to rule out underlying alloantibodies. For more information, see Chapter 14 and Methods 3-20 and 4-8 through 4-10.

Cold Autoantibodies

Cold autoantibodies may be clinically benign or pathologic. In either case, potent cold autoantibodies that are reactive with all red cells at room temperature or below, including the patient's own, can create special problems—especially if the reactivity persists at temperatures above room temperature and into the IAT phase of antibody identification. Such situations make it difficult to detect and identify potential clinically significant alloantibodies that are being masked by the cold autoantibody reactivity. The detection of cold autoantibodies can be dependent on the test method used. Gel-column tests can give a mixed-field appearance even though only one cell population is present. Solid-phase tests are designed to minimize their detection. There are different approaches to testing sera with potent cold autoagglutinins. Once the presence of a cold autoantibody has been confirmed, the goal in most situations is to circumvent or remove the interfering cold autoagglutinin reactivity in order to detect underlying and potentially clinically significant antibodies. Procedures to accomplish this include the following:

1. Omitting the room-temperature and/or immediate-spin phase of testing using test tube methods if one was performed.
2. The use of anti-IgG rather than polyspecific AHG reagent for the IAT phase of antibody identification when using test tube methods.
3. Cold auto- or allogeneic adsorption of the patient's serum or plasma to remove autoantibodies but not alloantibodies (Method 4-5 and 3-20).
4. Prewarming techniques in which reagent red cells and patient serum or plasma are prewarmed to 37 C separately before they are combined (Method 3-6).
5. Adsorption with rabbit erythrocytes or rabbit erythrocyte stroma.[36,37]

The use of the last two procedures listed is controversial for the purposes of circumventing cold autoantibodies. Notes on and limitations of the procedures can be found within their respective method descriptions or references.

In some situations, the goal of testing is not to circumvent the cold autoantibody but rather to define its serologic characteristics (eg, specificity, thermal amplitude, titer). This may be requested and useful if the patient's clinical situation is suggestive of a pathologic cold autoagglutinin. See Chapter 14 for a more detailed discussion of immune-mediated hemolysis caused by some cold autoantibodies.

Delayed Serologic/Hemolytic Transfusion Reactions

Delayed transfusion reactions are defined by the development of a new alloantibody in a patient following transfusion that results in laboratory evidence (serologic) or laboratory and clinical evidence (hemolytic) of the destruction of incompatible transfused red cells that were compatible at the time of infusion. If a patient has received transfusion in the last 3 months and the autocontrol is positive in the IAT phase, there may be antibody-coated donor red cells in the patient's circulation, resulting in a positive DAT result that can show mixed-field reactivity. An elution should be performed, especially when tests on plasma or serum are inconclusive. For example, a recent transfusion recipient may have a positive autocontrol and show weak reactivity with most, but not all, Fy(a+) red cells. It may be possible to confirm anti-Fy^a specificity in an eluate because more antibody is often bound to donor red cells, and importantly, the preparation of an eluate concentrates the antibody. It is rare for transfused red cells to make the autocontrol positive at a phase other than IAT, but this can occur, especially with a newly developing or cold-reacting alloantibody. If the DAT result does have a mixed-field appearance and the plasma or serum is reactive with all cells tested, a transfusion reaction caused by an alloantibody to a high-prevalence antigen should be considered (Fig 13-2).

Antibodies to High-Prevalence Antigens

If all reagent red cells are reactive in the same test phase and with uniform strength but the autocontrol is nonreactive, an alloantibody to a high-prevalence antigen should be considered. Antibodies to high-prevalence antigens can be identified by testing selected red cells of rare phenotypes and by typing the patient's autologous red cells with antisera to high-prevalence antigens. Knowing the ethnic or ancestral origin of the antibody producer can be helpful when selecting additional tests to perform (Table 13-6).[5] Chemically modified and/or enzyme-modified red cells (eg, DTT/AET-treated or ficin-treated red cells) can give characteristic reactivity patterns that help limit possible specificities (Table 13-7). Testing rare red cells that lack all antigens in a blood group system [eg, K_0, Rh_{null}, or Lu(a–b–) cells] can localize the reactivity to that blood group system if nonreactive.

If red cells negative for a particular high-prevalence antigen are not available, red cells that are positive for the lower prevalence antithetical antigen can sometimes be helpful. For example, if a sample contains anti-Co^a, weaker reactions may be observed with Co(a+b+) red cells than with Co(a+b–) red cells because of a dosage effect.

Antibodies to high-prevalence antigens may be accompanied by antibodies to common antigens, which can make identification much more difficult. In such cases, it may be necessary to determine the patient's phenotype for common antigens, choose a phenotypically similar red cell sample (ie, one that lacks the same common antigens as the patient's red cells) that is incompatible with the patient's serum, and adsorb the antibody to the high-prevalence antigen onto that red cell sample. This approach leaves antibodies to common red cell antigens in the adsorbed plasma or serum, where they can be identified with a routine selected red cell panel. Because the identification of antibodies to high-prevalence antigens is complicated, it may be necessary to refer such specimens to an IRL.

Ancestry of Antibody Maker

Antibodies such as anti-U, -McC^a, -Sl^a, -Js^b, -Hy, -Jo^a, -Tc^a, -Cr^a, and -At^a should be considered if the sample is from an individual of African ancestry because the antigen-negative phenotypes occur almost exclusively in this population. Individuals with anti-Kp^b are almost always of European ancestry. Anti-Di^b is usually found among populations of Asian, South American Indian, and Native American ancestry. Other examples are found in Table 13-6.

Serologic Clues

Knowing the serologic characteristics of particular antibodies to high-prevalence antigens may help with identification.

1. Reactivity in tests at room temperature suggests anti-H, -I, -IH, -P, -$PP1P^k$ (-Tj^a), -En^a, -LW (some), -Ge (some), -Sd^a, or -Vel.
2. Lysis of reagent red cells during testing with fresh serum is characteristic of anti-Vel, -P, -$PP1P^k$ (-Tj^a), -Jk3, and some examples of anti-H and -I. Serum instead of plasma must be used in tests to see lysis.
3. Reduced or absent reactivity with enzyme-treated red cells occurs with anti-Ch, -Rg, -En^a, -In^b, -JMH, -Ge2, and some examples of anti-Yt^a.
4. Weak nebulous reactions in the IAT phase are often associated with anti-Kn^a, -McC^a, -Yk^a, and -Cs^a. KN system antigens are labile during storage: antibodies may be more reactive with donor red cells and fresher reagent red cells.
5. Complement-binding autoantibodies, such as anti-I and -IH, or alloantibodies, such as anti-$PP1P^k$ and -Vel, may give stronger results when a polyspecific AHG reagent is used.

Antibody to High-Prevalence Antigen vs Warm Autoantibody

When a patient produces an antibody to a high-prevalence antigen after transfusion, the patient's posttransfusion red cell sample may have a positive DAT result, and both serum or plasma

TABLE 13-6. High-Prevalence Antigens Absent in Certain Populations*

Phenotype	Population
AnWj–	Transient in any population>Israeli Arabs (inherited type)
At(a–)	Blacks
Cr(a–)	Blacks
Di(b–)	South Americans>Native Americans>Japanese
Fy(a–b–)	Blacks>Arabs/Jews>Mediterraneans>Whites
Ge:–2,–3 (Gerbich phenotype)	Papua New Guineans>Melanesians>Whites>any
Ge:–2,3 (Yus phenotype)	Mexicans>Israelis>Mediterraneans>any
Ge:–2,–3,–4 (Leach phenotype)	Any
Gy(a–)	Eastern Europeans (Romany)>Japanese
hr^B–	Blacks
hr^S–	Blacks
Hy–	Blacks
In(b–)	Indians>Iranians>Arabs
Jk(a–b–)	Polynesians>Finns>Japanese>any
Jo(a–)	Blacks
Jr(a–)	Japanese>Asians>Europeans>Bedouin Arabs>any
Js(b–)	Blacks
k–	Whites>any
Kn(a–)	Whites>Blacks>any
Kp(b–)	Whites>Japanese
Lan–	Whites>Japanese>Blacks>any
Lu(a–b–)	Any
LW(a–b–)	Transient in any>inherited type in Canadians

(Continued)

TABLE 13-6. High-Prevalence Antigens Absent in Certain Populations* (Continued)

Phenotype	Population
LW(a–)	Balts
O$_h$ (Bombay)	Indians>Japanese>any
Ok(a–)	Japanese
P–	Japanese>Finns>Israelis>any
PP1P^k–	Swedes>Amish>Israelis>Japanese>any
Sl(a–)	Blacks>Whites>any
Tc(a–b+c–)	Blacks
U– and S–s–U+^{var}	Blacks
Vel–	Swedes>any
WES(b–)	Finns>Blacks>any
Yk(a–)	Whites>Blacks>any
Yt(a–)	Arabs>Jews>any

*Adapted with permission from Reid et al.[5]

and the eluate may be reactive with all reagent red cells tested. Because this pattern of reactivity is identical to that of many warm-reacting autoantibodies that appear after transfusion, the two scenarios can be very difficult to differentiate. A posttransfusion DAT result that is significantly weaker than the serum or plasma reactivity would be more characteristic of an alloantibody to a high-prevalence antigen than a warm autoantibody, because only the transfused cells are coated with the alloantibody. The DAT result in a posttransfusion sample containing a

TABLE 13-7. Alterations of Antigens by Various Agents*

Agent	Antigens Usually Denatured or Altered†
Proteolytic enzymes‡	M, N, S, Fy^a, Fy^b, Yt^a, Ch, Rg, Pr, Tn, Mg, Mi^a/Vw, Cl^a, Je^a, Ny^a, JMH, Xg^a, some Ge, and In^b
Dithiothreitol (DTT) or 2-aminoethylisothiouronium bromide (AET)	Yt^a; JMH; Kn^a; McC^a; Yk^a; LW^a; LW^b; all KEL, LU, DO, CROM, and IN blood group antigens

*Appropriate controls should be used with modified red cells.
†Some antigens listed may be weakened rather than completely denatured.
‡Different proteolytic enzymes may have different effects on certain antigens.

new alloantibody to a high-prevalence antigen would be expected to give a mixed-field appearance (ie, some red cells agglutinated among many unagglutinated red cells), again because only the transfused red cells would be coated with antibody. In practice, however, weak sensitization and mixed-field agglutination can be difficult to differentiate. If a pretransfusion specimen is not available, it may be helpful to perform a red cell genotype or to use red cell separation procedures to isolate autologous red cells for testing. Performing a DAT on autologous red cells, testing the posttransfusion sample or the eluate with DAT-negative autologous red cells, or both may help distinguish an autoantibody from an alloantibody. If a DAT result from autologous red cells is negative, the reactivity is consistent with an alloantibody. If the posttransfusion serum or plasma is reactive with DAT-negative autologous red cells, the reactivity is consistent with an autoantibody. (See Chapter 14 and Fig 13-2.)

Antibodies to Low-Prevalence Antigens

If a sample is reactive only with a single donor or reagent red cell sample after alloantibody exclusions are complete, an antibody to a low-prevalence antigen should be suspected. To identify such an antibody, a panel of reagent red cells that express low-prevalence antigens can be tested with the serum. Alternatively, the one reactive red cell sample can be tested with known antibodies to low-prevalence antigens. Unfortunately, sera that contain antibodies to low-prevalence antigens often contain multiple antibodies to low-prevalence antigens. Although low-prevalence antigens are rare by definition, naturally occurring antibodies that recognize some of them are much less rare. Many antibodies to low-prevalence antigens are reactive only at temperatures below 37 C and therefore have doubtful clinical significance. To confirm the suspected specificities, one may need the expertise and resources of an IRL. Some IRLs, however, do not attempt to identify antibodies to low-prevalence antigens because many of these antibodies are not clinically meaningful, and compatible units are readily available.

If an antibody to a low-prevalence antigen is suspected and all common alloantibody specificities have been excluded, transfusion should not be delayed if identification studies are performed. Because antisera to type donor units for low-prevalence antigens are rarely available, it is usually necessary to rely on the crossmatch to avoid transfusion of antigen-positive units. When the serum is reactive with only one donor unit or reagent red cell sample, the most likely cause is an antibody to a low-prevalence antigen; however, some other possible explanations are that the red cells may be ABO incompatible, have a positive DAT result, or are polyagglutinable (ie, red cells that have cryptic antigens exposed and react with all normal adult serum).

Antibodies to Low-Prevalence Antigens in Pregnancy

An antibody to a low-prevalence antigen may also be suspected when a maternal antibody screen is nonreactive but her ABO-compatible newborn has a positive DAT result and/or unexplained decrease in red cell survival. A positive result when testing the mother's serum or plasma, or an eluate from the infant's DAT+ red cells, against the father's red cells can implicate an antibody to a low-prevalence antigen as the probable cause, even if the specificity is unknown. This testing can be performed only if the mother's sample is ABO compatible with the father's red cells or if the eluate from the infant's red cells does not contain anti-A or -B that would react with his red cells, or if the ABO antibodies are removed from the serum or eluate by adsorption.

Drug-Dependent Antibodies

Certain drugs induce the formation of antibodies in some patients. These drug-dependent antibodies may cause positive antibody detection/identification tests typically at the IAT phase and/or a positive DAT result. Actual immune hemolytic anemia caused by drugs is a rare event, with an estimated incidence of about one in a million.[38] Prompt correlation between clinical course, drug history, and serologic findings gives opportunity for timely recognition of the event and provision of potentially lifesaving information to the patient's clinician. When antibodies to a drug or drug/red cell membrane complexes are detected in routine serology, additional and sometimes complex testing may be needed to rule out the presence of alloantibodies and exclude the possibility of a transfusion reaction (delayed or serologic) occurring in the patient. Testing for drug-dependent antibodies and information on drug-induced immune hemolytic anemia may be found in Chapter 14.

Antibodies to Reagent Components

Antibodies to a variety of drugs and chemicals in testing reagents can cause positive results in antibody detection and identification tests. The offending component may be found in the suspending media of the reagent red cells or maybe a constituent of the antibody enhancement medium that is added to the test system. Most of these anomalous reactions are in-vitro phenomena and have no clinical significance in transfusion therapy, other than causing laboratory problems that delay transfusions. A systematic comparison of the sample's reactivity with cells or enhancement media sourced from different manufacturers, with washed red cells vs cells in original diluent, or with red cells from commercial sources vs donor blood may identify the offending component. For a more complete discussion, see the suggested reading by Garratty at the end of this chapter as well as listed references.[39-41]

Rouleaux

Rouleaux formation is one of the most commonly encountered anomalous serologic reactions. It is an in-vitro phenomenon that is produced by abnormal patient serum/plasma protein concentrations. Problems with rouleaux are more prevalent when using plasma, which has become the sample of choice for blood bank testing often due to automation requirements. Rouleaux formation is caused by aggregates of red cells that can be mistaken for agglutination upon macroscopic examination. It can occur in any test that contains patient plasma and reagent red cells at the time of reading. If viewed microscopically, rouleaux red cell aggregates will often look like a stack of coins. It may be difficult to detect antibodies by direct agglutination in a test plasma that contains rouleaux-producing proteins. Rouleaux formation itself is not observed in the IAT phase of testing because the washing steps remove the majority of implicated plasma proteins. Patient plasma samples exhibiting rouleaux are, however, prone to incomplete washing at the IAT phase and potentially false-negative results. Fortunately, such false-negative results caused by incomplete washing should easily be recognized by the failed antihuman globulin control cell step of the IAT. The saline replacement technique can be used to detect direct-agglutinating antibodies in the presence of rouleaux and confirm the suspected reactivity to be rouleaux if it is dispersed by the procedure (Method 3-7).

Other Anomalous Serologic Reactions

Antibodies that react only with red cells freshly washed in saline, red cells that are aged (in vitro or in vivo), and red cells that have been stored in some plastic containers, among others, have also been described. These types of anomalous reactions are less frequently encountered but are entertained as possibilities after close scrutiny of unexplained reactivity. Additional information can be found in the suggested reading by Garratty.

SELECTED PROCEDURES

Although the same method used for antibody detection tests is routinely used for basic antibody identification, alternative techniques and methods may be needed to resolve complex antibody identification problems. Some of the procedures described in this section are used routinely by many laboratories; others are used selectively and may apply only in special circumstances. It is important to remember that no single method is optimal for detecting all antibodies. When routine methods fail to indicate specificity, or the presence of an antibody is suspected but cannot be confirmed, the use of other enhancement techniques or procedures may be helpful. Techniques involving enzyme treatment of red cells, testing at lower temperatures, or testing with various additive solutions should, whenever possible, include an autocontrol to ensure proper interpretation of results.

Obtaining Autologous Red Cell Phenotype

It may be difficult to determine the patient's phenotype if the individual received transfusion in the past 3 months. A pretransfusion specimen, if available, should be used to determine the phenotype. If a pretransfusion sample is not available, the patient's newly formed autologous red cells can be separated from the transfused red cells and then typed (Method 2-22). Separation of young red cells by centrifugation is based on the difference in the densities of new and mature red cells. Separation is most successful when 3 days have elapsed since the last transfusion, which will provide time for new autologous red cell production. New autologous red cells must be isolated from the sample while it is fresh. The technique is ineffective and can often result in false-positive typing if the sample is too old (>24 hours) or the patient is not producing new red cells.

Sickle cells are quite dense, making centrifugation an ineffective technique for separating the autologous red cells from the transfused donor red cells in a patient with sickle cell disease. Autologous sickle cells may be separated from donor red cells using washes with hypotonic saline (Method 2-23). Sickle cells containing hemoglobin SS are resistant to lysis by hypotonic saline, whereas donor red cells containing hemoglobin AA are lysed.

Cold and warm autoantibodies may also complicate antigen typing because of the immunoglobulins coating the patient's red cells. It may be possible to remove cold autoantibodies with warm (37 C) saline washes (Method 2-17). If the cold autoantibodies are very potent, it may be necessary to treat the red cells with 0.01M dithiothreitol (DTT) to dissociate IgM molecules that cause spontaneous agglutination (Method 2-18). When red cells are coated with IgG autoantibodies, it is not possible to perform antigen typing with reagents that require an IAT (eg, Fy^a, Fy^b) without first removing the bound IgG.

However, it is often possible to type antibody-coated red cells with direct-agglutinating antisera, such as IgM monoclonal reagents. With rare exceptions, most direct-agglutinating monoclonal reagents give valid phenotyping results despite a positive DAT result.[42] Common techniques for removing IgG antibodies, when needed, include gentle heat elution (Method 2-19), treatment with chloroquine diphosphate (Method 2-20), and treatment with acid glycine/EDTA (Method 2-21).

LISS and PEG

PEG techniques are used to enhance reactivity and reduce incubation time compared to testing in the absence of an additive solution. LISS allows for reduced incubation time and may be used to suspend test red cells for use in tube or column agglutination tests or as an additive medium for tube or solid-phase tests. Commercially prepared LISS additives or PEG additives may contain additional enhancing agents. Care should be taken to closely follow the instructions in the manufacturer's product insert to ensure that the appropriate proportion of serum to LISS or PEG is achieved. Generic LISS and PEG procedures, as well as the principles and special considerations for each technique, can be found in Methods 3-4 and 3-5. Because LISS and PEG enhance autoantibodies, their use may complicate alloantibody identification in samples that also contain autoantibodies.[43-44]

Temperature Reduction

Some antibodies (eg, anti-M, -N, -P1, $-Le^a$, $-Le^b$, and -A1) react better at room temperature or below, and their specificity may be apparent only at a temperature <22 C. An autocontrol is especially important for tests at low temperatures because many sera also contain autoanti-I or other cold-reactive autoantibodies.

Increased Serum-to-Cell Ratio

Increasing the volume of serum incubated with a standard volume of red cells may enhance the reactivity of antibodies that are present in low concentrations. One acceptable procedure involves mixing 4 volumes (drops) of serum or plasma with 1 volume of a 2% to 5% saline suspension of red cells and incubating the mixture for 60 minutes at 37 C. Periodic mixing during the incubation promotes contact between the red cells and the antibodies. It is helpful to remove the serum before washing the cells for an IAT because the standard three to four washes may be insufficient to remove all of the unbound immunoglobulin if increased amounts of serum or plasma are used. More than four washes are not recommended because bound antibody molecules may dissociate. Increasing the serum-to-red-cell ratio is not appropriate for tests using LISS or commercial PEG, which may be manufactured by dissolving the PEG in LISS. Tests performed in a low-ionic-strength medium require specific proportions of serum or plasma and additive.

Increased Incubation Time

For some antibodies, the routine incubation period (typically 10 to 15 minutes minimum for some additive solutions, and 30 minutes for tests with no additive solutions) may not be sufficient to achieve maximum antibody binding; therefore, the reactions may be negative or weak, particularly in saline or albumin media. Extending the incubation time to between 30 and 60 minutes for albumin or saline tests often improves the reactivity and helps clarify the pattern of reactions. Extended incubation may be contraindicated when LISS or PEG is used. If the incubation period exceeds the recommended times for these methods, the reactivity may be diminished or lost. Care must be taken to use all reagents according to the manufacturers' directions.

Alteration in pH

Altering the pH of the test system can change the reactivity of certain antibodies, enhancing the reactivity of some and decreasing that of others.

Some examples of anti-M are enhanced when the pH of the test system is lowered to 6.5.[45] If anti-M is suspected because the only reactive red cells are M+N−, a definitive pattern (ie, reactivity with M+N+ red cells also) may be seen if the serum is acidified. The addition of 1

volume of 0.1 N HCl to 9 volumes of serum or plasma lowers the pH to approximately 6.5. The acidified serum should be tested with known M-negative red cells to control for nonspecific agglutination.

Lowering the pH, however, significantly decreases the reactivity of other antibodies.[46] If unbuffered saline with a pH <6.0 is used to prepare red cell suspensions or for washing in an IAT, antibodies in the RH, FY, JK, and MNS blood groups may lose reactivity. Phosphate-buffered saline (Method 1-8) can be used to control the pH and enhance the detection of antibodies that are poorly reactive at a lower pH.[47]

Enzyme Modification/Destruction of Blood Group Antigens on Red Cells

Ficin and papain are the most frequently used enzymes for complex antibody identification. They destroy or weaken antigens such as M, N, S, Fy[a], Fy[b], JMH, Ch, Rg, and Xg[a] (Table 13-7). Antibodies to these antigens are nonreactive with treated red cells. Conversely, ficin- and papain-treated red cells show persistent or enhanced reactivity with other antibodies (eg, those to antigens of the RH, P1PK, I, JK, and LE systems). For this reason, enzyme techniques may be used to separate mixtures of antibodies. For example, if a serum sample contains anti-Fy[a] and anti-Jk[a], many of the red cell samples on the initial panel would be reactive. If a panel of enzyme-treated red cells were tested, the anti-Jk[a] reactivity would persist and perhaps increase in reactivity, whereas the anti-Fy[a] reactivity would no longer be detected because its target antigen was destroyed by the enzyme treatment. Procedures for the preparation and use of proteolytic enzymes are given in Methods 3-8 to 3-13.

Additional enzymes that are commonly used in advanced IRLs include trypsin, α-chymotrypsin, and pronase. Depending on the enzyme and method used, other antigens may be altered or destroyed. Antigens that are inactivated by one proteolytic enzyme may not be inactivated by other enzymes. Trypsin treatment has been used to remove CD38 from red cells, thereby avoiding the interference of anti-CD38 immunotherapy.[48] The clinical significance of antibodies that are reactive only with enzyme-treated cells is questionable; such "enzyme-only" antibodies may not have clinical significance.[49]

Chemical Modification/Destruction of Blood Group Antigens on Red Cells

Certain blood group antigens can be destroyed or weakened by chemical treatment of the cells (Table 13-7). Modified red cells can be useful for both confirming the presence of suspected antibodies and detecting additional antibodies. The use of modified red cells can be especially helpful if a sample contains an antibody to a high-prevalence antigen because antigen-negative red cells are rare. Sulfhydryl reagents such as 2-aminoethylisothiouronium bromide (AET), 2-mercaptoethanol (2-ME), or DTT cleave disulfide bonds that are responsible for the conformation of certain blood group antigens and therefore can be used to weaken or destroy antigens in the KEL system and some other antigens (Method 3-18).[50,51] DTT treatment will also destroy CD38 on red cells and has commonly been used to mitigate the interference of anti-CD38 immunotherapy on serology testing.[22,23] ZZAP reagent, which contains both a proteolytic enzyme and DTT, denatures antigens that are sensitive to DTT (eg, all KEL system antigens) as well as antigens that are sensitive to enzymes (Method 4-8).[52] Glycine-HCl/EDTA treatment of red cells destroys Bg and KEL system antigens as well as the Er[a] antigen (Methods 2-21 and 4-2).[53] Chloroquine diphosphate can be used to weaken the expression of Class I HLA antigens (Bg antigens) on red cells.[54] Chloroquine treatment also weakens some other antigens, including Rh antigens (Method 2-20).

Inhibition Techniques

Soluble forms of some blood group antigens exist in body fluids, such as saliva, urine, and plasma. These substances are also present in other natural sources, or they can be prepared synthetically. Soluble substance can be used to inhibit the reactivity of the corresponding antibody that could mask the presence of underlying nonneutralizable antibodies. Also, inhibition of the reactivity by a soluble substance can help with the identification of the specificity of the antibody. For example, if a suspected anti-P1 does not produce a definitive pattern of agglutination, the loss of reactivity after the addition of soluble P1 substance strongly suggests that the specificity is anti-P1 if a parallel dilution control with saline remains reactive. Inhibition results can be interpreted only when the test is nonreactive and the dilution control that substitutes an equal volume of saline for the soluble substance is reactive.

The most commonly used substances for inhibition include the following:

1. *LE (Lewis) substances.* Le[a] substances, Le[b] substances, or both are present in the saliva of individuals who possess the LE gene (*FUT3*). Le[a] substance is present in the saliva of Le(a+b−) individuals, and both Le[a] and Le[b] substances are present in the saliva of Le(a−b+) individuals (Method 2-8). Commercially prepared LE substance is available.
2. *P1 substance.* Soluble P1 substance is present in hydatid cyst fluid and the ovalbumin of pigeon eggs. Commercially prepared P1 substance is available.
3. *Sd[a] substance.* Soluble Sd[a] blood group-substance is present in various body fluids, but urine has the highest concentration of Sd[a].[55] To confirm the presence of anti-Sd[a] in a serum sample, urine from a known Sd(a+) individual (or a pool of urine specimens) can be used to inhibit the antibody reactivity (Method 3-19).
4. *CH/RG (Chido and Rodgers) substances.* CH/RG antigens are epitopes on the fourth component of human complement (C4).[56,57] Most normal red cells have a trace amount of C4 on their surface. Anti-Ch and anti-Rg are reactive with this C4 in an IAT. A useful test to identify anti-Ch and anti-Rg is inhibition of the antibodies with plasma from Ch+, Rg+ individuals (Method 3-17). Although not an inhibition technique, soluble Ch and Rg substance in plasma can also be used to coat red cells in vitro with excess C4d. Such coated

red cells will directly agglutinate anti-Ch and -Rg, allowing for their rapid identification.[58]

Denaturation of Immunoglobulins

Sulfhydryl reagents, such as DTT and 2-ME, can also be used to cleave the disulfide bonds that join the monomeric subunits of the IgM pentamer. Intact 19S IgM molecules are cleaved into 7S immunoglobulin subunits, which have altered serologic reactivity.[59] The interchain bonds of 7S immunoglobulin monomers are relatively resistant to such cleavage.

Uses of sulfhydryl reagents to denature immunoglobulins include the following:

1. Determining the immunoglobulin class of an antibody (Method 3-16). In a pregnant woman's sample, IgG antibody indicates the potential for HDFN.
2. Identifying antibodies in a mixture of IgM and IgG antibodies, particularly when an agglutinating IgM antibody masks the presence of IgG antibodies. It is important to note that when treated plasma is used for IgG antibody identification, the effect of the dilution caused by the treatment should be considered.
3. Determining the relative amounts of IgG and IgM components of a given specificity (eg, anti-A or -B).
4. Dispersing red cell agglutinates caused by IgM autoantibodies (Method 2-18).
5. Removing IgG antibodies from red cells using a mixture of DTT and proteolytic enzyme (ZZAP reagent) (Method 4-8).

Adsorption

Antibody can be removed from a serum sample by adsorption onto red cells that express the corresponding antigen. After the antibody attaches to the membrane-bound antigens, the antibody remains attached to the red cells when serum/plasma and cells are separated. It may be possible to harvest the bound antibody by elution or examine the adsorbed serum or plasma for antibody(ies) remaining after the adsorption process.

Adsorption techniques are useful for the following purposes:

1. Separating multiple antibodies present in a single serum.
2. Removing autoantibody to permit the detection or identification of underlying alloantibodies. (See Chapter 14 for more information.)
3. Removing unwanted antibody (often anti-A, anti-B, or both) from serum that contains an antibody suitable for reagent use.
4. Confirming the presence of specific antigens on red cells by their ability to remove antibody of corresponding specificity from previously characterized serum.
5. Confirming the specificity of an antibody by showing that it can be adsorbed onto red cells of only a particular blood group phenotype.

Adsorption serves different purposes in different situations; no single procedure is satisfactory for all purposes (Methods 4-5, 4-8, 4-9, and 4-10). A basic procedure for antibody adsorption can be found in Method 3-20. The usual serum/plasma-to-cell ratio is 1 volume of serum or plasma to an equal volume of washed red cell blood component. To enhance antibody removal, a larger volume of red cells increases the proportion of antigen. The incubation temperature should be that at which the antibody is optimally reactive. Pretreating red cells with a proteolytic enzyme may enhance antibody uptake and reduce the number of adsorptions required to remove an antibody completely. Because enzymes destroy some antigens, antibodies directed against those antigens are not removed by enzyme-treated red cells. To ensure that an adsorption process is complete (ie, that no unadsorbed antibody remains), it is essential to confirm that the adsorbed serum is nonreactive with a sample of the adsorbing red cells that was not used for adsorption. Adsorption requires a substantial volume of red cells, and vials of reagent 3% to 4% red cell suspensions are usually not sufficient. Blood samples from donor units are the most convenient sources.

When separating mixtures of antibodies, the selection of red cells of the appropriate phenotype is extremely important. If one or more antibodies have been previously identified, red cells that express the corresponding antigens can be used to remove the known antibodies. For example, if a person who types K+k–, Fy(a–b+) has produced anti-k, it may be necessary to adsorb the anti-k onto K–k+, Fy(a–b+) red cells to remove the anti-k. Then, the adsorbed sample can be tested with common K–k+, Fy(a+b–) red cells to detect or exclude anti-Fy^a.

Elution

Elution dissociates antibodies from sensitized red cells. Bound antibody may be released by changing the thermodynamics of antigen-antibody reactions, neutralizing or reversing forces of attraction that hold antigen-antibody complexes together, or disturbing the structure of the antigen-antibody binding site. The usual objective is to recover bound antibody in a usable form.

Selected elution procedures are given in Methods 4-1 through 4-4. No single method is best for all situations. Heat or freeze-thaw elution techniques are usually restricted to the investigation of HDFN caused by ABO incompatibility because these elution procedures rarely work well for other antibodies. Acid or organic solvent methods are used for eluting warm-reactive auto- and alloantibodies. Commercial kits are available for performing elution. (See Chapter 14, Table 14-2 for a list of elution methods and their uses, advantages, and disadvantages.)

Elution techniques are useful for the following:

1. Investigation of a positive DAT result (Chapter 14).
2. Concentration and purification of antibodies, detection of weakly expressed antigens, and identification of multiple antibody specificities. Such studies are used in conjunction with an appropriate adsorption technique, as described below and in Method 2-7.

3. Preparation of antibody-free red cells for autologous adsorption studies (Methods 4-5 and 4-8).

Technical factors that influence the outcome of elution procedures include the following:

1. *Incomplete washing.* Sensitized red cells should be thoroughly washed before an elution to prevent contamination of the eluate with unbound residual antibody. Six washes with saline are usually adequate, but more washes may be needed if the serum contains a high-titer antibody. (The considerations in item 3 below should be kept in mind.) To confirm the efficacy of the washing process, supernatant fluid from the final wash should be tested for antibody activity and found to be nonreactive.
2. *Binding of protein to glass surfaces.* If an eluate is prepared in the test tube that was used during the sensitization or washing phases, antibody that nonspecifically binds to the test tube surface may dissociate during the elution. Similar binding can also occur from a whole blood sample when a patient has a positive DAT result and has free antibody in the serum. To avoid such contamination, red cells used to prepare an eluate should be transferred to a clean test tube before washing and then to another clean tube before the elution procedure is initiated.
3. *Dissociation of antibody before elution.* IgM antibodies, such as anti-A or anti-M, or low-affinity IgG may spontaneously dissociate from the red cells during the wash phase. To minimize the loss of bound antibody, cold (4 C) saline or wash solution provided by the manufacturer should be used for washing.
4. *Incorrect technique.* Such factors as incomplete removal of organic solvents or failure to correct the tonicity or pH of an eluate may cause the reagent red cells used to test the eluate to hemolyze or appear "sticky." The presence of stromal debris may interfere with the reading of test results. Careful technique

and strict adherence to procedures should eliminate such problems.

5. *Instability of eluates.* Diluted protein solutions, such as those obtained by elution into saline, are unstable. Eluates should be tested as soon as possible after preparation. Alternatively, bovine albumin may be added to a final concentration of 6% weight/volume, and the preparation may be frozen during storage. Eluates can also be prepared in antibody-free plasma, 6% albumin, or a similar protein medium. When commercial elution kits are used, the manufacturer's instructions for preparation and storage should be followed.

Combined Adsorption-Elution

Combined adsorption-elution tests can be used to separate a mixture of antibodies in a single-serum sample, detect weakly expressed antigens on red cells, or help identify weakly reactive antibodies. The process consists of first incubating serum with selected red cells and then eluting antibody from the adsorbing red cells.

Care must be taken when selecting the adsorbing cells to separate a mixture of antibodies. The cells should express only one of the antigens corresponding to an antibody in the mixture so that the eluate from the cells will contain only that antibody. Both the eluate and adsorbed serum can be used for further testing. Unmodified red cells are generally used for adsorptions when subsequent elutions are being prepared.

Titration

The titer of an antibody is usually determined by testing serial twofold dilutions of the serum with selected red cells. Results are expressed as the reciprocal of the highest serum dilution that shows macroscopic agglutination. Titration values can provide information about the relative amount of antibody present in a sample or the relative strength of antigen expression on red cells.

Titration studies are useful for the following purposes:

1. *Prenatal studies.* When the antibody has a specificity that is known to cause HDFN, or the antibody's clinical significance is unknown, the results of titration studies may contribute to the decision about performing additional procedures (eg, Doppler sonography or amniocentesis). (See Chapter 23 and Method 5-3.)

2. *Antibody identification.* Some antibodies that agglutinate virtually all reagent red cells may give an indication of specificity by demonstrating reactivity of different strengths with different red cell samples in titration studies. For example, potent undiluted autoanti-I may be reactive with both adult and umbilical cord blood red cells, but titration studies may reveal reactivity with adult I+ red cells at a higher dilution than with cord blood I+^{w} red cells. The reactivity of most antibodies weakens progressively with serial dilutions (ie, a 2+ reaction becomes 1+ in the next dilution), and weak antibodies (<1+) may lose their reactivity when diluted. Yet, some antibodies that have weak reactions when they are undiluted continue to react at dilutions as high as 1 in 2048. Such antibodies include anti-Ch, -Rg, -Cs^a, -Yk^a, -Kn^a, -McC^a, and -JMH. Titration studies may be performed on a sample showing unexplained weak IAT reactions to determine whether the reactivity is consistent with the antibodies in this group; however, not all examples of these antibodies demonstrate such high-titer, low-avidity characteristics. Thus, the serologic characteristics may suggest certain specificities, but failure to do so does not eliminate these possibilities. The antibodies listed above are not expected to cause shortened red cell survival, although there are examples of other antibodies (eg, anti-Lu^b, -Hy, and -Yt^a) that may mimic these serologic characteristics and cause shortened red cell survival. Anti-CD38 may also show high-titer reactivity and is generally nonreactive with Lu(a–b–) cells.[48,60] If administration of this therapy to the patient

is not disclosed to laboratory staff, the investigation may conclude the sample contains an antibody to a high-prevalence LU system antigen. Details about titration are given in Method 3-15.

3. *Separating multiple antibodies.* Titration results may suggest that one antibody is reactive at higher dilutions than another antibody. That information can allow the serum to be diluted before it is tested with a red cell panel, which effectively removes one antibody and allows the other to be identified. For example, if a serum contains anti-Jk^a that is reactive to a titer of 2 and anti-c that is reactive to a titer of 16, it may be possible to dilute the serum 1:8 (ie, one volume of serum in a final volume of 8) to clearly detect and identify only the anti-c. This can be useful when the selection of reagent red cells is limited by resource availability or by the antibody specificities present in the patient's serum.

Other Methods

Methods other than traditional tube, gel, or solid-phase techniques may be used for antibody identification. Some methods are especially useful for testing small volumes of samples or reagents. Such methods include testing in capillary tubes, microplates, or enzyme-linked immunosorbent assays. Other methods that are useful in laboratories with specialized equipment include immunofluorescence, flow cytometry, and immunoblotting.

CONSIDERATIONS FOLLOWING ANTIBODY IDENTIFICATION

Unexpected red cell antibodies are revealed in antibody detection tests and characterized through antibody identification testing. Information obtained from this process is then used to help determine the potential clinical significance of the unexpected antibody for the purpose of providing an effective transfusion of red cell components or to identify the need for further monitoring for HDFN.

Significance of Identified Antibodies

The phases in which an antibody is identified and its specificity are the two primary means used to predict an unexpected antibody's potential clinical significance. Antibodies that are reactive at 37 C, in an IAT, or both are potentially clinically significant. Antibodies that are reactive at room temperature and below are usually not clinically significant; however, there are many exceptions. For example, anti-Vel, -P, and -PP1P^k (-Tj^a) may be reactive only at cold temperatures, yet may cause red cell destruction in vivo. Anti-Ch, anti-Rg, and many of the KN and COST antibodies have little or no clinical significance despite their reactivity in an IAT. Reported experience with examples of antibodies with the same specificity can be used in assessing the clinical significance.

Table 13-5 summarizes the expected reactivity and clinical significance of commonly encountered alloantibodies. For some antibodies, little or no data exist, and the decision about clinical significance has to be based on the premise that clinically significant antibodies are those that are active at 37 C, in an IAT, or both.

Certain laboratory tests have been used to predict the clinical significance of antibodies. The monocyte monolayer assay, which quantifies phagocytosis, adherence of antibody-coated red cells, or both, can be used to predict the in-vivo clinical significance of some antibodies.[61,62] The test for antibody-dependent cellular cytotoxicity, which measures lysis of antibody-coated red cells, and the chemiluminescence assay, which measures the respiratory release of oxygen radicals after phagocytosis of antibody-coated red cells, have been helpful in predicting in-vivo antibody significance—particularly for predicting the severity of HDFN. For cold-reactive antibodies, in-vitro thermal amplitude studies may be able to predict the likelihood of in-vivo hemolysis.[63]

In-vivo tests may also be used to evaluate the significance of an antibody. The most common technique is a red cell survival study in which radiolabeled, antigen-positive red cells (usually labeled with ^{51}Cr) are infused into the patient. After a specified period has elapsed, a sample of blood from the patient is tested for radioactivity. With this technique, it is possible to measure the survival of 1 mL of infused cells. Another in-vivo technique, flow cytometry, can also be used to measure the survival of infused red cells, but a larger aliquot of red cells (about 10 mL) is usually required. Interpretation of in-vivo survival test results is complicated by the fact that small aliquots of incompatible red cells may have a faster rate of destruction than an entire transfused unit of Red Blood Cells (RBCs). Comparison with documented cases in the literature and consultation with an IRL should provide guidance about previous examples of similar specificities.

Subsequent Antibody Identification in Patients with a Known History of Antibodies

Once a clinically significant antibody has been identified, the patient must receive red cells negative for the corresponding antigen if at all possible, so it is rarely necessary to routinely repeat the identification of known antibodies in subsequent pretransfusion testing. AABB *Standards* states that in patients with previously identified clinically significant antibodies, testing methods should be used that identify *additional* clinically significant antibodies.[9(p37)] Each laboratory should define policies and methods for the detection of additional antibodies in these patients.

Selection of Donor Units for Patients Whose Serum Contains Antibodies

Antigen-Negative Blood

RBC units selected for transfusion to a patient with potentially clinically significant antibodies should be negative for the corresponding antigen(s). Even if the antibodies are no longer detectable, all subsequent RBC transfusions to that patient should lack the antigen to prevent a secondary immune response. The transfusion service must maintain records of all patients in whom clinically significant antibodies have been previously identified, and an IAT cross-

match procedure is required if the sample contains—or has previously contained—a clinically significant antibody.[9(pp38,77)] Exceptions to these practices should be made only in extreme clinical emergencies under the direction of a physician.

A potent example of the antibody should be used to identify antigen-negative RBC units. Often, the antibody is a commercial antiserum, but to save expensive or rare reagents, units can be tested first (often referred to as screened) for compatibility with the patient's serum. Then, the absence of the antigen in compatible units can be confirmed with commercial reagents. If the antibody is unusual and commercial antiserum is not available, a stored sample from the sensitized patient may be used to select units for transfusion at a later time, especially if the patient's later samples lose reactivity. If any patient serum or plasma is used as a typing reagent, referred to as a single-source antibody, the antibody reactivity should be well characterized and retain reactivity after storage. Appropriate negative and weak-positive controls (eg, from heterozygous donors) should be used at the time of the testing. The following criteria, established by the FDA for licensing some reagents, should be used as guidelines for human-source reagents used in lieu of commercial reagents[64]:

1. Anti-K, -k, -Jk^a, -Fy^a, and -C^w: dilution of 1:8 must produce at least a 1+ reaction.
2. Anti-S, -s, -P1, -M, -I, -c (saline), -e (saline), and -A1: dilution of 1:4 must produce at least a 1+ reaction.
3. Most other specificities: undiluted reagent must produce at least a 2+ reaction.

When selecting units for patients with clinically significant antibodies, some serologists recommend typing the units with antibodies from two different sources, but others consider this step unnecessary—especially when potent commercial reagents are available and an IAT crossmatch will be performed. Different lots of antibody from the same manufacturer and even different reagents from different manufacturers may have been prepared from the same source material because manufacturers often acquire these resources from the same entity.

If a donor unit is tested for selected antigens and labeled by the blood center, the use of licensed (commercial) reagents, if available, is required. If no licensed reagent is available, the unit must be labeled with appropriate wording (eg, "Tested and found negative for XX antigen using unlicensed typing reagents").[65] Except for results of ABO and D typing, there is no requirement that the hospital repeat testing of donor minor antigen typing if the results are on the label or on an attached tag.[9(p36)] Minor antigen typing results on packing slips or not physically attached to the donor unit should be confirmed by the hospital, if possible, when the unit is intended for transfusion to a patient with the corresponding alloantibody.

Crossmatch for Compatibility

For certain antibodies, typing the donor units may not be necessary, and the patient's serum can be used to select serologically compatible RBC units. This is especially true for antibodies that characteristically are reactive below 37 C (eg, anti-M, -N, -P1, -Le^a, -Le^b, and -A1) and that do not ordinarily produce a secondary immune response following the transfusion of antigen-positive RBC units.

Phenotype-Matched Blood

Sometimes it may be best practice to provide phenotypically matched, antigen-negative RBC units as a prophylactic measure. For example, when a patient of the R_1R_1 phenotype produces anti-E, some serologists suggest that RBC units should be negative for both the E and c antigens. This recommendation is based on the assumption that the stimulus to produce anti-E may also have stimulated anti-c or anti-cE that remains undetected by routine tests.[66] Similarly, for an R_2R_2 patient with demonstrable anti-C, the use of e-negative donor blood may be considered.

It may be prudent to select RBC units that are phenotypically matched with the patient for clinically significant antigens when a patient has a potent warm autoantibody or is receiving monoclonal antibody therapy and compatibility

cannot be demonstrated by routine testing. This is also true when an antibody has not been specifically demonstrated but decreased survival of transfused cells is observed.

For patients needing chronic transfusion therapy for sickle cell disease or thalassemia, limited antigen-matching, specifically for Rh antigens (generally C and E) and K is becoming common practice to prevent or mitigate alloimmunization. Transfusion of phenotypically matched RBC units, however, does not prevent formation of all new alloantibodies.

When Uncommon or Rare Blood Is Needed

Rare blood includes units that are negative for high-prevalence antigens (<1:1000 units) or are negative for a combination of many common antigens (<1:100). When a patient has multiple antibodies, it is helpful to determine the prevalence of compatible donors. To calculate this prevalence, one must multiply the prevalence of donors who are negative for one antigen by the prevalence of donors who are negative for each of the other antigens. The steps are outlined in Table 13-8, using the example of a group O patient's serum that contains anti-c, anti-Fy^a, and anti-S. As shown, only 1.3% of the general population would be a compatible donor for a group O patient with anti-c, anti-Fy^a, and anti-S.

If any of these antibodies is present alone, finding compatible blood is not very difficult, but the combination requires a large number of units in order to find one compatible unit (ie, 1.3 compatible donors out of 100, or approximately 1 out of 80). The calculation in the table uses the prevalence in populations of European ancestry, and prevalence may be different in populations of non-European ancestry. In calculating the probability of compatible donors, one should use the antigen prevalence that corresponds with the racial composition of the donor population, if available.

When units of rare or uncommon phenotypes are needed, the local IRL should be contacted. Local IRLs that reside within or are associated with blood centers typically have an inventory (fresh and/or frozen) of RBC units of

TABLE 13-8. Calculating Prevalence of Compatible Donors Required to Find Antigen-Negative Units

Step	Example
Identify the prevalence of antigen-negative individuals for each of the applicable antigens	18% c−, 34% Fy(a−), and 45% S−
Calculate the prevalence of units negative for all antigens combined	$0.18 \times 0.34 \times 0.45 = 0.028$, or 2.8%
Identify the prevalence of ABO-compatible donors so that it can be factored into the calculation	45%*
Calculate the prevalence of ABO-compatible antigen-negative units	$0.028 \times 0.45 = 0.013$, or 1.3%

*Prevalence of group O donors.

uncommon phenotypes and sometimes rare phenotypes. When the local IRL does not have RBCs of the necessary phenotype, they typically have a mechanism for searching for the required units. (See IRL section below.)

If the clinical situation allows, autologous RBC transfusions should be considered for patients with rare phenotypes who are expected to need blood in the future. Additionally, family members are another potential source of rare blood donors. The absence of high-prevalence antigens is usually associated with the inheritance of the same rare recessive blood group gene from each heterozygous parent. Children from the same parents have one chance in four of inheriting the same two rare genetic mutations, making siblings much more likely than the general population to have the rare blood type. In most cases, blood from the patient's parents, children, and half of the patient's siblings express only one rare gene. If transfusion is essential and there is no alternative to transfusing incompatible blood, these heterozygous (single-dose) donors may be preferable to random donors. For infants with HDFN resulting from multiple antibodies or an antibody to a high-prevalence antigen, the mother (if she is ABO compatible) is often the logical donor.

IMMUNOHEMATOLOGY REFERENCE LABORATORIES

IRLs typically have the skilled staff, procedures, and, most importantly, resources (such as frozen aliquots of fully phenotyped rare red cells lacking high-prevalence antigens) to investigate and resolve many or most complex antibody problems. IRLs can also provide consultation and information to laboratories about unfamiliar or infrequently encountered complex antibody problems. Additionally, IRLs often help facilities procure units of specific phenotypes when such units cannot be found in a routine transfusion service. Many IRLs also have access to the American Rare Donor Program (ARDP), which provides a network for finding RBC units with rare phenotypes throughout the United States and also has connection to similar programs worldwide (See Method 3-21).

KEY POINTS

1. A clinically significant red cell antibody is an antibody that is frequently associated with HDFN, hemolytic transfusion reactions, or a notable decrease in the survival of transfused red cells.

2. It is important to consider the patient's medical history (transfusions, pregnancies, transplantations, diagnoses, drugs, and biologic therapies/immunotherapies) before starting antibody identification testing.

3. Biologic therapies are expanding beyond IVIG and RhIG. Monoclonal antibodies developed as immunotherapeutic agents [eg, daratumumab (anti-CD38)] may also interfere with serologic results. Novel therapies may affect serologic testing in the future.

4. The autologous control, in which serum and autologous red cells are tested under the same conditions as the serum and reagent red cells, is an important part of antibody identification. The autologous control is not the same as a DAT.

5. An antibody may be tentatively excluded or ruled out if an antigen is present on a reagent cell and the patient's serum or plasma is not reactive with it.

6. The phenotype of the patient's autologous red cells is an important part of antibody identification. When an antibody has been tentatively identified, the corresponding antigen is expected to be absent from the autologous red cells, although exceptions can occur. Discrepancies between autologous phenotype and antibody specificity may indicate alloantibody in a patient having a variant or partial antigen.

7. Genotyping is an accepted method for obtaining red cell phenotype information. DNA-based methods are also used to resolve conflicting results in antibody identification or in serologic-vs genotyping-based phenotype discrepancies.

8. Common clinically significant alloantibodies that should be considered in the process of exclusion during antibody identification testing are, at a minimum, anti-D, -C, -E, -c, -e, -K, -Fy^a, -Fy^b, -Jk^a, -Jk^b, -S, and -s.

9. Based on probability, the use of two reactive and two nonreactive red cell samples is the very minimum acceptable for antibody confirmation.

10. The use of DTT or 2-ME to determine the immunoglobulin class of plasma/serum reactivity is useful in the prenatal setting, where detection of IgG antibody would indicate the ability of the antibody to cross the placenta and the potential for HDFN.

11. Elution dissociates antibodies from sensitized red cells. Bound antibody may be released by changing the thermodynamics of an antigen-antibody reaction, neutralizing or reversing forces of attraction that hold antigen-antibody complexes together, or disturbing the structures of the antigen-antibody binding site.

12. RBC units selected for transfusion to a patient with a potentially clinically significant antibody should be negative for the corresponding antigen(s). Even if the antibody is no longer detectable, all subsequent RBC transfusions to the patient should lack the antigen to prevent a secondary immune response.

REFERENCES

1. Tremi A, King K. Red blood cell alloimmunization: Lessons from sickle cell disease. Transfusion 2013;53:692-5.

2. Chou ST, Jackson T, Vege S, et al. High prevalence of red blood cell alloimmunization in sickle cell disease despite transfusion from Rh-matched minority donors. Blood 2013;122:1062-71.

3. Spanos T, Karageorga M, Ladis V, et al. Red cell alloantibodies in patients with thalassemia. Vox Sang 1990;58:50-5.

4. Issitt PD, Anstee DJ. Applied blood group serology. 4th ed. Durham, NC: Montgomery Scientific Publications, 1998.

5. Reid ME, Lomas-Francis C, Olsson M. The blood group antigens factsbook. 3rd ed. London: Elsevier Academic Press, 2012.

6. Malyska H, Kleeman JE, Masouredis SP, Victoria EJ. Effects on blood group antigens from storage at low ionic strength in the presence of neomycin. Vox Sang 1983;44:375-84.

7. Westhoff CM, Sipherd BD, Toalson LD. Red cell antigen stability in K3EDTA. Immunohematology 1993;9:109-11.

8. Van Thof L, ed. Standards for immunohematology reference laboratories. 11th ed. Bethesda, MD: AABB, 2019.

9. Gammon R, ed. Standards for blood banks and transfusion services. 32nd ed. Bethesda, MD: AABB, 2020.

10. Casina TS. In search of the holy grail: Comparison of antibody screening methods. Immunohematology 2006;22:196-202.

11. Winters JL, Richa EM, Bryant SC, et al. Polyethylene glycol antiglobulin tube versus gel microcolumn: Influence on the incidence of delayed hemolytic transfusion reactions and delayed serologic transfusion reactions. Transfusion 2010; 50:1444-52.

12. Bunker ML, Thomas CL, Geyer SJ. Optimizing pretransfusion antibody detection and identification: A parallel, blinded comparison of tube PEG, solid-phase, and automated methods. Transfusion 2001;41:621-6.

13. Pisacka M, Kralova M, Sklenarova M. Solid-phase-membrane only antibodies—reactive only in Capture-R Ready but nonreactive by Capture-R Select and in other techniques (abstract). Transfusion 2011;51(Suppl 3):175A.

14. Lang N, Sulfridge DM, Hulina J, et al. Solid phase reactive only antibodies (abstract). Transfusion 2011;51(Suppl 3):172A.

15. Liu C, Grossman BJ. Antibody of undetermined specificity: frequency, laboratory features, and natural history. Transfusion 2013;53:931-8.

16. Miller NM, Johnson ST, Carpenter E, et al. Patient factors associated with unidentified reactivity in solid-phase and polyethylene glycol antibody detection methods. Transfusion 2017;57: 1288-93.

17. Howard JE, Winn LC, Gottlieb CE, et al. Clinical significance of anti-complement component of antiglobulin antisera. Transfusion 1982;22: 269-72.

18. Nedelcu E, Hall C, Stoner A, et al. Interference of anti? CD47 therapy with blood bank testing (abstract). Transfusion 2017;57(S3):148A.

19. Velliquette RW, Degtyaryova D, Hong H, et al. Serological observations in patients receiving Hu5F9? G4 monoclonal anti-CD47 therapy (abstract). Transfusion 2017;57(S3):159A.

20. Howard-Menk C, Crane J, Doshi L, Papari M. HU5F9? G4 monoclonal anti-CD47 therapy: A first experience with interference in antibody identification (abstract). Transfusion 2018; 58(S2):177A.

21. Howie HL, Delaney M, Wang X. Serological blind spots for variants of human IgG3 and IgG4 by a commonly used anti-immunoglobulin reagent. Transfusion 2016;56:2953-62.

22. Oostendorp M, Lammerts van Bueren JJ, Doshi P, et al. When blood transfusion medicine becomes complicated due to interference by monoclonal antibody therapy. Transfusion 2015; 55:1555-62.

23. Chapuy CL, Nicholson RT, Aguad MD, et al. Resolving the daratumumab interference with blood compatibility testing. Transfusion 2015; 55:1545-54.

24. Anani WQ, Duffer K, Kaufman RM, et al. How do I work up pretransfusion samples containing anti-CD38? Transfusion 2017;57:1337-42.

25. Carreno-Tarrogona G, Cedena T, Montejano L, et al. Papain-treated panels are a simple method for the identification of alloantibodies in multiple myeloma patients treated with anti-CD38 based therapies. Transfus Med 2019;29(3):193-6.

26. Velliquette RW, Shakarian G, Lomas-Francis C, Westhoff CM. Testing samples from patients receiving anti-CD38 therapy with commercial papain treated reagent red cells (abstract). Transfusion 2018;58(S2):196A.

27. Velliquette RW, Kirkegaard J, Jones D, et al. Monoclonal anti-CD38 and anti-CD47 therapy interference with platelet antibody screen test methods (abstract). Transfusion 2018;58(S2): 51A.

28. Judd WJ, Steiner EA, Oberman HA, Nance S. Can the reading for serologic reactivity following 37 degrees C incubation be omitted? Transfusion 1992;32:304-8.

29. Reid ME, Øyen R, Storry J, et al. Interpretation of RBC typing in multi-transfused patients can be unreliable (abstract). Transfusion 2000;40 (Suppl):123S.

30. Lomas-Francis C, DePalma H. 2007 Rock Øyen Symposium. DNA-based assays for patient testing: Their application, interpretation, and correlation of results. Immunohematology 2008; 24:180-90.

31. Fisher RA. Statistical methods and scientific inference. 2nd ed. Edinburgh, Scotland: Oliver and Boyd, 1959.

32. Harris RE, Hochman HG. Revised p values in testing blood group antibodies: Fisher's exact test revisited. Transfusion 1986;26:494-9.

33. Kanter MH, Poole G, Garratty G. Misinterpretation and misapplication of p values in antibody identification: The lack of value of a p value. Transfusion 1997;37:816-22.

34. Moulds JM, Zimmerman PA, Doumbo OK, et al. Molecular identification of Knops blood group polymorphisms found in long homologous region D of complement receptor 1. Blood 2001; 97:2879-85.

35. Arndt PA, Leger RM, Garratty G. Serologic findings in autoimmune hemolytic anemia associated with immunoglobulin M warm autoantibodies. Transfusion 2009;49:235-42.

36. Waligora SK, Edwards JM. Use of rabbit red cells for adsorption of cold autoagglutinins. Transfusion 1983;23:328-30.

37. Yuan S, Fang A, Davis R, et al. Immunoglobulin M red blood cell alloantibodies are frequently adsorbed by rabbit erythrocyte stroma. Transfusion 2010;50:1139-43.

38. Arndt PA, Garratty G. The changing spectrum of drug-induced immune hemolytic anemia. Semin Hematol 2005;42:137-44.

39. Judd WJ, Steiner EA, Cochran RK. Paraben-associated autoanti-Jka antibodies: Three examples detected using commercially prepared low-ionic strength saline containing parabens. Transfusion 1982;22:31-5.

40. Judd WJ, Storry JR, Annesley TD, et al. The first example of a paraben-dependent antibody to an Rh protein. Transfusion 2001;41:371-4.

41. Dube VE, Zoes C, Adesman P. Caprylate-dependent auto-anti-e. Vox Sang 1977;33:359-63.

42. Rodberg K, Tsuneta R, Garratty G. Discrepant Rh phenotyping results when testing IgG-sensitized RBCs with monoclonal Rh reagents (abstract). Transfusion 1995;35(Suppl):67S.

43. Reisner R, Butler G, Bundy K, Moore SB. Comparison of the polyethylene glycol antiglobulin test and the use of enzymes in antibody detection and identification. Transfusion 1996;36:487-9.

44. Issitt PD, Combs MR, Bumgarner DJ, et al. Studies of antibodies in the sera of patients who have made red cell autoantibodies. Transfusion 1996;36:481-6.

45. Beattie KM, Zuelzer WW. The frequency and properties of pH-dependent anti-M. Transfusion 1965;5:322-6.

46. Bruce M, Watt AH, Hare W, et al. A serious source of error in antiglobulin testing. Transfusion 1986;26:177-81.

47. Rolih S, Thomas R, Fisher F, Talbot J. Antibody detection errors due to acidic or unbuffered saline. Immunohematology 1993;9:15-18.

48. Velliquette RW, Shakarian G, Jhang J, et al. Daratumumab-derived anti-CD38 can be easily mistaken for clinically significant antibodies to Lutheran antigens or to Knops antigens (abstract). Transfusion 2015;55(3S):26A.

49. Issitt PD, Combs MR, Bredehoeft SJ, et al. Lack of clinical significance of "enzyme-only" red cell alloantibodies. Transfusion 1993;33:284-93.

50. Advani H, Zamor J, Judd WJ, et al. Inactivation of Kell blood group antigens by 2-aminoethylisothiouronium bromide. Br J Haematol 1982; 51:107-15.

51. Branch DR, Muensch HA, Sy Siok Hian AL, Petz LD. Disulfide bonds are a requirement for Kell and Cartwright (Yta) blood group antigen integrity. Br J Haematol 1983;54:573-8.

52. Branch DR, Petz LD. A new reagent (ZZAP) having multiple applications in immunohematology. Am J Clin Pathol 1982;78:161-7.

53. Liew YW, Uchikawa M. Loss of Er^a antigen in very low pH buffers. Transfusion 1987;27:442-3.

54. Swanson JL, Sastamoinen R. Chloroquine stripping of HLA A,B antigens from red cells. Transfusion 1985;25:439-40.

55. Morton JA, Pickles MM, Terry AM. The Sd^a blood group antigen in tissues and body fluids. Vox Sang 1970;19:472-82.

56. O'Neill GJ, Yang SY, Tegoli J, et al. Chido and Rodgers blood groups are distinct antigenic components of human complement C4. Nature 1978;273:668-70.

57. Tilley CA, Romans DG, Crookston MC. Localisation of Chido and Rodgers determinants to the C4d fragment of human C4. Nature 1978;276:713-15.

58. Judd WJ, Kraemer K, Moulds JJ. The rapid identification of Chido and Rodgers antibodies using C4d-coated red blood cells. Transfusion 1981; 21:189-92.

59. Freedman J, Masters CA, Newlands M, Mollison PL. Optimal conditions for use of sulphydryl compounds in dissociating red cell antibodies. Vox Sang 1976;30:231-9.

60. Aye T, Arndt PA, Leger RM, et al. Myeloma patients receiving daratumumab (anti-CD38) can appear to have an antibody with Lutheran-related specificity (abstract). Transfusion 2015; 55(3S):28A.

61. Nance SJ, Arndt P, Garratty, G. Predicting the clinical significance of red cell alloantibodies us-

ing a monocyte monolayer assay. Transfusion 1987;27:449-52.

62. Arndt PA, Garratty G. A retrospective analysis of the value of monocyte monolayer assay results for predicting the clinical significance of blood group alloantibodies. Transfusion 2004;44: 1273-81.

63. Petz LD, Garratty G. Immune hemolytic anemias. 2nd ed. Philadelphia: Churchill Livingstone, 2004.

64. Code of federal regulations. Title 21, CFR Parts 660.25 and 660.26. Washington, DC: US Government Publishing Office, 2019 (revised annually).

65. Food and Drug Administration. 7342.001: Inspection of licensed and unlicensed blood banks, brokers, reference laboratories, and contractors. Compliance Program guidance manual. Silver Spring, MD: CBER Office of Compliance and Biologics Quality, 2010:50-3. [Available at https://www.fda.gov/media/84887/download.]

66. Shirey RS, Edwards RE, Ness PM. The risk of alloimmunization to c (Rh4) in R1R1 patients who present with anti-E. Transfusion 1994;34: 756-8.

SUGGESTED READINGS

Daniels G. Human blood groups. 3rd ed. Hoboken, NJ: Wiley-Blackwell, 2013.

Daniels G, Poole J, de Silva M, et al. The clinical significance of blood group antibodies. Transfus Med 2002;12:287-95.

Engelfriet CP, Overbeeke MA, Dooren MC, et al. Bioassays to determine the clinical significance of red cell antibodies based on Fc receptor-induced destruction of red cells sensitized with IgG. Transfusion 1994;34:617-26.

Garratty G. In vitro reactions with red blood cells that are not due to blood group antibodies: A review. Immunohematology 1998;14:1-11.

Hamilton J, Johnson ST, Rudmann SV. Antibody identification: Art or science? A case study approach. Bethesda, MD: AABB, 2013.

Hamilton J, Johnson ST, Rudmann SV. Investigating positive DAT results: A case study approach. Bethesda, MD: AABB, 2016.

Harmening DM. Modern blood banking and transfusion practices. 6th ed. Philadelphia: FA Davis, 2012.

Issitt PD, Anstee DJ. Applied blood group serology. 4th ed. Durham, NC: Montgomery Scientific Publications, 1998.

Judd WJ, Johnson S, Storry J. Judd's methods in immunohematology. 3rd ed. Bethesda, MD: AABB Press, 2008.

Van Thof L, ed. Standards for immunohematology reference laboratories. 11th ed. Bethesda, MD: AABB, 2019.

Kanter MH. Statistical analysis. In: Busch MP, Brecher ME, eds. Research design and analysis. Bethesda, MD: AABB, 1998:63-104.

Klein HG, Anstee DJ. Mollison's blood transfusion in clinical medicine. 12th ed. Oxford, UK: Wiley-Blackwell, 2014.

Menitove JE. The Hardy-Weinberger principle: Selection of compatible blood based on mathematic principles. In: Fridey JL, Kasprisin CA, Chambers LA, Rudmann SV, eds. Numbers for blood bankers. Bethesda, MD: AABB, 1995:1-11.

Gammon R, ed. Standards for blood banks and transfusion services. 32nd ed. Bethesda, MD: AABB, 2020.

Reid ME, Lomas-Francis C, Olsson M. The blood group antigen factsbook. 3rd ed. London: Elsevier Academic Press, 2012.

Rolih S. A review: Antibodies with high-titer, low-avidity characteristics. Immunohematology 1990;6: 59-67.

Rudmann SV, ed. Serologic problem-solving: A systematic approach for improved practice. Bethesda, MD: AABB Press, 2005.

Weisbach V, Kohnhauser T, Zimmermann R, et al. Comparison of the performance of microtube column systems and solid-phase systems and the tube low-ionic-strength solution additive indirect antiglobulin test in the detection of red cell alloantibodies. Transfus Med 2006;16:276-84.

Westhoff C. 2007 Rock Øyen Symposium. Potential of blood group genotyping for transfusion medicine practice. Immunohematology 2008;24:190-5.

CHAPTER 14

The Positive Direct Antiglobulin Test and Immune-Mediated Hemolysis

P. Dayand Borge Jr, MD, PhD, and Paul M. Mansfield, MT(ASCP)^{CM}SBB

HEMOLYTIC ANEMIA IS THE shortening of red cell survival. The normal life span of red cells is approximately 110 to 120 days. In healthy individuals, 1% of red cells are removed by the reticuloendothelial system each day, but this is matched by red cell production in the marrow. Normal marrow can increase red cell production to compensate for blood loss. Thus, in the absence of bleeding, an increased reticulocyte count is an indirect measure of hemolysis. If the marrow is able to adequately compensate, a reduced red cell survival may not result in anemia.

Immune-mediated hemolysis, the subject of this chapter, is only one cause of hemolytic anemia, and many causes of hemolysis are unrelated to immune reactions. Immune hemolytic anemia is the result of an immune response that targets red cells. The diagnosis of hemolytic anemia rests on clinical findings and laboratory data, such as hemoglobin or hematocrit values; reticulocyte count; red cell morphology; and bilirubin, haptoglobin, and lactate dehydrogenase (LDH) levels.

In some cases, the destruction of red cells takes place in the intravascular space with the release of free hemoglobin into the plasma. The red cells are ruptured following activation of the classical complement cascade. The characteristic features of this rare type of hemolysis are hemoglobinemia and, when the plasma hemoglobin level exceeds the renal threshold, hemoglobinuria. Conversely and more commonly, extravascular hemolysis results when macrophages in the spleen and liver phagocytose red cells completely or partially (producing spherocytes) or destroy red cells by cytotoxic events, resulting in an increase in serum bilirubin. This distinction is a simplification, however, because hemoglobin can also be released into the plasma following extravascular destruction if hemolysis is brisk.

The serologic investigations carried out in the blood bank help determine whether the hemolysis has an immune basis and, if so, what type of immune hemolytic anemia is present. This is important because the treatment for each type is different but generally involves some type of immunomodulatory therapy. Although there is no evidence-based algorithm for therapy, treatment options can include corticosteroids, intravenous immunoglobulin (IVIG), splenectomy, rituximab, and other more potent immunosuppressive medications.[1] As more patient outcome data with different treatment modalities become available, the determination of what is considered first-line therapy will change. For example, although rituximab is considered

P. Dayand Borge Jr, MD, PhD, Chief Medical Officer, East Division; and Paul M. Mansfield, MT(ASCP)^{CM}SBB, Manager, IRL, Penn-Jersey Region and National Reference Laboratory for Blood Group Serology, American Red Cross Blood Services, Philadelphia, Pennsylvania
The authors have disclosed no conflicts of interest.

to be first-line therapy for cold agglutinin syndrome (CAS), eculizumab, an antibody that mitigates complement-mediated hemolysis, may be more effective in patients with acute, brisk hemolysis.[2]

The direct antiglobulin test (DAT) is a simple test used to determine if red cells have been coated in vivo with immunoglobulin, complement, or both. The DAT is used primarily for the investigation of hemolytic transfusion reactions (HTRs), hemolytic disease of the fetus and newborn (HDFN), autoimmune hemolytic anemia (AIHA), and drug-induced immune hemolytic anemia (DIIHA). A positive DAT result may or may not be associated with immune-mediated hemolysis. As shown in Table 14-1, there are many causes of a positive DAT result.

THE DAT

The DAT should be performed on every patient in whom the presence of hemolysis has been established to distinguish immune from nonimmune hemolytic anemia. The DAT should also be performed when a positive autocontrol is found in antibody identification studies (see Chapter 13), but there is no benefit to performing a DAT (or autocontrol) as part of routine pretransfusion testing. The DAT should not be performed as a screening test for hemolytic anemia. The predictive value of a positive DAT result is 83% in a patient with hemolytic anemia, but only 1.4% in a patient without hemolytic anemia.[3]

Small amounts of immunoglobulin G (IgG) and complement that are lower than the detection limit of routine testing techniques appear to be present on all red cells. Using sensitive testing techniques, 5 to 90 IgG molecules/red cell[4] and 5 to 40 C3d molecules/red cell[5] have been detected in healthy individuals. Depending on the technique and reagents used, the DAT can detect 100 to 500 molecules of IgG/red cell and 400 to 1100 molecules of C3d/red cell. Positive DAT results are reported in 1 in 1000 to 1 in 14,000 blood donors and 1% to 15% of hospital patients.[6] These large differences in incidence are probably related to the different DAT techniques used.

Most blood donors with a positive DAT result appear to be healthy, and most patients with positive DAT results have no obvious signs of hemolytic anemia. However, a careful evaluation may show evidence of increased red cell destruction. Studies suggest that a positive DAT result in a healthy blood donor may be a marker of risk of future development of malignancy.[7,8]

A positive DAT result in a patient with hemolytic anemia indicates that the most likely diagnosis is one of the immune hemolytic anemias. However, the DAT result can be positive, coincidentally, in patients with hemolytic anemia that is not immune mediated. Conversely, some patients with immune hemolytic anemia have a negative DAT result. (See "DAT-Negative AIHA.")

TABLE 14-1. Some Causes of a Positive DAT Result

• Autoantibodies to intrinsic red cell antigens
• Hemolytic transfusion reactions
• Hemolytic disease of the fetus and newborn
• Drug-induced antibodies
• Passively acquired alloantibodies (eg, from donor plasma, derivatives, or immunoglobulin)
• Nonspecifically adsorbed proteins (eg, hypergammaglobulinemia, high-dose intravenous immune globulin, or modification of red cell membrane by some drugs)
• Complement activation due to bacterial infection, autoantibodies, or alloantibodies
• Antibodies produced by passenger lymphocytes (eg, in transplanted organs or hematopoietic components)

DAT = direct antiglobulin test.

The DAT can also be positive for IgG or complement without a clear correlation with anemia in patients with sickle cell disease, beta-thalassemia, renal disease, multiple myeloma, autoimmune disorders, AIDS, or other diseases associated with elevated serum globulin or blood urea nitrogen levels.[9-11] The interpretation of a positive DAT result should take into consideration the patient's history, clinical data, and results of other laboratory tests.

Initial transfusion reaction investigations include a DAT on a posttransfusion specimen. In the presence of immune-mediated hemolysis, the DAT result may be positive if sensitized red cells have not been destroyed, or negative if hemolysis and rapid clearance have occurred. Preparation and testing of an eluate from DAT-positive posttransfusion-reaction red cells is indicated. Even if the DAT result is only weakly positive or negative, testing of an eluate may be informative. If the DAT result is positive on the postreaction specimen, a DAT should also be performed on the pretransfusion specimen for comparison and appropriate interpretation.

The Principles of the DAT

The DAT is based on the test developed by Coombs, Mourant, and Race[12] for the detection of antibodies attached to red cells that do not produce direct agglutination. This test, an indirect antiglobulin test (IAT), was initially used to demonstrate antibody in serum, but it was later applied to demonstrate the in-vivo coating of red cells with antibody or complement components (the DAT).

Most of the antiglobulin reactivity is directed at the heavy chains (eg, Fc portion of the sensitizing antibody) or the complement component, thus bridging the gap between adjacent red cells to produce visible agglutination. The strength of the observed agglutination is usually proportional to the amount of bound protein.

The DAT is performed by testing freshly washed red cells directly with antiglobulin reagents containing anti-IgG and anti-C3d. In the United States, only polyspecific anti-IgG,-C3d and monospecific anti-IgG, anti-C3d, and anti-C3b,-C3d reagents are currently licensed. The red cells need to be washed to remove free plas-

ma globulins and complement; otherwise, the antiglobulin reagent can be neutralized, leading to a false-negative result. The saline used for washing the red cells should be at room temperature; washing red cells with warm (eg, 37 C) saline can result in the loss of red-cell-bound, low-affinity IgG. Washing should be uninterrupted, especially if performing manual washing, and red cells should be tested immediately after washing to prevent false-negative results caused by the elution of IgG. Performing a DAT using a column agglutination test (eg, gel test) does not require washing of the red cells before testing because plasma proteins do not neutralize detection of red-cell-bound reactivity. This may represent a positive bias for detection of red-cell-bound low-affinity IgG.

Although any red cells may be tested, EDTA-anticoagulated blood samples are preferred. The EDTA prevents in-vitro fixation of complement by chelating the calcium that is needed for C1 activation. If red cells from a clotted blood sample have a positive DAT result due to complement, the results should be confirmed on red cells from freshly collected blood kept at 37 C or an EDTA-anticoagulated specimen if these results are to be used for diagnostic purposes.

The DAT can be initially performed with a polyspecific antihuman globulin (AHG) reagent that is capable of detecting both IgG and C3d. (See Method 3-14.) If the results are positive, tests with monospecific reagents (anti-IgG and anti-complement separately) need to be performed to appropriately characterize the immune process involved and determine the diagnosis. Because polyspecific reagents are usually blended, and testing conditions for optimally detecting IgG and C3d on red cells may differ, some laboratories perform the DAT initially with anti-IgG and anti-C3d reagents separately. If the polyspecific reagent is polyclonal, proteins other than IgG or C3d (eg, IgM, IgA, or other complement components) can occasionally be detected; however, specific reagents to distinguish these other proteins by serologic techniques are not readily available. If umbilical cord blood samples are to be tested, it is appropriate to use anti-IgG only, because HDFN results from fetal red cell sensitization with maternally derived

IgG antibody, and complement activation rarely occurs.[6]

It is important to follow the reagent manufacturer's instructions and recognize any product limitations. False-negative or weaker results can be obtained if the washed red cells are allowed to sit before they are tested with anti-IgG or if the reading of the results is delayed. Some anti-complement reagents, in contrast, demonstrate stronger reactivity if centrifugation is delayed for a short time after the reagent has been added. When the DAT result is positive with both anti-IgG and anti-C3, the red cells should be tested with an inert control reagent (eg, 6% albumin or saline). Lack of agglutination of the red cells in the control reagent provides some assurance that the test results are accurately interpreted. If the control is reactive, the DAT result is invalid. [See sections below on warm AIHA (WAIHA) and CAS.] Reactivity with this control reagent can indicate spontaneous agglutination caused by heavy coating of IgG or rare warm-reactive IgM, or it can indicate IgM cold autoagglutinins that were not dissociated during routine washing.

Evaluation of a Positive DAT Result

A positive DAT result alone is not diagnostic of hemolytic anemia. Understanding the significance of this positive result requires knowledge of the patient's diagnosis; recent drug, pregnancy, transfusion, and hematopoietic transplantation history; and the presence of acquired or unexplained hemolytic anemia. Dialogue with the attending physician is important. Clinical considerations together with laboratory data should dictate the extent to which a positive DAT result is evaluated.

Patient History

The following situations may warrant further investigation of a positive DAT result.

1. *Evidence of in-vivo hemolysis (ie, red cell destruction).* If a patient with anemia who has a positive DAT result shows evidence of hemolysis, testing to evaluate a possible immune etiology is appropriate. Reticulocytosis; spherocytes observed on the peripheral blood film; hemoglobinemia; hemoglobinuria; decreased serum haptoglobin; and elevated levels of serum unconjugated (indirect) bilirubin or LDH, especially LDH1, may be associated with increased red cell destruction. These factors are indicative of hemolytic anemia but not specifically immune hemolytic anemia. *If there is no evidence of hemolytic anemia, no further studies are necessary* unless the patient requires a red cell transfusion and the serum contains incompletely identified antibodies to red cell antigens. Testing an eluate may be helpful for antibody identification. (See "Elution" section below and Chapter 13.)

2. *Recent transfusion.* When a patient has recently received transfusion, a positive DAT result may be the first indication of a developing immune response. Developing antibody sensitizes the transfused red cells that have the corresponding antigen, and the DAT result becomes weakly positive (usually <2+). The antibody may not be present in sufficient quantity to be detected in the serum. Antibody may appear as early as 7 to 10 days after transfusion in a primary immunization or as early as 1 to 2 days in a secondary response.[6,13] These alloantibodies could shorten the survival of red cells that have already been transfused or are administered in subsequent transfusions. A mixed-field appearance in the posttransfusion DAT result (ie, agglutination of donor red cells and no agglutination of the patient's red cells) may or may not be observed.

3. *Administration of drugs associated with immune-mediated hemolysis.* Many drugs have been reported to cause a positive DAT result and/or immune-mediated hemolysis, but this occurrence is not common.[14] (See "Drug-Induced Immune Hemolytic Anemia" section.)

4. *History of hematopoietic progenitor cell or organ transplantation.* Passenger lymphocytes of donor origin produce antibodies

directed against ABO or other blood group antigens on the recipient's red cells, causing a positive DAT result.[6]

5. *Administration of IVIG or intravenous (IV) anti-D.* IVIG may contain ABO antibodies, anti-D, or sometimes other antibodies.[15] IV anti-D used to treat immune thrombocytopenia (previously known as "immune thrombocytopenic purpura") causes Rh-positive patients to develop a positive DAT result.[16]

6. *Administration of potentially interfering therapeutic agents that may react with target antigen on red cells.* For example, anti-CD38 administered to treat myeloma (ie, daratumumab) causes reactivity with all red cells because of the presence of low amounts of CD38 on red cells.[17,18] The DAT may or may not be positive. A complete history (eg, diagnosis, medications) is important in these cases.

Serologic Investigation

Three investigative approaches are helpful in the evaluation of a positive DAT result.

1. Test the DAT-positive red cells with anti-IgG and anti-C3d reagents to characterize the type of protein(s) coating the red cells. This will help to classify an immune-mediated hemolytic anemia.

2. Test the serum/plasma to detect and identify clinically significant antibodies to red cell antigens. Additional tests that are useful in classifying the immune hemolytic anemias and procedures for detecting alloantibodies in the presence of autoantibodies are described later in this chapter.

3. Test an eluate prepared from the DAT-positive red cells with reagent red cells to determine whether the coating protein has red cell antibody specificity. When the only coating protein is complement, the eluate is likely to be nonreactive. However, an eluate from the patient's red cells coated only with complement should be tested if there is clinical evidence of antibody-mediated hemolysis, for example, after transfusion. The eluate preparation can concentrate small amounts of IgG that may not be detectable in routine testing of the patient's plasma.

Results of these tests combined with the patient's history and clinical data should assist in classification of the problem involved.

Elution

Elution can be informative in the following situations:

- Clinical signs and symptoms of immune hemolysis are present.
- Serum test results are negative or inconclusive for a patient who has recently received transfusion.
- HDFN is suspected but no alloantibodies were detected in the maternal plasma.

Performing an elution routinely on the red cells of all patients who have a positive DAT result is not recommended. The majority of pretransfusion patients with a positive DAT result have a nonreactive eluate that is often associated with an elevated serum globulin level.[9-11]

Elution frees antibody from sensitized red cells and recovers antibody in a usable form. Multiple elution methods have been described and reviewed.[19] Many laboratories use commercial acid elution kits, primarily for ease of use and decreased exposure to potentially harmful chemicals; these kits are suitable to recover antibody in most cases. False-positive eluate results associated with high-titer antibodies have been reported when the low-ionic wash solution supplied with the commercial acid eluates was used.[20] Because no single elution method is ideal in all situations, an alternative elution method (eg, an organic solvent) may be used in some high-complexity reference laboratories when a nonreactive acid eluate result is not in agreement with clinical data.[21]

Table 14-2 lists the uses of some common elution methods. Typically, eluates are tested only at the antiglobulin phase. If an IgM antibody is being investigated or suspected, however, centrifugation and reading after the 37 C

TABLE 14-2. Antibody Elution Methods

Method	Use	Comments
Lui freeze-thaw	ABO HDFN	Quick; small volume of red cells needed; poor recovery of other antibodies
Heat (56 C)	ABO HDFN, IgM agglutinating antibodies	Easy; poor recovery of IgG allo- and autoantibodies
Acid elution kits (commercial)	Warm auto- and alloantibodies	Easy; possible false-positive eluate results when high-titer antibody is present[20]
Chemical/organic solvent	Warm auto- and alloantibodies	Chemical hazards—eg, flammability, toxicity, or carcinogenicity

HDFN = hemolytic disease of the fetus and newborn; IgM = immunoglobulin M.

incubation should be performed. Technical considerations for elution are discussed in Chapter 13.

In cases of HTR or HDFN, specific antibody (or antibodies) is usually detected in the eluate that may or may not be detectable in the serum. For transfusion reactions, newly developed antibodies that are initially detectable only in the eluate are usually detectable in the serum after about 14 to 21 days.[22] If the eluate is nonreactive and a non-group-O patient has received plasma containing anti-A or anti-B (as a result of the transfusion of group O platelets, for example) and the recipient appears to have immune hemolysis, the eluate should be tested against A_1 and/or B cells. It may be appropriate to test the eluate against red cells from recently transfused donor units, which could have caused immunization to a low prevalence antigen on the donor red cell. For cases of HDFN when no maternal antibody has been detected and paternal red cells are ABO incompatible with maternal plasma, testing an eluate prepared from the infant's red cells with the paternal red cells may detect a maternally derived antibody to a low-prevalence antigen.

When the eluate reacts with all cells tested, autoantibody is the most likely explanation, especially if the patient has not had a recent transfusion. However, if the patient has recently received a transfusion, an antibody to a high-prevalence antigen should be considered. When no unexpected antibodies are present in the se-

rum and the patient has not recently received a transfusion, no further serologic testing of an autoantibody detected only in the eluate is necessary.

The patient's complete history, including the presence of potential passive antibodies, needs to be reviewed when the serologic test results are evaluated. If both the serum and eluate are nonreactive, there is evidence of immune hemolysis, and the patient has received a drug reported to have caused immune-mediated hemolysis, testing to demonstrate drug-related antibodies should be considered. Finally, if the eluate is disproportionately weaker than the strength of the positive DAT (eg, eluate is 2+ but DAT is 4+), along with clinical evidence of immune hemolysis, and the patient is receiving a drug therapy known to cause immune-mediated hemolysis, drug-induced immune hemolytic anemia is also a possibility. (See "Laboratory Investigation of Drug-Induced Immune Hemolysis" below.)

AUTOIMMUNE HEMOLYTIC ANEMIA

Immune hemolytic anemias can be classified in various ways. One classification system is shown in Table 14-3. The AIHAs are subdivided into the major types: WAIHA, CAS, mixed- or combined-type AIHA, and paroxysmal cold hemoglobinuria (PCH). Other classification

TABLE 14-3. Classification of Immune Hemolytic Anemias

Autoimmune hemolytic anemia (AIHA)
● Warm AIHA
● Cold agglutinin syndrome
● Mixed-type AIHA
● Paroxysmal cold hemoglobinuria
Alloimmune hemolytic anemia
● Hemolytic transfusion reaction
● Hemolytic disease of the fetus and newborn
Drug-induced immune hemolytic anemia

schemes consider PCH as one of the cold-reactive AIHAs. Not all cases fit neatly into these categories. Table 14-4 shows the typical serologic characteristics of the AIHAs. Drugs (discussed in the "Drug-Induced Immune Hemolytic Anemia" section) may also induce immune hemolysis; the effects of drug-induced autoantibodies are serologically indistinguishable from WAIHA.

Warm Autoimmune Hemolytic Anemia

The majority of AIHA cases are caused by warm-reactive autoantibodies that are optimally reactive with red cells at 37 C. The autoantibody is usually IgG, but it can be IgM or IgA.

Serologic Characteristics

The DAT result may be positive because of IgG plus complement (67% of cases), IgG without complement (20%), or complement without IgG (13%).[6] Performing an elution at initial diagnosis and/or during pretransfusion testing is useful to demonstrate that the IgG coating the patient's red cells is auto-reactive.

Typically, in WAIHA, the eluate is reactive with virtually all red cells tested, and reactivity is enhanced in tests against enzyme-treated red cells, with polyethylene glycol (PEG) enhancement, or in column agglutination and solid-phase tests. The eluate usually has no serologic activity if the only protein coating the red cells is complement.

If the autoantibody has been adsorbed by the patient's red cells in vivo, the serum may not contain detectable free antibody. The serum contains free antibody when the amount of

TABLE 14-4. Typical Serologic Findings in AIHA

	WAIHA	CAS	Mixed-Type AIHA	PCH
DAT (routine)	IgG IgG + C3 C3	C3 only	IgG + C3 C3	C3 only
Ig type	IgG	IgM	IgG, IgM	IgG
Eluate	IgG antibody	Nonreactive	IgG antibody	Nonreactive
Serum	By IAT, 35% agglutinate untreated red cells at 20 C	IgM agglutinating antibody, titer ≥1000 (60%) at 4 C, reactive at 30 C	IgG IAT-reactive antibody plus IgM agglutinating antibody reactive at 30 C	Negative routine IAT result, IgG biphasic hemolysin in Donath-Landsteiner test
Specificity	Broadly reactive, multiple specificities reported	Usually anti-I	Usually unclear	Anti-P

AIHA = autoimmune hemolytic anemia; WAIHA = warm AIHA; CAS = cold agglutinin syndrome; PCH = paroxysmal cold hemoglobinuria; DAT = direct antiglobulin test; IgG = immunoglobulin G; IgM = immunoglobulin M; IAT = indirect antiglobulin test.

autoantibody exceeds the available binding sites on the patient's red cells; thus, serum autoantibody reactivity is "left over," that is, what was not adsorbed by the patient's red cells in vivo. The DAT result in such cases is usually strongly positive.

Autoantibody in the serum typically is reactive against all cells by an IAT. Approximately 60% of patients with WAIHA have serum antibodies that react with untreated saline-suspended red cells. When tested with PEG, enzyme-treated red cells, column agglutination, or solid-phase methods, >90% of these sera can be shown to contain autoantibody. Agglutination at room temperature is present in about one-third of patients with WAIHA, but these cold agglutinins have normal titers at 4 C and are nonreactive at 30 C and 37 C. Thus, these cold agglutinins are nonpathogenic and the patient does not have CAS in addition to WAIHA.[6]

An unusual subcategory of WAIHA is associated with IgM agglutinins in the plasma that are reactive at 37 C.[6,23] This type of WAIHA is characterized by severe hemolysis, and the prognosis for these patients can be poor. The red cells are typically spontaneously agglutinated in the DAT; that is, the washed red cells are reactive with all reagents tested, including a control, such as 6% albumin or saline. (See "Serologic Problems" section.) Complement is usually detected on the red cells; IgG or IgM may or may not be detected. IgM agglutinins are often detected in an eluate (eg, acid) when it is inspected for agglutination after the 37 C incubation and before the antiglobulin test is conducted. Some serum IgM warm autoagglutinins may be difficult to detect; some are enhanced in the presence of albumin or at low pH. Optimal reactivity of the agglutinin sometimes occurs between 20 C and 30 C rather than at 37 C. These antibodies have low titers at 4 C, usually <64, which easily differentiates this IgM warm autoantibody from those in CAS. To prevent misinterpretation of titration results, titrations at different temperatures (eg, 37 C, 30 C, room temperature, and 4 C) need to be carried out with separate sets of tubes to avoid carryover agglutination.[6,23] Testing for the presence of a warm hemolysin can sometimes define the AIHA as consistent with a warm IgM AIHA.[23]

Serologic Problems

Warm autoantibodies can cause technical difficulties during red cell testing. Spontaneous agglutination can occur if the red cells are heavily coated with IgG and the reagent contains a potentiator, such as albumin. This has been observed when high-protein Rh typing sera are used. If the control reagent provided by the manufacturer for these antisera is reactive, the typing is invalid. IgG can less commonly cause spontaneous agglutination in lower-protein reagents (eg, monoclonal typing sera); this reactivity is often weaker or more fragile than true agglutination and may not be detected by a 6% albumin control.[24] Spontaneous agglutination caused by red cells heavily coated with IgG is less frequently observed.

Warm-reactive IgM agglutinins can also cause spontaneous agglutination, resulting in ABO and Rh typing problems and/or reactivity with the negative control reagent for the DAT.[23] In these cases, treatment with dithiothreitol (DTT) or 2-mercaptoethanol (2-ME) (Method 2-18) to disrupt the IgM agglutinin is required to accurately interpret typing and DAT results. When the spontaneous agglutination is disrupted, the control reagent is nonreactive.

When the DAT result is positive due to IgG, antiglobulin-reactive typing reagents cannot be used unless the red-cell-bound IgG is first removed. (See Methods 2-20 and 2-21.) An alternative is to use low-protein antisera (eg, monoclonal reagents) that do not require an antiglobulin test. (Refer to the manufacturer's instructions for the detection of spontaneous agglutination.) It is helpful to know which of the common red cell antigens are lacking on the patient's red cells to predict which clinically significant alloantibodies the patient may have produced or may produce in the future. Antigens absent from autologous cells could well be the target of present or future alloantibodies. The patient's phenotype for the common antigens can be determined serologically or predicted using DNA-based methods.

The presence of autoantibody in the serum increases the complexity of the serologic evaluation and the time needed to complete pretransfusion testing. If a patient who has warm-reactive autoantibodies in the serum needs a transfusion, it is important to determine whether alloantibodies are also present. Some alloantibodies may make their presence known by reacting more strongly or at different phases than the autoantibody, but quite often, routine testing may not suggest the existence of masked alloantibodies.[25,26]

Methods to detect alloantibodies in the presence of warm-reactive autoantibodies are used to attempt to remove, reduce, or circumvent the autoantibody. Antibody detection methods that use PEG, enzymes, column agglutination, or solid-phase red cell adherence usually enhance autoantibodies. Antibody detection tests using low-ionic-strength saline (LISS) or saline tube methods may not detect autoantibodies but they do detect most clinically significant alloantibodies. Other procedures involve adsorption; two widely used adsorption approaches are discussed below.

Adsorption with Autologous Red Cells

In a patient who has not recently received transfusion, adsorption with autologous red cells (autologous adsorption; see Method 4-8) is the best way to detect alloantibodies in the presence of warm-reactive autoantibodies. Only autoantibodies are removed, and alloantibodies, if present, remain in the serum.

Autologous adsorption typically requires some initial preparation of the patient's red cells. At 37 C, in-vivo adsorption has occurred, and all antigen sites on the patient's own red cells may be blocked. A gentle heat elution at 56 C for 3 to 5 minutes can dissociate some of the bound IgG. This can be followed by treatment of the autologous red cells with proteolytic enzymes to increase their capacity to adsorb autoantibody. (Treatment with proteolytic enzyme alone does not remove IgG coating the red cells.) Treatment of the red cells with ZZAP, a mixture of papain or ficin and DTT, accomplishes both of these actions in one step. It is proposed that the sulfhydryl component makes the IgG molecules more susceptible to the protease and dissociates the antibody molecules from the cell.[27] Multiple sequential autologous adsorptions with new aliquots of red cells may be necessary if the se-

rum contains high levels of autoantibody. Once autoantibody has been removed, the adsorbed serum is tested for alloantibody reactivity.

Autologous adsorption is not recommended for patients who have received transfusion within the last 3 months because a blood sample may contain some transfused red cells that might adsorb alloantibody. Red cells normally survive for about 110 to 120 days. In patients with AIHA, autologous and transfused red cells can be expected to have shortened survival. However, determining how long transfused red cells remain in circulation in patients who need repeated transfusions is not feasible. It has been demonstrated that very small amounts (<10%) of antigen-positive red cells are capable of removing alloantibody reactivity in in-vitro studies.[28] Therefore, it is recommended to wait for 3 months after transfusion before performing autologous adsorptions.

Adsorption with Allogeneic Red Cells

The use of allogeneic red cells for adsorption (allogeneic adsorption) may be helpful when the patient has recently received transfusion or when insufficient autologous red cells are available. The goal is to remove autoantibody and leave the alloantibody in the adsorbed serum. The adsorbing red cells must not have the antigens against which the alloantibodies are reactive. Because the alloantibody specificity is unknown, red cells of different phenotypes are usually used to adsorb several aliquots of the patient's serum.

Given the number of potential alloantibodies, the task of selecting the red cells may appear formidable. However, red cell selection is based only on those few antigens for which alloantibodies of clinical significance are likely to be present. These include the common Rh antigens (D, C, E, c, and e), K, Fy^a and Fy^b, Jk^a and Jk^b, and S and s. Red cell selection is made easier by the fact that some of these antigens can be destroyed by appropriate pretreatment (eg, with enzymes or ZZAP) before use in adsorption procedures. (See Chapter 13, Table 13-5.) Antibodies to high-prevalence antigens cannot be excluded by allogeneic adsorptions because the adsorbing red cells are expected to express the antigen and adsorb the alloantibody along with autoantibody.

When the patient's phenotype is not known, group O red cell samples of three different Rh phenotypes (R_1R_1, R_2R_2, and rr) should be selected. (See Method 4-9.) One sample should lack Jk^a, and another, Jk^b. As shown in Table 14-5, ZZAP or enzyme pretreatment of the adsorbing red cells reduces the phenotype requirements. Untreated red cells may be used, but the adsorbing red cells must include at least one sample that is negative for the S, s, Fy^a, Fy^b, and K antigens in addition to the Rh and JK (Kidd) phenotype requirements stated above.

If the patient's phenotype is known or can be determined, adsorption with a single sample of red cells may be possible. Red cells can be selected that match the patient's phenotype or at least match the Rh and JK phenotypes if ZZAP treatment is used. For example, if a patient's phenotype is E–, K–, S–, Fy(a–), Jk(a–), untreated adsorbing red cells need to lack all five antigens, but enzyme-treated red cells only need to be E–, K–, Jk(a–) because enzyme treatment denatures Fy^a antigen, and ZZAP-treated red cells

only need to be E–, Jk(a–) because the 2-ME or DTT in ZZAP denatures K, and ficin or papain denatures Fy^a. Caution should be used when matching red cells with the patient's phenotype, as the patient may possess variant antigens; an antibody directed against variant antigen specificities not expressed by the patient may be adsorbed out and not detected.

Adsorption using untreated red cells in the presence of PEG (Method 4-10) or LISS[29,30] is a modification that has been used to decrease the incubation time for adsorptions and increase efficiency. Adsorptions performed with the addition of PEG have been reported to result in unexpected nondetection of alloantibodies in some cases.[31,32]

Testing of Adsorbed Serum

In some cases, each aliquot of serum may need to be adsorbed two or three times to remove the autoantibody. The fully adsorbed aliquots are then tested against reagent red cells known to either lack or carry common antigens of the RH, MNS, KEL, FY, and JK blood group systems (eg,

---

TABLE 14-5. Selection of Red Cells for Allogeneic Adsorption

Step 1. Select red cells for each Rh phenotype.

R_1R_1
R_2R_2
rr

Step 2. On the basis of the red cell treatment or lack of treatment (below), at least one of the Rh-phenotyped cells should be negative for the antigens listed below.

ZZAP-Treated Red Cells	Enzyme-Treated Red Cells	Untreated Red Cells
Jk(a–)	Jk(a–)	Jk(a–)
Jk(b–)	Jk(b–)	Jk(b–)
	K–	K–
		Fy(a–)
		Fy(b–)
		S–
		s–

antibody detection cells). If an adsorbed aliquot is reactive, the aliquot should be tested to identify the antibody. Adsorbing several aliquots with different red cell samples provides a battery of potentially informative specimens. For example, if the aliquot adsorbed with Jk(a–) red cells subsequently is reactive only with Jk(a+) red cells, the presence of alloanti-Jk^a can be inferred confidently.

Sometimes, autoantibody is not completely removed by three sequential adsorptions. Additional adsorptions can be performed, but the performance of multiple adsorptions has the potential to dilute the serum. If the adsorbing cells do not appear to remove the antibody, the autoantibody may have an unusual specificity that is not reactive with the red cells used for adsorption. For example, autoantibodies with KEL, LW, or En^{a}FS specificity are not removed by ZZAP-treated red cells. (See Table 14-5 for which antigens will be expressed on treated adsorbing cells.) The possibility that the sample contains an auto- or alloantibody to a high-prevalence antigen should always be considered when adsorption fails to remove the reactivity.

Autoantibodies sometimes have patterns of reactivity that suggest the presence of alloantibody. For example, the serum of a D– patient may have apparent anti-C reactivity. The anti-C reactivity may reflect warm-reactive autoantibody even if the patient's red cells lack C. The apparent alloanti-C would, in this case, be adsorbed by C– red cells, both autologous and allogeneic. This is unlike the behavior of a true alloanti-C, which would be adsorbed only by C+ red cells. In one study, the serum adsorbed with autologous red cells often retained autoantibodies that mimicked alloantibodies in addition to the true alloantibody(ies) present, whereas serum adsorbed with allogeneic red cells most often contained only alloantibodies.[33] This reflects an inefficiency of autologous adsorption that is caused primarily by limited volumes of autologous red cells available for removing all of the autoantibody reactivity from the serum.

Specificity of Autoantibody

In many cases of WAIHA, no autoantibody specificity is apparent. The patient's serum reacts with all red cell samples tested. If testing is performed with cells of rare Rh phenotypes, such as D– – or Rh$_{null}$, some autoantibodies are weakly reactive or are nonreactive, and the autoantibody appears to have broad specificity in the RH system. Apparent specificity for simple Rh antigens (D, C, E, c, and e) is occasionally seen, especially in saline or LISS IATs. A "relative" specificity based on stronger reactivity with cells of certain phenotypes may also be seen; relative specificity may also be apparent after adsorption. Autoantibody specificities can be clearer in the serum than in the eluate.

Apart from RH specificity, warm autoantibodies with many other specificities have been reported (eg, specificities in the LW, KEL, JK, FY, and DI systems).[34,35] Patients with autoantibodies of KEL, RH, LW, GE, SC, LU, and LAN specificities may have transiently depressed expression of the respective antigen, and the DAT result may be negative or very weakly positive.[35] In these cases, the autoantibody may initially appear to be alloantibody. Proof that it is truly autoantibody is demonstration that after the antibody and hemolytic anemia subside, the antigen strength returns to normal, and stored serum containing antibody is reactive with the patient's red cells.

Tests against red cells of a rare phenotype and by special techniques to determine autoantibody specificity have limited clinical or practical application. If the autoantibody reacts with all red cells except those of a rare Rh phenotype (eg, Rh$_{null}$), compatible donor blood is unlikely to be available. Such blood, if available, should be reserved for alloimmunized patients of that uncommon phenotype.

Selection of Blood for Transfusion

The most important consideration is to exclude the presence of potentially clinically significant alloantibodies *before* selecting Red Blood Cell (RBC) units for transfusion. There are multiple reports in the literature demonstrating that patients who have warm autoantibodies in their sera have a higher rate of alloimmunization (eg,

12% to 40%, with a mean of 32%).[25,36-39] Although these patients present a serologic challenge, they deserve the same protection from HTRs as any other patient. Autoantibodies that react with all reagent red cells, even weakly, are capable of masking alloantibody reactivity (ie, reactivity of red cells with both alloantibody and autoantibody may not be any stronger than with autoantibody alone).[25,26]

It is the exclusion of newly formed alloantibodies that is of concern. Because of the presence of autoantibodies, all crossmatches are incompatible. This is unlike the case of clinically significant alloantibodies without autoantibodies, where a compatible crossmatch with antigen-negative red cells is possible. Monitoring for evidence of red cell destruction caused by *alloantibodies* is difficult in patients who already have AIHA; these patients' own red cells and transfused red cells have shortened survival.

If no alloantibodies are detected in adsorbed serum nor are previously identified, random units of the appropriate ABO group and Rh type may be selected for transfusion unless there are contrary indications in the patient file. If clinically significant alloantibodies are present, the transfused cells should lack the corresponding antigen(s). For patients facing long-term transfusion support, it is prudent to obtain an extended phenotype or predicted phenotype by genotyping. Consideration can then be given to transfusion with donor units that are antigen-matched for clinically significant blood group antigens to avoid additional alloimmunization and potentially decrease the number of adsorptions required and the complexity of pretransfusion workup.

If the autoantibody has clear-cut specificity for a single antigen (eg, anti-e) and active hemolysis is ongoing, blood lacking that antigen should be selected according to the patient's history, availability of the unit, and medical observation. A good practice is to verify the allele to avoid alloimmunization. There is evidence that such transfused red cells survive longer than the patient's own red cells.[6] If the autoantibody shows broader reactivity—reacting with all cells but showing some relative specificity (eg, preferentially reacting with e+ red cells), whether to transfuse blood lacking the corresponding anti-

gen is debatable. In the absence of hemolysis or evidence of compromised survival of transfused cells, autoantibody specificity is not important. However, donor units that are negative for the antigen may be chosen because this is a simple way to circumvent the autoantibody and detect potential alloantibodies.

It may be undesirable to expose the patient to Rh antigens absent from autologous cells, especially D and especially in females of childbearing potential, merely to improve serologic compatibility testing results with the autoantibody. (For example, when a D– patient has autoanti-e, available e– units are likely to be D+; D–e– units are extremely rare.) Referral of the sample for molecular investigation to determine the risk for allo- or autoantibody production will aid in decision-making in these complex cases and potentially improve patient care.

Some laboratories use the adsorbed serum to screen and select nonreactive units (units that are antigen-negative for clinically significant alloantibodies, if detected) for transfusion. Other laboratories do not perform a crossmatch with the adsorbed serum because all units will be incompatible in vivo due to the autoantibody. Issuing a unit that is serologically compatible with adsorbed serum may provide some assurance that the correct unit has been selected and avoid incompatibility because of additional antibodies (eg, anti-Wr[a]), but this practice can also provide a false sense of security about the safety of the transfusion for these patients.

A transfusion management protocol using prophylactic antigen-matched units for patients with warm autoantibodies, where feasible, in combination with streamlined adsorption procedures has been described.[40] The same antigens for the commonly occurring, clinically significant antibodies (D, C, E, c, e, K, Fy[a], Fy[b], Jk[a], Jk[b], S, and s) are taken into account, as discussed in the previous section on adsorptions. The ability to implement such a protocol depends on the ability of the transfusion service, and more often the blood supplier, to maintain an adequate inventory of phenotyped units to meet the antigen-matching needs. In recent years, molecular technologies have been applied to red cell genotyping for patients with warm autoantibodies to determine which common alloantibodies the patient can make. DNA tests are attractive for determining the predicted phenotype of patients with a positive DAT (IgG) result because IgG is not always successfully removed and some red cell antigens are sensitive to IgG removal treatment.[41,42] Recent transfusions do not interfere with molecular testing. It must be remembered that genotyping may not accurately predict the phenotype if uncommon or rare silencing mutations are present or the patient has received a stem cell transplant.

Some experts propose that an electronic crossmatch can be safely used for patients with autoantibodies when the presence of common, clinically significant alloantibodies has been excluded.[43,44] This approach circumvents the need to issue units that are labeled "incompatible"; however, as discussed above, this practice can also lead to a false sense of security.

Although resolving serologic problems for these patients is important, delaying transfusion in the hope of finding serologically compatible blood may, in some cases, cause greater danger to the patient. Only clinical judgment can resolve this dilemma; therefore, having a dialogue with the patient's physician is important.

Transfusion of Patients with Warm-Reactive Autoantibodies

Patients with warm-reactive autoantibodies may have no apparent hemolysis or may have life-threatening anemia. Patients with little or no evidence of significant hemolysis tolerate transfusion quite well. The risk of transfusion is somewhat increased in these patients because of the difficulties with pretransfusion testing. The duration of survival of the transfused red cells is about the same as that of the patient's own red cells.

In patients with active hemolysis, transfusion may increase hemolysis, and the transfused red cells may be destroyed more rapidly than the patient's own red cells. This is related to the increased red cell mass available from the transfusion and the kinetics of red cell destruction.[6] Destruction of transfused cells may increase hemoglobinemia and hemoglobinuria. Disseminated intravascular coagulation can develop in patients with severe posttransfusion hemolysis.

The transfusion of patients with AIHA is a clinical decision that should be based on the balance between the risks and clinical need. Transfusion should not be withheld solely because of serologic incompatibility. The volume transfused should usually be the smallest amount required to maintain adequate oxygen delivery and not necessarily the amount required to reach an arbitrary hemoglobin level.[6] The patient should be carefully monitored throughout the transfusion.

DAT-Negative AIHA

Clinical and hematologic evidence of WAIHA is present in some patients whose DAT result is negative. The most common causes of AIHA associated with a negative DAT result are red-cell-bound IgG below the detection threshold of the antiglobulin test, red-cell-bound IgM and IgA that are not detectable by routine AHG reagents, and low-affinity IgG that is washed off the red cells during the washing phase for the DAT.[6,45]

Nonroutine tests can be applied in these situations. Unfortunately, these assays require standardization and many have a low predictive value. One of the easier tests is for low-affinity antibodies. Washing with ice-cold (eg, 4 C) saline or LISS may help retain antibody on the cells; a control (eg, 6% albumin) is necessary to confirm that cold autoagglutinins are not causing the positive results.[6,45] Methods that have been used to detect lower levels of red-cell-bound IgG include the complement fixation antibody consumption assay, the enzyme-linked antiglobulin test, radiolabeled anti-IgG, flow cytometry, solid-phase testing, the direct PEG test, the direct Polybrene test, column agglutination, and concentrated eluates.[43]

Anti-IgG, anti-C3d, and the combined anti-C3b,-C3d reagents are the only licensed products available in the United States for use with human red cells. AHG reagents that react with IgA or IgM are available commercially but probably have not been standardized for use with red cells in agglutination tests. They must be used cautiously, and their hemagglutination reactivity must be carefully standardized by the user.[6] Outside the United States, AHG reagents for the detection of IgM and IgA in tube tests or column agglutination tests may be available.

Cold Agglutinin Syndrome

CAS, which is less common than WAIHA, is the hemolytic anemia that is most commonly associated with autoantibodies that react preferentially in the cold. CAS occurs as an acute or chronic condition. The acute form is often secondary to *Mycoplasma pneumoniae* infection. The chronic form is often seen in elderly patients and is sometimes associated with lymphoma, chronic lymphocytic leukemia, or Waldenström macroglobulinemia. Acrocyanosis and hemoglobinuria may occur in cold weather; thus, patients should be advised to avoid cold. CAS is often characterized by agglutination, at room temperature, of red cells in an EDTA specimen, sometimes to the degree that the red cells appear to be clotted.

Serologic Characteristics

Complement is the only protein detected on red cells in almost all cases of CAS. If the red cells have been collected properly and washed at 37 C, there will be no immunoglobulin on the cells and no reactivity in the eluate. If other proteins are detected, a negative control for the DAT (eg, 6% albumin or saline) should be tested to ensure that the cold autoagglutinin is not causing a false-positive result. The cold-reactive autoagglutinin is usually IgM, which binds to red cells in the lower temperature of the peripheral circulation of an individual and causes complement components to attach to the red cells. As the red cells circulate to warmer areas, the IgM dissociates but the complement remains.

IgM cold-reactive autoagglutinins associated with immune hemolysis usually react at 30 C, and 60% have a titer of ≥1000 when tested at 4 C.[6] If 22% to 30% bovine albumin is included in the test system, pathologic cold agglutinins will react at 30 C or 37 C.[6] On occasion, pathologic cold agglutinins have a lower titer (ie, <1000), but they have a high thermal amplitude (ie, reactive at 30 C with or without the addition of albumin). The thermal amplitude of the antibody has greater significance than the titer. Hemolytic activity against untreated red cells

can sometimes be demonstrated at 20 C to 25 C. Except in rare cases with anti-Pr specificity, enzyme-treated red cells are hemolyzed in the presence of adequate complement.

To determine the true thermal amplitude or titer of the cold autoagglutinin, the specimen is collected and maintained strictly at 37 C until the serum and red cells are separated to avoid in-vitro autoadsorption. Alternatively, plasma can be used from an EDTA-anticoagulated specimen that has been warmed for 10 to 15 minutes at 37 C (with repeated mixing) and then separated from the cells, ideally at 37 C. This process should release autoadsorbed antibody back into the plasma.

In chronic CAS, the IgM autoagglutinin is usually a monoclonal protein with kappa light chains. In the acute form induced by *Mycoplasma* or viral infections, the antibody is polyclonal IgM with normal kappa and lambda light-chain distribution. Rare examples of IgA and IgG cold-reactive autoagglutinins have also been described.[6]

Serologic Problems

Problems with ABO and Rh typing and other tests are not uncommon. Often, it is only necessary to maintain the blood sample at 37 C immediately after collection and to wash the red cells with warm (37 C) saline before testing. Alternatively, an EDTA sample can be warmed to 37 C for about 10 minutes, after which the red cells are washed with warm saline. It is helpful to perform a parallel control test with 6% bovine albumin to determine whether autoagglutination persists. If the control test result is nonreactive, the results obtained with anti-A and anti-B are usually valid. If autoagglutination still occurs, it may be necessary to treat the red cells with sulfhydryl reagents. Because cold-reactive autoagglutinins are almost always IgM and sulfhydryl reagents denature IgM molecules, reagents (such as 2-ME or DTT) can be used to abolish autoagglutination. (See Method 2-18.) The red cells can also be treated with ZZAP reagent, as in the preparation for adsorptions. (See Method 4-8.)

When the serum agglutinates group O reagent red cells, ABO serum tests are invalid. Repeating the tests using prewarmed serum and group A_1, B, and O red cells and allowing the red cells to "settle" after incubation at 37 C for 1 hour (instead of centrifuging the sample) often resolves any discrepancy. (See Method 2-11.) By eliminating the centrifugation step, interference by cold-reactive autoantibodies might be avoided. Weak anti-A and/or -B in some patients' sera may not react at 37 C. Alternatively, adsorbed serum (either autoadsorbed or adsorbed with allogeneic group O red cells) can be used. Serum adsorbed with rabbit erythrocyte stroma should not be used for ABO serum tests because anti-B and anti-A1 may be removed.[46,47]

Detection of Alloantibodies in the Presence of Cold-Reactive Autoantibodies

Cold-reactive autoagglutinins rarely mask clinically significant alloantibodies if serum tests are conducted at 37 C and IgG-specific reagents are used for the antiglobulin phase. The use of potentiators (eg, albumin or PEG) is not recommended because they may increase the reactivity of the autoantibodies. In rare instances, it may be necessary to perform autologous adsorption at 4 C. (See Method 4-5.) Achieving the complete removal of potent cold-reactive autoagglutinins is very time-consuming and usually unnecessary. Sufficient removal of cold autoagglutinins may be facilitated by treating the patient's cells with enzymes or ZZAP before adsorption. One or two cold autologous adsorptions should remove enough autoantibody to make it possible to detect alloantibodies at 37 C that were otherwise masked by the cold-reactive autoantibody. As an alternative, the allogeneic adsorption process used for WAIHA can be performed at 4 C. Rabbit erythrocyte stroma, which removes autoanti-I and -IH from sera, should be used with caution because this method can remove clinically significant alloantibodies—notably anti-D, -E, and -Vel, and IgM antibodies regardless of blood group specificity.[48,49]

Specificity of Autoantibody

The autoantibody specificity in CAS is most often anti-I but is usually of academic interest only. Anti-i is found less commonly, and it is usual-

ly associated with infectious mononucleosis. On rare occasions, other specificities are seen.

Autoantibody specificity is not diagnostic for CAS. Autoanti-I may be seen in healthy individuals as well as in patients with CAS. The nonpathologic forms of autoanti-I, however, rarely react at titers above 64 at 4 C and are usually nonreactive with I– (cord i and adult i) red cells at room temperature. In contrast, the autoanti-I of CAS may react quite strongly with I– red cells in tests at room temperature, and equal or even stronger reactions occur with I+ red cells. Autoanti-i reacts in the opposite manner, demonstrating stronger reactions with I– red cells than with red cells that are I+. Anti-I^T, originally thought to recognize a transition state of i to I (explaining the designation "I^T"), reacts strongly with cord red cells, weakly with normal adult I red cells, and most weakly with the rare adult i red cells. In rare cases, the cold agglutinin specificity may be anti-Pr, which reacts equally well with untreated red cells of I or i phenotypes but does not react with enzyme-treated red cells. Procedures to determine the titer and specificity of cold-reactive autoantibodies are given in Methods 4-6 and 4-7. Typical reactivity patterns of cold autoantibodies are shown in the table in Method 4-6.

Mixed-Type AIHA

Although about one-third of patients with WAIHA have nonpathologic IgM antibodies that agglutinate at room temperature, another group of patients with WAIHA have cold agglutinins that react at or above 30 C. This latter group is referred to as having "mixed" or "combined warm and cold" AIHA and can be subdivided into patients with high-titer, high-thermal-amplitude IgM cold antibodies (the rare WAIHA plus classic CAS) and patients with normal-titer (<64 at 4 C), high-thermal-amplitude cold antibodies.[50-52] Patients with mixed-type AIHA often present with hemolysis and complex serum reactivity in all phases of testing.

Serologic Characteristics

In mixed-type AIHA, both IgG and C3 are usually detectable on patients' red cells; however, C3, IgG, or IgA alone may be detectable on the red cells.[6] An eluate contains a warm-reactive IgG autoantibody. Both warm-reactive IgG autoantibodies and cold-reactive, agglutinating IgM autoantibodies are present in the serum. These autoantibodies usually result in reactivity at all phases of testing and with virtually all cells tested. The IgM agglutinating autoantibody reacts at 30 C or above. If adsorptions are performed to detect alloantibodies, it may be necessary to perform them at both 37 C and 4 C.

Specificity of Autoantibodies

The unusual cold-reactive IgM agglutinating autoantibody can have specificities that are typical of CAS (ie, anti-I or -i) but often has no apparent specificity.[50,51] The warm-reactive IgG autoantibody often appears to be serologically indistinguishable from autoantibodies encountered in typical WAIHA.

Transfusion for Patients with Mixed-Type AIHA

If blood transfusions are necessary, the considerations for the exclusion of alloantibodies and the selection of blood for transfusion are identical to those described for patients with acute hemolysis caused by WAIHA and CAS. (See above.)

Paroxysmal Cold Hemoglobinuria

PCH is the rarest form of DAT-positive AIHA. Historically, PCH was associated with syphilis, but this association is now unusual.[53] More commonly, PCH presents as an acute transient condition that is secondary to a viral infection, particularly in young children. In such cases, the biphasic hemolysin may be only transiently detectable. PCH can also occur as an idiopathic chronic disease in older people.

Serologic Characteristics

PCH is caused by a cold-reactive IgG complement-binding antibody. As with IgM cold-reactive autoagglutinins, reactivity occurs with red cells in colder areas of the body (usually the extremities) and causes C3 to bind irreversibly to red cells. The antibody then dissociates from the red cells as the blood circulates to warmer parts of the body. Red cells washed in a routine manner

for the DAT are usually coated only with complement, but IgG may be detectable on cells that have been washed with cold saline and tested with cold anti-IgG reagent.[6] Keeping the test system close to its optimal binding temperature allows the cold-reactive IgG autoantibody to remain attached to its antigen. Because complement components are usually the only globulins present on circulating red cells, eluates prepared from the red cells of patients with PCH are almost always nonreactive.

The IgG autoantibody in PCH is classically described as a biphasic hemolysin because binding to red cells occurs at low temperatures, but hemolysis does not occur until the complement-coated red cells are warmed to 37 C. This is the basis of the diagnostic test for the disease, the Donath-Landsteiner test. (See Method 4-11.) The autoantibody may agglutinate normal red cells at 4 C but rarely to titers >64. Because the antibody rarely reacts above 4 C, pretransfusion antibody detection tests are usually nonreactive, and the serum is usually compatible with random donor cells by routine crossmatch procedures.

Specificity of Autoantibody

The autoantibody of PCH has most frequently been shown to have P specificity. The autoantibody reacts with all red cells by the Donath-Landsteiner test (including the patient's own red cells), except those of the very rare p or P^k phenotypes.

Transfusion for Patients with PCH

Transfusion is rarely necessary for adult patients with PCH, unless their hemolysis is severe. In young children, the thermal amplitude of the antibody tends to be much wider than in adults and hemolysis is often more brisk, so transfusion may be required as a lifesaving measure. Although there is some evidence that p red cells survive longer than P (P1+ or P1−) red cells, the prevalence of p blood is approximately 1 in 200,000, and the urgent need for transfusion usually precludes attempts to obtain this rare blood. Transfusion of donor blood should not be withheld from patients with PCH whose need is urgent. Transfusion of red cells that are negative for the P antigen should be considered only for those patients who do not respond adequately to randomly selected units of donor blood.[6]

DRUG-INDUCED IMMUNE HEMOLYTIC ANEMIA

Drugs rarely cause immune hemolytic anemia; the estimated incidence is 1 in 1 million people.[54] Many drugs have been implicated in hemolytic anemia over the years, as can be seen in the list provided in Appendix 14-1 and reviewed elsewhere.[14]

Drugs sometimes induce the formation of antibodies against the drug, red cell membrane components, or an antigen formed by the drug and the red cell membrane. These antibodies may cause a positive DAT result, immune red cell destruction, or both.[14,54] In some instances, a positive DAT result can be caused by nonimmunologic protein adsorption (NIPA) onto the red cell, which is caused by the drug.[14]

Theoretical Mechanisms of Drug-Induced Antibodies

Numerous theories have been suggested to explain how drugs induce immune responses and what relation such responses may have to the positive DAT result and immune-mediated cell destruction observed in some patients.[6] For many years, drug-associated positive DAT results were classified by four mechanisms: drug adsorption (penicillin-type), immune complex formation, autoantibody production, and NIPA. This classification has been useful serologically, but many aspects lack definitive proof. In addition, some drugs demonstrate serologic reactivity that appears to involve more than one mechanism. A more comprehensive approach, termed a "unifying hypothesis," is shown in Fig 14-1. One or more populations of antibodies may be present. In addition, NIPA, which is independent of antibody production, appears to play a role in drug-induced immune hemolytic anemia.[14]

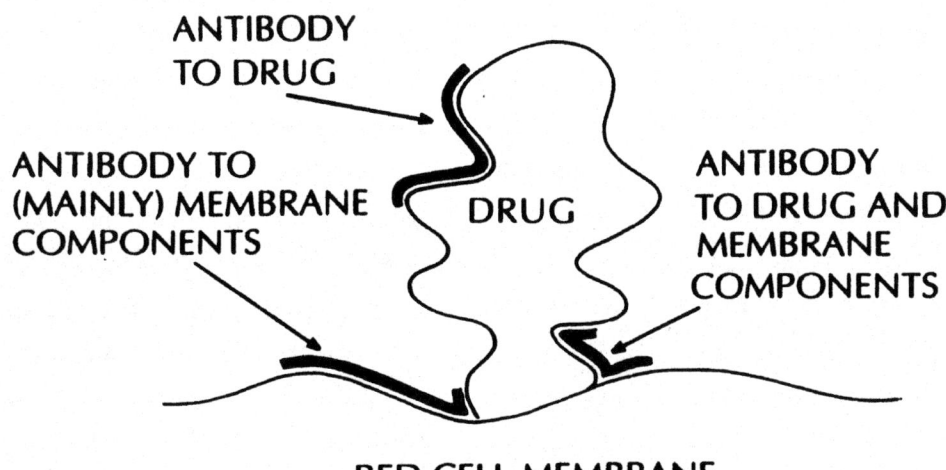

FIGURE 14-1. Proposed unifying theory of drug-induced antibody reactions (based on a cartoon by Habibi as cited by Garratty[34]). The thicker lines represent antigen-binding sites for the Fab region of the drug-induced antibody. Drugs (haptens) bind loosely or firmly to cell membranes, and antibodies may be made to 1) the drug [producing in-vitro reactions typical of a drug adsorption (penicillin-type) reaction]; 2) membrane components or mainly membrane components (producing in-vitro reactions typical of autoantibody); or 3) part-drug, part-membrane components (producing an in-vitro reaction typical of antibody reactive in the presence of a drug).[34(p55)]

Serologic Classification

Drug-induced antibodies can be classified into two groups: drug dependent (those that require the presence of the drug in the test system to be detected) and drug independent (those that do not require the in-vitro addition of the drug for detection).[6] Drug-dependent antibodies are subdivided into those that react with drug-treated red cells (eg, antibodies to penicillin and some cephalosporins) and those that react with untreated red cells in the presence of a solution of the drug (eg, antibodies to quinine and ceftriaxone). Drug-independent antibodies (eg, autoantibodies induced by methyldopa and fludarabine) have serologic reactivity that is independent of the drug despite the fact that the drug originally induced the immune response. Because the drug does not need to be added to the test system, drug-independent antibodies behave like autoantibodies that are serologically indistinguishable from idiopathic warm autoantibodies.

If a patient is suspected of having DIIHA, the suspected drug should be stopped. Laboratory testing to detect drug-dependent antibodies can be performed, but DIIHA caused by drug-independent antibodies or NIPA can be suggested only by showing a temporal association of the drug administration and hemolysis.

The historical details of penicillin- and methyldopa-induced antibodies are not described in this chapter but have been extensively reviewed elsewhere.[6,54] DIIHA caused by high-dose intravenous penicillin therapy is no longer seen, and methyldopa, the prototype for drug-independent antibodies, is not used as frequently as in the past. Currently, the drugs most commonly associated with DIIHA are piperacillin, ceftriaxone, and cefotetan; there has also been a small increase in DIIHA caused by drugs in the platinum family.[14]

Drug-Dependent Antibodies Reactive with Drug-Treated Red Cells

Some drugs (eg, penicillin, ampicillin, and many cephalosporins) covalently bind to red cells, thus making it possible to coat red cells in the laboratory with the drug. Antibodies directed to these drugs will react with the drug-treated red cells but not with untreated red cells (ie, no re-

action unless the patient also has alloantibodies to red cell antigens present on these cells).

Penicillin and the cephalosporins are beta-lactam antibiotics. It was thought for some time that antibodies to any drug in the penicillin and cephalosporin families could be detected by testing red cells with drug-treated cells using methods previously described for penicillin and cephalothin. It is now known that this is not the case. Synthetic penicillins and newer cephalosporins cannot be assumed to have the same red-cell-binding characteristics as penicillin and cephalothin (a first-generation cephalosporin). Cefotetan (a second-generation cephalosporin) binds very well to red cells, and antibodies caused by cefotetan typically react to very high titers with cefotetan-treated red cells. However, ceftriaxone (a third-generation cephalosporin) does not bind well to red cells; therefore, antibodies to ceftriaxone cannot be tested by this method.[55] Piperacillin, a semisynthetic penicillin, binds to red cells at high pH. However, a large percentage of plasma from healthy blood donors and patients reacts with piperacillin-treated red cells, so this method is not recommended for testing for piperacillin antibodies.[53] For drug-dependent antibodies detected using drug-treated red cells, the following are expected:

- The DAT result is usually positive for IgG, but complement may also be present.
- Serum contains an antibody that reacts with drug-treated red cells but not untreated red cells.
- Antibody eluted from the patient's red cells reacts with drug-treated red cells but not untreated red cells.

Hemolysis develops gradually but may be life-threatening if the etiology is unrecognized and drug administration is continued. The patient may or may not have been previously exposed to the drug, and in the case of cefotetan, even only a single dose given prophylactically can result in severe hemolysis. Normal plasma has been shown to react with some drug-treated red cells (eg, red cells treated with cefotetan, piperacillin, or oxaliplatin),[55] suggesting prior exposure to these drugs through environmental routes.

Drug-Dependent Antibodies Reactive with Untreated Red Cells in the Presence of Drug

Antibodies to many drugs that have been reported to cause immune hemolytic anemia are detected by testing untreated red cells in the presence of the drug. Piperacillin and some of the second- and third-generation cephalosporins react by this method; anti-ceftriaxone has been detected only by testing red cells in the presence of drug.[55] The following observations are characteristic:

- IgG and complement are detected but complement may be the only protein present.
- Serum antibody can be IgM, IgG, or IgM with IgA.
- A drug (or metabolite) must be present in vitro for the antibody in the patient's serum to be detected. Antibodies may cause hemolysis, agglutination, and/or sensitization of red cells in the presence of the drug.
- The patient need only take a small amount of the drug (eg, a single dose).
- Acute intravascular hemolysis with hemoglobinemia and hemoglobinuria is the usual presentation. Renal failure is quite common.
- Once antibody has been formed, severe hemolytic episodes may recur after exposure to very small quantities of the drug.

On occasion, it appears that a patient's serum contains an "autoantibody" in addition to a drug antibody reacting in the presence of the drug. Rather than a true autoantibody, it is believed that this reactivity results from the presence of circulating drug or drug-plus-antibody complexes.[55] In these cases, an eluate is usually nonreactive when the drug is not present in the system. However, in some cases, especially those involving piperacillin, the eluate reacts while the patient is still taking the drug. A sample collected several days after the drug has been discontinued will be nonreactive. A true warm autoantibody is expected to be reactive in an eluate prepared from the patient's red cells, and autoantibody in the serum persists. Consequently, DIIHA can be misdiagnosed as WAIHA, especially if the eluate reacts. Differentiation of warm-reactive autoantibody from DIIHA is important for clinical management.[53]

Drug-Independent Antibodies: Autoantibody Production

Some drugs induce autoantibodies that appear serologically indistinguishable from those of WAIHA. Red cells are coated with IgG, and the eluate as well as the serum react with virtually all cells tested in the absence of the drug. The antibody has no direct or indirect in-vitro interaction with the drug. As mentioned earlier, the prototype drug for such cases is methyldopa, which is now used much less frequently than in the past. Currently, fludarabine, used to treat chronic lymphocytic leukemia, is the most commonly used drug that produces drug-independent antibodies and AIHA.[54]

Nonimmunologic Protein Adsorption

The positive DAT result associated with some drugs is caused by modification of the red cell membrane by the drug and is independent of antibody production. Hemolytic anemia associated with this mechanism is rare.

Cephalosporins (primarily cephalothin) are the drugs with which positive DAT results and NIPA were originally associated. In vitro, red cells coated with cephalothin in pH 9.8 buffer and incubated with normal plasma adsorb albumin, IgA, IgG, IgM, C3, and other proteins in a nonimmunologic manner. For this reason, the IAT result with virtually all plasma will be positive. Other drugs that cause NIPA and a positive DAT result include diglycoaldehyde, cisplatin, oxaliplatin, and beta-lactamase inhibitors (clavulanic acid, sulbactam, and tazobactam).[14]

NIPA should be suspected when a patient's plasma/serum and most normal plasma/sera are reactive in an IAT with drug-treated red cells but the eluate from the patient's red cells is nonreactive with the drug-treated cells.

Laboratory Investigation of Drug-Induced Immune Hemolysis

The drug-related problems that are most commonly encountered in the blood bank are those associated with a positive DAT result and a nonreactive eluate. Recent red cell transfusions and/or dramatic hemolysis may result in a weak DAT result by the time hemolysis is suspected. When other, more common causes of immune-mediated hemolysis have been excluded *and* a temporal relationship exists between the administration of a drug and the hemolytic anemia, a drug antibody investigation should be pursued.

The patient's serum should be tested for unexpected antibodies by routine procedures. If the serum does not react with untreated red cells, the tests should be repeated with the drug(s) suspected of causing the problem.[55] Some drug formulations contain inert ingredients (eg, pill or capsule forms), and other drugs are combinations of two drugs (eg, piperacillin plus tazobactam). Although it would seem logical to test the patient's serum with the actual drug that the patient received, inert ingredients or drug combinations can make preparation of drug-treated red cells difficult or make the results confusing. It is preferable to test serum using pure drug formulations as well as separate components of combination drugs.

If the drug has already been reported to cause hemolytic anemia, testing methods may be described in the case reports. Far more drug-dependent antibodies are detected by testing serum in the presence of drug; therefore, when a previous report of antibodies to a drug is not available, an initial screening test can be performed with a solution of the drug at a concentration of approximately 1 mg/mL in phosphate-buffered saline.[55] (See Method 4-13.) Serum, rather than plasma, is the preferred specimen for testing for hemolysis to be observed; this also allows for the addition of fresh normal serum (as a source of complement) to the test system. The addition of the fresh complement increases the sensitivity of the test for the detection of in-vitro hemolysis resulting from complement activation.

If these tests are not informative, attempts can be made to coat normal red cells with the drug.[55] The patient's serum and an eluate from the patient's red cells can be tested against the drug-treated red cells. (See Method 4-12.) This is the method of choice when cephalosporins (except for ceftriaxone) are thought to be implicated. Results that are definitive for a drug-induced positive DAT result are reactivity of the eluate with drug-treated red cells and absence of reactivity with untreated red cells.

Drug-treated red cells should always be tested with saline and normal serum (or plasma) as negative controls. This approach ensures that the observed reactivity with the patient's serum/plasma is appropriately interpreted. Antibodies reactive with red cells treated with some drugs (eg, beta-lactams and platinums) have been detected in the plasma from blood donors and patients without hemolytic anemia and are thought to be caused by environmental exposure. Therefore, misinterpretation of reactivity in a patient's serum is possible.[55]

Whenever possible, a positive control should be tested with drug-treated red cells. Negative results of a patient's serum and eluate without a positive control can be interpreted only as showing that antibodies to that drug were not detected. The drug may or may not be bound to the test red cells.

If the drug in question is known to cause NIPA, the patient's serum and the controls (negative and positive) should also be tested at a dilution of 1 in 20. Normal sera at this dilution do not usually contain enough protein for NIPA to be detected.

When a patient is receiving more than one drug that has a temporal relationship to hemolysis, the coadministered drugs should be tested. Antibodies to more than one drug have been reported in cases where chemotherapeutics have been administered multiple times.[56] In addition, an immune response may be caused by a metabolite of a drug rather than the drug itself. If the clinical picture is consistent with immune-mediated hemolysis and the above tests are non-informative, it may be helpful to test metabolites of the parent drug that are present in the serum or urine of an individual who is taking that drug.[57] Antibodies to some nonsteroidal anti-inflammatory drugs have required testing in the presence of metabolite.[58] The metabolism and half-life of the drug determines when the drug metabolite should be collected. Pharmacology information for the metabolite(s) detectable in serum or urine, as well as previous reports for the drug under investigation should be consulted.

KEY POINTS

1. The DAT is used to determine whether red cells have been coated in vivo with immunoglobulin, complement, or both. The DAT is used primarily for the investigation of hemolytic transfusion reactions, HDFN, AIHA, and drug-induced immune hemolysis.
2. The DAT should be used to determine whether a hemolytic anemia has an immune etiology.
3. A positive DAT result may or may not be associated with hemolysis.
4. Performance of the DAT on postreaction specimens is part of the initial investigation of a transfusion reaction. The DAT result may be positive if sensitized red cells have not been destroyed, or may be negative if hemolysis and rapid clearance have occurred.
5. The DAT is performed by testing freshly washed red cells directly with antiglobulin reagents containing anti-IgG and anti-C3d. False-negative or weaker results can be obtained if the washed red cells are allowed to sit before testing with anti-IgG or if the reading is delayed.
6. When the DAT result is positive with both anti-IgG and anti-C3, the red cells should be tested with an inert control reagent (eg, 6% albumin or saline). If the control is reactive, the DAT result is invalid, possibly indicating spontaneous agglutination from heavy coating of IgG or rare warm-reactive IgM. The invalid DAT result could also be caused by IgM cold autoagglutinins that were not dissociated during routine washing.
7. A positive DAT result alone is not diagnostic of hemolytic anemia. The interpretation of the significance of this positive result requires additional patient-specific information. Dialogue with the attending physician is important. Clinical considerations together with laboratory data should dictate the extent to which a positive DAT result is evaluated.
8. The following situations may warrant further investigation of a positive DAT result:
   - Evidence of in-vivo red cell destruction.
   - Recent transfusion.
   - Administration of drugs that have previously been associated with immune-mediated hemolysis.
   - History of hematopoietic progenitor cell or organ transplantation.
   - Administration of IVIG or intravenous anti-D.
   - Administration of therapeutic monoclonal antibodies that may react with target antigen on red cells.
9. Elution frees antibody from sensitized red cells and recovers antibody in a usable form. Elution is useful in certain situations for implicating an autoantibody, detecting specific antibodies that may not be detectable in the serum, and deciding to test the patient's serum for drug-dependent antibodies.
10. AIHAs are subdivided into the major types: WAIHA, CAS, mixed- or combined-type AIHA, and PCH. Drugs may also induce immune hemolysis.

REFERENCES

1. Zanella A, Barcellini W. Treatment of autoimmune hemolytic anemias. Haematologica 2014; 99:1547-54.

2. Shapiro R, Chin-Yee I, Lam S. Eculizumab as a bridge to immunosuppressive therapy in severe cold agglutinin disease of anti-Pr specificity. Clin Case Rep 2015;3:942-4.

3. Kaplan HS, Garratty G. Predictive value of direct antiglobulin test results. Diagnostic Med 1985;8:29-32.

4. Garratty G. The significance of IgG on the red cell surface. Transfus Med Rev 1987;1:47-57.

5. Freedman J. The significance of complement on the red cell surface. Transfus Med Rev 1987;1:58-70.

6. Petz LD, Garratty G. Immune hemolytic anemias. 2nd ed. Philadelphia: Churchill-Livingstone, 2004.

7. Rottenberg Y, Yahalom V, Shinar E, et al. Blood donors with positive direct antiglobulin tests are at increased risk for cancer. Transfusion 2009; 49:838-42.

8. Hannon JL. Management of blood donors and blood donations from individuals found to have a positive direct antiglobulin test. Transfus Med Rev 2012;26:142-52.

9. Toy PT, Chin CA, Reid ME, Burns MA. Factors associated with positive direct antiglobulin tests in pretransfusion patients: A case control study. Vox Sang 1985;49:215-20.

10. Heddle NM, Kelton JG, Turchyn KL, Ali MAM. Hypergammaglobulinemia can be associated with a positive direct antiglobulin test, a nonreactive eluate, and no evidence of hemolysis. Transfusion 1988;28:29-33.

11. Clark JA, Tanley PC, Wallas CH. Evaluation of patients with positive direct antiglobulin tests and nonreactive eluates discovered during pretransfusion testing. Immunohematology 1992; 8:9-12.

12. Coombs RRA, Mourant AE, Race RR. A new test for the detection of weak and "incomplete" Rh agglutinins. Br J Exp Pathol 1945;26:255-66.

13. Heddle NM, Soutar RL, O'Hoski PL, et al. A prospective study to determine the frequency and clinical significance of alloimmunization posttransfusion. Br J Haematol 1995;91:1000-5.

14. Garratty G, Arndt PA. Drugs that have been shown to cause drug-induced immune hemolytic anemia or positive direct antiglobulin tests: Some interesting findings since 2007. Immunohematology 2014;30:66-79.

15. Desborough MJ, Miller J, Thorpe SJ, et al. Intravenous immunoglobulin-induced haemolysis: A case report and review of the literature. Transfus Med 2014;24:219-26.

16. Rushin J, Rumsey DH, Ewing CA, Sandler SG. Detection of multiple passively acquired alloantibodies following infusions of IV Rh immune globulin. Transfusion 2000;40:551-4.

17. Chapuy CI, Nicholson RT, Aguad MD, et al. Resolving the daratumumab interference with blood compatibility testing. Transfusion 2015; 55:1545-54.

18. Oostendorp M, Lammerts van Bueren JJ, Doshi P, et al. When blood transfusion medicine becomes complicated due to interference by monoclonal antibody therapy. Transfusion 2015;55:1555-62.

19. Judd WJ. Elution—dissociation of antibody from red blood cells: Theoretical and practical considerations. Transfus Med Rev 1999;13:297-310.

20. Leger RM, Arndt PA, Ciesielski DJ, Garratty G. False-positive eluate reactivity due to the low-ionic wash solution used with commercial acid-elution kits. Transfusion 1998;38:565-72.

21. Judd WJ, Johnson ST, Storry JR. Judd's methods in immunohematology. 3rd ed. Bethesda, MD: AABB Press, 2008.

22. Judd WJ, Barnes BA, Steiner EA, et al. The evaluation of a positive direct antiglobulin test (autocontrol) in pretransfusion testing revisited. Transfusion 1986;26:220-4.

23. Arndt PA, Leger RM, Garratty G. Serologic findings in autoimmune hemolytic anemia associated with immunoglobulin M warm autoantibodies. Transfusion 2009;49:235-42.

24. Rodberg K, Tsuneta R, Garratty G. Discrepant Rh phenotyping results when testing IgG-sensitized RBCs with monoclonal Rh reagents (abstract). Transfusion 1995;35(Suppl):67S.

25. Leger RM, Garratty G. Evaluation of methods for detecting alloantibodies underlying warm autoantibodies. Transfusion 1999;39:11-16.

26. Church AT, Nance SJ, Kavitsky DM. Predicting the presence of a new alloantibody underlying a warm autoantibody (abstract). Transfusion 2000;40(Suppl):121S.

27. Branch DR, Petz LD. A new reagent (ZZAP) having multiple applications in immunohematology. Am J Clin Pathol 1982;78:161-7.

28. Laine EP, Leger RM, Arndt PA, et al. In vitro studies of the impact of transfusion on the detection of alloantibodies after autoadsorption. Transfusion 2000;40:1384-7.

29. Chiaroni J, Touinssi M, Mazet M, et al. Adsorption of autoantibodies in the presence of LISS to detect alloantibodies underlying warm autoantibodies. Transfusion 2003;43:651-5.

30. Magtoto-Jocom J, Hodam J, Leger RM, Garratty G. Adsorption to remove autoantibodies using allogeneic red cells in the presence of low ionic strength saline for detection of alloantibodies (abstract). Transfusion 2011;51(Suppl):174A.

31. Judd WJ, Dake L. PEG adsorption of autoanti-bodies causes loss of concomitant alloantibody. Immunohematology 2001;17:82-5.

32. Combs MR, Eveland D, Jewet-Keefe B, Telen MJ. The use of polyethylene glycol in adsorptions: More evidence that antibodies may be missed (abstract). Transfusion 2001;41(Suppl):30S.

33. Issitt PD, Combs MR, Bumgarner DJ, et al. Studies of antibodies in the sera of patients who have made red cell autoantibodies. Transfusion 1996;36:481-6.

34. Garratty G. Target antigens for red-cell-bound autoantibodies. In: Nance SJ, ed. Clinical and basic science aspects of immunohematology. Arlington, VA: AABB, 1991:33-72.

35. Garratty G. Specificity of autoantibodies reacting optimally at 37° C. Immunohematology 1999;15:24-40.

36. Branch DR, Petz LD. Detecting alloantibodies in patients with autoantibodies (editorial). Transfusion 1999;39:6-10.

37. Young PP, Uzieblo A, Trulock E, et al. Autoantibody formation after alloimmunization: Are blood transfusions a risk factor for autoimmune hemolytic anemia? Transfusion 2004;44:67-72.

38. Maley M, Bruce DG, Babb RG, et al. The incidence of red cell alloantibodies underlying pan-reactive warm autoantibodies. Immunohematology 2005;21:122-5.

39. Ahrens N, Pruss A, Kähne A, et al. Coexistence of autoantibodies and alloantibodies to red blood cells due to blood transfusion. Transfusion 2007;47:813-16.

40. Shirey RS, Boyd JS, Parwani AV, et al. Prophylactic antigen-matched donor blood for patients with warm autoantibodies: An algorithm for transfusion management. Transfusion 2002;42:1435-41.

41. Hillyer CD, Shaz BH, Winkler AM, Reid M. Integrating molecular technologies for red blood cell typing and compatibility testing into blood centers and transfusion services. Transfus Med Rev 2008;22:117-32.

42. Denomme GA. Prospects for the provision of genotyped blood for transfusion. Br J Haematol 2013;163:3-9.

43. Lee E, Redman M, Burgess G, Win N. Do patients with autoantibodies or clinically insignificant alloantibodies require an indirect antiglobulin test crossmatch? Transfusion 2007;47:1290-5.

44. Richa EM, Stowers RE, Tauscher CD, et al. The safety of electronic crossmatch in patients with warm autoantibodies (letter). Vox Sang 2007;93:92.

45. Leger RM, Co A, Hunt P, Garratty G. Attempts to support an immune etiology in 800 patients with direct antiglobulin test-negative hemolytic anemia. Immunohematology 2010;26:156-60.

46. Waligora SK, Edwards JM. Use of rabbit red cells for adsorption of cold autoagglutinins. Transfusion 1983;23:328-30.

47. Dzik WH, Yang R, Blank J. Rabbit erythrocyte stroma treatment of serum interferes with recognition of delayed hemolytic transfusion reaction (letter). Transfusion 1986;26:303-4.

48. Mechanic SA, Maurer JL, Igoe MJ, et al. Anti-Vel reactivity diminished by adsorption with rabbit RBC stroma. Transfusion 2002;42:1180-3.

49. Storry JR, Olsson ML, Moulds JJ. Rabbit red blood cell stroma bind immunoglobulin M antibodies regardless of blood group specificity (letter). Transfusion 2006;46:1260-1.

50. Sokol RJ, Hewitt S, Stamps BK. Autoimmune haemolysis: An 18-year study of 865 cases referred to a regional transfusion centre. Br Med J 1981;282:2023-7.

51. Shulman IA, Branch DR, Nelson JM, et al. Autoimmune hemolytic anemia with both cold and warm autoantibodies. JAMA 1985;253:1746-8.

52. Garratty G, Arndt PA, Leger RM. Serological findings in autoimmune hemolytic anemia (AIHA) associated with both warm and cold autoantibodies (abstract). Blood 2003;102(Suppl):563a.

53. Eder AF. Review: Acute Donath-Landsteiner hemolytic anemia. Immunohematology 2005;21:56-62.

54. Garratty G. Immune hemolytic anemia associated with drug therapy. Blood Rev 2010;24:143-50.

55. Leger RM, Arndt PA, Garratty G. How we investigate drug-induced immune hemolytic anemia. Immunohematology 2014;30:85-94.

56. Leger RM, Jain S, Nester TA, Kaplan H. Drug-induced immune hemolytic anemia associated with anti-carboplatin and the first example of anti-paclitaxel. Transfusion 2015;55:2949-54.

57. Salama A, Mueller-Eckhardt C, Kissel K, et al. Ex vivo antigen preparation for the serological detection of drug-dependent antibodies in immune haemolytic anaemias. Br J Haematol 1984;58:525-31.

58. Johnson ST, Fueger JT, Gottschall JL. One center's experience: The serology and drugs associated with drug-induced immune hemolytic anemia—a new paradigm. Transfusion 2007;47:697-702.

APPENDIX 14-1
Drugs Associated with Immune Hemolytic Anemia

Drug	Method of Detection			
Aceclofenac			+Drug	
Acetaminophen			+Drug	
Acyclovir		DT		
Alemtuzumab	AA			
Aminopyrine		DT		
Amoxicillin		DT		
Amphotericin B			+Drug	
Ampicillin		DT	+Drug	
Antazoline			+Drug	
Azapropazone	AA	DT		
Bendamustine	AA			
Butizide			+Drug	
Carbimazole	AA	DT	+Drug	
Carboplatin	AA	DT	+Drug	NIPA
Carbromal		DT		
Cefamandole		DT		
Cefazolin		DT		
Cefixime		DT	+Drug	
Cefotaxime		DT	+Drug	
Cefotetan	AA	DT	+Drug	NIPA
Cefoxitin	AA	DT	+Drug	
Cefpirome			+Drug	
Ceftazidime	AA	DT	+Drug	
Ceftizoxime		DT	+Drug	
Ceftriaxone			+Drug	
Cefuroxime		DT		
Cephalexin		DT		
Cephalothin		DT	+Drug	NIPA
Chloramphenicol	AA	DT		
Chlorinated hydrocarbons	AA	DT	+Drug	
Chlorpromazine	AA		+Drug	
Chlorpropamide			+Drug	

APPENDIX 14-1
Drugs Associated with Immune Hemolytic Anemia (Continued)

Drug		Method of Detection		
Cimetidine		DT	+Drug	
Ciprofloxacin			+Drug	
Cisplatin		DT	+Drug	NIPA
Cladribine	AA			
Clavulanate				NIPA
Cyanidanol	AA	DT	+ Drug	
Cyclofenil	AA		+ Drug	
Cyclosporine		DT		
Diclofenac	AA	DT	+ Drug	
Diethylstilbestrol			+ Drug	
Diglycoaldehyde				NIPA
Dipyrone		DT	+ Drug	
Erythromycin		DT		
Etodolac			+ Drug	
Fenoprofen	AA		+ Drug	
Fluconazole		DT	+ Drug	
Fludarabine	AA			
Fluorescein		DT	+ Drug	
Fluorouracil			+ Drug	
Furosemide			+ Drug	
Hydralizine		DT		
Hydrochlorothiazide		DT	+ Drug	
Hydrocortisone		DT	+ Drug	
9-Hydroxy-methyl-ellipticinium			+ Drug	
Ibuprofen			+Drug	
Imatinib mesylate		DT		
Insulin		DT		
Isoniazid		DT	+ Drug	
Levodopa	AA			
Levofloxacin		DT	+Drug	

(Continued)

APPENDIX 14-1
Drugs Associated with Immune Hemolytic Anemia (Continued)

Drug		Method of Detection		
Mefenamic acid	AA			
Mefloquine		DT	+ Drug	
Melphalan			+ Drug	
6-Mercaptopurine		DT		
Methadone		DT		
Methotrexate	AA	DT	+ Drug	
Methyldopa	AA			
Nabumetone			+Drug	
Nafcillin		DT		
Naproxen			+ Drug	
Oxaliplatin		DT	+ Drug	NIPA
Paclitaxel		DT	+ Drug	
p-Aminosalicylic acid			+ Drug	
Pemetrexed			+ Drug	
Penicillin G		DT		
Phenacetin			+ Drug	
Phenytoin		DT		
Piperacillin		DT	+ Drug	
Probenicid			+ Drug	
Procainamide	AA			
Propyphenazone			+ Drug	
Pyrazinamide		DT	+ Drug	
Pyrimethamine		DT		
Quinidine		DT	+ Drug	
Quinine			+ Drug	
Ranitidine		DT	+ Drug	
Rifabutin			+ Drug	
Rifampicin		DT	+ Drug	
Sodium pentothal/thiopental			+ Drug	
Stibophen			+ Drug	
Streptokinase		DT		

APPENDIX 14-1
Drugs Associated with Immune Hemolytic Anemia (Continued)

Drug	Method of Detection			
Streptomycin	AA	DT	+Drug	
Sulbactam				NIPA
Sulfamethoxazole			+Drug	
Sulfasalazine			+Drug	
Sulfisoxazole			+Drug	
Sulindac	AA	DT	+Drug	
Suprofen	AA		+Drug	
Tazobactam				NIPA
Teicoplanin	AA		+Drug	
Teniposide	AA		+Drug	
Tetracycline		DT		
Ticarcillin	AA	DT		
Tolbutamide		DT		
Tolmetin	AA		+Drug	
Triamterene		DT	+Drug	
Trimethoprim			+Drug	
Vancomycin			+Drug	
Vincristine		DT	+Drug	
Zomepirac	AA		+Drug	

AA = drug-independent autoantibody; DT = testing with drug-treated red cells; +Drug = testing in the presence of drug; NIPA = nonimmunologic protein adsorption.

CHAPTER 15
Platelet and Granulocyte Antigens and Antibodies

David F. Stroncek, MD, and Ralph R. Vassallo, MD, FACP

THIS CHAPTER DISCUSSES ANTIGENS expressed on platelets and granulocytes and the antibodies formed by sensitized individuals. These antigens and the immune responses to them are of importance in alloimmune, autoimmune, and drug-induced immune syndromes involving platelets and granulocytes.

PLATELET ANTIGENS AND ANTIBODIES

Platelets express a variety of antigenic markers on their surface. Some of these antigens are shared with other cells, such as ABH and HLA determinants, whereas others are essentially platelet specific, such as human platelet alloantigens (HPAs).

HPA

Platelets play roles in inflammation, immune responses, cardiovascular disease, and even cancer.[1-3] However, their primary function is hemostasis. Platelets perform all these functions through multiple ligand-receptor interactions involving glycoproteins expressed on their cell surface membranes.

Platelet membrane glycoproteins are expressed in different forms as a result of single nucleotide polymorphisms (SNPs) in the genes that encode them. The amino acid changes resulting from these SNPs in turn result in glycoprotein structural and antigenic changes capable of eliciting alloantibody responses after pregnancy or transfusion. Currently, 35 different HPAs expressed on six different platelet membrane glycoproteins (GPs)—GPIIb, GPIIIa, GPIbα, GPIbβ, GPIa, and CD109—have been formally recognized (Table 15-1).[4] These antigens are often referred to as "platelet specific" and, although some are found on cells other than platelets (especially leukocytes and endothelial cells), their chief clinical importance appears to be linked to their presence on platelets.

Twelve antigens are clustered into six important biallelic groups (HPA-1, HPA-2, HPA-3, HPA-4, HPA-5, and HPA-15). The nomenclature for HPAs consists of numbering the antigens in their order of discovery, with the higher-frequency antigens designated "a" and the lower-frequency antigens designated "b."[5] HPAs for which antibodies against only one of the two antithetical (non-wild-type) antigens have been detected are labeled with a "w" for "workshop," such as HPA-6bw. New low-frequency HPAs continue to be discovered but have not yet been confirmed in the Immuno Polymorphism Database (https://www.ebi.ac.uk/ipd/hpa/).[6-8]

15

David F. Stroncek, MD, Director, Center for Cellular Engineering, Department of Transfusion Medicine, Clinical Center, National Institutes of Health, Bethesda, Maryland; and Ralph R. Vassallo, MD, FACP, Executive Vice President/Chief Medical and Scientific Officer, Vitalant, Scottsdale, Arizona

D. Stroncek has disclosed no conflicts of interest. R. Vassallo has disclosed a financial relationship with Cerus Corp and Terumo BCT.

TABLE 15-1. Human Platelet Alloantigens

Current Nomenclature	Legacy Nomenclature	Phenotypic Frequency*	Glycoprotein	Amino Acid Change	Gene/ Nucleotide Change
HPA-1a	Zw^a, Pl^{A1}	72% a/a			
HPA-1b	Zw^b, Pl^{A2}	26% a/b 2% b/b	GPIIIa	Leu33Pro	*ITGB3* *176T>C*
HPA-2a	Ko^b	85% a/a			
HPA-2b	Ko^a, Sib^a	14% a/b 1% b/b	GPIba	Thr145Met	*GPIBA* *482C>T*
HPA-3a	Bak^a, Lek^a	37% a/a			
HPA-3b	Bak^b	48% a/b 15% b/b	GPIIb	Ile843Ser	*ITGA2B* *2621T>G*
HPA-4a	Yuk^b, Pen^a	>99.9% a/a			
HPA-4b	Yuk^a, Pen^b	<0.1% a/b <0.1% b/b	GPIIIa	Arg143Gln	*ITGB3* *506G>A*
HPA-5a	Br^b, Zav^b	88% a/a			
HPA-5b	Br^a, Zav^a, Hc^a	20% a/b 1% b/b	GPIa	Glu505Lys	*ITGA2* *1600G>A*
HPA-6bw	Ca^a, Tu^a	<1% a/b or b/b	GPIIIa	Arg489Gln	*ITGB3* *1544G>A*
HPA-7bw	Mo^a	<1% a/b or b/b	GPIIIa	Pro407Ala	*ITGB3* *1297C>G*
HPA-8bw	Sr^a	<1% a/b or b/b	GPIIIa	Arg636Cys	*ITGB3* *1984C>T*
HPA-9bw (assoc. with HPA-3b)	Max^a	<1% a/b or b/b	GPIIb	Val837Met	*ITGA2B* *2602G>A*
HPA-10bw	La^a	<1% a/b or b/b	GPIIIa	Arg62Gln	*ITGB3* *263G>A*
HPA-11bw	Gro^a	<1% a/b or b/b	GPIIIa	Arg633His	*ITGB3* *1976G>A*
HPA-12bw	Iy^a	<1% a/b or b/b	GPIbβ	Gly15Glu	*GPIBB* *119G>A*
HPA-13bw	Sit^a	<1% a/b or b/b	GPIa	Met799Thr	*ITGA2* *2483C>T*
HPA-14bw (assoc. with HPA-1b)	Oe^a	<1% b/b	GPIIIa	Lys611del	*ITGB3* *1909-1911delAAG*
HPA-15a	Gov^b	35% a/a			
HPA-15b	Gov^a	42% a/b 23% b/b	CD109	Ser682Tyr	*CD109* *2108C>A*

TABLE 15-1. Human Platelet Alloantigens (Continued)

Current Nomenclature	Legacy Nomenclature	Phenotypic Frequency*	Glycoprotein	Amino Acid Change	Gene/ Nucleotide Change
HPA-16bw	Duvᵃ or Duvᵃ⁺	<1% a/b or b/b	GPIIIa	Thr140Ile	*ITGB3 497C>T*
HPA-17bw	Vaᵃ	<1% a/b or b/b	GPIIIa	Thr195Met	*ITGB3 662C>T*
HPA-18bw	Cabᵃ	<1% a/b or b/b	GPIa	Gln716His	*ITGA2 2235G>T*
HPA-19bw	Sta	<1% a/b or b/b	GPIIIa	Lys137Gln	*ITGB3 487A>C*
HPA-20bw	Kno	<1% a/b or b/b	GPIIb	Thr619Met	*ITGA2B 1949C>T*
HPA-21bw	Nos	<1% a/b or b/b	GPIIIa	Glu628Lys	*ITGB3 1960G>A*
HPA-22bw	Sey	<1% a/b or b/b	GPIIb	Lys164Thr	*ITGA2B 584A>C*
HPA-23bw	Hug	<1% a/b or b/b	GPIIIa	Arg622Trp	*ITGB3 1942C>T*
HPA-24bw	Cab2ᵃ⁺	<1% a/b or b/b	GPIIb	Ser472Asn	*ITGA2B 1508G>A*
HPA-25bw	Swiᵃ	<1% a/b or b/b	GPIa	Thr1087Met	*ITGA2 3347C>T*
HPA-26bw	Secᵃ	<1% a/b or b/b	GPIIIa	Lys580Asn	*ITGB3 1818G>T*
HPA-27bw	Cab3ᵃ⁺	<1% a/b or b/b	GPIIb	Leu841Met	*ITGA2B 2614C>A*
HPA-28bw	War	<1% a/b or b/b	GPIIb	Val740Leu	*ITGA2B 2311G>T*
HPA-29bw	Khaᵇ	<1% a/b or b/b	GPIIIa	Thr7Met	*ITGB3 98C>T*

*Phenotypic frequencies are for people of European ancestry who live in North America. Human platelet alloantigen (HPA) frequencies in other races and ethnic groups can be found in the Immuno Polymorphism Database at http://www.ebi.ac.uk/ipd/hpa/freqs_1.html.

Platelet Alloantigens on GPIIb/IIIa

HPA-1a is the platelet alloantigen that was discovered first and is most familiar.[9] Originally named "Zwᵃ" and more commonly referred to as "Pl^{A1}," it is expressed on GPIIIa, the β-subunit of the integrin GPIIb/IIIa (α_{IIb}/b_3) complex.

Integrins are a broadly distributed family of adhesion molecules consisting of an α and a β chain held together by divalent cations in a heterodimeric complex.[10] Integrins are essential for platelet adhesion and aggregation because they serve as receptors for ligands, such as fibrinogen, collagen, fibronectin, von Willebrand factor (vWF), and other extracellular matrix proteins.

Postactivation binding of fibrinogen by GPIIb/IIIa results in platelet aggregation, which forms the "platelet plug" to stop bleeding. GPIIb/IIIa's hemostatic importance is demonstrated by the serious bleeding in patients with Glanzmann thrombasthenia, a rare disorder that is caused by congenital absence or dysfunction of the GPIIb/IIIa genes *ITGA2B* and/or *ITGB3*.[11] Patients with Glanzmann thrombasthenia who are exposed to normal platelets by transfusion or pregnancy can make isoantibodies against GPIIb/IIIa.

GPIIb/IIIa is the most abundantly expressed (50,000-80,000 molecules/platelet) glycoprotein complex on the platelet membrane, making it highly immunogenic.[12] Antibodies against HPA-1a account for the vast majority (>80%) of the HPA-specific platelet antibodies detected in the sera of alloimmunized people of European ancestry. HPA-1a antibodies are produced by the 2% of individuals with the platelet type HPA-1b/1b.

Twenty-five of the 35 recognized HPAs are carried by GPIIb (8) and GPIIIa (17). Like HPA-1a/1b, the HPA-4a/4b antigens are also expressed on GPIIIa and have been implicated in fetal and neonatal alloimmune thrombocytopenia (FNAIT), posttransfusion purpura (PTP), and platelet transfusion refractoriness. The low-frequency HPA-4b antigen is more common in populations of Japanese and Chinese ancestry.[12]

The HPA-3a/3b antigens are expressed on GPIIb but, despite the relatively high rate of homozygosity of the low-frequency antigen in the general population, detection of HPA-3 antibodies is uncommon. Some HPA-3 antibodies are difficult to detect in monoclonal antigen capture assays (ACAs), such as the modified antigen capture enzyme-linked immunosorbent assay (MACE) and monoclonal antibody-specific immobilization of platelet antigens (MAIPA), in which GPIIb is extracted from platelets with detergents that can denature the antigenic epitopes recognized by various HPA-3 antibodies.[13,14]

In addition to HPA-1b, -3b, and -4b, 19 other low-frequency platelet antigens are expressed on either GPIIb or GPIIIa (Table 15-1). These antigens were all discovered in cases of FNAIT by specific antibodies in maternal sera reactive solely with paternal GPIIb/IIIa. The vast majority of these antigens are private antigens restricted to the single families in which they were discovered. HPA-6bw and HPA-21bw are exceptions, having antigen frequencies of 1% and 2%, respectively, in people of Japanese ancestry, and HPA-9bw has been implicated in several cases of FNAIT.[15-18]

Platelet Alloantigens on GPIb/V/IX

The GPIb/V/IX complex forms the vWF receptor on platelets, and platelets express approximately 12,500 copies of this seven-unit complex.[12] Following vascular injury, binding of the GPIb/V/IX complex to vWF facilitates platelet adhesion to vascular subendothelium and initiates signaling events within adherent platelets that lead to platelet activation, aggregation, and hemostasis. GPIb is composed of two α (GPIbα) and two β (GPIbβ) subunits (25,000 surface copies) that form noncovalent associations with two GPIX and one GPV. GPIbα carries HPA-2a/2b, and GPIbβ carries HPA-12bw. Antibodies against HPA-2a, -2b, and -12bw have all been implicated in FNAIT.

Deficiency of the entire GPIb/V/IX complex can occur from mutations in the encoding genes *GPIBA*, *GPIBB*, or *GP9*, and is the cause of Bernard Soulier syndrome (BSS). BSS is a disorder characterized by prolonged bleeding time, thrombocytopenia, and the presence of "giant platelets," and affects approximately one person per million.[19] BSS patients whose platelets are devoid of GPIb/V/IX can produce isoantibodies when they are exposed to the protein complex on normal platelets through transfusions or pregnancy.[19]

Platelet Alloantigens on GPIa/IIa

The integrin GPIa/IIa, also known as integrin a_2b_1, is a major collagen receptor on platelets. The GPIa protein carries the HPA-5a/5b antigens. Antibodies against HPA-5 antigens are the second most frequently detected, after anti-HPA-1a, in patients with FNAIT and are also frequently detected in patients with PTP and transfusion refractoriness. About 3000 to 5000 molecules of the GPIa/IIa heterodimeric complex are expressed on platelets.[20] HPA-13bw, -18bw, and -25bw are low-frequency antigens that are also expressed on GPIa and have all been implicated in FNAIT. Interestingly, the HPA-13bw polymorphism has been reported to cause functional defects that reduce platelet responses to collagen-induced aggregation and spreading on collagen-coated surfaces.[5]

Platelet Alloantigens on CD109

CD109 is a glycosylphosphatidylinositol (GPI)-linked protein and a member of the a_2-macroglobulin/complement superfamily. Its function is still not completely understood, but CD109 has been reported to bind to and negatively regulate the signaling of transforming growth factor beta. CD109 is also expressed on activated T lymphocytes, CD34+ hematopoietic cells, and endothelial cells, and it carries the HPA-15 antigens.

Platelets express an average of 2000 molecules of CD109, although interindividual copy numbers vary significantly.[21] Studies show the presence of HPA-15 antibodies in 0.22% to 4% of maternal sera in patients with suspected FNAIT, and several reports suggest that HPA-15 antibodies are more frequently detected in sera from patients with immune platelet refractoriness.[21-24]

Other Antigens on Platelets

ABO and Other Blood Groups

Most of the ABH antigen on platelets is carried on saccharides attached to the major platelet membrane glycoproteins (Table 15-2). GPIIb and platelet endothelial cell adhesion molecule 1 (PECAM-1/CD31) carry the largest amounts of A and B antigens.[25] Platelet A and B antigen levels are quite variable from individual to individual, with 5% to 10% of non-group-O individuals expressing extremely high levels of A or B on their platelets.[25,26] These "high expressers" have highly active glycosyltransferases, which are much more efficient at attaching A or B antigens.[25]

Interestingly, although individuals with the subgroup A_2 red cell phenotype express lower levels of A on their red cells than A_1 individuals, they do not express detectable A antigens on their platelets. As a result, A_2 platelets may be successfully transfused to group O patients with high-titer immunoglobulin G (IgG) anti-A or -A,B who are refractory to non-group-O platelets.[27]

Although platelets are often transfused without regard to ABO compatibility, the use of major-mismatched platelets (eg, A or B platelets into group O recipients) frequently results in lower posttransfusion recovery rates, while minor mismatches (eg, O platelets into A or B

TABLE 15-2. Other Platelet Antigens

Antigen	Phenotypic Frequency	Glycoprotein (GP)*	Amino Acid Change[†]	Encoding Gene	Nucleotide Change[‡]
ABO	Same as for red cells	GPIIb/IIIa, IV, Ia/IIa, GPIb/V/IX, CD31	Multiple	*ABO*	Multiple
HLA-A, -B, and -C	Same as for leukocytes	Class I HLA	Multiple	*MHC*	Multiple
GPIV	90%-97% (African ancestry) 90%-97% (Asian ancestry) 99.9% (European ancestry)	CD36	Tyr325Thr* Pro90Ser*	*CD36*	1264T>G* 478C>T* Exons 1-3 del
GPVI	N/A	GPVI	N/A	*GP6*	N/A

*ABO saccharides are attached to platelet GPs during their glycosylation.
[†] Only the most common changes are shown.
[‡] Only the most common mutations are shown.

recipients) do not.[28,29] Clinical trials comparing ABO-identical to -unmatched platelets in patients with cancer who require multiple platelet transfusions have suggested that rates of refractoriness are significantly higher when unmatched components are used.[30] Although other red cell antigens (eg, Le[a], Le[b], I, i, P, P[k], and Cromer) are also present on platelets, there is no evidence that these antigens significantly reduce platelet survival in vivo.[31,32]

GPIV/CD36

Platelets, monocytes/macrophages, and nucleated erythrocytes are the only blood cells that express GPIV/CD36 (Table 15-2). GPIV belongs to the Class B scavenger receptor family and binds a number of different ligands, including low-density lipoprotein cholesterol, thrombospondin, types I and IV collagen, and malaria-infected red cells. A number of mutations in *CD36* have been described that result in a complete lack of protein expression on both platelets and monocytes in populations of Asian and African ancestry.[30-32] CD36-deficient individuals exposed to normal platelets can produce antibodies to CD36 that have been reported to cause FNAIT, PTP, and platelet transfusion refractoriness.[31,33-37]

GPVI

GPVI is a major collagen receptor on platelets and a member of the immunoglobulin superfamily. GPVI interactions with collagen exposed on the extracellular matrix result in platelet activation and aggregation. To date, no HPAs have been identified on GPVI, but platelet autoantibodies formed against GPVI have been reported to cause a mild form of autoimmune thrombocytopenia.[38,39] Interestingly, GPVI autoantibodies induce shedding of GPVI from platelets, resulting in reduced collagen binding and clinically significant bleeding.

HLA

HLA is present on all nucleated cells of the body. (See Chapter 16.) HLA associated with platelets is the main source of Class I HLA in whole blood.[40] Most Class I HLA on platelets is expressed as integral membrane proteins, whereas smaller amounts may be adsorbed from surrounding plasma. HLA-A and -B locus antigens are significantly represented, but there appears to be only minimal platelet expression of HLA-C.[41] With rare exceptions, Class II HLA is not present on the platelet membrane.

Transfusion-associated HLA alloimmunization appears to be influenced by the underlying disease, immunosuppressive effects of treatment regimens, and whether the blood components contain a significant amount of leukocytes. Widespread use of leukocyte-reduced blood components has considerably reduced HLA alloimmunization from transfusion.[42] Despite white cell inactivation by pathogen inactivation technologies, pathogen-reduced platelet transfusions are associated with more HLA alloimmunization and immune transfusion refractoriness.[43,44] HLA antibodies also commonly develop following pregnancy and are present in the sera of >32% of women who have had four or more pregnancies.[45] HLA antibodies have also been identified in 1.4% to 3.3% of women who have never been pregnant or received transfusion and men with no previous transfusions, and not all such antibodies recognize only denatured bead-coating antigens.[46] Sensitization to HLA antigens becomes important in platelet transfusion recipients when HLA antibodies cause destruction of allogeneic platelets, contributing to platelet transfusion refractoriness.

Alloimmune Platelet Disorders

Platelet Transfusion Refractoriness

A less-than-expected increase in platelet count occurs in about 25% to 70% of patients with thrombocytopenia who have received multiple transfusions.[47] Patients treated for malignant hematopoietic disorders are particularly likely to become refractory to platelet transfusions. Responses to platelet transfusions are often determined 10 to 60 minutes after transfusion by calculating either a corrected platelet count increment (CCI) or a percentage platelet recovery (PPR), both of which normalize transfusion responses for patient blood volume and platelet dose. (See Chapter 19 for more on CCIs.) Most experts would agree that a 1-hour posttransfusion CCI of <5000 to 7500 or a PPR of platelets transfused or a PPR <30% after two consecutive transfusions adequately defines the refractory state.

HLA sensitization is the most common immune cause of refractoriness and can be diagnosed by demonstration of significant levels of antibodies to Class I HLA in the refractory patient's serum. (See Chapter 16 for more information on detecting HLA antibodies.) Other immune causes to be considered include antibodies to HPA, ABO incompatibility, and drug-induced antibodies.

Poor platelet recovery (1-hour CCI) is usually caused by antibody-mediated destruction, severe splenic sequestration, massive bleeding, or a combination of nonimmune factors affecting platelet survival (18- to 24-hour CCI). Some of the most commonly cited nonimmune factors associated with refractoriness are listed in Table 15-3. Even when possible immune causes of refractoriness are identified, nonimmune factors are often simultaneously present.[48,49]

Selection of Platelets for Transfusion in Patients with Alloimmune Refractoriness

Several strategies may be considered when selecting platelets for transfusion to patients with alloimmune refractoriness. When HLA antibodies are present, a widely used approach is to supply apheresis platelets from donors whose HLA-A and -B antigens match those of the patient. A pool of 1000 to 3000 or more HLA-typed apheresis donors is generally necessary to find HLA-identical donors for most patients.[50]

When exact matches are unavailable, it is useful to directly determine the specificity of the patient's HLA antibodies and select donors whose platelets lack the corresponding antigens.[48,49,51] This antibody specificity prediction (ASP) method is at least as effective as selection by HLA matching or platelet crossmatching and is superior to random selection of platelets. Furthermore, many more potential HLA-typed donors are identified by the ASP method than are available using traditional HLA-matching criteria.[51]

A popular, although outmoded, system graded components by their degree of mismatch, that is, within or outside so-called cross-reactive groups (CREGs). An "A grade" was a perfect four-out-of-four match for the HLA-A and HLA-B alleles. A BU/B2U grade contained a single mismatch with one or two antigens, respectively. A BX grade had a single mismatch, with one antigen cross-reactive with a known antibody within a CREG. C and D grade matches had three

TABLE 15-3. Causes of Platelet Refractoriness[48]

Nonimmune	Immune
Fever	HLA antibodies
Medications (eg, amphotericin, vancomycin)	ABO incompatibility
Hepatic or splenic sequestration	Human platelet antigen (HPA) antibodies
Sepsis	Drug-dependent autoantibodies
Disseminated intravascular coagulation	Autoantibodies secondary to lymphoproliferative disease
Hemorrhage	Immune thrombocytopenia
Graft-vs-host disease	
Prolonged platelet storage	
Thrombotic microangiopathy (TTP; HUS, drug-induced)	

TTP = thrombotic thrombocytopenia; HUS = hemolytic uremic syndrome.

and four mismatched alleles, respectively. Since the advent of the single-bead assay, the importance of CREGs has diminished, as antigen-specific reactivity is known (see Chapter 16 for more detail).

A best-mismatch estimation can also be performed in a more automated fashion by comparing donor and recipient immunogenic epitopes, stereochemical amino acid "eplets," on exposed quaternary HLA protein structures. An Excel spreadsheet is available that computes the total number of mismatches between donor and recipient HLA antigens, with <11 mismatches resulting in better posttransfusion CCIs.[52]

Pretransfusion crossmatching of the patient's serum against platelets from potential donors is an additional approach to provide effective platelet transfusions to patients with alloimmune refractoriness.[53] Each potential platelet unit is tested in the crossmatch assay with a current sample of the patient's serum. The solid-phase red cell adherence (SPRCA) test is the most widely used method.[54] Although less successful than published HLA-identical or antigen-negative success rates, crossmatching is more widely available and significantly faster than waiting for HLA test results.[53] It avoids exclusion of HLA-mismatched but compatible donors and has the added advantage of facilitating the selection of platelets when platelet-specific antibodies are present.

Platelet crossmatching, however, will not always be successful, particularly when patients are highly alloimmunized or have interfering ABO antibodies, which can make finding sufficient amounts of compatible platelets problematic. Although the incidence of platelet-specific antibodies causing patients to be transfusion-refractory is very small, this possibility should be investigated when most of the crossmatches are unexpectedly incompatible or when HLA-matched transfusions fail. If platelet-specific antibodies are present, donors of known platelet antigen phenotype or family members, who may be more likely to share the patient's phenotype, should be tested. Platelet crossmatching or HPA genotyping should be considered for patients who do not respond to ABO- and HLA-compatible platelets.

HLA-selected and -crossmatched platelets should be irradiated to prevent transfusion-associated graft-vs-host disease (TA-GVHD).[55(p41)] Because these platelets are selected to minimize incompatible antigens, they are more likely to cause TA-GVHD because the recipient's immune system may fail to recognize donor T lymphocytes as foreign. Irradiation prevents the lymphocyte proliferation required for TA-GVHD.

Fetal and Neonatal Alloimmune Thrombocytopenia

FNAIT (also known as neonatal alloimmune thrombocytopenia and abbreviated as NATP or NAIT) is a syndrome involving immune destruction of fetal platelets by maternal antibody analogous to red cell destruction in hemolytic disease of the fetus and newborn. During pregnancy, a mother may become sensitized to an incompatible paternal antigen on fetal platelets. IgG specific for the platelet antigen crosses the placenta, causing immune platelet destruction and thrombocytopenia.

FNAIT is the most common cause of severe fetal/neonatal thrombocytopenia, and affected infants are at risk of major bleeding complications, especially intracranial hemorrhage. The most commonly implicated platelet antigen incompatibility in FNAIT is HPA-1a, but all HPAs identified to date have been implicated.[56] A serologic diagnosis of FNAIT may be made by: 1) testing maternal serum for platelet antibodies using assays that can differentiate platelet-specific from non-platelet-specific reactivity, and 2) performing platelet genotyping on parental DNA.[57] Demonstration of both a platelet-specific (HPA) antibody in the maternal serum and the corresponding incompatibility for the antigen in the parental platelet types confirms the diagnosis.

Treatment of acutely thrombocytopenic newborns includes the administration of intravenous immune globulin (IVIG) with or without antigen-compatible platelet transfusions, occasionally provided by the mother as washed components when higher-frequency antigen-negative donors are unavailable.[58] When antigen-negative platelets are not available, random units may also be effective.[59] Once the diagnosis of FNAIT has been made in a family, subsequent fetuses are at risk. Antenatal treatment with IVIG with or without steroids has proven to be an effective means of moderating fetal thrombocytopenia and preventing intracranial hemorrhage.[60] (For a more in-depth discussion of FNAIT, see Chapter 23.)

Posttransfusion Purpura

PTP is a rare syndrome characterized by the development of dramatic, sudden, and self-limiting thrombocytopenia 5 to 10 days after a blood transfusion in patients with a previous history of HPA sensitization by pregnancy or transfusion.[61] Coincident with the thrombocytopenia is the recrudescence of a potent platelet-specific alloantibody, usually anti-HPA-1a, in the patient's plasma. Other specificities have been implicated; these are almost always associated with antigens on GPIIb/IIIa. The patient's own antigen-negative platelets as well as transfused platelets are destroyed. The pathogenesis of autologous platelet destruction is not fully understood. Mounting evidence suggests the development of transient platelet autoantibodies along with the alloantibodies.[62] These panreactive autoantibodies often target the same glycoprotein that expresses the allo-targeted HPA.

Platelet antibody assays usually reveal serum antibody specificity, usually anti-HPA-1a. Genotyping documents the absence of HPA-1a or other platelet-specific antigens. IVIG is first-line therapy, successfully elevating platelet counts in days. Plasma exchange, which is less effective than the primary therapy, is employed in the 10% to 15% of IVIG failures.[61] Antigen-negative platelets transfused following the institution of treatment appear to survive somewhat better than unselected units.[63]

After recovery, future platelet transfusions should be from antigen-negative donors. Interestingly, the frequency of PTP has significantly decreased with the introduction of leukocyte-reduced blood components.[64] Although no data have been reported to explain this trend, use of leukocyte-reduced components may also be of benefit in reducing the risk of PTP.

Drug-Induced Thrombocytopenia

Thrombocytopenia caused by drug-induced platelet antibodies is a recognized complication of drug therapy. Drugs commonly implicated include quinine, sulfa drugs, vancomycin, piperacillin, GPIIb/IIIa antagonists, and heparin.[65,66] Both drug-dependent antibodies and non-drug-dependent antibodies may be produced. Non-drug-dependent antibodies, although stimulated by drugs, do not require the continued presence of the drug to be reactive with platelets and are serologically indistinguishable from other platelet autoantibodies.

Although several mechanisms for drug-induced antibody formation have been described, most clinically relevant drug-dependent platelet antibodies are thought to result when a drug interacts with platelet membrane glycoproteins, inducing conformational changes recognized by the humoral immune system and development of drug-dependent antibodies.[67,68] These antibodies can cause the sudden, rapid onset of thrombocytopenia that usually resolves within 3 to 4 days after drug discontinuation.

Immune responses triggered by exposure to heparin are particularly important because of both the widespread use of this anticoagulant and the devastating thrombotic complications associated with the heparin-induced thrombocytopenia (HIT) syndrome.[69] The incidence rate of HIT is unknown, but it may develop in up to 5% of patients treated with unfractionated heparin. Low-molecular-weight heparin is less likely to be associated with HIT than unfractionated heparin.

A reduction in baseline platelet count by 30% to 50% generally occurs within 5 to 14 days after primary exposure to heparin, or sooner if the patient has been exposed to heparin within the last 3 months. The platelet count is often <100,000/µL but usually recovers within 5 to 7 days upon discontinuation of heparin. More than 50% of patients with HIT develop thrombosis, which can occur in the arterial or venous system, or both.[70] Patients may develop sometimes-fatal stroke, myocardial infarction, limb or other organ ischemia, or deep venous thrombosis. It is thus of critical importance to discontinue heparin therapy when a diagnosis of HIT is suspected. Moreover, strong consideration should be given to using an alternative (nonheparin) anticoagulant (eg, a direct thrombin inhibitor) to prevent thrombosis.[70]

The mechanism of HIT involves formation of a complex between heparin and platelet factor 4 (PF4), a tetrameric protein released from platelet α granules. IgG antibodies to the complex attach secondarily to platelet FcγRIIa receptors via their Fc region, resulting in platelet activation, thrombin generation, and thrombosis.

Autoimmune or Immune Thrombocytopenia

Immune thrombocytopenia (ITP) is an immune platelet disorder in which autoantibodies are directed against platelet antigens, resulting in platelet destruction.[71,72] Chronic ITP, which is most common in adults, is characterized by an insidious onset and moderate thrombocytopenia that may exist for months to years before diagnosis. Females are twice as likely to be affected as males.

Spontaneous remissions are rare, and treatment is usually required to raise the platelet count. First-line therapy consists of steroids or IVIG followed by more potent immunosuppressive agents and, less frequently, splenectomy in nonresponders.[73] Many other therapies have been used in patients who do not respond to splenectomy, with variable results.

Chronic ITP may be idiopathic or associated with other conditions, such as human immunodeficiency virus infection, malignancy, or other autoimmune diseases. Acute ITP is mainly a childhood disease characterized by the abrupt onset of severe thrombocytopenia and bleeding symptoms, often after a viral infection. The majority of cases resolve spontaneously over a 2- to 6-month period. If treatment is required, IVIG or anti-D immunoglobulin infusions given to D-positive patients are usually effective in raising platelet counts. Ostensibly blockading reticuloendothelial system Fc receptors, these modalities may have additional mechanisms of action.[74] Steroids are used less often because of their serious side effects in children. Splenecto-

my, if used, is reserved for children whose disease is severe and lasts >6 months; this condition is similar to chronic ITP in adults. Rituximab and various thrombopoietin receptor agonists have been used as second-line therapies for acute ITP.[72,73]

Studies of both sera and washed platelets from patients with ITP have identified IgG, IgM, and IgA autoantibodies that are reactive with a number of platelet surface-membrane structures that most often include GP complexes IIb/IIIa, Ia/IIa, and Ib/IX but can also include GPIV, GPV, and GPVI.[75] In the majority of cases, platelet-associated autoantibodies are reactive with two or more platelet glycoproteins.[76] There is no compelling evidence to date suggesting that a patient's profile of autoantibody specificities correlates with the severity of the disease or predicts that patient's response to therapy.

Testing for Platelet Antigens and Antibodies

Laboratory detection of platelet antibodies provides important results to aid in clinical diagnosis of an immune platelet disorder. A comprehensive workup for platelet antibodies requires the use of multiple test methods, including a glycoprotein-specific assay, a test employing intact/whole platelets, and HPA genotyping.[57,77] Glycoprotein-specific assays are the most sensitive and specific for identifying the HPA specificity of serum antibodies (Fig 15-1).

The inclusion of assays that use intact platelet targets is critical for detection of antibodies that can be missed by glycoprotein-specific tests because the process of platelet lysis with detergent and capture of glycoprotein with a specific monoclonal antibody can disrupt HPA epitopes recognized by some antibodies. HPA genotyping by DNA methods is helpful to confirm the HPA specificity of the alloantibodies and for prenatal typing of a fetus in suspected cases of FNAIT. The test methods that follow are examples of the current state-of-the-art methods used by reference laboratories. For in-depth descriptions of platelet antibody and antigen testing, readers should consult recent reviews.[57,78,79]

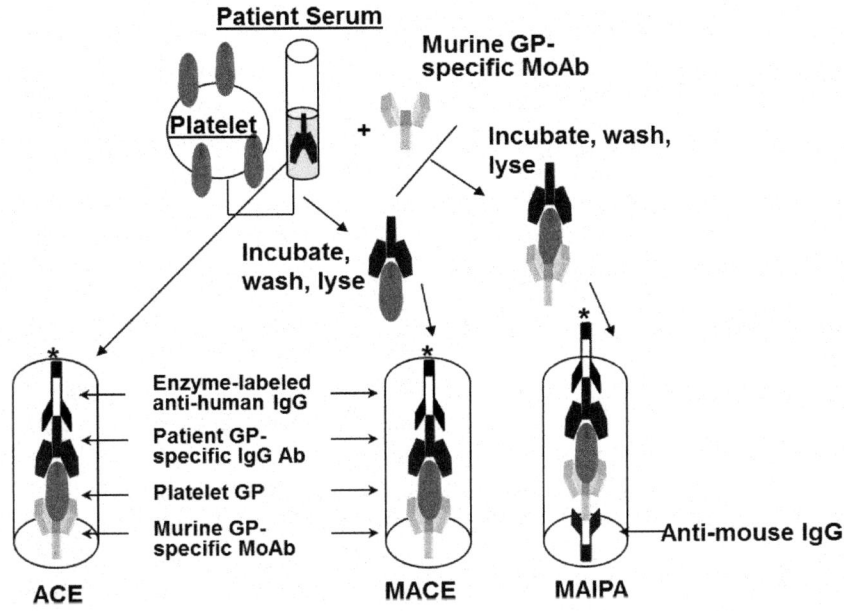

FIGURE 15-1. Enzyme-linked immunosorbent assay (ELISA) testing. Antigen capture ELISA (ACE) employs microtiter well plates precoated with adherent glycoproteins (GPs) to screen patient serum for GP-specific antibody (Ab). It can be modified (modified-ACE, or MACE) by preincubation of patient serum with target platelets, followed by washing and lytic solubilization of platelet GPs. The lysate is added to microtiter plate wells for capture of platelet GP by a specific mouse immunoglobulin G (IgG) monoclonal antibody (MoAb). Platelet GP-specific IgG Ab in the patient's serum bound to the GP is detected by the addition of an enzyme-labeled goat antihuman IgG and chromogenic substrate. The monoclonal Ab immobilization of platelet antigens (MAIPA) assay is very similar to the MACE, but the patient's serum and MoAb are incubated with platelets before washing and platelet GP solubilization, and the patient GP-specific Ab/GP/MoAb complex is captured by goat antimouse IgG adherent to the well bottom. There is a progressive increase in test sensitivity from ACE to MAIPA.

Assays Using Intact Platelets

An assay that is widely used for the detection of platelet-specific antibodies and for platelet cross-matching is the SPRCA assay.[54] Intact platelets are immobilized in round-bottomed wells of a microtiter plate and are then incubated with the patient's serum. After washing, detector red cells coated with antihuman IgG are added, and the mixture is centrifuged and examined visually. The method's main limitations are its subjective endpoint and failure to distinguish platelet-specific (ie, platelet glycoprotein-directed/HPA) from non-platelet-specific antibodies (ie, ABO or HLA antibodies). Antibodies to glycoproteins with low surface copy numbers may also be difficult to detect.

Flow cytometry is commonly used for immunofluorescent detection of platelet antibodies using intact platelets.[57] Following incubation of platelets with the patient's serum, platelet-bound antibodies are detected with a fluorescently labeled antiglobulin reagent specific for human IgG or IgM. The results can be expressed as a ratio of mean or median channel fluorescence of platelets sensitized with patient serum to that of platelets incubated with negative control serum. Platelet autoantibodies coating patient platelets can also be detected in a direct flow cytometry assay.[80]

Flow cytometry has proven to be a very sensitive method for detection of antibodies to platelets. Alloantibodies specific for labile epitopes and unreliably detected by ACAs can be detected with intact platelets using flow cytometry.[13] Flow cytometry does not differentiate between platelet-specific and non-platelet-specific antibodies. This is a drawback when investigating FNAIT or PTP because more relevant platelet-specific antibodies can be obscured by non-platelet-specific reactivity.

Antigen Capture and Other Assays

Platelet glycoprotein ACAs are used to determine the HPA that is recognized by platelet antibodies in a patient's serum. Commonly employed assays include enzyme-linked immunosorbent assays (ACE, MACE, and MAIPA) (Fig 15-1).[57,81] The assays require the use of monoclonal antibodies that recognize the target antigens of interest but do not compete with the patient's antibody. These assays capture specific platelet glycoproteins on plastic wells of a microplate after sensitization with the patient's serum. The patient's bound antibody is detected with an enzyme-labeled antihuman globulin. Because only the glycoproteins of interest are immobilized, interference by reactions from non-platelet-specific antibodies, especially anti-HLA, is eliminated. A different solid-phase assay affixes HPA antigens to microbeads that are exposed first to patient serum and then a fluorescently labeled antihuman globulin. Specific binding can be detected with the use of a Luminex mini-flow platform.[82,83] Care must be taken when using commercial ACAs that antibodies to the HPAs most commonly associated with specific disease states are detectable by the assay.

Platelet Genotyping

Genotyping for the SNPs in the genes encoding HPA can be performed by any of the myriad molecular methods available. Allele-specific polymerase chain reaction (PCR) and restriction fragment length polymorphism analysis are two methods that have been used successfully.[77]

These techniques are reliable, but they are also laborious and time consuming. Higher-throughput methods have been developed, such as real-time PCR, melting curve analysis, allele-specific fluorescent beadchip probes, and next-generation sequencing.[78,84]

Testing for Platelet Autoantibodies

Numerous assays have been developed to detect platelet autoantibodies in patients with ITP. Although many tests are quite sensitive, particularly in detecting cell-surface, platelet-associated immunoglobulins, none has been sufficiently specific to be particularly useful in either the diagnosis or the management of ITP. The American Society of Hematology practice guidelines for ITP state that serologic testing is unnecessary, assuming that the clinical findings are compatible with the diagnosis.[71] However, platelet antibody tests may be helpful in the evaluation of patients suspected of having ITP when nonimmune causes may be present. The goal of serologic testing in ITP is to detect autoantibody bound to the patient's own platelets with or without demonstration of similar reactivity in patient plasma.

Newer assays are designed to detect immunoglobulin binding to platelet-specific epitopes found on platelet GPIIb/IIIa, GPIa/IIa, and/or GPIb/V/IX complexes. These solid-phase, GP-specific assays appear to have improved specificity in distinguishing ITP from nonimmune thrombocytopenia, but this benefit is often balanced by a decrease in sensitivity.[76,85] One commercially available test uses eluates prepared from the patient's washed platelets.[76] The eluates are tested against a panel of monoclonal-antibody-immobilized platelet glycoprotein complexes, and platelet antibodies are detected using an enzyme-linked antihuman globulin. In the indirect phase of the assay, patient plasma is tested against the same glycoprotein panel. Although autoantibodies are most often detected in the eluates, they are infrequently detected (in approximately 17% of cases) in the plasma. Patients with ITP may have antibodies that are reactive with one or several GP targets.[76]

Testing for Drug-Dependent Platelet Antibodies

Any platelet serology test used to detect platelet-bound immunoglobulin can be modified to detect drug-dependent antibodies. Each patient serum sample should be tested against normal platelets in the presence and absence of the drug. Moreover, at least one normal serum sample should be tested with and without the drug to control for nonspecific antibody binding that may occur in the drug's presence. A positive control sample known to be reactive with the drug being assayed should be tested with and without the drug to complete the evaluation. A positive result demonstrates greater reactivity against normal platelets in the presence of the drug than without and demonstrates that the drug did not nonspecifically cause a positive result with normal serum controls. Flow cytometry is the most sensitive and most commonly used method to detect both IgG and IgM drug-dependent antibodies.[57,86] Limitations to detection of drug-dependent platelet antibodies include the following: 1) for many drugs, the optimal concentration for antibody detection has not been determined, and hydrophobic drugs are difficult to solubilize; 2) the presence of nondrug antibodies can mask drug-related antibodies; and 3) a patient may be sensitized to a drug metabolite and not the native drug.

Assays for heparin-dependent antibodies include ELISA using microtiter wells coated with complexes of PF4 and heparin or heparin-like molecules (eg, polyvinyl sulfonate).[87] Optical density values above cutoff that can be inhibited by added high-dose heparin confirms the presence of heparin-dependent antibodies. Although IgG antibodies are the most clinically relevant antibodies, a few patients with HIT appear to have only IgM or IgA antibodies detectable in variants of this assay.

These assays are sensitive but not specific for the subset of antibodies that result in clinically significant platelet activation and thrombosis. The ^{14}C-serotonin release assay (SRA) is a functional assay for detection of this type of antibody.[88] Other functional tests include heparin-induced platelet aggregation and various other measures of platelet activation (adenosine tri-phosphate release, phosphatidylserine exposure, etc). In asymptomatic patients receiving heparin or anticipating its use, neither PF4 ELISA nor functional tests are sufficiently predictive of HIT to warrant use as screening tests.[89]

GRANULOCYTE ANTIGENS AND ANTIBODIES

Antibodies against granulocyte (neutrophil) antigens are implicated in the following clinical syndromes: neonatal alloimmune neutropenia (NAN), transfusion-related acute lung injury (TRALI), febrile transfusion reactions, primary or secondary autoimmune neutropenia (AIN), refractoriness to granulocyte transfusion, transfusion-related alloimmune neutropenia, and immune neutropenia after hematopoietic progenitor cell (HPC) transplantation. To date, 10 neutrophil antigens carried on five different glycoproteins have been characterized and given human neutrophil alloantigen (HNA) designations by the Granulocyte Antigen Working Party of the International Society of Blood Transfusion (Table 15-4).[90] This nomenclature system follows a convention similar to that used for HPA nomenclature. Several of the antigens on granulocytes are shared with other cells and are not granulocyte specific.

HNA

Antigens on FcγRIIIb

The first granulocyte-specific antigen detected was NA1, later named HNA-1a. Five alleles of HNA-1 have now been identified, encoding three antigens: HNA-1a, HNA-1b, and HNA-1c, which are located on the protein FcγRIIIb (CD16b).[90] Recently, another epitope on HN-1b, termed HNA-1d, was described.[91] FcγRIIIb is a GPI-linked protein receptor for the Fc region of IgG and is present only on the surfaces of neutrophils. Three alleles encode HNA-1b: one encoding HNA-1b alone, one along with HNA-1c, and another with HNA-1d.[91] Neutrophils express 100,000 to 200,000 molecules of FcγRIIIb, but there are rare individuals (approximately 0.1%) whose neutrophils express no FcγRIIIb (CD16 null) and who can produce anti-

TABLE 15-4. Human Neutrophil Antigens

Antigen	Phenotypic Frequency*	Glycoprotein	Amino Acid Change	Encoding Gene	Nucleotide Change
HNA-1a	12% a/a	CD16b	Multiple[†]	FCGR3B	Multiple[†]
HNA-1b	54% a/b				
	46% b/b				
HNA-1c	5%				
HNA-2	97% CD177+	CD177	N/A	CD177	N/A
HNA-2 null	3% CD177−				
HNA-3a	56%-59% a/a	CTL2	Arg152Gln	SLC44A2	455G>A
HNA-3b	34%-40% a/b				
	3%-6% b/b				
HNA-4a	78.6% a/a	CD11b	Arg61His	ITGAM	230G>A
HNA-4b	19.3% a/b				
	2.1% b/b				
HNA-5a	54.3% a/a	CD11a	Arg766Thr	ITGAL	2466G>C
HNA-5b	38.6% a/b				
	7.1% b/b				

	Nucleotide Changes						Amino Acid Changes					
	141	147	227	266	277	349	36	38	65	78	82	106
HNA-1a	G	C	A	C	G	G	Arg	Leu	Asn	Ala	Asp	Val
HNA-1b	C	T	G	C	A	A	Ser	Leu	Ser	Ala	Asn	Ile
HNA-1c	C	T	G	A	A	A	Ser	Leu	Ser	Asp	Asn	Ile

*Phenotypic frequencies are for people of European ancestry who live in North America.
[†]HNA-1 amino acid and nucleotide changes are shown in a separate section of the table.
HNA = human neutrophil antigen; N/A = not applicable.

bodies that are reactive with FcγRIIIb when they are exposed to it through transfusion or pregnancy.[92,93] Antibodies to HNA-1a and -1b have been implicated in TRALI, NAN, and AIN, and antibodies to HNA-1c and -1d have resulted in NAN.[91,94,95]

Antigens on CD177

HNA-2 (previously known as NB1) is not an alloantigen because HNA-2 antibodies are isoantibodies that recognize common epitopes on CD177 protein, which is missing from the neutrophils of immunized individuals. Neutrophils from approximately 1% to 11% of people lack expression of CD177.[94-96] The genetic basis of CD177 deficiency is SNPs leading to truncated mRNAs with premature stop codons.[97] Interestingly, CD177 is expressed only on a neutrophil subpopulation in CD177-positive individuals.[98] The proportion of the CD177-positive neutrophil population ranges from 0% to 100%, with a median of 60%.[99,100] Among individuals homozygous for CD177, neutrophil subpopulations are due to the epigenetic silencing of either the maternal or paternal allele, with both alleles inactivated in some neutrophils.[100] Both CD177 alleles are expressed in hematopoietic stem cells, but one of the two alleles is silenced during neutrophil differentiation.[100] This explains the increased CD177 subpopulation size in healthy people given granulocyte colony-stimulating factor (G-CSF) and in patients with polycythemia vera.

In neutrophils, CD177 is physically associated with the neutrophil serine proteinase 3 (PR3) and the b_2 integrin Mac-1 (CD11b/CD18). CD177 recognizes platelet and endothelial cell adhesion molecule 1 (PECAM-1), an immunoglobulin family molecule expressed on endothelial cells, platelets, and some leukocytes. The migration, through human umbilical vein endothelial cells, of neutrophils that express CD177 is more efficient than that of CD177-negative neutrophils due to a PECAM-1-dependent mechanism. Recent studies have shown that CD177 signals in a b_2-integrin-dependent manner, which leads to impaired neutrophil migration.[101]

Antibodies against HNA-2 have been implicated in NAN, TRALI, AIN, and neutropenia in hematopoietic stem cell transplant recipients.[102-104] Interestingly, autoantibodies directed against the CD177-associated protein PR3 are found in patients with antineutrophil cytoplasmic antibody (ANCA)-associated vasculitis. Patients with ANCA vasculitis have been found to have a larger mean CD177 subpopulation size than healthy people.[100]

Antigens on CTL2

HNA-3a and HNA-3b are carried on the choline transporter-like protein 2 (CTL2), and an SNP in the gene (*SLC44A2*) accounts for the polymorphism (Table 15-4).[105,106] CTL2 is also expressed on both T and B lymphocytes, platelets, and vascular endothelium. HNA-3a antibodies are usually agglutinins. They occasionally develop in women after pregnancy, and HNA-3a antibodies are the most frequent cause of fatal TRALI, in addition to causing febrile reactions and NAN.[107] HNA-3b antibodies are rarely detected,

but several have been found during screening of the serum of multiparous blood donors and recently reported to result in NAN.[108]

Antigens on CD11a and CD11b

HNA-4a/4b and HNA-5a antigens are present on monocytes and lymphocytes as well as granulocytes. HNA-4a is carried on the CD11b/18 (Mac-1, CR3, $\alpha_m b_2$) glycoprotein.[90] CD11b/18 plays a role in neutrophil adhesion to endothelial cells and phagocytosis of C3bi opsonized microbes. There is some evidence showing that pathogenic alloantibodies against HNA-4a interfere with CD11b/18-dependent neutrophil adhesion and enhance neutrophil respiratory burst.[109] Antibodies against HNA-4a and -4b have been implicated in NAN, and autoantibodies against CD11b/18 have also been described.[110,111]

HNA-5a is carried on CD11a/18 (LFA-1, $\alpha_L b_2$) glycoprotein.[112] CD11a/18, like CD11b/18, plays a role in neutrophil adhesion to endothelial cells. Antibodies that are reactive with HNA-5a have been found in a chronic transfusion recipient with aplastic anemia and have also been reported to be associated with NAN.[111,113]

Other Neutrophil Antigens

Neutrophils do not express ABH or other red cell group antigens, but they do express modest amounts of HLA Class I, as well as HLA Class II upon activation.

Immune Neutrophil Disorders

Neonatal Alloimmune Neutropenia

NAN is caused by maternal antibodies against the antigens on fetal neutrophils; the most frequent specificities are those against HNA-1a, HNA-1b, and HNA-2 antigens, although HNA-1c, -1d, -3a, -3b, -4a, -4b, and -5a have caused this syndrome. NAN may also occur in the children of women who lack the FcγRIIIb protein. Neutropenia in NAN can occasionally be life-threatening because of increased susceptibility to infection.[114] Management with antibiotics, IVIG, G-CSF, and/or plasma exchange may be helpful.

TRALI

TRALI is an acute, often life-threatening reaction characterized by respiratory distress, hypotension or hypertension, and noncardiogenic pulmonary edema that occurs within 6 hours of a blood component transfusion.[115] TRALI represented 30% of transfusion-associated fatalities reported to the US Food and Drug Administration over the last 5 reported fiscal years, second only to circulatory overload fatalities.[116] In severe TRALI, causative antibodies are most often found in the plasma of blood donors. When these antibodies are transfused, they cause activation of primed neutrophils that are sequestered in the lungs of certain patients. The activated neutrophils undergo oxidative burst, releasing toxic substances that damage pulmonary endothelium and resulting in capillary leak and pulmonary edema. HNA and Class II HLA antibodies are thought to be more pathogenic than Class I HLA antibodies.[117] (For a more in-depth discussion of TRALI, see Chapter 22.)

Autoimmune Neutropenia

AIN may occur in adults or in infants. When present in adults, it is generally persistent and may be idiopathic or secondary to autoimmune diseases, malignancies, or infections.[118] In AIN of infancy, the autoantibody has neutrophil antigen specificity (usually HNA-1a, but occasionally -1b or -4a) in about 60% of patients.[114] This condition is generally self-limiting and relatively benign, with recovery usually occurring in 7 to 24 months.[119]

Testing for Granulocyte Antibodies and Antigens

Granulocyte antibody testing is technically complex and labor-intensive. The inability to maintain the integrity of granulocytes at room temperature, in refrigerated conditions, or by cryopreservation requires that cells be isolated from fresh blood on each day of testing. This demands that readily available blood donors typed for the various granulocyte antigens be available. Class I HLA antibodies that are often present in patient sera complicate detection and identification of granulocyte antibodies. For these reasons, it is critical that granulocyte antibody and antigen testing be performed by an experienced laboratory using appropriate controls.

Granulocyte Agglutination Test

This was one of the first tests developed for the detection of granulocyte antibodies. It is typically performed by overnight incubation of small volumes of isolated fresh neutrophils with the patient's serum in a microplate. The wells are viewed under an inverted phase microscope for neutrophil agglutination or aggregation.

Granulocyte Immunofluorescence Test

This test also requires fresh target cells that are incubated, usually at room temperature for 30 minutes, and washed in EDTA and phosphate-buffered saline. Neutrophil-bound antibodies are then detected with fluorescein-isothiocyanate-labeled antihuman IgG or IgM using either a fluorescence microscope or a flow cytometer.[120] A combination of agglutination and immunofluorescence tests is beneficial.[106] Other methods include chemiluminescence, SPRCA, and the monoclonal antibody-specific immobilization of granulocyte antigens (MAIGA) assay, which is similar to the MAIPA assay but uses monoclonal antibodies to capture the various glycoproteins that express HNA. The MAIGA assay is used to differentiate between HLA- and HNA-specific antibodies.

Luminex-Based Antibody Identification

Microbeads coated with HNA antigens have been developed that can detect anti-HNA-1a, -1b, -1c, -2, -3a, -3b, -4a, -5a, and -5b antibodies.[121] Although rates of false positives remain high (5.5%), for anti-HNA-1a, -1b, -1c, -2, and -3a, sensitivity has been reported to be ≥90%.[121]

HNA Typing

As with HPA, typing for HNA is performed largely using molecular methods to detect the allelic variants that determine the antigens. Any methods used in HPA typing can be applied to HNA typing with simple modifications to the primer and probe sequences. Readers are referred to several publications on this subject.[122,123] Because the molecular defect that results in CD177 deficiency is variable, typing for HNA-2/CD177 has traditionally required serologic testing on freshly isolated neutrophils using specific monoclonal antibodies. Testing may evolve as the SNPs responsible for some individuals' loss of expression are confirmed.[97]

KEY POINTS

1. Platelets express a variety of antigenic markers on their surfaces. Some of these types of antigens, such as ABH and HLA, are shared with other cells, whereas HPAs are essentially platelet specific. There are currently 35 numbered HPAs carried on six platelet glycoproteins.

2. HLA Class I sensitization is the most common immune cause of platelet refractoriness and can be diagnosed by the demonstration of significant levels of antibodies to HLA-A and -B in patient serum. When antibodies to HLA antigens are demonstrated, widely used treatment approaches supply apheresis platelets from HLA-identical donors, those without antigens to which the recipient is sensitized, or crossmatch-compatible platelets.

3. Presumed-compatible HLA mismatches perform least-well. HLA-selected platelets should be irradiated to prevent transfusion-associated GVHD.

4. HPA antibodies are less commonly responsible for platelet transfusion refractoriness, but in such cases, genotypically matched or crossmatch-compatible apheresis platelets are required.

5. Sensitization to HPA is the most common cause of FNAIT, a syndrome involving immune destruction of fetal platelets by maternal antibody. Platelet-specific antibodies are also involved in PTP, a rare syndrome characterized by severe thrombocytopenia that occurs 5 to 10 days after a blood transfusion. The most commonly implicated antibody in both conditions is anti-HPA-1a. Serologic testing using intact platelets and antigen capture assays together with HPA genotyping is used to confirm both diagnoses.

6. Autoantibodies directed against platelet antigens may result in ITP. Chronic ITP, which is most common in adults, is characterized by an insidious onset and moderate thrombocytopenia that may be present for months to years before diagnosis. Females are twice as likely to be affected as males. The goal of serologic testing in ITP is to detect autoantibody bound to the patient's own platelets, although testing infrequently affects management.

7. Granulocyte (neutrophil) antigens are implicated in the clinical syndromes NAN, TRALI, febrile transfusion reactions, AIN, refractoriness to granulocyte transfusion, transfusion-related alloimmune neutropenia, and immune neutropenia after HPC transplantation.

8. Granulocyte antibody testing remains low-throughput and requires both immunofluorescence and agglutination methods supplemented by MAIGA to fully evaluate patient sera for antibodies.

REFERENCES

1. Deppermann C, Kubes P. Start a fire, kill the bug: The role of platelets in inflammation and infection. Innate Immun 2018;24(6):335-48.

2. Franco AT, Corken A, Ware J. Platelets at the interface of thrombosis, inflammation and cancer. Blood 2015;126:582-8.

3. Pasalic L, Wang SS, Chen VM. Platelets as biomarkers of coronary artery disease. Semin Thromb Hemost 2016;42:223-33.

4. Immuno polymorphism database. All HPA genetic information. Hinxton, UK: European Bioinformatics Institute, 2019. [Available at http://

www.ebi.ac.uk/ipd/hpa/table2.html (accessed June 7, 2019).]

5. Metcalfe P, Watkins NA, Ouwehand WH, et al. Nomenclature of human platelet antigens. Vox Sang 2003;85:240-5.

6. Jallu V, Beranger T, Bianchi F, et al. Cab4b, the first human platelet antigen carried by glycoprotein IX discovered in a context of severe neonatal thrombocytopenia. J Thromb Hemost 2017; 15:1646-54.

7. Sullivan MJ, Kuhlmann R, Peterson JA, Curtis BR. Severe neonatal alloimmune thrombocytopenia caused by maternal sensitization against a new low-frequency alloantigen (Dom[b]) located on platelet glycoprotein IIIa. Transfusion 2017; 57:1847-8.

8. Wihadmadyatami H, Heidinger K, Roder L, et al. Alloantibody against new platelet alloantigen (Lap[a]) on glycoprotein IIb is responsible for a case of fetal and neonatal alloimmune thrombocytopenia. Transfusion 2015;55:2920-9.

9. Aster RH, Newman PJ. HPA-1a/b(PlA1/ A2,Zwa/b): The odyssey of an alloantigen system. Immunohematology 2007;23:2-8.

10. Bennett JS, Berger BW, Billings PC. The structure and function of platelet integrins. J Thromb Haemost 2009;7(Suppl 1):200-5.

11. Nurden AT, Pillois X, Wilcox DA. Glanzmann thrombasthenia: State of the art and future directions. Semin Thromb Hemost 2013;39:642-55.

12. Lucas GF, Metcalfe P. Platelet and granulocyte glycoprotein polymorphisms. Transfus Med 2000;10:157-74.

13. Harrison CR, Curtis BR, McFarland JG, et al. Severe neonatal alloimmune thrombocytopenia caused by antibodies to human platelet antigen 3a (Bak[a]) detectable only in whole platelet assays. Transfusion 2003;43:1398-402.

14. Socher I, Zwingel C, Santoso S, Kroll H. Heterogeneity of HPA-3 alloantibodies: Consequences for the diagnosis of alloimmune thrombocytopenic syndromes. Transfusion 2008;48:463-72.

15. Koh Y, Ishii H, Amakishi E, et al. The first two cases of neonatal alloimmune thrombocytopenia associated with the low-frequency platelet antigen HPA-21bw (Nos) in Japan. Transfusion 2012;52:1468-75.

16. Peterson JA, Pechauer SM, Gitter ML, et al. The human platelet antigen-21bw is relatively common among Asians and is a potential trigger for neonatal alloimmune thrombocytopenia. Transfusion 2012;52:915-16.

17. Peterson JA, Balthazor SM, Curtis BR, et al. Maternal alloimmunization against the rare platelet-specific antigen HPA-9b (Max[a]) is an important cause of neonatal alloimmune thrombocytopenia. Transfusion 2005;45:1487-95.

18. Kaplan C, Porcelijn L, Vanlieferinghen P, et al. Anti-HPA-9bw (Max[a]) fetomaternal alloimmunization, a clinically severe neonatal thrombocytopenia: Difficulties in diagnosis and therapy and report on eight families. Transfusion 2005;45: 1799-803.

19. Andrews RK, Berndt MC. Bernard-Soulier syndrome: An update. Semin Thromb Hemost 2013;39:656-62.

20. Corral J, Rivera J, Gonzalez-Conejero R, Vicente V. The number of platelet glycoprotein Ia molecules is associated with the genetically linked 807 C/T and HPA-5 polymorphisms. Transfusion 1999;39:372-8.

21. Ertel K, Al-Tawil M, Santoso S, Kroll H. Relevance of the HPA-15 (Gov) polymorphism on CD109 in alloimmune thrombocytopenic syndromes. Transfusion 2005;45:366-73.

22. Mandelbaum M, Koren D, Eichelberger B, et al. Frequencies of maternal platelet alloantibodies and autoantibodies in suspected fetal/neonatal alloimmune thrombocytopenia, with emphasis on human platelet antigen-5 alloimmunization. Vox Sang 2005;89:39-43.

23. Berry JE, Murphy CM, Smith GA, et al. Detection of Gov system antibodies by MAIPA reveals an immunogenicity similar to the HPA-5 alloantigens. Br J Haematol 2000;110:735-42.

24. Vassallo RR. Recognition and management of antibodies to human platelet antigens in platelet transfusion-refractory patients. Immunohematology 2009;25:119-24.

25. Curtis BR, Edwards JT, Hessner MJ, et al. Blood group A and B antigens are strongly expressed on platelets of some individuals. Blood 2000;96: 1574-81.

26. Ogasawara K, Ueki J, Takenaka M, Furihata K. Study on the expression of ABH antigens on platelets. Blood 1993;82:993-9.

27. Skogen B, Rossebø Hansen B, Husebekk A, et al. Minimal expression of blood group A antigen on thrombocytes from A2 individuals. Transfusion 1988;28:456-9.

28. Slichter SJ, Davis K, Enright H, et al. Factors affecting posttransfusion platelet increments, platelet refractoriness, and platelet transfusion intervals in thrombocytopenic patients. Blood 2005;105:4106-14.

29. Triulzi DJ, Assmann SF, Strauss RG, et al. The impact of platelet transfusion characteristics on post-transfusion platelet increments and clinical bleeding in patients with hypo-proliferative thrombocytopenia. Blood 2012;119:5553-62.
30. Heal JM, Rowe JM, Blumberg N. ABO and platelet transfusion revisited. Ann Hematol 1993;66:309-14.
31. Dunstan RA, Simpson MB. Heterogeneous distribution of antigens on human platelets demonstrated by fluorescence flow cytometry. Br J Haematol 1985;61:603-9.
32. Spring FA, Judson PA, Daniels GL, et al. A human cell-surface glycoprotein that carries Cromer-related blood group antigens on erythrocytes and is also expressed on leucocytes and platelets. Immunology 1987;62:307-13.
33. Ghosh A, Murugusan G, Chen K, et al. Platelet CD36 surface expression levels affect functional responses to oxidized LSL and are associated with inheritance of specific genetic polymorphisms. Blood 2011;117:6355-66.
34. Curtis BR, Ali S, Glazier AM, et al. Isoimmunization against CD36 (glycoprotein IV): Description of four cases of neonatal isoimmune thrombocytopenia and brief review of the literature. Transfusion 2002;42:1173-9.
35. Rac ME, Safranow K, Poncyljusz W. Molecular basis of human CD36 gene mutations. Mol Med 2007;13:288-96.
36. Bierling P, Godeau B, Fromont P, et al. Post-transfusion purpura-like syndrome associated with CD36 (Nak^a) isoimmunization. Transfusion 1995;35:777-82.
37. Ikeda H, Mitani T, Ohnuma M, et al. A new platelet-specific antigen, Nak^a, involved in the refractoriness of HLA-matched platelet transfusion. Vox Sang 1989;57:213-17.
38. Boylan B, Chen H, Rathore V, et al. Anti-GPVI-associated ITP: An acquired platelet disorder caused by autoantibody-mediated clearance of the GPVI/FcRγ-chain complex from the human platelet surface. Blood 2004;104:1350-5.
39. Akiyama M, Kashiwagi H, Todo K, et al. Presence of platelet-associated anti-glycoprotein (GP)VI autoantibodies and restoration of GPVI expression in patients with GPVI deficiency. J Thromb Haemost 2009;7:1373-83.
40. Bialek JW, Bodmer W, Bodmer J, Payne R. Distribution and quantity of leukocyte antigens in the formed elements of the blood. Transfusion 1966;6:193-204.
41. Saito S, Ota S, Seshimo H, et al. Platelet transfusion refractoriness caused by a mismatch in HLA-C antigens. Transfusion 2002;42:302-8.
42. Seftel MD, Growe GH, Petraszko T, et al. Universal prestorage leukoreduction in Canada decreases platelet alloimmunization and refractoriness. Blood 2004;103:333-9.
43. Estcourt LJ, Malouf R, Hopewell S, et al. Pathogen-reduced platelets for the prevention of bleeding. Cochrane Database Syst Rev 2017;7:CD009072.
44. Saris A, Kerkhoffs JL, Norris PJ, et al. The role of pathogen-reduced platelet transfusions on HLA alloimmunization in hemato-oncological patients. Transfusion 2019;59:470-81.
45. Triulzi DJ, Kleinman S, Kakaiya RM, et al. The effect of previous pregnancy and transfusion on HLA alloimmunization in blood donors: Implications for a transfusion-related acute lung injury risk reduction strategy. Transfusion 2009;49:1825-35.
46. Vassallo RR, Hsu S, Einarson M, et al. A comparison of two robotic platforms to screen platelet-pheresis donors for HLA antibodies as part of a transfusion-related acute lung injury mitigation strategy. Transfusion 2010;50:1766-77.
47. Kerkhoffs JL, Eikenboom JC, Van De Watering LM, et al. The clinical impact of platelet refractoriness: Correlation with bleeding and survival. Transfusion 2008;48:1959-65.
48. Hod E, Schwartz J. Platelet transfusion refractoriness. Br J Haematol 2008;142:348-60.
49. Vassallo RR Jr. New paradigms in the management of alloimmune refractoriness to platelet transfusions. Curr Opin Hematol 2007;14:655-63.
50. Bolgiano DC, Larson EB, Slichter SJ. A model to determine required pool size for HLA-typed community donor apheresis programs. Transfusion 1989;29:306-10.
51. Petz LD, Garratty G, Calhoun L, et al. Selecting donors of platelets for refractory patients on the basis of HLA antibody specificity. Transfusion 2000;40:1446-56.
52. Brooks EG, MacPherson BR, Fung MK. Validation of HLAMatchmaker algorithm in identifying acceptable HLA mismatches for thrombocytopenic patients refractory to platelet transfusions. Transfusion 2008;48:2159-66.
53. Vassallo RR, Fung M, Rebulla P, et al. Utility of cross-matched platelet transfusions in patients with hypoproliferative thrombocytopenia: A systematic review. Transfusion 2014;54:1180-91.

54. Rachel JM, Summers TC, Sinor LT, Plapp FV. Use of a solid phase red blood cell adherence method for pretransfusion platelet compatibility testing. Am J Clin Pathol 1988;90:63-8.

55. Gammon R, ed. Standards for blood banks and transfusion services. 32nd ed. Bethesda, MD: AABB, 2020.

56. Curtis BR. Recent progress in understanding the pathogenesis of fetal and neonatal alloimmune thrombocytopenia. Br J Haematol 2015;171:671-82.

57. Curtis B, McFarland J. Detection and identification of platelet antibodies and antigens in the clinical laboratory. Immunohematol 2009;25:125-35.

58. Peterson JA, McFarland JG, Curtis BR, Aster RH. Neonatal alloimmune thrombocytopenia: Pathogenesis, diagnosis and management. Br J Haematol 2013;161:3-14.

59. Kiefel V, Bassler D, Paes B, et al. Antigen-positive platelet transfusion in neonatal alloimmune thrombocytopenia (NAIT). Blood 2006;107:3761-3.

60. Pacheco LD, Berkowitz RL, Moise KJ Jr, et al. Fetal and neonatal alloimmune thrombocytopenia: A management algorithm based on risk stratification. Obstet Gynecol 2011;118:1157-63.

61. McFarland JG. Posttransfusion purpura. In: Popovsky MA, ed. Transfusion reactions. 4th ed. Bethesda, MD: AABB Press, 2012:263-87.

62. Taaning E, Tonnesen F. Pan-reactive platelet antibodies in post-transfusion purpura. Vox Sang 1999;76:120-3.

63. Brecher ME, Moore SB, Letendre L. Posttransfusion purpura: The therapeutic value of Pl^A1-negative platelets. Transfusion 1990;30:433-5.

64. Bolton-Maggs PHB, ed, Poles D, et al on behalf of the Serious Hazards of Transfusion (SHOT) Steering Group. The 2015 Annual SHOT Report. Manchester, UK: SHOT Office, 2016. [Available at https://www.shotuk.org/wp-content/uploads/myimages/SHOT-2015-Annual-Report-Web-Edition-Final-bookmarked-1.pdf (accessed October 16, 2019).]

65. Drug-induced immune thrombocytopenia: Results of the testing for drug-dependent platelet-reactive antibodies by the BloodCenter of Wisconsin, 1995-2015. Linked from: George JN. Platelets on the web: Drug-induced thrombocytopenia. Oklahoma City, OK: OUHSC, 2015. [Available at http://www.ouhsc.edu/platelets/ditp.html (accessed June 7, 2019).]

66. Reese JA, Li X, Hauben M, et al. Identifying drugs that cause acute thrombocytopenia: An analysis using 3 distinct methods. Blood 2010;116:2127-33.

67. Aster RH, Bougie DW. Drug-induced immune thrombocytopenia. N Engl J Med 2007;357:580-7.

68. Bougie DW, Wilker PR, Aster RH. Patients with quinine-induced immune thrombocytopenia have both "drug-dependent" and "drug-specific" antibodies. Blood 2006;108:922-7.

69. Greinacher A, Selleng K, Warkentin TE. Autoimmune heparin-induced thrombocytopenia. J Thromb Haemost 2017;15:2099-114.

70. Linkins LA, Dans AL, Moores LK, et al. Treatment and prevention of heparin-induced thrombocytopenia: Antithrombotic therapy and prevention of thrombosis. 9th ed. American College of Chest Physicians evidence-based clinical practice guidelines. Chest 2012;141(Suppl 2):e495S-530S.

71. Neunert C, Lim W, Crowther M, et al. The American Society of Hematology 2011 evidence-based practice guideline for immune thrombocytopenia. Blood 2011;117:4190-207.

72. Lambert MP, Gernsheimer TB. Clinical updates in adult immune thrombocytopenia. Blood 2017;128:2829-35.

73. Chaturvedi S, Arnold DM, McCrae KR. Splenectomy for immune thrombocytopenia: Down but not out. Blood 2018;131:1172-82.

74. Lazarus AH, Crow AR. Mechanism of action of IVIG and anti-D in ITP. Transfus Apher Sci 2003;28:249-55.

75. McMillan R. Antiplatelet antibodies in chronic immune thrombocytopenia and their role in platelet destruction and defective platelet production. Hematol Oncol Clin North Am 2009;23:1163-75.

76. Davoren A, Bussel J, Curtis BR, et al. Prospective evaluation of a new platelet glycoprotein (GP)-specific assay (PakAuto) in the diagnosis of autoimmune thrombocytopenia (AITP). Am J Hematol 2005;78:193-7.

77. Wu GG, Kaplan C, Curtis BR, Pearson HA. Report on the 14th International Society of Blood Transfusion Platelet Immunology Workshop. Vox Sang 2010;99:375-81.

78. Veldhuisen B, Porcelijn L, van der Schoot CE, de Haas M. Molecular typing of human platelet and neutrophil antigens (HPA and HNA). Transfus Apher Sci 2014;50:189-99.

79. Reil A, Bux J. Geno- and phenotyping of human neutrophil antigens. Methods Mol Biol 2015; 1310:193-203.

80. Christopoulos CG, Kelsey HC, Machin SJ. A flow-cytometric approach to quantitative estimation of platelet surface immunoglobulin G. Vox Sang 1993;64:106-15.

81. Kiefel V, Santoso S, Weisheit M, Mueller-Eckhardt C. Monoclonal antibody-specific immobilization of platelet antigens (MAIPA): A new tool for the identification of platelet-reactive antibodies. Blood 1987;70:1722-6.

82. Porcelijn L, Huiskes E, Comijs-van Osselen I, et al. A new bead-based human platelet antigen antibodies detection assay versus the monoclonal antigen immobilization of platelet antigens assay. Transfusion 2014;54:1486-92.

83. Cooper N, Bein G, Heidinger K, et al. A bead-based assay in the work-up of suspected platelet alloimmunization. Transfusion 2016;56:115-18.

84. Davey S, Navarrete C, Brown C. Simultaneous human platelet antigen genotyping and detection of novel single nucleotide polymorphisms by targeted next-generation sequencing. Transfusion 2017;57:1497-504.

85. McMillan R, Tani P, Millard F, et al. Platelet-associated and plasma anti-glycoprotein autoantibodies in chronic ITP. Blood 1987;70:1040-5.

86. Curtis BR, McFarland JG, Wu GG, et al. Antibodies in sulfonamide-induced immune thrombocytopenia recognize calcium-dependent epitopes on the glycoprotein IIb/IIIa complex. Blood 1994;84:176-83.

87. McFarland J, Lochowicz A, Aster R, et al. Improving the specificity of the PF4 ELISA in diagnosing heparin-induced thrombocytopenia. Am J Hematol 2012;87:776-81.

88. Sheridan D, Carter C, Kelton JG. A diagnostic test for heparin-induced thrombocytopenia. Blood 1986;67:27-30.

89. Favaloro EJ, McCaughan G, Pasalic L. Clinical and laboratory diagnosis of heparin induced thrombocytopenia: An update. Pathology 2017; 49:346-55.

90. Flesch BK, Curtis BR, de Haas M, et al. Update on the nomenclature of human neutrophil antigens and alleles. Transfusion 2016;56:1477-9.

91. Reil A, Sach UJ, Siahanidou T, et al. HNA-1d: A new human neutrophil antigen located on Fcγ receptor IIb associated with neonatal immune neutropenia. Transfusion 2013;53:2145-51.

92. de Haas M, Kleijer M, van Zwieten R, et al. Neutrophil Fc gamma RIIIb deficiency, nature,

and clinical consequences: A study of 21 individuals from 14 families. Blood 1995;86:2403-13.

93. Stroncek DF, Skubitz KM, Plachta LB, et al. Alloimmune neonatal neutropenia due to an antibody to the neutrophil Fc-γ receptor III with maternal deficiency of CD16 antigen. Blood 1991; 77:1572-80.

94. Muschter S, Bertold T. Greinacher A. Developments in the definition and clinical impact of human neutrophil antigens. Curr Opin Hematol 2011;18:452-60.

95. Moritz E, Norcia AMMI, Cardone JDB, et al. Human neutrophil alloantigens systems. An Acad Bras Cienc 2009;81:559-69.

96. Sachs UJ, Andrei-Selmer CL, Maniar A, et al. The neutrophil-specific antigen CD177 is a counter-receptor for platelet endothelial cell adhesion molecule-1 (CD31). J Biol Chem 2007; 282:23603-12.

97. Li Y, Mair DC, Schuller RM, et al. Genetic mechanism of human neutrophil antigen 2 deficiency and expression variations. PLoS Genet 2015;11:e1005255.

98. Moritz E, Chiba AK, Kimura EY, et al. Molecular studies reveal that A134T, G156A and G133A SNPs in the CD177 gene are associated with atypical expression of human neutrophil antigen-2. Vox Sang 2010;98:160-6.

99. Matsuo K, Lin A, Procter JL, et al. Variations in the expression of granulocyte antigen NB1. Transfusion 2000;40:654-62.

100. Eulenberg-Gustavus C, Bahring S, Maass PG, et al. Gene silencing and a novel monoallelic expression pattern in distinct CD177 neutrophil subset. J Exp Med 2017;214:2089-101.

101. Bai M, Grieshaber-Bouyer R, Wang J, et al. CD177 modulates human neutrophil migration through activation-mediated integrin and chemoreceptor regulation. Blood 2017;130:2092-100.

102. Lalezari P, Murphy GB, Allen FH Jr. NB1, a new neutrophil-specific antigen involved in the pathogenesis of neonatal neutropenia. J Clin Invest 1971;50:1108-15.

103. Bux J, Becker F, Seeger W, et al. Transfusion-related acute lung injury due to HLA-A2-specific antibodies in recipient and NB1-specific antibodies in donor blood. Br J Haematol 1996;93:707-13.

104. Stroncek DF, Shapiro RS, Filipovich AH, et al. Prolonged neutropenia resulting from antibodies to neutrophil-specific antigen NB1 following

marrow transplantation. Transfusion 1993;33: 158-63.

105. Curtis BR, Cox NJ, Sullivan MJ, et al. The neutrophil alloantigen HNA-3a (5b) is located on choline transporter-like protein 2 and appears to be encoded by an R>Q154 amino acid substitution. Blood 2010;115:2073-6.

106. Greinacher A, Wesche J, Hammer E, et al. Characterization of the human neutrophil alloantigen-3a. Nat Med 2010;16:45-8.

107. Reil A, Keller-Stanislawski B, Gunay S, Bux J. Specificities of leucocyte alloantibodies in transfusion-related acute lung injury and results of leucocyte antibody screening of blood donors. Vox Sang 2008;95:313-17.

108. Lopes LB, Abbas SA, Moritz E, et al. Antibodies to human neutrophil antigen HNA-3b implicated in cases of neonatal alloimmune neutropenia. Transfusion 2018;58:1264-70.

109. Sachs UJ, Chavakis T, Fung L, et al. Human alloantibody anti-Mart interferes with Mac-1-dependent leukocyte adhesion. Blood 2004;104: 727-34.

110. Fung YL, Pitcher LA, Willett JE, et al. Alloimmune neonatal neutropenia linked to anti-HNA-4a. Transfus Med 2003;13:49-52.

111. Hartman KR, Wright DG. Identification of autoantibodies specific for the neutrophil adhesion glycoproteins CD11b/CD18 in patients with autoimmune neutropenia. Blood 1991;78: 1096-104.

112. Simsek S, van der Schoot CE, Daams M, et al. Molecular characterization of antigenic polymorphisms (Ond(a) and Mart(a)) of the beta 2 family recognized by human leukocyte alloantisera. Blood 1996;88:1350-8.

113. Porcelijn L, Abbink F, Terraneo L, et al. Neonatal alloimmune neutropenia due to immuno-globulin G antibodies against human neutrophil antigen-5a. Transfusion 2011;51:574-7.

114. Farruggia P. Immune neutropenias of infancy and childhood. World J Pediatr 2016;12:142-8.

115. Kleinman S, Caulfield T, Chan P, et al. Toward an understanding of transfusion-related acute lung injury: Statement of a consensus panel. Transfusion 2004;44:1774-89.

116. Food and Drug Administration. Fatalities reported to FDA following blood collection and transfusion: Annual summary for fiscal year 2017. Silver Spring, MD: CBER Office of Communication, Outreach, and Development, 2017. [Available at https://www.fda.gov/media/124796/download (accessed October 16, 2019).]

117. Toy P, Gajic O, Bacchetti P, et al. Transfusion-related acute lung injury: Incidence and risk factors. Blood 2012;119:1757-67.

118. Afzal W, Owlia MB, Hasni S, Newman KA. Autoimmune neutropenia updates: Etiology, pathology, and treatment. South Med J 2017;110: 300-7.

119. Audrain M, Martin J, Fromont P, et al. Autoimmune neutropenia in children: Analysis of 116 cases. Pediatr Allergy Immunol 2011;22:494-6.

120. Clay ME, Schuller RM, Bachowski GJ. Granulocyte serology: Current concepts and clinical significance. Immunohematology 2010;26:11-21.

121. Schulz U, Reil A, Kiefel V, et al. Evaluation of a new microbeads assay for granulocyte antibody detection. Transfusion 2017;57:70-81.

122. Stroncek DF, Fadeyi E, Adams S. Leukocyte antigen and antibody detection assays: Tools for assessing and preventing pulmonary transfusion reactions. Transfus Med Rev 2007;21:273-86.

123. Bux J. Molecular genetics of granulocyte polymorphisms. Vox Sang 2000;78(Suppl 2):125-30.

CHAPTER 16
The HLA System

Jeremy Ryan Peña, MD, PhD; Arthur B. Eisenbrey III, MD, PhD; and
Patricia M. Kopko, MD

THE HLA SYSTEM IS COMPOSED OF a complex array of genes located within the human major histocompatibility complex (MHC) on the short arm of chromosome 6. Their protein products, the HLA antigens, contribute to the recognition of self and nonself, the immune responses to antigenic stimuli, and the coordination of cellular and humoral immunity.

HLA molecules play a key role in antigen presentation and the initiation of the immune response. The HLA system is generally viewed as second in importance only to the ABO antigens in influencing the survival of transplanted solid organs. In hematopoietic stem cell transplantation (HSCT), the HLA system is paramount with regard to graft rejection and graft-vs-host disease (GVHD). HLA antigens and antibodies are also important in complications of transfusion therapy, such as platelet refractoriness, febrile nonhemolytic transfusion reactions (FNHTRs), transfusion-related acute lung injury (TRALI), and transfusion-associated GVHD (TA-GVHD).

The biologic roles of the genes in the MHC continue to be identified (neither transfusion nor transplantation are natural events), and the tremendous polymorphism of the HLA genes is used outside of transplantation. Studies correlating HLA genes with disease susceptibility and disease resistance began soon after serologic techniques for HLA Class I typing were developed and have resurged with the adoption of molecular methods. (Historically significant methods of identifying HLA polymorphisms using antibody binding to surface antigens and mixed lymphocyte culture reactions have been discussed in previous editions of the *Technical Manual*, and the reader is encouraged to review those methods for perspective.)

Understanding the relationships between the polymorphisms of the HLA genes and antigen presentation by the HLA molecules has permitted the analysis of peptide-binding restriction parameters needed for effective vaccine development. The MHC and HLA genetic polymorphisms have been used by anthropologists and population geneticists as accurate tools for population studies. Because of the complexity of the MHC and the extent of polymorphism in the HLA genes, a complex nomenclature was developed (and continues to evolve) to define unique allele sequences based on the relationship of each allele's protein sequence to the serologic specificity of the corresponding antigen.[1,2]

BIOCHEMISTRY, TISSUE DISTRIBUTION, AND STRUCTURE

Characteristics of Class I and Class II Antigens

Class I antigens (HLA-A, -B, and -C) have a molecular weight of approximately 57,000 Daltons

Jeremy Ryan Peña, MD, PhD, Assistant Professor of Pathology, Harvard Medical School, and Director, HLA Laboratory, Beth Israel Deaconess Medical Center, Boston, Massachusetts; Arthur B. Eisenbrey III, MD, PhD, Associate Professor of Pathology, University of Toledo College of Medicine, Toledo, Ohio, and Associate Professor of Pathology, Wayne State University School of Medicine, Detroit, Michigan; and Patricia M. Kopko, MD, Professor of Pathology, University of California San Diego Medical Center, San Diego, California
The authors have disclosed no conflicts of interest.

and consist of two protein chains: a glycoprotein heavy chain (45,000 Daltons) encoded on the short arm of chromosome 6 and, as a light chain, the β_2-microglobulin molecule (12,000 Daltons) encoded by a gene on chromosome 15. The heavy chain penetrates the cell membrane, whereas β_2-microglobulin does not. Rather, β_2-microglobulin associates (noncovalently) with the heavy chain through the latter's nonvariable ($\alpha 3$) domain. (See Fig 16-1.) The external portion of the heavy chain consists of three amino acid domains ($\alpha 1$, $\alpha 2$, and $\alpha 3$), of which the outermost domains, $\alpha 1$ and $\alpha 2$, contain the majority of polymorphic regions conferring serologic HLA antigen specificity.

The "classical" HLA Class I molecules (HLA-A, -B, and -C) are present on platelets and most nucleated cells in the body, with some exceptions that include neurons, corneal epithelial cells, trophoblasts, and germinal cells. Only vestigial amounts remain on mature red cells, with certain allotypes better expressed than others. These Class I types were independently recognized as red cell antigens by serologists and designated as "Bennett-Goodspeed" (Bg) antigens. The specificities called "Bg^a," "Bg^b," and "Bg^c" are actually HLA-B7, HLA-B17 (B57 or B58),

and HLA-A28 (A68 or A69), respectively. Platelets express primarily HLA-A and HLA-B antigens. HLA-C antigens are present at very low levels, and Class II antigens are generally not present on platelets.

Class II antigens (HLA-DR, -DQ, and -DP) have a molecular weight of approximately 63,000 Daltons and consist of two structurally similar glycoprotein chains (α and β), both of which traverse the membrane. (See Fig 16-1.) The extramembranous portion of each chain has two amino acid domains, of which the outermost contains the variable regions of the Class II alleles. The expression of Class II antigens is more restricted than that of Class I antigens. Class II antigens are expressed constitutively on B lymphocytes, monocytes, macrophages, dendritic cells, intestinal epithelium, and early hematopoietic cells. There is also constitutive expression of Class II antigens on some endothelial cells, especially those lining the microvasculature. However, in general, endothelium, particularly that of larger blood vessels, is negative for Class II antigen expression, although Class II antigen expression can be readily induced (for instance, by interferon-gamma during immune activation). Resting T lymphocytes are normally

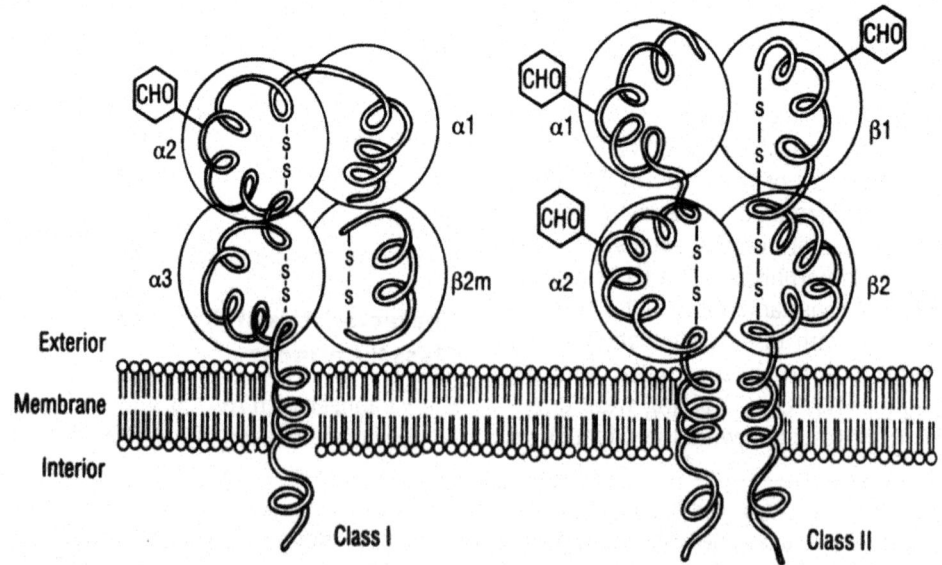

FIGURE 16-1. Stylized diagram of Class I and Class II major histocompatibility complex molecules showing α and β polypeptide chains, their structural domains, and attached carbohydrate units.

negative for Class II antigen expression and become positive when activated.

Soluble HLA Class I and Class II antigens shed from cells are present in blood and body fluids and may play a role in modulating immune reactivity.[3] Levels of soluble HLA increase with infection [including with human immunodeficiency virus (HIV)], inflammatory disease, and transplant rejection, but HLA levels decline with progression of some malignancies. Levels of soluble HLA in blood components are proportional to the number of residual donor leukocytes and the duration of storage. Soluble HLA in blood components may be involved in the immunomodulatory effect of blood transfusion.[4]

Configuration

A representative three-dimensional structure of Class I and Class II molecules can be obtained by x-ray crystallographic analysis of purified HLA antigens. (See Fig 16-2.) The outer domains, which contain the regions of greatest amino acid variability and the antigenic epitopes of the molecules, form a structure known as the "peptide-binding groove." Alleles that are defined by polymorphisms in the HLA gene sequences encode unique amino acid sequences and therefore form unique binding grooves, each of which is able to bind peptides of differ-

ent sequences. The peptide-binding groove is critical for the functional aspects of HLA molecules. (See "Biologic Function" section below.)

Nomenclature for HLA Antigens

An international committee sponsored by the World Health Organization (WHO) establishes the nomenclature of the HLA system. This nomenclature is updated regularly to incorporate new HLA alleles.[2] HLA antigens are designated by a number following the letter that denotes the HLA series (eg, HLA-A1 or HLA-B8). Previously, antigenic specificities that were not fully confirmed carried the prefix "w" (eg, HLA-Aw33) for "workshop." When the antigen's identification became definitive, the WHO Nomenclature Committee dropped the "w" from the designation. (The committee meets regularly to update nomenclature by recognizing new specificities or genetic loci.) The "w" prefix is no longer applied in this manner and is now used only for the following: 1) Bw4 and Bw6, to distinguish such "public" antigens (see "'Public' Antigens" section below) from other B-locus alleles; 2) all serologically defined C-locus specificities, to avoid confusion with components of the complement system; and 3) Dw specificities that were defined by mixed leukocyte reactions but are now known to be caused by *HLA-DR*, *HLA-DQ*, and *HLA-DP* polymorphisms. The nu-

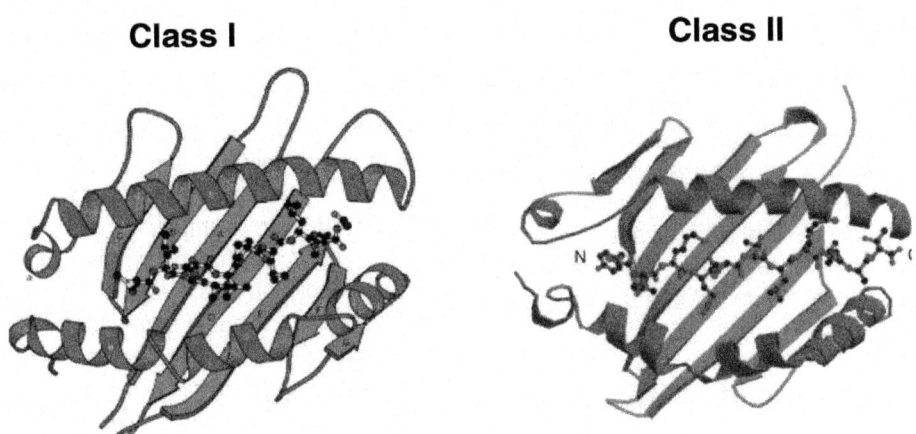

FIGURE 16-2. Ribbon diagram of HLA Class I and Class II molecules. Note the peptide in the groove of each molecule.

meric designations for the HLA-A and HLA-B specificities are assigned according to the order of their official recognition.

Splits and Cross-Reactive Groups

Refinement of serologic methods permitted antigens that were previously believed to represent a single specificity to be "split" into specificities that were recognized as serologically (and, later, genetically) distinct. The designation for an individual antigen that was split from an earlier recognized antigen often includes the number of the parent antigen in parentheses [eg, HLA-B44 (12)].

In addition to "splits," certain apparently distinct HLA antigens may have other epitopes in common. Antibodies that are reactive with these shared determinants often cause cross-reactions in serologic testing. The collective term for a group of HLA antigens that exhibit such cross-reactivity is "cross-reactive epitope group" (CREG).

"Public" Antigens

In addition to splits and CREGs, HLA antibodies may recognize epitopes present across many different HLA specificities. Called "public" antigens, these common amino acid sequences appear to represent less variable portions of the HLA molecule. Two well-characterized public antigens, HLA-Bw4 and HLA-Bw6, are present in almost all HLA-B molecules.[5] The HLA-A locus molecules A23, A24, A25, and A32 also have a Bw4-like epitope.

Public antigens are clinically important because patients exposed to them through pregnancy, transfusion, or transplantation can make antibodies to these antigens. A single antibody, when directed against a public antigen, can resemble multiple discrete alloantibodies, and this has significant consequences for identifying compatible donors for transplantation and platelet transfusion.

Nomenclature for HLA Alleles

Nucleotide sequencing has replaced serologic methods for investigating the HLA system, and increasing numbers of HLA alleles are being identified, many of which share common serologic phenotypes. The minimum requirement for designation of a new allele is the sequence of exons 2 and 3 for HLA Class I and exon 2 for HLA Class II. These exons encode the variable amino acids that confer HLA antigen specificity and much of the biologic function of the HLA molecule.

A uniform nomenclature has been adopted that takes into account the locus, major serologic specificity, and allele group determined by molecular typing techniques. For example, although many alleles have been sequenced only for exons 2 and 3, nucleotide sequencing has identified at least 300 unique amino acid sequence variants (alleles) of HLA-DR4 as of late 2019 (see http://hla.alleles.org/alleles/class2.html).[2] The first HLA-DR4 variant is designated DRB1*04:01, indicating the locus (DR), protein (β1 chain), major serologic specificity (04 for HLA-DR4), and sequence 2 variation allele number (variant 01). The asterisk indicates that an allele name follows (and that the typing was determined by molecular techniques). There may be up to four sets of digits after the asterisk; each set of digits is separated by a colon and is called a field. The digits in the first field correspond to the antigen's serologic specificity in most cases. The digits in the second field make up the code for a unique amino acid sequence in exon 2 (Class II) or exons 2 and 3 (Class I), with numbers being assigned in the order in which the DNA sequences were determined. Therefore, B*27:04 represents the HLA-B locus, has a serologic specificity of B27, and was the fourth unique exon 2 and 3 sequence allele described in this family. (See Table 16-1.) A third field in the allele name is added for alleles that differ only by synonymous ("silent") nucleotide substitutions in exons 2 and 3 for Class I or in exon 2 for Class II. For example, A*01:01:02 differs from A*01:01:01 only in that the codon for isoleucine in position 142 is ATT instead of ATC. A fourth field in the allele name can be added for alleles that differ only in sequences within introns or in 3' or 5' untranslated regions. Finally, the nomenclature accommodates alleles with null or low expression or other characteristics by the addition of an "N" or "L," respectively, or another letter as appropriate to the end of the al-

TABLE 16-1. Current HLA Nomenclature

Species	Locus		Antigen Equivalent		Allele		Silent Mutation		Outside Exon	Expression Modifier
HLA	DRB1	*	04	:	01	:	01	:	02	N,L,S,Q

Examples:
    DR4   - Serology
    DRB1*04:xx   - Serologic Equivalent
    DRB1*04:02   - Allele
    DRB1*04:01:01; DRB1*04:01:02 - Silent Mutations
    A*02:15N;   DRB4*01:03:01:02N - Null Alleles (exon, intron)
    A*24:02:01:02L
    B*44:02:01:02S   > - Expression Modifiers
    B*32:11Q

lele name. The other official expression modifiers are as follows: S (secreted, not on cell surface), Q (expression level questionable), A (unknown but aberrant expression, perhaps null), and C (cytoplasmic expression only). The last two have not been used to date.

Biologic Function

The essential function of the HLA system is self/nonself discrimination, which is accomplished by the interaction of T lymphocytes with peptide antigens presented by HLA proteins. T lymphocytes interact with peptide antigens only when the T-cell receptor (TCR) for antigen engages both an HLA molecule and the antigenic peptide contained within the TCR's peptide-binding groove. This limitation is referred to as "MHC restriction."[6]

In the thymus, T lymphocytes with TCRs that bind to self HLA molecules are selected (positive selection), with the exception of those with TCRs that also bind to a peptide derived from a self-antigen, in which case the T lymphocytes are deleted (negative selection). Some self-reactive T cells escape negative selection and, if not functionally inactivated (for instance, by the mechanism of anergy), may become involved in an autoimmune process.

Role of Class I Molecules

Class I molecules are synthesized, and peptide antigens are inserted into the peptide-binding groove, in the endoplasmic reticulum. Peptide antigens that fit into the Class I peptide-binding groove are typically eight or nine amino acids in length and are derived from proteins made by the cell (endogenous proteins). Such endogenous proteins—which may be normal self-proteins; altered self-proteins, such as those in cancer cells; or viral proteins, such as those in virus-infected cells—are degraded in the cytosol by a large multifunctional protease (LMP) and are transported to the endoplasmic reticulum by a transporter associated with antigen processing (TAP). The LMP and TAP genes are both localized to the MHC.

Class I molecules are transported to the cell surface, where the molecules are available to interact with CD8-positive T lymphocytes. If the TCR of a CD8 cell can bind the antigenic peptide in the context of the specific Class I molecule displaying it, then TCR binding activates the cytotoxic properties of the T cell, which attacks the cell, characteristically eliciting an inflammatory response. The presentation of antigen by Class I molecules is especially important in host defense against viral pathogens and malignant transformation. Tumor cells that do not express Class I antigens escape this form of immune surveillance.

Role of Class II Molecules

Like Class I molecules, Class II molecules are synthesized in the endoplasmic reticulum, but peptide antigens are not inserted into the peptide-binding groove there. Instead, an invariant chain (Ii) is inserted as a placeholder. The Class II-invariant chain complex is transported to an endosome, where the invariant chain is removed by a specialized Class II molecule called "DM." The *DM* locus is also localized to the MHC. A Class II antigenic peptide is then inserted into the peptide-binding groove.

Peptide antigens that fit into the Class II peptide-binding groove are typically 12 to 25 amino acids in length and are derived from proteins that are taken up by the cell through endocytosis (of exogenous proteins). Exogenous proteins, which may be normal self-proteins or proteins derived from pathogens, such as bacteria, are degraded to peptides by enzymes in the endosomal pathway. Class II molecules are then transported to the cell surface, where the molecules are available to interact with CD4-positive T lymphocytes, which secrete immunostimulatory cytokines in response. That mechanism is especially important for the production of antibodies.

GENETICS OF THE MHC

Class I and II HLA molecules are cell-surface glycoproteins and are products of closely linked genes mapped to the p21.3 band on the short arm of chromosome 6 (Fig 16-3). That genomic region, the MHC, is usually inherited en bloc as a haplotype. Each of the many loci has multiple alleles with codominant expression of the products from each chromosome. The HLA system is the most polymorphic genetic system described in humans.[7]

The genes *HLA-A*, *HLA-B*, and *HLA-C* encode the corresponding Class I A, B, and C antigens. The genes *HLA-DRA1*, *-DRB1*, *-DRB3*, *-DRB4*, *-DRB5*; *HLA-DQA1*, *-DQB1*; and *HLA-DPA1* and *-DPB1* encode the corre-

sponding Class II antigens. Located between the Class I and Class II genes is a group of non-HLA genes that code for molecules that include the complement proteins C2, Bf, C4A, and C4B; a steroid enzyme (21-hydroxylase); and a cytokine (tumor necrosis factor) and other genes involved in immune responses. This non-HLA region is referred to as "MHC Class III" even though it does not contain any HLA genes.

Organization of HLA Genetic Regions

The HLA Class I region contains (in addition to the classical genes *HLA-A*, *HLA-B*, and *HLA-C*) other gene loci designated *HLA-E*, *HLA-F*, *HLA-G*, *HLA-H*, *HFE*, *HLA-J*, *HLA-K*, *HLA-L*, *MICA*, and *MICB*. The latter genes encode nonclassical, or Class Ib, HLA proteins, which have limited polymorphism, low levels of expression, and limited distribution of tissue expression.[8] Some Class Ib genes express nonfunctional proteins or no proteins whatsoever (termed "pseudogenes" and are presumed evolutionary dead ends). Other, expressed, nonclassical HLA proteins have been associated with a variety of functions. For example, HLA-E is associated with the surveillance system of one subset of natural killer cells. HLA-G is expressed by the trophoblast and may be involved in the development of maternal immune tolerance of the fetus.

The genomic organization of the MHC Class II (*HLA-D*) region is more complex. An MHC Class II molecule consists of a noncovalent complex of two structurally similar chains: the α-chain and the β-chain. Both of these chains are encoded within the MHC. The polymorphism of HLA Class II molecules results from differences in both the α-chain and the β-chain; this polymorphism depends on the Class II isoform. For example, with HLA-DR, the α-chain is essentially monomorphic, but the β-chain is very polymorphic. Multiple loci code for the α- and β-chains of the Class II MHC proteins.

Different haplotypes have different numbers of Class II genes and pseudogenes. The proteins coded by *DRA1* and *DRB1* result in HLA-DR1 through HLA-DR18 antigens. The products of *DRA1* and *DRB3* (if present) express HLA-DR52; those of *DRA1* and *DRB4* (if present) express HLA-DR53; and those of *DRA1* and *DRB5*

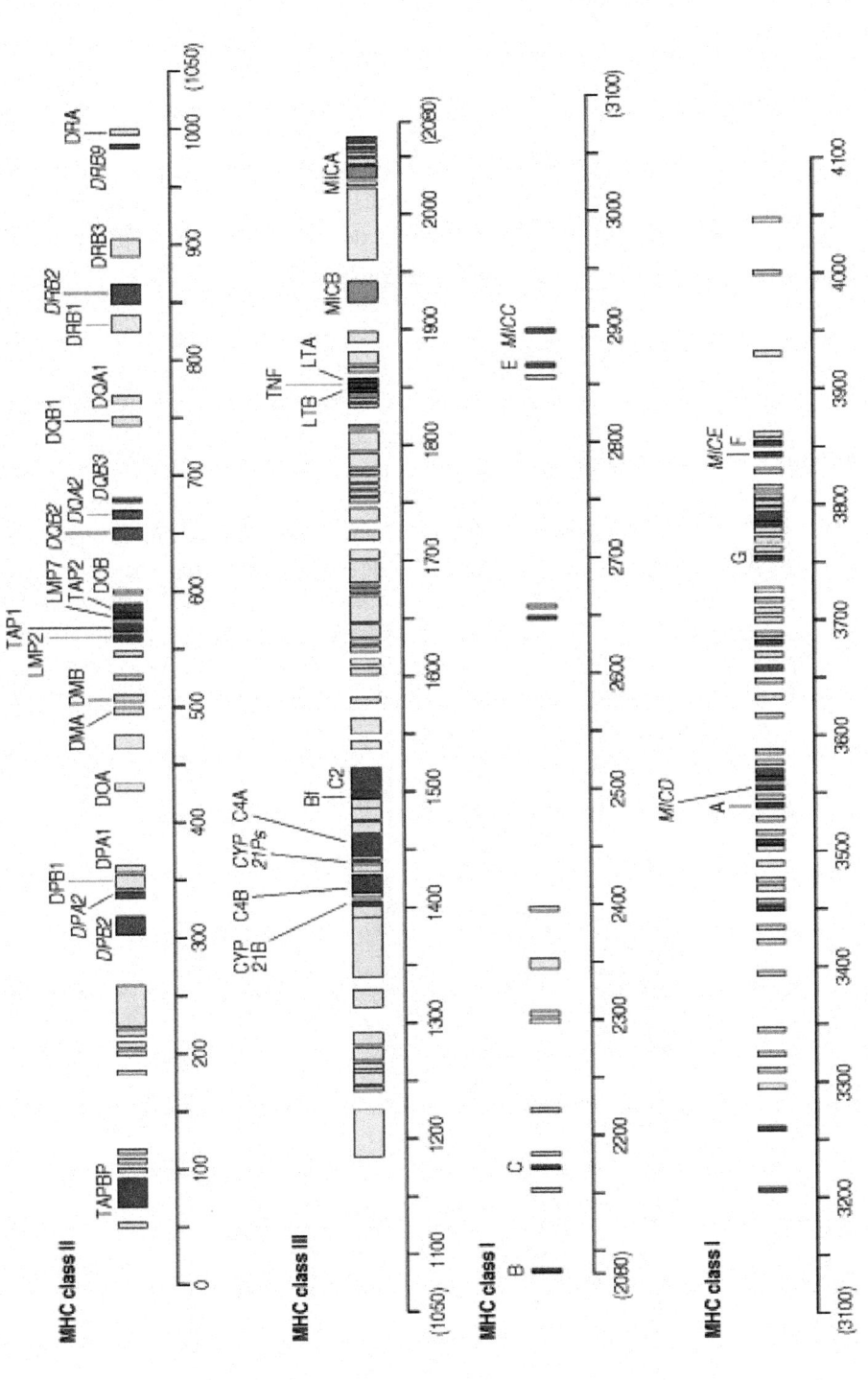

FIGURE 16-3. The HLA complex is located on the short arm of chromosome 6. The centromere is to the top left of the figure, the telomere to the bottom right. The organization of the Class I, II, and III regions is shown. (See also http://hla.alleles.org/alleles/index.html.) Used with permission from Janeway CA, Travers P, Walport M, et al. The immune system in health and disease. 5th ed. New York: Garland Science, 2001.

(if present) express HLA-DR51. The HLA-DQ1 through DQ9 antigens are expressed on the glycoproteins coded by *DQA1* and *DQB1* in the DQ cluster. Many of the other genes of the DQ cluster are likely pseudogenes. A similar organization is found in the HLA-DP gene cluster.

Although not generally considered part of the HLA system, the MHC Class III region contains four complement genes with alleles that are typically inherited together as a unit, termed a "complotype." More than 10 different complotypes are inherited in humans. Two of the Class III genes, *C4A* and *C4B*, encode for variants of the C4 molecule and antigens of the Chido/Rodgers blood group system. These variants have distinct protein structures and functions; the C4A molecule (if present) carries the Rg antigen, and the C4B molecule (if present) carries the Ch antigen. Both of these antigens are adsorbed onto the red cells of individuals who possess the gene(s).

Patterns of Inheritance

Although MHC organization is complicated, its inheritance follows the established principles of Mendelian genetics. Every person has two different copies of chromosome 6 and possesses two HLA haplotypes, one from each parent. The combination of HLA alleles inherited from both parents constitutes the genotype. The expressed HLA genes then result in the phenotype, both of which can be determined by typing for HLA antigens or alleles. Because HLA genes are autosomal and codominant, the phenotype represents the combined expression of both haplotypes. However, to define haplotypes, parents (and possibly other family members) also need to be typed to determine which alleles are inherited together. Figure 16-4 illustrates inheritance of haplotypes and demonstrates that four possible combinations of haplotypes are possible in the offspring, assuming no recombination occurs. The chance that two siblings will be phenotypically HLA identical is 25%. The chance that any one patient with "n" siblings will have at least one HLA-identical sibling is $1 - (3/4)^n$. Having two siblings provides a 44% chance of finding an HLA-identical sibling, and having three siblings provides a 58% chance.

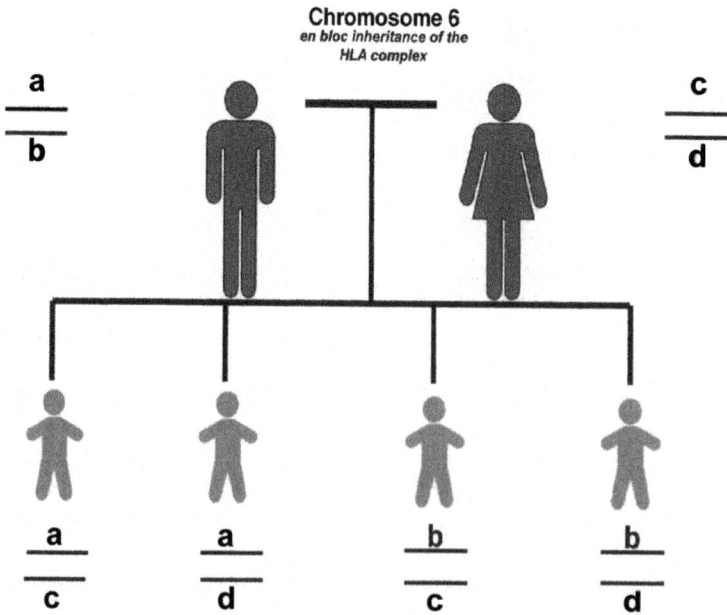

FIGURE 16-4. The designations a/b and c/d represent paternal and maternal HLA haplotypes, respectively. Except for crossovers, the HLA complex is transmitted en bloc from parent to offspring.

Absence of Antigens

Before the advent of molecular-based HLA typing, the absence of an antigen in serologic phenotyping results was attributed to homozygosity at a locus (eg, inheritance of A1 from both parents, which in reality represented only an apparent absence of the antigen as a result of limitations of phenotyping methods) or to a null (nonexpressed) allele. With DNA sequencing and other molecular HLA typing methods, homozygosity can now be presumed with a higher degree of confidence. However, proving homozygosity requires family studies or methods permitting hemizygous typing (ie, typing of an individual haplotype). A null allele is characterized by one or more DNA sequence changes, within or outside the gene's coding region, that prevent expression of a functional protein at the cell surface. Such inactivation of a gene may be caused by nucleotide substitutions, deletions, or insertions that lead to a premature cessation in the protein's synthesis. In the absence of a family study, a phenotyping study revealing a single allele at any locus offers only presumptive evidence for homozygosity. In this situation, the allele should be listed only once because it is unknown whether that allele is present twice (a true homozygote) or there is another allele not detected by the available method.

Crossovers

The genes of the HLA region occasionally demonstrate chromosome crossover, in which segments containing linked genetic material are exchanged between the two chromosomes during meiosis or gametogenesis. The recombinant chromosomes are then transmitted as new haplotypes to the offspring. Crossover frequency is related partly to the physical distance between the genes and partly to the resistance or susceptibility of specific A, B, and DR antigens to recombination. (See below.) The *HLA-A*, *HLA-B*, and *HLA-DR* loci are close together, with 0.8% crossover between the *A* and *B* loci and 0.5% between the *B* and *DR* loci. Crossovers between the *HLA-B* and *HLA-C* loci or between the *HLA-DR* and *HLA-DQ* loci are extremely rare, whereas crossovers between the *DQ* and *DP* loci are relatively common.[9] In family studies and relationship evaluations, the possibility of recombination should always be considered.

Linkage Disequilibrium

The MHC system is so polymorphic that the number of possible unique HLA phenotypes is theoretically greater than that of the global human population. Moreover, new HLA alleles are constantly being discovered and characterized. As of August 2018, 4340 HLA-A alleles, 5212 HLA-B alleles, 2593 DRB1 alleles, and 1257 DQB1 alleles had been identified.[2,10] Usually, HLA genes are inherited together as haplotypes. Many HLA alleles are overrepresented compared with what would be expected if the distribution of HLA genes were random. The phenomenon of linkage disequilibrium describes the discrepancy between expected and observed HLA allele frequencies.

Expected frequencies for HLA alleles are derived by multiplication of the frequencies of each allele. For example, in individuals of European ancestry, the overall frequency of HLA-A1 is 0.15 and that for HLA-B8 is 0.10; therefore, 3.0% ($0.15 \times 0.10 \times 2$) of all HLA haplotypes in people of European ancestry would be expected to contain both HLA-A1 and HLA-B8 if the alleles were randomly distributed. The actual haplotype frequency of the A1 and B8 combination, however, is 7% to 8% in that population.

Certain allelic combinations occur with increased frequency in different racial groups and constitute common haplotypes in those populations. These common haplotypes are called "ancestral haplotypes" because they appear to be inherited from a single common ancestor or to be conserved within the population, because of either survival advantage of carriers or resistance to recombination. The most common ancestral haplotype in people of Northern European ancestry—*A1, B8, DR17 (DRB1*03:01), DQ2*—includes both Class I and Class II regions.

Some alleles in apparent linkage disequilibrium may represent relatively young haplotypes that have not had sufficient time to undergo recombination, whereas some old haplotypes are resistant to recombination because of selection or physical limitations. For example, the *A1, B8, DRB1*03:01* haplotype appears to be resistant to recombination because of deletion of the complement C4A gene, which results in decreased distance between HLA-B and HLA-DRB1 in those individuals. Linkage disequilibrium affects the likelihood of finding suitable unrelated donors for HLA-matched platelet transfusions and HSCT.

HLA TYPING

Clinical identification of HLA antigens and alleles is now performed almost exclusively by molecular methods. Historically, serologic (antibody-based) and cell-based assays were also used. The reader is referred to previous editions of the AABB *Technical Manual* and Bontadini[11] for detailed descriptions of the use of the lymphocytotoxicity method.

Detailed procedures for commonly used assays are available from reagent and kit manufacturers and have been summarized in reviews of available methodology.[11] Depending on the clinical situation, a particular HLA antigen/allele detection or typing method may be preferable to determine the HLA genotype or phenotype. (See Table 16-2.) Current molecular (DNA-based)

HLA typing has several advantages over past serologic assays: 1) high sensitivity and specificity, 2) use of small sample volumes, and 3) no need for cell-surface-antigen expression or cell viability. Although serologic methods can identify a limited number of HLA specificities, high-resolution DNA-based methods have the potential capability to identify all known alleles as well as new alleles.

Polymerase chain reaction (PCR) technology allows amplification of large quantities of a particular target segment of genomic DNA. Low- to intermediate-resolution typing detects the HLA serologic equivalents with great accuracy (eg, it distinguishes DR15 from DR16), whereas high-resolution typing distinguishes individual alleles (eg, *DRB1*01:01:01* from *DRB1*01:02:01*). Several molecular methods are PCR-based; the most common molecular methods for HLA typing are described below.

Oligonucleotide Probes

Sequence-specific oligonucleotide probes (SSO or SSOP) use arrays of labeled oligonucleotide probes to detect HLA nucleotide sequences present in immobilized DNA.[11] Reverse SSO (rSSO) has been widely adopted and uses probes

TABLE 16-2. HLA Typing Methods and Appropriate Applications

Method	Clinical Application	Resolution
SSP (PCR)	Solid-organ and HSCT	Serologic to allele level, higher resolution with large number of primers
Forward SSOP hybridization	Solid-organ and HSCT (can accommodate high-volume testing)	Serologic to allele level
Reverse SSOP hybridization	Solid-organ and HSCT	Serologic, higher resolution with larger number of probes
DNA sequencing	Unrelated HSCT, resolution of typing problems with other methods, characterization of new alleles	Allele level
Lymphocytotoxicity	Supplemental testing for DNA-based HLA typings without defined HLA antigen assignments, and research support for HLA allele and antigen designation	Serologic specificity

SSP = sequence-specific primer; PCR = polymerase chain reaction; HSCT = hematopoietic stem cell transplantation; SSOP = sequence-specific oligonucleotide probe.

individually attached to a solid-phase matrix (for example, each probe may be attached to a different microbead). DNA from a target locus is then amplified and labeled in PCR reactions, and the binding to the different probes is evaluated. Commercially available microbead array assays use rSSO methods for HLA Class I and Class II low-to-high-resolution tissue typing and computer proprietary algorithms to match binding patterns to allele databases.[12]

Sequence-Specific Primers

A second major technique uses sequence-specific primer (SSP) pairs that target and amplify a particular DNA sequence.[11] This sequence-specific method requires the performance of multiple PCR assays in which each reaction is selected for a particular allele or group of alleles. The amplification products are directly visualized after agarose gel electrophoresis. Because SSPs have specific targets, the amplified material indicates the presence of the allele or alleles that have that sequence. The pattern of positive and negative PCR amplifications is examined to determine the HLA allele(s) present. Primer pair sets are commercially available that can determine HLA-A, -B, -C, -DR, -DQA1, -DQB1, and -DPB1 phenotypes and may be combined to determine common alleles.

Sequence-Based Typing ("Sequencing")

High-resolution typing is necessary for assignment of HLA alleles.[13] Sanger-chemistry sequence-based typing (SBT) can be used to identify known alleles and characterize new alleles.[11] Although SBT is considered the "gold standard" for HLA typing, ambiguities occur when two different base pairs are found at the same position and can result in two different possible combinations of alleles. These ambiguities occur because SBT evaluates both maternal and paternal HLA genes (haplotypes) simultaneously. Pairs of single nucleotide substitutions can be encountered in which *cis* (same parental haplotype) or *trans* (nucleotide assignment of the second polymorphic site is on the other haplotype) can give ambiguous results when those nucleotide combina-

tions are assigned to different alleles. The haplotype to assign individual base pairs in polymorphic combinations may be determined with additional results from selected SSP or SSO reactions.

Next-Generation Sequencing

Massively parallel sequencing ("next-generation sequencing," or NGS) has allowed for sequencing of whole genes and reduced the frequency of the ambiguities that occur with Sanger-chemistry SBT of HLA because NGS sequences single strands of DNA. HLA typing kits are commercially available for both clinical and research instruments.[14] NGS methods obtain sequences, from libraries, formed from fractured pre- or post-PCR cellular DNA. The very large number of sequences obtained allow for identification of overlapping sequences and arrangement of the resulting sequences through computer analysis (requiring very powerful processors, large sequence databases, and complex programming).

Two families of NGS are sequencing by synthesis and sequencing by hybridization and ligation. Sequencing by synthesis has three methodologies: pyrosequencing; ion semiconductor sequencing; and fluorescently labeled, reversible nucleotide terminator chemistry. Nucleotide sequence detection is by photon release from dideoxynucleotide incorporation, detection of hydrogen ion release, or laser interrogation of dye terminator incorporation. A much less common method is matrix-assisted laser desorption/ionization time-of-flight mass spectrometry (MALDI-TOF MS). NGS is rapidly evolving, and selection of methods and instrumentation should be determined by individual laboratory needs.

OTHER NON-HLA HISTOCOMPATIBILITY DETERMINANTS

Although HLA and ABO remain the most important histocompatibility systems in transplantation, the following is a brief review of some non-HLA factors with emerging relevance to transplantation. Clinical testing for these markers is most commonly performed in the HLA laboratory.

Non-HLA in Solid-Organ Transplantation

Even in identical twins or HLA-matched donor-recipient pairs, allograft rejection has been observed, suggesting the role of non-HLA determinants.[15] In solid-organ transplantation these other non-HLA antigens can elicit an antibody response from the recipient. Some of the better-studied targets include MICA (major histocompatibility class I chain related gene A), AT1R (angiotensin II type I receptor), ETAR (endothelin type A receptor), vimentin, and perlecan (LG3).[16] With the exception of MICA, these antigens are often targets of autoantibody responses. It is estimated that <3% of antibody-mediated rejection is due to non-HLA antibodies.[17] The two best-studied antibodies for which there are commercial clinical assays currently in use are MICA and AT1R.

Non-HLA Hematopoietic Stem Cell Transplantation

In HSCT, killer immunoglobulin-like receptor (KIR) typing of donors is becoming increasingly more common. Natural killer (NK) cells use KIR to recognize self vs nonself through interactions mediated by KIR ligands on target cells.[18] By selecting donors with more activating KIR alleles (called group B KIR) and/or by giving the recipients who lack the ligands that signal, there may be increased graft-vs-leukemia effect and improved HSCT outcomes.

CROSSMATCHING AND DETECTION OF HLA ANTIBODIES

Cell-Based Assays

Compatibility testing similar to the red cell crossmatch has been performed by lymphocytotoxicity for over 50 years[19] and is best referred to as "lymphocyte crossmatching." Crossmatching consists of incubating serum from a potential recipient with lymphocytes (unfractionated or separated into T and B lymphocytes) from prospective donors. Variations of the lymphocytotoxicity test include extended incubations, inclusion of wash steps, and use of an antiglobulin reagent. Flow cytometry has largely replaced the cytotoxicity crossmatch method with greater sensitivity than the antiglobulin-enhanced crossmatch.

Solid-Phase Assays

The current approach to identify HLA antibodies relies on the use of beads or microparticles (ie, solid-phase methodology) coated either with clusters of HLA Class I or Class II antigens from cultured lymphocytes (ie, an HLA phenotype) or with individually purified or recombinant HLA antigens (single-antigen beads).[19] Antibody-binding is detected by staining with fluorescently labeled antihuman globulin (AHG). The presence of antibody is detected with flow cytometry, flow microarrays, or enzyme-linked immunosorbent assay (ELISA). Only an ELISA method is FDA-approved for donor screening (August 2018). Flow cytometry and flow microarray methods are more sensitive than lymphocytotoxicity and focus on the detection of IgG antibodies. The use of single-antigen bead assays are of particular importance for highly sensitized patients where multiple HLA antibody specificities cannot be reliably distinguished and identified with either cell-based cytotoxic assays or solid-phase assays using clusters of HLA molecules.

Although HLA antibody has been demonstrated in transplantation population studies to be detrimental to transplanted organ and patient survival, the clinical significance of low-level antibodies detectable only by solid-phase assays cannot be predicted for individual patients. Newer adaptations of the solid-phase technology can determine whether the antibodies do or do not fix complement and may improve the predictive value of testing for individual patients.

THE HLA SYSTEM AND TRANSFUSION

HLA system antigens and antibodies play important roles in a number of transfusion-related events, including platelet refractoriness, FNHTRs, TRALI, and TA-GVHD. HLA antigens are highly immunogenic. In response to pregnancy, transfusion, or transplantation, immunologically competent individuals are more likely to form antibodies to HLA antigens than to any other antigens.

Platelet Refractoriness

The incidence of HLA alloimmunization and platelet refractoriness has been substantially reduced by the implementation of nearly universal transfusion of leukocyte-reduced cellular blood components in Canada and the United States.[20] The refractory state exists when a transfusion of suitably preserved platelets fails to increase the recipient's platelet count. Platelet refractoriness may be caused by clinical factors, such as sepsis, high fever, disseminated intravascular coagulopathy, bleeding, medications, hypersplenism, complement-mediated destruction, or a combination of these factors; alternatively, it may have an immune basis.[21]

Antibody Development

Antibodies against HLA Class I antigens are a common cause of immune-mediated platelet refractoriness, but antibodies to platelet-specific or ABH antigens may also be involved. Although platelets express HLA Class I antigens, the most likely cause of HLA sensitization from transfusion is the leukocytes in the blood component. This is demonstrated by the development of antibodies to HLA Class II antigens, which are not expressed on platelets. Leukocyte reduction to $<5 \times 10^6$ per component was shown to reduce alloimmunization from 19% to 7% and alloimmune platelet refractoriness from 14% to 4% in patients undergoing chemotherapy for acute leukemia or stem cell transplantation.[20]

Identifying Compatible Donors

Selected donor platelets may be either HLA-matched (identical or zero-mismatch), antigen-negative (antibody avoidance), or crossmatch-compatible units. A perfect antigen-matched unit (HLA identical) might yield no significant posttransfusion count increment because the majority of allogeneic units have been typed only at low resolution, and some patients display allele-specific antibodies. The authors strongly believe that in the age of molecular HLA typing and single-antigen testing for HLA antibodies, the antigen-match grade system (A, BU, B2U, BX, C, and D matches) is obsolete and should no longer be used. In this older, HLA-match grade system, a grade A match represents a donor who has identical HLA-A and -B antigens with the patient. The assumption is that the patient should not have any antibodies to an A match. With the advent of molecular typing, a BU or B2U match should also be equally compatible (as an A match) with the recipient because, unlike serologic methods, molecular typing methods should not "miss" an antigen. However, a BX match could be incompatible if a patient makes antibodies to the cross-reactive antigen present on the donor platelets. Conversely, a grade C or D match may be compatible if the patient does not have antibody against any of the donor antigens.[22]

Single-antigen testing for Class I HLA antibodies allows for the selection of antigen-negative units. This practice has been shown to be as effective as using HLA-matched units for refractory patients, and in many cases, it can be easier to find antigen-negative units than a perfect four-locus match. However, when patients are highly alloimmunized with multiple specificities, it may be necessary to honor only the strongest [highest mean-fluorescent-intensity (MFI)] antibodies. Finally, the provision of crossmatch-compatible units is a useful alternative when the HLA type and antibody profile of a patient is not yet known.

Febrile Nonhemolytic Transfusion Reactions

HLA, granulocyte, and platelet-specific antibodies have been implicated in the pathogenesis of

FNHTRs. The recipient's antibodies, reacting with transfused antigens, elicit the release of cytokines (eg, interleukin-1) that are capable of causing fever. Serologic investigation, if undertaken, may require multiple techniques and target cells from a number of different donors. Cytokines in stored cellular blood components, particularly non-leukocyte-reduced components, are also a cause of FNHTRs.[23] (See Chapter 22.)

TRALI

In TRALI, a potentially fatal transfusion reaction that may occur with transfusion of plasma-containing blood components, acute noncardiogenic pulmonary edema develops in response to transfusion. The pathogenesis of TRALI appears to reflect the presence of HLA or neutrophil antibodies in donor blood that react with the target antigens in the recipient. Studies have shown that 2% (male donors) to 17% (female donors) of blood components can contain detectable amounts of HLA antibodies.[24] If present, such antibodies can be reactive with and fix complement to the recipient's granulocytes, leading to severe capillary leakage and pulmonary edema. Rarely, the recipient's HLA antibodies are reactive with transfused leukocytes from the donor (reverse TRALI). (See Chapter 22 for more on TRALI.)

Chimerism and TA-GVHD

"Chimerism" refers to the presence of two cell populations, such as transfused or transplanted donor cells and recipient cells, in an individual. Persistent chimerism after blood transfusion may lead to the development of TA-GVHD in the recipient. The development of TA-GVHD depends on the following factors: 1) the degree to which the recipient is immunocompromised, 2) the number and viability of lymphocytes in the transfused component, and 3) the number of HLA alleles shared by the donor and recipient. The development of TA-GVHD with the use of fresh blood components from blood relatives has highlighted the pathogenic role of the HLA system.

Figure 16-5 illustrates the conditions for increased risk of TA-GVHD. The parents have one HLA haplotype in common. Each child, therefore, has one chance in four of inheriting the same haplotype from each parent, and child 1 is homozygous for the shared parental HLA haplotype. Transfusion of blood from child 1 to an unrelated recipient with different haplotypes would have no untoward consequences. If, however, child 1 were a directed donor for a relative who was heterozygous for that haplotype (eg, one of the parents or child 3), the recipient's body would fail to recognize the antigens on the transfused lymphocytes as foreign and would not eliminate them. The donor cells would recognize the recipient's other haplotype as foreign and would become activated, proliferate, and attack the host.

To avoid this situation, it is recommended that all cellular components from blood relatives be irradiated before transfusion. Irradiation causes damage to nucleic acids of residual lymphocytes in blood components, which prevents them from dividing, thereby preventing them from attacking the host. (See Chapter 17.) Other specially chosen donor units, including HLA-matched platelets, may also present an increased risk of TA-GVHD and should be irradiated. Rarely, TA-GVHD has occurred after the transfusion of blood from an unrelated donor, usually within populations in which shared HLA haplotypes are common.

Chimerism is proposed to be responsible for the maintenance of tolerance in some organ transplant recipients as well as for the maintenance of HLA sensitization.[25] It has been postulated that scleroderma is a form of GVHD resulting from chimeric cells derived from fetal cells transferred across the placenta during pregnancy.[26] Furthermore, the persistence of donor lymphocytes originally present in and transplanted with a solid-organ allograft has been documented to cause fatal GVHD in recipients of these organs.[27] Although donor lymphocytes are potentially detectable by molecular typing for HLA in all but HLA-identical transplants, current standards require chimerism testing for marrow engraftment monitoring using a different method. The test for chimerism after transplantation involves identifying the genetic profiles of the recipient and donor and then evaluating the extent of mixture in the recipient after transplantation. The technique commonly employed uses DNA analysis of short tandem repeat (STR)

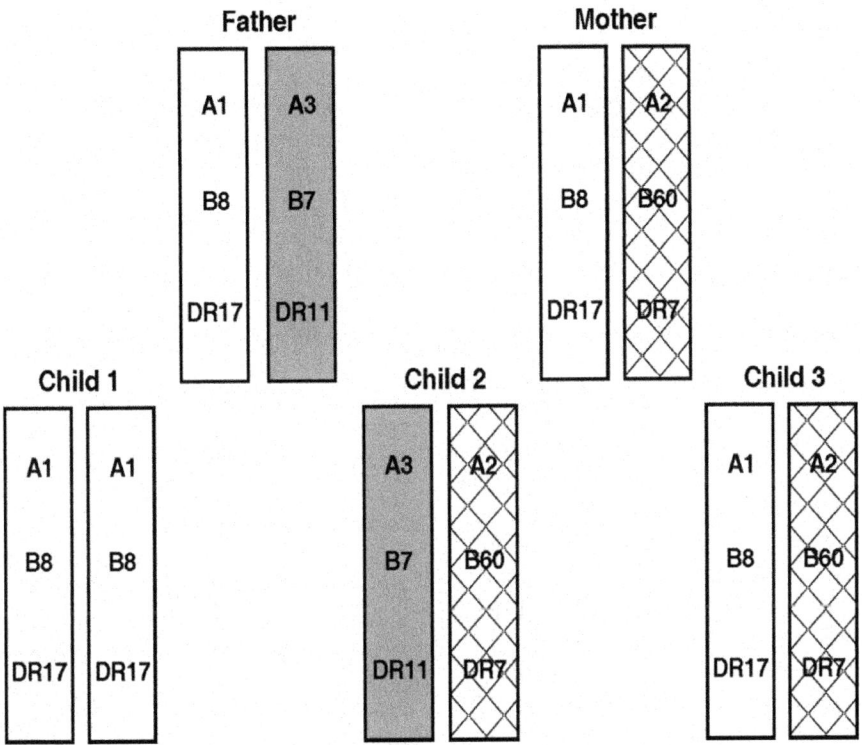

FIGURE 16-5. HLA haplotypes in a family at risk for transfusion-associated graft-vs-host disease (GVHD). In contrast to the family shown in Fig 16-4, each parent shares a common HLA haplotype, *HLA-A1,B8,DR17.* Child 1 is homozygous for the haplotype shared by the parents and by child 3. The lymphocytes of child 1 are capable of producing posttransfusion GVHD if they are transfused to either parent or to child 3.

sequences that are amplified, separated by capillary electrophoresis, and evaluated by the DNA fragment sizes.[28]

HLA incompatibility has rarely been implicated in shortened red cell survival in patients with antibodies to HLA antigens, such as Bg[a] (B7), Bg[b] (B17-B57 or B58), and Bg[c] (A28-A68 or A69). These antigens are expressed, although weakly, on red cells. Such incompatibility may not be detected by conventional pretransfusion testing.

HLA TESTING AND TRANSPLANTATION

HLA testing is an integral part of solid-organ and HSCT. The extent of testing differs depending on the type of transplantation. (See Chapter 26.)

Hematopoietic Stem Cell Transplants

It has long been recognized that disparity within the HLA system is a significant barrier to successful HSCT.[29] HLA similarity and compatibility between the donor and the recipient are required for engraftment and to reduce the risk of GVHD. However, some degree of rejection or GVHD is a common problem for recipients of allogeneic stem cells, despite immunosuppressive conditioning.

The goal of HLA typing is to match the alleles of the prospective donor and recipient at the *HLA-A, -B, -C, -DRB1,* and *-DQB1* loci.[30] Some transplant programs also attempt to match donors and recipients for HLA-DP alleles. When matched stem cell donors are unavailable, haploidentical stem cell transplants are considered for patients with high-risk hematologic malignancies.[31]

Although HLA-identical sibling donors remain the best choice for HSCT, there is increasing use of unrelated donors identified by searching the files of more than 20 million donors listed in the National Marrow Donor Program's registry of volunteer donors, cord blood registries, and international registries.[30]

Kidney Transplants

ABO and lymphocyte crossmatch compatibility remain the most important factors in determining the immediate outcomes of kidney transplantations. ABO- or crossmatch-incompatible transplantations may be facilitated using protocols that include various combinations of antibody suppression, splenectomy, plasmapheresis, infusion of intravenous immune globulin (IVIG), and other treatments to remove preexisting antibodies and promote accommodation of the transplanted organ.

Unlike in HSCT, renal transplants are not routinely HLA matched. Analogous to red cell transfusions, in renal transplantation the donor and recipient need to be compatible, meaning that the donor does not express preformed antibodies (ABH or HLA) directed against antigens on the donor kidney. Recipients and donors are routinely typed for ABO and HLA. Recipients are typed for HLA-A, -B, and -DR at a minimum. Donors are typed for HLA-A, -B, -C, -DRB, -DQA, -DQB, and -DPB antigens by molecular methods. Before transplantation, a crossmatch between recipient serum and donor lymphocytes is required. Clinical Laboratory Improvement Amendments (CLIA) regulations [*Code of Federal Regulations* (CFR) Title 42, Part 493.1278(e)] and US federal Organ Procurement and Transplant Network regulations require a sensitive crossmatch method.[32] Flow cytometry is the most sensitive method and has been credited with predicting early acute rejection and delayed graft function, both of which are strong predictors of chronic rejection (if results are positive) and long-term allograft survival (if results are negative).[33]

HLA antibody levels are dynamic and change with new immunologic challenges, including inflammatory conditions. Serum used for crossmatching is often obtained within 48 hours of surgery for sensitized potential recipients and may be retained in the frozen state for any subsequent testing. An incompatible crossmatch with unfractionated or T lymphocytes is typically a contraindication to kidney transplantation. A positive B-cell crossmatch is significant when caused by donor-specific HLA Class I or Class II antibodies.

Sera from patients awaiting deceased-donor kidney transplant surgery are tested at regular intervals to screen for HLA antibodies and to determine the specificities of the detected antibodies. If an antibody with a defined HLA specificity is identified in a recipient, a common practice is to avoid donors who express the corresponding HLA antigen(s). Such antigens are deemed "unacceptable." Using a standardized algorithm involving the HLA frequencies from 12,000 HLA-typed donors, a calculated "panel-reactive antibody" (cPRA) is obtained and is a more specific measure of the sensitization of the patient and the percentage of probability of encountering incompatible or "unacceptable" random donors.[34] Frozen serum samples used for periodic antibody testing are often stored so that "historical" samples with the greatest reactivity can be used in addition to a preoperative sample for pretransplantation crossmatching.

Prospective crossmatching is often not performed for recipients for whom HLA antibodies are not detected (ie, cPRA = 0%) after repeat testing. Prompt transplantation with reduced cold-ischemia time for the renal allograft may provide greater benefit to the patient than prospective crossmatching, provided that 1) a very sensitive method for antibody detection, such as flow cytometry or microarrays, has been used, and 2) it is certain that the patient has had no additional sensitizing event (ie, immunizations or transfusions in the 2 weeks before or at any time after the serum was screened).[35] "Virtual crossmatching" for renal transplantation requires careful review of the patient history and HLA antibody test results and is similar to the concept of an "electronic crossmatch" for red cell transfusion. In other words, a virtual crossmatch is an inferred crossmatch that involves a determination of the presence or absence of donor HLA-specific antibodies in a patient by comparing the patient's HLA antibody specificity profile to the HLA type of the proposed donor without carrying out a physical crossmatch such as a complement-dependent cytotoxicity or flow-cytometric crossmatch.

Long-term allograft survival is longer with living donors than deceased organ donors. One-year graft survival rates from living and deceased renal donors were 97% and 91.3%, respectively, and the half-lives of living-donor and deceased-donor renal allograft recipients were 14.2 years and 9.9 years, respectively.[36]

The significantly better graft survival rate for recipients of living- vs deceased-donor renal allografts, even when donors and recipients are completely unrelated, coupled with inadequate numbers of deceased-organ donors has led to kidney paired donations (KPD), which permit patients with an ABO- or HLA-incompatible potential living donor to exchange their donor for the donor of other patients in the same situation.[37] KPDs have been facilitated through local and national registries. As a simple example, a blood group A transplant candidate with an incompatible blood group B potential living kidney donor could exchange that donor for the incompatible blood group A living kidney donor of a blood group B transplant candidate. Patients with HLA-incompatible potential donors have similar possibilities for donor exchange, and multiple "pairs" can be involved in one continuous exchange (chain) process.

The introduction of altruistic donors (ie, individuals who choose to donate a kidney without having a specific intended recipient) can significantly expand KPD options. Briefly, an altruistic donor donates a kidney to a patient with an incompatible potential living donor, who then donates to a different recipient with an incompatible donor, starting a chain with the possibility of a large number of living-donor transplants. A chain of 10 transplants has been reported.[38]

Other Solid-Organ Transplants

For liver, heart, lung, and heart/lung transplants, ABO compatibility remains the primary immunologic concern for donor selection, and pretransplantation determination of ABO compatibility between the donor and recipient is required. Young pediatric heart or liver transplant recipients, who have low levels of ABO isoagglutinins, have had successful outcomes with ABO-incompatible hearts or livers.[39,40] HLA antibody screening and typing of potential recipients of nonrenal organs is recommended to improve deceased-donor organ transplantation outcomes. Likewise, a crossmatch should be available before transplantation when the recipient has demonstrated HLA antibody, except for emergency situations. Although the degree of HLA compatibility correlates with graft survival after heart, lung, small-intestine, and liver transplantations, prospective HLA matching is generally not performed for these procedures because of the relative scarcity of donors. Pancreas transplantation generally follows the same guidelines as kidney transplantation.

OTHER CLINICALLY SIGNIFICANT ASPECTS OF HLA

For some conditions, especially those believed to have an autoimmune etiology, an association exists between HLA phenotype and the occurrence of, or resistance to, clinical disease.[41-44] (See Table 16-3.) HLA-associated disease suscep-

TABLE 16-3. HLA-Associated Diseases

Disease	HLA	RR[40-43]
Celiac disease	DQ2	>250
Ankylosing spondylitis	B27	>150
Narcolepsy	DQ6	>38
Subacute thyroiditis	B35	14
Type 1 diabetes	DQ8	14
Multiple sclerosis	DR15, DQ6	12
Rheumatoid arthritis	DR4	9
Juvenile rheumatoid arthritis	DR8	8
Grave disease	DR17	4

RR = relative risk.

tibilities are known or suspected to be inherited, and the diseases display a clinical course with acute exacerbations and remissions and usually have characteristics of autoimmune disorders.

Although linkage to disease-susceptibility genes was favored as an explanation for the HLA associations with individual diseases, evidence has been accumulating that implicates the HLA molecules themselves. The most frequently stated hypothesis is abnormal presentation of peptides by particular HLA molecules that result in autoreactivity from presentation of cross-reactive nonself peptides or improper presentation of self peptides. The ancestral haplotype HLA-A1, B8, DR17 (DRB1*03:01), DQ2, discussed in the "Linkage Disequilibrium" section above, is associated with susceptibility to type 1 diabetes, systemic lupus erythematosus, celiac disease, common variable immunodeficiency, immunoglobulin A (IgA) deficiency, and myasthenia gravis.[43] This haplotype is also associated with an accelerated course of HIV infection. A problem with the abnormal peptide presentation hypothesis is the lack of commonality in the associated disease processes.[44]

One of the first disease associations identified was between HLA-B27 and ankylosing spondylitis. Although >90% of patients of European ancestry with ankylosing spondylitis express HLA-B27 (most commonly HLA-B*27:02 or -B*27:05), the test's specificity is low; only 20% of individuals with B27 develop ankylosing spondylitis. One of the strongest associations between an HLA allele and a medical condition is narcolepsy and the HLA-DQ6 HLA allele DQB1*06:02.[45] As with HLA-B27 and ankylosing spondylitis, >90% of individuals with narcolepsy are positive for HLA-DQB1*06:02, but only a minority of the individuals with the allele develop the disease. For some autoimmune diseases, the specific peptide that might trigger the autoimmune response has been at least tentatively identified: a gluten peptide, gliadin, for celiac disease; cyclic citrullinated peptides for rheumatoid arthritis; and a peptide from glutamic acid decarboxylase for type 1 diabetes.[46-48] Resistance to cerebral malaria seems to result from a strong cytotoxic T-cell response to particular malarial peptides that are restricted by (ie, fit into the peptide-binding grooves of) two specific HLA molecules.[49]

Peptide-binding specificity is important to consider in the development of vaccines. For example, a vaccine to enhance immune responses to melanoma using a melanoma-specific peptide that binds only to the cells of individuals with the HLA type HLA-A*02:01 was selected for development because A*02:01 is the most common allele in virtually all populations.[50]

Some HLA alleles have been noted to be associated with increased risk for hypersensitivity reactions, such as toxic epidermal necrolysis (TEN), with certain drugs. Among the growing list of associations are HLA-B*57:01 with abacavir, HLA-B*15:02 with carbamazepine, and HLA-B*58:01 with allopurinol.[51] The use of molecular genetics in pharmacology is called pharmacogenetics.

The degree of association between a given HLA type and a disease is often described in terms of relative risk (RR), which is a measure of how much more frequently a disease occurs in individuals with a specific HLA type than in individuals not having that HLA type. Calculation of RR is usually based on the cross-product ratio of a 2×2 contingency table. However, because the HLA system is so polymorphic, there is an increased possibility of finding an association between an HLA antigen and a disease by chance alone. Therefore, calculating RRs for HLA disease associations is more complex and is typically accomplished by use of Haldane's modification of Woolf's formula.[52,53] The RR values for some diseases associated with HLA types are shown in Table 16-3.

HLA testing was previously used to establish relationships or for forensic testing purposes. However, HLA typing has been replaced by analysis of STR polymorphisms at numerous well-defined polymorphic loci for relationship and other forensic testing. STR analysis is sometimes used to confirm that an apparent twin who is HLA-identical to the recipient is a true monozygotic twin through an analysis of these loci on other chromosomes. These reliable methods and established population databases allow exclusion or identification of individuals using extremely small samples of DNA-containing biologic material such as body fluids and tissues.

STR analysis may also be used to identify unlabeled or mislabeled surgical pathology samples.

CLINICAL CONSULTATION IN HLA

Clinical consultation in HLA is essential yet underutilized. Not unlike transfusion medicine and blood banking, the field of clinical histocompatibility requires expertise in laboratory methods, interpretation, and clinical application of test results, combined with an understanding of overarching regulatory processes, to resolve issues. According to CLIA (42 CFR 493.1455), a "clinical consultant must be qualified to consult with and render opinions to the laboratory's clients concerning the diagnosis, treatment and management of patient care," and be a licensed physician or meet the CLIA requirements to be a laboratory director. This training is not a part of most routine postgraduate medical education (or clinical laboratory technologist education). Marques et al[54] have provided an excellent review of the role and importance of a laboratory-medicine-trained expert.

It is imperative that the HLA laboratory director, technical supervisor, and clinical consultant (HLA expert) develop relationships with transplantation surgeons, physicians, and other clinical care staff (eg, transplantation coordinators). Implicit in consultation is that the referring physician is seeking the advice of the HLA expert in either developing a treatment plan or managing care, with assistance in selecting or interpreting HLA tests.

One major distinction between the practice of transfusion medicine and HLA practice is the assignment of clinical relevance of antibodies. In general, blood banks will avoid transfusion of antigen-positive red cell units to a patient who has (ever) had an antibody against that antigen, in order to mitigate hemolytic transfusion reactions. For all the major red cell antibodies, the mere concern for presence is considered clinically significant. In contrast, HLA antibodies are not treated the same way. HLA antibodies targeting donor allograft/tissue are referred to as donor-specific antibodies (DSAs). The presence of DSAs can adversely impact long-term allograft

outcomes. There is still debate as to what level of HLA antibody is clinically significant, especially in the era of solid-phase immunoassays,[55] but it is not uncommon to transplant organs despite the low-level (low concentration) presence of DSAs. This practice can result in risk for an anamnestic response in the recipient. This risk is often minimized by increasing or altering the patient's immunosuppressive regimen. The decision to proceed with transplantation despite the presence of DSAs is predicated upon assigning clinical relevance to the DSAs, and the procedure can be performed only in the context of a particular recipient and donor pair.

Consultation in HSCT

The primary role of the HLA expert in HSCT is in allogeneic donor selection. Donor selection is straightforward when fully matched related donors are available. Queries from the transplantation team may be made when multiple HLA-matched donors are available and the question becomes, which is the better/best one? Conversely, the consult question of which is the least problematic arises when only mismatched donors are available. In both cases, the HLA expert might consider the role of low-expressed HLA antigens,[56] permissive mismatches,[57,58] or other factors such as age, gender, and CMV status.[59] For mismatched allogeneic donors (including haploidentical and cord donors), identifying DSAs against any donors is critical for successful HSCT.[60]

Consultation in Solid-Organ Transplantation

The most commonly transplanted solid organ is the kidney; therefore, renal transplantation consultation is used as a model here. In pretransplantation consultation, the general approach to kidney transplantation is to determine if an intended donor is compatible—that is, are there HLA immunologic barriers that make the transplant undesirable? For patients awaiting deceased-donor kidneys, there is a requirement to test patients for HLA antibodies and to determine whether any preexisting antibodies are an impediment to future transplantations. The HLA director (or clinical consultant) plays a critical role in assigning clinically relevant antibodies because this determines which future donors will be viable for a patient. In the United States, the computer program that assigns donor kidneys to potential recipients excludes "matches" when "unacceptable antigens" are present. The unacceptable antigens are assigned by the patient's transplantation program and HLA laboratory. If assignments are ill-assigned (ie, listing too many unacceptable antigens), donor kidneys may be excluded that may have provided functioning allografts. Conversely, failure to list clinically relevant antibodies may result in unexpectedly incompatible crossmatches, delayed transplantations, and potential for accelerated rejection. After transplantation, there may be programmatic or clinically directed screening or monitoring for DSA formation to help guide management[61] or as an adjunct for the diagnosis of rejection.[62]

REGULATORY ASPECTS OF CLINICAL HISTOCOMPATIBILITY

The field of clinical histocompatibility (also known as HLA) is a highly regulated field, and has similarities to blood banking and transfusion medicine. The CFR has requirements (42 CFR 493.1278) that apply to laboratories performing histocompatibility testing,[63] and the Centers for Medicare and Medicaid Services (CMS) has given select US organizations deemed status for accrediting laboratories that perform histocompatibility testing, such as the College of American Pathologists (CAP) and the American Society for Histocompatibility and Immunogenetics (ASHI). In addition to the rules governing clinical laboratories, clinical transplantation programs also adhere to guidelines set by organizations as a requirement for membership, participation, and reimbursement by CMS. For solid-organ transplantation, the United Network for Organ Sharing (UNOS) holds the federal contract for the Organ Procurement Transplant Network (OPTN). The National Marrow Donor Program (NMDP) oversees HSCT, and the Foundation for the Accreditation of Cellular Therapy (FACT) accredits HSCT programs.

FUTURE DIRECTIONS

The role of HLA in medicine has historically been focused on transplantation and limited to studies of the traditional structural HLA antigens (ie, HLA-A, -B, -C, and -DR, and more recently, -DQ and -DP). As biomedical knowledge increases as a result of the acceleration in technologies like NGS and computational methods, understanding of the role of HLA in health and disease will continue to grow, and the role of the HLA expert and HLA laboratory will continually evolve.

Individual immune responses to HLA antigens and alleles remain difficult to predict. Observations that patients exposed to only a few alloantigens can become highly sensitized, even against antigens to which they have not been exposed, are contrasted with those of other organ recipients whose donors are complete HLA mismatches, yet no detectable alloresponses are made. Some of these phenomena may be due to epitopes and/or eplets (immunogenic determinants) shared by seemingly disparate HLA antigens (even from different loci). In the first case, exposure to an allogeneic but common epitope results in alloreactivity to all antigens that carry that epitope. In the latter case, it may be a result of shared epitopes between mismatched antigens that prevent an alloresponse. Although not widely used, there is some evidence to suggest that eplet/epitope-based matching (vs antigen-matching) may result in better outcomes.[64] A limitation of eplet/epitope-based matching is that eplet/epitope identification requires high-resolution typing. In the United States, HLA typing for transplantation must be by molecular methods, but only low-resolution (antigen-equivalent) typing is required for solid-organ transplantation. As NGS becomes more widely available and demand for eplet/epitope-matching increases, it is possible that high-resolution HLA typing for solid-organ transplantation will become the standard of care same as it currently is for HSCT.

SUMMARY

In conclusion, the HLA system is a complex and highly polymorphic set of genes that are collectively involved in all aspects of the immune response. The recent development of molecular tools to explore this genetic oasis is providing additional information, such as the elucidation of additional unrecognized polymorphisms within the HLA complex (ie, single nucleotide polymorphisms, or SNPs). In the future, the translation of this basic information will undoubtedly lead to new clinical applications in transplantation, autoimmune diseases, vaccine development, pharmacogenetics, and infectious diseases.

KEY POINTS

1. Genes encoded by the major histocompatibility complex (HLA complex in humans) are critical components of the immune system and play a major role in distinguishing self from nonself.
2. HLA genes are located within multiple highly polymorphic loci on the short arm of chromosome 6.
3. HLA genes encode multiple Class I (eg, HLA-A, -B, and -C) and Class II (eg, HLA-DR, -DQ, and -DP) cell-surface proteins.
4. Class I proteins are expressed ubiquitously; Class II proteins have restricted tissue distribution.
5. HLA genes are normally inherited as haplotypes—a linked set of HLA genes from the mother and father—referred to as the maternal haplotype and paternal haplotype, respectively.
6. Together, the maternal and paternal haplotypes are referred to as the genotype. The cell-surface expression of proteins encoded by the HLA genes is referred to as the phenotype.
7. Class I and Class II HLA proteins are strongly immunogenic and can induce an immune response—for example, formation of HLA antibodies and reactive T cells.
8. Donor-specific HLA antibodies are associated with graft dysfunction and/or loss.
9. Solid-phase assays (eg, flow cytometry and flow microarrays) have become the gold standard for detecting and identifying HLA antibodies.
10. Identification of HLA antibodies in donations from directed donors can be used to perform a virtual (in-silico) crossmatch.

REFERENCES

1. Marsh SG, Albert ED, Bodmer WF, et al. Nomenclature for factors of the HLA system, 2010. Tissue Antigens 2010;75:291-455.
2. Robinson J, Halliwell JA, Hayhurst JD, et al. The IPD and IMGT/HLA database: Allele variant databases. Nucleic Acids Res 2015;43:D423-31.
3. Tabayoyong WB, Zavazava N. Soluble HLA revisited. Leuk Res 2007;31:121-5.
4. Ghio M, Contini P, Mazzei C, et al. Soluble HLA class I, HLA class II, and Fas ligand in blood components: A possible key to explain the immunomodulatory effects of allogeneic blood transfusions. Blood 1999;93:1770-7.
5. Voorter CE, van der Vlies S, Kik M, et al. Unexpected Bw4 and Bw6 reactivity patterns in new alleles. Tissue Antigens 2000;56:363-70.
6. Zinkernagel RM, Doherty PC. The discovery of MHC restriction. Immunol Today 1997;18:14-17.
7. Mungall AJ, Palmer SA, Sims SK, et al. The DNA sequence and analysis of human chromosome 6. Nature 2003;425:805-11.
8. Horton R, Wilming L, Rand V, et al. Gene map of the extended human MHC. Nat Rev Genet 2004;5:889-99.
9. Buchler T, Gallardo D, Rodriguez-Luaces M, et al. Frequency of HLA-DPB1 disparities detected by reference strand-mediated conformation analysis in HLA-A, -B, and -DRB1 matched siblings. Hum Immunol 2002;63:139-42.
10. IPD-IMGT/HLA: Statistics. Hinxton, UK: European Molecular Biology Laboratory/European Bioinformatics Institute, 2019. [Available at

http://www.ebi.ac.uk/ipd/imgt/hla/stats.html (accessed October 18, 2019).]

11. Bontadini A. HLA techniques: Typing and antibody detection in the laboratory of immunogenetics. Methods 2012;56:471-6.

12. Erlich H. HLA DNA typing: Past, present, and future. Tissue Antigens 2012;80:1-11.

13. Nunes E, Heslop H, Fernandez-Vina M, et al. Definitions of histocompatibility typing terms. Blood 2011;118:e180-3.

14. De Santis D, Dinauer D, Duke J, et al. 16(th) IHIW: Review of HLA typing by NGS. Int J Immunogenet 2013;40:72-6.

15. Opelz G; Collaborative Transplant Study. Non-HLA transplantation immunity revealed by lymphocytotoxic antibodies. Lancet 2005;365:1570-6.

16. Delville M, Charreau B, Rabant M, et al. Pathogenesis of non-HLA antibodies in solid organ transplantation: Where do we stand? Hum Immunol 2016;77:1055-62.

17. Amico P, Honger G, Bielmann D, et al. Incidence and prediction of early antibody-mediated rejection due to non-human leukocyte antigen-antibodies. Transplantation 2008;85:1557-63.

18. Rajalingam R. The basics of KIR-HLA complexity. ASHI Quarterly 2015;39:22-7.

19. Terasaki PI. A personal perspective: 100-year history of the humoral theory of transplantation. Transplantation 2012;93:751-6.

20. Klein HG, Anstee DJ. Immunology of leucocytes, platelets and plasma components. In: Mollison's blood transfusion in clinical medicine. 12th ed. Oxford, UK: Wiley-Blackwell, 2014:549-610.

21. Hod E, Schwartz J. Platelet transfusion refractoriness. Br J Haematol 2008;142:348-60.

22. Kopko PM, Warner P, Kresie L, et al. Methods for the selection of platelet products for alloimmune-refractory patients. Transfusion 2015;55:235-44.

23. Davenport RD, Kunkel SL. Cytokine roles in hemolytic and nonhemolytic transfusion reactions. Transfus Med Rev 1994;8:157-68.

24. Triulzi DJ, Kleinman S, Kakaiya RM, et al. The effect of previous pregnancy and transfusion on HLA alloimmunization in blood donors: Implications for a transfusion-related acute lung injury risk reduction strategy. Transfusion 2009;49:1825-35.

25. SivaSai KS, Jendrisak M, Duffy BF, et al. Chimerism in peripheral blood of sensitized patients waiting for renal transplantation: Clinical implications. Transplantation 2000;69:538-44.

26. Artlett CM, Smith JB, Jimenez SA. Identification of fetal DNA and cells in skin lesions from women with systemic sclerosis. N Engl J Med 1998;338:1186-91.

27. Pollack MS, Speeg KV, Callander NS, et al. Severe, late-onset graft-versus-host disease in a liver transplant recipient documented by chimerism analysis. Hum Immunol 2005;66:28-31.

28. Clark JR, Scott SD, Jack AL, et al. Monitoring of chimerism following allogeneic haematopoietic stem cell transplantation (HSCT): Technical recommendations for the use of short tandem repeat (STR) based techniques, on behalf of the United Kingdom National External Quality Assessment Service for Leucocyte Immunophenotyping Chimerism Working Group. Br J Haematol 2015;168:26-37.

29. Thomas ED. Bone marrow transplantation: A review. Semin Hematol 1999;36:95-103.

30. Petersdorf EW. Optimal HLA matching in hematopoietic cell transplantation. Curr Opin Immunol 2008;20:588-93.

31. Ricci MJ, Medin JA, Foley RS. Advances in haplo-identical stem cell transplantation in adults with high-risk hematological malignancies. World J Stem Cells 2014;6:380-90.

32. Organ Procurement and Transplant Network. Policy 4: Histocompatibility. Rockville, MD: Health Resources and Services Administration, 2017.

33. Bryan CF, Baier KA, Nelson PW, et al. Long-term graft survival is improved in cadaveric renal retransplantation by flow cytometric cross-matching. Transplantation 1998;66:1827-32.

34. Cecka JM. Calculated PRA (CPRA): The new measure of sensitization for transplant candidates. Am J Transplant 2010;10:26-9.

35. Gebel HM, Bray RA. Sensitization and sensitivity: Defining the unsensitized patient. Transplantation 2000;69:1370-4.

36. Scientific Registry of Transplant Recipients; Organ Procurement and Transplantation Network. SRTR/OPTN 2012 annual data report. [Available at https://srtr.transplant.hrsa.gov/.]

37. Terasaki PI, Cecka JM, Gjertson DW, et al. High survival rates of kidney transplants from spousal and living unrelated donors. N Engl J Med 1995;333:333-6.

38. Rees MA, Kopke JE, Pelletier RP, et al. A nonsimultaneous, extended, altruistic-donor chain. N Engl J Med 2009;360:1096-101.

39. Daebritz SH, Schmoeckel M, Mair H, et al. Blood type incompatible cardiac transplantation

in young infants. Eur J Cardiothorac Surg 2007; 31:339-43; discussion, 43.

40. Heffron T, Welch D, Pillen T, et al. Successful ABO-incompatible pediatric liver transplantation utilizing standard immunosuppression with selective postoperative plasmapheresis. Liver Transpl 2006;12:972-8.

41. Thorsby E. Invited anniversary review: HLA associated diseases. Hum Immunol 1997;53:1-11.

42. Pile KD. Broadsheet number 51: HLA and disease associations. Pathology 1999;31:202-12.

43. Price P, Witt C, Allcock R, et al. The genetic basis for the association of the 8.1 ancestral haplotype (A1, B8, DR3) with multiple immunopathological diseases. Immunol Rev 1999;167: 257-74.

44. Holoshitz J. The quest for better understanding of HLA-disease association: Scenes from a road less travelled by. Discov Med 2013;16:93-101.

45. Pelin Z, Guilleminault C, Risch N, et al. HLA-DQB1*0602 homozygosity increases relative risk for narcolepsy but not disease severity in two ethnic groups. US Modafinil in Narcolepsy Multicenter Study Group. Tissue Antigens 1998;51:96-100.

46. Cinova J, Palova-Jelinkova L, Smythies LE, et al. Gliadin peptides activate blood monocytes from patients with celiac disease. J Clin Immunol 2007;27:201-9.

47. van Gaalen FA, van Aken J, Huizinga TW, et al. Association between HLA class II genes and autoantibodies to cyclic citrullinated peptides (CCPs) influences the severity of rheumatoid arthritis. Arthritis Rheum 2004;50:2113-21.

48. Mayr A, Schlosser M, Grober N, et al. GAD autoantibody affinity and epitope specificity identify distinct immunization profiles in children at risk for type 1 diabetes. Diabetes 2007;56:1527-33.

49. Hill AV. The immunogenetics of resistance to malaria. Proc Assoc Am Physicians 1999;111: 272-7.

50. Slingluff CL Jr, Yamshchikov G, Neese P, et al. Phase I trial of a melanoma vaccine with gp100(280-288) peptide and tetanus helper peptide in adjuvant: Immunologic and clinical outcomes. Clin Cancer Res 2001;7:3012-24.

51. Pavlos R, Mallal S, Phillips E. HLA and pharmacogenetics of drug hypersensitivity. Pharmacogenomics 2012;13:1285-306.

52. Haldane JB. The estimation and significance of the logarithm of a ratio of frequencies. Ann Hum Genet 1956;20:309-11.

53. Woolf B. On estimating the relation between blood group and disease. Ann Hum Genet 1955;19:251-3.

54. Marques MB, Anastasi J, Ashwood E, et al. The clinical pathologist as consultant. Am J Clin Pathol 2011;135:11-12.

55. Bettinotti MP, Zachary AA, Leffell MS. Clinically relevant interpretation of solid phase assays for HLA antibody. Curr Opin Organ Transplant 2016;21:453-8.

56. Fernandez-Vina MA, Klein JP, Haagenson M, et al. Multiple mismatches at the low expression HLA loci DP, DQ, and DRB3/4/5 associate with adverse outcomes in hematopoietic stem cell transplantation. Blood 2013;121:4603-10.

57. Fleischhauer K, Shaw BE, Gooley T, et al. Effect of T-cell-epitope matching at HLA-DPB1 in recipients of unrelated-donor haemopoietic-cell transplantation: A retrospective study. Lancet Oncol 2012;13:366-74.

58. Fernandez-Vina MA, Wang T, Lee SJ, et al. Identification of a permissible HLA mismatch in hematopoietic stem cell transplantation. Blood 2014;123:1270-8.

59. Spellman SR, Eapen M, Logan BR, et al. A perspective on the selection of unrelated donors and cord blood units for transplantation. Blood 2012;120:259-65.

60. Yoshihara S, Taniguchi K, Ogawa H, et al. The role of HLA antibodies in allogeneic SCT: Is the 'type-and-screen' strategy necessary not only for blood type but also for HLA? Bone Marrow Transplant 2012;47:1499-506.

61. Tait BD, Susal C, Gebel HM, et al. Consensus guidelines on the testing and clinical management issues associated with HLA and non-HLA antibodies in transplantation. Transplantation 2013;95:19-47.

62. Haas M, Loupy A, Lefaucheur C, et al. The Banff 2017 Kidney Meeting report: Revised diagnostic criteria for chronic active T cell-mediated rejection, antibody-mediated rejection, and prospects for integrative endpoints for next-generation clinical trials. Am J Transplant 2018; 18:293-307.

63. Code of federal regulations. Standard: Histocompatibility. Title 42, CFR Part 493.1278. Washington, DC: US Government Publishing Office, 2019 (revised annually).

64. Wiebe C, Pochinco D, Blydt-Hansen TD, et al. Class II HLA epitope matching—A strategy to minimize de novo donor-specific antibody development and improve outcomes. Am J Transplant 2013;13:3114-22.

CHAPTER 17

Transfusion-Service-Related Activities: Pretransfusion Testing and Storage, Monitoring, Processing, Distribution, and Inventory Management of Blood Components

Caroline R. Alquist, MD, PhD, and Sarah K. Harm, MD

HOSPITAL-BASED TRANSFUSION SERvice activities ensure transfusion of pure, potent, safe, and efficacious blood components to recipients needing this life-sustaining therapy. Safe transfusion practice begins at the bedside with proper recipient identification, sample collection, and labeling; continues with pretransfusion testing; and culminates in the selection and distribution of compatible blood and blood components that have been appropriately processed, tested, monitored, and stored.

SAMPLES AND REQUESTS

Transfusion Requests

All requests for blood and blood components must be legible, accurate, and complete, with two independent identifiers for correct recipient identification.[1(pp38-39)] Requests should include the type and amount of component requested,

any special needs (eg, irradiation) or special processing required (eg, volume reduction) and the name of the ordering physician or authorized health professional. Additional useful information to guide testing and/or product/component selection may include the recipient's gender, age, weight, diagnosis, and transfusion and/or pregnancy history.

Recipient Identification and Sample Labeling

Collection of a properly labeled pretransfusion blood sample from the intended recipient is critical to safe blood transfusion. At the time of sample collection, the phlebotomist must 1) accurately identify the potential transfusion recipient before collecting the pretransfusion sample and 2) ensure that the correct recipient information is placed on the sample label before the sample leaves the side of the recipient.[1(p38)] A mechanism must be in place to identify the phlebotomist, as well as the date and time of

Caroline R. Alquist, MD, PhD, Section Head of Clinical Pathology, Department of Pathology and Laboratory Medicine, Ochsner Health System, and Assistant Professor, Ochsner Clinical School, University of Queensland School of Medicine, New Orleans, Louisiana; and Sarah K. Harm, MD, Medical Director of Blood Bank, University of Vermont Medical Center, and Associate Professor, Department of Pathology, Robert Larner MD College of Medicine, Burlington, Vermont
The authors have disclosed no conflicts of interest.

sample collection.[1(p38)] ABO-incompatible Red Blood Cell (RBC) transfusions should never occur, but when they do, they most commonly result from misidentification of recipients or pretransfusion sample labeling errors.[2] These errors could result in wrong blood in tube (WBIT), a situation where the blood in the tube is not that of the recipient identified on the sample label.[3] The risk of WBIT when using manual methods of patient identification is reported to be at least 1 in 3000 samples.[4]

Because of the risk for WBIT, for allogeneic transfusions, two determinations of a transfusion recipient's ABO group are required. Electronic identification systems that use machine-readable information (eg, bar codes or embedded radio-frequency-emitting chips) are available to perform and integrate many functions, including recipient identification, sample labeling, blood unit identification, and linkage of blood components to their intended recipient(s).[5-7] The use of an electronic patient identification system at the time of pretransfusion sample collection significantly decreases the risk of WBIT to about 1 in 15,000 samples.[4]

Confirming Sample Linkage

When a pretransfusion sample is received in the laboratory, laboratory personnel must confirm that the information on the sample label and the information on the pretransfusion testing request are in agreement. If there is any doubt about the identity of the recipient or the labeling of the sample, a new sample must be obtained.[1(p38)] One study found that samples failing to meet acceptability criteria were 40 times more likely to have a blood grouping discrepancy, and a larger multicenter study found a WBIT rate of approximately 1 in 30 mislabeled (rejected) samples.[4,8] Thus, adherence to a strict policy of rejecting incorrectly labeled samples for testing should help avoid blood grouping errors and decrease the risk for transfusion of ABO-incompatible blood components.

PRETRANSFUSION TESTING OF RECIPIENT BLOOD

Serologic Testing Overview

The recipient's ABO group and RhD type must be determined before transfusion, with the exception of emergent situations (discussed later in this chapter). In addition, testing for unexpected antibodies to red cell antigens (eg, antibody detection test or screen) is required before transfusion of Whole Blood, RBCs, and Granulocytes.[1(p39)] Results of testing on the current sample must be compared with previous transfusion service records to identify any discrepancy between previous and current determinations of ABO group and RhD type.[1(p41)] Current testing results must also be compared to previous records to identify any history of clinically significant antibodies, adverse events to transfusion, or special transfusion requirements.[1(p41)] Crossmatch testing is required on any blood component containing ≥2 mL of red cells. Unless the need for blood is urgent or emergent, a crossmatch must be performed before a Whole Blood or RBC transfusion. Crossmatching is also required before granulocyte transfusion and platelet transfusions unless the component is prepared by a method known to result in a component containing <2 mL of red cells.[1(p42)] When clinically significant antibodies are not detected using current antibody detection tests and there is no record of previous detection of such antibodies, then a method must be used to detect ABO incompatibility.[1(p42)] The advantages and limitations of various pretransfusion testing schemes are shown in Table 17-1.

Serologic Testing Principles

The basis of pretransfusion testing using test tube methods, solid phase, or column agglutination is the detection of in-vitro red cell antigen/antibody reactions by observation of agglutination or hemolysis. Agglutination is a reversible chemical reaction that occurs in two stages: 1) sensitization, in which the antibody attaches to the red cell antigen, and 2) agglutination, in which the sensitized red cells are bridged to form a macroscopically detectable lattice. The

TABLE 17-1. Pretransfusion Testing Schemes

Test Scheme	Tests Performed	Advantages	Limitations
Hold	None	A sample has been collected.	ABO, RhD, and antibody detection testing are *not* performed.
Type and hold	ABO and RhD	A sample has been collected; the recipient's ABO group and RhD type are known.	Antibody detection testing is *not* performed.
Type and screen	ABO, RhD, and antibody detection test/identification	Most of the pretransfusion testing has been performed; compatible blood can be provided in most situations.	Does *not* include crossmatch.
Type and screen with crossmatch*	ABO, RhD, antibody detection test/identification, Red Blood Cell unit selection or phenotyping, and crossmatch	Routine pretransfusion testing has been performed; compatible blood can be provided in most situations.	Units are removed from general inventory and may not be available for timely use by other recipients.

*"Prepare" (or other term) may be used instead of the word "crossmatch" by some hospital electronic ordering systems.

antihuman globulin (AHG) phase, or indirect antiglobulin test (IAT, sometimes referred to as the indirect Coombs test), detects bound red cell antibodies that do not produce direct agglutination. AHG reagent consists of immunoglobulin M (IgM) antibodies directed against the Fc portion of IgG molecules.[9] In the past, AHG sera were produced primarily by injecting animals with human globulins to stimulate antibody production against the foreign human protein. Now AHG is most often manufactured from hybridoma cell lines as a monoclonal antibody. This antiserum attaches to and causes agglutination of red cells sensitized with human globulins, as illustrated in Fig 17-1. Causes of false-positive and false-negative results in antiglobulin tests using test tube methods are listed in Appendices 17-1 and 17-2.

Various factors may enhance or decrease sensitization and agglutination, including temperature, immunoglobulin class, and interactions between antigen configuration and the antigen-binding fragment site of the antibody. These fac-

tors affect the incubation time necessary to achieve the detectable endpoint. The strength of agglutination or degree of hemolysis, or both, observed during serologic testing should be recorded immediately after reading. Refer to Method 1-9 for details on the grading and scoring of serologic test reactions.

Test Methods

Pretransfusion testing may be performed using the traditional tube method or with other automated and semiautomated testing platforms using column-agglutination (sometimes called "gel" or "beads"), microplate solid-phase, or hemagglutination-microplate technologies. Fluid-phase and solid-phase assays are discussed in greater detail in Chapter 8. Automated testing systems require validation before implementation and after any alteration in software functionality. Molecular testing is not routinely performed for pretransfusion testing. However, testing by molecular methods may be employed to resolve ABO group and/or RhD typing discrepancies

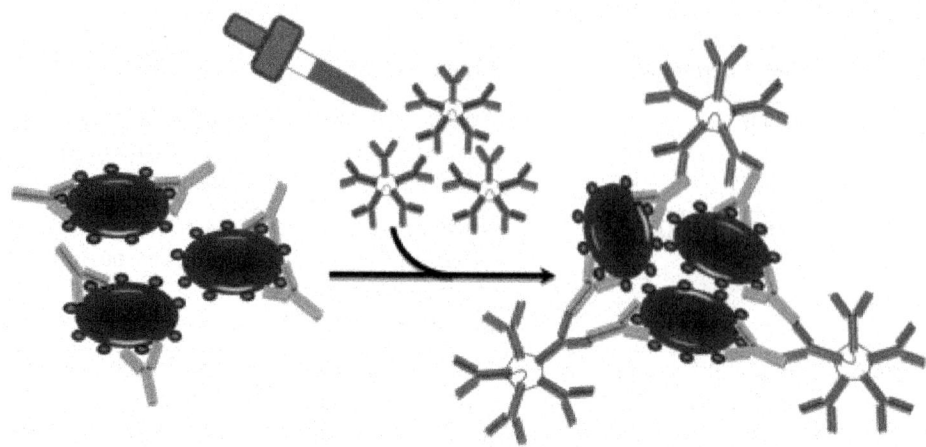

FIGURE 17-1. The antihuman globulin (AHG) reaction. AHG (IgM anti-IgG) molecules are shown reacting with the Fc portion of human IgG coating adjacent red cells. (Image courtesy of J. O'Connor.)

and to determine red cell antigen genotyping when serologic typing cannot be performed. Molecular testing is discussed in greater detail in Chapter 8. Additionally, platelet crossmatch compatibility testing may also occur in the pretransfusion setting, using commercial solid-phase adherence assays when patients have antibodies to HLA or human platelet antigen (HPA) identified in their serum. Further information on selection of HLA-matched, HLA-antigen-negative, or crossmatch-compatible platelet units for the treatment of platelet refractoriness is covered in Chapters 16 and 19.

Sample Requirements

Pretransfusion testing uses recipient red cells and either serum or plasma. Because the endpoint of pretransfusion testing is the visualization of agglutination, the use of hemolyzed or lipemic samples may create difficulties in evaluating test results. Plasma is often the preferred sample, as incompletely clotted serum samples may contain small fibrin clots that trap red cells into aggregates, which may cause false-positive results. In addition, clotting may be incomplete in anticoagulated serum samples, such as those from recipients who have been treated with heparin; addition of thrombin or protamine sulfate to the sample may correct this problem.

(See Method 1-3.) At times, it may be necessary to obtain a pretransfusion blood sample from the same extremity in which there is an intravenous infusion. If this is the case, steps should be taken to avoid dilution of the sample, which might result in a failure to detect unexpected red cell antibodies. Plasma is also preferred for automated methods to avoid fibrin interference and clots.

Sample Age

When pretransfusion testing is performed for a recipient who has been pregnant or received transfusion within the previous 3 months, or when pregnancy and/or transfusion history are uncertain, the pretransfusion sample used for testing must be no more than 3 days old at the time of the intended transfusion because a recent transfusion or pregnancy may stimulate production of unexpected antibodies. The day of collection is counted as day 0; therefore, a sample collected on a Monday can be used for a transfusion until 11:59 pm on Thursday of the same week.[1(p40)] Although the specification of 3 days is arbitrary, the 3-day requirement was created as a practical approach to ensure that the sample used for testing reflects the recipient's current immunologic status.[10] If the histories of transfusion and pregnancy are known with certainty and if no transfusion or pregnancy has occurred in the previous 3 months, pretransfusion testing may be completed in advance of a scheduled surgical procedure. Pretransfusion testing is performed at some centers up to 45 days before a scheduled surgical procedure to reduce delays and cancellations associated with unexpected antibodies identified when samples are drawn on the day of surgery.[11]

ABO Group and RhD Typing

To determine the recipient's ABO group, the recipient's red cells must be tested with anti-A and anti-B reagent (forward or front typing). In addition, the recipient's serum or plasma must be tested against A_1 and B red cells (reverse or back typing). (See Method 2-2.) Donor red cells must be ABO compatible with the recipient's plasma. Any discrepant ABO typing results must be resolved before type-specific blood can be given (Method 2-4). If urgent or emergent transfusion is necessary before ABO typing can be completed, the recipient should receive group O red cells.[1(p39)] Group O RBC unit selection should be continued, as needed, until the patient's ABO group can be confirmed by two determinations.[1(pp40-41)]

A second determination can be accomplished as follows:

- Testing a second sample collected at a time different from the first sample, including a new verification of patient identification.

- Comparison with previous records.
- Retesting the same sample if patient identification was verified using a validated electronic identification system.

Routine testing for ABO and resolution of ABO discrepancies are described in greater detail in Chapter 10. Table 17-2 lists blood component selection criteria for ABO groups when ABO-identical components are not available.

To determine the recipient's RhD type, the recipient's red cells must be tested for the RhD antigen using anti-D reagent (Method 2-13).[1(pp39-40)] Weak RhD testing is not required for recipient samples except when assessing the red cells of an infant born to an RhD-negative mother (Method 2-15).[1(p51)] If problems in RhD typing arise, especially if the recipient is a female of childbearing potential, it is prudent to limit transfusion to blood components containing red cells that are RhD negative, at least until the problem is resolved. Testing for the RhD antigen is described in greater detail in Chapter 11.

Detection of Unexpected Antibodies

Antibody detection tests, also known as antibody screens, are designed to detect clinically significant (predominantly IgG) antibodies, including those associated with hemolytic disease of the fetus and newborn (HDFN), hemolytic transfusion reactions, or notably decreased survival of transfused red cells. The procedure uses

TABLE 17-2. Blood Component ABO Requirements

Whole Blood	Must be identical to that of the recipient. Low-titer group O Whole Blood may be used for emergent transfusions.
Red Blood Cells	Must be compatible with the recipient's plasma.
Granulocytes	Must be compatible with the recipient's plasma.
Plasma	Selected to be compatible with the recipient's red cells. Some centers are using thawed group A plasma for emergent transfusions.
Platelets	All ABO groups are acceptable. Although ABO-identical platelets are preferred, components that are compatible with the recipient's red cells are recommended.
Cryoprecipitated Antihemophilic Factor	All ABO groups are acceptable.

the IAT method to demonstrate in-vitro reactions between red cells with known antigen expression and any antibodies that might be present in the patient. The recipient serum or plasma is incubated with unpooled reagent antibody-screening cells. Panels of two, three, or four screening cells may be used. Following incubation at 37 C, the cells are then washed to remove unbound globulins. The presence of agglutination with the addition of AHG reagent indicates antibody binding to a specific red cell antigen.

When reactivity is identified in the antibody detection test (screen), additional testing is performed to identify the target red cell antigen(s). Additional testing strategies used for antibody identification may include use of enhancement media [albumin additive, low-ionic-strength saline (LISS), polyethylene glycol (PEG)] and/or enzyme or chemical treatment of the panel screening cells. Antibody identification is discussed in greater detail in Chapter 13.

Recipients with clinically significant red cell antibodies or a history of such antibodies must receive crossmatch-compatible Whole Blood, RBCs, or Granulocytes that lack the corresponding antigen. Clinically significant red cell alloantibodies may become undetectable in a recipient's plasma over time. Between 30% and 35% of antibodies are undetectable within 1 year, and nearly 50% are undetectable after 10 or more years.[12] Failure to detect a weakly reactive red cell alloantibody can be followed by a rapid anamnestic production of antibody and/or a delayed hemolytic transfusion reaction.[13]

Immediate-Spin Crossmatch

The immediate-spin (IS) crossmatch method is the serologic method used to detect ABO incompatibility between donor red cells and recipient serum. This method can be used as the sole crossmatch method *only* if the recipient has no present or previously detected, clinically significant antibodies.[1(p42)] When IS crossmatch is used for recipients with a negative antibody detection test result, the risk of an overt hemolytic reaction from an undetected alloantibody is low.[14] The potential benefits of using an IS crossmatch instead of a full AHG crossmatch in recipients

with a negative antibody screen include reductions in turnaround time, workload, and reagent costs.

In the IS saline technique, recipient serum or plasma is mixed with saline-suspended donor red cells at room temperature. The tube is centrifuged immediately and observed for the presence of agglutination. Failure to properly perform the IS crossmatch test can lead to false-negative results and the failure to detect ABO-incompatible RBC units.[15] This technique is described in greater detail in Method 3-1.

Computer/Electronic Crossmatch

ABO compatibility may be verified alternatively by using a computerized/electronic crossmatch, provided that the following conditions have been met[1(pp42-43)]:

- The computer system has been validated on-site to ensure that only ABO-compatible Whole Blood or RBCs are selected for transfusion.
- The computer system contains the donation identification number (DIN), component name, ABO group, and RhD type of the component; the ABO group confirmation of the component; the two unique recipient identifiers; the ABO group and RhD type of the recipient and the results of the antibody screen; and the interpretation of compatibility.
- A method exists to verify correct entry of data before the release of blood components.
- The system contains logic to alert the user 1) to discrepancies between the donor ABO group/RhD type on the unit label and the ABO group/RhD type determined by blood group confirmatory tests and 2) to ABO incompatibility between the recipient and donor unit.

This method can be used as the sole crossmatch method *only* if the recipient has no present or previously detected, clinically significant antibodies.[1(pp42-43)] Potential advantages of a computer crossmatch include decreased workload, reduced sample volume required for testing, reduced exposure of personnel to blood samples, and better use of blood inventory.[16]

Antiglobulin Crossmatch

Blood lacking relevant antigens should be selected for transfusion in a recipient with a clinically significant antibody identified currently or historically, even if the antibody is presently nonreactive.[1(p41)] This crossmatch includes incubation at 37 C and the IAT (AHG test). The AHG crossmatch may be performed using tube, column-agglutination ("gel" or "beads"), or solid-phase systems. For a routine tube AHG crossmatch, the donor red cells obtained from a segment of tubing that was originally attached to the donor unit to be transfused are washed and resuspended to between 2% and 5% concentration in saline. Recipient serum or plasma is then mixed with the washed donor red cells. Following incubation at 37 C, the cells are again washed to remove unbound immunoglobulins. The presence of agglutination with the addition of AHG reagent indicates incompatibility (Method 3-2).

Interpretation of Antibody Detection Testing (Screening) and Crossmatch Results

Most samples tested have a negative antibody detection test and are crossmatch compatible with the donor RBC units selected. However, a negative antibody screening result does not guarantee that the serum or plasma does not contain clinically significant red cell antibodies; it shows only that the sample contains no detectable antibodies that are reactive with the screening cells or techniques used. Furthermore, a compatible crossmatch does not guarantee normal red cell survival. See Appendix 17-3 for a summary of positive pretransfusion test results and their possible causes. Requirements for compatibility testing for neonates/infants <4 months of age are discussed in Chapter 24.

BLOOD AND BLOOD COMPONENT STORAGE AND MONITORING

General Considerations

Transport and storage requirements must be followed to optimize the safety and efficacy of blood and blood components. Transport requirements must be adhered to anytime blood components are transferred between locations, including 1) from the collection site to the processing facility, 2) from the supplier to the blood bank, 3) from the blood bank to the recipient, and 4) back to the blood bank if not transfused. Storage requirements and expiration dates vary by component type and are based on factors such as in-vitro red cell metabolism for RBC components in various storage solutions or coagulation protein stabilization solutions for plasma components (Table 17-3). Failure to adhere to these storage and expiration requirements can result in decreased component potency and/or safety.

Temperature requirements during transport of blood components differ from those during storage.[17] (See Table 17-3.) Shipping from the supplier to the hospital blood bank is considered transport, and applicable temperature requirements must be met. When blood components are issued from the blood bank to the recipient-care area, maintenance of appropriate temperature requirements allows for the possibility of returning the components to inventory if they are not transfused.

Refrigerators, freezers, and platelet incubators for blood and blood component storage can be equipped with continuous-temperature-monitoring devices to allow detection of temperature deviations before components are affected. Automated electronic monitoring devices that are available include 1) weekly pen-and-chart recorders, 2) sets of hard-wired or radio-frequency temperature-recording devices, and 3) centralized temperature-monitoring systems.

Thermometers or thermocouples should be strategically placed in the equipment for optimal temperature monitoring. If an automated temperature-recording device is not used, temperatures of the blood storage environment must be recorded manually every at least every 4 hours.[1(p16)] This requirement includes ambient room temperature monitoring of platelets that are not stored in a platelet chamber or incubator.

Recorded temperatures should be checked daily to ensure proper operation of the equipment and recorder. Deviations from acceptable

TABLE 17-3.   Reference Standard 5.1.8A—Requirements for Storage, Transportation, and Expiration*[1]

Item No.	Component	Storage	Transport[†]	Expiration[‡]	Additional Criteria
Whole Blood Components					
1	Whole Blood	1-6 C	1-10 C	CPD/CP2D: 21 days CPDA-1: 35 days	
2	Whole Blood Irradiated	1-6 C	1-10 C	Original expiration or 28 days from date of irradiation, whichever is sooner	
3	Whole Blood Leukocytes Reduced	1-6 C	1-10 C	CPD/CP2D: 21 days CPDA-1: 35 days Open system: 24 hours	
Red Blood Cell Components, Whole-Blood-Derived or Apheresis-Derived					
4	Red Blood Cells (RBCs)	1-6 C	1-10 C	ACD/CPD/CP2D: 21 days CPDA-1: 35 days Additive solution: 42 days Open system: 24 hours	
5	Deglycerolized RBCs	1-6 C	1-10 C	Open system: 24 hours Closed system: 14 days or as FDA approved	
6	Frozen RBCs 40% Glycerol[§]	−65 C or colder if 40% glycerol or as FDA approved	Maintain frozen state	10 years (A policy shall be developed if rare frozen units are to be retained beyond this time)	Frozen within 6 days of collection unless rejuvenated Frozen before Red Blood Cell expiration if rare unit
7	RBCs Irradiated	1-6 C	1-10 C	Original expiration or 28 days from date of irradiation, whichever is sooner	

#	Component	Storage Temperature	Transport Temperature	Expiration	Notes
8	RBCs Leukocytes Reduced	1-6 C	1-10 C	ACD/CPD/CP2D: 21 days CPDA-1: 35 days Additive solution: 42 days Open system: 24 hours	AS-1: freeze after rejuvenation
9	Rejuvenated RBCs	1-6 C	1-10 C	CPD, CPDA-1: 24 hours	
10	Deglycerolized Rejuvenated RBCs	1-6 C	1-10 C	24 hours or as approved by FDA	
11	Frozen Rejuvenated RBCs§	−65 C or colder	Maintain frozen state	CPD, CPDA-1: 10 years AS-1: 3 years (A policy shall be developed if rare frozen units are to be retained beyond this time)	
12	Washed RBCs	1-6 C	1-10 C	24 hours	

Platelet Components◊,¶

#	Component	Storage Temperature	Transport Temperature	Expiration
13	Platelets	20-24 C with continuous gentle agitation#	As close as possible to 20-24 C** Maximum time without agitation: 30 hours	24 hours to 5 days, depending on collection system
14	Platelets Cold Stored††	1-6 C (agitation optional)	1-10 C	According to manufacturer's written instructions
15	Platelets Irradiated	20-24 C with continuous gentle agitation#	As close as possible to 20-24 C** Maximum time without agitation: 30 hours	No change from original expiration date

(Continued)

TABLE 17-3. Reference Standard 5.1.8A—Requirements for Storage, Transportation, and Expiration*[1] (Continued)

Item No.	Component	Storage	Transport†	Expiration‡	Additional Criteria
16	Platelets Leukocytes Reduced	20-24 C with continuous gentle agitation#	As close as possible to 20-24 C** Maximum time without agitation: 30 hours	Open system: 4 hours Closed system: No change in expiration	
17	Pooled Platelets Leukocytes Reduced	20-24 C with continuous gentle agitation#	As close as possible to 20-24 C** Maximum time without agitation: 30 hours	4 hours after pooling or 5 days following collection of the oldest unit in the pool	
18	Pooled Platelets (in open system)	20-24 C with continuous gentle agitation#	As close as possible to 20-24 C** Maximum time without agitation: 30 hours	Open system: 4 hours	
19	Apheresis Platelets	20-24 C with continuous gentle agitation#	As close as possible to 20-24 C** Maximum time without agitation: 30 hours	24 hours or 5 days, depending on collection system	
20	Apheresis Platelets Irradiated	20-24 C with continuous gentle agitation#	As close as possible to 20-24 C** Maximum time without agitation: 30 hours	No change from original expiration date	
21	Apheresis Platelets Leukocytes Reduced	20-24 C with continuous gentle agitation#	As close as possible to 20-24 C** Maximum time without agitation: 30 hours	Open system: within 4 hours of opening the system Closed system: 5 days or 7 days#	

#	Component	Storage Temperature	Transportation	Expiration	Special Notes
22	Apheresis Platelets Platelet Additive Solution Added Leukocytes Reduced	20-24 C with continuous gentle agitation#	As close as possible to 20-24 C** Maximum time without agitation: 30 hours	5 days	
23	Apheresis Platelets Pathogen Reduced	20-24 C with continuous gentle agitation#	As close as possible to 20-24 C** Maximum time without agitation: 30 hours	5 days	
Granulocyte Components					
24	Apheresis Granulocytes	20-24 C	As close as possible to 20-24 C	24 hours	Transfuse as soon as possible; Standard 5.28.10 applies
25	Apheresis Granulocytes Irradiated	20-24 C	As close as possible to 20-24 C	No change from original expiration date	Transfuse as soon as possible; Standard 5.28.10 applies
Plasma Components					
26	Cryoprecipitated AHF§	−18 C or colder	Maintain frozen state	12 months from original collection	Thaw the FFP at 1-6 C Place cryoprecipitate in the freezer within 1 hour after removal from refrigerated centrifuge
27	Cryoprecipitated AHF (after thawing)	20-24 C	As close as possible to 20-24 C	Single unit: 6 hours	Thaw at 30-37 C
28	Pooled Cryoprecipitated AHF (pooled before freezing)§	−18 C or colder	Maintain frozen state	12 months from earliest date of collection of product in pool	Thaw the FFP at 1-6 C Place cryoprecipitate in the freezer within 1 hour after removal from refrigerated centrifuge

(Continued)

TABLE 17-3. Reference Standard 5.1.8A—Requirements for Storage, Transportation, and Expiration *1 (Continued)

Item No.	Component	Storage	Transport†	Expiration‡	Additional Criteria
29	Pooled Cryoprecipitated AHF (after thawing)	20-24 C	As close as possible to 20-24 C	Pooled in an open system: 4 hours / If pooled using a sterile connection device: 6 hours	Thaw at 30-37 C
30	Fresh Frozen Plasma (FFP) §,§§	−18 C or colder or −65 C or colder	Maintain frozen state	−18 C or colder: 12 months from collection / −65 C or colder: 7 years from collection	Placed in freezer within 8 hours of collection or as stated in FDA-cleared operator's manuals/package inserts / Storage at −65 C or colder requires FDA approval if product is stored for longer than 12 months
31	FFP (after thawing)§§	1-6 C	1-10 C	If issued as FFP: 24 hours	Thaw at 30-37 C or by using an FDA-cleared device
32	Plasma Frozen Within 24 Hours After Phlebotomy (PF24)§,§§	−18 C or colder	Maintain frozen state	12 months from collection	
33	Plasma Frozen Within 24 Hours After Phlebotomy (after thawing)§§	1-6 C	1-10 C	If issued as PF24: 24 hours	Thaw at 30-37 C or by using an FDA-cleared device
34	Plasma Frozen Within 24 Hours After Phlebotomy Held at Room Temperature Up to 24 Hours After Phlebotomy (PF24RT24)§	−18 C or colder	Maintain frozen state	12 months from collection	

35	Plasma Frozen Within 24 Hours After Phlebotomy Held at Room Temperature Up to 24 Hours After Phlebotomy (after thawing)	1-6 C	1-10 C	If issued as PF24RT24: 24 hours	Thaw at 30-37 C or by using an FDA-cleared device
36	Thawed Plasma§§	1-6 C	1-10 C	5 days from date product was thawed or original expiration, whichever is sooner	Shall have been collected and processed in a closed system
37	Plasma Cryoprecipitate Reduced§	−18 C or colder	Maintain frozen state	12 months from collection	Shall be refrozen within 24 hours of thawing the FFP from which it was derived
38	Plasma Cryoprecipitate Reduced (after thawing)	1-6 C	1-10 C	If issued as Plasma Cryoprecipitate Reduced: 24 hours	Thaw at 30-37 C
39	Thawed Plasma Cryoprecipitate Reduced	1-6 C	1-10 C	If issued as Thawed Plasma Cryoprecipitate Reduced: 5 days from date product was thawed or original expiration, whichever is sooner	Shall have been collected and processed in a closed system
40	Liquid Plasma	1-6 C	1-10 C	5 days after expiration of Whole Blood	21 CFR 610.53(b)
41	Recovered Plasma (liquid or frozen)	Refer to short supply agreement	Refer to short supply agreement	Refer to short supply agreement	Requires a short supply agreement∞
42	Plasma Pathogen Reduced§	−18 C or colder	Maintain frozen state	12 months from original collection	

(Continued)

TABLE 17-3.   Reference Standard 5.1.8A—Requirements for Storage, Transportation, and Expiration*[1] (Continued)

Item No.	Component	Storage	Transport[†]	Expiration[‡]	Additional Criteria
Tissue and Derivatives					
43	Tissue	Conform to source manufacturer's written instructions	Conform to manufacturer's written instructions	Conform to manufacturer's written instructions	21 CFR 1271.3(b), 21 CFR 1271.3(bb), and 21 CFR 1271.15(d)
44	Derivatives	Conform to manufacturer's written instructions	Conform to manufacturer's written instructions	Conform to manufacturer's written instructions	

*Products may be pathogen reduced if approved by the FDA.

[†]For products being transported between the collection and processing site, Standards 5.6.5 and 5.6.5.1 apply.

[‡]If the seal is broken during processing, components stored at 1 to 6 C shall have an expiration time of 24 hours, and components stored at 20 to 24 C shall have an expiration time of 4 hours, unless otherwise indicated. This expiration shall not exceed the original expiration date or time.

[§]If a liquid freezing bath is used, the container shall be protected from chemical alteration.

[◌]The platelet storage system shall be FDA-cleared or -approved for the conditions specified.

[¶]The temperature range decided upon at the time of manufacturing shall be maintained. 21 CFR 640.24(d).

[#]21 CFR 640.25(a).

[**]21 CFR 610.53(b).

[††]Applies to modified, unmodified, apheresis, and whole-blood-derived platelet products

[‡‡]May be stored for 7 days only if: 1) storage containers are cleared or approved by FDA for 7-day platelet storage and 2) labeled with the requirement to test every product stored beyond 5 days with a bacteria detection device cleared by FDA and labeled as a "safety measure."

[§§]These lines could apply to apheresis plasma or whole-blood-derived plasma.

[∞]21 CFR 601.22.

temperature ranges should be documented and explained (including any actions taken and an assessment of blood component acceptability for transfusion), dated, and initialed by the person noting the deviation.

Most blood component-storage devices are equipped with audible alarms to alert personnel that temperature ranges are approaching unacceptable levels. Central alarm monitoring allows facilities that do not have personnel in the vicinity of the equipment to alert designated staff at another location when an alarm is activated. Because platelets must be gently agitated during storage, typically using horizontal flatbed or elliptical rotators, alarm systems should also emit alerts when the platelet agitator has malfunctioned.

Transfusion services may place blood storage refrigerators in other areas of the hospital to allow immediate access to blood in emergency situations. Such a practice requires that the same blood component storage monitoring standards be met in these other areas.

If an equipment failure occurs and prevents acceptable temperature ranges from being maintained, the facility should have policies, processes, and procedures in place to relocate blood and blood components. The secondary storage location may be another on- or off-site refrigerator or freezer, qualified storage boxes, or coolers used with a validated process that has been shown to maintain required temperatures during storage. Because the safety, purity, potency, and quality of the blood components could be affected by delays in relocation to a secondary storage location, it is recommended that the relocation occur *before* upper or lower acceptable storage temperatures are exceeded. This can be accomplished by setting the alarm points of the storage devices so that an alarm sounds before the unacceptable temperature limit is reached.

In some facilities, temperature-monitoring indicators may be used for each blood component container. Such indicators monitor the liquid temperature of the immediate inner bag, not the liquid core temperature in the unit, which may be cooler. Policies, processes, and procedures should specify how the facility will determine the disposition of blood components when using temperature-monitoring indicators.

Specific Considerations

Holding blood components that have been dispensed from the blood bank to other hospital areas before transfusion is considered "storage." If the blood components are not kept in a monitored device, they must be stored in containers (eg, boxes or coolers) validated to maintain the correct temperature during storage (Table 17-3). If the temperature of the blood or blood component exceeds the temperature range, it must be discarded.

Red Blood Cells

RBC components are stored in plastic bags of different types with various added anticoagulants and additive solutions that modify the cellular and protein environment. The storage temperature of RBC units must be maintained at 1 to 6 C throughout the duration of storage (Table 17-3).

During storage of RBC units, biochemical and morphologic changes to the red cells occur that collectively have been referred to as the "storage lesion." These changes include cell membrane shape change and microvesiculation; decreased pH, adenosine triphosphate, and 2,3-diphosphoglycerate; and increased lysophospholipids, potassium, and free hemoglobin.[18] In addition to decreased posttransfusion in-vivo red cell recovery, the red cell storage lesion directly affects how long RBC units may be stored. Product approval by the Food and Drug Administration (FDA) requires in-vivo labeling studies demonstrating that at least 75% of the transfused red cells are present in circulation 24 hours after transfusion with less than 1% hemolysis. Although the in-vitro observations of the storage lesion are well described, there is emerging evidence that red cell storage duration does not correlate with worse clinical outcomes.[19-21] One situation where evidence supports the use of fresher RBC units is large-volume transfusions (>25 mL/kg) in neonates.[22]

Whole Blood

Whole Blood, which contains red cells, plasma, and platelets, is collected and stored in plastic collection bags that contain various anticoagulant and storage solutions approved for Whole Blood donations. The storage temperature must be maintained at 1 to 6 C throughout the duration of storage (Table 17-3). Whole Blood units are subject to the same storage lesion changes as described above for RBC components, and the expiration date of the unit depends on the storage solution used during collection.

Platelets

Platelet metabolic, morphologic, and functional changes associated with storage define the shelf life and storage conditions of platelet components. Metabolic changes include the glycolytic production of lactic acid and the oxidative metabolism of free fatty acids, resulting in carbon dioxide production. Platelet pH is maintained above 6.2 via buffering of lactic acid by bicarbonate and promotion of oxidative metabolism facilitated by the diffusion of oxygen and carbon dioxide across a gas-permeable storage bag undergoing gentle agitation.[23] The maximum total time for platelets to be without agitation is 30 hours (Table 17-3). Platelets are stored at 20 to 24 C. Investigation of cold-stored and cryopreserved platelets is ongoing.

Platelet shelf life is also limited by increased risk of bacteria growth due to room-temperature storage. Blood banks and transfusion services are required to have methods to detect or inactivate bacteria in all platelet components.[1(p12)] Recent changes have allowed platelet shelf life to be extended from 5 days to 7 days if the platelets are stored in bags approved for 7-day storage, are stored in 100% plasma, and have screened negative for bacterial contamination with an FDA-approved "safety measure" test. At the time of writing, the shelf life of platelets stored in platelet additive solution or treated with pathogen inactivation systems in the United States cannot exceed 5 days.

Plasma and Cryoprecipitate

Plasma and cryoprecipitate storage conditions and shelf life affect coagulation factor activity.[24,25] Fresh Frozen Plasma (FFP), Plasma Frozen Within 24 Hours After Phlebotomy (PF24), Plasma Frozen Within 24 Hours After Phlebotomy Held At Room Temperature Up To 24 Hours After Phlebotomy (PF24RT24), and Plasma Cryoprecipitate Reduced must be stored at −18 C or colder (Table 17-3). Frozen plasma and cryoprecipitate must be thawed before transfusion as described in the "Pretransfusion Processing" section below.

Granulocytes

Granulocytes should be transfused as soon as possible after receipt from the supplier. Granulocytes are stored at 20 to 24 C (Table 17-3), should not be agitated, and must never be leukocyte reduced. In addition, granulocyte components should be irradiated because recipients who require granulocytes are severely immunocompromised.

PRETRANSFUSION PROCESSING

Thawing Plasma and Cryoprecipitate

Frozen plasma (FFP, PF24, PF24RT24, Plasma Cryoprecipitate Reduced) must be thawed at 30 to 37 C using a waterbath or other FDA-approved device. Thawing in a waterbath requires the frozen component to be in a plastic overwrap before submersion into the water to prevent contamination of the container entry ports. Once thawed, plasma is stored at 1 to 6 C and expires 24 hours after thawing (Table 17-3).

Thawed FFP, PF24, and PF24RT24 must be relabeled as "Thawed Plasma" if stored for longer than 24 hours. Although not licensed by the FDA, Thawed Plasma is included in the AABB *Standards for Blood Banks and Transfusion Services*[1(p30)] and the *Circular of Information for the Use of Human Blood and Blood Components*.[25] Thawed Plasma is stored at 1 to 6 C and expires 5 days after it was originally thawed. Facilities may label such components as

"Thawed Plasma" at the initial time of thawing. By maintaining a Thawed Plasma inventory, transfusion services may decrease wastage of thawed plasma components and have plasma immediately available for emergent need such as for trauma recipients.[26]

Levels of labile coagulation factors (Factor V and Factor VIII) and stable factors are well above 50% of immediate post-thaw levels in Thawed Plasma that has been stored for up to 5 days.[27] Thawed Plasma does, however, contain reduced concentrations of Factor V, Factor VII, and Factor VIII as compared to thawed FFP, PF24, and PF24RT24. For this reason, Thawed Plasma is not suitable for single-factor replacement when antihemophilic factor derivatives are unavailable.

Cryoprecipitate is thawed at 30 to 37 C and gently resuspended; it can be pooled for ease of transfusion using small quantities of 0.9% sodium chloride injection (USP) to rinse the contents of the bag into the final container by the transfusion service (Method 6-11) or pooled before storage by the blood supplier. Thawed cryoprecipitate is stored at 20 to 24 C and expires within 4 hours of pooling if it is pooled in an open system, or within 6 hours for single units, prestorage-pooled units, or units pooled using an FDA-cleared sterile connection device.[25]

Thawing and Deglycerolizing RBCs

RBC units may be frozen and stored for up to 10 years following the addition of glycerol as a cryopreservation agent (Methods 6-6 and 6-7).[28,29] Frozen RBC units can be thawed using a 37 C dry heater or 37 C waterbath. After units are thawed, the glycerol must be removed before the component is transfused. Commercial instruments for batch or continuous-flow washing are available for deglycerolization. The manufacturer's instructions should be followed to ensure maximal red cell recovery and minimal hemolysis. Measurement of free hemoglobin in the final wash can be used to confirm adequate free hemoglobin removal and as a surrogate marker for adequate deglycerolization (Method 6-8).

Integrally attached tubing must be filled with the deglycerolized red cells and sealed appropri-ately so that a segment may be detached and available for ABO/RhD confirmation and cross-match testing.

The shelf life of Deglycerolized RBCs depends on the type of system used. Closed-system devices allow storage for up to 14 days, and components prepared using open systems expire within 24 hours of the start of the deglycerolization process.

Platelet Gel Production

Platelet gel is produced when thrombin and calcium are added to platelet-rich plasma to produce a glue-like substance for surgical application.[30] This product is typically prepared at the bedside immediately before use. Facilities involved in the production of this component should refer to the current edition of the AABB *Standards for Perioperative Autologous Blood Collection and Administration* for guidance and quality oversight of this manufacturing process.

Irradiation

Irradiation of cellular components is intended to prevent transfusion-associated graft-vs-host disease (TA-GVHD), which is caused by proliferation of donor T lymphocytes. People at increased risk of TA-GVHD include profoundly immunocompromised recipients; recipients of intrauterine transfusion; recipients undergoing marrow, umbilical cord blood, or peripheral blood stem cell transplantation; and recipients of cellular components from blood relatives or donors selected for HLA compatibility or platelet crossmatch compatibility.

Sources of ionizing radiation include gamma rays (cesium-137 or cobalt-60 radioisotopes) and x-rays. The required irradiation dose for either source needed to prevent proliferation of donor T lymphocytes in the recipient is a minimum of 25 Gy (2500 cGy/rad) to the central point of the blood container and 15 Gy (1500 cGy/rad) to any other part of the container.[1(p27)] Confirmation that the blood container has received an adequate radiation dose can be achieved with the use of commercially available radiographic film indicators.

Irradiation is associated with damage to the red cell membrane, which may result in increases in extracellular free hemoglobin and potassium during component storage. For this reason, the expiration date of irradiated RBCs is 28 days after irradiation or the original expiration date, whichever is earlier.[25]

Hospital transfusion services may purchase irradiated blood components from their supplier or perform irradiation within the blood bank using approved and monitored radiation devices. Hospitals that perform their own irradiation may irradiate their inventory on demand or in batches. Maintenance of a dual inventory (irradiated and nonirradiated) requires policies and procedures to ensure that transfusion recipients receive the appropriate component for their clinical situation.

Leukocyte Reduction

Prestorage leukocyte reduction is the preferred method for leukocyte reduction because it prevents accumulation of cytokines during component storage. Quality control of bedside filtration is challenging, and the process has been associated with hypotensive transfusion reactions.[31]

Poststorage leukocyte reduction can be performed by the blood bank before issuing a component using a leukocyte reduction filter attached by a sterile connection. It can also be performed at the bedside during transfusion using a blood-administration filter designed for this purpose. Leukocyte reduction filters are designed to remove >99.9% of white cells (3-log reduction) and meet the AABB standard of <5 × 10^6 leukocytes in 95% of sampled units for RBCs and Apheresis Platelets, and <8.3 × 10^5 leukocytes in ≥95% of sampled units for whole-blood-derived platelets.[1(p27)] The manufacturer's instructions must be followed for the filtration device used to achieve acceptable leukocyte reduction.

Volume Reduction

Volume reduction results when plasma and additive solutions are partially removed from RBC or platelet components, typically following centrifugation. This process may be used to aggressively manage volume in recipients at risk of transfusion-associated circulatory overload, re-

duce exposure to plasma proteins or additives, or achieve a target hematocrit level.

Volume reduction of platelets is described in Method 6-13. The speed of centrifugation may affect the degree of platelet loss. Higher g forces are associated with better platelet retention but raise the theoretical concern of platelet damage and activation as platelets are forced against the container wall. When platelet component volumes are reduced, platelets should rest at room temperature for 20 to 60 minutes following centrifugation and before resuspension in remaining plasma or added saline. The manufacturer's instructions must be followed regarding the minimum volume necessary to maintain proper air exchange across the gas-permeable platelet-storage bag. The shelf life of volume-reduced platelets is 4 hours. In addition to centrifugation, RBC units can be volume reduced through settling by gravity overnight with the ports of the unit facing upward and simple removal of the overlying plasma and preservative solution. The shelf life of volume-reduced RBC units is 24 hours when stored at 1 to 6 C.

Washing

Cellular components may be washed to remove plasma proteins. Washing is also performed to remove glycerol from frozen RBC units after thawing. Indications for washing RBC or platelet components include a recipient history of severe allergic reactions to components containing plasma, the presence of antibodies against immunoglobulin A (IgA) in an IgA-deficient recipient when IgA-deficient cellular components are not available, the presence of maternal antibodies to human platelet antigens (eg, HPA-1a, when using maternal blood for a neonatal transfusion), and the need for complement removal for recipients experiencing posttransfusion purpura. RBC units for intrauterine transfusions may be washed to remove some of the preservative solutions and excess potassium that accumulates during storage.

Washing is accomplished with the use of 1 to 2 L of sterile normal saline (preferably using automated equipment). As with volume reduction, washed platelets should rest at room temperature for 20 to 60 minutes without agitation between centrifugation and resuspension with normal saline. Up to 20% of the red cell yield or 33% of the platelet yield may be lost during washing. Because washing creates an "open system" and removes anticoagulant-preservative solutions, washed RBC units expire 24 hours after the start of washing, and washed platelet units expire 4 hours after the start of washing. It is recommended that hospitals performing washing comply with the manufacturer's recommendations regarding minimum volumes needed for component storage bags to maintain optimal storage conditions unless the component is used shortly thereafter.

Pooling

Certain blood components (whole-blood-derived platelets, cryoprecipitate, or reconstituted Whole Blood) may need to be pooled to provide clinically effective transfusion therapy without the need to transfuse multiple single components.

Pooled whole-blood-derived platelets may contain a significant number of red cells, and therefore ABO compatibility and risk for RhD alloimmunization in the recipient must be considered. If whole-blood-derived platelets are pooled using an open system, the expiration time is 4 hours from the start of pooling. A commercially available, FDA-cleared, prestorage, whole-blood-derived platelet pooling system allows storage for up to 5 days and the ability to perform culture-based bacteria testing.[32] When this system is used, the pool maintains the expiration date of the earliest collected component in the pool.

Single cryoprecipitate units are pooled after thawing in a manner similar to that used for platelets (Method 6-11). The expiration time of cryoprecipitate pools depends on the method used for pooling. Cryoprecipitate pooled in an open system expires within 4 hours of the start of pooling. Thawed single concentrates and pooled concentrates using sterile connection devices expire 6 hours after thawing. Thawed cryoprecipitate is stored at 20 to 24 C. As an alternative, the blood center may pool single concentrates before freezing.

Reconstituted Whole Blood consists of ABO/RhD-compatible RBCs combined with ABO-compatible plasma. This component can be used for neonatal exchange transfusion. The conventional approach is to combine group O RBCs (RhD compatible with the neonate) and group AB plasma to achieve a 50% ± 5% hematocrit of the final product. The volumes of the two components before pooling can be adjusted to achieve a desired hematocrit level. Following recombination, the component can be stored at 1 to 6 C for up to 24 hours. US sites performing this manufacturing step are required to register with the FDA.

Current FDA uniform guidelines should be followed when pooled components are labeled.[33] A unique pool number should be affixed to the final container, and all units in the pool must be documented in electronic or manual records.

Aliquoting

Recipients requiring low-volume transfusions may receive aliquots of smaller volumes derived from the original unit via an FDA-cleared sterile connection device or integrated transfer bags. Available products designed for use with sterile connection devices include transfer packs, smaller-volume bags, and tubing with integrally attached syringes.

The expiration date of the aliquot and minimum residual volumes that must be maintained depend on the storage container used. Hospital transfusion services must develop policies and procedures for aliquot preparation and storage that comply with manufacturer specifications. The use of aliquots for neonatal transfusion has been shown to result in a decreased number of donor exposures.[34] The process of preparing aliquots for small-volume transfusion in neonates and children is discussed in greater detail in Chapter 24. Lower-volume components (split units) may also be prepared for adult recipients who require slow rates of transfusion because of concerns about fluid overload. Split units are recommended when the component volume cannot be transfused at a rate that ensures completion of the transfusion within 4 hours or for small volume transfusions (ie, for pediatric and neonatal patients.) Split units, especially apheresis platelet split units, may also be considered during times of inventory shortages, depending on the clinical situation of the patient and under the guidance of the blood bank medical director. Split units are discussed in greater detail in the "Inventory Management" section.

DISTRIBUTION

Inspection

Visual inspection of the blood component unit is a critical control point in blood component manufacturing and must occur before labeling, before shipping, upon receipt, and before issue for transfusion. Proper documentation of this process includes the 1) date of inspection, 2) DIN, 3) description of any visible abnormalities, 4) action(s) taken, and 5) identity of the staff member performing the inspection. Visible abnormalities may include discoloration of the segments, component, or supernatant fluid or the presence of visible clots, particulate matter, or other foreign bodies. Detection of any such abnormalities should result in component quarantine for further investigation that may include returning the component to the supplier.

If a component is determined to be bacterially contaminated, the component manufacturer must be notified so that an immediate investigation can take place. Other components prepared from that collection should be quarantined until the investigation is complete. If the component (or co-component) has been transfused, the recipient's attending physician should be notified, and consultation with the medical director is recommended.

Shipping

Blood components may be transported between blood centers, between hospitals, and between blood centers and hospitals. All containers used to transport blood components must be qualified before use to ensure that the proper component transport temperature is maintained. The shipping transit time, mode of transport, and climate conditions must also be validated. All components should be inspected upon receipt to confirm appropriate transport conditions, component appearance, and expiration date. Any deviation from routine shipping or component conditions should be reported to the shipping facility and documented according to each location's policies, processes, and procedures.

Whole Blood, RBCs, and Thawed Plasma Components

Whole Blood, RBCs, and thawed plasma components must be transported at a temperature of 1 to 10 C. A variety of options exist for maintaining transport temperature, including bagged wet ice, commercial cooling packs, and specially designed containers. All transport coolers must be qualified to maintain the transport temperature when packed using a validated process.

Blood components transported at 1 to 10 C and stored at 1 to 6 C may need to be temporarily removed from those temperatures for entry into inventory, irradiation, or other processing. The maximum number of units that can be manipulated before the component reaches an unacceptable temperature should be determined and not exceeded. Validation of this process may be accomplished using manual temperature monitoring indicators affixed to the blood components or electronic devices that can measure the temperature of the blood components.

Platelets, Thawed Cryoprecipitate, and Granulocytes

Platelets, thawed Cryoprecipitate, and Granulocytes must be transported at a temperature as close to 20 to 24 C as possible (Table 17-3). All transport coolers must be qualified to maintain this transport temperature when packed using a validated process. For platelets, the total maximum time without agitation is 30 hours.

Frozen Components

Frozen components should be packaged to minimize breakage and maintain a frozen state. Dry ice in a suitable container has historically been used for shipping these components. Any dry ice alternative should be qualified in the properly packed shipping container. All transport coolers must be qualified to maintain the transport temperature when packed using a validated process.

Receiving

The receiving facility should notify the shipping facility and provide documentation of any deviation from usual shipping container packing or the usual appearance of the shipped blood components. Any blood component not in compliance with the facility's policies, processes, and procedures should be quarantined. Only after investigation of the deviation and determination that the component meets acceptance criteria may the component be removed from quarantine and released into the general inventory.

Blood components should be fully traceable from collection to final disposition. Electronic or manual records indicating compliance with policies, processes, and procedures should be generated and maintained for the applicable record-retention time. Any deviation must be recorded, and blood components not meeting requirements should be quarantined. Deviations must be investigated to determine appropriate component disposition and possible corrective action. The results of any corrective action should be reported to the blood supplier as needed. Inventory management should consist of routine determination that all blood components are accounted for and transfused or appropriately discarded.

Component Testing

Before transfusion, the ABO group of all units and RhD type of any units labeled "Rh negative" must be confirmed by serologic testing for all red-cell-containing components (RBCs, Whole Blood, and Granulocytes). Any typing discrepancies identified must be reported immediately to the supplier and resolved before the component is issued for transfusion.[1(p39)]

Retention and Storage of Donor Samples

IS crossmatch and AHG/IAT crossmatch are both performed using the recipient's serum or plasma and donor red cells, which must be obtained from a segment of tubing that was inte-grally attached to the donor unit to be trans-fused.

The recipient's sample and a segment from any red cell-containing component must be stored at refrigerated temperatures for at least 7 days after each transfusion.[1(p39)] Retaining both the recipient's sample and donor unit segment containing red cells allows for repeat and/or additional testing if the recipient has a transfusion reaction. Testing of stored samples should be based on the sample storage limitations in the reagent manufacturer's package insert.

Lack of appropriate storage space may limit the length of time that samples are stored. Institutions that limit the use of pretransfusion recipient samples to those that have been stored for no more than 3 days frequently store these samples for 10 days (ie, 3 days + 7 days). Institutions that permit the testing of pretransfusion samples that have been stored for >3 days need to ensure that each pretransfusion sample is retained for at least 7 additional days after the transfusion for which the sample was used for donor selection.

Donor red cells may be obtained from the remainder of the segment used in the crossmatching or from a segment removed before the blood was issued. If the opened crossmatching segment is saved, it should be placed in a tube labeled with the unit number and then sealed or stoppered.

ISSUING OF COMPONENTS

Donor RBC Unit Selection

The results of compatibility testing, as well as a visual inspection, should guide donor unit selection (see "Transfusion Documentation and Recipient Identification" section below). Compatibility considerations vary according to ABO, RhD, and other blood group antigens of the recipient.

ABO Group Compatibility

Whenever possible, recipients should receive ABO-identical blood components; however, occasionally it may be necessary to select alternative components. If the component to be transfused contains ≥2 mL of red cells, the donor's red cells must be ABO compatible with the recipient's plasma.[1(p42)] Because plasma-containing components can also affect the recipient's red cells, anti-A and/or anti-B antibodies in plasma for routine transfusions should be compatible with the recipient's red cells when feasible.[35] However, it is not uncommon for blood banks and transfusion services to transfuse incompatible plasma-containing blood components during emergent transfusion situations or platelet inventory shortages. Some centers use thawed group A plasma for emergent transfusions because of the relative scarcity of group AB plasma.[36] Low-titer group O Whole Blood is now part of trauma resuscitation protocols due to the evidence supporting a balanced ratio approach to massive hemorrhage.[37] As a result of frequent platelet shortages, ABO-incompatible platelet components are often transfused. Requirements for components and acceptable alternative choices are summarized in Table 17-2.

RhD Type

RhD-positive blood components should be routinely selected for RhD-positive recipients. RhD-negative units are compatible with RhD-positive recipients but should be reserved for RhD-negative recipients. RhD-negative recipients (especially females of childbearing potential) should receive red cell-containing components that are RhD-negative to avoid alloimmunization to the RhD antigen and prevent the potential for possible HDFN. When ABO-compatible, RhD-negative components are not available for an RhD-negative recipient, the blood bank physician and the recipient's physician should weigh alternative courses of action. The risk of alloimmunization to the RhD antigen in hospitalized RhD-negative recipients of RhD-positive RBC units is approximately 22%, while the incidence of alloimmunization after apheresis platelet transfusion is 0 to 1.4%.[38-41] Depending on the clinical situation (especially childbearing potential) of the recipient and the volume of red cells transfused, it may be desirable to administer Rh Immune Globulin to an RhD-negative recipient who is given RhD-positive blood components.[42] In order to help hospitals manage the

limited group O, RhD-negative RBC inventory, AABB and the Choosing Wisely campaign have emphasized selective use of group O RhD-negative RBCs in known group O, RhD-negative patients and for emergency transfusions for females of childbearing potential. Group O, RhD-positive RBCs should be used for emergency transfusions to males and females who are not of childbearing potential.[43] The patient should be switched to type-specific blood as soon as the patient's ABO/RhD type is known and confirmed (see "Emergent Transfusion" below).

Other Blood Groups

Antigens other than ABO and RhD are not routinely considered in the selection of units of blood for transfusion to nonalloimmunized recipients. However, for recipients with certain medical conditions, such as sickle cell disease, some institutions may elect to transfuse RBC units that are phenotypically matched to various degrees, to prevent alloimmunization in a population of frequent transfusion recipients.[44] One study showed that North American hospital transfusion service laboratories most commonly match for the C, E, and K antigens when phenotype-matched RBCs are transfused to nonalloimmunized recipients with sickle cell disease.[45] Matching for more than three antigens may be of incremental benefit, although sustaining an inventory of such components may be extremely challenging.

If the recipient has clinically significant and unexpected antibody(ies), blood lacking the corresponding antigen(s) should be selected for crossmatching. If there is an adequate quantity of the recipient's serum or if another recipient's serum with the same antibody specificity is available, and if that antibody reacts well with antigen-positive red cells, that serum may be used to screen for antigen-negative donor RBC units. When red cells are found to be antigen negative, this result must be confirmed with a licensed reagent when such a reagent is available. When licensed reagents are not available (eg, anti-Lan or anti-Yt[a]), expired reagents or stored serum samples from recipients or donors may be used, provided that the results of controls tested on the day of use are acceptable.[46] When crossmatch-compatible units cannot be found, the transfusion service's attending physician should be involved in the decision about how to manage the recipient. Antigen-negative donor RBC units are not usually provided for recipients whose antibodies are not clinically significant.

Transfusion Documentation and Recipient Identification

The recipient's medical record must include accurate and complete documentation of all transfusions. For each transfusion, this documentation must contain the transfusion order, consent for transfusion, component name, DIN, date and time of transfusion, pre- and posttransfusion vital signs, volume transfused, identification of the transfusionist, and, if applicable, any transfusion-related adverse events.

Ensuring that the correct blood component is transfused to the correct recipient is paramount for transfusion safety. All requests for blood components must contain at least two independent identifiers so that the intended recipient can be uniquely identified. Recipient compatibility testing records must also be reviewed. Current testing results must be compared with historical records, if available, and any discrepancies must be resolved before component selection.

Personnel must visually inspect and document that the selected component is acceptable for use. This inspection must include confirmation that the component does not have an abnormal color or appearance and that the container is intact. Once selected for transfusion, the blood component must have an attached label or tie tag that contains the intended recipient's two independent identifiers, the DIN, the donor ABO/RhD type, and the compatibility test result interpretation, if performed. At the time of issue, there must be a final check of each unit that includes the following[1(pp46-47)]:

- Intended recipient's two independent identifiers, ABO group, and RhD type.
- DIN, donor ABO group, and, if required, RhD type.
- Interpretation of the crossmatch test results, if performed.

- Special transfusion requirements [eg, cytomegalovirus (CMV)-reduced-risk, irradiated, or antigen-negative components], if applicable.
- Expiration date and, if applicable, time.
- Date and time of issue.
- Visual inspection of the product.

The transfusion service must confirm that the recipient identifying information, transfusion request, testing records, and blood component labeling and compatibility are accurate and in agreement. Any discrepancies identified must be resolved before issue. Additional records that may be useful include those that identify the person issuing the blood, the person to whom the blood was issued, and the unit's destination. After the transfusion, a record of the transfusion becomes part of the recipient's permanent electronic or paper medical record. Records must contain the identity of the person(s) performing the crossmatch and, if blood is issued before the resolution of compatibility problems, the final serologic findings.

Final identification of the transfusion recipient and blood component rests with the transfusionist(s). The Joint Commission requires hospitals to use a two-person verification process before initiating a blood or blood component transfusion. Alternatively, an automated ID technology (eg, bar coding) may be used in place of one of the individuals.[47] The individual(s) must identify the recipient and donor unit and certify that the identifying information on forms, tags, and labels is in agreement.

Special Clinical Situations

Emergent Transfusion

When blood is urgently or emergently needed, the recipient's physician must weigh the risk of transfusing uncrossmatched or partially compatible blood against the risk of delaying transfusion until compatibility testing is complete or fully compatible blood components are identified. A transfusion service physician should be available for consultation as needed.

If transfusion is deemed medically necessary and blood is released before pretransfusion testing is complete, the records must contain a signed statement from the requesting physician indicating that the clinical situation was sufficiently urgent to require release of blood components before completion of compatibility testing.[1(p48)] Such a statement does not need to be obtained before a lifesaving transfusion takes place, and it does not absolve blood bank personnel from their responsibility to issue properly labeled donor blood that is ABO compatible with the recipient.

When emergency release is requested, blood bank personnel should take the following actions:

- Issue uncrossmatched group O RBCs, or low-titer group O Whole Blood (see note below), if the recipient's ABO group is unknown. It is preferable to give RhD-negative RBCs if the recipient is a female of childbearing potential, while other recipients may receive group O, RhD-positive RBCs.
- Issue blood that is ABO and Rh compatible if there has been time to test a current sample.
- Indicate in a conspicuous fashion on the tag or label attached to the unit that compatibility testing was *not* completed at the time the unit was issued.
- Begin compatibility tests and complete them promptly (for massive transfusion, see below). If incompatibility is detected, the recipient's physician and the transfusion service physician should be notified as soon as possible.

Note: The use of low-titer group O Whole Blood for emergent transfusion of recipients whose ABO group is not known requires the blood bank/transfusion service to define low-titer group O Whole Blood and have policies, processes, and procedures for its use, the maximum volume allowed, and patient monitoring for adverse effects.[1(p48)]

Massive Transfusion

There are several different definitions of massive transfusion. In this chapter, it is defined as the administration of greater than 8 RBC units in an adult recipient in <24 hours or acute administration of more than 4 RBC units within 1 hour.

Exchange transfusion of a neonate/infant is also considered a massive transfusion.

Many hospitals have developed massive transfusion protocols to standardize the response to hemorrhage.[48,49] Massive transfusion protocols are designed to rapidly provide blood components in a balanced ratio of plasma and platelets to RBCs, particularly when laboratory testing is not rapid enough to guide transfusion support. Typical ratios of plasma and platelets to RBCs range from 1:2 to 1:1, with evidence that there is no statistically significant difference in recipient survival in the trauma setting if a 1:2 or a 1:1 ratio is used.[50] Additional studies are needed to clarify whether the use of these protocols is associated with improved recipient outcomes.

To ensure the ability to accurately interpret ABO group testing results, the recipient sample should be obtained for testing as early as possible during massive transfusion. If the recipient ABO group cannot be determined, continued support with group O RBCs is required, and consideration can be given to using group A plasma rather than AB plasma. Unexpected and significant usage of group O RBCs in the setting of massive transfusion should be considered when determining component inventory levels. In massive transfusion situations where large amounts of blood may be required, policies may be developed to provide RhD-positive RBCs to select RhD-negative recipients, such as all adult males and females without childbearing potential.

In the massive transfusion setting, an abbreviated crossmatch, such as IS crossmatch, should be performed, if possible, to confirm the ABO compatibility of the units administered. If the recipient has no transfusion testing history, collection of a second sample is recommended to verify the ABO group and RhD type, which may allow for the use of electronic/computer crossmatching. If the recipient qualifies for electronic/computer crossmatching (two separate ABO group and RhD typings, current negative antibody screen, no history of clinically significant antibodies), electronic crossmatching can save significant amounts of time when issuing blood components in an emergency. If a more limited pretransfusion testing protocol is used, the protocol should be described in a written standard operating procedure. The transfusion service should have a policy that addresses compatibility testing in recipients of massive transfusion, such as abbreviation or omission of crossmatching.[1(p45)]

Blood Administration after Non-Group-Specific Transfusion

Once a sample is received and the recipient's ABO group and RhD type are determined, the recipient can begin receiving transfusions of group-specific components. Group O RBC units stored in additive solution contain minimal residual plasma, which minimizes concerns regarding passive transfusion of A and B antibodies. Therefore, switching to ABO-identical RBC components can be done safely, although an occasional recipient may exhibit a transient positive direct antiglobulin test (DAT) result. In some cases, such as when large volumes of RBCs are transfused or small children or infants receive transfusions, passively acquired anti-A and/or anti-B may be detected in the recipient's serum or plasma.[51] In these cases, a transfusion medicine physician should be consulted before switching to type-specific blood components. Transfusion of RBCs that lack the corresponding A and/or B antigen(s) may be indicated.

RhD-negative RBC units should be selected if the recipient is a female of childbearing potential and RhD type is unknown, or if the recipient, regardless of gender, has anti-D or a history of anti-D. In massive transfusion situations where large amounts of blood may be required, policies may be developed to provide D-positive RBCs to select recipients. If a recipient receives blood of an RhD type that is different from that of his or her own blood, it may become difficult to determine the recipient's true RhD type. If there is any question about the recipient's true RhD type, it may be prudent to administer RhD-negative blood, especially if the recipient is a female of childbearing potential.

INVENTORY MANAGEMENT

General Considerations

A sufficient number of units of varying ABO and RhD specificities should be available to meet routine hospital needs, allow for unanticipated increases in utilization from emergency situations, and minimize component expiration and wastage. Factors that influence determination of blood bank component inventory levels include historic usage patterns, expiration/wastage rates, and distance from suppliers. Inventory levels should be periodically evaluated in response to institutional changes that may affect component usage, including expansion of inpatient beds or operating rooms; implementation of new surgical procedures; or changes in hospital guidelines or medical practice that may influence transfusion behavior.

The blood bank should also maintain a reserve of universally compatible RBCs for emergency use and have a reliable emergency delivery system to ensure adequate availability of blood components in unexpected situations when demand exceeds supply. Although the practice is not universally adopted, many transfusion services choose to use only leukocyte-reduced RBC inventories to decrease transfusion-associated alloimmunization and subsequent platelet refractoriness, as well as to reduce the incidence of febrile nonhemolytic transfusion reactions.[52,53] In times of platelet inventory shortage, medical directors may approve the splitting of apheresis platelet units (split units) or pooling of 3 whole-blood-derived platelet units (vs the usual adult dose of 4-6 pooled units) for prophylactic transfusion orders to conserve inventory. This practice is rooted in the findings of the platelet-dose trial called PLADO, which identified that prophylactic doses ranging from 1.1 to 4.4×10^{11} platelets per square meter had no difference in effect on subsequent patient bleeding.[54] Standard platelet doses traditionally range from 3 to 6×10^{11} platelets, but have not been shown to be superior to lower dosing for prophylactic hemostasis.[55,56] Using this logic, many pediatric centers also routinely utilize platelet splitting to better ration platelet supplies. Inventory conservation strategies, particularly for use in disaster plans, should be developed and tested periodically.

Routine inventory levels should be monitored daily to facilitate timely ordering from blood suppliers and maintain adequate inventory levels. This can be particularly challenging for platelets because of their limited shelf life. Inventory management plans should also take into consideration desirable inventory levels of special products, such as leukocyte-reduced (ie, CMV-reduced-risk) and irradiated components. Antigen-negative RBC units as well as HLA-matched, HLA-selected, or crossmatched platelets may be ordered on an as-needed basis from suppliers, but clear communication between the clinical team and the blood bank is required to anticipate patient needs given procurement delays inherent in the process and component expiration.

Surgical Blood Ordering Practices

Component outdate rates are influenced by surgical ordering practices. For example, when RBC units are crossmatched for surgical recipients, they are unavailable to other recipients and have a greater likelihood of expiring if the component is not promptly returned to the uncrossmatched inventory. The crossmatch-to-transfusion (C:T) ratio is the number of RBC units crossmatched divided by the number of RBC units actually transfused and is most useful in determining individual physician or specialty-specific ordering practices. When C:T ratios are monitored, a C:T ratio of >2.0 may indicate excessive ordering of crossmatched blood and may identify instances when a preoperative type and screen order is more appropriate.

One approach to reducing excessive C:T ratios is to identify procedures that do not typically require blood, and use this information to develop guidelines for the use of type and screen orders or hold-sample orders (samples that are received in the transfusion service but do not have any testing orders) instead of crossmatch orders. Maximum surgical blood order schedules (MSBOSs) for common elective procedures can also be developed based on local transfusion utilization patterns.[57] The MSBOS serves as a guideline not only for how many units should

be available, but also for which surgical procedures require a type and screen or not. The advent of IS and electronic crossmatching have decreased the utility of the MSBOS, and this practice is useful now primarily in hospital transfusion services that lack the ability to perform electronic crossmatching. A discussion with the clinician and the blood bank staff should occur to determine how many units to crossmatch for recipients undergoing elective surgery who are known to have clinically significant alloantibodies and require crossmatch-compatible, antigen-negative blood. If an MSBOS has been established, the transfusion service routinely crossmatches the predicted number of units for each recipient undergoing the designated procedures. Routine orders may need to be modified for recipients with anemia, bleeding disorders, or other conditions in which increased blood use is anticipated. As with other circumstances that require rapid availability of blood components, the transfusion service staff should be prepared to provide additional blood components if the need arises.

Unfortunately, it is not uncommon for an initial pretransfusion sample to be received by the transfusion service laboratory on the morning of a same-day-admission surgical procedure, which gives the laboratory limited time to complete pretransfusion red cell compatibility testing.[58] Up to 9% of type and screen samples may not be tested completely until *after* the recipient's surgery has begun. Such testing may offer the first and only opportunity for a laboratory to determine a recipient's ABO group and RhD type. In addition, approximately 3% of samples received have a serologic finding that requires further investigation.[59] The discovery of a serologic finding in the immediate preoperative or perioperative period requiring further investigation may cause dangerous delays in blood availability for a recipient. Thus, each recipient's blood sample should be received in the laboratory in advance of the scheduled procedure, and sufficient time must be available to complete all preoperative pretransfusion testing before surgery begins. Collection of a type and screen sample days or even weeks in advance of surgery, with collection of a second sample on the morning of a scheduled surgery, is one approach to mitigate the problem.

Return of Blood Components and Reissue

The transfusion service may receive back into inventory units that meet acceptance specifications. These conditions include the following[1(p47)]:

- The container closure has not been disturbed.
- The component has been maintained at the appropriate temperature.
- At least one sealed segment remains integrally attached to the container, if RBCs.
- Documentation indicates that the component has been inspected and is acceptable for reissue.

Individual-unit temperature indicators or temperature-reading devices can be used to determine the acceptability of components for return to inventory. Blood and blood components may also be transported or stored in qualified containers using a validated process that has been shown to maintain acceptable temperatures for a defined interval. If time frames are used to determine the acceptability of a component's return to inventory, the time frame must be validated by the individual facility. The validation should demonstrate that for the defined period, the appropriate temperature of the component has been maintained.

Components meeting the acceptance criteria may be returned to the general blood inventory and reissued. Components not meeting the acceptance criteria must be quarantined for further investigation or discarded in a biohazard container to prevent inadvertent return to inventory.

KEY POINTS

1. Two independent recipient identifiers are required for pretransfusion samples. A mechanism must be in place to identify the time and date of collection, as well as the identity of the phlebotomist who drew each blood sample tube.
2. Laboratory personnel must confirm that the information on the pretransfusion testing sample label and the information on the pretransfusion testing request are in agreement. If there is any doubt about the identity of the recipient or about the labeling of the sample, a new sample must be obtained.
3. Pretransfusion testing, including ABO group, RhD type, antibody detection, and crossmatching, is performed to prevent transfusion of incompatible RBCs. ABO and RhD test results on a current sample must be compared with previous transfusion service records, if available, or confirmed with second sample. Discrepant ABO group results should be resolved before blood is given. If transfusion is necessary before confirmation of ABO group or resolution of discrepant results, the recipient should receive group O RBCs.
4. If a recipient has been pregnant or received transfusion within the previous 3 months, or if the pregnancy history and transfusion history are uncertain, the pretransfusion sample used for testing must be no more than 3 days old at the time of intended transfusion, because recent transfusion or pregnancy may stimulate production of unexpected antibodies.
5. At the time of blood component issue, labeling information must be complete and be checked against blood bank records. Any discrepancies identified must be resolved before components are issued or transfused.
6. Visual inspection of the blood component is a critical control point in the manufacturing process and must occur at distribution, before labeling, before shipping, upon receipt, and before issue for transfusion.
7. Refrigerators, freezers, and platelet incubators for blood component storage must be monitored to ensure that proper storage conditions are maintained. Because the safety, purity, potency,

and quality of the blood components may be affected by improper storage, alarm settings should be configured to notify necessary personnel *before* the upper or lower acceptable storage temperatures are exceeded.

8. Temperature requirements during transport of blood components differ from those during storage. Blood components held outside the blood bank before transfusion are considered to be in storage. Validated processes must ensure that acceptable storage temperatures are maintained.

9. Acceptable time frames for returning blood components to inventory after issue should be validated by individual facilities. Individual-unit temperature indicators or temperature-reading devices may be used to determine component acceptability for return to inventory.

10. Thawed FFP, PF24, and PF24RT24 expire within 24 hours of thawing. These components may be labeled as "Thawed Plasma" to allow for a 5-day shelf life (from the date the component was thawed) if they were originally collected in a closed system.

REFERENCES

1. Gammon R, ed. Standards for blood banks and transfusion services. 32nd ed. Bethesda, MD: AABB, 2020.

2. Linden JV, Wagner K, Voytovich AE, Sheehan J. Transfusion errors in New York state: An analysis of 10 years' experience. Transfusion 2000; 40:1207-13.

3. Bolton-Maggs PH, Wood EM, Wiersum-Osselton JC. Wrong blood in tube—potential for serious outcomes: Can it be prevented? Br J Haematol 2015;168:3-13.

4. Kaufman RM, Dinh A, Cohn CS, et al for the BEST Collaborative. Electronic patient identification for sample labeling reduces wrong blood in tube errors. Transfusion 2019;59(3):972-80.

5. Knels R, Ashford P, Bidet F, et al for the Task Force on RFID of the Working Party on Information Technology; International Society of Blood Transfusion. Guidelines for the use of RFID technology in transfusion medicine. Vox Sang 2010;98(Suppl 2):1-24.

6. Askeland RW, McGrane S, Levitt JS, et al. Improving transfusion safety: Implementation of a comprehensive computerized bar code-based tracking system for detecting and preventing errors. Transfusion 2008;48:1308-17.

7. Murphy MF, Fraser E, Miles D, et al. How do we monitor hospital transfusion practice using an end-to-end electronic transfusion management system? Transfusion 2012;52:2502-12.

8. Lumadue JA, Boyd JS, Ness PM. Adherence to a strict specimen-labeling policy decreases the incidence of erroneous blood grouping of blood bank specimens. Transfusion 1997;37:1169-72.

9. Coombs RRA, Mourant AE, Race RR. A new test for the detection of weak and "incomplete" Rh agglutinins. Br J Exp Pathol 1945;26:255-66.

10. Shulman IA. When should antibody screening tests be done for recently transfused recipients? Transfusion 1990;30:39-41.

11. Boisen ML, Collins RA, Yazer MH, Waters JH. Pretransfusion testing and transfusion of uncrossmatched erythrocytes. Anesthesiology 2015;122:191-5.

12. Ramsey G, Smietana SJ. Long-term follow-up testing of red cell alloantibodies. Transfusion 1994;34:122-4.

13. Hendrickson JE, Hillyer CD. Noninfectious serious hazards of transfusion. Anesth Analg 2009; 108:759-69.

14. Shulman IA, Odono V. The risk of overt acute hemolytic transfusion reaction following the use of an immediate-spin crossmatch. Transfusion 1994;34:87-8.

15. Shulman IA, Calderon C. Effect of delayed centrifugation or reading on the detection of ABO incompatibility by the immediate-spin crossmatch. Transfusion 1991;31:197-200.

16. Mazepa MA, Raval JS, Park YA; Education Committee of the Academy of Clinical Laboratory Physicians and Scientists. Pathology consultation on electronic crossmatch. Am J Clin Pathol 2014;141:618-24.

17. Nunes E. Transport versus storage: What is the difference? AABB News 2013;15(2):4-5.

18. Klein HG, Spahn DR, Carson JL. Red blood cell transfusion in clinical practice. Lancet 2007; 370:415-26.

19. Fergusson DA, Hebert P, Hogan DL, et al. Effect of fresh red blood cell transfusions on clinical outcomes in premature, very low-birth-weight infants: The ARIPI randomized trial. JAMA 2012;308:1443-51.

20. Lacroix J, Hebert P, Fergusson DA, et al. Age of transfused blood in critically ill adults. N Engl J Med 2015;372:1410-18.

21. Steiner ME, Ness PM, Assmann SF, et al. Effects of red-cell storage duration on recipients undergoing cardiac surgery. N Engl J Med 2015; 372:1419-29.

22. Strauss RG. Data-driven blood banking practices for neonatal RBC transfusions. Transfusion 2000;40:1528-40.

23. Shrivastava M. The platelet storage lesion. Transfus Apher Sci 2009;41:105-13.

24. Scott E, Puca K, Heraly JC, et al. Evaluation and comparison of coagulation factor activity in fresh-frozen plasma and 24-hour plasma at thaw and after 120 hours of 1 to 6 C storage. Transfusion 2009;49:1584-91.

25. AABB, American Red Cross, America's Blood Centers, Armed Services Blood Program. Circular of information for the use of human blood and blood components. Bethesda, MD: AABB, 2017.

26. Werhli G, Taylor NE, Haines, AL, et al. Instituting a thawed plasma procedure: It just makes sense and saves cents. Transfusion 2009;49: 2625-30.

27. Tholpady A, Monson J, Radovancevic R, et al. Analysis of prolonged storage on coagulation Factor (F)V, FVII, and FVIII in thawed plasma: Is it time to extend the expiration date beyond 5 days? Transfusion 2013;53:645-50.

28. Meryman HT, Hornblower M. A method for freezing and washing RBCs using a high glycerol concentration. Transfusion 1972;12:145-56.

29. Valeri CR, Ragno G, Pivacek LE, et al. A multicenter study of in vitro and in vivo values in human RBCs frozen with 40-percent (wt/vol) glycerol and stored after deglycerolization for 15 days at 4 degrees C in AS-3: Assessment of RBC processing in the ACP 215. Transfusion 2001; 41:933-9.

30. Borzini P, Mazzucco L. Platelet gels and releasates. Curr Opin Hematol 2005;12:473-9.

31. Cyr M, Hume H, Sweeney JD, et al. Anomaly of the des-Arg9-bradykinin metabolism associated with severe hypotensive reactions during blood transfusions: A preliminary report. Transfusion 1999;39:1084-8.

32. Benjamin RJ, Kline L, Dy BA, et al. Bacterial contamination of whole-blood-derived platelets: The introduction of sample diversion and prestorage pooling with culture testing in the American Red Cross. Transfusion 2008;48: 2348-55.

33. Food and Drug Administration. Guidance: United States industry consensus standard for the uniform labeling of blood and blood components using ISBT 128. (June 2014) Silver Spring, MD: CBER Office of Communication, Outreach, and Development, 2014.

34. Liu EA, Mannino FL, Lane TA. Prospective, randomized trial of the safety and efficacy of a limited donor exposure transfusion program for premature neonates. J Pediatr 1994;125:92-6.

35. Fung M, Downes KA, Shulman IA. Transfusion of platelets containing ABO-incompatible plasma: A survey of 3,156 North American laboratories. Arch Pathol Lab Med 2007;131:909-16.

36. Dunbar NM, Yazer MH; Biomedical Excellence for Safer Transfusion Collaborative. A possible new paradigm? A survey-based assessment of the use of thawed group A plasma for trauma resuscitation in the United States. Transfusion 2016;56:125-9.

37. Sehault JN, Bahr M, Anto V, et al. Safety profile of uncrossmatched, cold-stored, low-titer, group O+ whole blood in civilian trauma patients. Transfusion 2018;58(10):2280-8.

38. Yazer MH, Triulzi DJ. Detection of anti-D in D- recipients transfused with D+ red blood cells. Transfusion 2007;47:2197-201.

39. Cid J, Lozano M, Ziman A, et al. Low frequency of anti-D alloimmunization following D+ platelet transfusion: The Anti-D Alloimmunization after D-incompatible Platelet Transfusions (ADAPT) study. Br J Haematol 2015;168:598-603.

40. O'Brien KL, Haspel RL, Uhl L. Anti-D alloimmunization after D-incompatible platelet transfusions: A 14-year single-instiution retrospective review. Transfusion 2014;54:650-4.

41. Weinstein R, Simard A, Ferschke J, et al. Prospective surveillance of D- recipients of D+ apheresis platelets: Alloimmunization against D is not detected. Transfusion 2015;55:1327-30.

42. Pollack W, Ascari WQ, Crispen JF, et al. Studies on Rh prophylaxis II: Rh immune prophylaxis after transfusion with Rh-positive blood. Transfusion 1971;11:340-4.

43. Callum JL, Waters JH, Shaz BH, et al. The AABB recommendations for the Choosing Wisely campaign of the American Board of Internal Medicine. Transfusion 2014;54:2344-52.

44. Afenyi-Annan A, Brecher ME. Pre-transfusion phenotype matching for sickle cell disease recipients. Transfusion 2004;44:619-20.

45. Osby M, Shulman IA. Phenotype matching of donor red blood cell units for nonalloimmu-

nized sickle cell disease recipients: A survey of 1182 North American laboratories. Arch Pathol Lab Med 2005;129:190-3.

46. Food and Drug Administration. Compliance Program guidance manual. Chapter 42 - Blood and blood components. Silver Spring, MD: FDA, 2013. [Available at https://www.fda.gov/media/84887/download.]

47. 2020 National patient safety goals. Oakbrook Terrace, IL: The Joint Commission, 2019. [Available at http://www.jointcommission.org/standards_information/npsgs.aspx (accessed November 6, 2019).]

48. Young PP, Cotton BA, Goodnough LT. Massive transfusion protocols for recipients with substantial hemorrhage. Transfus Med Rev 2011; 25:293-303.

49. Hendrickson JE, Shaz BH, Pereira G, et al. Implementation of a pediatric trauma massive transfusion protocol: One institution's experience. Transfusion 2012;52:1228-36.

50. Holcomb JB, Tilley BC, Baraniuk S, et al. Transfusion of plasma, platelets, and red blood cells in a 1:1:1 vs a 1:1:2 ratio and mortality in recipients with severe trauma: The PROPPR randomized clinical trial. JAMA 2015;313:471-82.

51. Garratty G. Problems associated with passively transfused blood group alloantibodies. Am J Clin Pathol 1998;109:169-77.

52. Seftel MD, et al. Universal prestorage leukoreduction in Canada decreases platelet alloimmunization and refractoriness. Blood 2004;103(1): 333-9.

53. King KE, et al. Universal leukoreduction decreases the incidence of febrile nonhemolytic

transfusion reactions to RBCs. Transfusion 2004;44(1):25-9.

54. Slichter SJ, Kaufman RM, Assmann SF, et al. Dose of prophylactic platelet transfusions and prevention of hemorrhage. N Engl J Med 2010: 362(7):600-13.

55. Tinmouth A, Tannock IF, Crump M, et al. Low? dose prophylactic platelet transfusions in recipients of an autologous peripheral blood progenitor cell transplant and patients with acute leukemia: A randomized controlled trial with a sequential Bayesian design. Transfusion 2004; 44:1711-19.

56. Heddle NM, Cook RJ, Tinmouth A, et al. A randomized controlled trial comparing standard- and low-dose strategies for transfusion of platelets (SToP) to patients with thrombocytopenia. Blood 2009;113:1564-73.

57. Boral LI, Dannemiller FJ, Standard W, et al. A guideline for anticipated blood usage during elective surgical procedures. Am J Clin Pathol 1979;71:680-4.

58. Friedberg RC, Jones BA, Walsh MK. Type and screen completion for scheduled surgical procedures: A College of American Pathologists Q-Probes study of 8941 type and screen tests in 108 institutions. Arch Pathol Lab Med 2003; 127:533-40.

59. Saxena S, Nelson JM, Osby M, et al. Ensuring timely completion of type and screen testing and the verification of ABO/Rh status for elective surgical recipients. Arch Pathol Lab Med 2007;131:576-81.

APPENDIX 17-1
Sources of False-Positive Results in Antiglobulin Testing

Cells Agglutinated before Washing

If potent agglutinins are present, agglutinates may not disperse during washing. Observe red cells before the addition of antihuman globulin (AHG) or use a control tube and substitute saline for AHG. Reactivity before the addition of AHG or in the saline control invalidates AHG results.

Particles of Contaminants

Dust or dirt in glassware may cause clumping (not agglutination) of red cells. Fibrin or precipitates in test serum may produce red cell clumps that mimic agglutination.

Improper Procedures

Overcentrifugation may pack cells so tightly that they do not easily disperse and they appear to be positive.

Centrifugation of the sample with polyethylene glycol or positively charged polymers before washing may create clumps that do not disperse.

Cells That Have a Positive Direct Antiglobulin Test (DAT) Result

Cells that are positive by DAT will be positive in any indirect antiglobulin test. Procedures for removing IgG from DAT-positive cells are given in Methods 2-20 and 2-21.

Complement

Complement components, primarily C4, may bind to cells from clots or from citrate-phosphate-dextrose-adenine-1 donor segments during storage at 4 C and occasionally at higher temperatures. For DAT, use red cells anticoagulated with EDTA, acid-citrate-dextrose, or citrate-phosphate-dextrose.

Samples collected in tubes containing silicone gel may have spurious complement attachment.[1]

Complement may attach to red cells in samples collected from infusion lines used to administer dextrose-containing solutions. Reactions are strongest when large-bore needles are used or sample volume is <0.5 mL.[2]

1. Geisland JR, Milam JD. Spuriously positive direct antiglobulin tests caused by silicone gel. Transfusion 1980;20:711-13.
2. Grindon AJ, Wilson MJ. False-positive DAT caused by variables in sample procurement. Transfusion 1981;21:313-14.

APPENDIX 17-2

Sources of False-Negative Results in Antiglobulin Testing

Neutralization of Antihuman Globulin (AHG) Reagent

Neutralization of AHG reagent may result from failure to wash cells adequately to remove all serum or plasma. Fill tube at least three-quarters full of saline for each wash. Check volume dispensed by automated washers.

If increased serum volumes are used, routine washing may be inadequate. Wash additional times or remove serum before washing.

The AHG might be contaminated by extraneous protein. Using contaminated droppers or the wrong reagent dropper can neutralize an entire bottle of AHG. Do not use a finger or hand to cover the tube.

If the concentration of IgG paraproteins in test serum is high, protein may remain even after multiple washes.[1]

Interruption in Testing

Bound IgG may dissociate from red cells and leave too little IgG to detect or neutralize AHG reagent.

Agglutination of IgG-coated red cells will weaken. Centrifuge and read results immediately.

Improper Reagent Storage

AHG reagent may lose reactivity if it is frozen.

Excessive heat or repeated freezing or thawing may cause loss of reactivity of test serum.

Reagent red cells may lose antigen strength during storage. Other subtle cell changes may cause loss of reactivity.

Improper Procedures

Overcentrifugation may pack red cells so tightly that the agitation required to resuspend red cells breaks up agglutinates. Undercentrifugation may not be optimal for agglutination.

Failure to add test serum, enhancement medium, or AHG may cause a negative test result.

Red cell suspensions that are too heavy may mask weak agglutination. Suspensions that are too light may be difficult to read.

Improper or insufficient serum:cell ratios can adversely affect results.

Complement

Rare antibodies, notably some anti-Jk^a or anti-Jk^b, may be detected only when polyspecific AHG is used and active complement is present.

Saline

The low pH of saline solution can decrease the sensitivity of the test.[2] The optimal pH of saline wash solution for most antibodies is 7.0 to 7.2.

Some antibodies may require saline to be at a specific temperature to retain antibody on the cell. Use 37 C or 4 C saline.

1. Ylagen ES, Curtis BR, Wildgen ME, et al. Invalidation of antiglobulin tests by a high thermal amplitude cryoglobulin. Transfusion 1990;30:154-7.

2. Rolih S, Thomas R, Fisher E, Talbot J. Antibody detection errors due to acidic or unbuffered saline. Immunohematology 1993;9:15-18.

APPENDIX 17-3

Causes of Positive Pretransfusion Test Results*

Negative Antibody Detection Test Result and Incompatible Immediate-Spin Crossmatch
Donor red cells are ABO incompatible.
Donor red cells are polyagglutinable.
Anti-A1 is in the serum of an individual with A_2 or A_2B.
Other alloantibodies (eg, anti-M) are reactive at room temperature.
Rouleaux have formed.
Autoantibodies (eg, anti-I) are cold-reactive.
Anti-A or anti-B has been passively acquired.
Negative Antibody Detection Test Result and Incompatible Antiglobulin Crossmatch
Donor red cells have a positive direct antiglobulin test result.
Antibody is reactive only with red cells having strong expression of a particular antigen (eg, dosage) or variation in antigen strength (eg, P1).
An antibody to a low-prevalence antigen is present on the donor red cells.
Anti-A or anti-B has been passively acquired.
Positive Antibody Detection Test Result and Compatible Crossmatches
Autoanti-HI (-H) or anti-Le^{bH} and non-group-O units are selected.
Antibodies are dependent on the reagent red cell diluent used.
Antibodies demonstrating dosage and donor red cells are from heterozygotes (ie, expressing a single dose of antigen).
Donor unit lacks corresponding antigen.
Positive Antibody Detection Test Result, Incompatible Crossmatches, and Negative Autocontrol
Alloantibody(ies) are present.
Positive Antibody Detection Test Result, Incompatible Crossmatches, Positive Autocontrol, and Negative Direct Antiglobulin Test Result
An antibody is present to an ingredient in the enhancement media, or an enhancement-dependent autoantibody is present.
Rouleaux have formed.
Positive Antibody Detection Test Result, Incompatible Crossmatches, Positive Autocontrol, and Positive Direct Antiglobulin Test Result
Alloantibody is causing a delayed serologic or hemolytic transfusion reaction.
Passively acquired autoantibody (eg, intravenous immune globulin, therapeutic monoclonal antibody) is present.
Cold- or warm-reactive autoantibody is present.

*Causes depend on serologic methods used.

CHAPTER 18

Administration of Blood Components

Melanie Jorgenson, RN, BSN, LSSGB

T HE SAFE ADMINISTRATION OF BLOOD and its components requires a multidisciplinary collaboration among clinical and ancillary services and clinicians. Policies and procedures must be developed with input from transfusionists, the transfusion service, surgeons, anesthesiology care providers, primary-care physicians, and transport personnel. The medical director of the transfusion service or designee will review and approve the policies and procedures on an annual basis. The transfusionist typically provides the last line of defense in the detection of errors before the transfusion commences. All personnel involved in preparing, delivering, and administering a transfusion must be given appropriate training to ensure the provision of the safest transfusion possible.

EVENTS AND CONSIDERATIONS BEFORE DISPENSING COMPONENTS

Before a transfusion begins, thoughtful consideration, planning, and preparation are required. The following areas are discussed in detail throughout this chapter:

1. The recipient's consent to transfuse, along with transfusion risks, benefits, and alternatives.
2. Recipient history and education.
3. Baseline assessment of the recipient.
4. The provider's orders for blood components and administration.
5. Pretransfusion sample.
6. Preparation of ordered units for transfusion.
7. Prophylactic medications.
8. Equipment.
9. Intravenous (IV) access.
10. Readiness to transfuse.
11. Delivery of blood components.
12. Infusion sets and compatible IV solutions.
13. Verification of the recipient's identification, and other verifications at the time of administration.
14. Rates of transfusion.
15. Monitoring during the transfusion.
16. Suspected transfusion reactions.
17. Documentation of the transfusion.
18. Unique transfusion settings.

Recipient Consent

The AABB *Standards for Blood Banks and Transfusion Services (Standards)* states, "The blood bank or transfusion service medical director shall participate in the development of policies, processes, and procedures regarding recipient consent for transfusion."[1(p49)] Recipient informed consent must address indications for; risks, benefits, and possible side effects of; and alternatives to transfusions of allogeneic blood components. Some state laws require certain additional elements in the recipient consent.

The recipient has the right to choose or refuse a transfusion and must have an opportunity to ask questions of a learned professional before providing consent. Documentation of the consent process must be entered into the recipient's

Melanie Jorgenson, RN, BSN, LSSGB, Client Delivery Lead, Accumen, San Diego, California
The author has disclosed no conflicts of interest.

18

medical record. Some facilities require an institution-approved signed consent form to document that the consent process has occurred and that the risks, benefits, and alternatives of transfusion were discussed with the recipient or legal representative. Each institution must have a process for recording a patient's refusal to receive blood or blood components in the patient's medical record. Institutional policies must identify health-care providers who are permitted to obtain consent and must indicate the length of time and range of recipient care (eg, in- and outpatient) for which a consent remains valid.

Consent for transfusion must be obtained from recipients who have the requisite capacity to make such decisions. If a recipient is unable to give consent, a legally authorized representative or surrogate may do so (depending on local and state laws). If no one is available to provide consent and the need for transfusion is considered a medical emergency, the blood component may be administered based on the doctrine of implied consent. Individual state and local laws governing requirements for implied consent may vary, but the emergent need for transfusion must be carefully documented in the medical record.[2] Informed consent for transfusion may or may not include the name of the health-care provider who obtained consent, and hospital policy may require the consenter to include an entry into the medical record that documents the conversation.

Recipient History and Education

It is important to collect a history from the recipient before the component is ordered to assess whether the recipient is at increased risk of a transfusion reaction. This history includes previous transfusions and any adverse reactions. If the recipient has had previous reactions to a transfusion, the medical team must determine whether the recipient needs to receive prophylactic medications before transfusion and whether special processing of the component is indicated to mitigate unnecessary exposure and the risk of an adverse reaction. Premedication orders should be carefully timed with the anticipated administration of the unit. (See Chapter

17 for greater detail on pretransfusion processing.)

The transfusionist must educate the recipient about reporting any symptoms that may be indicative of a reaction and indicate how long the transfusion will take. The recipient's questions must be answered before the transfusion is started.

Baseline Assessment of Recipient

A baseline physical assessment must include measurement of vital signs, including blood pressure, heart rate, temperature, and respiratory rate. Many institutions also routinely measure oxygen saturation using oximetry. The pretransfusion assessment must include symptoms, such as shortness of breath, rash, pruritus, wheezing, and chills, as a basis for comparison after the transfusion is initiated.

It is important to consider a patient's baseline assessment when preparing to transfuse a blood component. A recipient with renal or cardiopulmonary disease may require a slower infusion rate to prevent transfusion-associated circulatory overload (TACO). A recipient with an elevated temperature may destroy cellular components at an increased rate.[3] Moreover, if the recipient presents with an elevated temperature before the transfusion, it may be difficult to determine later whether an additional increase in temperature was caused by a transfusion reaction. Administration of an antipyretic may be considered in such cases.

Orders to Prepare and to Transfuse Blood and Blood Components

A licensed provider often writes two orders for the components to be administered. The first order requests appropriate laboratory testing and preparation of the ordered blood component and notes special processing requirements. The second order explains to the transfusionist how to administer the components, including the transfusion rate. Recipient name and another independent identifier (eg, date of birth or medical record number must be included). ideally, orders should include sufficient specific information for clarity, such as:

- Component [eg, Red Blood Cells (RBCs) or Apheresis Platelets] to prepare or to administer.
- Special processing required (eg, leukocyte reduction, irradiation, or washing).
- Number of units or volume to administer.
- Date and time for the infusion.
- Flow rate or duration for administering the component.
- Indication for transfusion.

It is important to note that it is appropriate for the rate and duration of the transfusion (eg, not to exceed 4 hours from the time the container is entered until completion)[4] to be described in a policy approved by the hospital's medical staff. The policy might also make considerations for comorbidities (eg, renal disease, cardiac disease) that impact the rate/duration.

When the health-care team is considering transfusion, orders for various laboratory tests (eg, ABO/Rh testing, type and screen, type and crossmatch) may be written by the health-care provider to prepare for a possible transfusion. To administer the intended blood components, administration orders are written.

The transfusionist has the responsibility, as with any other order, to critically think through the order. As with medication orders, the transfusionist must determine the orders are for the right recipient, for the right blood component, for the right reasons, in the right amount, and at the appropriate rate. The ordering provider and the transfusionist must ensure the order does not conflict with any facility-specific transfusion guidelines. If the transfusionist has concern about any of these areas, a conversation with the ordering provider is essential before carrying out the order. Any deviations from the guidelines must be documented in the recipient medical record by the ordering provider and/or transfusionist as appropriate.

Pretransfusion Sample

In nonemergent situations, a pretransfusion blood sample is required before all RBC transfusions. In some hospitals where a historical ABO type is known, a pretransfusion sample might not be required for plasma and platelet transfusions, because these components do not require a crossmatch except in rare cases (eg, unit of platelets with excessive red cell content). Typically, the sample is obtained within 3 days of transfusion, with the draw date considered to be day 0.[1(p40)]

Institutional policies may vary regarding the sample outdate. If the recipient has not had a transfusion or been pregnant in the preceding 90 days, the sample may be acceptable for longer than 3 days for testing purposes. In emergent cases in which the patient's survival is in jeopardy, blood components may be dispensed without completing pretransfusion testing, and retrospective testing may be performed once sample collection can be achieved.[1(p48)]

Containers used for blood specimens must be labeled in the presence of the recipient.[5] The sample must be labeled at the recipient's side with at least two unique identifiers (eg, the recipient's name, date of birth, or identification number). The identification of the person collecting the sample and the date the sample was collected must be traceable.[1(p38)] Some policies may also require documentation of the time the sample was collected.

All those involved in the pretransfusion sample collection and recipient verification must be taught that their utmost attention is absolutely necessary to avoid mislabeling of samples leading to ABO mismatches with potentially fatal outcomes. These types of errors are referred to as "wrong blood in tube" (WBIT).

In some institutions, computer-assisted positive recipient identification and collection of confirmatory ABO samples are additional methods used to further mitigate recipient identification errors. Additional information about pretransfusion samples may be found in Chapter 17.

Preparation of Ordered Units for Transfusion

Pretransfusion testing of the recipient's blood sample, including evaluation for unexpected antibodies to red cell antigens, is described in detail in Chapters 13 and 17. The time interval from sample receipt to availability of the requested component can vary greatly. A positive antibody detection test result requires further investigation, and it takes time to definitively identify clinically significant red cell antibodies. If clinically significant red cell antibodies are present, identification of corresponding antigen-negative or crossmatch-compatible units may require additional time, especially when external suppliers must be consulted to locate an appropriate unit. For recipients with multiple or rare antibodies, additional hours and sometimes days may be required to find a crossmatch-compatible unit. If the need for transfusion is urgent, the ordering licensed provider must weigh the risks and benefits of administering least-incompatible or uncrossmatched units, ideally in consultation with the transfusion service's medical staff.

Some components require thawing, pooling, relabeling, or other preparation before release. All these factors necessitate timely communication between transfusion service staff and transfusionists. Components that are pooled or require thawing may also have a shortened shelf life after being prepared (4-24 hours); transfusionists must be made aware when the time available to complete a transfusion of such components is decreased.[1(pp56-64)]

Prophylactic Medications Given before Transfusion

Recent evidence indicates use of premedication does not minimize transfusion-related adverse events. In a Cochrane review[6] of studies on premedication, the evidence from three randomized controlled trials (RCTs) involving 462 recipients indicated no pretransfusion medication regimen reduces the risk of allergic reaction or febrile nonhemolytic transfusion reaction (FNHTR). However, the conclusion is based on the evidence from three trials of low to moderate quality. A better-powered RCT is necessary to evaluate the role of pretransfusion medication in the prevention of allergic reactions and FNHTR.

Overall, as Duran[7] states, "in the absence of definitive evidence-based studies, pretransfusion medication to prevent transfusion reactions should not be encouraged." Yet for patients with a history of moderate to severe allergic reactions, premedication with antihistamines (diphenhydramine and/or H2 blockers) may help reduce the incidence or decrease the severity of future reactions. Corticosteroids may also be useful. Premedication may not prevent an anaphylactic transfusion reaction; therefore, close observation is required when transfusing patients at high risk for anaphylaxis.

Although antipyretics (eg, acetaminophen) are commonly administered to reduce the risk of FNHTRs, their effectiveness is limited and should be discouraged, as they can mask a transfusion-related adverse event.[8] For patients with a history of FNHTR with rigors, meperidine may be used to premedicate, although its efficacy in this setting has not been studied.

If premedication is required, it must be administered before obtaining the component from the transfusion service. Oral premedication should be administered 30 minutes before the start of the transfusion. Intravenous medications should be given 10 minutes before the transfusion is initiated. Corticosteroids require significant time to exert their effect, but the optimal timing for their use has not been established in the transfusion setting.[9,10]

Nonpharmacologic methods have been shown to reduce the incidence of common transfusion reactions. Prestorage leukocyte reduction reduces the incidence of febrile reactions. The removal or reduction of plasma proteins, by either washing, volume reduction, or dilution with platelet additive solution, can reduce the incidence and severity of allergic reactions. For anaphylactic reactions, all cellular components should be washed, and plasma lacking the cognate allergen [such as immunoglobulin A (IgA)-deficient plasma] should be used. Pooled solvent/detergent-treated plasma may also be used to mitigate the risk of an allergic reaction. (For further discussion of noninfectious adverse events, see Chapter 22.)

Equipment

Blood Warmers

Infusions of cold components can cause hypothermia and cardiac complications, increasing morbidity and mortality.[11] The likelihood of clinically important hypothermia is increased when blood is transfused through a central venous device directly into the right atrium.

Blood warmers are rarely needed during routine transfusions. However, they are used when rapid transfusion of components is required, especially in trauma or surgery settings. Blood warmers are also advantageous during transfusions to neonates, where hypothermia can cause serious adverse effects. Opinions vary on the utility of blood warmers in recipients with cold agglutinins.[12,13] Blood warmers are contraindicated for platelet transfusions, but may be used for other blood components; the manufacturer's suggestions should be followed.

AABB *Standards*[1(p7)] states that "warming devices shall be equipped with a temperature-sensing device and a warning system to detect malfunctions and prevent hemolysis or other damage to blood or blood components." Warming blood to temperatures >42 C may cause hemolysis.[14] The transfusion service must collaborate with departments using blood warmers to ensure the devices are cleared and approved by the Food and Drug Administration (FDA) for infusion of components. Warming devices must be validated, and maintenance, testing of alarms, and equipment use must be performed according to the manufacturer's suggestions. As with any medical equipment, education and competency assessment for the user must be completed and documented. Blood components must not be warmed by placing them in a microwave, on a heat source, or in hot water, or by using devices that are not approved by the FDA specifically for blood warming.

Infusion Systems

Infusion pumps or systems are used to administer fluids, medications, blood, and blood components through clinically accepted routes of administration. These devices allow for a controlled infusion rate over a desired period; the devices also provide an alarm system to notify clinicians of problems with the infusion. Consequently, the use of infusion pumps or systems may be preferred over simple gravity-based administration. However, there is potential for hemolysis of the cellular components infused through these pumps. The manufacturer of the pump must be consulted to determine whether the pump is approved for the infusion of blood components. If it is not approved, the institution must establish a validation plan to confirm the pump will not damage cellular components before using. Most infusion devices require the use of a compatible blood administration set with an in-line filter.

Syringe Infusion Pumps

A syringe infusion pump may be used for small-volume transfusions to neonatal or pediatric recipients. The transfusion service must have established policies for preparing blood in syringes for administration. For more details, see Chapter 24.

Pressure Devices

The use of an externally applied pneumatic compression device may achieve flow rates of 70 to 300 mL per minute, depending on the pressure applied. The device must have a gauge to monitor the pressure, which must be applied evenly over the entire bag. Any pressure >300 mm Hg may cause the seams of the blood component bag to leak or rupture. When a pressure device is used, a large-gauge cannula must be employed to prevent hemolysis.

The application of an external pressure device to the blood bag to expedite the transfusion of RBC units causes minimal damage to the red cells and is a safe practice in the majority of recipients.[15] However, the use of pressure devices has been reported to provide only a small increase in component flow rates. When rapid infusion is desired, an increase in IV catheter or cannula size typically provides better results. Pressure devices are contraindicated for platelet transfusions.

Availability of Emergency Equipment

The transfusionist must be prepared to obtain and initiate emergency interventions when needed. Items used to respond to a transfusion reaction include the following:

- A new bag of 0.9% sodium chloride IV solution and a new administration set to keep an IV line open.

- Appropriate medications to treat a reaction, along with a mechanism to obtain emergency medications prescribed to treat the sequelae of transfusion reactions.
- A mechanism to activate emergency resuscitation measures in the event of a severe reaction.
- Ventilatory assistance and an oxygen source.

Intravenous Access

Acceptable IV catheter sizes for use in transfusing cellular blood components range from 25 to 14 gauge.[16,17] A 20- to 18-gauge IV catheter is suitable for the general adult population and provides adequate flow rates without excessive discomfort to the recipient. When an infant or a toddler receives transfusion, a 25- to 24-gauge IV catheter may be suitable, but a constant flow rate using an infusion device must be applied.[18] (See Chapter 24.)

When using smaller-gauge catheters, it is recommended that the transfusion rate be slowed. The pressure or force used during the transfusion is more likely than the needle gauge to cause hemolysis of red cells.[19]

In some circumstances when IV access cannot be achieved, intraosseous infusions may be warranted.

Readiness to Transfuse

After notification that the ordered units are available, in order to reduce the time the blood component is outside of the controlled laboratory environment, the transfusionist should request components for delivery to the recipient location only after the following items have been addressed:

1. The ordered component is available.
2. Informed consent for transfusion has been completed and documented.
3. IV access is available, patent, and appropriate for transfusion.
4. The order is appropriate for the clinical situation of the recipient.
5. A transfusionist or an appropriate designee is available to properly monitor the recipient

throughout the transfusion in accordance with the institutional policy.
6. The recipient has received any ordered prophylactic medications.
7. The necessary equipment is available and functioning.

Occasionally, despite the best attempts at planning, the blood component arrives at the patient's bedside but there is a significant delay in the start of transfusion due to unanticipated circumstances. In this situation there must be a process for prompt return of the blood component to the transfusion service for proper storage. Transfusion services must ensure every hospital department is aware of the requirement for returning components if a transfusion is delayed.

BLOOD COMPONENT TRANSPORTATION AND DISPENSING

There must be a process to correctly identify the intended recipient and component and attached transfusion record at the time of the request to issue the component. To verify the correct unit is being issued to the correct recipient, transfusion services must allow the issue of only 1 unit at a time unless it is an emergent or large-volume transfusion. Upon dispensation, a final clerical comparison of transfusion service records with each unit or component must be performed and documented. Verification must include[1(pp46-47)]:

1. The type of component (red cells, plasma, platelets, cryoprecipitate, granulocytes, whole blood).
2. The intended recipient's two independent identifiers (name, date of birth, or recipient identification number and/or unique identifier given at the time the crossmatch sample is drawn), ABO group, and Rh type.
3. The donation identification number (DIN), donor ABO group, and, if required, donor Rh type.

4. The interpretation of results of crossmatch tests, if performed.

5. Special transfusion or blood component processing requirements.

6. The component's expiration date and, if applicable, time.

7. The date and time of issue.

Before issuing the unit, transfusion service personnel must visually inspect it for abnormal appearance (significant color change, cloudiness, clots, clumps, or loss of bag integrity). The component must not be used if abnormal appearance is noted.[4]

Institutions may use dedicated personnel or automated delivery systems (eg, validated pneumatic tube systems, validated transport coolers, automated blood delivery robots, or blood dispensing kiosks in remote sites) to facilitate the delivery of components to their final destination. Provision of RBCs via automated blood vending machines (remote, automated, computer-controlled blood storage and dispensing refrigerators) at the point of care may help prevent delays in transportation. The use of a remote dispensing solution employs an electronic issuance process and requires confirmation of the absence of clots, clumps, or loss of bag integrity before stocking the dispensing refrigerator. In all methods of delivery of blood components, institutions must have a process in place to ensure that the appropriate component is delivered to the intended recipient.

BLOOD ADMINISTRATION

Infusion Sets

Components must be administered through special IV tubing with a filter designed to remove blood clots and particles that are potentially harmful to the recipient.[1(p50)] Standard blood administration tubing typically has a 170- to 260-micron (macroaggregate) filter, but this particular micron size is not mandated or required. The tubing can be primed with either 0.9% sodium chloride or the component itself. The manufacturer's instructions must be reviewed for proper use.

Microaggregate Filters

Microaggregate filters are not used for routine blood administration. These second-generation filters were originally developed to remove leukocytes and to complement or replace the clot screen used in the 1970s.[20] They have since been replaced by more efficient leukocyte reduction filters.[21] Microaggregate filters have a screen filter depth of 20 to 40 microns and retain fibrin strands and clumps of dead cells. Red cells, which are 8 microns in diameter, can flow through the filters. Microaggregate filters are typically used for the reinfusion of shed autologous blood collected during or after surgery.

Leukocyte Reduction Filters

Leukocyte reduction filters are designed to reduce the number of leukocytes to $<5 \times 10^6$ per RBC unit, resulting in the removal of >99.9% of the leukocytes. Leukocyte reduction decreases the incidence of FNHTRs, risk of HLA alloimmunization, and transmission of cytomegalovirus (CMV) by cellular blood components.[20,21] (See Chapter 7.) These filters are provided by various manufacturers for prestorage use shortly after collection of the units or for poststorage use at the recipient's bedside.

Prestorage leukocyte reduction is more effective than bedside leukocyte reduction, results in lower levels of cytokines in storage, and can promote ready access to an adequate inventory of leukocyte-reduced components.[22] In contrast, the use of bedside leukocyte reduction filters has been associated with dramatic hypotension in some individuals, often in the absence of other symptoms. This happens more frequently with recipients taking angiotensin-converting enzyme inhibitors. The use of components that were filtered in the blood center or transfusion service before storage decreases the incidence of such reactions.[23] Incorporating prestorage leukocyte reduction into the blood component manufacturing process greatly reduces the need for bedside leukocyte reduction.

It is important to verify the leukocyte reduction filter used is compatible with the component transfused (RBCs or platelets) and to note the maximum number of units that can be administered through one filter. Filters designed for RBCs or platelets may not be used inter-changeably. The manufacturer's instructions must be followed for priming and administering blood components through the filter. Otherwise, leukocyte removal may be ineffective or an air lock may develop, preventing passage of the component through the filter. Leukocyte filters must never be used to administer granulocytes or hematopoietic progenitor cells.

Compatible IV Solutions

No medications or solutions other than 0.9% so-dium chloride injection, USP, must be adminis-tered with blood components through the same tubing at the same time. Solutions containing only dextrose may cause red cells to swell and lyse. Lactated Ringer solution or other solutions containing high levels of calcium may overcome the buffering capacity of the citrate anticoagu-lant in the blood preservative solution and cause clotting of the component.[24] If other medica-tions or fluids are used, the tubing must be flushed with 0.9% sodium chloride solution be-fore or after transfusion.

AABB *Standards* allows exceptions to the above restrictions when 1) the drug or solution has been approved by the FDA for use with blood administration, or 2) there is documenta-tion available to show the addition is safe and does not adversely affect the blood or compo-nent.[1(p50)]

Acceptable solutions according to these crite-ria include ABO-compatible plasma, 5% albu-min, or plasma protein fraction. Certain solu-tions are compatible with blood or blood components as noted in the package inserts re-viewed by the FDA, including Normosol-R pH 7.4 (Hospira), Plasma-Lyte-A injection pH 7.4 (Baxter Healthcare), and Plasma-Lyte 148 injec-tion (Multiple Electrolytes Injection, Type 1, USP, Baxter Healthcare). It is important to note there are several formulations of Plasma-Lyte that are not isotonic or that contain calcium; package inserts must be checked to confirm their compatibility with blood components.

Recipient Verification at the Time of Administration

Proper bedside identification of the recipient is the final step to prevent the administration of an incorrect blood component to a recipient. Al-though individuals are often concerned about the possibility of exposure to infectious agents from transfusion, equal concern must focus on the inadvertent transfusion of incompatible blood. Approximately 1 in every 15,000 to 19,000 units of RBCs is transfused to the wrong recipient each year; 1 in 76,000 to 80,000 transfusions results in an acute hemolytic trans-fusion reaction; and 1 in 1.8 million units of transfused RBCs results in death from an acute hemolytic transfusion reaction.[25]

To prevent the potentially fatal consequences of misidentification, specific systems have been developed and marketed. These include identifi-cation bracelets with bar codes and/or radio-frequency identification devices, biometric scan-ning, mechanical or electronic locks that prevent access to bags assigned to other unintended re-cipients, and handheld computers suitable for transferring blood request and administration data from the recipient's bedside to the transfu-sion service information system in real time. Each system provides a method to bring staff to-ward self-correction during the procedure.[26,27] Studies show that rates of positive recipient iden-tification can be increased by such systems. How-ever, none of these systems negates the need for good quality management, such as standard oper-ating procedures, regular training, periodic com-petency assessment, and system monitoring.

Verifications before the Start of Transfusion

- *Identification of recipient and unit.* The transfusionist must verify that the recipient's two independent identifiers (eg, name and identification number) present on the pa-tient's armband match the information on the unit label or attached tag. The require-ments of the institution for recipient identifi-cation must be satisfied.

- *Donation identification number.* The DIN and donor ABO/Rh type on the blood component label must match the attached tag.
- *Blood type.* The recipient's ABO group (and Rh type if required) must be compatible with that of the unit. Interpretation of any crossmatch tests (if performed) must also be verified.
- *Medical order and consent to transfuse.* The transfusionist must verify the component matches the provider's order and that any special processing requested in the order was performed. The consent must be present on the patient's record.
- *Expiration date (and time, if applicable).* The transfusion of the unit must start before the expiration date or time has passed.

The transfusion must not be initiated if any discrepancy or abnormality is found.

Starting the Transfusion

The unit identifiers and compatibility result must remain appended to the blood unit until the completion of the transfusion. Once the identification of the unit and the recipient is verified, the unit is spiked using an aseptic technique. At institutions using Joint Commission hospital accreditation, Joint Commission requirements for the transfusionist (HR.01.02.01) apply[28]: "If blood transfusions and intravenous medications are administered by staff other than doctors of medicine or osteopathy, the staff members must have special training for this duty."

The blood administration tubing must be primed with either 0.9% sodium chloride or the blood component itself. If any solution or medication other than 0.9% sodium chloride is infused before component administration, the tubing must be flushed with 0.9% sodium chloride immediately before the blood infusion.

The infusion for all routine (nonemergent) administrations of blood components must start slowly, at approximately 2 mL per minute, for the first 15 minutes while the transfusionist remains near the recipient. Some policies may require "direct observation of the recipient" during this time. Severe reactions may occur af-

ter as little as 10 mL has been transfused. Potentially life-threatening reactions most commonly occur within 10 to 15 minutes of the start of a transfusion. The recipient must be reassessed, and vital signs must be obtained, to evaluate the recipient's tolerance of the transfusion.[29]

Rates of Transfusion

After the first 15 minutes of the transfusion of the ordered blood component, if no adverse events are suspected, the rate of transfusion must be increased to the ordered rate. Transfusions of a blood component must be completed within 4 hours of the start of transfusion.[4] However, the recipient's size, blood volume, and hemodynamic condition should be taken into consideration in determining the flow rate. (See Table 18-1.) Special attention must be made to ensure the completion of the unit within the 4-hour window while avoiding transfusion of the unit too rapidly in relation to the recipient's cardiac and/or respiratory status. If the recipient is unable to tolerate completion of the entire transfusion dose in the 4-hour timeframe, a request to the transfusion service can be made to issue an aliquot or a split component of a smaller volume to allow for the transfusion dose to be infused over two separate transfusions.

The advantages of using relatively rapid transfusion rates (eg, 240 mL/hour) include correction of deficiency as rapidly as possible as well as reduced recipient and nursing time dedicated to transfusion. Disadvantages include the potential to cause reactions (eg, volume overload) or increase the severity of a reaction (eg, FNHTRs, septic reactions, or allergic reactions). Many FNHTRs, as well as septic, allergic, and respiratory complications, and even some hemolytic reactions, may not be evident within the first 15 minutes.

If, at any time, an adverse reaction is suspected, the transfusion must be halted and the transfusion service notified. Saline may be used to keep the line open.

Monitoring during the Transfusion

The transfusionist must continue to periodically monitor the recipient throughout the infusion, including the IV site and flow rate. If the IV rate

TABLE 18-1. Blood Component Transfusions in Nonemergent Settings

Component	Suggested Adult Flow Rates		Special Considerations	ABO Compatibility	Filter
	First 15 Minutes	After 15 Minutes			
Red Blood Cells (RBCs)	1-2 mL/min (60-120 mL/hour)	As rapidly as tolerated; approximately 4 mL/minute or 240 mL/hour	Infusion duration must not exceed 4 hours Generally administered over 1-2 hours for hemodynamically stable recipients For recipients at risk of fluid overload, may adjust flow rate to as low as 1 mL/kg/hour	Whole Blood: ABO identical RBCs: ABO compatible with recipient's plasma Crossmatch required	In-line (170-260 micron) Leukocyte reduction if indicated
Platelets	2-5 mL/min (120-300 mL/hour)	300 mL/hour or as tolerated	Usually given over 1-2 hours For recipients at risk of fluid overload, use slower flow rate (see RBCs)	Crossmatch not required ABO/Rh compatibility preferable but not required May be HLA matched	In-line (170-260 micron) Leukocyte reduction if indicated
Plasma	2-5 mL/min (120-300 mL/hour)	As rapidly as tolerated; approximately 300 mL/hour	Time for thawing may be needed before issue For recipients at risk of fluid overload, use slower flow rate (see RBCs)	Crossmatch not required ABO compatibility with recipient red cells	In-line (170-260 micron)
Granulocytes	1-2 mL/min (60-120 mL/hour)	120-150 mL/hour or as tolerated	Over approximately 2 hours Infuse as soon as possible after collection/release of component; irradiate	Crossmatch required Must be compatible with recipient's plasma May be HLA matched	In-line (170-260 micron) Do not use leukocyte reduction or microaggregate filters
Cryoprecipitated AHF	As rapidly as tolerated		Infuse as soon as possible after thawing; pooling is preferred	Crossmatch and ABO compatibility not required	In-line (170-260 micron)

has slowed down, the transfusionist must take one or more of the following actions: 1) verify that the IV is patent and there are no signs of infiltration; 2) raise or elevate the unit; 3) examine the filter for air, excessive debris, or clots; 4) attempt to administer the component through an infusion pump; or 5) consider the addition of 0.9% sodium chloride as a diluent if the unit is too viscous. Frequent recipient monitoring during the infusion helps alert the transfusionist to a possible transfusion reaction and allows for early intervention.

Vital signs must be taken within 15 minutes of beginning the transfusion and then according to institutional policy. There is little evidence to support a best practice related to the frequency of vital-sign monitoring other than at baseline, soon after the start of the transfusion, and after transfusion.[30] AABB *Standards* requires that the medical record include vital signs taken before, during, and after transfusion.[1(p50)] Vital signs must be taken immediately if there is a suspected transfusion reaction or a change in the clinical condition of the recipient.

Suspected Transfusion Reactions

The transfusionist must be knowledgeable of the signs and symptoms indicative of an adverse reaction and be able to act quickly. (See Chapter 22.) Visual observation and recipient reporting of any changes must be used to determine if a reaction has occurred, as the recipient may experience symptoms before changes occur in vital signs. If a transfusion reaction is suspected, the transfusion must be stopped. The patency of the IV must be maintained with new IV tubing and a new bag of 0.9% saline attached near the IV insertion site to prevent infusion of any residual blood component to the recipient.

The component unit identification information must be rechecked. Prompt notification of the transfusion service and a licensed provider for treatment of suspected transfusion reactions is needed. The protocol for collection of a post-transfusion specimen and evaluation of adverse reaction must be initiated. For serious adverse events, notification of the hospital's rapid response team must be considered. Institutions must provide ready access to descriptions of common transfusion reactions, including signs and symptoms as well as immediate steps to be taken or interventions to anticipate.

As soon as possible, the transfusion service must be notified of a suspected transfusion reaction, and institutional policy must be followed for returning the component bag and/or to order the laboratory studies needed to evaluate the reaction. Documentation of the suspected transfusion reaction must be completed per institution policy.

Completing the Transfusion

The recipient is assessed at the completion of the transfusion, and the following information is documented: his or her vital signs and the date, time, and volume transfused. If the transfusion was uneventful, the blood unit bag and tubing are discarded in a biohazard container. The 0.9% saline bag must be discarded per institution policy.

Because recipients can experience transfusion reactions several hours to days after the transfusion is complete, clinical staff must continue to monitor the recipient periodically after the end of the transfusion to detect febrile or pulmonary reactions potentially associated with the blood administration. If the recipient is not under direct clinical supervision after a transfusion, clinical staff must provide written instructions to the recipient and caregiver regarding transfusion reaction signs and symptoms. This information must also include a contact person and phone number to report signs and symptoms.

DOCUMENTATION OF THE TRANSFUSION

The transfusion must be documented in the recipient's medical record. At a minimum, AABB *Standards* requires documentation of the following[1(p50)]:

1. Transfusion order.
2. Recipient consent.
3. Component name.
4. Donation identification number.
5. Donor ABO/RH type.

6. Date and time of transfusion.
7. Vital signs before, during, and after transfusion.
8. Volume transfused.
9. Identification of the transfusionist.
10. Transfusion-related adverse events, if applicable.

It should be noted that although AABB *Standards* does not specify documentation of start and end times for transfusions, the *Circular of Information for the Use of Human Blood and Blood Components* requires that transfusions be completed within 4 hours.[4] Documentation would be necessary to demonstrate compliance with this requirement and is also required by the College of American Pathologists (CAP). If additional units are to be transfused, the institution's policy and/or manufacturer's recommendations must be followed to determine whether the same blood administration tubing may be used. If there are no contraindications from the manufacturer, institutions frequently allow additional units to be transfused with the same blood administration set within 4 hours of the start of the initial transfusion.

UNIQUE TRANSFUSION SETTINGS

See Chapter 19 for information on massive transfusion and Chapter 24 for transfusion in neonatal and pediatric recipients.

Rapid Infusions

If components need to be administered rapidly, the use of rapid-infusion/warming devices, large-bore administration tubing, and large-bore IV catheters, including central venous or intraosseous access, can decrease the infusion time without inducing hemolysis.[31-33] Some tubing sets with appropriate filters are specifically designed for rapid blood administration and may be used alone or with specific devices. Flow rates as fast as 10 to 25 mL/second (600-1500 mL/minute) have been reported with such tubing. Rapid infusion of multiple blood components can lead to hypothermia, coagulopathy, and electrolyte imbalances. Use of a blood/fluid warming device can lessen the incidence of hypothermia.[34]

Hypocalcemia has been noted with rapid transfusions. This is usually transient and dependent on the amount and rate of citrate infused. Calcium replacement may be administered based on the recipient's ionized serum calcium level and the rate of citrate administration.[35] Transfusion-associated hyperkalemic cardiac arrest has been reported with rapid administration of RBCs. It may develop with rapid RBC administration even with a modest transfusion volume such as 1 unit (in a neonate). Contributing factors are acidosis, hypoglycemia, hypocalcemia, and hypothermia at the time of cardiac arrest.[35]

If components are urgently needed and a delay in transfusion could be detrimental to the recipient, the transfusion service must have a process to provide components before all pretransfusion compatibility testing is completed. In such cases, uncrossmatched units are released with a signed statement from the requesting provider indicating the clinical situation requires urgent release before the completion of testing.[1(pp47-48)]

If components in the transfusion service inventory are not immediately accessible to a trauma unit or operating room, a supply of group O red cells may be maintained in an appropriate remote storage device in these areas. The transfusion service must ensure proper storage of components at these satellite storage sites.

Out-of-Hospital Transfusion

Transfusion of blood in a non-hospital setting requires a well-planned program incorporating all the relevant aspects of the hospital setting and emphasizing safety considerations.[36]

Out-of-hospital settings for blood transfusion can include dialysis centers, medical transport vehicles, skilled nursing facilities, outpatient surgery centers, and even recipients' homes. The proper documentation and maintenance of records is part of a well-designed program. Transfusionists must be competent in performing blood administration procedures, recipient monitoring, and recognition and reporting of suspected transfusion reactions. To optimize the care of these recipients, proper arrangements for treatment of suspected transfusion reactions must be made. Blood administration outside the hospital must be performed by personnel with substantial experience in blood administration in this setting.

Transfusion in the home generally allows close monitoring of the transfusion event because the personnel-to-recipient ratio is 1:1. The disadvantage is that no trained assistant is available in the event of a severe adverse reaction. Issues to consider when preparing for a transfusion in the home include availability of the following[36]:

- A competent adult in the home to assist in recipient identification and to summon medical assistance if needed.
- A mechanism to obtain immediate provider consultation.
- A telephone to contact emergency personnel, and easy access for emergency vehicles.

- Documentation of prior transfusions with no history of severe reactions.
- A way to properly dispose of medical waste.

CONCLUSION

Transfusion of blood components and the creation of blood administration procedures and policies must be recipient centric. Policies and procedures must follow best practice and provide the transfusionist with information to competently perform transfusions and recognize and report suspected transfusion reactions. Close monitoring and early intervention when transfusion reactions occur can make a critical difference in recipient outcomes. Audits of the blood administration process to identify areas for improvement, instances of nonconformance, and analysis of their causes are needed for optimal transfusion safety. Periodical auditing of all segments of the blood administration process is strongly suggested for continuous process improvement.

KEY POINTS

1. Blood administration involves the process of informed consent, preparation of the recipient, administration of the appropriate component to the correct recipient, and monitoring of the recipient during and after the transfusion for any adverse reaction. All steps must be appropriately documented in the recipient's medical record.
2. The recipient must be informed of the need for a transfusion and educated about the transfusion of the blood component. Informed consent for the transfusion must be obtained from the recipient.
3. A licensed care provider must initiate requests for blood administration with an order for the appropriate blood component testing and preparation and an order for the administration of the component(s).
4. Transfusionists must be educated on appropriate clinical indications for transfusion and proper safety steps involved in a successful transfusion process.
5. Before planned transfusion, the transfusionist must verify available, appropriate, and patent venous access; administer any ordered prophylactic medications; and gather required equipment (eg, blood warmer, infusion pump, pressure devices, and emergency equipment).
6. Vital signs and a baseline assessment of the recipient must be performed for subsequent comparison.
7. Institutions must identify appropriate blood and blood component issue and delivery mechanisms to ensure the transfusionist receives the components in a timely manner.
8. Transfusion services must ensure all departments are aware of the requirement for returning components if a transfusion is delayed.

9. At the recipient's bedside, verification of recipient and component identification must be performed. The following items must be verified: 1) recipient's two independent identifiers and ABO/Rh type, 2) DIN and donor ABO group, and if required, Rh type, 3) interpretation of crossmatch tests, if performed, 4) special transfusion requirements are met, if applicable, and 5) expiration date/time of the component.

10. Components must be administered through the appropriate infusion sets and filters. Only compatible IV solutions (usually 0.9% sodium chloride injection, USP) may be administered through the same tubing unless the tubing has been flushed with 0.9% sodium chloride, USP, immediately before and after the transfusion.

11. The infusion must start slowly at approximately 2 mL per minute for the first 15 minutes.

12. During this time, the transfusionist must remain near the recipient. If no sign of reaction appears, the infusion rate can be increased. The transfusionist monitors the recipient throughout the infusion and stops the infusion in the event of an adverse reaction.

13. Infusions must be completed within 4 hours of the start of transfusion. After completion, the transfusionist takes the recipient's vital signs. If the recipient will not be under direct clinical supervision after the transfusion, the recipient and caregiver must receive instructions regarding signs and symptoms to report and to whom to report these reactions.

14. The following information, at a minimum, regarding the transfusion must be documented in the recipient's medical record: 1) the transfusion order, 2) recipient consent for transfusion, 3) name of component, 4) DIN and donor ABO group, and if required, Rh type, 5) date and time of infusion, 6) vital signs before, during, and after transfusion, 7) volume transfused, 8) identity of the transfusionist, and 9) any adverse reaction(s).

REFERENCES

1. Gammon R. Standards for blood banks and transfusion services. 32nd ed. Bethesda, MD: AABB, 2020.

2. Stowell CP, Sazama K, eds. Informed consent in blood transfusion and cellular therapies: Patients, donors, and research subjects. Bethesda, MD: AABB Press, 2007.

3. Klein H, Anstee D. Mollison's blood transfusion in clinical medicine. 12th ed. Oxford: Wiley-Blackwell, 2014.

4. AABB, American Red Cross, America's Blood Centers, Armed Services Blood Program. Circular of information for the use of human blood and blood components. Bethesda, MD: AABB, 2017.

5. 2020 National patient safety goals. Oakbrook Terrace, IL: The Joint Commission, 2019. [Available at http://www.jointcommission.org/standards_information/npsgs.aspx (accessed October 24, 2019).]

6. Marti-Carvajal AJ, Sola I, Gonzalez LE, et al. Pharmacological interventions for the prevention of allergic and febrile non-haemolytic transfusion reactions. Cochrane Database Syst Rev 2010;(6):CD007539.

7. Duran J. Effects of leukoreduction and premedication with acetaminophen. J Pediatr Oncol Nurs 2014;31:223-9.

8. Ezidiegwu CN, Lauenstein KJ, Rosales LG, et al. Febrile nonhemolytic transfusion reactions. Management by premedication and cost implications in adult patients. Arch Pathol Lab Med 2004;128:991-5.

9. Patterson BJ, Freedman J, Blanchette V, et al. Effect of premedication guidelines and leukoreduction on the rate of febrile nonhaemolytic platelet transfusion reactions. Transfus Med 2000;10:199-206.

10. Goss JE, Chambers CE, Heupler FA, et al. Systemic anaphylactoid reactions to iodinated contrast media during cardiac catheterization procedures: Guidelines for prevention, diagnosis, and treatment. Cath Cardiovasc Diagn 1995;34:99-104.

11. Boyan CP, Howland WS. Cardiac arrest and temperature of bank blood. JAMA 1963;183:58-60.

12. Donham JA, Denning V. Cold agglutinin syndrome: Nursing management. Heart Lung 1985;14:59-67.

13. Iserson KV, Huestis DW. Blood warming: Current applications and techniques. Transfusion 1991;31:558-71.

14. Hirsch J, Menzebach A, Welters ID, et al. Indicators of erythrocyte damage after microwave warming of packed red blood cells. Clin Chem 2003;49:792-9.

15. Frelich R, Ellis MH. The effect of external pressure, catheter gauge, and storage time on hemolysis in RBC transfusion. Transfusion 2001; 41:799-802.

16. Stupnyckyj C, Smolarek S, Reeves C, et al. Changing blood transfusion policy and practice. Am J Nurs 2014;114:50-9.

17. Makic MB, Martin SA, Burns S, et al. Putting evidence into nursing practice: Four traditional practices not supported by the evidence. Crit Care Nurse 2013;33:28-42.

18. Barcelona SL, Vilich F, Coté CJ. A comparison of flow rates and warming capabilities of the Level 1 and Rapid Infusion System with various-size intravenous catheters. Anesth Analg 2003;97: 358-63.

19. Miller MA, Schlueter AJ. Transfusions via handheld syringes and small-gauge needles as risk factors for hyperkalemia. Transfusion 2004;44: 373-81.

20. Wortham ST, Ortolano GA, Wenz B. A brief history of blood filtration: Clot screens, microaggregate removal, and leukocyte reduction. Transfus Med Rev 2003;17:216-22.

21. Lane TA. Leukocyte reduction of cellular blood components: Effectiveness, benefits, quality control, and costs. Arch Pathol Lab Med 1994; 118:392-404.

22. Cushing M, Bandarenko N, eds. Blood transfusion therapy: A handbook. 13th ed. Bethesda, MD: AABB, 2020 (in press).

23. Zoon KC, Jacobson ED, Woodcock J. Hypotension and bedside leukocyte reduction filters. Int J Trauma Nurs 1999;5:121-2.

24. Dickson DN, Gregory MA. Compatibility of blood with solutions containing calcium. S Afr Med J 1980;57:785-7.

25. Vamvakas EC, Blajchman MA. Transfusion-related mortality: The ongoing risks of allogeneic blood transfusion and the available strategies for their prevention. Blood 2009;113:3406-17.

26. Pagliaro P, Rebulla P. Transfusion recipient identification. Vox Sang 2006;91:97-101.

27. Koshy R. Navigating the information technology highway: Computer solutions to reduce errors and enhance patient safety. Transfusion 2005; 45(Suppl 4):189S-205S.

28. Comprehensive accreditation manual for hospitals. Oakbrook Terrace, IL: The Joint Commission, 2020.

29. Bradbury M, Cruickshank JP. Blood transfusion: Crucial steps in maintaining safe practice. Br J Nurs 2000;9:134-8.

30. Oldham J, Sinclair L, Hendry C. Right patient, right blood, right care: Safe transfusion practice. Br J Nurs 2009;18:312, 314, 316-20.

31. Davis DT, Johannigman JA, Pritts TA. New strategies for massive transfusion in the bleeding trauma patient. J Trauma Nurs 2012;19:69-75.

32. ACS TQIP massive transfusion in trauma guidelines. Chicago, IL: American College of Surgeons, 2014.

33. Shaz B, Hillyer C. Massive transfusion. In: Shaz B, Hillyer C, Roshal M, Abrams C, eds. Transfusion medicine and hemostasis. 2nd ed. London: Elsevier Science, 2013.

34. Hrovat TM, Passwater M, Palmer RN, for the Scientific Section Coordinating Committee. Guidelines for the use of blood warming devices. Bethesda, MD: AABB, 2002.

35. Hayter MA, Pavenski K, Baker J. Massive transfusion in the trauma patient: Continuing professional development. Can J Anaesth 2012:59: 1130-45.

36. Benson K. Home is where the heart is: Do blood transfusions belong there too? Transfus Med Rev 2006;20:218-29.

CHAPTER 19
Hemotherapy Decisions and Their Outcomes

Nadine Shehata, MD, FRCP, and Yunchuan Delores Mo, MD

A S WITH ALL MEDICAL INTERVEN-tions, the risks and benefits of blood transfusion must be weighed carefully. This chapter provides an overview of the scientific literature supporting the use of transfusion therapy in adult patients.

RED BLOOD CELL TRANSFUSION

Red Blood Cells (RBCs) are transfused to increase oxygen-carrying capacity in patients with anemia in whom physiologic compensatory mechanisms are inadequate to maintain normal tissue oxygenation. There are myriad causes of anemia; one classification scheme is shown in Table 19-1. In patients with chronic, stable anemia, RBC transfusion is often unnecessary. In a patient with well-compensated anemia from iron deficiency, for example, replacing iron is the appropriate maneuver to correct the anemia. Conversely, RBC transfusion may be life-saving in individuals with anemia where physiologic compensatory mechanisms are inadequate to maintain tissue oxygenation, such as in individuals with trauma-induced hemorrhage. Signs and symptoms of anemia that should prompt

consideration of RBC transfusion include hemodynamic instability, chest pain of cardiac origin, dyspnea, and tachycardia at rest. In nonbleeding patients, the hemoglobin concentration is used to help guide RBC transfusion decisions because 98% of blood oxygen is hemoglobin bound, the hemoglobin is easy to measure, and no better physiologic measurements to support RBC transfusion are currently available. As discussed below, current RBC transfusion thresholds (ie, hemoglobin concentrations used for RBC transfusion) are lower than those used previously.

Liberal vs Restrictive Transfusion Strategies

The first high-quality study investigating the clinical use of RBC transfusions was the Transfusion Requirements in Critical Care (TRICC) trial.[1] In the TRICC trial, 838 hemodynamically stable, critically ill patients with a hemoglobin level <9 g/dL were randomly assigned to receive RBC transfusion for a hemoglobin <10 g/dL (liberal group) or <7 g/dL (restrictive group). The primary endpoint, 30-day all-cause mortality, did not significantly differ between the study groups. Significantly better survival was observed in the restrictive group in younger

Nadine Shehata, MD, FRCP, Associate Professor, Departments of Medicine and Laboratory Medicine and Pathobiology, University of Toronto, Hematologist, Division of Hematology, and Director, Transfusion Medicine Laboratory, Mount Sinai Hospital, Toronto, Ontario, Canada; and Yunchuan Delores Mo, MD, Associate Medical Director of Transfusion Medicine, Division of Laboratory Medicine, Children's National Medical Center, and Assistant Professor, Department of Pathology, George Washington University, Washington, District of Columbia

N. Shehata has grant funding from the Canadian Institute for Health Research and Canadian Blood Services and chairs the International Collaboration for Transfusion Medicine. Y. Mo has disclosed no conflicts of interest.

19

TABLE 19-1. Classification of Anemia

Blood Loss	
Increased Red Cell Destruction (hemolysis)	**Decreased Red Cell Production**
Extrinsic to Red Cells	**Microcytic**
Immune	Iron deficiency
Alloantibody-mediated hemolytic anemia	Thalassemia
Warm autoimmune hemolytic anemia	Lead poisoning
Cold agglutinin syndrome	Anemia of chronic disease
Paroxysmal cold hemoglobinuria	Sideroblastic anemia
Paroxysmal nocturnal hemoglobinuria	
Drug-related hemolytic anemia	**Normocytic**
Nonimmune	Myelophthisic anemia
Mechanical cause (eg, mechanical heart valves)	Renal/low erythropoietin
Microangiopathic anemia	Anemia of chronic disease
	Marrow hypo/dys/aplasia
Intrinsic to Red Cells	
Hemoglobin disorders	**Macrocytic**
Membrane defects	*Megaloblastic*
Enzyme defects	B12 deficiency
	Folate deficiency
	Medication
	Nonmegaloblastic
	Marrow hypo/dys/aplasia
	Alcoholism
	Liver disease
	Hypothyroidism

patients (<55 years old) and in less acutely ill patients [Acute Physiology and Chronic Health Evaluation (APACHE) II score <20]. The 2011 trial known as FOCUS[2] was the second large randomized controlled trial (RCT) to examine the clinical consequences of adhering to a liberal vs restrictive RBC transfusion strategy in adult patients. In this study, 2016 patients age 50 years or older having hip-fracture surgery with a history of (or risk factors for) cardiovascular disease were randomly assigned to receive post-operative RBC transfusion for hemoglobin levels <10 g/dL (liberal group) vs 8 g/dL (restrictive group). FOCUS was designed as a superiority trial; the aim was to determine whether transfusing RBCs more liberally was associated with better functional outcomes following hip-fracture repair. There was no difference in the primary endpoint of death or the inability to walk across a room unassisted at 60 days after randomization. Smaller trials of liberal vs restrictive post-operative RBC transfusion in orthopedic surgical patients similarly failed to show a benefit of liberal transfusion.[3,4]

RCTs of various sizes comparing liberal vs restrictive RBC transfusion strategies have now been performed in several populations of hospitalized adult and pediatric patients,[5-7] including cardiac surgery,[8-12] septic shock,[13] acute upper gastrointestinal bleeding,[14,15] surgical oncology,[16] postpartum hemorrhage,[17] and traumatic brain injury.[18] More RCTs are in various stages of development. With a few exceptions,[16] these studies fail to demonstrate any clinical benefits of a liberal transfusion strategy. A 2016 meta-analysis[19] evaluated 31 trials comparing liberal vs restrictive transfusion strategies. A total of 12,587 patients in various clinical settings were included. Overall, using a restrictive RBC transfusion threshold (typically hemogloblin of 7.0-8.0 g/dL) reduced the proportion of patients exposed to blood components by 43%, without causing either harm or benefit as compared with a liberal transfusion strategy. On this basis, clinical practice guidelines, including a 2016 AABB guideline,[20] recommended that a restrictive RBC strategy should be used for hospitalized inpatients. A few points merit emphasis. First, clinical practice guidelines are not standards, nor can they substitute for clinical judgment. The RCTs in this area have tended to simplify the decision to transfuse RBCs by basing it on a single parameter, the patient's hemoglobin level. For individual patients, clinical signs and symptoms, comorbidities, and other factors should be integrated into the transfusion decision. That said, if an individual patient is clinically stable,

and the *only* factor driving the decision to transfuse RBCs is the patient's hemoglobin, then a restrictive approach should be followed. Second, the RCTs conducted to date have almost exclusively included hemodynamically stable, hospitalized, adult patients. Hemoglobin levels may be of limited utility in patients who are actively bleeding during the perioperative period. Also, it is often appropriate for providers to provide transfusion to ambulatory outpatients more liberally, for logistical reasons (eg, fewer clinic visits). Subjective quality-of-life (QOL) measures may vary based on a patient's hemoglobin, although a consistent relationship between hemoglobin and functional activity/QOL has been difficult to demonstrate.[21]

Acute coronary syndromes represent an indication distinct from those mentioned. Currently, the optimal transfusion strategy for patients with acute myocardial infarction (MI) or unstable angina remains unclear and is the subject of ongoing study.[22] In the TRICC study, patients with acute coronary syndromes were the only subgroup in which survival was poorer among patients assigned to the restrictive transfusion strategy. However, the survival advantage seen in the liberal transfusion group was not statistically significant.[1,23] In cardiac surgery, restrictive transfusion strategies were not found to be associated with increased adverse events. In the 2015 Transfusion Indication Threshold Reduction (TITRe2) trial,[10] 2007 adult patients having elective cardiac surgery were randomly assigned postoperatively to a liberal (hemoglobin <9 g/dL) vs restrictive (<7.5 g/dL) RBC transfusion strategy. There was no significant difference in the primary outcome of serious infection or ischemic events (eg, stroke or MI). A secondary analysis, however, revealed higher 90-day all-cause mortality among patients in the restrictive group [4.2% vs 2.6%; hazard ratio (HR), 1.64 (1.00-2.67)]. Nonetheless, the Transfusion Requirements in Cardiac Surgery (TRICS III) trial did not find a statistically significant difference in the composite primary outcome of mortality from any cause, MI, stroke, and new renal failure requiring dialysis at discharge or at 28 days following surgery or after 6 months. TRICS III randomly assigned 5243 patients to a restrictive RBC transfusion strategy (hemoglobin <7.5 g/dL from the induction of anesthesia) or a liberal strategy [<9.5 g/dL in the operating room or intensive care unit (ICU) or <8.5 g/dL in the non-ICU ward]. Mortality was 11.4% in the restrictive group vs 12.5% in the liberal group (p <0.001 for noninferiority) at discharge or at 28 days after surgery, and 17.4% vs 17.1% respectively (p = 0.006 for noninferiority) after 6 months.[11,12] A subgroup analysis suggested younger patients may benefit from more liberal thresholds and older patients may benefit from more restrictive thresholds.[12] Future trials need to confirm or refute these findings. For other patients such as those with acute coronary syndrome, severe thrombocytopenia, or chronic transfusion-dependent anemia, however, the AABB guideline noted that there was insufficient evidence to recommend a restrictive RBC transfusion strategy.[20] Patients with solid tumors with septic shock may also not benefit from restrictive strategies. In 300 such patients randomly assigned to hemoglobin thresholds of <7 g/dL or <9 g/dL only during their ICU stay, a trend toward an increased mortality with a restrictive strategy (56% vs 45%; p = 0.08) was observed.[24]

RBC Storage Duration

As described above, clinical trials have typically failed to demonstrate a benefit of RBC transfusion for most patients with moderate anemia. Likely, this reflects the ability of physiologic compensatory mechanisms to ensure adequate tissue oxygenation at hemoglobin levels in the range where transfusion is often considered. An alternate hypothesis potentially explaining the apparent lack of benefit of RBC transfusion relates to the RBC "storage lesion." In the United States, RBC units may be refrigerated for up to 42 days, and various biochemical and morphologic changes are known to occur. For example, extracellular potassium increases; 2,3-diphosphoglycerate (2,3-DPG), a key regulator of oxygen offloading, declines; and free hemoglobin and free iron increase. Observational studies suggested that RBCs stored for longer durations might be associated with adverse clinical outcomes.[25] The impact of RBC storage duration on clinical outcomes in various patient populations

has been examined in several RCTs, including ARIPI[26] (neonates), ABLE[27] and TRANSFUSE[28] (patients in ICU), RECESS[29] (cardiac surgery patients), TOTAL[30] (children with severe anemia, mainly from malaria), and INFORM[31] (hospitalized adult patients). No differences in clinical outcomes were seen in any of these trials. At this time, no clinical practice changes based on RBC storage duration are indicated.

Donor Characteristics and Transfusion Recipient Outcomes

The effect of blood donor characteristics on recipient outcomes was not explored for RBCs until recently.[32-34] In one study, increased risk of death was associated with receipt of blood from younger donors (17 to <20 years old) compared to donors 40 to <50 years old [adjusted HR, 1.08; 95% confidence interval (CI), 1.06-1.10].[34] Younger donors were found to have a similar effect on recipient death in another database study, but the effect of age was no longer significant when other confounding factors were considered.[33] Male recipients of RBCs from female donors had a higher risk of mortality,[32,34,35] but this risk has not been consistently described.[33] Because other factors could potentially explain the association, aside from pregnancy, and the physiologic mechanisms are not understood, RBCs are not selected according to donor gender or age.

Emergency Transfusion of RBCs

RBC transfusions are typically matched for ABO (Table 19-2) as well as RhD blood group antigens. In bleeding emergencies, there may be insufficient time to complete standard pretransfusion testing. Uncrossmatched group O RBC units are used in situations where RBCs must be transfused immediately, before any patient testing is completed. Group O, RhD-negative units are the component of choice for females of childbearing potential. Group O, RhD-positive units are used for men and for postmenopausal women and in some centers when the inventory cannot support RhD negative units for females. Approximately 4% of recipients are expected to have one or more non-ABO red cell

TABLE 19-2. ABO Matching

Recipient ABO Type	ABO-Compatible RBC Units	ABO-Compatible Plasma or Platelet Units
O	O	A, B, O, AB
A	A, O	A, AB
B	B, O	B, AB
AB	A, B, O, AB	AB

RBC = Red Blood Cell.

alloantibodies; nonetheless, in practice, clinically significant hemolytic reactions to uncrossmatched type O units are rare (0.06%; 95% CI, 0.01-0.21%).[36] Occasionally, for bleeding emergencies, patients with known red cell alloantibodies may need RBC transfusion before antigen-negative units can be identified and crossmatched. Close communication between the primary service (eg, the emergency room or operating room staff) and a transfusion medicine physician is important in such cases. Clinicians may have concerns about transfusing units that are not proven to be "fully compatible." However, most non-ABO antibodies will not cause immediate, intravascular hemolysis, as can occur with a major-ABO-mismatched transfusion. Rather, most non-ABO red cell alloantibodies will cause delayed, extravascular hemolysis. Thus, transfusing units that may be, or are known to be, incompatible is still preferable to exsanguination or life-threatening severe anemia. A brief summary of approaches to massive transfusion is provided toward the end of this chapter.

RBC Transfusion for Thalassemia and Sickle Cell Disease

Two hemoglobin disorders, thalassemia and sickle cell disease, are among the most commonly inherited syndromes. The thalassemia syndromes involve the reduced production of α or β globin as a result of gene mutations. β-thalassemia ma-jor is characterized by severe anemia secondary to ineffective erythropoiesis, and extramedullary hematopoiesis. Individuals with thalassemia major often begin a regular RBC transfusion program in childhood if there is poor growth or evidence of extramedullary hematopoiesis resulting in bony abnormalities, and/or if the hemoglobin level is <7 to 9 g/dL.[37,38] RBC transfusion is used to treat anemia and reduce the risk of morbidity from extramedullary hematopoiesis. RBCs are provided every 2 to 4 weeks to maintain a pretransfusion hemoglobin of 9 to 10 g/dL.[37] Alloimmunization, which is reported to occur in 20% to 30% of patients with thalassemia, can be reduced by selecting RBCs matched for Cc, Ee, and K antigens, in addition to the usual matching for ABO and RhD in patients who do not have alloantibodies.[39]

The sickle cell syndromes include hemoglobin SS, hemoglobin SC, hemoglobin Sβ⁰ and Sβ⁺. Hemoglobin S results from a single amino acid substitution (valine for glutamic acid) in position 6 of the β globin protein. Hemoglobin S polymerizes in relatively deoxygenated regions of the circulation, causing abnormal red cell morphology, subsequent occlusion of the microvasculature, and acute and chronic organ dysfunction. Sickled red cells cause microvasculature occlusion not only because of their rigidity but also because they tend to adhere to other blood cells and the endothelium.[40,41] RBC transfusions in patients with sickle cell disease decrease the incidence of acute and chronic complications by reducing the proportion of circulating sickle cells. However, allogeneic RBCs are also associated with risk, and RBC transfusion requires balancing risks and benefits. In patients with sickle cell disease, the prevalence of alloimmunization remains approximately 20%.[42,43] Alloimmunization rates are high in sickle cell disease partially because of antigen disparity between donors and sickle cell disease patients and because of variant Rh alleles.[44] Additionally, the inflammatory response that occurs with vaso-occlusive crises may predispose to alloimmunization.[45] In addition to alloimmunization, the risk of hemolytic transfusion reactions secondary to alloantibodies and the risk of iron overload and hyperhemolysis secondary to

RBC transfusion also need to be balanced against the benefits of transfusion.

Hyperhemolysis refers to the development of severe anemia where the hemoglobin level following transfusion is lower than that before transfusion. Hyperhemolysis may be acute or delayed. It may be associated with a new alloantibody or a previous antibody that was not detected with antibody screening, or it may not be associated with an alloantibody. The transfused cells as well as the patient's own cells are hemolyzed, resulting in a reduction of hemoglobin to levels below the pretransfusion hemoglobin and characteristic reticulocytopenia. Subsequent RBC transfusion is also likely to result in hyperhemolysis.[46,47] Transfusion avoidance, intravenous immune globulin (IVIG), corticosteroids, and erythropoiesis-stimulating agents for anemia and reticulocytopenia have been used to treat hyperhemolysis.[48,49] Other interventions that have been described include the use of rituximab to prevent subsequent delayed hemolytic transfusion reactions in the presence of alloantibodies and potentially eculizumab for the treatment of hyperhemolysis.[49]

Hemoglobin substitutes, or hemoglobin-based oxygen carriers (HBOCs), have also been described in the treatment of sickle cell patients with contraindications to RBC transfusions, including those with rare blood types or extensive alloimmunization resulting in widespread donor incompatibility, as well as in individuals who refuse blood because of religious beliefs. Although the safety profile of early HBOCs resulted in premature withdrawal of select agents, a number of second-generation products may be better tolerated.[50] Case reports[51] have demonstrated clinical benefits in recipients, leading to growing interest in expanding the applications of HBOCs, especially in the sickle cell population. Currently, the availability of such products in the United States is confined to pharmaceutical clinical trials or expanded access (compassionate use) granted by the Food and Drug Administration (FDA).

To reduce the risk of alloimmunization, patients with sickle cell disease, similar to patients with thalassemia, often receive selected RBC units (ie, units matched for Cc, Ee, K) in addition to the usual matching for ABO and RhD.[52,53] Nonetheless, alloimmunization may still occur in these patients despite phenotypic matching, due to genetic variants and heterogeneous epitope expression for any given Rh antigen. In one study, 38% of alloantibodies occurred in recipients who phenotypically expressed the corresponding Rh antigen.[44,54,55] Genotyping for red cell antigens has additional costs; however, the cost of genotyping needs to be balanced against the need to avoid alloimmunization in those at high risk who require frequent transfusions. For patients who have developed an alloantibody, extended-matched RBCs (ie, including antigens of the FY and JK systems, and S) are also often used.[39]

RBCs can be administered to patients with SCD as a simple transfusion, by manual exchange, or by automated exchange. Automated exchange transfusion can readily deliver more volume, thereby significantly reducing hemoglobin S levels and reducing the risk of iron overload. RBCs are administered acutely or chronically as prophylaxis or for various indications, such as pulmonary hypertension.[41] Clear indications for the use of RBCs are provided by RCT evidence and, in the absence of RCTs, from clinical guidelines. Table 19-3 summarizes RBC transfusion recommendations in sickle cell disease from a recent National Heart, Lung, and Blood Institute (NHLBI) guideline.[41] The 1998 Stroke Prevention Trial in Sickle Cell Anemia (STOP trial) showed that chronic RBC transfusions significantly reduced the incidence of stroke in sickle cell patients determined to be at high risk based on transcranial Doppler (TCD) ultrasonography (middle cerebral artery or internal carotid artery flow velocity of 200 cm/sec or higher).[56] The subsequent STOP2 trial showed that discontinuing chronic transfusion in this patient population results in a reversion to baseline risk of abnormal flow velocities and stroke.[57] In the recent TCD With Transfusions Changing to Hydroxyurea (TWITCH) trial, children with sickle cell disease and abnormal TCD velocities were randomly assigned to monthly transfusion or hydroxycarbamide (hydroxyurea) for 1 year. Hydroxycarbamide was found to be noninferior to chronic transfusion for the primary outcome of stroke but was associated with an increased risk of vaso-occlusive crises.[58] RBCs are not

TABLE 19-3. The Use of RBC Transfusion for Sickle Cell Disease Complications*

Complication	Transfusion Method (strength of recommendation)
Symptomatic severe acute chest syndrome (defined by an oxygen saturation <90% despite supplemental oxygen)	Exchange (strong)
Acute splenic sequestration and severe anemia	Simple (strong)
Acute stroke in children and adults: Initiate a program of monthly transfusions	Simple or exchange (strong)
Hepatic sequestration	Simple or exchange (moderate)
Intrahepatic cholestasis	Exchange or simple (consensus)
Multisystem organ failure	Exchange or simple (consensus)
Aplastic crisis	Simple (consensus)
Symptomatic anemia	Simple (consensus)
Child with transcranial Doppler reading >200 cm/sec	Exchange or simple (strong)
Adults or children with previous clinically overt stroke	Exchange or simple (moderate)

*Adapted from Yawn et al.[41]

generally indicated in an uncomplicated painful vaso-occlusive crisis or asymptomatic anemia. Guidance from sickle cell experts is suggested for patients with sickle cell disease requiring surgery with general anesthesia, as these individuals may require simple or exchange transfusion.[41]

RBC Transfusion in Autoimmune Hemolytic Anemia

Autoimmune hemolytic anemia can be categorized as warm autoimmune hemolytic anemia (WAIHA) secondary to an immunoglobulin G (IgG) autoantibody (60%), cold autoimmune hemolytic anemia secondary to an IgM autoantibody (30%), or mixed disease (both IgG and IgM autoantibodies; 8%), with the remainder producing negative results in the direct antiglobulin test.[59] The mainstay of therapy for autoimmune hemolytic anemia is immunosuppression, although RBC transfusions play a key supportive role. Combination therapies and avoidance of cold is often beneficial for patients with cold autoimmune hemolytic anemia. Red cell autoantibodies are often broadly reactive; thus, finding compatible RBCs for patients with WAIHA or mixed disease may be problematic.[60] Autoantibodies demonstrating in-vitro panreactivity may also mask the presence of one or more clinically significant alloantibodies. Alloantibodies have been reported to occur in 20% to 40% of patients with warm autoantibodies.[61,62] For patients who have not received transfusion in the past 120 days, autologous adsorption is the preferred method of removing the autoantibody to permit alloantibody identification. For recent transfusion recipients, allogeneic (heterologous) adsorptions may be performed to identify underlying alloantibodies. Selecting phenotypically or genotypically matched RBCs is an option to attempt to reduce the risks of alloimmunization and the need for additional adsorption procedures in these patients.[63,64] In some WAIHA cases, the autoantibody will demonstrate relative antigenic specificity. For example, the autoantibody may appear to react more strongly in vitro with RhD-positive units compared to RhD-negative units. In such cases, there may be some benefit in providing units that are negative for the "mimicking" autoantibody specificity to prolong survival of transfused red cells.[65] However, it is more important to avoid exposure to antigens to which the patient has preformed underlying alloantibodies than to provide units matched for the relative specificity of the autoantibody.

In many WAIHA cases and in those with mixed disease, fully crossmatch-compatible RBC units will never be available if the patient's autoantibody reacts in vitro with all tested red cells. However, hemolysis in some cases progresses extremely rapidly, and RBC transfusions should not be withheld from patients with potentially life-threatening anemia. Clinicians should be reassured that even if RBCs are incompatible in vitro, the transfused units may not be destroyed. Sufficient volumes of red cells should be transfused to relieve signs and symptoms of anemia (eg, air hunger, tachycardia at rest, chest pain). Such transfusions, which are considered lifesaving, should not be avoided, particularly for patients who have not received transfusion or been pregnant and thus are highly unlikely to have alloantibodies. Frequent monitoring of the transfusion recipient is warranted, and close communication between the transfusion service and primary clinical service is critical.[60]

RBC Transfusion for Patients Receiving Anti-CD38 and Anti-CD47 Monoclonal Antibodies

CD38 is a transmembrane glycoprotein expressed at low levels on lymphoid and myeloid cells, red cells, and some nonhematopoietic tissues. In patients with multiple myeloma, CD38 is overexpressed on neoplastic plasma cells.[66] Daratumumab and other related human monoclonal antibodies are directed against specific CD38 epitopes, and are offered to some patients with relapsed multiple myeloma and non-Hodgkin lymphoma. Anti-CD38 monoclonal antibodies interfere with blood bank compatibility testing due to binding to CD38 expressed on the surface of reagent red cells. This may result in variable, nonspecific reactivity (including panagglutination) with all serologic testing methods, requiring the use of antihuman globulin (AHG; eg, antibody screen, AHG crossmatch). The direct antiglobulin test is typically negative but may demonstrate reactivity with IgG alone, and ABO/Rh typing is unaffected unless AHG reagents are used for the latter. Significant hemolysis does not typically occur in patients, as daratumamab has been demonstrated to result in the loss of CD38 expression from red cells.[67]

CD47—a cellular protein expressed on all cells, including red cells and platelets, with its ligand signal regulatory protein α (SIRPα)—inhibits phagocytosis.[68,69] CD47 is overexpressed in hematologic malignancies and some solid tumors.[70] Monoclonal antibodies targeting CD47 that are intended to enhance phagocytosis are currently in clinical trials.[70] Use of one of these antibodies, Hu5F9-G4, interfered with antibody screening, reverse typing, and crossmatching of red cells.[71] The direct antiglobulin test is negative, but eluates may be reactive depending on the reagent.[71]

Options for safely providing RBCs for patients receiving daratumumab include performing antibody detection testing with reagent cells pretreated with dithiothreitol (DTT)[72] or selection of phenotypically or genotypically matched RBCs.[73,74] DTT is a reducing agent that causes CD38 but not CD47 denaturation on the cell surface by destruction of disulfide bonds, resulting in elimination of daratumumab binding and enabling detection of underlying red cell alloantibodies (with the exception of antigens also sensitive to DTT such as KEL antigens). If RBC transfusion is anticipated and pretreatment of reagent cells with DTT is unavailable, or for CD47 antibodies, a preliminary type and screen and serologic phenotype should be obtained before the patient receives the first dose. The extended phenotype can be obtained using molecular techniques. Close communication between treating physicians and the transfusion service is essential to ensure safe transfusion practices for these patients.

PLATELET TRANSFUSION

Prophylactic Platelet Transfusions for Therapy-Induced Hypoproliferative Thrombocytopenia

Most platelet transfusions are administered to nonbleeding patients with hypoproliferative thrombocytopenia resulting from chemotherapy or stem cell transplantation. This practice began in the 1960s, at a time when fatal intracerebral hemorrhage was a frequent cause of death among severely thrombocytopenic patients receiving chemotherapy. In the 1990s a seminal study[75] demonstrated that days of gross hemorrhage increased at lower platelet counts, although a clear threshold for increased bleeding risk was not identified. Nevertheless, it became standard practice to transfuse platelets prophylactically for a platelet count <20,000/μL. The threshold for platelet prophylaxis was subsequently lowered to 10,000/μL on the basis of both observational studies[76,77] and RCTs.[78-80] An observational study suggested that an even lower platelet count threshold, 5000/μL, would be safe,[81] but the threshold of 10,000/μL has been used most commonly and is currently recommended by several clinical practice guidelines.[82-84]

Since the year 2000, a number of RCTs have been performed to determine the best approach to platelet transfusion. In many cases, the primary endpoint used has been bleeding at World Health Organization (WHO) Grade 2 score or higher. A summary of the WHO scale is provid-

ed in Table 19-4. Because of the tremendous advances in the care of patients with cancer since the 1960s, severe bleeding is now extremely rare. Consequently, two RCTs challenged the necessity of providing prophylactic platelet transfusions at all.[85-87] In a study by Wandt and colleagues,[87] 391 patients receiving chemotherapy for acute myelogenous leukemia (AML) or undergoing autologous hematopoietic stem cell transplantation (HSCT) were randomly assigned to receive or not receive prophylactic platelet transfusions for a morning platelet count at or below 10,000/μL. Patients in the no-prophylaxis arm received platelets only if bleeding occurred. WHO Grade 2 or higher bleeding was observed among 42% of patients in the no-prophylaxis arm vs 19% of patients receiving prophylactic platelet transfusions (p <0.0001). The risk of bleeding was much higher among patients receiving chemotherapy for AML compared to the autologous HSCT patients: 27 out of 28 (96%) Grade 3 or Grade 4 bleeding episodes occurred among patients receiving chemotherapy for AML. In the Trial of Prophylactic Platelets (TOPPS) study,[85,86] 600 patients receiving chemotherapy or autologous HSCT were randomly assigned to platelet prophylaxis or no-prophylaxis for a morning platelet count <10,000/μL. Grade 2 or higher bleeding occurred in 50% of the no-prophylaxis patients vs 43% of those receiving prophylaxis. As in the study of Wandt and colleagues, the benefits of platelet prophylaxis were much stronger among patients receiving chemotherapy compared to autologous HSCT recipients. These two RCTs were included in a recent meta-analysis that concluded that providing platelet prophylaxis in the setting of hypoproliferative thrombocytopenia is associated with a significant reduction in Grade 2 or higher bleeding (odds ratio, 0.53; 95% CI, 0.32-0.87).[88] Thus, prophylactic platelet transfusions continue to be standard, although some individual facilities are contemplating a therapeutic-platelet-transfusion-only strategy for adult autologous HSCT recipients. It needs to be emphasized that the usual platelet transfusion threshold used, 10,000/μL, is intended for hospitalized patients only. Outpatients are typically given platelet transfusions more liberally, for practical reasons (ie, to permit fewer clinic vis-

TABLE 19-4. Summary of WHO Bleeding Scale*

WHO Bleeding Grade	Examples
1	Oropharyngeal bleeding ≤30 minutes in 24 hours
	Epistaxis ≤30 minutes in previous 24 hours
	Petechiae of oral mucosa or skin
	Purpura ≤1 inch in diameter
	Positive stool occult blood test
2	Epistaxis >30 minutes in 24 hours
	Purpura >1 inch in diameter
	Hemoptysis
	Melanotic stool
	Gross/visible hematuria
	Visible blood in body cavity fluid
	Bleeding at invasive sites
3	Bleeding requiring RBC transfusion over routine needs
	Bleeding associated with moderate hemodynamic instability
4	Bleeding associated with severe hemodynamic instability
	CNS bleeding on imaging study
	Fatal bleeding

*Modified from Kaufman et al.[82]

WHO = World Health Organization; RBC = Red Blood Cell; CNS = central nervous system.

its). Nonetheless, the optimal approach to prophylaxis in outpatients has not yet been formally studied.

The optimal platelet dose for transfusion has also been investigated. A provocative 1985 study[89] suggested that although most platelets will circulate for their normal life span (approximately 8-10 days), a relatively small, fixed number of platelets, estimated to be approximately $7100/\mu L$ per day, are used to promote vascular integrity. This population of platelets is thought to be cleared in an age-independent fashion. With this hypothesis in mind, Hersh et al[90] proposed that perhaps only a low dose of platelets is all that is needed for prophylaxis, and published a mathematical model suggesting that providing low-dose platelets (3 units of platelet concentrates vs 6) would, over time, result in an overall 22% savings in the number of platelets transfused. Subsequently, a small number of RCTs examined the question of the optimal dose of platelets to transfuse for prophylaxis in the setting of therapy-related hypoproliferative thrombocytopenia.[88] The largest of these was the PLADO study (on platelet dose),[91] in which 1272 hospitalized hematology-oncology patients with hypoproliferative thrombocytopenia were randomly assigned to receive low-dose (1.1 × 10^{11} platelets/m^2), medium-dose (2.2 × 10^{11} platelets/m^2), or high-dose platelets (4.4 × 10^{11} platelets/m^2) for a morning platelet count of <10,000/μL. The medium-dose arm was meant to approximate one apheresis platelet unit, the current standard at the time. The primary endpoint, the proportion of patients in each arm with Grade 2 or higher bleeding, was not significantly different (71%, 69%, and 70%, respectively), demonstrating that low-dose platelets are a safe alternative to the standard dose. Consistent with the prediction from the Hersh model, fewer overall platelets were transfused in the low-dose arm. However, because patients receiving low-dose platelets had a lower increment, it was necessary to provide them with transfusions more often (average of five transfusions per patient vs three for patients in the medium- or high-dose arms.) To date, low-dose platelets have not been widely adopted as standard, although low-dose platelets are sometimes used to stretch inventories during shortages. When low-dose platelets are used, it is necessary to consider not only the number of platelets being transfused but also the recipient's body surface area.[90]

Platelet Transfusions as Prophylaxis for Invasive Procedures

Platelet transfusions are often administered before minor (ie, bedside) and major (ie, surgical) procedures to try to reduce the bleeding risk in patients with quantitative or qualitative platelet deficiencies. The published evidence supporting the use of platelet transfusions in these settings is limited. In 2015, AABB published a clinical practice guideline on platelet transfusion; these recommendations are summarized in Table 19-5.[82] This guideline was based on a systematic review of the literature.[88] Except for one recommendation (platelet prophylaxis for therapy-related hypoproliferative thrombocytopenia), all other recommendations are weak and based on

low- or very-low-quality evidence. For central venous catheter placement, AABB suggests that prophylactic platelet transfusion may be considered for a platelet count <20,000/μL. A prophylactic platelet count threshold of 50,000/μL is suggested for lumbar puncture and for major elective nonneuraxial surgery. A 2018 American Society of Clinical Oncology (ASCO) Clinical Practice Guideline Update[84] contained similar recommendations for oncology patients. The recommendations included a minimum platelet count of 40,000 to 50,000/μL for major invasive procedures and a lower threshold of 20,000/μL for less-invasive procedures, including central venous catheter insertion or removal and marrow aspirations and biopsies. Recent Cochrane Reviews[92,93] examining the role of prophylactic platelet transfusions before invasive procedures did not identify significant new evidence from interim RCTs or nonrandomized studies. Although the platelet count is important to consider, it is also relevant to note that this does not provide information on platelet function or endothelial dysfunction. Clinical judgment, rather than a specific platelet count threshold, is of primary importance when deciding whether to transfuse platelets in these settings.

Platelet Transfusions to Treat Active Bleeding

In thrombocytopenic patients who are bleeding, it is often recommended that platelets should be transfused to maintain a platelet count above 50,000/μL. In bleeding patients with qualitative platelet dysfunction (eg, patients taking antiplatelet medications or after cardiopulmonary bypass), platelet transfusion has been suggested even at a normal platelet count. Interestingly, a multicenter RCT examining the effect of platelet transfusion on 190 patients with acute intracerebral hemorrhage after antiplatelet therapy found, in fact, an increased risk of death, functional disability, or serious adverse outcomes in the transfusion group compared to the control group.[94] Although the authors were unable to identify a clear explanation for their findings, they hypothesized that platelet transfusion may have led to higher rates of thromboembolic

TABLE 19-5. Summary of AABB Recommendations for Prophylactic Platelet Transfusion in Adults[82]

Clinical Setting	Platelet Transfusion May Be Indicated for:	Strength of Recommendation	Quality of Evidence
Therapy-related hypoproliferative thrombocytopenia	Platelet count ≤10,000/μL	Strong	Moderate
Central venous catheter placement	Platelet count <20,000/μL	Weak	Low
Diagnostic lumbar puncture	Platelet count <50,000/μL*	Weak	Very low
Major elective nonneuraxial surgery	Platelet count <50,000/μL	Weak	Very low
Cardiac surgery with bypass	Perioperative bleeding with thrombocytopenia and/or evidence of platelet dysfunction. Routine platelet prophylaxis not recommended.	Weak	Very low
Intracranial hemorrhage on antiplatelet therapy	Insufficient evidence for recommendation	Uncertain	Very low

*Clinical judgment should be used for patients with platelet counts between 20,000 and 50,000/μL.

complications or exacerbation of cerebral ischemia in cases of misdiagnosed infarction with hemorrhagic conversion.

ABO and RhD Matching for Platelets

ABO matching is not an absolute requirement for platelets (or plasma) as it is for RBCs. But platelets do express ABH antigens, often at high levels.[95,96] Preformed anti-A or anti-B in the recipient may destroy transfused major-mismatched platelets (eg, group A donor, group O recipient).[95-98] Transfusion of major-mismatched platelets usually results in lower platelet increments.[99] Conversely, transfusing ABO-minor-mismatched platelets (eg, O donor, B recipient) can cause hemolytic transfusion reactions, albeit rarely in adults, resulting from passive administration of anti-A or anti-B in the plasma.[100] Several studies have investigated the impact of ABO matching on various outcomes,[97,99-103] including mortality, bleeding, transfusion reactions, platelet count increment,

and refractoriness. Mortality, bleeding, and transfusion reaction rates were not definitively shown to be improved by ABO matching, but the platelet count increment did increase with ABO matching. Two controlled trials[103,104] demonstrated a 40% to 60% reduction in refractoriness with ABO matching, but because definitions of refractoriness differed, the absolute benefit could not be determined. In practice, ABO-identical or -compatible platelets may be transfused whenever permitted by available inventory, although practices may differ by institution, patient population, and clinical setting. If ABO-matched units are unavailable, plasma reduction or selection of units with low anti-A or anti-B titers may mitigate the risk of hemolytic transfusion reactions associated with ABO-minor-incompatible platelets.

Platelets do not express Rh antigens,[105] but platelet units do contain minute quantities of "contaminating" red cells. As few as 0.03 mL of RhD-positive red cells are believed to be required to cause alloimmunization resulting in anti-D. Apheresis platelet units now typically contain only microliter quantities of red cells (0.00043 mL),[106-108] although whole-blood-derived units may contain up to 100-fold-higher amounts (approximately 0.036 mL).[109] However, platelets are often administered to immunocompromised patients, who may be less capable of becoming sensitized. Thus, the overall frequency of alloimmunization from RhD-positive platelet units in both immunocompetent and immunocompromised patients is less than 2%, as demonstrated in a large, multicenter retrospective review.[109] This low risk can essentially be eliminated by administering Rh Immune Globulin (RhIG) within 72 hours of transfusion of RhD-positive platelets to an RhD-negative recipient. Nonetheless, the decision to administer RhIG to prevent RhD alloimmunization when the rate of antibody formation is low should include consideration of risks and benefits and the potential clinical impact of alloimmunization (ie, in females of childbearing potential or before stem cell transplantation).

Platelet Refractoriness

Platelet refractoriness represents a consistent failure to achieve an appropriate platelet count increment following platelet transfusion. In most cases, platelet refractoriness is thought to have a nonimmune cause such as sepsis, disseminated intravascular coagulation (DIC), bleeding, hypersplenism, drug effects, or other platelet-consumptive states. Approximately 20% of cases of platelet refractoriness are thought to have an immune etiology.[110] Some possible causes of platelet refractoriness are listed in Chapter 15. (See Table 15-3.)[111]

If a typical apheresis platelet unit (~4×10^{11} platelets) is transfused to an average-size, relatively healthy recipient, the expected 1-hour posttransfusion increment is ~30,000 to 60,000/μL.[112] In severely thrombocytopenic patients receiving platelet prophylaxis, it is common for the observed platelet increment to be smaller and for the transfused platelets to have a shorter survival. The prevailing hypothesis explaining this observation is that the lower the pretransfusion platelet count, the higher the proportion of platelets needed to maintain vascular integrity.[89]

There has not been agreement on a precise definition of platelet refractoriness. Published studies of platelet transfusion have often used a platelet refractoriness definition of repeated 1-hour corrected count increments (CCIs) <7500, although some groups have used an alternative CCI threshold of 5000.[113] The CCI attempts to adjust the absolute platelet increment observed for the number of platelets transfused ($\times 10^{11}$) and the size of the recipient as reflected by body surface area [BSA (m^2)]:

$$\frac{\text{Platelet increment} \times \text{BSA (m}^2)}{\text{Platelets transfused } (\times 10^{11})}$$

Example: A patient with a BSA of 2.0 m^2 and a platelet count of 5000/μL receives a unit of apheresis platelets containing 4×10^{11} platelets, and the posttransfusion platelet count is 25,000/μL. The CCI may be calculated as follows:

$$\text{CCI} = \frac{20,000 \times 2.0}{4.0} = 10,000$$

CCIs are not used in routine clinical practice, because the number of platelets transfused is usually unavailable. Rather, the unadjusted platelet count increment is used to judge whether the patient's platelet count increased appropriately. To evaluate a patient for immune refractoriness, platelet counts should be obtained between 10 and 60 minutes after transfusion. Poor increments (eg, <10,000/μL) on at least two posttransfusion counts may be attributable to immune refractoriness.[111] Alternatively, if the platelet count increases appropriately 1 hour after transfusion but then declines to baseline at 24 hours, a nonimmune cause of platelet refractoriness is likely (eg, consumption).

Immune refractoriness is usually caused by antibodies that target HLA[114,115] and cause rapid clearance of transfused platelets. Less commonly, immune refractoriness is attributable to antibodies directed against platelet-specific glycoproteins known as human platelet antigens (HPAs). Transfusion recipients may become alloimmunized to platelet HLA antigens either by prior pregnancy, organ transplantation, or transfusion. Platelets express HLA Class I antigens, but they are relatively poor immunogens. When immune refractoriness occurs in platelet transfusion recipients, the HLA antibody response is mainly provoked by "contaminating" white cells in the unit rather than the platelets themselves.[116] The Trial to Reduce Alloimmunization to Platelets (TRAP) confirmed that leukocyte reduction significantly reduces the risk of HLA alloimmunization.[113] Pregnancy is by far the most important risk factor for primary HLA sensitization.[117] In the era of leukocyte-reduced blood components, immune refractoriness, often reflecting a secondary immune response to HLA antigens, is a particular problem in multiparous women.[118]

Identifying HLA antibodies is a second important step in approaching immune refractoriness. HLA antibody detection is most commonly performed using flow cytometry of multiantigen-coated beads, although other methods (eg, lymphocytotoxicity assays, enzyme-linked immunosorbent assays) are also used. Laboratories historically reported a panel-reactive antibody (PRA) score based on the number of reactive wells observed on cytotoxicity assays to determine the degree of HLA alloimmunization,[116] but this practice has been largely replaced by determination of the calculated PRA (cPRA) based on antigen frequencies in the United Network for Organ Sharing (UNOS) network.[119] There is no standard definition of a meaningful cPRA score, and thresholds for defining platelet refractoriness may vary by institution.

Maneuvers to mitigate platelet immune refractoriness were recently reviewed.[118,120] Options to manage immune refractoriness include providing HLA-matched platelets, HLA-antibody avoidance (ie, identifying HLA-antibody specificity and providing antigen-negative platelet units, analogous to similar strategies with RBC units), and platelet crossmatching.[121] When providing HLA-matched platelet units, donor units with closely matching Class I A and B antigens (see Chapters 15 and 16 for more information on platelet matching) have been demonstrated to result in improved transfusion response, although a failure to achieve a good increment is still seen in 20% of cases.[121] A recent systematic

review[118] examined the efficacy of providing HLA-matched platelet units for refractory patients. Most of the existing data come from observational studies performed before 2000, before the routine use of current HLA antibody testing methods. Posttransfusion increments were the most common outcome reported among immune-refractory patients receiving HLA-matched platelets, with varying degrees of success. A 2014 single-center observational study[122] found that providing HLA-matched units was associated with a successful increment in only 29% of transfusions to refractory patients. Although better than providing random units, transfusing HLA-matched platelets was of only limited utility. Studies powered to examine the effect of HLA-selected platelets on bleeding outcomes have not yet been performed.

When HLA-matched platelets are not available for immune-refractory patients, prophylactic transfusions of random units are unlikely to result in an effective incremental response and may cause further sensitization to additional HLA antigens. In cases of bleeding complications in such patients, unmatched HLA units may provide temporary hemostatic benefit and should not be withheld to avoid alloimmunization. IVIG and other therapeutic modalities used to treat immune thrombocytopenia (ITP) have not been demonstrated to be effective in reducing the degree of alloimmunization in both randomized and nonrandomized studies but may be effective in patients who have ITP secondary to their underlying hematologic disorder.[84] Other measures that may be considered include antifibrinolytic agents.

A minority of refractory patients who do not have an HLA alloantibody or have a poor response to HLA-matched platelet transfusions may harbor alloantibodies directed against HPAs.[119] In addition to platelet refractoriness, HPA antibodies are also associated with fetal/neonatal alloimmune thrombocytopenia (FNAIT) and posttransfusion purpura (PTP). (See Chapters 15 and 23.) Such patients may benefit from additional testing such as HPA antigen typing and HPA antibody determination. These assays may not be available outside of major blood collection centers or specialized reference laboratories, although a select number of commercial kits are available. Blood suppliers are limited in their ability to provide a wide variety of HPA-matched platelets due to the relatively small pool of HPA-typed donors. However, donors known to be negative for specific HPA antigens implicated in FNAIT (eg, HPA-1a) may be recruited for patients with refractory thrombocytopenia and HPA antibodies.

As pathogen inactivation technology has become more widely available, multiple studies have reported an increased risk of platelet refractoriness secondary to HLA alloimmunization in patients receiving pathogen-reduced platelet concentrates. The majority of observations have been described with use of the INTERCEPT system, although similar findings were also noted in a Mirasol study,[123] and alloimmunization rates continue to be monitored as secondary outcomes in ongoing clinical trials. The exact etiology is unclear, although higher rates of alloimmunization may be related to smaller post-transfusion increments and therefore increased numbers of platelet transfusions (and donor exposures) in patients receiving pathogen-reduced vs standard platelets.

PLASMA TRANSFUSION

Plasma Prophylaxis for Invasive Procedures

Before performing invasive procedures, physicians often transfuse plasma to patients with modest abnormalities in coagulation tests [eg, prothrombin time/international normalized ratio (PT/INR) or activated partial thromboplastin time (aPTT)], with the goal of reducing the bleeding risk. In most cases, this practice exposes patients to all of the risks of plasma transfusion without providing true benefits, because 1) mild-to-moderate coagulation marker abnormalities fail to predict bleeding in nonbleeding individuals[124]; 2) modest elevations in PT/INR are usually not corrected into the normal range by plasma transfusion alone[125]; and 3) RCTs and observational studies have failed to demonstrate that prophylactic plasma transfusions affect bleeding outcomes.[126-130] The lack of conclusive

evidence for prophylactic plasma transfusions to date[131,132] has led to widely divergent practices and highlights the need for additional data from large, multicenter RCTs in order to establish the ideal role of plasma transfusion in this setting.

Plasma Transfusions to Treat Bleeding and Other Conditions

Plasma transfusion is indicated for bleeding patients with multiple coagulation factor deficiencies (eg, liver disease, DIC). It is also indicated to manage patients with specific plasma-protein deficiencies (eg, Factor V deficiency) for which a licensed coagulation factor concentrate is not available. Studies examining the impact of plasma transfusions in bleeding patients undergoing cardiac surgery have been mostly limited to non-RCTs[131]; the clinical efficacy of plasma transfusion in this setting has yet to be defined. A systematic review of plasma transfusion in patients with central nervous system hemorrhage by an expert consensus panel advised against plasma transfusion in the absence of coagulopathy or vitamin K antagonist therapy, given the potential for cardiopulmonary complications and serious adverse reactions following transfusion.[133] Systematic reviews conducted in 2004[134] and 2012[135] revealed an emphasis on prophylactic rather than therapeutic use of fresh plasma in the available literature as well as a paucity of evidence-based plasma transfusion practices.

Therapeutic plasma exchange is considered first-line therapy for treatment of thrombotic thrombocytopenic purpura (TTP). Plasma is the replacement fluid of choice for repletion of ADAMTS13 (**A D**isintegrin **A**nd **M**etalloproteinase with a **T**hrombo**S**pondin type 1 motif, member 13) in order to restore von Willebrand factor (vWF)-cleaving activity. Although the efficacy of plasma exchange has been clearly demonstrated for treatment of TTP, the optimal type of plasma component (ie, Fresh Frozen Plasma vs Plasma Cryoprecipitate Reduced or solvent/detergent-treated plasma) has not been definitively established; all appear efficacious.[136] Plasma may also be used in conjunction with (or in place of) albumin as replacement fluid for patients with underlying coagulopathy or bleeding (eg, diffuse alveolar hemorrhage) who require therapeutic exchange.

Vitamin K Antagonist Reversal

During clot formation, several coagulation factors such as Factors II, VII, IX, and X associate with the surface of activated platelets via hydrophobic protein domains called gamma-carboxyglutamic acid (Gla) domains. Gla domains help ensure that, when activated, coagulation factors localize where they are needed to provide hemostatic function. To form Gla domains, specific glutamic acid (Glu) residues must undergo posttranslational gamma-carboxylation. The reduced form of vitamin K is required to contribute electrons to these carboxylation reactions. In the process, vitamin K becomes oxidized. Enzymes called vitamin K epoxide reductases serve to recycle vitamin K back to its "useful" reduced form so that it can participate in subsequent gamma-carboxylation reactions. Warfarin and other types of vitamin K antagonists (VKAs) are structurally similar to vitamin K, resulting in competitive inhibition of epoxide reductases when present. Thus, VKA intake results in deficiency of reduced vitamin K, which in turn leads to decreased functional activity of Factors II (thrombin), VII, IX, and X, as well as antithrombotic factors protein C and protein S.[137]

There are several methods available to reverse the effect of VKAs. For patients in whom urgent reversal is needed (eg, bleeding or emergent indication for invasive surgery), the treatment of choice is a four-factor prothrombin complex concentrate (PCC). PCCs contain high levels of Factors II, VII, IX, and X in the nonactivated state, as well as proteins C and S. Three-factor PCCs containing smaller quantities of Factor VII are also available and were used off-label before FDA approval of four-factor PCCs specifically for VKA reversal.[138] Several studies directly comparing three-factor to four-factor PCCs have demonstrated a slight advantage of four-factor over three-factor products.[138,139] A recent RCT demonstrated that reversal was more rapid and reliable in bleeding patients taking warfarin who received a PCC compared to those who received plasma.[140,141] Both products had a similar profile for thromboembolic events.[142] Concur-

rent vitamin K administration is also recommended during reversal to ensure a sustained effect. Selection of the route of administration for supplemental vitamin K is dependent on clinical urgency, because intravenous formulations take effect within 6 to 12 hours, compared to 12 to 24 hours for oral formulations.[143]

Plasma may be used if PCCs are contraindicated, such as in patients who have had heparin-induced thrombocytopenia (because some PCCs contain heparin) or in situations where PCCs may be unavailable. Given the transient effect of plasma and the relatively large dose required (15-20 mL/kg) for effective reversal, patients should be closely monitored for evidence of fluid overload, especially those with particular volume sensitivity (eg, cardiac and/or renal insufficiency).

In the absence of specific reversal agents for the direct oral anticoagulants (as in the case of idarucizumab for dabigatran or andexanet alfa for Factor Xa inhibitors), four-factor PCCs have been found to be superior to plasma for reversal of Factor Xa inhibitors, although the evidence is limited to a small number of studies.[144]

Types of Plasma

Several varieties of plasma are available for transfusion, including Fresh Frozen Plasma (FFP), Plasma Frozen Within 24 Hours After Phlebotomy (PF24), Plasma Cryoprecipitate Reduced, and solvent/detergent-treated plasma (SD plasma). By definition, FFP is frozen within 8 hours of collection and transfused within 24 hours of thawing, to preserve levels of the most heat-labile coagulation factors, Factors V and VIII. Many transfusion services provide Thawed Plasma, which is plasma that has been thawed and maintained in a closed system at 1 to 6 C for up to 5 days. Thawed Plasma is not currently regulated by the FDA but is included in both the *Circular of Information for the Use of Blood and Blood Components*[145] and AABB *Standards for Blood Banks and Transfusion Services (Standards)*.[146] Advantages of Thawed Plasma include immediate availability in bleeding emergencies and reduced wastage due to its longer shelf life. The activity of individual coagulation factors, such as Factor VIII, may decline at variable rates over time, but overall factor activities have been shown to remain within the normal range during 5-day refrigerated storage.[147] Differences in clinical outcome among recipients of various types of plasma have not been demonstrated, and many transfusion services currently use Thawed Plasma from any original source (FFP, PF24, SD plasma, etc) interchangeably with freshly thawed FFP. SD plasma provides an extra measure of safety with respect to transmission of enveloped viruses and other pathogens[148] but is significantly more expensive than untreated plasma components, as it is a pooled, treated product. Primary indications include severe allergic transfusion reactions or the need for reduced risk of infectious disease transmission in those requiring large-volume plasma transfusions on a chronic basis (eg, TTP).[136] Although the first-generation SD plasma was noted to have 20% to 30% lower Factor V levels compared to FFP, second-generation Octaplas LG appears to contain levels similar to other plasma products and may therefore be used interchangeably for treatment of congenital or acquired Factor V deficiency.[149]

CRYOPRECIPITATE TRANSFUSION

Cryoprecipitate is a plasma derivative that is relatively enriched for fibrinogen, Factor VIII, vWF, fibronectin, and Factor XIII. There are limited indications for cryoprecipitate, as there are pathogen-reduced and recombinant products available for several of the indications where cryoprecipitate was used previously. Cryoprecipitate is suggested for fibrinogen replacement for acquired hypofibrinogenemic conditions such as liver transplantation and postpartum hemorrhage.[150-152] Pathogen-reduced concentrates are standard-of-care to treat congenital hypofibrinogenemia, dysfibrinogenemia, and von Willebrand disease. Congenital Factor XIII deficiency, associated with a delayed bleeding phenotype, is extremely rare, and there is now a recombinant Factor XIII concentrate available. Fibronectin is not currently used as a therapeutic agent. Thus, cryoprecipitate is used primarily to replace fi-

brinogen in patients who are bleeding or having invasive procedures.

Pregnancy is associated with an increase in fibrinogen concentration above the laboratory levels of normal (approximately 6 g/L in the third trimester compared to 2-4 g/L in the non-pregnant state).[153] A low fibrinogen concentration among women with postpartum hemorrhage has been reported to be independently associated with severe bleeding.[154,155] To restore hemostasis, fibrinogen replacement has been advocated.[156] Plasma, cryoprecipitate, and fibrinogen concentrate are all sources of fibrinogen. However, the volume of plasma needed is considerably larger than that of cryoprecipitate to achieve the same replacement dose of fibrinogen (eg, 300-400 mg of fibrinogen can be replaced with 250 mL of plasma or with only 10-15 mL of cryoprecipitate). Fibrinogen concentrate is also a low-volume option, and it has the additional advantages of being pathogen reduced and requiring no thawing time. To date, cryoprecipitate and fibrinogen concentrate have not been directly compared in RCTs in adults. In a small retrospective study of women with postpartum hemorrhage, similar outcomes were achieved among patients receiving either cryoprecipitate or fibrinogen concentrate.[151] In the 2015 Fibrinogen Concentrate as Initial Treatment for Postpartum Haemorrhage (FIB-PPH) trial,[157] women with postpartum hemorrhage were randomly assigned to receive 2 g of fibrinogen concentrate or placebo. No difference in clinical outcomes was observed (20% of patients in the fibrinogen concentrate group received RBCs vs 22% of controls). However, only a small proportion of patients had severe postpartum hemorrhage in this trial. In two other small trials in patients with acquired hypofibrinogenemia (ie, through surgery or bleeding), mortality, bleeding, and transfusion requirements did not differ when using cryoprecipitate or fibrinogen concentrate.[158]

Cardiac surgery is associated with acquired hemostatic defects secondary to cardiopulmonary bypass that lead to excess bleeding.[159-161] Individuals undergoing cardiac surgery are at high risk of receiving blood transfusion.[162] The use of prophylactic fibrinogen is intended to reduce the risk of bleeding and consequently the exposure to blood components, because a lower fibrinogen concentration following cardiac surgery was associated with a higher bleeding risk.[163] In a small, single-center, placebo-controlled, double-blinded RCT, prophylactic fibrinogen concentrate administered after protamine administration reduced blood component usage among nonanemic cardiac surgery patients. Patients randomly assigned to fibrinogen concentrate vs placebo were significantly less likely to receive any allogeneic blood component (67% vs 45%; p = 0.015). Postoperative bleeding was significantly (although modestly) lower in the fibrinogen concentrate group (median blood loss of 300 mL vs 355 mL; p = 0.042).[164] Nonetheless, further studies are needed to define the role of fibrinogen replacement and its effects on bleeding, mortality, blood component utilization, and adverse events,[165] specifically in comparison to cryoprecipitate.[166] A more recent placebo-controlled multicenter RCT comparing fibrinogen concentrate to placebo in postoperative cardiac surgery patients showed no benefit, and patients receiving fibrinogen concentrate actually received significantly more allogeneic blood components.[167] Fibrinogen replacement using either cryoprecipitate or fibrinogen concentrate has not been associated with increased mortality or thromboembolic events.

GRANULOCYTE TRANSFUSION

Prolonged severe neutropenia with intensive chemotherapy for hematologic malignancies or in the setting of HSCT (defined as an absolute neutrophil count of <500/μL) predisposes patients to life-threatening bacterial and fungal infections despite aggressive antimicrobial therapy.[168] Granulocyte transfusions are believed to reduce the risk of morbidity and mortality associated with such infections. Donors are stimulated with corticosteroids and/or granulocyte colony-stimulating factor (G-CSF), allowing large numbers of granulocytes to be collected by apheresis. Granulocyte components are stored at room temperature and should be transfused as soon as possible within 24 hours of collection

per AABB *Standards*.[146(p60)] Studies have shown that granulocytes may maintain functional activity for up to 48 hours if stored at 10 C, although the percentage of recovered cells decreases by approximately 50% after the first 24 hours.[169,170] Because of their short shelf life, granulocyte components may be released from the collection facility before results of donor infectious disease tests are complete. Therefore, granulocyte donors are often selected from a pool of pre-screened or frequent, long-term apheresis donors who have undergone recent testing. Granulocyte components contain a significant number of red cells and require crossmatching unless they contain <2 mL of red cells.[146(p42)] To prevent acute hemolytic reactions, granulocyte components are matched to the recipient according to ABO-matching rules for RBCs (Table 19-2). Alternatively, red cells may be removed from ABO-incompatible units with methods such as gravity sedimentation for donations, using hydroxyethyl starch (HES).[171] Similarly, the recipient should receive HLA-matched components when HLA alloantibodies are present. Consideration may also be given to the cytomegalovirus (CMV) status of the donor if the recipient is CMV negative, although there is limited evidence for proven transmission of CMV to seronegative recipients after granulocyte transfusion.[172,173] Furthermore, CMV-seronegative granulocytes may not always be available in a timely manner, particularly if the recipient has stringent ABO or HLA antigen restrictions or if the donor population has a high prevalence of CMV infection.[174] In these cases, the clinical urgency for granulocyte therapy should be weighed against the risks of a CMV infection and/or transfusing a mismatched component. All granulocyte components must be irradiated to prevent transfusion-associated graft-vs-host disease.[175] Leukocyte reduction filters should never be used for administration. Recipients should be closely monitored during granulocyte infusions, as febrile cytokine reactions, volume overload, and pulmonary toxicity due to localization of granulocytes to the lungs may occur.

However, a survival benefit of transfusing granulocytes to septic, neutropenic patients has not been definitively demonstrated.[176] This lack of benefit may be due to the inability to provide an adequate number of granulocytes for transfusion.[168,177] In a systematic review of 10 RCTs, prophylactic granulocyte transfusion was not associated with a difference in morbidity or mortality secondary to infections; however, intermediate-dose granulocyte transfusions (1-4 × 10^10 granulocytes per day) were associated with a reduction in the number of patients with infections after 30 days [relative risk (RR), 0.4; 95% CI, 0.26-0.63] and the number of patients with bacteremia and fungemia (RR, 0.45; 95% CI, 0.30-0.65).[177] Trials of therapeutic granulocyte transfusion in septic immunocompromised patients have also shown inconsistent results.[168] For example, in the multicenter Resolving Infection in Neutropenia with Granulocytes (RING) trial,[176] neutropenic patients with proven or likely infection were randomly assigned to receive standard antimicrobial therapy or standard antimicrobial therapy plus granulocytes collected from donors stimulated with G-CSF and dexamethasone. Overall, no benefit was observed from transfusing granulocytes. Nonetheless, the RING study was underpowered, having enrolled only 50% of the predefined sample size required to detect a difference in the primary composite outcome of survival and microbial clearance after 42 days. Also, the target dose of >4 × 10^10 granulocytes per transfusion (0.6 × 10^9 cells/kg) was achieved in only 70% of transfusions.[178] A secondary analysis suggested that patients who received higher doses of granulocytes tended to have better outcomes than patients who received lower doses.[176] Currently, the role of granulocyte transfusion remains undefined, and clinical judgment is required. If granulocyte transfusions are used, higher doses of granulocytes, as typically obtained from donors stimulated with G-CSF (or a combination of G-CSF and corticosteroids) compared to corticosteroids alone, may be more effective.[179]

MASSIVE TRANSFUSION PROTOCOLS

"Massive transfusion" is most often defined as transfusion of 10 or more RBC units in a 24-hour period in adults, although other definitions are also used (eg, 4 RBC units in 1 hour).[180] In the past, trauma patients with substantial blood loss were typically treated with RBC transfusions plus crystalloid, with hemostatic blood components such as platelets, plasma, and cryoprecipitate administered based on laboratory test results. In recent years, this approach has been largely superseded by a more aggressive and empiric approach, whereby the initial resuscitation of trauma patients is focused on early transfusion with plasma, platelets, and RBCs in a fixed ratio (eg, 1:1:1; note: for platelets, the "1" refers to a single whole-blood-derived platelet concentrate and not 1 apheresis platelet unit). These fixed ratios are intended to approximate the transfusion of whole blood through a combination of components in order to prevent dilutional coagulopathy. The fixed ratio or "formula-based" approach was devised by military physicians during the Iraq and Afghanistan wars of the 2000s. The publication credited with sparking interest in this approach[181] described 246 injured soldiers in Iraq who were retrospectively grouped by the ratio of plasma to RBCs received. Patients in the low plasma-to-RBC group (median of 1 unit of plasma for every 8 RBC units) had a 65% mortality rate, as compared with a 19% mortality rate among patients in the high plasma-to-RBC group (median of 1 unit of plasma for every 1.4 RBC units). Although striking, this study and multiple other subsequent retrospective studies were highly confounded. Trauma patients who die from their injuries due to blood loss tend to do so very early (ie, often in less than an hour after hospital arrival).[182] It was unclear whether early and aggressive plasma transfusion led to better survival, or whether plasma transfusion was available for the less-severely injured patients who survived (ie, there was time to thaw and transfuse frozen plasma in cases where patients did not die rapidly on arrival).[183,184]

Two recent multicenter studies examined transfusion management of massively bleeding trauma patients. The Prospective, Observational, Multicenter, Major Trauma Transfusion (PROMMTT) study[185] was a prospective observational study of adult trauma patients treated at 1 of 10 civilian trauma centers in the United States. Study staff performed direct bedside observation as patients were resuscitated. To reduce potential survivor bias, patients dying within the first 30 minutes of arrival were excluded. Patients who received plasma to RBCs in a 1:1 ratio had significantly better 6-hour survival than patients receiving a lower ratio of plasma to RBCs. However, survival at later time points did not differ significantly. A subsequent RCT, called the Pragmatic Randomized Optimal Platelet and Plasma Ratios (PROPPR) trial,[186] compared outcomes among 680 adult civilian trauma patients who were randomly assigned to be resuscitated using a 1:1:1 vs 1:1:2 ratio of plasma to platelets to RBCs. The primary outcomes, 24-hour and 30-day survival, did not significantly differ between the study groups. Currently, it is common for blood banks to incorporate fixed ratios of blood components (ie, 1:1:1 or 1:1:2) into their local massive transfusion protocols (MTPs). Although it is difficult to judge the effectiveness of this approach from the published data, it does improve the speed and simplicity of the initial response. Laboratory-based, targeted transfusion of specific components is often used after the patient has stabilized. It is important to note that although much of the data on MTPs relates to trauma, in civilian hospitals, massive transfusions are actually more likely to occur among other patient populations (eg, solid-organ transplantation patients and cardiac surgery patients).[187,188]

Group AB plasma is the preferred blood component in trauma MTPs before blood group determination because it lacks both anti-A and anti-B. However, because AB plasma is in short supply due to the low prevalence of type AB donors (~4%), group A plasma has been used in several centers as an alternate to AB plasma. The use of relatively plentiful group A units allows for routine availability of a prethawed inventory for immediate use without wastage of a precious resource (ie, group AB plasma) if thawed components are not used during their 5-day shelf life.[189] Studies of group B and AB trauma patients who have received group A plasma support the safety of this practice.[190,191]

Early use of plasma has been advocated to reduce the risk of trauma-associated coagulopathy. Two recent RCTs examined the use of prehospital plasma resuscitation for civilian trauma and yielded divergent results for the benefit of this strategy.[192,193] The Prehospital Air Medical Plasma (PAMPer) trial randomly assigned trauma patients at risk of hemorrhagic shock to either 2 units of thawed plasma (group AB or group A with a low anti-B antibody titer) or standard trauma care during air medical transport.[192] The 30-day mortality rate was lower in the 230 patients who received plasma (23.2%) compared with that of the 271 patients (33%) who received standard trauma care (p = 0.03).[192] The Control of Major Bleeding After Trauma Trial (COMBAT) randomly assigned trauma patients to 2 units of frozen AB plasma (75 patients) or saline (69 patients) and did not find a statistically significant difference in 28-day mortality (15% in the plasma group and 10% in the control group; p = 0.37) and was thus terminated early (144 of 150 patients had been enrolled).[193] The difference in outcomes may be due to the injury severity of the trauma patients and prehospitalization use of red cells and ventilation in the PAMPer trial. Future studies are needed to clarify the role of early resuscitation with plasma.

Whole blood resuscitation in the absence of blood component availability is currently employed in military settings and is regaining acceptance for civilian trauma. Concerns regarding the functionality of platelets stored in the cold as part of refrigerated whole blood, and plasma incompatibility have largely been surmounted. Cold-storage platelets arguably demonstrate superior hemostatic effect (including increased adhesion, aggregation, and clot strength), albeit inferior in-vivo survival and posttransfusion recovery, compared with platelets stored at room temperature.[194] AABB *Standards*[146] now permits transfusion of ABO-compatible whole blood rather than requiring ABO-identical whole blood, facilitating the use of low-titer group O whole blood for civilian trauma resuscitation. Thus far, early studies have not demonstrated a significant risk of hemolysis[195] or evidence of inferior clinical outcomes compared to traditional component therapy.[196] However, determination of specific titer thresholds and other selection criteria for whole blood components have not yet been defined, and current practices are highly variable from institution to institution. Whole blood has the advantages of smaller volumes than the combination of RBCs, plasma, and platelets; early plasma and platelet resuscitation for effective management of coagulopathy; and fewer donor exposures by combining all components into a single product.[197] Experience is gaining in the use of whole blood for civilian trauma, but whole blood has not yet become standard for these patients nor for other patients with massive hemorrhage.

KEY POINTS

1. In deciding to transfuse RBCs, it is important to consider the patient's clinical status; comorbidities; etiology and time course of anemia; and hemoglobin level. In hemodynamically stable inpatients, when hemoglobin level is the sole consideration, then a restrictive transfusion approach (hemoglobin threshold of 7-8 g/dL) should be used.
2. Currently, insufficient evidence is available to recommend a restrictive RBC transfusion approach for patients with acute coronary syndrome, severe thrombocytopenia, or chronic transfusion-dependent anemia.
3. In patients with sickle cell disease at high risk for stroke based on transcranial Doppler ultrasonography, chronic RBC transfusion (or hydroxyurea) reduces stroke risk. RBC transfusion is not recommended to treat patients with sickle cell disease with uncomplicated painful vaso-occlusive crises, or asymptomatic anemia.
4. Neonatal, pediatric, and adult patients may receive RBC units of any storage age within the licensed storage period.
5. When clinically indicated, RBC transfusion should not be withheld in cases of WAIHA, even though units are incompatible because of the autoantibody. Efforts should be made to detect and avoid underlying clinically significant alloantibodies, and sufficient RBCs should be transfused to relieve signs and symptoms of anemia.
6. In hospitalized patients with hypoproliferative thrombocytopenia, prophylactic platelet transfusions reduce the risk of spontaneous bleeding. For this patient group, a prophylactic platelet transfusion threshold of 10,000/μL is appropriate.
7. Most cases of platelet refractoriness are nonimmune in origin. Patients with immune refractoriness may benefit from a trial of HLA-matched, antigen-negative, or crossmatched platelet units.
8. Plasma transfusion is indicated for bleeding patients with multiple coagulation factor deficiencies and in massive transfusion protocols. Urgent warfarin reversal is best achieved using a four-factor prothrombin complex concentrate (PCC).
9. Cryoprecipitate is used for fibrinogen replacement. Fibrinogen concentrate may be used as an alternative.
10. Granulocytes are at times transfused to treat severe refractory bacterial or fungal infections in neutropenic patients. The utility of granulocyte transfusions remains unclear. If granulocytes are used, high doses should be administered.

REFERENCES

1. Hébert PC, Wells G, Blajchman MA, et al. A multicenter, randomized, controlled clinical trial of transfusion requirements in critical care. Transfusion Requirements in Critical Care Investigators, Canadian Critical Care Trials Group. N Engl J Med 1999;340:409-17.
2. Carson JL, Terrin ML, Noveck H, et al. Liberal or restrictive transfusion in high-risk patients after hip surgery. N Engl J Med 2011;365:2453-62.
3. Grover M, Talwalkar S, Casbard A, et al. Silent myocardial ischaemia and haemoglobin concentration: A randomized controlled trial of transfu-

sion strategy in lower limb arthroplasty. Vox Sang 2006;90:105-12.

4. So-Osman C, Nelissen R, Te Slaa R, et al. A randomized comparison of transfusion triggers in elective orthopaedic surgery using leucocyte-depleted red blood cells. Vox Sang 2010;98:56-64.

5. Carson JL, Carless PA, Hébert PC. Transfusion thresholds and other strategies for guiding allogeneic red blood cell transfusion. Cochrane Database Syst Rev 2012;(4):CD002042.

6. Holst LB, Petersen MW, Haase N, et al. Restrictive versus liberal transfusion strategy for red blood cell transfusion: Systematic review of randomised trials with meta-analysis and trial sequential analysis. BMJ 2015;350:h1354.

7. Lacroix J, Hébert PC, Hutchison JS, et al; TRIPICU Investigators; Canadian Critical Care Trials Group; Pediatric Acute Lung Injury and Sepsis Investigators Network. Transfusion strategies for patients in pediatric intensive care units. N Engl J Med 2007;356(16):1609-19.

8. Bracey AW, Radovancevic R, Riggs SA, et al. Lowering the hemoglobin threshold for transfusion in coronary artery bypass procedures: Effect on patient outcome. Transfusion 1999;39:1070-7.

9. Hajjar LA, Vincent JL, Galas FR, et al. Transfusion requirements after cardiac surgery: The TRACS randomized controlled trial. JAMA 2010; 304:1559-67.

10. Murphy GJ, Pike K, Rogers CA, et al. Liberal or restrictive transfusion after cardiac surgery. N Engl J Med 2015;372:997-1008.

11. Mazer CD, Whitlock RP, Fergusson DA, et al; TRICS Investigators and Perioperative Anesthesia Clinical Trials Group. Restrictive or liberal red-cell transfusion for cardiac surgery. N Engl J Med 2017;377:2133-44.

12. Mazer CD, Whitlock RP, Shehata N. Restrictive versus liberal transfusion for cardiac surgery. N Engl J Med 2018;379(26):2576-7.

13. Holst LB, Haase N, Wetterslev J, et al. Lower versus higher hemoglobin threshold for transfusion in septic shock. N Engl J Med 2014;371: 1381-91.

14. Villanueva C, Colomo A, Bosch A, et al. Transfusion strategies for acute upper gastrointestinal bleeding. N Engl J Med 2013;368:11-21.

15. Jairath V, Kahan BC, Gray A, et al. Restrictive versus liberal blood transfusion for acute upper gastrointestinal bleeding (TRIGGER): A pragmatic, open-label, cluster randomised feasibility trial. Lancet 2015;386:137-44.

16. de Almeida JP, Vincent J-L, Galas FRBG, et al. Transfusion requirements in surgical oncology patients: A prospective, randomized controlled trial. Anesthesiology 2015;122:29-38.

17. Prick BW, Jansen A, Steegers E, et al. Transfusion policy after severe postpartum haemorrhage: A randomised non-inferiority trial. BJOG 2014;121:1005-14.

18. Robertson CS, Hannay HJ, Yamal J-M, et al. Effect of erythropoietin and transfusion threshold on neurological recovery after traumatic brain injury. JAMA 2014;312:36-47.

19. Carson JL, Stanworth SJ, Roubinian N, et al. Transfusion thresholds and other strategies for guiding allogeneic red blood cell transfusion. Cochrane Database Syst Rev 2016;10: CD002042.

20. Carson JL, Guyatt G, Heddle NM, et al. Clinical practice guidelines from the AABB: Red Blood Cell transfusion thresholds and storage. JAMA 2016;316:2025-35.

21. So-Osman C, Nelissen R, Brand R, et al. Postoperative anemia after joint replacement surgery is not related to quality of life during the first two weeks postoperatively. Transfusion 2011;51:71-81.

22. Carson JL, Brooks MM, Abbott JD, et al. Liberal versus restrictive transfusion thresholds for patients with symptomatic coronary artery disease. Am Heart J 2013;165(6):964-71.e1.

23. Hébert PC, Yetisir E, Martin C, et al. Is a low transfusion threshold safe in critically ill patients with cardiovascular diseases? Crit Care Med 2001;29:227-34.

24. Bergamin FS1, Almeida JP, Landoni G, et al. Liberal versus restrictive transfusion strategy in critically ill oncologic patients: The Transfusion Requirements in Critically Ill Oncologic Patients Randomized Controlled Trial. Crit Care Med 2017;45(5):766-73.

25. Koch CG, Li L, Sessler DI, et al. Duration of red-cell storage and complications after cardiac surgery. N Engl J Med 2008;358:1229-39.

26. Fergusson DA, Hébert P, Hogan DL, et al. Effect of fresh red blood cell transfusions on clinical outcomes in premature, very low-birth-weight infants: The ARIPI randomized trial. JAMA 2012;308:1443-51.

27. Lacroix J, Hébert PC, Fergusson DA, et al. Age of transfused blood in critically ill adults. N Engl J Med 2015;372:1410-18.

28. Cooper DJ, McQuilten ZK, Nichol A, et al; TRANSFUSE Investigators and the Australian and New Zealand Intensive Care Society Clini-

cal Trials Group. Age of red cells for transfusion and outcomes in critically ill adults. N Engl J Med 2017;377:1858-67.

29. Steiner ME, Ness PM, Assmann SF, et al. Effects of red-cell storage duration on patients undergoing cardiac surgery. N Engl J Med 2015;372:1419-29.

30. Dhabangi A, Ainomugisha B, Cserti-Gazdewich C, et al. Effect of transfusion of Red Blood Cells with longer vs shorter storage duration on elevated blood lactate levels in children with severe anemia. JAMA 2015;314:2514-23.

31. Heddle NM, Cook RJ, Arnold DM, et al. Effect of short-term vs. long-term blood storage on mortality after transfusion. N Engl J Med 2016;375:1937-45.

32. Chassé M, McIntyre L, English SW, et al. Effect of blood donor characteristics on transfusion outcomes: A systematic review and meta-analysis. Transfus Med Rev 2016;30:69-80.

33. Edgren G, Ullum H, Rostgaard K, et al. Association of donor age and sex with survival of patients receiving transfusions. JAMA Intern Med 2017;177:854-60.

34. Chassé M, Tinmouth A, English SW, et al. Association of blood donor age and sex with recipient survival after Red Blood Cell transfusion. JAMA Intern Med 2016;176:1307-14.

35. Caram-Deelder C, Kreuger AL, Evers D, et al. Association of blood transfusion from female donors with and without a history of pregnancy with mortality among male and female transfusion recipients. JAMA 2017;318:1471-8.

36. Fiorellino J, Elahie AL, Warkentin TE. Acute haemolysis, DIC and renal failure after transfusion of uncross-matched blood during trauma resuscitation: Illustrative case and literature review. Transfus Med 2018;28(4):319-25.

37. Rachmilewitz EA, Giardina PJ. How I treat thalassemia. Blood 2011;118:3479-88.

38. Goss C, Giardina P, Degtyaryova D, et al. Red blood cell transfusions for thalassemia: Results of a survey assessing current practice and proposal of evidence-based guidelines. Transfusion 2014;54:1773-81.

39. Compernolle V, Chow ST, Tanael S, et al for the International Collaboration for Transfusion Medicine Guidelines (ICTMG). Red cell specifications for patients with hemoglobinopathies: A systematic review and guideline. Transfusion 2018;58:1555-66.

40. Bunn HF. Pathogenesis and treatment of sickle cell disease. N Engl J Med 1997;337:762-9.

41. Yawn BP, Buchanan GR, Afenyi-Annan AN, et al. Management of sickle cell disease: Summary of the 2014 evidence-based report by expert panel members. JAMA 2014;312:1033-48.

42. Rosse WF, Gallagher D, Kinney TR, et al. Transfusion and alloimmunization in sickle cell disease. The Cooperative Study of Sickle Cell Disease. Blood 1990;76:1431-7.

43. Yazdanbakhsh K, Ware RE, Noizat-Pirenne F. Red blood cell alloimmunization in sickle cell disease: Pathophysiology, risk factors, and transfusion management. Blood 2012;120:528-37.

44. Chou ST, Jackson T, Vege S, et al. High prevalence of red blood cell alloimmunization in sickle cell disease despite transfusion from Rh-matched minority donors. Blood 2013;122:1062-71.

45. Fasano RM, Booth GS, Miles M, et al. Red blood cell alloimmunization is influenced by recipient inflammatory state at time of transfusion in patients with sickle cell disease. Br J Haematol 2015;168:291-300.

46. Danaee A, Inusa B, Howard J, Robinson S. Hyperhemolysis in patients with hemoglobinopathies: A single-center experience and review of the literature. Transfus Med Rev 2015;29:220-30.

47. Win N. Hyperhemolysis syndrome in sickle cell disease. Expert Rev Hematol 2009;2:111-15.

48. Win N, Sinha S, Lee E, Mills W. Treatment with intravenous immunoglobulin and steroids may correct severe anemia in hyperhemolytic transfusion reactions: Case report and literature review. Transfus Med Rev 2010;24:64-7.

49. Pirenne F, Yazdanbakhsh K. How I safely transfuse patients with sickle-cell disease and manage delayed hemolytic transfusion reactions. Blood 2018;131:2773-81.

50. Alayash AI. Hemoglobin-based blood substitutes and the treatment of sickle cell disease: More harm than help? Biomolecules 2017;7(1). pii: E2.

51. Davis JM, El-Haj N, Shah NN, et al. Use of the blood substitute HBOC-201 in critically ill patients during sickle cell crisis: A three-case series. Transfusion 2018;58:132-7.

52. Kacker S, Ness PM, Savage WJ, et al. Cost-effectiveness of prospective red blood cell antigen matching to prevent alloimmunization among sickle cell patients. Transfusion 2014;54:86-97.

53. Vichinsky EP, Luban NL, Wright E, et al. Prospective RBC phenotype matching in a stroke-prevention trial in sickle cell anemia: A multi-

center transfusion trial. Transfusion 2001;41: 1086-92.

54. Tournamille C, Meunier-Costes N, Costes B, et al. Partial C antigen in sickle cell disease patients: Clinical relevance and prevention of alloimmunization. Transfusion 2010;50:13-19.

55. The American Society of Hematology 2020 clinical practice guideline for sickle cell disease. Blood 2020 (in press).

56. Adams RJ, McKie VC, Hsu L, et al. Prevention of a first stroke by transfusions in children with sickle cell anemia and abnormal results on transcranial Doppler ultrasonography. N Engl J Med 1998;339:5-11.

57. Adams RJ, Brambilla D; STOP2 Trial investigators. Discontinuing prophylactic transfusions used to prevent stroke in sickle cell disease. N Engl J Med 2005;353:2769-78.

58. Ware RE, Davis BR, Schultz WH, et al. Hydroxycarbamide versus chronic transfusion for maintenance of transcranial doppler flow velocities in children with sickle cell anaemia—TCD With Transfusions Changing to Hydroxyurea (TWiTCH): A multicentre, open-label, phase 3, non-inferiority trial. Lancet 2016;387:661-70.

59. Barcellini W, Fattizzo B, Zaninoni A, et al. Clinical heterogeneity and predictors of outcome in primary autoimmune hemolytic anemia: A GIMEMA study of 308 patients. Blood 2014; 124(19):2930-6.

60. Petz LD. A physician's guide to transfusion in autoimmune haemolytic anaemia. Br J Haematol 2004;124:712-16.

61. Issitt PD, Combs MR, Bumgarner DJ, et al. Studies of antibodies in the sera of patients who have made red cell autoantibodies. Transfusion 1996;36:481-6.

62. Laine ML, Beattie KM. Frequency of alloantibodies accompanying autoantibodies. Transfusion 1985;25:545-6.

63. Shirey RS, Boyd JS, Parwani AV, et al. Prophylactic antigen-matched donor blood for patients with warm autoantibodies: An algorithm for transfusion management. Transfusion 2002;42: 1435-41.

64. El Kenz H, Efira A, Le PQ, et al. Transfusion support of autoimmune hemolytic anemia: How could the blood group genotyping help? Transl Res 2014;163:36-42.

65. Petz LD, Garratty G. Immune hemolytic anemias. Philadelphia: Churchill Livingstone, 2004.

66. de Weers M, Tai YT, van der Veer MS, et al. Daratumumab, a novel therapeutic human CD38 monoclonal antibody, induces killing of multiple myeloma and other hematological tumors. J Immunol 2011;186:1840-8.

67. Sullivan HC, Gerner-Smidt C, Nooka AK, et al. Daratumumab (anti-CD38) induces loss of CD38 on red blood cells. Blood 2017;129: 3033-7.

68. Oldenborg PA, Zheleznyak A, Fang YF, et al. Role of CD47 as a marker of self on red blood cells. Science 2000;288(5473):2051-4.

69. Olsson M, Bruhns P, Frazier WA, et al. Platelet homeostasis is regulated by platelet expression of CD47 under normal conditions and in passive immune thrombocytopenia. Blood 2005; 105(9):3577-82.

70. Russ A, Hua AB, Montfort WR, et al. Blocking "don't eat me" signal of CD47-SIRPα in hematological malignancies, an in-depth review. Blood Rev 2018;32(6):480-9.

71. Velliquette RW, Aeschlimann J, Kirkegaard J, et al. Monoclonal anti-CD47 interference in red cell and platelet testing. Transfusion 2019; 59(2):730-7.

72. Chapuy CI, Nicholson RT, Aguad MD, et al. Resolving the daratumumab interference with blood compatibility testing. Transfusion 2015; 55(6 Pt 2):1545-54.

73. Hannon JL, Clarke G. Transfusion management of patients receiving daratumumab therapy for advanced plasma cell myeloma. Transfusion 2015;55(11):2770.

74. Mitigating the anti-CD38 interference with serologic testing. Association Bulletin, #16-02. Bethesda, MD: AABB, 2016.

75. Gaydos LA, Freireich EJ, Mantel N. The quantitative relation between platelet count and hemorrhage in patients with acute leukemia. N Engl J Med 1962;266:905-9.

76. Wandt H, Frank M, Ehninger G, et al. Safety and cost effectiveness of a 10 x 10(9)/L trigger for prophylactic platelet transfusions compared with the traditional 20 x 10(9)/L trigger: A prospective comparative trial in 105 patients with acute myeloid leukemia. Blood 1998;91:3601-6.

77. Slichter SJ, Harker LA. Thrombocytopenia: Mechanisms and management of defects in platelet production. Clin Haematol 1978;7:523-39.

78. Heckman KD, Weiner GJ, Davis CS, et al. Randomized study of prophylactic platelet transfusion threshold during induction therapy for adult acute leukemia: 10,000/microL versus 20,000/microL. J Clin Oncol 1997;15:1143-9.

79. Rebulla P, Finazzi G, Marangoni F, et al. The threshold for prophylactic platelet transfusions in adults with acute myeloid leukemia. Gruppo Italiano Malattie Ematologiche Maligne dell'Adulto. N Engl J Med 1997;337:1870-5.

80. Zumberg MS, del Rosario MLU, Nejame CF, et al. A prospective randomized trial of prophylactic platelet transfusion and bleeding incidence in hematopoietic stem cell transplant recipients: 10,000/L versus 20,000/microL trigger. Biol Blood Marrow Transplant 2002;8:569-76.

81. Gmür J, Burger J, Schanz U, et al. Safety of stringent prophylactic platelet transfusion policy for patients with acute leukaemia. The Lancet 1991;338:1223-6.

82. Kaufman RM, Djulbegovic B, Gernsheimer T, et al. Platelet transfusion: A clinical practice guideline from the AABB. Ann Intern Med 2015;162:205-13.

83. Nahirniak S, Slichter SJ, Tanael S, et al. Guidance on platelet transfusion for patients with hypoproliferative thrombocytopenia. Transfus Med Rev 2015;29:3-13.

84. Schiffer CA, Bohlke K, Delaney M, et al. Platelet transfusion for patients with cancer: American Society of Clinical Oncology clinical practice guideline update. J Clin Oncol 2018;36(3):283-99.

85. Stanworth SJ, Estcourt LJ, Llewelyn CA, et al. Impact of prophylactic platelet transfusions on bleeding events in patients with hematologic malignancies: A subgroup analysis of a randomized trial. Transfusion 2014;54:2385-93.

86. Stanworth SJ, Estcourt LJ, Powter G, et al. A no-prophylaxis platelet-transfusion strategy for hematologic cancers. N Engl J Med 2013;368:1771-80.

87. Wandt H, Schaefer-Eckart K, Wendelin K, et al. Therapeutic platelet transfusion versus routine prophylactic transfusion in patients with haematological malignancies: An open-label, multicentre, randomised study. Lancet 2012;380:1309-16.

88. Kumar A, Mhaskar R, Grossman BJ, et al. Platelet transfusion: A systematic review of the clinical evidence. Transfusion 2014;55:1116-27.

89. Hanson SR, Slichter SJ. Platelet kinetics in patients with bone marrow hypoplasia: Evidence for a fixed platelet requirement. Blood 1985;66:1105-9.

90. Hersh JK, Hom EG, Brecher ME. Mathematical modeling of platelet survival with implications for optimal transfusion practice in the chronically platelet transfusion-dependent patient. Transfusion 1998;38:637-44.

91. Slichter SJ, Kaufman RM, Assmann SF, et al. Dose of prophylactic platelet transfusions and prevention of hemorrhage. N Engl J Med 2010;362:600-13.

92. Estcourt LJ, Malouf R, Hopewell S, et al. Use of platelet transfusions prior to lumbar punctures or epidural anaesthesia for the prevention of complications in people with thrombocytopenia. Cochrane Database Syst Rev 2018;4:CD011980.

93. Estcourt LJ, Malouf R, Doree C, et al. Prophylactic platelet transfusions prior to surgery for people with a low platelet count. Cochrane Database Syst Rev 2018;9:CD012779.

94. Baharoglu MI, Cordonnier C, Salman RA, et al. Platelet transfusion versus standard of care after acute stroke due to spontaneous cerebral haemorrhage associated with antiplatelet therapy (PATCH): A randomized, open-label, phase 3 trial. Lancet 2016;387:2605-13.

95. Cooling L. ABO and platelet transfusion therapy. Immunohematology 2007;23:20-33.

96. Kelton JG, Hamid C, Aker S, Blajchman MA. The amount of blood group A substance on platelets is proportional to the amount in the plasma. Blood 1982;59:980-5.

97. Julmy F, Ammann RA, Taleghani BM, et al. Transfusion efficacy of ABO major-mismatched platelets (PLTs) in children is inferior to that of ABO-identical PLTs. Transfusion 2009;49:21-33.

98. Aster RH. Effect of anticoagulant and ABO incompatibility on recovery of transfused human platelets. Blood 1965;26:732-43.

99. Lee EJ, Schiffer CA. ABO compatibility can influence the results of platelet transfusion. Results of a randomized trial. Transfusion 1989;29:384-9.

100. Kaufman RM. Platelet ABO matters. Transfusion 2009;49:5-7.

101. Triulzi DJ, Assmann SF, Strauss RG, et al. The impact of platelet transfusion characteristics on posttransfusion platelet increments and clinical bleeding in patients with hypoproliferative thrombocytopenia. Blood 2012;119:5553-62.

102. Kaufman RM, Assmann SF, Triulzi DJ, et al. Transfusion-related adverse events in the Platelet Dose study. Transfusion 2015;55:144-53.

103. Heal J, Rowe J, McMican A, et al. The role of ABO matching in platelet transfusion. Eur J Haematol 1993;50:110-17.

104. Carr R, Hutton J, Jenkins J, et al. Transfusion of ABO-mismatched platelets leads to early platelet refractoriness. Br J Haematol 1990;75:408-13.

105. Dunstan RA, Simpson MB, Rosse WF. Erythrocyte antigens on human platelets: Absence of Rh, Duffy, Kell, Kidd, and Lutheran antigens. Transfusion 1984;24:243-6.

106. Molnar R, Johnson R, Geiger TL. Absence of D alloimmunization in D- pediatric oncology patients receiving D-incompatible single-donor platelets. Transfusion 2002;42:177-82.

107. Culibrk B, Stone E, Levin E, et al. Application of the ADVIA cerebrospinal fluid assay to count residual red blood cells in blood components. Vox Sang 2012;103:186-93.

108. Santana JM, Dumont LJ. A flow cytometric method for detection and enumeration of low-level, residual red blood cells in platelets and mononuclear cell products. Transfusion 2006; 46:966-72.

109. Cid J, Lozano M, Ziman A, et al. Low frequency of anti-D alloimmunization following D+ platelet transfusion: The Anti-D Alloimmunization after D-incompatible Platelet Transfusions (ADAPT) study. Br J Haematol 2015;168:598-603.

110. Doughty HA, Murphy MF, Metcalfe P, et al. Relative importance of immune and non-immune causes of platelet refractoriness. Vox Sang 1994; 66:200-5.

111. Hod E, Schwartz J. Platelet transfusion refractoriness. Br J Haematol 2008;142:348-60.

112. Aster RH. Pooling of platelets in the spleen: Role in the pathogenesis of "hypersplenic" thrombocytopenia. J Clin Invest 1966;45(5):645-57.

113. Slichter SJ. Leukocyte reduction and ultraviolet B irradiation of platelets to prevent alloimmunization and refractoriness to platelet transfusions. The Trial to Reduce Alloimmunization to Platelets Study Group. N Engl J Med 1997;337: 1861-9.

114. Yankee RA, Grumet FC, Rogentine GN. Platelet transfusion: The selection of compatible platelet donors for refractory patients by lymphocyte HL-A typing. N Engl J Med 1969;281:1208-12.

115. Slichter SJ. Factors affecting posttransfusion platelet increments, platelet refractoriness, and platelet transfusion intervals in thrombocytopenic patients. Blood 2005;105:4106-14.

116. Claas FH, Smeenk RJ, Schmidt R, et al. Alloimmunization against the MHC antigens after platelet transfusions is due to contaminating leukocytes in the platelet suspension. Exp Hematol 1981;9:84-9.

117. Triulzi DJ, Kleinman S, Kakaiya RM, et al. The effect of previous pregnancy and transfusion on HLA alloimmunization in blood donors: Implications for a transfusion-related acute lung injury risk reduction strategy. Transfusion 2009;49: 1825-35.

118. Pavenski K, Rebulla P, Duquesnoy R, et al. Efficacy of HLA-matched platelet transfusions for patients with hypoproliferative thrombocytopenia: A systematic review. Transfusion 2013;53: 2230-42.

119. Kopko PM, Warner P, Kresie L, Pancoska C. Methods for the selection of platelet products for alloimmune-refractory patients. Transfusion 2015;55:235-44.

120. Stanworth SJ, Navarrete C, Estcourt L, Marsh J. Platelet refractoriness - practical approaches and ongoing dilemmas in patient management. Br J Haematol 2015;171:297-305.

121. Moroff G, Garratty G, Heal JM, et al. Selection of platelets for refractory patients by HLA matching and prospective crossmatching. Transfusion 1992;32:633-40.

122. Rioux-Massé B, Cohn C, Lindgren B, et al. Utilization of cross-matched or HLA-matched platelets for patients refractory to platelet transfusion. Transfusion 2014;54:3080-7.

123. Escourt LJ, Malouf R, Hopewell S, et al. Pathogen-reduced platelets for the prevention of bleeding. Cochrane Database Syst Rev 2017; 30(7):CD009072.

124. Holland L, Sarode R. Should plasma be transfused prophylactically before invasive procedures? Curr Opin Hematol 2006;13:447-51.

125. Abdel-Wahab O, Healy B, Dzik W. Effect of fresh-frozen plasma transfusion on prothrombin time and bleeding in patients with mild coagulation abnormalities. Transfusion 2006;46:1279-85.

126. Karam O, Tucci M, Combescure C, et al. Plasma transfusion strategies for critically ill patients. Cochrane Database Syst Rev 2013;12: CD010654.

127. Murad MH, Stubbs JR, Gandhi MJ, et al. The effect of plasma transfusion on morbidity and mortality: A systematic review and meta-analysis. Transfusion 2010;50:1370-83.

128. Segal JB, Dzik WH. Paucity of studies to support that abnormal coagulation test results predict bleeding in the setting of invasive procedures: An evidence-based review. Transfusion 2005; 45:1413-25.

129. Yang L, Stanworth S, Hopewell S, et al. Is fresh-frozen plasma clinically effective? An update of

a systematic review of randomized controlled trials. Transfusion 2012;52:1673-86.

130. Jia Q, Brown MJ, Clifford L, et al. Prophylactic plasma transfusion for surgical patients with abnormal preoperative coagulation tests: A single-institution propensity-adjusted cohort study. Lancet Haematol 2016;3:e139-48.

131. Desborough M, Sandu R, Brunskill SJ, et al. Fresh frozen plasma for cardiovascular surgery. Cochrane Database Syst Rev 2015;7:CD007614.

132. Huber J, Stanworth SJ, Doree C, et al. Prophylactic plasma transfusion for patients undergoing non-cardiac surgery (protocol). Cochrane Database Syst Rev 2017;8:CD012745.

133. Shander A, Michelson EA, Sarani B, et al. Use of plasma in the management of central nervous system bleeding: Evidence-based consensus recommendations. Adv Ther 2014;31:66-90.

134. Stanworth SJ, Brunskill SJ, Hyde CJ, et al. Is fresh frozen plasma clinically effective? A systematic review of randomized controlled trials. Br J Haematol 2004;126:139-52.

135. Yang L, Stanworth S, Hopewell S, et al. Is fresh frozen plasma clinically effective? An update of a systematic review of randomized controlled trials. Transfusion 2012;52:1673-86.

136. O'Shaughnessy DF, Atterbury C, Bolton-Maggs P, et al. Guidelines for the use of fresh-frozen plasma, cryoprecipitate, and cryosupernatant. Br J Haematol 2004;126:11-28.

137. Presnell SR, Stafford DW. The vitamin K-dependent carboxylase. Thromb Haemost 2002; 87:937-46.

138. Jones GM, Erdman MJ, Smetana KS, et al. 3-Factor versus 4-factor prothrombin complex concentrate for warfarin reversal in severe bleeding: A multicenter, retrospective, propensity-matched pilot study. J Thromb Thrombolysis 2016;42:19-26.

139. Al-Majzoub O, Rybak E, Reardon DP, et al. Evaluation of warfarin reversal with 4-factor prothrombin complex concentrate compared to 3-factor prothrombin complex concentrate at a tertiary academic medical center. J Emerg Med 2016;50(1):7-13.

140. Sarode R, Milling TJ, Refaai MA, et al. Efficacy and safety of a four-factor prothrombin complex concentrate (4F-PCC) in patients on vitamin K antagonists presenting with major bleeding: A randomized, plasma-controlled, Phase IIIb study. Circulation 2013;128:1234-43.

141. Goldstein JN, Refaai MA, Milling TJ Jr, et al. Four-factor prothrombin complex concentrate

versus plasma for rapid vitamin K antagonist reversal in patients needing urgent surgical or invasive interventions: A phase 3b, open-label, non-inferiority, randomised trial. Lancet 2015; 385:2077-87.

142. Milling TJ Jr, Refaai MA, Sarode R, et al. Safety of a four-factor prothrombin complex concentrate versus plasma for vitamin K antagonist reversal: An integrated analysis of two Phase IIIb clinical trials. Acad Emerg Med 2016;23(4): 466-75.

143. Meehan R, Tavares M, Sweeney J. Clinical experience with oral versus intravenous vitamin K for warfarin reversal. Transfusion 2013;53:491-8.

144. Tornkvist M, Smith JG, Labaf A. Current evidence of oral anticoagulant reversal. Thromb Res 2018;162:22-31.

145. AABB, American Red Cross, America's Blood Centers, Armed Services Blood Program Office. Circular for the use of human blood and blood components. Bethesda, MD: AABB, 2017.

146. Gammon R, ed. Standards for blood banks and transfusion services. 32nd ed. Bethesda, MD: AABB, 2020.

147. Downes KA, Wilson E, Yomtovian R, Sarode R. Serial measurement of clotting factors in thawed plasma stored for 5 days. Transfusion 2001;41: 570.

148. Benjamin RJ, McLaughlin LS. Plasma components: Properties, differences, and uses. Transfusion 2012;52(Suppl 1):9S-19S.

149. Cushing MM, Asmis L, Calabia C, et al. Efficacy of solvent/detergent plasma after storage at 2-8 °C for 5 days in comparison to other plasma products to improve factor V levels in factor V deficient plasma. Transfus Apher Sci 2016; 55:114-19.

150. Levy JH, Goodnough LT. How I use fibrinogen replacement therapy in acquired bleeding. Blood 2015;125:1387-93.

151. Ahmed S, Harrity C, Johnson S, et al. The efficacy of fibrinogen concentrate compared with cryoprecipitate in major obstetric haemorrhage—an observational study. Transfus Med 2012;22:344-9.

152. Pavord S, Maybury H. How I treat postpartum hemorrhage. Blood 2015;125:2759-70.

153. Reger B, Peterfalvi A, Litter I, et al. Challenges in the evaluation of D-dimer and fibrinogen levels in pregnant women. Thromb Res 2013;131: e183-7.

154. Charbit B, Mandelbrot L, Samain E, et al. The decrease of fibrinogen is an early predictor

of the severity of postpartum hemorrhage. J Thromb Haemost 2007;5:266-73.

155. Cortet M, Deneux-Tharaux C, Dupont C, et al. Association between fibrinogen level and severity of postpartum haemorrhage: Secondary analysis of a prospective trial. Br J Anaesth 2012; 108:984-9.

156. Abdul-Kadir R, McLintock C, Ducloy A-S, et al. Evaluation and management of postpartum hemorrhage: Consensus from an international expert panel. Transfusion 2014;54:1756-68.

157. Wikkelso AJ, Edwards HM, Afshari A, et al. Preemptive treatment with fibrinogen concentrate for postpartum haemorrhage: Randomized controlled trial. Br J Anaesth 2015;114:623-33.

158. Jensen NH, Stensballe J, Afshari A. Comparing efficacy and safety of fibrinogen concentrate to cryoprecipitate in bleeding patients: A systematic review. Acta Anaesthesiol Scand 2016;60: 1033-42.

159. Besser MW, Klein AA. The coagulopathy of cardiopulmonary bypass. Crit Rev Clin Lab Sci 2010; 47:197-212.

160. Besser MW, Ortmann E, Klein AA. Haemostatic management of cardiac surgical haemorrhage. Anaesthesia 2014;70:87-95.

161. Woodman R, Harker LA. Bleeding complications associated with cardiopulmonary bypass. Blood 2003;76:1680-97.

162. Bennett-Guerrero E, Zhao Y, O'Brien SM, et al. Variation in use of blood transfusion in coronary artery bypass graft surgery. JAMA 2010;304: 1568-75.

163. Kindo M, Hoang Minh T, Gerelli S, et al. Plasma fibrinogen level on admission to the intensive care unit is a powerful predictor of postoperative bleeding after cardiac surgery with cardiopulmonary bypass. Thromb Res 2014;134:360-8.

164. Ranucci M, Baryshnikova E, Crapelli GB, et al. Randomized, double-blinded, placebo-controlled trial of fibrinogen concentrate supplementation after complex cardiac surgery. J Am Heart Assoc 2015;4:e002066.

165. Wikkelso A, Lunde J, Johansen M, et al. Fibrinogen concentrate in bleeding patients. Cochrane Database Syst Rev 2013;8:CD008864.

166. Maeda T, Miyata S, Usui A, et al. Safety of fibrinogen concentrate and cryoprecipitate in cardiovascular surgery: Multicenter database study. J Cardiothorac Vasc Anesth 2019;33:321-7.

167. Rahe-Meyer N, Levy JH, Mazer CD, et al. Randomized evaluation of fibrinogen vs placebo in complex cardiovascular surgery (REPLACE): A double-blind Phase III study of haemostatic therapy. Br J Anaesth 2016;117:41-51.

168. Strauss RG. Role of granulocyte/neutrophil transfusions for haematology/oncology patients in the modern era. Br J Haematol 2012;158: 299-306.

169. Hubel K, Rodger E, Gaviria JM, et al. Effective storage of granulocytes collected by centrifugation leukapheresis from donors stimulated with granulocyte-colony-stimulating factor. Transfusion 2005;45(12):1876-89.

170. Drewniak A, Boelens JJ, Vrielink H, et al. Granulocyte concentrates: Prolonged functional capacity during storage in the presence of phenotypic changes. Haematologica 2008;93(7): 1058-67.

171. Bryant BJ, Yau YY, Byrne PJ, et al. Gravity sedimentation of granulocytapheresis concentrates with hydroxyethyl starch efficiently removes red blood cells and retains neutrophils. Transfusion 2010;50:1203-9.

172. Narvios A, Pena E, Han X, Lichtiger B. Cytomegalovirus infection in cancer patients receiving granulocyte transfusions. Blood 2002;99: 390-1.

173. Nichols WG, Price T, Boeckh M. Cytomegalovirus infections in cancer patients receiving granulocyte transfusions (comment). Blood 2002; 99(9):3483-4.

174. Diaz R, Soundar E, Hartman SK, et al. Granulocyte transfusions for children with infections and neutropenia or granulocyte dysfunction. Pediatr Hematol Oncol 2014;31(5):425-34.

175. West K, Gea-Banacloche J, Stroncek D, Kadri SS. Granulocyte transfusions in the management of invasive fungal infections. Br J Haematol 2017;177:357-74.

176. Price TH, Boeckh M, Harrison RW, et al. Efficacy of transfusion with granulocytes from G-CSF/dexamethasone-treated donors in neutropenic patients with infection. Blood 2015; 126:2153-61.

177. Estcourt LJ, Stanworth S, Doree C, et al. Granulocyte transfusions for preventing infections in people with neutropenia or neutrophil dysfunction. Cochrane Database Syst Rev 2015;6: CD005341.

178. Cancelas JA. Granulocyte transfusion: Questions remain. Blood 2015;126:2082-3.

179. Marfin AA, Price TH. Granulocyte transfusion therapy. J Int Care Med 2015;30(2):79-88.

180. Moren AM, Hamptom D, Diggs B, et al. Recursive partitioning identifies greater than 4 U of packed red blood cells per hour as an improved

massive transfusion definition. J Trauma Acute Care Surg 2015;79:920-4.

181. Borgman M, Spinella P, Perkins J, et al. The ratio of blood products transfused affects mortality in patients receiving massive transfusions at a combat support hospital. J Trauma 2007;63: 805-13.

182. Acosta JA, Yang JC, Winchell RJ, et al. Lethal injuries and time to death in a level I trauma center. J Am Coll Surg 1998;186:528-33.

183. Stansbury LG, Dutton RP, Stein DM, et al. Controversy in trauma resuscitation: Do ratios of plasma to red blood cells matter? Transfus Med Rev 2009;23:255-65.

184. Callum JL, Nascimento B, Tien H, Rizoli S. "Formula-driven" versus "lab-driven" massive transfusion protocols: At a state of clinical equipoise (editorial). Transfus Med Rev 2009;23:247-54.

185. Holcomb JB, del Junco DJ, Fox EE, et al. The Prospective, Observational, Multicenter, Major Trauma Transfusion (PROMMTT) study. JAMA Surgery 2013;148:127-36.

186. Holcomb JB, Tilley BC, Baraniuk S, et al. Transfusion of plasma, platelets, and red blood cells in a 1:1:1 vs a 1:1:2 ratio and mortality in patients with severe trauma: The PROPPR randomized clinical trial. JAMA 2015;313:471-82.

187. Dzik WS, Ziman A, Cohen C, et al. Survival after ultramassive transfusion: A review of 1360 cases. Transfusion 2016;56:558-63.

188. Johnson DJ, Scott AV, Barodka VM, et al. Morbidity and mortality after high-dose transfusion. Anesthesiology 2016;124:387-95.

189. Dunbar NM, Yazer MH. A possible new paradigm? A survey-based assessment of the use of thawed group A plasma for trauma resuscitation in the United States. Transfusion 2016;56:125-9.

190. Chhibber V, Greene M, Vauthrin M, et al. Is group A thawed plasma suitable as the first option for emergency release transfusion? Transfusion 2014;54:1751-5.

191. Dunbar NM and Yazer MH. Safety of the use of group A plasma in trauma: The STAT study. Transfusion 2017;57:1879-84.

192. Sperry JL, Guyette FX, Brown JB, et al; PAMPer Study Group. Prehospital plasma during air medical transport in trauma patients at risk for hemorrhagic shock. N Engl J Med 2018; 379(4):315-26.

193. Moore HB, Moore EE, Chapman MP, et al. Plasma-first resuscitation to treat haemorrhagic shock during emergency ground transportation in an urban area: A randomised trial. Lancet 2018;392(10144):283-91.

194. Stubbs JR, Tran SA, Emery RL, et al. Cold platelets for trauma-associated bleeding: Regulatory approval, accreditation approval, and practice implementation – just the "tip of the iceberg." Transfusion 2017;57:2836-44.

195. Seheult JN, Bahr M, Anto V, et al. Safety profile of uncrossmatched, cold-stored, low-titer, group O+ whole blood in civilian trauma patients. Transfusion 2018;58(10):2280-8.

196. Seheult JN, Anto V, Alarcon AH, et al. Clinical outcomes among low-titer group O whole blood recipients compared to recipients of conventional components in civilian trauma resuscitation. Transfusion 2018;58:1838-45.

197. Yazer MH, Cap AP, Spinella PC, et al. How do I implement a whole blood program for massively bleeding patients? Transfusion 2018;58:622-8.

CHAPTER 20
Patient Blood Management

Steven M. Frank, MD, and Nicole R. Guinn, MD

BLOOD TRANSFUSIONS CAN BE LIFE-saving but are also associated with risks and complications.[1] Growing attention by professional associations and health-care organizations to the wide variation in transfusion practice[2] and overuse of blood[3] has intensified the need for more appropriate utilization. Furthermore, efforts to lower health-care costs and improve quality of care and patient safety have led to increased focus on reducing unnecessary transfusions.

Accordingly, many institutions have implemented patient blood management (PBM) strategies and related activities. The 2017 National Blood Collection and Utilization Survey[4] reported that more than one-third of hospitals had a PBM program and that even more facilities had implemented one or more interventions to improve care and reduce unnecessary transfusions. These initiatives have resulted in a steady decline in blood and blood component transfusions in the United States.[5]

DEFINITION AND SCOPE OF PATIENT BLOOD MANAGEMENT

PBM is an evidence-based, multidisciplinary approach to optimizing the care of patients who might need a transfusion. Although evidence-based transfusion guidelines are fundamental, PBM goes beyond appropriate blood component utilization. It encompasses the entire course of care, from before the patient enters the hospital to after treatment is completed. The primary aim of PBM is to improve patient safety and clinical outcomes by appropriately managing the patient's own blood. PBM entails a proactive approach in which clinicians strive to reduce or avoid unnecessary transfusions by using evidence-based pharmacologic, medical, and surgical modalities to manage anemia, optimize hemostasis, and minimize blood loss in a patient-specific manner. In addition, when a transfusion is the only appropriate intervention, PBM requires that transfusion decisions be based on best practices and that the amount given be the appropriate amount to improve patient outcome.

Although the term "patient blood management" may be fairly new, the concepts have developed over time in parallel with medical advances. A full discussion of the history is beyond the scope of this chapter. However, three examples illustrate the shared drivers of blood transfusion and PBM. One example is the influence of wartime injuries. The discoveries of blood groups, crossmatching, and blood storage in the early years of the 20th century enabled the use of banked blood to treat exsanguinating wounds suffered in armed conflicts. Yet, transporting blood was difficult, and battlefield surgeons de-

---

Steven M. Frank, MD, Professor, Department of Anesthesiology/Critical Care Medicine, Medical Director, Johns Hopkins Health Systems Blood Management Program, and Faculty, Armstrong Institute for Patient Safety and Quality, The Johns Hopkins Medical Institutions, Baltimore, Maryland; and Nicole R. Guinn, MD, Associate Professor, Department of Anesthesiology, and Medical Director, Center for Blood Conservation, Duke University Medical Center, Durham, North Carolina

S. Frank has disclosed a financial relationship with Haemonetics, Medtronic, and Baxter International. N. Guinn has disclosed no conflicts of interest.

20

veloped techniques to treat casualties when no transfusion was possible. A second example is the influence of Jehovah's Witnesses, who cite biblical passages as the foundation for not accepting blood transfusions. By the middle of the 20th century, when blood transfusion had become universally accepted as a medical treatment for a wide range of indications, Jehovah's Witness patients had to seek out those few physicians and hospitals that would provide medical and surgical care without transfusions. These surgeons and hospitals became increasingly used by Jehovah's Witnesses and others who wished to avoid transfusions, and blood conservation programs began to flourish. Third, the high risk of viral transmission for human immunodeficiency virus (HIV) and hepatitis B and C peaked in the early 1980s, along with an increasing awareness of, and concern about, transfusion-transmitted infectious disease. With an emphasis on an individualized, patient-centric approach, these issues led the way toward the PBM movement seen today.

Although the focus is frequently on surgical patients, PBM encompasses the entire scope of any patient's hospital experience. It includes:

1. Efforts to identify and manage anemia and bleeding risks before any treatment begins.
2. Use of blood-sparing surgical techniques and intraoperative blood recovery methods.
3. Adjunctive strategies during intensive care unit (ICU) stays and postoperative care that decrease the need for transfusion.
4. Blood utilization review for transfusion guideline compliance and feedback to ordering physicians.
5. PBM education for all health-care providers involved in patient care.

RESOURCES TO SUPPORT A PBM PROGRAM

One of the most appealing concepts of PBM is that it can reduce risk, improve outcomes, and save money, all at the same time. Furthermore, by improving quality and reducing costs, PBM increases the value of health care delivered. De-

pending on the baseline degree of transfusion overuse, a successful PBM program can often pay for itself several times over by reducing transfusion-related costs.[6-9] Given that the bundled payment system makes reimbursement for blood poor to nonexistent in the United States, and that the overhead costs of transfusion are approximately three- to fourfold the blood acquisition costs,[10] a solid PBM program will easily be self-supporting.

The first step toward developing a successful program is to generate a business plan that sets financial goals and engages the hospital's administration to gain financial support. The program's leaders will need salary support to buy time to get the work done. Personnel cannot develop a successful program on nights and weekends, or in their spare time. Depending on the size of the hospital, some portion of time should be supported for a medical director (physician), a full-time nurse coordinator or transfusion safety officer, administrative support, and a data manager. For smaller hospitals, it is entirely possible that 5% of blood acquisition costs will be needed to support the personnel to operate the program. For larger hospitals or health systems, perhaps 2% to 3% of the annual blood acquisition budget will be needed to support the program. To justify this expense, one must consider the potential return on investment from the reduction in blood acquisition cost, which has been reported to be as much as 400%—indicating five dollars saved for every one dollar spent.[9] Not to be ignored are the substantial time and effort required from the information technology team to collect and analyze data on compliance with transfusion guidelines, format dashboards, and report results. Such activities are critical to improving performance. Of course, electronic records help in the data collection process, but skilled programmers are often in high demand, and these individuals are essential to the success of the PBM efforts. Without dedicated support, the programmers will likely not put PBM high on their priority list.

The best PBM programs have representation from many departments within the hospital and thus are truly multidisciplinary. For example, members should be included from hospital administration, nursing, hospitalists, surgical services, quality and safety, the blood bank, information technology, hematology, critical care, anesthesiology, pharmacy, and finance. Presentation of the business plan to the top administrators is helpful to gain financial support and buy-in from leadership.

Support for PBM often falls into the category of safety and quality efforts. If the institution has a safety and quality institute or division, one can make the case that, given the risks and expenses of transfusion and the potential return on investment in reduced blood-acquisition costs, PBM is an important effort to support. If one considers the medical, legal, and financial implications of giving the wrong unit to a patient and the associated risks of a life-threatening hemolytic reaction, the initiative is even more likely to attract support from the safety and quality division. PBM can also fall into the category of "supply chain management," which is designed to optimize and reduce spending on equipment and supplies—in this case the blood-acquisition cost and other activities related to transfusion.

PATIENT BLOOD MANAGEMENT STANDARDS AND CERTIFICATION

The AABB *Standards for a Patient Blood Management Program (PBM Standards)* was created and is updated by a consensus panel of experts in the field.[11] The *PBM Standards* forms the basis for a PBM certification process for hospitals that is jointly offered by AABB and The Joint Commission. Certification is provided on three levels, according to the extent of PBM-related activity at a facility. As indicated in Table 20-1, level 3 status is achieved when the top 17 requirements are met; level 2 with the top 20; and level 1 with all 24. To receive level 1 certification, hospitals must have the capacity to perform autologous blood recovery (use of a cell-saver device); have a formal program to render quality care to those patients who will not accept transfusion (also called a bloodless program); and use methods to identify and manage preoperative anemia in both medical and surgical patients. Other standards have been released by other societies, such as the Society for Ad-

vancement of Blood Management (SABM).[12] These standards include similar requirements to operate a high-quality PBM program.

METHODS OF PATIENT BLOOD MANAGEMENT

Education

The general methods used to implement and sustain a strong PBM program are outlined in Table 20-2. It is intuitive that education is perhaps the most important component of any quality improvement effort. Even educated clinicians are unlikely to be familiar with each of the nine large randomized trials that have been published, most in the past decade,[13-21] all in support of a restrictive (Red Blood Cell) RBC transfusion strategy. Each of these studies supports a hemoglobin threshold lower than those traditionally used (Table 20-3). In fact, it is likely that more high-profile, prospective clinical trials have been conducted on hemoglobin transfusion thresholds than on almost any other practice in medicine. All nine of these studies were published in high-impact journals. Each of the trials supports a threshold of 7 g/dL, even for critically ill patients,[15-18,20] or 7.5 to 8 g/dL for those with cardiovascular disease.[13,14,19,21] When these restrictive thresholds were compared to the liberal thresholds of 9 to 10 g/dL, the clinical outcomes (including both primary and secondary outcomes) were the same in five of the studies,[13,14,16,19,20] meaning that the extra blood was not helpful. In the other four studies, outcomes were worse with liberal thresholds (either overall or in some subgroups),[15,17,18,21] meaning that the extra blood was actually harmful. Through simple educational efforts, clinicians can be made aware of these landmark studies. As a result, blood utilization will be reduced and patient outcomes improved with restrictive thresholds.

It should be noted that the randomized trials emphasize the hemoglobin "threshold," which is the level before transfusion, rather than the hemoglobin "target," a term that has been used to refer to the level achieved after the transfusion.[26] In Table 20-3, it is clear that in these

TABLE 20-1.   PBM Program Levels*[11]

Item	Responsibility	Activity Level 1	Activity Level 2	Activity Level 3
1	Evidence of institutional support for the patient blood management program at the hospital administration level.	X	X	X
2	Metrics regarding transfusion appropriateness in accordance with transfusion guidelines.	X	X	X
3	Documentation of transfusion including patient consent, observation, adverse events and outcomes.	X	X	X
4	Budgeting to the level of care required by the implementation of the AABB *Standards for a Patient Blood Management Program*	X	X	X
5	Pretransfusion patient testing and evaluation.	X	X	X
6	Patient- or case-specific assessment of potential blood usage.	X	X	X
7	Preprocedural blood ordering including completion of type and antibody testing before procedure start time with a plan for antibody-positive patients.	X	X	X
8	Preprocedure optimization of patient coagulation function.	X	X	X
9	Monitoring of blood components wastage and cause.	X	X	X
10	Minimize blood loss due to laboratory testing.	X	X	X
11	Process for managing the blood needs of unidentified patients and resolving their identification.	X	X	X
12	Processes to identify, prior to or upon admission, patients who may decline transfusion under any circumstances with notification to the appropriate individuals.	X	X	X
13	Massive transfusion protocol use and compliance.	X	X	X
14	Transfusion care and anemia management of pre-term, neonate, infant, and pediatric critical care patients, if applicable.	X	X	X
15	PBM for obstetric patients including postpartum hemorrhage protocol with evidence of its use, plan(s) for patients with known high bleeding risk (eg, placental abnormalities), and plans for patients where blood is not an option.	X	X	X
16	Single-unit transfusion strategies for defined patient population(s).	X	X	X
17	Manage acquired coagulopathy.	X	X	X
18	Blood conservation strategies for high blood usage service lines.	X	X	N/A
19	Processes and/or equipment to facilitate rapid decision making with regard to anemia and coagulation management.	X	X	N/A

TABLE 20-1.   PBM Program Levels*[11] (Continued)

Item	Responsibility	Activity Level 1	Activity Level 2	Activity Level 3
20	Evaluating and managing iron and micronutrient deficiencies in defined patients with Red Blood Cells ordered in the outpatient setting.	X	X	N/A
21	Evaluation and management of anemia in nonoperative patients.	X	N/A	N/A
22	Program to care for patients who decline use of blood or blood-derived products.	X	N/A	N/A
23	Identification and management of presurgical anemia before elective procedures for which type and screen or type and crossmatch is recommended.	X	N/A	N/A
24	Use of perioperative techniques consistent with current AABB *Standards for Perioperative Autologous Blood Collection and Administration.*	X	N/A	N/A

*A patient blood management program can be designated as a program activity level 1, 2, or 3 program. To be designated a specific activity level, the program shall be responsible for or have direct involvement with oversight and monitoring of the activities listed above. [Used with permission from **AABB** *Standards for a Patient Blood Management Program.*[11(pp3-5)]]

RBCs = Red Blood Cells.

trials, the target is about 1 g/dL higher than the threshold, and this difference should be considered when defining evidence-based transfusion practice. The actual dose of blood is the primary determinant of the target; thus, a popular PBM campaign called "Why give 2 when 1 will do?" was created to encourage single-unit RBC transfusions in nonbleeding, hemodynamically stable patients. In fact, eight of the nine clinical trials mentioned above specifically called for the use of single-unit RBC transfusions, followed by reassessment, before administration of additional units. The Choosing Wisely campaign, designed to reduce unnecessary tests and procedures, includes six different societies that have aims to reduce unnecessary transfusions. AABB, for example, emphasizes the evidence-based hemoglobin threshold of 7 to 8 g/dL and the importance of giving single-unit RBC transfusions in its Choosing Wisely aims.[27]

The various venues for education are many. A well-delivered lecture showing evidence from the randomized trials is probably the most effective method of education. Online tutorials, newsletters, and e-mails can be easily ignored or deleted and therefore are likely to be less effective than an in-person lecture. With regard to blood components other than RBCs, the evidence is less complete. For plasma, platelets, and cryoprecipitate, the primary outcome of concern is bleeding, which is difficult to measure and thus difficult to study. However, guidelines do exist for plasma[28] and platelets[29] that promote what evidence base there is, in terms of reducing unnecessary transfusions. But many of these recommendations are based on evidence rated as weak or very weak because adequate randomized trials on indications for these components are lacking.

The Johns Hopkins Health System has created an electronic tutorial to educate clinical providers on blood management principles. The tutorial covers everything from the definitions for type and screen and crossmatch and who needs them preoperatively, to the hospital guidelines for transfusion thresholds for RBCs, plasma, and platelets. It also covers transfusion reactions, how to properly label specimens for blood

TABLE 20-2. Methods for Implementing a Patient Blood Management Program*

1. Obtain support from health system leadership (business plan).
2. Assemble a multidisciplinary team of stakeholders.
3. Educate (with emphasis on the nine RCTs supporting restrictive transfusion).[13-21]
4. Harmonize transfusion guidelines.
5. Add decision support for computerized provider order entry (with best practice advisories).
6. Implement data acquisition/analytics.
7. Create dashboards.[22]
8. Provide transfusion guideline compliance audits with feedback (reports) to providers.
9. Implement methods to improve blood utilization:
• Evidence-based transfusion thresholds.
• "Why give 2 when 1 will do" Choosing Wisely campaign for RBCs.[23]
• Preoperative anemia management.[24]
• Antifibrinolytics (eg, aminocaproic acid, tranexamic acid).
• Intraoperative autologous blood recovery (Cell Saver[†] instrument).
• Anesthetic management (autologous normovolemic hemodilution, controlled hypotension, normothermia).
• Surgical methods (newer cautery methods, topical hemostatics, and sealants).
• Reduction of phlebotomy blood loss (smaller tubes, eliminate unnecessary testing).
• Point-of-care testing (eg, thromboelastography).

*Modified from Frank et al.[9]
†Haemonetics Corp.
RCT = randomized controlled trial; RBCs = Red Blood Cells.

preparation orders, and a short review of the ABO and Rh blood groups. It introduces the maximum surgical blood order schedule (MSBOS),[30] identifies where this list of surgical procedures can be found, and explains how it is used to determine appropriate preoperative blood orders.

Qualification/Competence

An area of debate is the use of qualifications or credentials to grant hospital privileges to individual providers for administering blood to patients. It has been said that historically, all one needed was a pen and paper, or now a computer and keyboard, to order blood for a patient, with little or no specific training. Some hospitals have required that new staff be trained in PBM, as de-

scribed above, before being granted generalized privileges to practice. Extremely few hospitals, however, have specific privileges for ordering a transfusion. Instead of stipulating specific credentials for transfusion, the *PBM Standards*[11] states that "individuals who order and/or transfuse blood shall meet facility defined requirements for education related to patient blood management."[11(p8)] This statement implies that hospitals should have some requisite education for providers who order transfusions.

Preoperative Strategies

Although PBM methods apply to both medical and surgical patients, for the latter they can be categorized according to their relevance in the

TABLE 20-3. Large Prospective Randomized Trials on RBC Transfusion Thresholds

Clinical Trial	Patient Population	Restrictive Strategy (Hb "trigger" to target), g/dL	Liberal Strategy (Hb "trigger" to target), g/dL	Reduction in Blood Utilization (with restrictive strategy)	Primary Outcomes			
					Event	Restrictive (incidence)	Liberal (incidence)	p Value
Hébert et al, 1999[15] (n = 838)	Critically ill (adults)	7 to 8.5	10 to 10.7	54% fewer RBC units transfused	30-day mortality	18.7%	23.3%	0.11
Hajjar et al, 2010[14] (n = 502)	Cardiac sur-gery (adults)	8 to 9.1	10 to 10.5	58% fewer RBC units transfused	Composite end-point	11%	10%	0.85
					• 30-day mortality	6%	5%	0.93
					• Cardiogenic shock	9%	6%	0.42
					• ARDS	2%	1%	0.99
					• Acute renal injury requiring dialysis	4%	5%	0.99
Carson et al, 2011[13] (n = 2016)	Femur fracture (elderly adults)	8.0 to 9.5	10.0 to 11.0	65% fewer RBC units transfused	Composite end-point	34.7%	35.2%	NS
					• 60-day mortality	28.1%	27.6%	NS
					• 60-day inability to walk	6.6%	7.6%	NS
Villanueva et al, 2013[18] (n = 921)	Gastrointesti-nal bleeding (adults)	7 to 9.2	9 to 10.1	59% fewer RBC units transfused	45-day all-cause mortality	5%	9%	0.02
Holst et al, 2014[20] (n = 998)	Septic shock (adults)	7 to 7.5	9 to 9.5	50% fewer RBC units transfused	90-day all-cause mortality	43.0%	45.0%	0.44

(Continued)

TABLE 20-3. Large Prospective Randomized Trials on RBC Transfusion Thresholds (Continued)

Clinical Trial	Patient Population	Restrictive Strategy (Hb "trigger" to target), g/dL	Liberal Strategy (Hb "trigger" to target), g/dL	Reduction in Blood Utilization (with restrictive strategy)	Primary Outcomes			
					Event	Restrictive (incidence)	Liberal (incidence)	p Value
Robertson et al, 2014[17] (n = 200)	Traumatic brain injury (adults)	7 to 9.7	9.5 to 11.4	74% fewer RBC units transfused	Glasgow outcome scale score (favorable)	42.5%	33%	0.28
Lacroix et al, 2007[16] (n = 637)	Critically ill (pediatric)	7 to 8.7	9.5 to 10.8	44% fewer RBC units transfused	Multiple organ dysfunction score	12%	12%	NS
Murphy et al, 2015[19] (n = 2007)	Cardiac surgery (adults)	7.5 to 9	9.0 to 10	40% fewer RBC units transfused	Serious infection or ischemic event at 90 days	35.1%	33.0%	0.30
Mazer et al, 2017[21] (n = 5243)	Cardiac surgery (adults)	7.5 to 9	9.5 to 10	33% fewer RBC units transfused	Death, MI, stroke, or renal failure w/ dialysis by day 28	11.4%	12.5%	NS

*Modified from Sadana et al.[25]

RBC = Red Blood Cell; Hb = hemoglobin; ARDS = acute respiratory distress syndrome; NS = not significant; MI = myocardial infarction.

pre-, intra-, and postoperative periods, as outlined in the sections below.

Preoperative Anemia Diagnosis and Treatment

One important and especially challenging area in PBM is the timely diagnosis and treatment of preoperative anemia. Treatment is especially important for patients who are undergoing elective surgery, as bringing such patients to the operating room with untreated anemia represents suboptimal care.[31-33] Anemia has been shown to be an independent predictor of increased perioperative morbidity and mortality[34] and should be considered a modifiable risk factor. Thus, elective surgery should be delayed when possible to allow for diagnosis and adequate treatment. Some centers have set up preoperative anemia clinics that are designed to optimize the condition of patients before surgery. Their goal is to improve outcomes and reduce overall costs.[24]

First, it is important to determine the cause of anemia. Simple iron deficiency can be treated with either oral or intravenous iron. Patient compliance with oral iron is low because of significant gastrointestinal side effects. Moreover, oral iron is both poorly and slowly absorbed. Therefore, many experts in the field advocate for intravenous iron therapy to allow for more rapid resolution of anemia.[35,36] The newer compounds can be administered in one or two high doses for complete iron repletion.[37,38] They also have a lower incidence of adverse events than the older iron compounds such as high-molecular-weight iron dextran. The specific formulation and dose should be determined by the patient's total iron deficit, institutional formulary, and also cost and coverage by insurance plans. For specific patients, erythropoiesis-stimulating agents (ESAs) may be indicated for treating preoperative anemia. Two concerns regarding the use of ESAs are difficulty with reimbursement and the Food and Drug Administration (FDA) "black box" warning about thrombotic events and promotion of tumor growth.[39,40] Use of pharmacologic therapy such as low-molecular-weight heparin for venous thrombosis prophylaxis may decrease the risk of thrombosis in postoperative patients, but ESAs should be used with caution in patients who have a history of thrombosis, ischemic stroke, uncontrolled hypertension, seizures, or cancer.[41] Hence, the risk/benefit ratio must be carefully considered when prescribing ESAs. Additionally, because ESAs cause functional iron deficiency, administration of concomitant iron therapy will help minimize the lowest effective total dose of ESAs needed to see an adequate response.[42]

One of the most challenging aspects of diagnosing and treating preoperative anemia is having enough time before surgery to achieve the goals. Often, preoperative laboratory tests are ordered 3 days before the surgery date, leaving little or no time to correct anemia. Of course, for semi-urgent surgeries, the options are limited, but for truly elective cases, the preoperative tests should be performed 4 or more weeks before the surgery date, giving adequate time for proper diagnosis and treatment of anemia.[31] Additionally, when appropriate, providers should rule out other medical causes of anemia, such as a gastrointestinal malignancy, when iron deficiency anemia is detected. Most patients will respond well to intravenous iron within 3 to 4 weeks, but they will respond even more dramatically and rapidly when ESAs are given along with the iron.[43]

Maximum Surgical Blood Order Schedule

One of the key components of a strong PBM program is a data-driven protocol for determining which patients need preoperative blood orders. The concept of the MSBOS was first developed in the mid-1970s to prevent the overordering of blood before surgery—hence, the term "maximum" surgical blood order schedule.[44] The main concern is that many institutions have an outdated MSBOS that is based on consensus opinions rather than on actual blood utilization data for specific surgical procedures. Now, with the popularity of electronic anesthesia records, actual institution-specific transfusion data can be used to generate a more accurate list of recommended preoperative blood orders. Using an algorithm that includes three variables—the percentage of patients who received transfusion, the median estimated blood loss, and the average number of units transfused per patient—

methods have been described for creating an institution-specific MSBOS derived from electronic data.[30] The actual document for that MSBOS, created as a guide for preoperative blood orders, includes 135 types of surgical procedures and the associated recommended blood order for each (Fig 20-1). Of course, these recommendations can be modified—for example, in patients with preoperative anemia or in those with red cell antibodies for whom compatible units may be difficult to find.

It has been shown that a data-driven MSBOS not only improves the blood ordering process but can also decrease costs by reducing unnecessary blood orders ($150,000-$300,000/year).[7] The crossmatch-to-transfusion ratio, a classic measure of blood-ordering efficiency, can be improved (decreased) by using an accurate MSBOS.[7] For those procedures in which blood is rarely or never transfused, the authors specify that no preoperative blood orders are needed. In the case of unexpected bleeding, the backup plan is emergency-release, uncrossmatched blood, which is much safer than many clinicians believe.[45]

Having an up-to-date MSBOS has other benefits as well. First, blood units will not be set aside unnecessarily for cases that have a low likelihood of transfusion. Overordering of preoperative crossmatches and setting aside RBC units leads to potential outdating and wastage. On the other extreme, patients who truly need blood prepared are more likely to have blood units ready when they are needed. When cases are identified that clearly should have blood ready to transfuse, the process of type and screen or type and crossmatch is best completed before the day of surgery, thereby decreasing the risk that surgery will begin before the blood is ready. The Joint Commission has recognized this particular problem as a potential performance measure,[46] and use of an MSBOS helps to reduce the problem by specifying which patients need blood prepared ahead of time. Many centers now use the 30-day time limit for expiration of the type and screen or crossmatch, as long as the patient has not been pregnant or received transfusion within the last 90 days.

Optimizing Coagulation

An important way to reduce blood loss and unnecessary transfusions is to optimize coagulation before surgery. For example, P2Y12 inhibitors such as clopidogrel should be discontinued, if possible, in time for their effect to subside before elective surgery. Often, a cardiac surgery patient needs 2 to 5 days off the medication for coagulation to normalize. Tests such as the Verify Now assay (Instrumentation Laboratories)[47] can detect residual P2Y12 inhibition, enabling the provider to determine the optimal time for surgery. Because the return to normal coagulation has significant variability when these drugs are discontinued, the test is important. Additionally, several over-the-counter herbal supplements, such as garlic, ginseng, and ginkgo, have been shown to affect coagulation and should be discontinued before elective surgery.[48]

Preoperative Autologous Blood Donation

Historically, preoperative autologous blood donation (PAD) was used in an attempt to avoid allogeneic blood. However, over the last decade, there has been a significant downward trend in the number of autologous units collected in the United States. In 2017, only 10,000 units were collected, representing approximately 0.08% of the total allogeneic RBC/whole blood collection and 62% fewer units than were collected in 2015.[4,49] Major factors contributing to this decline include the increased safety of and public confidence in the blood supply, adoption of intraoperative blood-conserving techniques, high wastage of PAD blood (>45% discarded), and a higher risk for preoperative anemia after donation.[49,50] Studies showed that although patients participating in a PAD program had lower exposure to allogeneic transfusions than did patients who did not participate, they had a higher likelihood of receiving any transfusion (allogeneic and/or autologous) as a result of donation-induced anemia.[49,51] Errors related to production and handling, delays in receipt of the units at the designated hospital, and increasing acquisition costs also added to the decrease in PAD.[52] The patient also may accrue additional cost in the form of lost wages if work time is required for the donation.

SURGICAL BLOOD ORDER SCHEDULE

Cardiac Surgery

Case Category	Rec
Heart or lung transplant	T/C 4U
Minimally invasive valve	T/C 4U
Revision sternotomy	T/C 4U
CABG/valve	T/C 4U
Valve	T/C 2U
Assist device	T/C 4U
Cardiac/major vascular	T/C 4U
Open ventricle	T/C 4U
CABG	T/C 2U
Cardiac wound surgery	T/C 2U
Percutaneous cardiac	T/C 2U
Pericardium	T/C 2U
Lead extraction	T/C 4U
AICD/pacemaker placement	T/S

General Surgery

Case Category	Rec
AP resection	T/C 2U
Intra-abdominal GI	T/C 2U
Whipple or pancreatic	T/C 2U
Liver resection	T/C 2U
Retroperitoneal	T/C 2U
Substernal	T/C 2U
Liver resection minor	T/S
Bone marrow harvest	T/S
Hernia – Ventral/Incisional	T/S
Hernia – Inguinal/Umbilical	No Sample
Appendectomy	No Sample
Abdomen/chest/soft tissue	No Sample
Lap. or open cholecystectomy	No Sample
Thyroid/parathyroid	No Sample
Central venous access	No Sample
Any Breast – except w/flaps	No Sample

Gynecological Surgery

Case Category	Rec
Uterus open (radical)	T/C 2U
Open pelvic	T/C 2U
Uterus/ovary open	T/S
Total vaginal hysterectomy	T/S
Hysterectomy robot/lap	T/S
Cystectomy robotic assisted	T/S
Cystoscopy	No Sample
External genitalia	No Sample
GYN cervix	No Sample
Hysteroscopy	No Sample
Superficial wound	No Sample

Neurosurgery

Case Category	Rec
Thoracic/Lumbar/Sacral fusion	T/C 4U
Spine tumor	T/C 2U
Posterior cervical spine fusion	T/C 2U
Spine Incision and Drainage	T/C 2U
Intracranial tumor / aneurysm	T/C 2U
Laminectomy/discectomy	T/S
Spine hardware removal/biopsy	T/S
ACDF	T/S
Extracranial	No Sample
Nerve procedure	No Sample
CSF/shunt procedure	No Sample

Updated Sept. 2018

Obstetrics

Case Category	Rec
Complex Cesarean (Accreta, Percreta, Previa, etc.)	T/C 4U
Repeat Cesarean	T/C 2U
Routine Primary Cesarean	T/S
Vaginal Delivery	T/S
D&C/D&E/Genetic Termination	T/S
Tubal Ligation	No Sample
Cerlage	No Sample

Orthopedic Surgery

Case Category	Rec
Thoracic/Lumbar/Sacral fusion	T/C 4U
Pelvic orthopedic	T/C 4U
Open hip	T/C 2U
Femur open (fracture)	T/C 2U
Above/below knee amputation	T/C 2U
Total hip arthroplasty	T/C 2U
Humerus open	T/S
Fasciotomy	T/S
Shoulder Incision & Drainage	T/S
Tibial/fibular	T/S
Total knee replacement	T/S
Shoulder open	T/S
Knee open	T/S
Thigh soft tissue	No Sample
Ortho external fixation	No Sample
Peripheral nerve/tendon	No Sample
Lower extremity I&D	No Sample
Hand orthopedic	No Sample
Upper extremity arthroscopy	No Sample
Upper extremity open	No Sample
Podiatry/Foot	No Sample
Hip closed/percutaneous	No Sample
Lower extremity arthroscopic	No Sample
Shoulder closed	No Sample
Tibial/fibular closed	No Sample

Otolaryngology Surgery

Case Category	Rec
Laryngectomy	T/C 2U
Facial reconstruction	T/C 2U
Cranial surgery	T/C 2U
Radical neck dissection	T/S
Carotid body tumor	T/C 2U
Mandibular surgery	T/S
Neck dissection	T/S
Mastoidectomy	No Sample
Parotidectomy	No Sample
Facial plastic	No Sample
Oral surgery	No Sample
Sinus surgery	No Sample
Thyroid/parathyroidectomy	No Sample
Suspension laryngoscopy	No Sample
Bronchoscopy	No Sample
Cochlear implant	No Sample
EGD	No Sample
External ear	No Sample
Inner ear	No Sample
Tonsillectomy/adenoidectomy	No Sample
Tympanomastoid	No Sample

Thoracic Surgery

Case Category	Rec
Esophageal open	T/C 2U
Sternal procedure	T/C 2U
Chest wall	T/C 2U
Thoracotomy	T/C 2U
Pectus repair	T/C 2U
VATS	T/S
Mediastinoscopy	T/S
EGD/FOB	No Sample
Central venous access	No Sample

Urology

Case Category	Rec
Cystoprostatectomy	T/C 2U
Urology open	T/C 2U
Nephrectomy open	T/C 2U
Lap/Robotic kidney/adrenal	T/S
RRP	T/S
Percutaneous nephrolithotomy	T/S
Robotic RRP	No Sample
External genitalia/Penile	No Sample
TURP	No Sample
Cysto/ureter/urethra	No Sample
TURBT	No Sample

Vascular/Transplant Surgery

Case Category	Rec
Liver transplant	T/C 6U
Thoracoabdominal aortic	T/C 12U
Major liver resection	T/C 4U
Major vascular	T/C 4U
Exploratory lap. vascular	T/C 4U
Kidney pancreas transplant	T/C 2U
Major endovascular	T/C 2U
Above/below knee amputation	T/S
Nephrectomy/kidney transplant	T/C 2U
Organ procurement	T/C 2U
Peripheral vascular	T/C 2U
Vascular wound I and D	T/C 2U
Carotid vascular	T/S
AV fistula	T/S
Peripheral endovascular	T/S
Angio/Arteriogram	No Sample
Peripheral wound I&D	No Sample
1st rib resection/thoracic outlet	No Sample
Superficial or skin	No Sample
Foot/toe amputation/debride	No Sample
Central venous access	No Sample

If the procedure you are looking for is not on this list, then choose the procedure that most closely resembles that procedure.

*Emergency Release blood is available for ALL cases and carries a risk of minor transfusion reaction of 1 in 1,000 cases.

FIGURE 20-1. An institution-specific maximum surgical blood order schedule (MSBOS) derived by collecting blood utilization data from an anesthesia information management system.[30] This list specifies recommended preoperative blood orders for different types of surgical procedures. (Modified from Frank et al.[30])
T/C = type and crossmatch; T/S = type and screen; U = unit.

Despite these concerns about efficacy, PAD can be a reasonable option for patients with rare blood types or multiple red cell alloantibodies. In these situations, advance planning and patient evaluation are crucial before PAD is attempted. To mitigate the anemia induced by PAD and to avoid allogeneic transfusions, efforts should focus on 1) timing of collections to allow 3 to 4 weeks between the last donation and planned surgery, 2) collecting the minimal amount, and 3) prescribing iron-replacement therapy with or without an ESA before donation.

Intraoperative Strategies

Autologous Blood Recovery

Intraoperative autologous blood recovery, one of the earliest blood conservation methods, became well established in the late 1970s.[53] The Cell Saver (Haemonetics) uses a specialized bowl to collect and wash debris from the shed blood. This method became popular in the 1980s, when patients strongly preferred to have their own blood rather than banked blood, primarily to avoid HIV.

In this procedure, shed blood is washed in a cone-shaped or cylindrical centrifuge bowl that concentrates the red cells, which are then transfused back to the patient. The resulting product has a hematocrit similar to that of RBCs from the blood bank and is devoid of plasma and platelets. If enough recovered blood is administered (approximately 5 or more units), the patient will begin to develop a dilutional coagulopathy. Nonetheless, for some vascular, transplant, orthopedic, and cardiac procedures, use of autologous recovered blood has become a standard of care for blood conservation.[54,55] A primary limitation of blood recovery is that a cavity where blood will pool is needed for optimal collection and recovery of shed blood. Additionally, blood collection can be inefficient when more than one suction source is used in the surgical field, causing blood to be routed to the waste suction and not the Cell Saver. Concerns also exist for potential contamination of the shed blood with microbes, tumor cells, or amniotic fluid during cesarean section. Washing and leukocyte reduction filters have been shown to re-

duce contamination risk significantly, however, and currently available literature does not show worse outcomes when recovered blood is used in these cases.[56] Another limitation is that some smaller hospitals do not have personnel on-site to operate the Cell Savers. Such institutions often need to call in an outside contractor, which requires advance planning and increased costs. One workaround for this limitation is to "collect only" with a collection reservoir and anticoagulant (citrate or heparin)[54]; then, when the qualified personnel are available, the shed blood can be processed through the machine. In some hospitals, the anesthesia or nursing staff are trained to operate the machines, but in others the perfusionists who operate the extracorporeal bypass equipment for cardiac surgery are responsible for processing recovered blood.

The use of autologous blood recovery has several advantages. Evidence shows that when one or more units are returned to the patient, intraoperative blood recovery adds economic value.[57,58] Additionally, recovered red cells are likely to be higher quality than stored (banked) RBCs.[59] Because recovered red cells do not suffer from "storage lesions," red cell membrane deformability[60] and 2,3-diphosphoglycerate levels are near normal,[61] whereas both of these parameters are decreased in stored blood. Use of autologous blood also eliminates the risk for viral transmission and alloimmunization. For all of these reasons, recovered red cells are usually preferred over allogeneic stored RBCs. More details on intraoperative blood recovery appear in AABB *Standards for Perioperative Autologous Blood Collection and Administration.*[62]

Reducing Intraoperative Blood Loss

Another strategy for reducing transfusions centers on decreasing intraoperative blood loss. Reducing intraoperative blood loss begins with meticulous surgical technique, but a number of other strategies to reduce bleeding have been developed (see Table 20-2). Simply maintaining normothermia by warming intravenous fluids and the patient directly (eg, forced-air warming) will reduce bleeding. Even mild hypothermia (35 C) increases bleeding by approximately 20% by inhibiting platelet function and the clotting cascade.[63] Another simple method of reducing intraoperative blood loss is controlled hypotension, which is especially effective in orthopedic and spine surgery. By increasing anesthetic depth and/or administering potent vasodilators, the provider can carefully reduce blood pressure while maintaining vital organ perfusion with a mean arterial blood pressure above the autoregulation threshold. Excess crystalloid should be avoided because the resulting hemodilution leads to decreased hemoglobin levels. Excess crystalloid can be avoided by administering colloid to expand intravascular volume (eg, albumin) and/or low-dose vasoconstrictors (eg, phenylephrine) to treat anesthetic-induced hypotension. Topical hemostatic agents, such as fibrin, thrombin, gelatin, collagen, and bone wax have been shown to aid in hemostasis.[64] Commercially available combination products such as Floseal (Baxter Healthcare Corp) contain bovine gelatin and human thrombin in the appropriate ratio to optimize hemostasis. Newer cautery methods, such as a saline-irrigated bipolar cautery, or the harmonic scalpel, which cauterizes vessels as it cuts, can also effectively reduce intraoperative bleeding.[65] Some evidence suggests that neuraxial anesthesia (spinal or epidural) may reduce bleeding by about 20%, perhaps by reducing venous and/or arterial blood pressures.[66]

Acute Normovolemic Hemodilution

Acute normovolemic hemodilution (ANH) is a technique that involves phlebotomy of 1-4 units of whole blood before the blood-loss portion of the surgery, and intentional hemodilution with crystalloid and/or colloid.[67,68] Because this process creates a state of intraoperative anemia, the shed blood contains fewer red cells. Near the end of the procedure, when most of the anticipated blood loss is complete, the phlebotomized blood is reinfused. For ANH to effectively reduce transfusion requirements, all three of the following conditions must be met: the preoperative hematocrit must be sufficiently high that the patient can tolerate the phlebotomy and hemodilution; the blood loss during surgery must be substantial enough to obtain the benefits; and the volume of phlebotomized blood must be

great enough to make a difference. Because these three requirements are not always present, whether the ANH technique reliably reduces the need for allogeneic transfusion remains controversial. A recent meta-analysis of 63 randomized trials showed that although ANH decreased the likelihood of transfusion by 26% and decreased the volume of allogeneic blood transfused by about 1 unit, possible publication bias may have led to an overestimate of the benefits.[69] Many small trials were included, and many lacked a transfusion protocol or threshold, which in these unblinded studies can lead to bias. The authors of an editorial concluded that ANH may be beneficial for specific cases that incorporate all three of the above-mentioned criteria and that patients might benefit most by receiving fresh coagulation factors and platelets in the whole blood that is reinfused. Thus, it might be most useful for patients undergoing major procedures, such as cardiac surgery, because it prevents the whole blood from being subjected to cooling and prevents potential damage to platelets by the cardiopulmonary bypass machine.[70]

Minimally Invasive Surgical Approaches

In the past two decades, new surgical approaches have been introduced, including laparoscopic, robotic, and endovascular techniques, that have dramatically reduced blood use. For instance, Johns Hopkins researchers found that only 1 in 800 patients undergoing robotic prostatectomy received a transfusion,[30] whereas historically, the vast majority of patients who underwent open prostatectomy received transfusion.[66,71] Similar impact has also been recognized with laparoscopic and robotic methods of gynecologic surgery, for example with hysterectomy and myomectomy procedures. Initially, robotic and other minimally invasive procedures were marketed for reducing pain and length of stay and enabling earlier return to work. However, these approaches have also dramatically reduced the need for transfusion.

Antifibrinolytic Medications

Antifibrinolytic drugs such as tranexamic acid and aminocaproic acid were introduced almost

50 years ago, but only in the past decade have they gained popularity for reducing perioperative blood loss and transfusion. Tranexamic acid, especially, has been called a "game changer" at some of the national orthopedic and blood management meetings. It is quickly becoming the standard of care for certain procedures, despite its use to reduce surgical bleeding being considered "off-label." Multiple studies have shown that antifibrinolytic drugs reduce bleeding, transfusion, and cost for spine surgery, hip and knee arthroplasty, and cardiac surgery.[72-75] Overall, compared to placebo, the studies collectively show that tranexamic acid reduces blood loss and transfusion requirements by approximately 30%. The drug is thought to stabilize clot that has already formed, by preventing its breakdown (fibrinolysis). The risk of deep venous thrombotic events does not appear to increase with these drugs, even in the three largest clinical trials with placebo control groups.[76-78] In studies of hemorrhaging trauma patients (the CRASH-2 Trial)[79] and postpartum hemorrhage (the WOMAN Trial),[78] each with 20,000 patients, investigators found a reduction in mortality when tranexamic acid was administered within 3 hours of bleeding onset; however, no benefit was observed after this 3-hour window.[80] The CRASH-2 trial showed a 9% reduction in overall mortality and a 15% reduction in mortality from hemorrhage. In the WOMAN trial, overall mortality decreased by 19%, and mortality from hemorrhage decreased by 31%. These studies included many hospitals in developing nations, and one limitation to consider is that blood is sometimes unsafe or unavailable in such areas, perhaps increasing the impact of tranexamic acid on mortality. Some centers use antifibrinolytics only when hyperfibrinolysis is evident based on data from viscoelastic testing. This practice seems appropriate but can delay treatment beyond the important 3-hour window of effectiveness. Dosing tranexamic acid is also somewhat controversial. A 1-g loading dose is now common for adult patients undergoing total joint replacement surgeries and was the dose used in the two above-mentioned trials. For longer surgeries, such as some spine procedures, this loading dose is often followed by a continuous infusion that ranges from 1 to 10 mg/kg/h.

However, the ideal dose has not yet been determined. Recent findings suggest that 3 to 5 mg/kg/h may provide a steady state and efficacious therapeutic level.[81,82] The contraindications to systemic tranexamic acid include uncontrolled seizures or an active thrombotic event, but a history of these conditions is not thought to be a contraindication. Some centers are applying tranexamic acid topically into the joint capsule in such patients undergoing hip and knee arthroplasty to minimize systemic levels of the drug. Efficacy with topical use has been demonstrated.[83]

Point-of-Care Testing

When turnaround times for laboratory tests are long, clinicians often decide to administer transfusion to the patient before receiving the test results. This is especially true with plasma or platelets because laboratory tests for coagulation and platelet counts take longer than hemoglobin measurements. With point-of-care testing, which has a rapid turnaround, the clinicians will not have to make blind decisions about whether or not to administer blood components. An example of point-of-care testing is thromboelastography (TEG) (Haemonetics) or rotational thromboelastometry (ROTEM) (Instrumentation Laboratories), which can give meaningful results on coagulation function within 10 to 15 minutes, or even faster with the rapid-TEG. The results from these tests reflect not only the number of platelets but also their functional integrity, which is more clinically relevant than a platelet count alone. Undoubtedly, point-of-care testing is an important component in a PBM program and can reduce unnecessary transfusions.[84]

Postoperative Strategies

Postoperative Blood Recovery

Postoperative blood recovery involves collecting and reinfusing blood from surgical drains and/or wounds. Adequate amounts of blood need to be collected and processed for this strategy to be effective. Thus, it is used mainly in trauma and vascular, cardiac, and complex orthopedic surgical cases for which the shed blood volume can be substantial (≥500 mL). Blood recovered postoperatively can be unwashed or washed. When unwashed recovered blood is used, shed blood is collected and filtered until a sufficient volume is reached; then it is transferred to an infusion bag for reinfusion. Alternatively, once sufficient shed blood is collected, it can be processed by washing and then transferred to a bag for reinfusion.

In the past, reinfusion of unwashed shed blood was popular as a blood conservation technique in joint replacement surgery. However, the growing use of antifibrinolytics has led to a decline in surgical bleeding, making postoperative blood recovery unnecessary.[85,86] In addition, unwashed shed blood is less desirable because it has a hematocrit of 20% to 30% and contains activated clotting and complement factors, inflammatory mediators, cytokines, and fat particles that can increase the risk for febrile reactions.[87,88] For patients with substantial postoperative blood loss, improved product quality and safety (eg, hematocrit of 60% to 80% with removal of contaminants) can be achieved with devices that wash and concentrate the postoperative wound-drainage blood. Maintaining the competency of nursing staff and the higher cost for these devices may be disadvantageous for some hospitals. However, for those centers engaged in complex, high-risk surgical cases, using postoperative autologous washed blood may reduce the need for allogeneic blood.

Reducing Phlebotomy Blood Loss

It is well recognized that patients are prone to iatrogenic blood loss from laboratory testing, especially when they are in the ICU, where frequent laboratory tests are ordered.[89,90] In addition, the easy access to blood draws when arterial and central venous catheters are present predisposes these ICU patients to lose approximately 1% or more of their circulating blood volume per day to testing. Approximately half the blood is lost when lines are cleared to draw an undiluted sample, and the rest is sent to the laboratory. Figure 20-2 shows the average amount of blood lost per day from laboratory testing for ICU patients in five different adult ICUs at Johns Hopkins Hospital. Smaller phlebotomy tubes are

useful for reducing blood loss, and in-line devices that return the wasted discard in a sterile fashion are also helpful. One of the ICUs, the neurocritical care unit, was able to cut blood loss in half by using an in-line return device (Fig 20-2). Simply eliminating unnecessary laboratory tests is also important, as for some patients, tests are ordered routinely with little or no clear rationale. In some cardiac surgery patients, up to 1 or 2 units of blood can be lost just from phlebotomy during longer ICU stays.[91]

Transfusion Thresholds

A patient's response to anemia is highly individualized and depends on ability to maintain adequate oxygen delivery to tissues. Tolerance depends on the patient's volume status, physiologic reserve (including cardiac, pulmonary, and renal function), and dynamics of the anemia. Patients with chronic anemia caused by chronic renal failure, slow gastrointestinal bleeding, or menorrhagia often adapt physiologically to a lower hemogloblin level by increasing cardiac output, heart rate, or stroke volume. However, rapid blood loss from surgical bleeding or trauma often results in hemodynamic instability, shock, and other symptoms that require more rapid volume replacement. Evidence suggests that the change in hemoglobin level (delta hemoglobin) is a better predictor of adverse outcomes than the absolute nadir hemoglobin during a hospital stay.[92] Thus, chronic anemia seems to be much better tolerated than acute anemia.

As discussed previously and according to the studies shown in Table 20-3, strong evidence supports using a restrictive transfusion strategy, with lower hemoglobin thresholds than were used historically (7-8 g/dL instead of 10 g/dL). However, the literature lacks evidence for applying a restrictive threshold to patients with substantial bleeding, those with cardiac or cerebral ischemia, and patients with hematologic malignancies undergoing chemotherapy and stem cell transplantation. More importantly, an arbitrary hemoglobin level or threshold should not be the sole driver for transfusion. Transfusion decisions should be individualized and based not only on the hemoglobin level but also on the

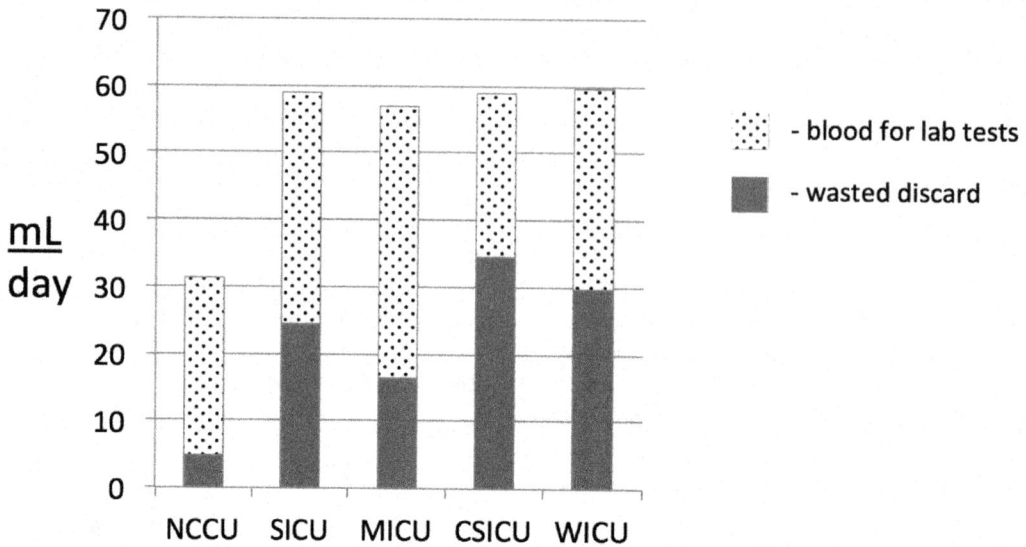

FIGURE 20-2. The bar graph illustrates the average volume of blood that patients lose as a result of laboratory testing in the five different adult intensive care units (ICUs) at the Johns Hopkins Hospital. The typical ICU patient loses approximately 60 mL/day, which is just over 1% of total blood volume in an average-size patient, or 2% of total blood volume for a small adult patient. In the NCCU, an in-line device is used to return the blood drawn to clear the saline from the lines. This device has reduced total blood loss by approximately 50%. NCCU = neurocritical care unit; SICU = surgical intensive care unit; MICU = medical intensive care unit; CSICU = cardiac surgical intensive care unit; WICU = Weinberg intensive care unit (primarily surgical patients).

patient's clinical signs and symptoms of anemia and ability to tolerate and compensate for the anemia.[93] For example, there is some evidence that bleeding is more likely in thrombocytopenic patients when the hematocrit is ≤25%,[94] although this has never been specifically studied in a randomized trial. Intravascular volume should also be carefully considered, as dilutional anemia from excess intravenous fluids can lead to unnecessary transfusions, and volume-depleted or actively bleeding patients may need transfusions at higher thresholds. More simply stated, the recommendation is to treat the whole patient and not just his or her laboratory values.

Single-Unit RBC Transfusions

Traditionally, physicians were strongly encouraged to order 2-unit RBC transfusions, a practice that evolved several decades ago when single-unit transfusions were extensively criticized.[95] A

unit of blood can have varying effects on hemoglobin and hematocrit, depending on the patient's total blood volume and fluid shifts. Often, a single RBC unit provides an adequate response and relieves symptoms. In 2014, when the AABB Choosing Wisely campaign[27] was launched, the first aim was "Don't transfuse more units of blood than absolutely necessary." This aim included a recommendation that physicians administer single-unit RBC transfusions to nonbleeding patients and then perform a clinical reassessment before giving additional units. Implementing a single-unit transfusion policy can have a significant impact and may reduce overall blood utilization more than monitoring hemoglobin thresholds.[96] The Johns Hopkins Health System launched a "Why give 2 when 1 will do?" campaign[23] that resulted in a 50% decrease in double-unit RBC transfusion orders and an overall 20% decrease in RBC utilization.[9] Even in leukemia patients who required multiple RBC transfusions, a single-unit policy was safe and effective in a small randomized pilot study.[97] One effective method of encouraging single-unit RBC orders was a custom-designed screen-saver image displayed on all health system computer workstations (Fig 20-3).

Transfusion Guidelines and Clinical Decision Support

Evidence-based transfusion guidelines are the basis for improving transfusion practice. Key physicians from various specialties should be involved in formulating these guidelines. For successful implementation, the guidelines must be combined with committed educational efforts. Issuing a memo of the transfusion guidelines to physicians without follow-up typically fails to reduce blood usage. Ideally the guidelines include indications for RBC, plasma, platelet, and

cryoprecipitate transfusions that are endorsed by the hospital's transfusion committee and medical executive committee. Concurrent reminders at the point of transfusion decision, such as pretransfusion checklists or order sets with the institution's transfusion guidelines and indications, can improve practice. Using computerized provider order entry (CPOE) systems with the capacity for clinical decision support (CDS), and requiring physicians to document the indication when outside of guidelines, facilitates adoption and improves transfusion practice.[6,98] An interruptive "pop-up alert," also known as a best practice advisory, can be built into the order set with logic to retrieve the most recent laboratory value. For example, the Johns Hopkins system advocates a hemoglobin threshold of 7 to 8 g/dL and single-unit RBC transfusions in patients who are hemodynamically stable and not actively bleeding (Fig 20-4). It has been shown that

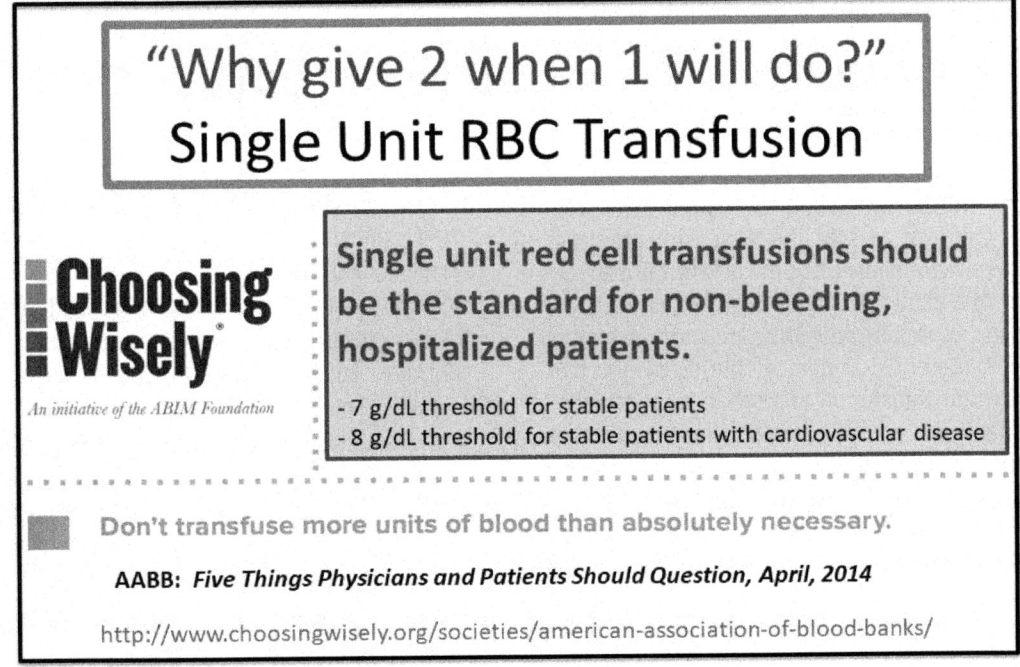

FIGURE 20-3. Image used for a "Why give 2 when 1 will do?" campaign to emphasize the importance of single-unit Red Blood Cell (RBC) transfusions in hemodynamically stable, nonbleeding patients. The image was displayed as a screen saver on workstations across the health system. This recommendation is backed by the AABB Choosing Wisely guidelines.[27] (Reprinted from Sadana et al.[25])

combining this alert with education is most efficacious. Embedding the published evidence into the alert with hyperlinks to the largest randomized trials is also important.[6,25] One limitation to electronic alerts is "alarm fatigue," meaning that clinicians become overwhelmed with these pop-ups and are more likely to ignore them.[99]

Audits with Provider Feedback

Auditing or monitoring physician practice is another useful intervention that reinforces evidence-based transfusion guidelines. Prospective or "real-time" audits (approval before issuing the component), in which the review is performed manually by laboratory staff, may be the most effective, but such reviews can be labor-intensive and time-consuming, and can create animosity. This process could also delay transfusions in hemorrhagic emergencies, and a process should be in place to avoid such delays.

In the authors' experience, monthly reports that compare blood utilization and transfusion guideline compliance rates of providers to those of peers in their own department are very effective. One method of presenting data to providers is the rank order bar graph, as shown in Fig 20-5.[2] When providers are compared directly to peers within their own specialty service, the individuals transfusing outside the evidence-based range will be compelled to change their practice. One can present the data with physician codes or with names, but the greatest impact occurs with names. In the authors' experience, clinicians, especially surgeons, are more receptive to data presented as hemoglobin thresholds and single-unit transfusion rates than as percentage of patients receiving transfusion or average number of units transfused per patient. For example, after the hemoglobin threshold rank order bar graph (Fig 20-5) was sent to surgeon #44, who had the highest threshold for transfusion, this surgeon's blood utilization in average number of units per patient decreased by more than 55%.

Another option for presenting the data is illustrated in Fig 20-6, in which the proportion of RBC orders is shown according to the hemoglobin threshold level. These hemoglobin thresholds were collected by looking for the most recent measured pretransfusion hemoglobin level and comparing time stamps of the laboratory tests and transfusion orders placed in the CPOE system. This rank order bar graph with an evidence-based, color-coded depiction of guideline compliance is easy to interpret and has improved practice by reducing unnecessary transfusions. The other feature of this type of data presentation is the length of each bar, which indicates the total number of transfused units for the 1-month period.

Audits should also be designed to detect "undertransfusion." With aggressive PBM programs, there is a possibility that some providers will avoid transfusions even when patients would indeed benefit. Providing feedback to providers on patients with very low postoperative hemoglobin levels is helpful for preventing undertransfusion.

DATA COLLECTION

Blood Utilization

In addition to the data described above, some metrics commonly collected to assess blood utilization include the following:

1. Average number of units transfused per patient or, alternatively, units transfused per 1000 patient days, which provides some degree of adjustment for case complexity. This measure is most classically associated with blood utilization as it correlates with transfusion cost adjusted for an institution's patient volume. This metric can be used to quantify the overall success of a PBM program, but it cannot be used to compare providers to one another unless they are performing similar procedures on similar patients.
2. Average number of units per transfusion recipient. This value is less useful than item 1 because it does not include the patient population that avoided transfusion, possibly as a result of successful blood conservation methods.
3. Percentage of patients who received transfusion. This metric may be useful for compar-

A.

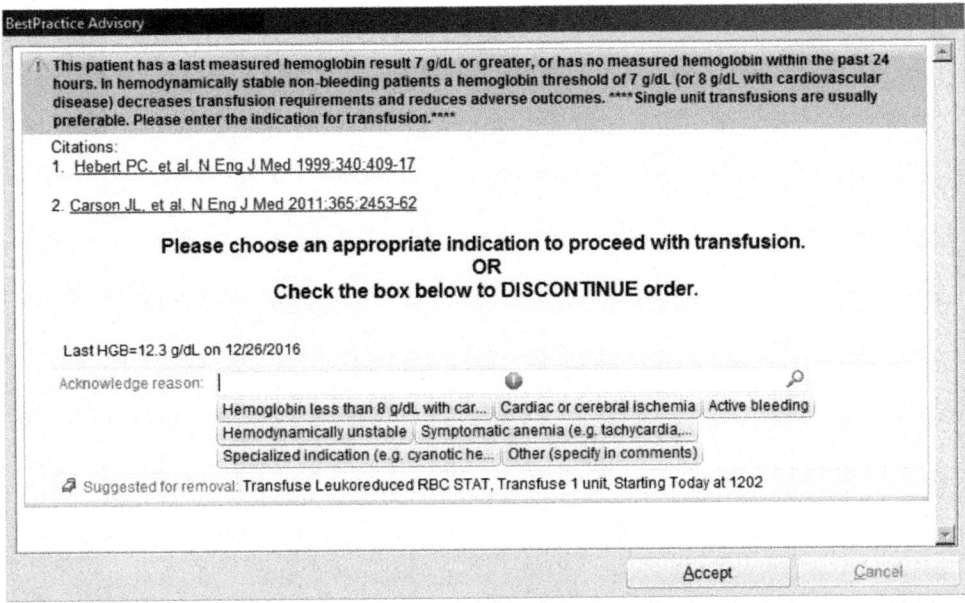

B.

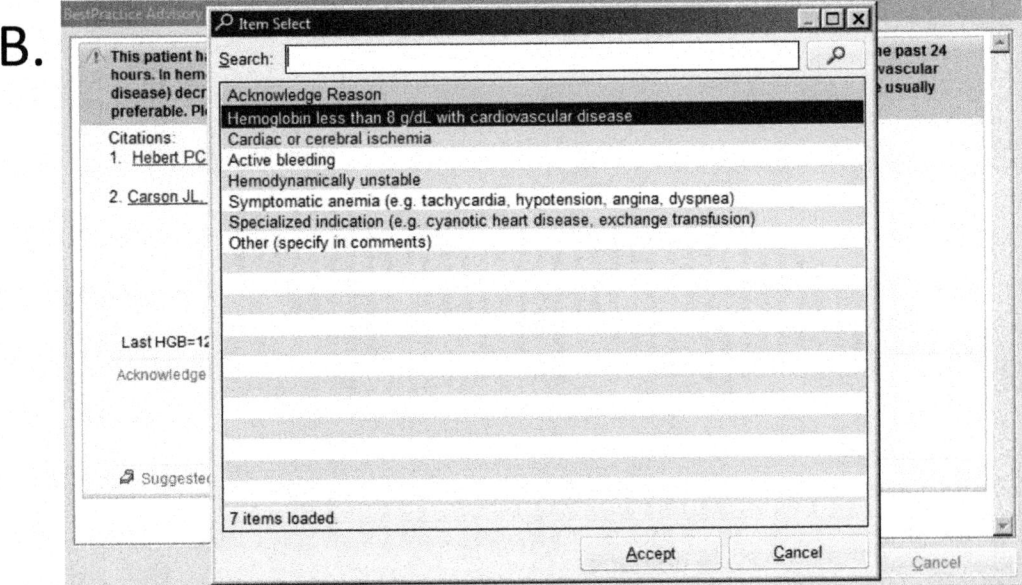

FIGURE 20-4. (A) The best practice advisory (BPA) shown is designed to display when a Red Blood Cell (RBC) order is placed for a patient whose preceding hemoglobin level is ≥7 g/dL or whose hemoglobin has not been measured in the past 24 hours. This BPA is used to remind clinicians to follow evidence-based transfusion guidelines in patients who are not actively bleeding and are hemodynamically stable. (B) The reasons to override the BPA and proceed with the RBC transfusion order are shown. One must be chosen to finalize the order. (Reprinted from Frank et al.[9])

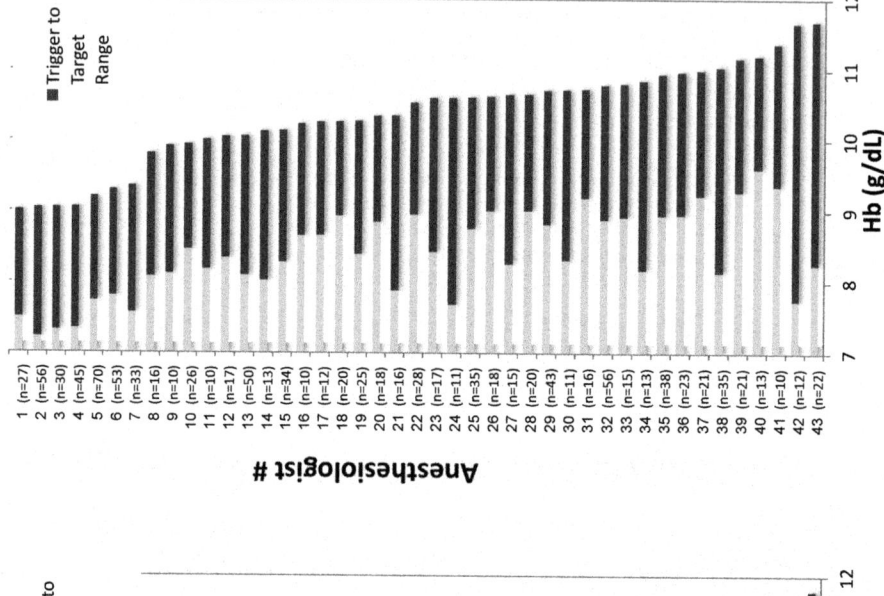

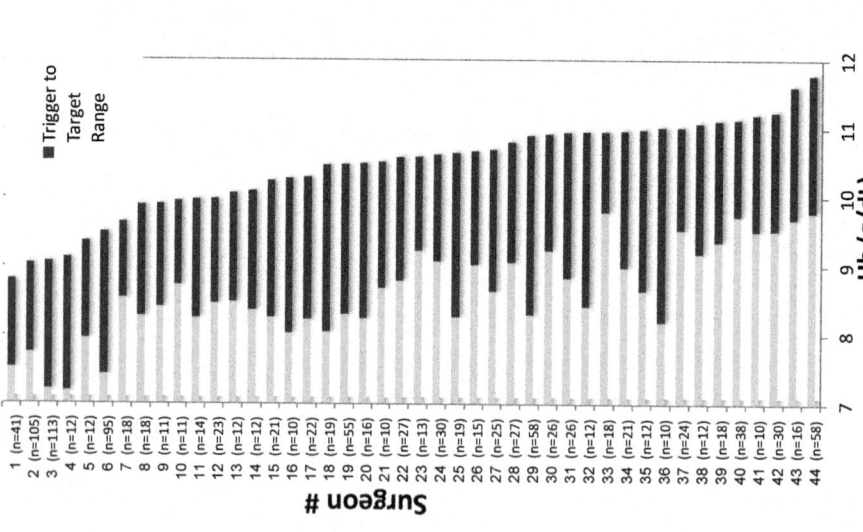

FIGURE 20-5. Comparison of mean transfusion hemoglobin thresholds and targets for all surgeons and anesthesiologists who had more than 10 patients in the database. The mean hemoglobin thresholds are designated by the left edge of the dark bars, and the mean hemoglobin targets by the right edge of the dark bars. The span between the lowest and highest hemoglobin thresholds was 2.6 g/dL for surgeons and 2.4 g/dL for anesthesiologists. The span between lowest and highest hemoglobin targets was 3.0 g/dL for surgeons and 2.7 g/dL for anesthesiologists. (Reprinted from Frank et al.[2])

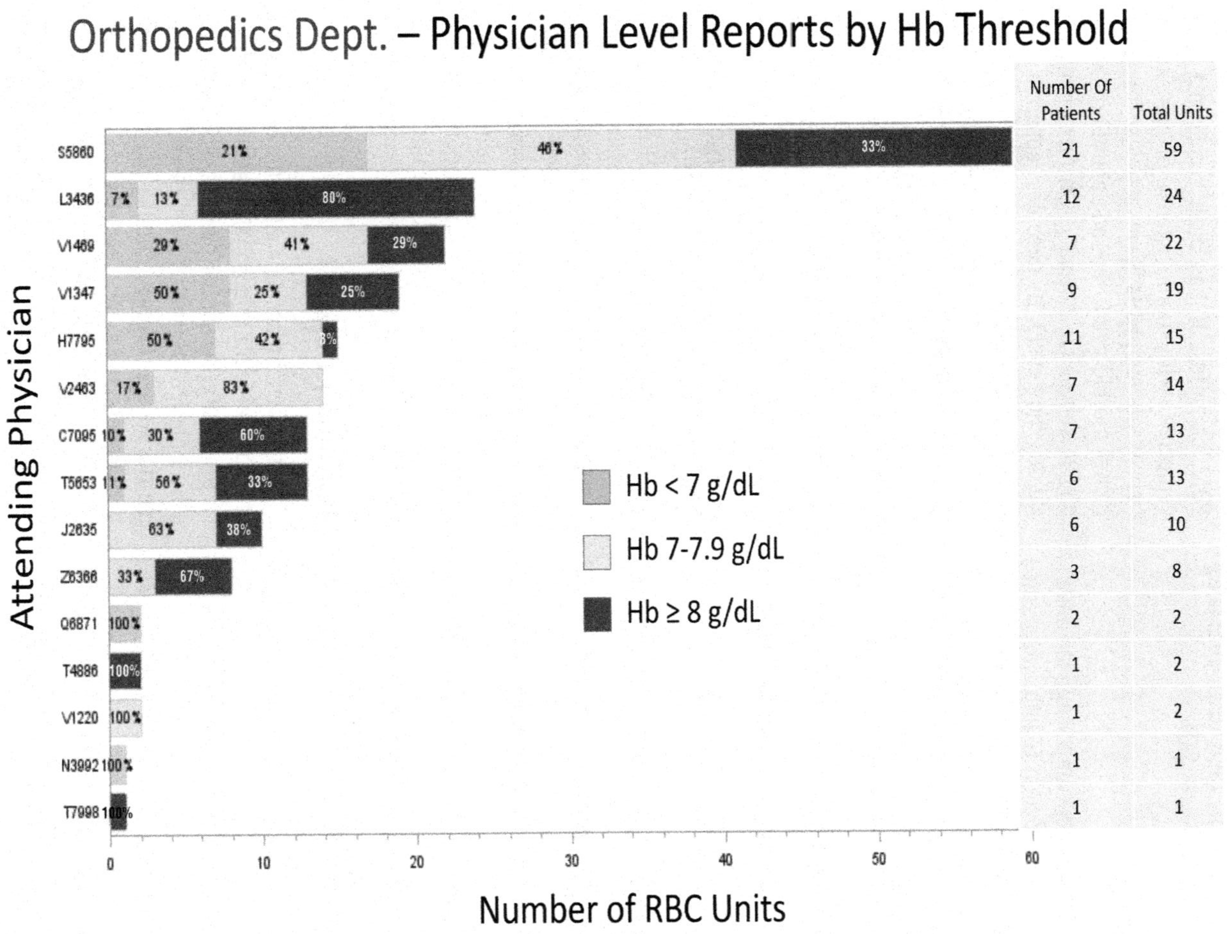

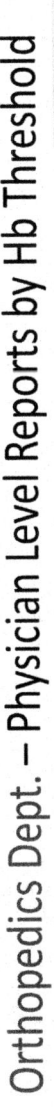

Orthopedics Dept. – Physician Level Reports by Hb Threshold

	Number Of Patients	Total Units
S5880	21	59
L3438	12	24
V1469	7	22
V1347	9	19
H7795	11	15
V2463	7	14
C7095	7	13
T0653	6	13
J2035	6	10
Z0366	3	8
Q0871	2	2
T4888	1	2
V1220	1	2
N3902	1	1
T7098	1	1

Legend:
- Hb < 7 g/dL
- Hb 7-7.9 g/dL
- Hb ≥ 8 g/dL

Number of RBC Units

Attending Physician

FIGURE 20-6. A typical monthly departmental blood utilization report. The number of Red Blood Cell (RBC) units administered by each attending physician on the orthopedic surgery service is depicted on the x-axis. Physicians are identified by a five-digit ID code on the y-axis. The proportion of RBC orders is shown according to the preceding hemoglobin (Hb) level. (Data were acquired from the computerized provider order entry system.)

ing providers to other providers who perform similar procedures on a similar population of patients. Again, it is less useful than item 1 because it disregards the number of units a patient receives; that is, whether a patient receives 1 or 10 units, the patient counts as only one transfusion recipient.

Clinical Outcomes

Clinical outcome data are important for determining how a PBM program is influencing the quality of patient care. Unfortunately, such data tend to be the most difficult to capture. Morbid events are commonly assessed in PBM programs, and examples of these are given in Table 20-4. Often, grouping these morbid events into larger categories (as shown in the table) can ease interpretation. Programs can also use a composite morbid event rate, which includes

TABLE 20-4. Clinical Outcomes to Follow in a Patient Blood Management Program

Thrombotic events
Disseminated intravascular coagulation
Deep venous thrombosis
Pulmonary embolus
Hospital-acquired infections
Surgical-site infection
Drug-resistant infection
Sepsis
Clostridium difficile
Ischemic events
Myocardial infarction
Transient ischemic attack
Cerebral vascular accident
Respiratory insufficiency/failure
Renal insufficiency/failure
Mortality
Length of stay

the occurrence of any one of these morbid events.

The in-hospital mortality rate is usually obtainable from the electronic medical record (EMR) (unlike 30-day or 1-year mortality) and is an important clinical outcome to measure in PBM programs. It has been recognized that, compared with nonrecipients of transfusion, transfusion recipients have about a threefold-higher morbid event rate and about a ninefold-higher in-hospital mortality. On further investigation, however, it becomes apparent that transfusion recipients have more comorbidities and undergo more complex procedures, thus demonstrating the need to risk-adjust retrospectively collected transfusion data. Otherwise, transfusion is so strongly associated with severity of illness and complexity of procedure that confounding by indication is commonplace in retrospective studies.[100]

One particularly worthwhile method of assessing outcomes is to use the ICD-9 or ICD-10 (International Classification of Diseases) codes from the billing database.[101-103] However, this method is dependent on the clinician charting the patient records accurately and the hospital coding team coding the charts correctly. Nonetheless, these codes can be very useful. Registry data can also be useful if an institution participates in programs such as the National Surgical Quality Improvement Program or the Society for Thoracic Surgeons database.

Benchmark Data

The ideal benchmark data allow the comparison of a hospital to other hospitals that perform similar procedures on similar patients. This comparison is particularly helpful for blood utilization metrics such as average number of units per patient undergoing a given procedure. This benchmark is useful for standardized procedures, such as a total hip arthroplasty, but less useful for cases such as spinal fusion, because the number of spinal levels is an important variable that often is not accounted for. When comparing blood use among hospitals, or even among providers (surgeons), one method of risk-adjustment that can be used is the case mix index. The case mix index has been shown to correlate directly to blood utilization, not only for RBCs but also for plasma and platelets.[104] The All Patients Refined-Diagnosis Related Groups (APR-DRG) weighted index (also called case mix index) is a good risk index that can be used to adjust for differences in procedure complexity and severity of illness for a group of patients or for an entire institution. These case mix index numbers are publically available on the Centers for Medicare and Medicaid Services website.[105]

EXTREMES OF TRANSFUSION

Bloodless Care

A good PBM program will ensure optimal care for patients who do not accept transfusion of allogeneic blood components for religious or other reasons. These patients receive what has been called "extreme blood management," whereby all the methods of blood conservation described above are used. Often, such care is delivered through a coordinated "bloodless program."[106] First, such patients need to be identified early in their hospital stay, or early in the preoperative period before surgery. Each individual patient may have different beliefs with regard to acceptance of fractionated blood components (minor fractions such as albumin, cryoprecipitate, and clotting factors) as well as procedures involving their own blood when kept in circuit (blood recovery, ANH). A knowledgeable provider should thoroughly discuss these options with the patient. Then the patient's decision should be well documented in the medical record and made available for all members of the health-care team, perhaps through use of alerts or a best practice advisory in the EMR. A transfusion consent form may further assist with this process.[107]

Protocols to diagnose and aggressively treat preoperative anemia are necessary for patients undergoing procedures with substantial blood loss and should include intravenous iron and ESAs when needed.[108,109] For this process, the institutional MSBOS can be used to determine the likelihood of significant blood loss and use this information to choose a hemoglobin target before elective surgery. Taken into account are the particular surgeon performing the procedure as well as the MSBOS category of "no sample," "type and screen," or "type and crossmatch" to indicate low-, medium-, and high-blood-loss surgical procedures, respectively. Providers also account for the patient's body mass, which reflects circulating blood volume.[110,111] For example, the optimal preoperative hemogloblin for a 40-kg patient would be substantially higher than that for an 80-kg patient, merely because the larger patient has a greater circulating blood volume and thus will tolerate a larger blood loss. A physician who is experienced in treating anemia with intravenous iron and ESAs can be very valuable to a bloodless program. Having autologous blood recovery equipment readily available and personnel to operate the machines is critical to safely managing patients who will not accept transfusion. One should also use rigorous methods to minimize blood loss and optimize hemoglobin levels and coagulation. For example, it is important to use small phlebotomy tubes and reduce the frequency of blood testing. Often, simply tolerating lower-than-usual hemoglobin levels is necessary when patients will not accept transfusions. Providing supplemental oxygen and minimizing myocardial demand may help decrease risk of ischemia. In cases of severe anemia, use of artificial oxygen carriers may be considered for emergency use through the FDA's Expanded Access (formerly called Compassionate Use) program.[112] In summary, rendering care for these bloodless-care patients entails all the best practices of PBM, often taking them to the extreme.[102,109]

It has been shown that when a carefully coordinated program implemented all of the above-mentioned PBM methods, the clinical outcomes for patients who did not accept transfusion were as good as or better than those of a carefully matched control patient group who did accept transfusion.[102] In addition, the hospital costs incurred to care for the bloodless-care patients were lower than those for the patients who accepted transfusion (total costs were 12% lower, and direct costs were 18% lower).[102]

Massive Transfusions

Providing optimal care for patients who receive massive transfusion is one goal of a good PBM program. Although the optimal ratio of blood components is somewhat controversial, recent evidence suggests that a 1:1:1 ratio of RBCs to plasma to platelets is ideal for those who require transfusion of an entire blood volume or more.[113] A hospital should have a system in place to thaw frozen plasma rapidly, and platelets and cryoprecipitate should be readily available to support massive transfusions. Some institutions are using viscoelastic testing (TEG or ROTEM) to guide the ratio of blood components. As discussed above, good evidence supports the use of antifibrinolytic drugs for reducing mortality in patients with trauma and postpartum hemorrhage. The rapid delivery of a balanced combination of blood components is important, and, as with any massive transfusion scenario, the provider should aggressively prevent hypothermia, which will increase bleeding. Massive transfusion can lead to citrate toxicity, which results in hypocalcemia that in turn causes hypotension from decreased cardiac contractility and vasomotor tone. Therefore, replacing calcium with calcium chloride or gluconate is important for patients with massive transfusions. Ionized calcium should be measured frequently and maintained above 1.0 mmol/L. It is important to recognize that plasma and platelets have approximately fivefold more citrate than RBCs for a given transfused volume. Consequently, when giving a 1:1:1 ratio of these components, the patient receives a large amount of citrate.[114]

Recently, clinical outcomes were reported after massive transfusion of patients, including those who received very high transfusion doses (up to and over 75 units of RBCs). It was found that for every 10 additional RBC units administered during the hospitalization, mortality increased by 10%, and after 50 RBC units, mortality reached 50% (the 50/50 rule).[103] Perhaps more importantly, hospital-acquired infections and thrombotic events were found to be four- to fivefold more common than renal, respiratory, or ischemic events in the massive transfusion recipients, and increases in the frequency of these events were also dose dependent. The researchers concluded that providers should be more vigilant to prevent, diagnose, and treat infections and thrombosis in massive transfusion recipients in order to optimize their outcomes. Dzik et al[115] reported a similar series of "ultramassive" transfusions (>20 RBC units over 48 hours), in which trauma patients had the highest mortality, followed by medicine patients; however, organ transplant, general, and cardiac surgery patients had lower mortality.

SUMMARY

Successfully implementing a PBM program requires planning, education, and teamwork. A PBM program is an important patient safety and quality measure that can also lead to cost savings. To implement a successful program, hospitals need sufficient resources to support the people who can accomplish the methods and techniques that are discussed above. However, the return on investment can be 400%.[9] Institutions also need sufficient information technology support to obtain the data required to improve practice. Education, evidence-based transfusion guidelines, and best practice advisories effectively encourage good practice and reduce unnecessary transfusions.

The specific activities performed by a PBM program can vary by institution and are defined by the executive management team of the facility. Guidance is available from various professional organizations, including AABB and SABM. The latter offers *Administrative and Clinical Standards for Patient Blood Management Programs*, which outlines 13 standards related to the activities of a PBM program. For the AABB/Joint Commission certification, a PBM program can be designated as an activity level 1, 2, or 3 program, as delineated in AABB's *Standards for a Patient Blood Management Program*. Information on this program and many other PBM resources may be found on the AABB website (aabb.org/pbm). With a successful PBM program, providers can reduce risk, improve outcomes, and reduce cost, which in combination increases the value of health care they deliver.

ACKNOWLEDGMENTS

The authors would like to thank Kathleen E. Puca, MD, MT(ASCP)SBB, Medical Director, BloodCenter of Wisconsin, and Associate Professor, Medical College of Wisconsin. Dr. Puca contributed as the author of the PBM chapter in the 19th edition of the *Technical Manual*, and portions of her chapter were used in the current version. The authors also wish to thank Claire F. Levine, MS, ELS, Scientific Editor, Department of Anesthesiology/Critical Care Medicine, Johns Hopkins Medicine, Baltimore, Maryland, for editorial assistance.

KEY POINTS

1. PBM is an evidence-based, multidisciplinary approach to optimizing the care of patients who might need transfusion.
2. Several factors have been drivers of PBM, including transfusion-associated risks, demand for improved quality of care, promotion of evidence-based practice, economic benefits, overutilization of blood components, patient autonomy and satisfaction, and a projected shrinking of the blood supply.
3. Elements of a PBM program include 1) financial support from the hospital administration; 2) management of anemia and bleeding risks before treatment begins; 3) intraoperative blood recovery, hemostatic pharmacologic agents, blood-sparing surgical techniques, and evidence-based transfusion guidelines; 4) ICU and postoperative strategies to reduce the need for transfusion; 5) blood utilization review; and 6) education of health-care providers.
4. PBM can provide benefit to medical as well as surgical patients.
5. Preoperative anemia is common. Identifying and treating preoperative anemia is one of the fundamentals of PBM.
6. Encouraging single-unit RBC transfusions in stable anemic patients is an effective method of reducing overuse. A Choosing Wisely "Why give 2 when 1 will do?" campaign can substantially reduce overall blood utilization.
7. PBM is more than just transfusion avoidance. It involves the use of pharmaceutical agents, blood recovery techniques, surgical tools to limit blood loss, limiting phlebotomy for laboratory testing, adherence to transfusion guidelines, and medical education.
8. A multidisciplinary team who will champion PBM is critical for the success, growth, and sustainability of the PBM program.
9. Ongoing blood utilization reviews that include audits and provider feedback, together with an emphasis on patient outcomes, are effective tools for a successful program.

REFERENCES

1. Carson JL, Triulzi DJ, Ness PM. Indications for and adverse effects of red-cell transfusion. N Engl J Med 2017;377:1261-72.
2. Frank SM, Savage WJ, Rothschild JA, et al. Variability in blood and blood component utilization as assessed by an anesthesia information management system. Anesthesiology 2012;117:99-106.
3. Proceedings from the National Summit on Overuse (July 8, 2013). Oakbrook Terrace, IL: The Joint Commission, 2013. [Available at https://www.jointcommission.org/overuse_summit/ (accessed November 29, 2019).]
4. Jones JM, Sapiano MRP, Savinkina AA, et al. Slowing decline in blood collection and transfusion in the United States—2017. Transfusion 2020;60(S2):S1-S9.
5. The 2016 AABB Blood Survey Fact Sheet. Bethesda, MD: AABB, 2019. [Available at: http://www.aabb.org/research/hemovigilance/bloodsurvey/Pages/default.aspx (accessed March 26, 2020).]

6. Zuckerberg GS, Scott AV, Wasey JO, et al. Efficacy of education followed by computerized provider order entry with clinician decision support to reduce red blood cell utilization. Transfusion 2015;55:1628-36.

7. Frank SM, Oleyar MJ, Ness PM, Tobian AA. Reducing unnecessary preoperative blood orders and costs by implementing an updated institution-specific maximum surgical blood order schedule and a remote electronic blood release system. Anesthesiology 2014;121:501-9.

8. Goodnough LT, Shieh L, Hadhazy E, et al. Improved blood utilization using real-time clinical decision support. Transfusion 2014;54:1358-65.

9. Frank SM, Thakkar RN, Podlasek SJ, et al. Implementing a health system-wide patient blood management program with a clinical community approach. Anesthesiology 2017;127:754-64.

10. Shander A, Hofmann A, Ozawa S, et al. Activity-based costs of blood transfusions in surgical patients at four hospitals. Transfusion 2010;50:753-65.

11. Frey K, ed. Standards for a patient blood management program. 3rd ed. Bethesda, MD: AABB, 2020.

12. SABM administrative and clinical standards for patient blood management programs. 5th ed. Englewood, NJ: Society for the Advancement of Blood Management, 2019. [Available at https://www.sabm.org/publications/ (accessed November 29, 2019).]

13. Carson JL, Terrin ML, Noveck H, et al. Liberal or restrictive transfusion in high-risk patients after hip surgery. N Engl J Med 2011;365:2453-62.

14. Hajjar LA, Vincent JL, Galas FR, et al. Transfusion requirements after cardiac surgery: The TRACS randomized controlled trial. JAMA 2010;304:1559-67.

15. Hébert PC, Wells G, Blajchman MA, et al. A multicenter, randomized, controlled clinical trial of transfusion requirements in critical care. N Engl J Med 1999;340:409-17.

16. Lacroix J, Hébert PC, Hutchison JS, et al. Transfusion strategies for patients in pediatric intensive care units. N Engl J Med 2007;356:1609-19.

17. Robertson CS, Hannay HJ, Yamal JM, et al. Effect of erythropoietin and transfusion threshold on neurological recovery after traumatic brain injury: A randomized clinical trial. JAMA 2014;312:36-47.

18. Villanueva C, Colomo A, Bosch A, et al. Transfusion strategies for acute upper gastrointestinal bleeding. N Engl J Med 2013;368:11-21.

19. Murphy GJ, Pike K, Rogers CA, et al. Liberal or restrictive transfusion after cardiac surgery. N Engl J Med 2015;372:997-1008.

20. Holst LB, Haase N, Wetterslev J, et al. Lower versus higher hemoglobin threshold for transfusion in septic shock. N Engl J Med 2014;371:1381-91.

21. Mazer CD, Whitlock RP, Fergusson DA, et al. Restrictive or liberal red-cell transfusion for cardiac surgery. N Engl J Med 2017;377:2133-44.

22. Wintermeyer TL, Liu J, Lee KH, et al. Interactive dashboards to support a patient blood management program across a multi-institutional healthcare system. Transfusion 2016;56:1480-1.

23. Podlasek SJ, Thakkar RN, Rotello LC, et al. Implementing a "Why give 2 when 1 will do?" Choosing Wisely campaign. Transfusion 2016;56:2164.

24. Guinn NR, Guercio JR, Hopkins TJ, et al. How do we develop and implement a preoperative anemia clinic designed to improve perioperative outcomes and reduce cost? Transfusion 2016;56:297-303.

25. Sadana D, Pratzer A, Scher LJ, et al. Promoting high-value practice by reducing unnecessary transfusions with a patient blood management program. JAMA Intern Med 2018;178:116-22.

26. Frank SM, Resar LM, Rothschild JA, et al. A novel method of data analysis for utilization of red blood cell transfusion. Transfusion 2013;53:3052-9.

27. Callum JL, Waters JH, Shaz BH, et al. The AABB recommendations for the Choosing Wisely campaign of the American Board of Internal Medicine. Transfusion 2014;54:2344-52.

28. Roback JD, Caldwell S, Carson J, et al. Evidence-based practice guidelines for plasma transfusion. Transfusion 2010;50:1227-39.

29. Kaufman RM, Djulbegovic B, Gernsheimer T, et al. Platelet transfusion: A clinical practice guideline from the AABB. Ann Intern Med 2015;162:205-13.

30. Frank SM, Rothschild JA, Masear CG, et al. Optimizing preoperative blood ordering with data acquired from an anesthesia information management system. Anesthesiology 2013;118:1286-97.

31. Shander A. Preoperative anemia and its management. Transfus Apher Sci 2014;50:13-15.

32. Elhenawy AM, Meyer SR, Bagshaw SM, et al. Role of preoperative intravenous iron therapy to correct anemia before major surgery: Study protocol for systematic review and meta-analysis. Syst Rev 2015;4:29.

33. Karkouti K, Wijeysundera DN, Beattie WS. Risk associated with preoperative anemia in cardiac surgery: A multicenter cohort study. Circulation 2008;117:478-84.

34. Mantilla CB, Wass CT, Goodrich KA, et al. Risk for perioperative myocardial infarction and mortality in patients undergoing hip or knee arthroplasty: The role of anemia. Transfusion 2011; 51:82-91.

35. Auerbach M. Oral or IV iron in inflammatory bowel disease. Am J Gastroenterol 2012;107: 950-1.

36. Auerbach M, Macdougall IC. Safety of intravenous iron formulations: Facts and folklore. Blood Transfus 2014;12:296-300.

37. Auerbach M, Pappadakis JA, Bahrain H, et al. Safety and efficacy of rapidly administered (one hour) one gram of low molecular weight iron dextran (INFeD) for the treatment of iron deficient anemia. Am J Hematol 2011;86:860-2.

38. Auerbach M. Intravenous iron in the perioperative setting. Am J Hematol 2014;89:933.

39. Fishbane S, Nissenson AR. The new FDA label for erythropoietin treatment: How does it affect hemoglobin target? Kidney Int 2007;72:806-13.

40. Fox JL. FDA likely to further restrict erythropoietin use for cancer patients. Nature Biotech 2007;25:607-8.

41. Robles NR. The safety of erythropoiesis-stimulating agents for the treatment of anemia resulting from chronic kidney disease. Clin Drug Investig 2016;36:421-31.

42. Roger SD, Tio M, Park HC, et al. Intravenous iron and erythropoiesis-stimulating agents in haemodialysis: A systematic review and meta-analysis. Nephrology 2017;22:969-76.

43. Goodnough LT, Skikne B, Brugnara C. Erythropoietin, iron, and erythropoiesis. Blood 2000; 96:823-33.

44. Friedman BA, Oberman HA, Chadwick AR, Kingdon KI. The maximum surgical blood order schedule and surgical blood use in the United States. Transfusion 1976;16:380-7.

45. Dutton RP, Shih D, Edelman BB, et al. Safety of uncrossmatched type-O red cells for resuscitation from hemorrhagic shock. J Trauma 2005; 59:1445-9.

46. Gammon HM, Waters JH, Watt A, et al. Developing performance measures for patient blood management. Transfusion 2011;51:2500-9.

47. Can MM, Tanboga IH, Turkyilmaz E, et al. The risk of false results in the assessment of platelet function in the absence of antiplatelet medication: Comparison of the PFA-100, multiplate electrical impedance aggregometry and verify now assays. Thromb Res 2010;125:e132-7.

48. Wang CZ, Moss J, Yuan CS. Commonly used dietary supplements on coagulation function during surgery. Medicines 2015;2:157-85.

49. Vassallo R, Goldman M, Germain M, Lozano M, for the BEST Collaborative. Preoperative autologous blood donation: Waning indications in an era of improved blood safety. Transfus Med Rev 2015;29:268-75.

50. Lee GC, Cushner FD. The effects of preoperative autologous donations on perioperative blood levels. J Knee Surg 2007;20:205-9.

51. Kennedy C, Leonard M, Devitt A, et al. Efficacy of preoperative autologous blood donation for elective posterior lumbar spinal surgery. Spine 2011;36:E1736-43.

52. Goldman M, Remy-Prince S, Trepanier A, Decary F. Autologous donation error rates in Canada. Transfusion 1997;37:523-7.

53. Waters JH. Indications and contraindications of cell salvage. Transfusion 2004;44:40S-4S.

54. Waters JH. Optimization of recovering shed blood when performing blood salvage. Anesth Analg 2009;108:1714-15.

55. Wang G, Bainbridge D, Martin J, Cheng D. The efficacy of an intraoperative cell saver during cardiac surgery: A meta-analysis of randomized trials. Anesth Analg 2009;109:320-30.

56. Esper SA, Waters JH. Intra-operative cell salvage: A fresh look at the indications and contraindications. Blood Transfus 2011;9:139-47.

57. Waters JH, Dyga RM, Waters JF, Yazer MH. The volume of returned red blood cells in a large blood salvage program: Where does it all go? Transfusion 2011;51:2126-32.

58. Frank SM. Who benefits from red blood cell salvage?—Utility and value of intraoperative autologous transfusion. Transfusion 2011;51:2058-60.

59. Salaria ON, Barodka VM, Hogue CW, et al. Impaired red blood cell deformability after transfusion of stored allogeneic blood but not autologous salvaged blood in cardiac surgery patients. Anesth Analg 2014;118:1179-87.

60. Frank SM, Abazyan B, Ono M, et al. Decreased erythrocyte deformability after transfusion and

the effects of erythrocyte storage duration. Anesth Analg 2013;116:975-81.

61. Scott AV, Nagababu E, Johnson DJ, et al. 2,3-Diphosphoglycerate concentrations in autologous salvaged versus stored red blood cells and in surgical patients after transfusion. Anesth Analg 2016;122:616-23.

62. Berg MP, ed. Standards for perioperative autologous blood collection and administration. 8th ed. Bethesda, MD: AABB, 2018.

63. Schmied H, Kurz A, Sessler DI, et al. Mild hypothermia increases blood loss and transfusion requirements during total hip arthroplasty. Lancet 1996;347:289-92.

64. Achneck HE, Sileshi B, Jamiolkowski RM, et al. A comprehensive review of topical hemostatic agents: Efficacy and recommendations for use. Ann Surg 2010;251:217-28.

65. Frank SM, Wasey JO, Dwyer IM, et al. Radiofrequency bipolar hemostatic sealer reduces blood loss, transfusion requirements, and cost for patients undergoing multilevel spinal fusion surgery: A case control study. J Orthop Surg Res 2014;9:50.

66. Shir Y, Raja SN, Frank SM, Brendler CB. Intraoperative blood loss during radical retropubic prostatectomy: Epidural versus general anesthesia. Urology 1995;45:993-9.

67. Goodnough LT. Acute normovolemic hemodilution. Vox Sang 2002;83(Suppl 1):211-15.

68. Shander A, Rijhwani TS. Acute normovolemic hemodilution. Transfusion 2004;44(12 Suppl):26S-34S.

69. Zhou X, Zhang C, Wang Y, et al. Preoperative acute normovolemic hemodilution for minimizing allogeneic blood transfusion: A meta-analysis. Anesth Analg 2015;121:1443-55.

70. Grant MC, Resar LM, Frank SM. The efficacy and utility of acute normovolemic hemodilution. Anesth Analg 2015;121:1412-14.

71. Monk TG, Goodnough LT, Brecher ME, et al. Acute normovolemic hemodilution can replace preoperative autologous blood donation as a standard of care for autologous blood procurement in radical prostatectomy. Anesth Analg 1997;85:953-8.

72. Benoni G, Fredin H, Knebel R, Nilsson P. Blood conservation with tranexamic acid in total hip arthroplasty: A randomized, double-blind study in 40 primary operations. Acta Orthop Scand 2001;72:442-8.

73. Irisson E, Hemon Y, Pauly V, et al. Tranexamic acid reduces blood loss and financial cost in primary total hip and knee replacement surgery.

Orthopaed Traumatol Surg Res 2012;98:477-83.

74. Zufferey PJ, Lanoiselee J, Chapelle C, et al. Intravenous tranexamic acid bolus plus infusion is not more effective than a single bolus in primary hip arthroplasty: A randomized controlled trial. Anesthesiology 2017;127:413-22.

75. Myles PS, Smith JA, Forbes A, et al. Tranexamic acid in patients undergoing coronary-artery surgery. N Engl J Med 2017;376:136-48.

76. Huang F, Wu D, Ma G, et al. The use of tranexamic acid to reduce blood loss and transfusion in major orthopedic surgery: A meta-analysis. J Surg Res 2014;186:318-27.

77. Gillette BP, DeSimone LJ, Trousdale RT, et al. Low risk of thromboembolic complications with tranexamic acid after primary total hip and knee arthroplasty. Clin Orthop Relat Res 2013;471:150-4.

78. WOMAN Trial Collaborators. Effect of early tranexamic acid administration on mortality, hysterectomy, and other morbidities in women with post-partum haemorrhage (WOMAN): An international, randomised, double-blind, placebo-controlled trial. Lancet 2017;389:2105-16.

79. Roberts I, Shakur H, Afolabi A, et al. The importance of early treatment with tranexamic acid in bleeding trauma patients: An exploratory analysis of the CRASH-2 randomised controlled trial. Lancet 2011;377:1096-101.

80. Gayet-Ageron A, Prieto-Merino D, Ker K, et al. Effect of treatment delay on the effectiveness and safety of antifibrinolytics in acute severe haemorrhage: A meta-analysis of individual patient-level data from 40 138 bleeding patients. Lancet 2018;391:125-32.

81. Johnson DJ, Johnson CC, Goobie SM, et al. High-dose versus low-dose tranexamic acid to reduce transfusion requirements in pediatric scoliosis surgery. J Pediatr Orthop 2017;37:e552-e7.

82. Goobie SM, Meier PM, Sethna NF, et al. Population pharmacokinetics of tranexamic acid in paediatric patients undergoing craniosynostosis surgery. Clin Pharmacokinet 2013;52:267-76.

83. Konig G, Hamlin BR, Waters JH. Topical tranexamic acid reduces blood loss and transfusion rates in total hip and total knee arthroplasty. J Arthroplasty 2013;28:1473-6.

84. Shore-Lesserson L, Manspeizer HE, DePerio M, et al. Thromboelastography-guided transfusion algorithm reduces transfusions in complex cardiac surgery. Anesth Analg 1999;88:312-19.

85. Oremus K, Sostaric S, Trkulja V, Haspl M. Influence of tranexamic acid on postoperative autologous blood retransfusion in primary total hip and knee arthroplasty: A randomized controlled trial. Transfusion 2014;54:31-41.

86. Springer BD, Odum SM, Fehring TK. What is the benefit of tranexamic acid vs reinfusion drains in total joint arthroplasty? J Arthroplasty 2016;31:76-80.

87. Munoz M, Garcia-Vallejo JJ, Ruiz MD, et al. Transfusion of post-operative shed blood: Laboratory characteristics and clinical utility. Eur Spine J 2004;13:S107-13.

88. Sinardi D, Marino A, Chillemi S, et al. Composition of the blood sampled from surgical drainage after joint arthroplasty: Quality of return. Transfusion 2005;45:202-7.

89. Thavendiranathan P, Bagai A, Ebidia A, et al. Do blood tests cause anemia in hospitalized patients? The effect of diagnostic phlebotomy on hemoglobin and hematocrit levels. J Gen Intern Med 2005;20:520-4.

90. Chant C, Wilson G, Friedrich JO. Anemia, transfusion, and phlebotomy practices in critically ill patients with prolonged ICU length of stay: A cohort study. Crit Care 2006;10:R140.

91. Koch CG, Reineks EZ, Tang AS, et al. Contemporary bloodletting in cardiac surgical care. Ann Thorac Surg 2015;99:779-84.

92. Spolverato G, Kim Y, Ejaz A, et al. Effect of relative decrease in blood hemoglobin concentrations on postoperative morbidity in patients who undergo major gastrointestinal surgery. JAMA Surg 2015;150:949-56.

93. Carson JL, Guyatt G, Heddle NM, et al. Clinical practice guidelines from the AABB: Red Blood Cell transfusion thresholds and storage. JAMA 2016;316:2025-35.

94. Uhl L, Assmann SF, Hamza TH, et al. Laboratory predictors of bleeding and the effect of platelet and RBC transfusions on bleeding outcomes in the PLADO trial. Blood 2017;130:1247-58.

95. Crispen JF. The single-unit transfusion. A continuing problem. Pa Med 1966;69:44-8.

96. Yang WW, Thakkar RN, Gehrie EA, et al. Single-unit transfusions and hemoglobin trigger: Relative impact on red cell utilization. Transfusion 2017;57:1163-70.

97. DeZern AE, Williams K, Zahurak M, et al. Red blood cell transfusion triggers in acute leukemia: A randomized pilot study. Transfusion 2016; 56:1750-7.

98. Hibbs SP, Nielsen ND, Brunskill S, et al. The impact of electronic decision support on transfusion practice: A systematic review. Transfus Med Rev 2015;29:14-23.

99. Mitka M. Joint Commission warns of alarm fatigue: Multitude of alarms from monitoring devices problematic. JAMA 2013;309:2315-6.

100. Carson JL, Hébert PC. Here we go again—blood transfusion kills patients?: Comment on "Association of blood transfusion with increased mortality in myocardial infarction: A meta-analysis and diversity-adjusted study sequential analysis." JAMA Intern Med 2013;173:139-41.

101. Kim Y, Spolverato G, Lucas DJ, et al. Red cell transfusion triggers and postoperative outcomes after major surgery. J Gastrointest Surg 2015; 19:2062-73.

102. Frank SM, Wick EC, Dezern AE, et al. Risk-adjusted clinical outcomes in patients enrolled in a bloodless program. Transfusion 2014;54:2668-77.

103. Johnson DJ, Scott AV, Barodka VM, et al. Morbidity and mortality after high-dose transfusion. Anesthesiology 2016;124:387-95.

104. Stonemetz JL, Allen PX, Wasey J, et al. Development of a risk-adjusted blood utilization metric. Transfusion 2014;54:2716-23.

105. Case mix index. Baltimore, MD: Centers for Medicare and Medicaid Services, 2019. [Available at https://www.cms.gov/Medicare/Medicare-Fee-for-Service-Payment/AcuteInpatientPPS/Acute-Inpatient-Files-for-Download-Items/CMS022630.html (accessed November 29, 2019).]

106. Resar LM, Wick EC, Almasri TN, et al. Bloodless medicine: Current strategies and emerging treatment paradigms. Transfusion 2016;56: 2637-47.

107. Jorgenson TD, Golbaba B, Guinn NR, Smith CE. When blood is not an option: The case for a standardized blood transfusion consent form. ASA Monitor 2017;81:48-50.

108. Guinn NR, Roberson RS, White W, et al. Costs and outcomes after cardiac surgery in patients refusing transfusion compared with those who do not: A case-matched study. Transfusion 2015;55:2791-8.

109. Resar LM, Frank SM. Bloodless medicine: What to do when you can't transfuse. Hematology Am Soc Hematol Educ Program 2014;2014:553-8.

110. Shander A, Rijhwani TS. Clinical outcomes in cardiac surgery: Conventional surgery versus bloodless surgery. Anesthesiol Clin North Am 2005;23:327-45.

111. Jassar AS, Ford PA, Haber HL, et al. Cardiac surgery in Jehovah's Witness patients: Ten-year experience. Ann Thorac Surg 2012;93:19-25.

112. Tan GM, Guinn NR, Frank SM, Shander A. Proceedings from the Society for Advancement of Blood Management Annual Meeting 2017: Management dilemmas of the surgical patient-when blood is not an option. Anesth Analg 2019;128(1):144-51.

113. Holcomb JB, Tilley BC, Baraniuk S, et al. Transfusion of plasma, platelets, and red blood cells in a 1:1:1 vs a 1:1:2 ratio and mortality in patients with severe trauma: The PROPPR randomized clinical trial. JAMA 2015;313:471-82.

114. Dzik WH, Kirkley SA. Citrate toxicity during massive blood transfusion. Transfus Med Rev 1988;2:76-94.

115. Dzik WS, Ziman A, Cohen C, et al for the Biomedical Excellence for Safer Transfusion Collaborative. Survival after ultramassive transfusion: A review of 1360 cases. Transfusion 2016;56:558-63.

CHAPTER 21

Approaches to Blood Utilization Auditing

Ira A. Shulman, MD; Jay Hudgins, DO; and Irina Maramica, MD, PhD, MBA

BLOOD TRANSFUSIONS ARE AMONG the most common procedures performed in hospitals in the United States but are also associated with significant risk for the patients. With millions of units of blood components transfused annually, quality organizations have focused on appropriate blood management as an area of opportunity to improve clinical outcomes through evidence-based standardization. Transfusion of blood components has also been identified as one of the most overused therapeutic interventions performed during patient hospitalizations.[1-4] Several clinical trials provide evidence that patient outcomes associated with a restrictive transfusion strategy are similar to, if not better, than patient outcomes associated with more liberal transfusion strategies.[5-7] Specifically, patients receiving fewer transfusions have a shorter length of stay, a lower incidence of infection, and lower readmission rates for postoperative complications.[8-10] With a growing evidence base linking transfusions with adverse clinical outcomes, a significant proportion of transfusions may be unwarranted.[11-13] In addition, the optimal use of blood components means not only avoiding overtransfusion or inappropriate transfusions but also making better transfusion decisions that would avoid undertransfusion.

To curtail inappropriate transfusions, several accreditation organizations have endorsed patient blood management (PBM) programs, which are based on multidisciplinary approaches to optimize the safety and outcomes in patients who are candidates for transfusion. By integrating evidence-based steps to reduce the probability of transfusions, PBM programs can reduce health-care costs while ensuring that blood components are available for patients who need them.[14]

However, successful implementation of a comprehensive PBM program requires the support of administrative and clinical leadership, who can remove obstacles to achieve interdepartmental consensus regarding existing gaps and goals of the program. This support is best achieved by developing a clear business case and enlisting clinical champions to highlight patient care benefits of the program. Central to this effort is the ability to audit transfusion practices and demonstrate measurable improvements in blood component utilization.[15] Furthermore, hospitals are required by accrediting agencies, such as The Joint Commission and AABB, to have blood utilization audit programs that monitor transfusions of all types of blood components.

Ira A. Shulman, MD, Director, USC Transfusion Medicine Services Group, Department of Pathology, University of Southern California, Los Angeles, California; Jay Hudgins, DO, Medical Director of Transfusion Medicine Services, Los Angeles County+USC Medical Center, Los Angeles, California; and Irina Maramica, MD, PhD, MBA, CLIA Laboratory Medical Director, Quest Diagnostics Nichols Institute, San Juan Capistrano, California
The authors have disclosed no conflicts of interest.

THE AUDITING PROCESS

Hospitals are allowed flexibility in designing the scope of the audit process; however, to satisfy this requirement, the review must be based on objective guidelines for assessing blood utilization and transfusion effectiveness. Institutional transfusion committees can provide oversight of PBM programs and take the first step in the development of the blood utilization review process by developing or adopting evidence-based guidelines for blood component use. This committee can also create auditing criteria for detecting outliers and targeting those practices requiring further evaluation. Audit criteria are designed to flag potentially inappropriate or questionable transfusion decisions. Such criteria are often institution-specific and may differ from clinical transfusion guidelines. However, the institutional guidelines are often based on national guidance. The 2013 AABB Blood Collection, Utilization, and Patient Blood Management Survey reported that the majority of hospitals (93%) use transfusion guidelines, most commonly developed by AABB (73%), the College of American Pathologists (32%), or the American Red Cross (12%).[16]

Monitoring of blood component ordering, transfusion, return, and wastage provides data for assessing an institution's transfusion efficiency.[17,18] Data must be collected, tabulated, and analyzed at regular, specified times. Blood utilization review ideally should be performed for all services that use blood, but the greatest impact of such a review is likely to be seen when auditing clinical services with high transfusion volumes (eg, surgery) and/or providing transfusion support to high-risk patients (eg, trauma victims, liver transplant recipients). Metrics reflecting the ordering and transfusion of all types of blood components used within the institution should form the basis for review of blood utilization. Data analysis should include trends in blood use throughout the institution, as well as by department; by patient population; by the protocol used, such as massive transfusion protocol (MTP); and by physician.

Data sources include electronic patient records, transfusion service records, and reports from the blood supplier(s). Clerical staff from the hospital's quality assurance department can be trained to process transfusion data and generate reports. Alternatively, with the help of the information systems department, hospitals can develop a blood transfusion dashboard to capture specific trends in transfusion practices and allow benchmarking with less effort and cost. These data should be further analyzed by members of the transfusion committee for inappropriate trends, with the goal of identifying areas for improvement. Aspects that may be useful for monitoring by the transfusion committee include the appropriateness of blood component ordering, specific quality indicators related to handling and dispensing blood components in both blood banks and satellite blood storage areas (including storage in or near the operating rooms), steps in blood component administration, and adverse events related to transfusions.[18,19] Metrics should also monitor undertransfusion of patients.[20] Hospital-based transfusion safety officers (TSOs) are used by some institutions. The TSO is a key person who supports the PBM program outside the laboratory through education, active surveillance of transfusion practices, and blood utilization review.[21]

In 2011, The Joint Commission published a performance measure set for PBM that focuses on transfusion appropriateness and clinical decision-making regarding blood component transfusion, as well as optimization of patient clinical status to reduce blood transfusion requirements.[22] Hospitals are encouraged to perform objective gap-analysis of Joint Commission PBM measures and identify areas for improvements.[23] AABB and The Joint Commission offer a joint PBM certification program that is based on the AABB *Standards for a Patient Blood Management Program (PBM Standards)*.[24,25] Certified programs are required to obtain and review at least quarterly (unless noted) the data summarized in Table 21-1.

In addition to any combined programs between AABB and The Joint Commission, institutions may adopt one or more of the following specific quality improvement objectives under the rubric of blood component stewardship:

- Promote reduced wastage of blood components that have been dispensed to the patient care area.
- Promote reduced wastage of blood components that are in the hospital inventory but never dispensed.
- Identify, develop, and promote the implementation of PBM to improve appropriate use of blood and blood components by health providers.
- Improve clinical outcomes and reduce the risk of adverse events from blood transfusion.

TABLE 21-1. Review Items Required by AABB and The Joint Commission for the PBM Certification Program

Data Review*
• Blood component use
• Blood component wastage and product expiration
• Crossmatch/transfusion (C/T) ratio
• Deviation from transfusion practices and protocols
• Transfusion reactions
• Intraoperative blood recovery use and quality control
• Informed consent for blood transfusion documentation
• Massive transfusion protocol effectiveness
• Blood infusion equipment and warmers maintenance program (annually)
• External assessment results (biannually)

*Quarterly except as noted.

DEFINING AUDIT CRITERIA

Before implementing an audit process, it is essential to define the criteria to which the audit should adhere. The *PBM Standards* provides a broad overview of areas to be monitored [eg, crossmatch/transfusion (C/T) ratio or MTP effectiveness] but the metrics mentioned are not necessarily the most effective ones to improve blood utilization. Programs like the joint certification program mentioned above provide a base by which an institution can begin the process of evaluating transfusion practices, and this process should be customized, either by expanding or narrowing criteria based on the practice at each medical center.

Defining an institution's audit criteria should, at a minimum, adhere to language similar to the previously mentioned quality improvement objectives for blood component stewardship, but the implementation of these recommendations must be institution specific. Other PBM program resources, such as the Patient Blood Management Guidelines from the National Blood Authority of Australia, give point-by-point recommendations for transfusion practices, covering MTPs, pediatrics, critical care, obstetrics, and perioperative care. Although these guidelines do not provide instruction on the optimal way to initiate auditing, they organize and present recommendations, practice points, and expert opinions based on a graded, evidence-based review in each area. Considering material in this manner can aid in the selection of areas for improvement at individual institutions.[26]

The impetus for PBM programs is primarily the improvement of patient outcomes, but they also aim to consistently and durably amend physician behaviors and improve adherence to guidelines.[27] Typically this is achieved by focusing on at least one of the following categories: education, feedback, cost awareness, rationing, or financial incentives. For the purposes of PBM, peer-to-peer education and feedback are likely to be the best options. From this point, the development and implementation of a multidisciplinary transfusion/blood utilization committee is the first and likely most important step to help define and develop institutional guidelines, by establishing physician champions who can support, defend, and help enforce guideline adherence at an institution.

In 2015, Yeh et al published the findings of their prospective interventional study that used a multimodal intervention as a strategy to reduce unnecessary transfusions in surgical intensive care unit (ICU) patients.[28] Authors used peer-to-peer feedback and monthly audits to increase adherence to restrictive transfusion guidelines defined in the TRICC trial. Specifically, during the 6-month intervention period, if a patient received transfusion outside of restrictive guidelines, the clinicians were notified by e-mail, and education from a surgical colleague was provided within 72 hours of the transfusion. They examined transfusion thresholds of hemoglobin levels greater than 8.0 g/dL and the rate of overtransfusion, defined as posttransfusion hemoglobin greater than 10.0 g/dL in the pre- and postintervention periods. As a result of these interventions, they saw a statistically significant decrease in both transfusions for hemoglobin greater than 8.0 g/dL (from 25% to 2%) and the rate of overtransfusion (from 11% to 3%). Monthly audits performed 6 months after the end of the intervention demonstrated durable improvements in the mean pretransfusion threshold and the overtransfusion rate. This study shows that peer-to-peer feedback, particularly when received from someone of the same subspecialty, can have a long-lasting effect on transfusion practices, which further highlights the need for diverse representation and participation with PBM.

Setting audit criteria is often a daunting process. Because of the specialized nature of medicine, each subspecialty often has specific guidelines to influence the way physicians conduct their practice. In contrast, transfusion/blood utilization committees often implement global transfusion guidelines for an institution, attempting to craft guidelines that would address the requirements of all clinical services in the hospital. These multidisciplinary committees may be better served by examining transfusion practices at their institutions and targeting certain areas, services, or specific documentation errors/omissions associated with transfusion. By narrowing focus, they limit the number of physicians, possibly address subspecialty-specif-

ic guidelines, and provide feedback based on subspecialty practices or appropriate documentation.

In 2017, Cauldwell et al performed a study to evaluate whether professional guidance promoting a policy of restrictive blood transfusion was being followed. They performed a retrospective analysis of postdelivery transfusion data from 17 maternity units in the United Kingdom and the United States from 1988 to 2000. They also performed an audit of women receiving transfusion at three centers 6 to 24 hours after delivery from 2013 to 2016. They found that in both time frames the rate of 2-unit transfusion in the postpartum period remained above 90%, though the median estimated blood loss remained the same between women who received 1 unit vs 2 units. In all institutions in the 2013-2016 period >85% of women receiving 2-unit transfusions had recorded pretransfusion hemoglobin >7.0 g/dL.[29] In this case, the findings for the obstetrics groups at these hospitals fall outside of accepted practice recommendations from the American College of Obstetricians and Gynecologists, which endorse the view of the American Board of Internal Medicine Foundation's Choosing Wisely Campaign that transfusion is not required if a patient is stable with a hemoglobin >7.0 g/dL.[30]

Another example of specialty-specific auditing was described by Lieberman and colleagues.[31] In this prospective study, they reviewed transfusions in the neonatal and pediatric ICU (NICU and PICU) populations, specifically in the use of plasma, cryoprecipitate, and recombinant Factor VIIa. The appropriateness of each order was independently evaluated using predefined transfusion criteria by two hematologists. The transfusion criteria for the use of plasma was developed based on a tool developed by Tinmouth et al,[32] while those for cryoprecipitate and recombinant Factor VIIa were developed by a team of five physicians trained in either transfusion medicine or hematology. They found that plasma was ordered as the fluid replacement in 7% of cases, to correct abnormal coagulation tests in 11% of cases, and for patients with minor or no bleeding in 46% of cases. Overall, they determined that 19% of plasma orders, 21% of cryoprecipitate orders, and 91%

of recombinant Factor VIIa orders were inappropriate. By performing an audit in this manner, they could identify areas of possible improvement that could be applied to a high-risk patient population.

When attempting to create audit criteria, prospective analysis of subspecialty practice can be an effective tool for change, particularly when physician "buy-in" is gained. In medical centers with many subspecialty practices, this approach may not be feasible because of the time or manpower necessary to perform the analysis. In such institutions, a more global approach may be needed that can overcome these limitations, such as harnessing automated electronic systems to monitor transfusion practices. One such system was described in 2006 by Grey and colleagues, who developed a system to electronically extract and collate large amounts of data from two laboratory information systems (LIS), ULTRA version 3.2 and TM, using standard information technology (IT) scripts.[33] The file from ULTRA captured hemoglobin values, and the file from the TM module extracted blood groups, antibody screens, crossmatches, and transfusion. Pre- and posttransfusion hemoglobin values were monitored 48 hours after the red cell transfusions. These data were imported into the MS ACCESS database, where they were linked with ICD-10 (International Classification of Diseases) clinical codes for surgical cases. This tool allowed monitoring of transfusion practices over an extended period, which helped define institution-specific transfusion guidelines and subsequently identified cases for peer review. In the years since this article was published, there have been advances in hospital electronic health records (EHRs) and LIS, and some information systems can serve as both clinical EHR and LIS. The use of an approach described here is predicated on having the resources available to develop these tools, but with the current goals of improving quality of care throughout medicine, it becomes more difficult to deny that methods such as these promote knowledge, transparency, and accountability in the era of data-driven quality assurance.

In defining audit criteria, institutions are not beholden to a homogenous approach to promoting adherence to transfusion guidelines. Until there is consensus, each hospital should examine its scope of practice to determine what guidelines are most appropriate for the patient population. Although several strategies can be employed to accomplish this goal, the following principles have emerged as integral to success:

- Identify resources that can provide basic metrics to initiate a PBM program.
- When forming a transfusion committee, identify physician champions from the clinical services to provide feedback while developing institutional guidelines.
- Make small changes at first and tailor toward a subspecialty practice.
- Employ a mechanism for feedback from a peer of the same subspecialty.
- When possible, use LIS/EHR systems to help guide the development of institution-specific guidelines and possibly automate the audit selection process.

TYPES OF BLOOD UTILIZATION REVIEW

AABB guidelines describe three methods of blood utilization review, which can be used individually or in combination depending on the institution's needs: prospective, concurrent, and retrospective.[18] Each method has advantages and shortcomings, which are summarized in Table 21-2.

Prospective Review

A prospective review of individual blood component orders occurs in real time before the component is distributed from the blood bank and immediately before transfusion. This proactive approach to blood utilization review provides an opportunity to intercept unnecessary transfusion and modify both component selection, as appropriate, and timing of administration. In academic institutions, a prospective review is often performed by clinical pathology residents under the supervision of a transfusion medicine physician. It requires vigilance by the blood bank staff to bring to the attention of residents all orders for blood components that fall outside established

TABLE 21-2. Types of Blood Utilization Review

Type of Review	Temporal Relation to Transfusion Event	Reviewer	Advantage	Disadvantage
Prospective	Real-time	• Residents • Medical director • Blood bank staff • CPOE	• Proactive • Improves patient care and saves blood in real time	• Labor-intensive • Potential to cause delays in issuing blood
Concurrent	Within 12-24 hours	• Residents • TSO	• Consultative opportunity • Training tool for residents	• Labor-intensive • Ineffective if no physician involvement
Retrospective internal	Days to weeks	• Quality assurance personnel • Medical director • Clinical peers	• Easiest approach • Provides data for trending and benchmarking	• Nonstandardized review • Difficult to use data for direct physician comparison
Retrospective external	Days to weeks	• Network of trained peer reviewers	• Objective, thorough, and standardized review • Produces directly comparable data	• Up-front expense that can be offset by savings in reduced blood usage

CPOE = computerized provider (physician) order entry; TSO = transfusion safety officer.

transfusion guidelines. Ideally, this review incorporates both laboratory values and clinical data obtained from patient records and/or direct communication with the clinical team. Prospective review improves patient care and saves blood components but is labor-intensive and can cause delays in situations requiring urgent transfusion support. Furthermore, increasing use of point-of-care testing in operating rooms allows clinicians to make real-time transfusion decisions based on results that are usually not available to transfusion services at the time of the request for blood components. Because of these considerations, most hospitals exempt the emergency department, labor and delivery departments, and operating rooms from a prospective review.

Examples of orders subject to prospective reviews include the following: requests for multiple doses of platelets without checking posttransfusion platelet counts in patients without acute hemorrhage, orders of inadequate doses of plasma components or cryoprecipitate, and orders for cytomegalovirus (CMV)-negative or irradiated components. In case of a disagreement between the ordering and reviewing physicians about the appropriateness of a blood order, the usual practice is to defer to ordering physicians, as they are more familiar with the patient's clinical condition, as long as the transfusion of the requested component does not have the potential for an immediate adverse effect on the patient. However, questionable blood component requests such as these may be subsequently referred to the transfusion committee for further review. Sometimes, the transfusion service physician may request additional testing to be performed before subsequent transfusions (eg, CMV testing for requests for CMV-negative blood).

Concurrent Review

The concurrent review process involves the review of transfusions administered within the previous 12 to 24 hours, thus avoiding the risk of delaying patient care. This allows the reviewer to judge the appropriateness of blood component use based on all pertinent laboratory and clinical data. If the transfusion episode appears to be out of line with good clinical practice, the review leads to an interaction with the transfusing clinician, who is still likely to remember events surrounding the transfusion. Concurrent review is a consultative opportunity, and the consultant should not be perceived as a gatekeeper. Rather, if properly conducted, this interaction can promote cooperative relationships between the transfusion service and medical staff, and influence transfusion practices.[19] Furthermore, performing these audits in academic institutions represents an excellent training tool for clinical pathology residents. Residents should be encouraged to document these reviews, evaluate them for efficacy, and present them in an educational format to other residents.

An example of a concurrent review that can result in consultative opportunity is a daily review of platelet transfusions along with pre- and posttransfusion platelet counts. In their audits of transfusion events that fall outside audit criteria for acceptable practice, residents should evaluate patient records for the presence of bleeding, deficiencies in platelet function, and the presence of medications known to affect platelet number or function. This review allows the identification of not only patients who may be receiving platelets outside of transfusion guidelines but also those who might be refractory.[34] Similarly, residents can perform plasma audits from daily reports that include pre- and posttransfusion prothrombin time/international normalized ratio (PT/INR) and activated partial thromboplastin time (aPTT) levels, using

evidence-based guidelines for plasma transfusion and evaluating additional information, such as the degree of abnormal result correction by plasma transfusion and the presence of drugs that may interfere with the coagulation system.[35,36] For example, cryoprecipitate audits can be based on fibrinogen levels, presence of bleeding, or Factor XIII deficiency.

However, in nonacademic institutions, if there is no TSO, a concurrent review might be too labor-intensive for the blood bank staff and allow only for review based on laboratory transfusion thresholds without the ability to evaluate the patient's clinical condition. Moreover, a concurrent review is effective only when the transfusion service physician or TSO is directly involved, resulting in a significant reduction in transfusions.[37-39] In contrast, concurrent review without physician involvement has failed to reduce blood usage.[40]

Retrospective Review

A retrospective review can be performed by those internal to, or external to, the organization. Such reviews are performed days to weeks following the transfusion event, usually at specified time intervals, using preset audit criteria that might differ from transfusion guidelines.

Internal Retrospective Review

Quality assurance personnel can perform the initial review. Cases that fall outside audit criteria can be referred to a transfusion medicine physician or a clinical peer of the physician whose transfusion decision is under review; this allows the closer evaluation to determine whether the patient's clinical condition justified the component request. This is the easiest approach to utilization review, providing valuable information about overall institutional transfusion practices and data for trending and benchmarking. However, one limitation of internal retrospective review is that patient data are often generated in a nonstandardized and inconsistent manner; thus, direct comparison of care provided by any two physicians can be difficult.

External Retrospective Review

This process uses an external third party that provides a network of trained physicians to serve as peer reviewers. Patient charts and transfusion decisions are evaluated using objective criteria in a thorough, critical, and standardized way, to produce directly comparable data. To be successful, it must allow review of all medical records, including all forms of paper and electronic data, and not require additional work on the part of the hospitals. Because a network of trained physicians provides the anonymous review of colleagues whose identity is blinded to the reviewers, the reviews are less likely to be biased; physicians often find it challenging to perform unbiased critical reviews of colleagues with whom they have social, economic, and political relationships.

Although retrospective reviews cannot change blood component usage in real time or effectively involve transfusing clinicians in the review process, they are excellent models of peer review.[19] They provide opportunities to mentor physicians on proper transfusion practices, such as correction of anemia, blood loss control, iron supplementation, evaluation of vital sign monitoring, and avoiding 2-unit transfusions without checking the response.[41] One effective indicator for retrospective monitoring of transfusion appropriateness is the transfusion recipient's discharge hemoglobin value.[42] Furthermore, if trends are identified in certain departments indicating frequent transfusion outside of transfusion guidelines, letters can be sent to clinicians and department heads, and representatives can be invited to transfusion committee meetings.

BLOOD UTILIZATION REVIEW OF TRANSFUSIONS TO HIGH-RISK PATIENTS

Uncontrolled hemorrhage requiring massive transfusion in patients with trauma or postpartum hemorrhage remains one of the leading causes of preventable death. It is now recognized that severe trauma-induced coagulopathy increases morbidity and mortality in these pa-tients and that early, aggressive, and ratio-based blood component resuscitation provides improved outcomes.[36] This is best achieved by protocol-driven care, now recommended by the National Partnership for Maternal Safety, National Institute for Health and Care Excellence policy, and Trauma Quality Improvement Program guidelines.[43,44] Development of MTPs that include point-of-care testing and hemostatic resuscitation requires careful planning and cooperation between various clinical teams, including surgery, anesthesia, and transfusion medicine. Review of transfusions is especially important in this high-risk patient population, as it offers an opportunity for continuous improvement of both the protocol and the delivery of care by the multidisciplinary team. Such reviews can yield important results as measured by improved patient outcomes and improved blood utilization. Because of the acuity of transfusion requirements, performing a prospective review of massive transfusions in real time can lead to delays in patient care and is often not feasible. This review is best achieved by concurrent or retrospective review of data on MTP availability, criteria for activation, timeliness of provision of components, and protocol effectiveness.[25,43,44]

THE ROLE OF A COMPUTERIZED PROVIDER ORDER ENTRY SYSTEM IN BLOOD UTILIZATION REVIEW

Application of health-care IT to transfusion medicine provides PBM programs with new tools for blood utilization review and for influencing physician ordering practices. Blood component order entry screens can incorporate clinical guidelines designed to guide physicians regarding the appropriateness of component orders.[45] Implementation of computerized provider order entry (CPOE) allows the creation of electronic reports that can be used for order auditing, assessment of blood utilization, and compliance monitoring.[5] In the 2013 AABB survey, 77.5% of institutions with transfusion guidelines incorporated them into paper or electronic order sets. Sixty-five percent reported that their CPOE system included transfusion guidelines. Of these, approximately half had guidelines with "hard stops," where the physician/provider must select a transfusion rationale before the order is accepted. Only 45.9% of these CPOE systems included an algorithm or clinical decision support to warn or alert the physician/provider when the blood component order is outside of guidelines. Most reporting hospitals (71.9%) required that a physician document the reason or clinical justification for transfusion in the medical record based on guidelines developed by the hospital transfusion or quality committee.[16]

In some hospitals, guidelines incorporated into the CPOE system do not result in hard stops, but rather, the indication for a blood component order is captured electronically and stored for later review. If the most recent laboratory value does not match the indication, an automatic message is provided to the clinician, requesting an indication for the "override." Component orders with overrides are collated electronically with other relevant information and are reviewed by transfusion committee members.

CPOE alone does not always improve blood use if only laboratory parameters are used for determining transfusion appropriateness, or if clinical users record inaccurate reasons for transfusion. Therefore, retrospective review remains important, even with CPOE, to evaluate transfusion appropriateness by reviewing clinical information. Additional functionality is achieved by incorporating a clinical decision support system (CDSS) into CPOE to guide transfusion ordering by providing clinicians with tailored treatment recommendations based on individual laboratory and clinical information, along with local transfusion guidelines.[1,46,47] For example, based on the clinical reason for transfusion selected by the clinician from a menu of choices, and the most recent laboratory values, the system could provide adaptive alerts, allowing the clinician to modify orders that do not fall within guidelines. This system is particularly useful if it requires physicians to enter the reason for overriding the system's recommendation. Subsequent analysis of reports, with reasons for the override, can be used to audit individual physician ordering practices. System-

atic reviews of the impact of an electronic CDSS found that it is a useful educational tool and its implementation improves RBC usage, increases provider compliance with guidelines, and results in cost savings.[48-50] Additional studies are needed to assess the effectiveness of the CDSS on ordering practices for other components and patient outcomes.[48,50]

USE OF "BIG DATA" TO ASSESS PERFORMANCE AND PROGRESS MEASURES IN TRANSFUSION MEDICINE

The advent of the EHR is opening up the field of "big data" in health care. Data collection and data mining through the linkage of different data sets within the EHR can provide a plethora of information, which can drive improvements in patient outcomes.[51,52] Examples of using big data in transfusion medicine are described below.

Benchmarking

Comparisons of blood usage between institutions and/or countries, performed with the aim of identifying best practices in transfusion medicine, were recently introduced.[53] Major challenges in developing meaningful benchmarking processes include defining best practices and developing cost-effective data collection methods. Often, hospitals do not have adequate IT support to develop data mining tools that enable transfusion services to collect uniform data across different hospitals. In the 2013 AABB survey, 41.9% of responding hospitals participated in performance benchmarking programs relating to transfusion medicine.[16]

Implementing benchmarking principles in transfusion medicine has improved practices on individual and organizational levels. Benchmarking can identify existing gaps that can become PBM program improvement targets and represents an instrument of learning, as it relies on communication, collaboration, and sharing of experiences. Benchmarking can identify opportunities for savings, which can be highlighted in presentations to hospital leadership. Furthermore, after the implementation of new practices, performance should be reevaluated, preferably by continuous data collection.

Three possible models of benchmarking in transfusion medicine have been described by Apelseth et al.[52] The ideal model according to these authors would be a regional benchmarking model, which requires a central coordinator who facilitates communication between institutions and manages the information flow to participants. In a sentinel model, data from a limited number of sites are collected into a central database, preferably by web-based reporting. This model is less costly and easier to implement and can be applied nationally and internationally. These two models gather information into a centralized database, whereas in a third, institutional model, all data are collected for the institution initiating the benchmarking process. The latter is least likely to succeed because it requires individual initiative, volunteer collaboration, and resources to be successful.

Benchmarking data can come from various sources, including medical record reviews, third-party gap assessments, blood bank inventory management, financial systems (eg, patient billing and budget), patient morbidity and mortality data, and observations or supportive statements from key stakeholders.[14] Several benchmarking databases exist that allow comparisons of PBM metrics with member hospitals nationwide or with other similarly sized hospitals.[53] Commonly used metrics are summarized in Table 21-3. In the 2013 AABB survey, the two most common metrics used by institutions to measure transfusion rate were 1) the total number of RBCs, platelets, and plasma units transfused (71.5%), and 2) the total number of components transfused (57.3%).[16] Other measures included the percentage of patients who received transfusion per hospital admission; the number of RBC units per transfusion recipient; transfused RBC units per 100 hospital admissions or discharges, per 1000 patient days, per adjusted patient days, or per adjusted or case mix index (CMI)-adjusted discharges; transfusions per surgical case; and transfusions per medical/surgical admission. For a meaningful comparison of transfusion rates between different institutions, it is important to use metrics that capture transfusions in both inpatient and outpatient settings; also, both the number of patients (eg, admissions or discharges) and

TABLE 21-3. PBM Metrics Used for Benchmarking

- Transfusion rate compared with that of comparably sized hospitals measured as one of the following:
  - Overall number of components transfused
  - Percentage of patients per admission who received transfusion
  - RBC units per transfusion recipient
  - Transfused RBC units per 100 hospital admissions or discharges
  - Transfused RBC units per 1000 patient days
  - Transfused RBC units per adjusted patient days
  - Transfused RBC units per adjusted or CMI-adjusted discharges
  - Transfusions per surgical case
  - Transfusions per medical/surgical admission

- Percentage of transfusions that fall outside of hospital or professional transfusion guidelines

---

- Transfusion administration compliance rates

- Reviews of wasted blood components

- Budget for transfusion services

RBC = Red Blood Cell; CMI = case mix index.

complexity of care (eg, CMI-adjusted discharges) affect the normalization of data for correlation between institutions.

Transfusion benchmarking described in the 2014-2015 AABB survey is another example of the sentinel model.[54] This benchmark report collated data sourced from 435 hospitals responding to the blood utilization survey. Hospitals were stratified into eight categories based on their 2014-2015 annual patient surgical volume. Transfusion and blood component expiration data were presented for each component as mean and median values for all categories. Using this report, hospitals can compare their data to other hospitals with similar annual inpatient surgical volumes. Benchmarking can contribute to evidence-based guidelines, especially when randomized controlled trials may be difficult or costly to perform. Examples of countries that reduced blood utilization using national PBM and benchmarking programs include Finland, Scotland, Spain, the Netherlands, Germany, the United Kingdom, Canada, and Australia.

Active Surveillance of Transfusion-Related Complications

An example of active surveillance of transfusion-related complications is searching large Medicare databases and linking the procedure code for transfusion with diagnostic codes to determine the rate of a recognized complication such as posttransfusion purpura, or using an automated electronic algorithm to detect transfusion-associated circulatory overload or transfusion-related acute lung injury and linking this to the transfusion episode.[51,55] Transfusion reaction tracking can help identify underrecognition or underreporting of transfusion-related adverse events. Once a problem is identified, education can be developed and implemented to improve staff knowledge and compliance with reporting of adverse events.[14]

Monitoring Patterns of Blood Use by Procedure over Time

Linking transfusion episode data with diagnostic and procedure codes allows monitoring of transfusion rates for specific types of cases (eg, hip replacement, cardiac surgery). These rates can be compared to national data or data in the literature. In the AABB survey, some hospitals reported using the percentage of patients who received transfusion per selected diagnosis code (eg, ICD-10), or average blood component use per surgical case category (eg, coronary artery bypass graft only or knee/hip replacement).[16]

Definition of Blood Order Schedules

A maximum surgical blood order schedule (MSBOS) for surgery can be developed by using data held within the anesthesia information management system.[56] Creating a data-driven MSBOS is useful in optimizing transfusion-ordering practices.[57] One metric used for assessing and benchmarking transfusion ordering practices is the C/T ratio, which may indicate overordering of crossmatched blood compared to actual transfusion when the ratio exceeds 2.0.[58] Duplicate type-and-screen procedures and unnecessary crossmatches for patients undergoing elective surgical procedures can be wasteful of transfusion service resources.[59] However, it is important to emphasize that should a patient have an active order for type and screen but be brought to the operating room for elective surgery before completing the ordered testing, such a practice could present both potential safety and quality issues in transfusion medicine.

KEY POINTS

1. Data-driven and multidisciplinary blood utilization auditing are central to establishing successful institutional and national evidence-based PBM programs.
2. Optimizing blood transfusions requires comprehensive review not only of transfusion appropriateness but also of processes for ensuring patient safety, best patient outcomes, and blood component stewardship.

3. Transfusion auditing can be performed as a prospective, concurrent, or retrospective review. Retrospective reviews may use either internal or external resources.

4. Different metrics have evolved over time to assess various aspects of transfusions and allow benchmarking of transfusion practices at different levels.

5. Various national organizations have developed educational resources and campaigns to promote the wise use of blood components. AABB and The Joint Commission, for example, have joined forces to produce a PBM certification program. These tools enable physicians to eliminate unnecessary blood transfusions and optimize transfusions in high-risk patients while reducing health-care costs and improving patient outcomes.

REFERENCES

1. Goodnough LT, Shah N. The next chapter in patient blood management: Real-time clinical decision support. Am J Clin Pathol 2014;142:741-7.

2. Morton J, Anastassopoulos KP, Patel ST, et al. Frequency and outcomes of blood products transfusion across procedures and clinical conditions warranting inpatient care: An analysis of the 2004 healthcare cost and utilization project nationwide inpatient sample database. Am J Med Qual 2010;25:289-96.

3. Ferraris VA, Davenport DL, Saha SP, et al. Surgical outcomes and transfusion of minimal amounts of blood in the operating room. Arch Surg 2012;147:49-55.

4. Carson JL, Carless PA, Hébert PC. Outcomes using lower vs higher hemoglobin thresholds for red blood cell transfusion. JAMA 2013;309:83-4.

5. Goodnough LT, Shah N. Is there a "magic" hemoglobin number? Clinical decision support promoting restrictive blood transfusion practices. Am J Hematol 2015;90:927-33.

6. Hébert PC, Wells G, Blajchman MA, et al. A multicenter, randomized, controlled clinical trial of transfusion requirements in critical care. Transfusion requirements in critical care investigators, Canadian Critical Care Trials Group. N Engl J Med 1999;340:409-17.

7. Carson JL, Brooks MM, Abbott JD, et al. Liberal or restrictive transfusion in high-risk patients after hip surgery. N Engl J Med 2011;365:2453-62.

8. Salpeter SR, Buckley JS, Chatterjee S. Impact of more restrictive blood transfusion strategies on clinical outcomes: A meta-analysis and systematic review. Am J Med 2014;127:124-31.

9. Goodnough LT, Maggio P, Hadhazy E, et al. Restrictive blood transfusion practices are associated with improved patient outcomes. Transfusion 2014;54(Pt 2):2753-9.

10. Rohde JM, Dimcheff DE, Blumberg N, et al. Health care-associated infection after red blood cell transfusion: A systematic review and meta-analysis. JAMA 2014;311:1317-26.

11. Goodnough LT, Verbrugge D, Vizmeg K, Riddell J. Identifying elective orthopedic surgical patients transfused with amounts of blood in excess of need: The transfusion trigger revisited. Transfusion 1992;32:648-53.

12. Shander A, Fink A, Javidroozi M, et al. Appropriateness of allogeneic red blood cell transfusion: The international consensus conference on transfusion outcomes. Transfus Med Rev 2011;25:232-46.

13. Spahn DR, Shander A, Hofmann A. The chiasm: Transfusion practice versus patient blood management. Best Pract Res Clin Anaesthesiol 2013;27:37-42.

14. Building a better patient blood management program: Identifying tools, solving problems and promoting patient safety (white paper). Bethesda, MD: AABB, 2015. [Available at http://www.aabb.org/pbm/Documents/AABB-PBM-Whitepaper.pdf (accessed December 1, 2019).]

15. Murphy MF, Yazer MH. Measuring and monitoring blood utilization. Transfusion 2013;53:3025-8.

16. Whitaker BI, Rajbhandary S, Harris A. The 2013 AABB blood collection, utilization, and patient blood management survey report. Bethesda, MD: AABB, 2015. [Available at http://www.aabb.org/research/hemovigilance/bloodsurvey/Pages/default.aspx (accessed December 1, 2019).]

17. Wagner J, AuBuchon JP, Saxena S, Shulman IA, for the Clinical Transfusion Medicine Committee. Guidelines for the quality assessment of transfusion. Bethesda, MD: AABB, 2006.

18. Becker J, Shaz B, for the Clinical Transfusion Medicine Committee and the Transfusion Medi-

cine Section Coordinating Committee. Guidelines for patient blood management and blood utilization. Bethesda, MD: AABB, 2011.

19. Saxena S, ed. The transfusion committee: Putting patient safety first. 2nd ed. Bethesda, MD: AABB Press, 2013.

20. Mair B, Agosti SJ, Foulis PR, et al. Monitoring for undertransfusion. Transfusion 1996;36:533-5.

21. Dunbar NM, Szczepiorkowski ZM. How do we utilize a transfusion safety officer? Transfusion 2015;55:2064-8.

22. Implementation guide for The Joint Commission Patient Blood Management Performance Measures 2011. Oakbrook Terrace, IL: The Joint Commission, 2011. [Available at https://www.jointcommission.org/assets/1/6/pbm_implementation_guide_20110624.pdf (accessed December 12, 2019).]

23. De Leon EM, Szallasi A. "Transfusion indication RBC (PBM-02)": Gap analysis of a Joint Commission Patient Blood Management Performance Measure at a community hospital. Blood Transfus 2014;12(Suppl 1):187-90.

24. Frey K, ed. Standards for a patient blood management program. 3rd ed. Bethesda, MD: AABB, 2020.

25. AABB, The Joint Commission. Patient blood management certification review process guide for health care organizations 2017. Oakbrook Terrace, IL: The Joint Commission, 2017. [Available at https://www.jointcommission.org/assets/1/18/2017_PBM_Org_RPG.pdf (accessed December 1, 2019).]

26. National Blood Authority Australia. Patient blood management guidelines. Canberra, Australia: National Blood Authority, 2019. [Available at https://www.blood.gov.au/pbm-guidelines (accessed December 1, 2019).]

27. Smith WR. Evidence for the effectiveness of techniques to change physician behavior. Chest 2000;118(2 Suppl):8SY17S.

28. Yeh DD, Naraghi L, Larentzakis A, et al. Peer-to-peer physician feedback improves adherence to blood transfusion guidelines in the surgical intensive care unit. J Trauma Acute Care Surg 2015;79:65-70.

29. Cauldwell M, Shamshirasz A, Wong TY, et al. Retrospective surveys of obstetric red cell transfusion practice in the UK and USA. Int J Gyenecol Obstet 2017;139:342-5.

30. Choosing Wisely. Washington, DC: American College of Obstetricians and Gynecologists, 2019. [Available at https://www.acog.org/About_ACOG/ACOG_Departments/Patient_Safety_and_Quality_Improvement/Choosing_Wisely (accessed December 1, 2019).]

31. Lieberman L, Lin Y, Cserti-Gazdewich C, et al, for the QUEST—Quality in Utilization Education and Safety in Transfusion—Research Collaborative. Utilization of frozen plasma, cryoprecipitate, and recombinant factor VIIa for children with hemostatic impairments: An audit of transfusion appropriateness. Pediatr Blood Cancer 2018;65(4).

32. Tinmouth A, Thompson T, Arnold DM, et al. Utilization of frozen plasma in Ontario: A province wide audit reveals a high rate of inappropriate transfusions. Transfusion 2013;53(10):2222-9.

33. Grey DE, Smith V, Villanueva G, et al. The utility of an automated electronic system to monitor and audit transfusion practice. Vox Sang 2006:90;316-24.

34. Kaufman RM, Djulbegovic B, Gernsheimer T, et al. Platelet transfusion: A clinical practice guideline from the AABB. Ann Intern Med 2015;162:205-13.

35. Roback JD, Caldwell S, Carson J, et al. Evidence-based practice guidelines for plasma transfusion. Transfusion 2010;50:1227-39.

36. Murad MH, Slubbs JR, Gandhi MJ, et al. The effect of plasma transfusion on morbidity and mortality: A systematic review and meta-analysis. Transfusion 2010;50:1370-83.

37. Silver H, Tahha HR, Anderson J, et al. A non-computer-dependent prospective review of blood and blood component utilization. Transfusion 1992;32:260-5.

38. Simpson MB. Prospective-concurrent audits and medical consultation for platelet transfusions. Transfusion 1987;27:192-5.

39. Hawkins TE, Carter JM, Hunter PM. Can mandatory pretransfusion approval programmes be improved? Transfus Med 1994;4:45-50.

40. Lam HT, Schweitzer SO, Petz L, et al. Effectiveness of a prospective physician self-audit transfusion-monitoring system. Transfusion 1997;37:577-84.

41. Paone G, Brewer R, Likosky DS, et al. Transfusion rate as a quality metric: Is blood conservation a learnable skill? Ann Thorac Surg 2013;96:1279-86.

42. Edwards J, Morrison C, Mohluddin M, et al. Patient blood transfusion management: Discharge hemoglobin level as a surrogate marker for red blood cell utilization appropriateness. Transfusion 2012;52:2445-51.

43. Stephens CT, Gumbert S, Holcomb JB. Trauma-associated bleeding: Management of massive transfusion. Curr Opin Anaesthesiol 2016;29:250-5.

44. Kacmar RM, Mhyre JM, Scavone BM, et al. The use of postpartum hemorrhage protocols in United States academic obstetric anesthesia units. Anesth Analg 2014;119:906-10.

45. Dzik S. Use of a computer-assisted system for blood utilization review. Transfusion 2007;47(2 Suppl):142S-4S.

46. Goodnough LT, Shieh L, Hadhazy E, et al. Improved blood utilization using real-time clinical decision support. Transfusion 2014;54:1358-65.

47. Rothschild JM, McGurk S, Honour M, et al. Assessment of education and computerized decision support interventions for improving transfusion practice. Transfusion 2007;47:228-39.

48. Hibbs SP, Nielsen ND, Brunskill S, et al. The impact of electronic decision support on transfusion practice: A systematic review. Transfus Med Rev 2015;29:14-23.

49. Cohn CS, Welbig J, Bowman R, et al. A data-driven approach to patient blood management. Transfusion 2014;54:316-22.

50. Dunbar NM, Szczepiorkowski ZM. Hardwiring patient blood management: Harnessing information technology to optimize transfusion practice. Curr Opin Hematol 2014;21:515-20.

51. Pendry K. The use of big data in transfusion medicine. Transfus Med 2015;25:129-37.

52. Apelseth TO, Molnar L, Arnold E, Heddle NM. Benchmarking: Applications to transfusion medicine. Transfus Med Rev 2012;26:321-32.

53. Carson JL, Guyatt G, Heddle NM, et al. Clinical practice guidelines from the AABB: Red blood cell transfusion thresholds and storage. JAMA 2016;316:2025-35.

54. Rajbhandary S, Whitaker B, Perez GE. The 2014-2015 AABB blood collection and utilization survey report. Bethesda, MD: AABB, 2018. [Available at http://www.aabb.org/research/hemovigilance/bloodsurvey/Pages/default.aspx (accessed December 1, 2019).]

55. Clifford L, Singh A, Wilson GA, Toy P. Electronic health record surveillance algorithms facilitate the detection of transfusion-related pulmonary complications. Transfusion 2013;53:1205-16.

56. Frank SM, Rothschild JA, Masear CG, Rivers RJ. Optimizing preoperative blood ordering with data acquired from an anesthesia information management system. Anesthesiology 2013;118:1286-97.

57. Cheng CK, Trethewey D, Brousseau P, Sadek I. Creation of a maximum surgical blood ordering schedule via novel low-overhead database method. Transfusion 2008;48:2268-9.

58. Dexter F, Ledolter J, Davis E, Witkowski TA. Systematic criteria for type and screen based on procedure's probability of erythrocyte transfusion. Anesthesiology 2012;116:768-78.

59. Compton ML, Szklarski PC, Booth G. Duplicate type and screen testing: Waste in the clinical laboratory. Arch Pathol Lab Med 2018;142:358-63.

CHAPTER 22

Noninfectious Complications of Blood Transfusion

Eldad A. Hod, MD, and Richard O. Francis, MD, PhD

STATISTICALLY, THE GREATEST RISK OF morbidity and mortality from transfusion is from the noninfectious complications. In fact, transfusion-associated circulatory overload (TACO), transfusion-related acute lung injury (TRALI), and hemolytic transfusion reactions (HTRs) are the three most commonly reported causes of transfusion-related mortality.[1]

HEMOVIGILANCE

Hemovigilance involves systematic surveillance for the complications of transfusion, analysis of these data, and subsequent data-driven improvements in transfusion practices. One of the main purposes of a hemovigilance program is to improve reporting of transfusion-related adverse events. It is widely believed that the major noninfectious complications are both underrecognized and underreported.

The National Healthcare Safety Network Hemovigilance Module was created via a collaboration between government and nongovernment organizations to implement a national surveillance of transfusion-related adverse events aimed at improving patient safety. Definitions and classification schemes are detailed in the appendices of the Hemovigilance Module Surveillance Protocol.[2]

RECOGNITION AND EVALUATION OF A SUSPECTED TRANSFUSION REACTION

Identification of a Transfusion Reaction

As with many medical therapies, adverse effects of transfusion usually cannot be accurately predicted or the risks completely avoided. Transfusing clinicians should be aware of such risks when discussing the need for transfusion with a patient. Informed consent for transfusion may include a discussion of the risks of infectious disease and serious noninfectious complications, such as TACO, TRALI, and HTRs. Furthermore, medical staff administering blood components should be well aware of the signs and symptoms of possible reactions. Staff should be prepared to mitigate any immediate episodes through appropriate procedures as well as to prevent future similar reactions whenever possible.

Many common clinical signs and symptoms are associated with more than one type of adverse reaction. (See Table 22-1.) Early recognition, prompt cessation of the transfusion, and further evaluation are key to a successful outcome. The signs and symptoms that may be

Eldad A. Hod, MD, Associate Professor; and Richard O. Francis, MD, PhD, Assistant Professor, Department of Pathology and Cell Biology, Columbia University Medical Center, New York, New York
The authors have disclosed no conflicts of interest.

TABLE 22-1. Categories of Adverse Transfusion Reactions and Their Management*

Type	Incidence[†]	Etiology	Presentation	Diagnostic Testing	Therapeutic/Prophylactic Approaches[‡]
Acute (<24 hours) Transfusion Reactions—Immunologic					
Hemolytic	ABO/Rh mismatch: 1:40,000 AHTR: 1:76,000 Fatal HTR: 1:1.8 million	Red cell incompatibility	Chills, fever, hemoglobinuria, hypotension, renal failure with oliguria, hemorrhage (DIC), back pain, pain along infusion vein, anxiety	Clerical check DAT Visual inspection (free Hb) Repeat patient ABO, pre- and posttransfusion sample Further tests as indicated to define possible incompatibility Further tests as indicated to detect hemolysis (LDH, bilirubin, etc)	Stop transfusion Keep urine output >1 mL/kg/hr with fluids and IV diuretic Analgesics Pressors for hypotension Hemostatic components (platelets, cryoprecipitate, or plasma) for bleeding
Febrile, nonhemolytic	0.1% to 1% with universal leukocyte reduction	Accumulated cytokines in platelet unit Antibody to donor WBCs	Fever, chills/rigors, headache, vomiting	Rule out hemolysis (DAT, inspect for hemoglobinemia, repeat patient ABO) Rule out bacterial contamination HLA antibody screen	Leukocyte-reduced blood Antipyretic premedication (acetaminophen, no aspirin) Washed cellular components if severe
Urticarial	1:100-1:33 (1%-3%)	Antibody to donor plasma proteins	Urticaria, pruritis, flushing, angioedema	None	Antihistamine In some cases after stopping transfusion, unit may be restarted slowly after antihistamine if symptoms resolve

Anaphylactic	1:20,000-1:50,000	Usually idiopathic and idiosyncratic Rarely, antibody to donor plasma proteins (includes IgA, haptoglobin, C4)	Hypotension, urticaria, angioedema, bronchospasm, stridor, abdominal pain	In appropriate setting, IgA and haptoglobin concentrations, anti-IgA, serum IgE concentrations if passively transfused	Stop transfusion IV fluids Epinephrine Antihistamines, corticosteroids, beta-2 agonists Modified components (eg, washed RBCs and platelets, SD plasma, IgA-deficient blood components if indicated)
TRALI	1:1200-1:190,000	WBC antibodies in donor (occasionally in recipient), other WBC-activating agents in components	Hypoxemia, respiratory failure, hypotension, fever, bilateral pulmonary edema	Rule out hemolysis (DAT, inspect for hemoglobinemia, repeat patient ABO) Rule out cardiogenic pulmonary edema HLA, HNA typing Anti-HLA, anti-HNA antibody screening Chest x-ray	Supportive care until recovery Deferral of implicated donors

Acute (<24 hours) Transfusion Reactions—Nonimmunologic

Transfusion-related sepsis	Varies by component (see Chapter 7 for discussion of platelets)	Bacterial contamination	Fever, chills, hypotension	Gram stain Culture of component Patient culture Rule out hemolysis (DAT, inspect for hemoglobinemia, repeat patient ABO)	Broad-spectrum antibiotics

(Continued)

TABLE 22-1. Categories of Adverse Transfusion Reactions and Their Management* (Continued)

Type	Incidence[†]	Etiology	Presentation	Diagnostic Testing	Therapeutic/Prophylactic Approaches[‡]
Hypotension associated with ACE inhibition	Dependent on clinical setting	Inhibited metabolism of bradykinin with infusion of bradykinin (negatively charged filters) or activators of prekallikrein	Flushing, hypotension	Rule out hemolysis (DAT, inspect for hemoglobinemia, repeat patient ABO)	Withdraw ACE inhibition Avoid albumin volume replacement for plasmapheresis Avoid bedside leukocyte filtration
Circulatory overload	1%	Volume overload	Dyspnea, orthopnea, cough, tachycardia, hypertension, headache	Chest x-ray Rule out TRALI	Upright posture Oxygen IV diuretic Phlebotomy (250-mL increments)
Nonimmune hemolysis	Rare	Physical or chemical destruction of blood (heating, freezing, hemolytic drug or solution added to blood)	Hemoglobinuria, hemoglobinemia	Rule out patient hemolysis (DAT, inspect for hemoglobinemia, repeat patient ABO) Test unit for hemolysis	Identify and eliminate cause if related to blood administration
Air embolus	Rare	Air infusion via line	Sudden shortness of breath, acute cyanosis, pain, cough, hypotension, cardiac arrhythmia	X-ray for intravascular air	Place patient on left side with legs elevated above chest and head

Hypocalcemia (ionized calcium; citrate toxicity)	Dependent on clinical setting	Rapid citrate infusion (massive transfusion of citrated blood, delayed metabolism of citrate, apheresis procedures)	Paresthesia, tetany, arrhythmia	Ionized calcium; Prolonged Q-T interval on electrocardiogram	Pause/reduce transfusion rate; Calcium supplementation
Hypothermia	Dependent on clinical setting	Rapid infusion of cold blood	Cardiac arrhythmia	Central body temperature	Employ blood warmer
Delayed (>24 hours) Transfusion Reactions—Immunologic					
Alloimmunization, red cell antigens	1:100 (1%)	Immune response to foreign antigens on red cells	Positive blood group antibody screening test, delayed serologic or hemolytic transfusion reaction, HDFN (maternal alloimmunization)	Antibody screen; DAT	Avoid unnecessary transfusions
Alloimmunization, HLA antigens	1:10 (10%)	WBCs and platelets (HLA)	Platelet refractoriness	Platelet antibody screen; HLA antibody screen	Avoid unnecessary transfusions; Leukocyte-reduced blood
Hemolytic	1:2500-11,000	Anamnestic immune response to red cell antigens	Fever, decreasing hemoglobin, new positive antibody screening test, mild jaundice	Antibody screen; DAT; Tests for hemolysis (visual inspection for hemoglobinemia, LDH, bilirubin, urinary hemosiderin as clinically indicated)	Identify antibody; Transfuse compatible RBCs as needed

(Continued)

TABLE 22-1. Categories of Adverse Transfusion Reactions and Their Management* (Continued)

Type	Incidence[†]	Etiology	Presentation	Diagnostic Testing	Therapeutic/Prophylactic Approaches[‡]
Graft-vs-host disease	Rare	Donor lymphocytes engraft in recipient and mount attack on host tissues	Erythroderma, vomiting, diarrhea, hepatitis, pancytopenia, fever	Skin biopsy HLA typing Molecular analysis for chimerism	Immunosuppression Irradiation, pathogen reduction, or other approved methods for blood components for patients at risk (including components from related donors and HLA-selected components)
Posttransfusion purpura	Rare	Recipient platelet antibodies (apparent alloantibody, usually anti-HPA-1a) destroy autologous platelets	Thrombocytopenic purpura, bleeding 8-10 days after transfusion	Platelet antibody screen and identification	IVIG HPA-1a-negative platelets Plasmapheresis

Delayed (>24 hours) Transfusion Reactions—Nonimmunologic

Type	Incidence[†]	Etiology	Presentation	Diagnostic Testing	Therapeutic/Prophylactic Approaches[‡]
Iron overload	After ≥20 RBC units	Multiple transfusions with obligate iron load in transfusion-dependent patient	Diabetes, cirrhosis, cardiomyopathy	Liver and cardiac iron concentration (MRI) Serum ferritin Liver enzymes Endocrine function tests	Iron chelators

*For platelet refractoriness, see Chapters 15 and 19; for septic transfusion reactions, see Chapter 7.
[†]Risk estimates may vary depending on study parameters. Readers are advised to carefully consult the literature.
[‡]For all acute reactions, the transfusion should be stopped to allow investigation, as explained in the text. The approaches listed do not represent comprehensive treatment recommendations.
AHTR = acute hemolytic transfusion reaction; HTR = hemolytic transfusion reaction; DIC = disseminated intravascular coagulation; DAT = direct antiglobulin test; Hb = hemoglobin; LDH = lactate dehydrogenase; IV = intravenous; WBCs = white blood cells; IgA = immunoglobulin A; RBCs = Red Blood Cells; SD plasma = solvent/detergent-treated plasma; TRALI = transfusion-related acute lung injury; HNA = human neutrophil antigen; ACE = angiotensin-converting enzyme; HDFN = hemolytic disease of the fetus and newborn; HPA = human platelet antigen; IVIG = intravenous immune globulin; MRI = magnetic resonance imaging.

indicators of a transfusion reaction include the following:

- Fever, generally defined as a ≥ 1 C rise in temperature to ≥ 38 C (the most common sign of an acute HTR).
- Chills with or without rigors.
- Respiratory distress, including wheezing, coughing, hypoxia, and dyspnea.
- Hyper- or hypotension.
- Abdominal, chest, flank, or back pain.
- Pain at the infusion site.
- Skin manifestations, including rash, flushing, urticaria, pruritus, and localized edema.
- Jaundice or hemoglobinuria.
- Nausea/vomiting.
- Abnormal bleeding.
- Oliguria/anuria.

Clinical Evaluation and Management of a Transfusion Reaction

The evaluation of a suspected transfusion reaction involves a two-pronged investigation combining clinical evaluation of the patient with laboratory verification and testing. The clinical team should discontinue the transfusion of the implicated component, and contact the blood bank for directions on the investigation. When an acute transfusion reaction is suspected, several steps must be taken immediately (below).

Patient-Focused Steps

1. Stop the transfusion immediately but keep the line open with normal saline, and preserve any residual component and the infusion set for further evaluation.
2. Document the clerical recheck between the patient and the component. The labels on the component, on patient records, and on patient identification should be examined for identification errors. Transfusing facilities may require repeat ABO and Rh typing of the patient using a new sample.
3. Consult the clinical team for a plan of care.
4. Identify the appropriate additional diagnostic tests to work up the case.

Component-Focused Steps

1. Contact the transfusion service for directions on investigating and documenting the potential causes of the reaction.
2. Obtain instructions concerning the return of any remaining component, associated intravenous fluid bags, and tubing.
3. The transfusion service determines whether the blood donor center should be notified of the acute transfusion reaction. The Food and Drug Administration (FDA) requires reporting to the blood center when the component is at fault for causing the reaction (eg, suspected problem with labeling or manufacturing or suspected bacterial contamination of the component). The FDA must be notified "as soon as possible" when a complication of transfusion is confirmed to be fatal [*Code of Federal Regulations* (CFR) Title 21, Part 606.170(b)].

Standard Laboratory Investigation of a Transfusion Reaction

When the laboratory receives notice of a possible transfusion reaction, the technologist should perform several steps:

1. Request return of any remaining component, associated intravenous fluid bags, and tubing for possible bacteria culture or Gram staining.
2. Request collection of a posttransfusion blood sample.
3. Perform a clerical check of the component bag, label, paperwork, and patient sample.
4. Repeat ABO testing on the posttransfusion sample.
5. Perform a visual check of pre- and posttransfusion samples for evidence of hemolysis (which may not be visible if <50 mg/dL of hemoglobin is present).
6. Perform a direct antiglobulin test (DAT) on a posttransfusion sample.
7. Report findings to the blood bank supervisor or transfusion service medical staff, who may

request additional studies or tests, request quarantine of co-components generated from the same donor collection, or impose transfusion restrictions/instructions.

The transfusion service must retain any patient records that are related to transfusion reactions, clinically significant antibodies, or special transfusion requirements. Transfusion services are able to share medical information on patient transfusion history. When a patient is cared for by different transfusion services, medical warning bracelets or wallet identification cards may benefit patients with red cell alloantibodies.

Specialized Laboratory Investigations for Selected Reactions

Additional laboratory evaluation may be required for investigations of some nonhemolytic transfusion reactions, such as anaphylaxis, sepsis, or TRALI, as described in their respective sections below.

ACUTE OR IMMEDIATE TRANSFUSION REACTIONS

Acute or immediate transfusion reactions occur within 24 hours of the administration of a component and often during the transfusion. Acute transfusion reactions include immune and nonimmune-mediated hemolysis, transfusion-related sepsis, TRALI, allergic reactions, TACO, sequelae of massive transfusion, air embolism, hypotensive reactions, febrile nonhemolytic transfusion reactions (FNHTRs), and hypothermia. The clinical significance of an acute transfusion reaction often cannot be determined by the patient's clinical history or signs and symptoms alone but requires laboratory evaluation.

Immune-Mediated Acute Hemolytic Transfusion Reactions

Presentation

Rapid hemolysis of as little as 10 mL of incompatible blood can produce symptoms of acute HTR (AHTR). The most common presenting symptom is fever with or without accompanying chills or rigors. A patient with a mild reaction may have abdominal, chest, flank, or back pain. If a patient has a severe AHTR, hypotension, dyspnea, and flank pain may be present and, in some cases, progress to shock with or without accompanying disseminated intravascular coagulation (DIC). Red or dark urine may be the first sign of intravascular hemolysis, particularly in an anesthetized or unconscious patient, who may also present with oliguria or, in rare cases, DIC. The severity of the symptoms of this reaction is related to the amount of incompatible blood transfused, antigen density, and antibody characteristics (eg, concentration, class, subclass). Prompt recognition of the reaction and immediate cessation of the transfusion can prevent grave consequences.

Differential Diagnosis

Many of the signs and symptoms of an immune-mediated AHTR also occur in other acute transfusion reactions. Fever with or without chills and accompanied by hypotension may also develop in transfusion-related sepsis and TRALI. However, hemolysis is not associated with TRALI, and respiratory difficulty is not typically a symptom of AHTRs. Fever or chills are more commonly caused by an FNHTR but cannot be distinguished initially from the more serious AHTR without an assessment of hemolysis. The patient's underlying disease process can also make the diagnosis of an AHTR difficult. Acute hemolysis may result from nonimmune mechanisms, as described in the "Nonimmune-Mediated Hemolysis" section below.

Pathophysiology

The interaction of preformed antibodies with red cell antigens is the immunologic basis for AHTRs. The most severe reactions are associated with transfusions of red cells that are ABO incompatible with the recipient, resulting in acute intravascular destruction of the transfused cells. Transfusion of ABO-incompatible antibodies, as can happen with minor-incompatible apheresis platelets or intravenous immune globulin (IVIG) infusion, may also cause hemolysis. The most common circumstance for hemolysis following platelet transfusion is when group O platelets from donors with high titers of anti-A are transfused to group A recipients.[3] Although these forms of acute hemolysis are not usually clinically significant or characterized by typical hemolytic symptoms, they can be severe if the transfused components have high titers of ABO antibodies. It should be noted that there are cases of hemolysis with low-titer antibodies, and that not all high-titer antibodies result in hemolysis, suggesting that donor/recipient characteristics may influence hemolysis risk.

When preformed immunoglobulin M (IgM) or IgG antibodies recognize corresponding red cell antigens, complement activation may occur, resulting in intravascular hemolysis, hemoglobinemia, and hemoglobinuria. IgM antibodies are strong activators of complement, and IgG antibodies, when present at sufficient concentrations and of the relevant subclass, may activate complement as well.

Complement activation involves C3 cleavage with the ensuing production of C3a, an anaphylatoxin that is released into the plasma, and C3b, which coats the red cells. If complement activation proceeds to completion, membrane attack complexes are assembled on the red cell surface, and intravascular lysis occurs. C5a, an anaphylatoxin that is 100 times more potent than C3a, is produced as part of this hemolysis. C3a and C5a promote the release of histamine and serotonin from mast cells, leading to vasodilation and smooth-muscle contraction, particularly of bronchial and intestinal muscles. C3a and C5a are recognized by many other cell types and are involved in the production and release of cytokines, leukotrienes, free radicals, and nitric oxide.[4] The end result may include wheezing, flushing, chest pain or tightness, and gastrointestinal symptoms. These symptoms may also be caused by release of bradykinin and norepinephrine resulting from antigen-antibody complex stimulation.

If complement activation does not proceed to completion, which is usually the case with non-ABO antibodies, the red cells can undergo extravascular hemolysis, where cells coated with C3b and/or IgG are rapidly removed from the circulation by phagocytes.[5] In extravascular hemolysis, the consequences of complement activation, including release of anaphylatoxins and opsonization of red cells, may still have adverse effects. Furthermore, it has been demonstrated in a hemolytic transfusion reaction mouse model that extravascular hemolysis can lead to cytokine release, which may play a role in producing the effects of acute hemolysis.[6]

Coagulation abnormalities that are associated with AHTRs may be caused by various mechanisms. The intrinsic pathway of the clotting cascade may be activated by antigen-antibody interaction, resulting in activation of Factor XII, also known as Hageman factor. Activation of the Hageman factor can result in hypotension through its effect on the kinin system. The kinin system produces bradykinin, which in turn increases vascular permeability and causes vasodilation.[7] Activated complement, tumor necrosis factor alpha (TNFα), and interleukin 1 (IL-1) may increase the expression of tissue factor. Tissue factor can activate the extrinsic pathway and is associated with the development of DIC. DIC is a potentially life-threatening consumptive coagulopathy. Its characteristics include microvascular thrombus formation with ischemic organ and tissue damage; consumption of platelets, fibrinogen, and coagulation factors; and activation of fibrinolysis with production of fibrin degradation products. The end result of these activations can vary from generalized oozing to uncontrolled bleeding.

Shock may also accompany AHTRs. Hypotension, caused by the release of vasoactive amines, kinins, and other mediators, produces a compensatory vasoconstrictive response that further aggravates organ and tissue damage. Renal failure may occur as well. Free hemoglobin impairs renal function, but compromised renal cortical blood supply is thought to be the major contributing factor in renal failure. In addition, antigen-antibody complex deposition, vasoconstriction, and thrombi formation contribute to the development of renal vascular compromise.

Frequency

The frequency of AHTRs is not easy to determine. The authors of a review article based on data from several surveillance systems estimated the risk of clinical or laboratory evidence of ABO

HTR to be 1 in 76,000 to 80,000 and the risk of a fatal ABO HTR to be 1:1.8 million.[8] Of the transfusion-related fatalities reported to the FDA from 2012 to 2016, 8% and 10% were caused by ABO and non-ABO HTRs, respectively.[1]

Treatment

Prompt recognition of an AHTR and immediate cessation of the transfusion are crucial. The unit of blood should be returned to the blood bank for investigation. Saline should be infused to maintain venous access, treat hypotension, and maintain renal blood flow, with a goal of a urine flow rate of >1 mL/kg/hour. Consultation with transfusion medicine, critical care, renal, and hematology experts should be considered.

The addition of the diuretic furosemide promotes increased urine output and further enhances renal cortical blood flow. If urine output remains diminished after a liter of saline has been infused, acute tubular necrosis may have occurred, and the patient may be at risk of developing pulmonary edema. Oliguric renal failure may be complicated by hyperkalemia and subsequent cardiac arrest. Metabolic acidosis and uremia often necessitate the institution of dialysis.

DIC is an equally serious component of an AHTR. DIC is difficult to treat and may be the first indication that hemolysis has occurred in an anuric or anesthetized patient. Traditional therapy for DIC includes treating or removing the underlying cause and providing supportive care via the administration of platelets, plasma, and cryoprecipitate.

Unconscious or anesthetized patients may receive multiple units of incompatible blood before acute hemolysis is recognized. Because the severity of an AHTR is related to the amount of incompatible red cells transfused, exchange transfusion may be considered. Some severe reactions to a single unit of strongly incompatible blood may require exchange transfusion as well. Antigen-negative blood must be used for the red cell exchange. Likewise, plasma and platelets that will not contribute to hemolysis should be chosen.

Finally, inhibiting the complement cascade may be beneficial, especially early in the hemolytic transfusion reaction. A single case report on the use of eculizumab, a monoclonal antibody that blocks the cleavage of complement component C5, suggests that this may be a useful strategy for preventing hemolysis of incompatible red cells.[9]

Prompt initiation of therapy to aggressively manage hypotension, renal blood flow, and DIC provides the greatest chance of a successful outcome. Furthermore, consultation with appropriate medical specialists early in the course of treatment will ensure that the patient receives hemodialysis, cardiac monitoring, and mechanical ventilation when needed.

Prevention

Clerical and human errors involving patient, sample, and blood unit identification are the most common causes of mistransfusion and, therefore, AHTRs. Reported estimates place the risk of a near-miss at 1:1000, wrong blood given at 1:15,000-19,000, ABO-incompatible transfusion at 1:40,000, and error that results in harm at 1:4500.[8,10] Institutional policies and procedures must be in place to minimize the likelihood of such errors, and corrective and preventive action programs should target continual reduction of such errors. However, no one method for reducing the number of errors is foolproof.[11] Products available to increase patient safety include technology-based solutions, such as radiofrequency identification chips, handheld bar-code scanners, and "smart" refrigerators similar to systems used for pharmacologic agents.

The prevention of potential hemolysis from the administration of minor-ABO-incompatible platelets remains a challenge with constrained platelet inventories. A number of options, including anti-A or anti-B titration of the component, limiting the total amount of incompatible plasma transfused from platelets, and volume reduction may offer some benefit.[12] The use of platelet additive solutions for reducing minor-incompatible hemolysis risk has not been clinically studied, although it decreases the titers of anti-A and anti-B in the components.

Nonimmune-Mediated Hemolysis

Transfusion-associated hemolysis can also result from several nonimmune causes. Longer duration of storage before issue is associated with increased hemolysis of storage-damaged red cells.[13] Furthermore, improper shipping or storage temperatures, as well as incomplete deglycerolization of frozen red cells, can lead to hemolysis. At the time of transfusion, using a needle with an inappropriately small bore size or employing a rapid-pressure infuser can cause mechanical hemolysis, which may be related to the use of roller pumps. Improper use of blood warmers or the use of microwave ovens or hot waterbaths can cause temperature-related hemolysis. AABB *Standards for Blood Banks and Transfusion Services (Standards)* allows for 0.9% sodium chloride to be added to blood during infusion.[14(p50)] Other fluids may be transfused with blood if "they have been approved for this use by the FDA" or "there is documentation available to show that the addition is safe and does not adversely affect the blood or blood component." Infusion of red cells simultaneously through the same tubing with hypotonic solutions or with certain pharmacologic agents may cause osmotic hemolysis. For safe administration, red cells and these solutions or agents should be given via alternate venous access locations. In rare cases, hemolysis may be caused by bacterial contamination of the Red Blood Cell (RBC) unit. Patients may also experience hemolysis as part of their underlying disease process. Although a negative DAT result usually indicates no evidence of an immune-mediated cause of hemolysis, complete destruction of incompatible transfused red cells may be associated with a negative DAT result.

When both immune and nonimmune causes of hemolysis have been excluded, the possibility of an intrinsic red cell membrane defect in the recipient or even in the transfused cells should be considered. Cells with these defects, such as G6PD deficiency,[15] are present in the blood supply; they have increased fragility when challenged with particular stressors and may undergo coincidental hemolysis.

Treatment

Hemolysis of nonimmune etiology may cause symptoms whose severity depends on the degree of hemolysis and amount of component transfused. In all cases, the transfusion should be discontinued and appropriate care should be administered. (See the earlier section on the treatment of AHTRs for details on managing hypotension and declining renal function.)

Prevention

Written procedures for all aspects of the manufacture and transfusion of blood and components should always be followed. Prompt recognition of nonimmune hemolysis and robust root cause analysis may prevent additional occurrences.

Transfusion-Related Sepsis

Presentation

Fever (particularly a temperature of ≥38.5 C or 101 F), chills, rigors, and hypotension during or shortly after transfusion are the most frequently presenting symptoms of transfusion-related sepsis. Gram-negative bacteria typically cause more severe symptoms, including shock, renal failure, and DIC. Gram-positive organisms may present with isolated fever in the patient and may present hours after the completion of transfusion. This reaction is observed most commonly with transfusion of platelets stored at room temperature.

Differential Diagnosis

The abruptness of onset and severity of the signs and symptoms associated with transfusion-related sepsis may be very similar to those of AHTRs. Mild cases may be confused with FNHTRs. Fever or bacteremia unrelated to transfusion may confound the diagnosis. The key to diagnosing transfusion-related sepsis is culturing the same organism from both the patient and the remainder of the component. The returned component should be visually examined in suspected cases of posttransfusion sepsis. The bag should be sampled aseptically from the residual component rather than the tubing to avoid retrograde contamination and false-positive cultures. Attention should be paid to any color changes, especially brown or purple discoloration in an RBC component and bubbles/frothiness in a platelet component. A Gram stain should be performed on the returned component.

Treatment

If transfusion-related sepsis is suspected, the transfusion should be stopped immediately, and supportive care and antibiotics should be initiated.

Prevention

Suspected septic transfusion reactions should be *immediately* reported to the blood collector so that co-components from the same donation can be intercepted to avoid exposing other patients to contaminated blood components.[16] Any co-components or aliquots from the same donation that are in the hospital's inventory should be *immediately* quarantined, pending investigation results. Bacteria detection tests and pathogen inactivation technologies are discussed in Chapter 7.

Febrile Nonhemolytic Transfusion Reactions

Presentation

An FNHTR is usually defined as the occurrence of a ≥1 C rise in temperature ≥38 C that is associated with transfusion and for which no other cause is identifiable. Accompanying symptoms may include rigors, chills, and respiratory changes. In some instances, the patient may be afebrile but have the remaining constellation of symptoms. Symptoms usually occur during transfusion but may occur up to 4 hours afterward. Although FNHTRs are self-limited, they may cause significant discomfort.

Differential Diagnosis

Recognition of an FNHTR requires diagnosis by exclusion. The symptoms associated with an FNHTR may be present in several other types of transfusion reactions, the most serious of which are HTRs, sepsis, and TRALI. Each of these other reactions has signs, symptoms, and associated laboratory results that help distinguish them from an FNHTR once an investigation is begun. Hemolysis and sepsis must be ruled out in a patient who experiences fever associated with transfusion. Fever may commonly occur as a manifestation of a patient's underlying illness. In a patient who has been experiencing spiking fevers during the course of admission, it may be difficult to rule out an FNHTR. Bacterial contamination of the component must always be considered to be a potential cause of a febrile reaction.

Pathophysiology

FNHTRs may be the result of accumulated cytokines in a cellular blood component. This mechanism may be particularly relevant in reactions that occur after the transfusion of platelets.[17] Whether passively transfused or generated by leukocytes in the recipient, pyrogenic cytokine release is the common event leading to symptoms of FNHTR. Recipient leukocyte antibodies may also cause febrile transfusion reactions.[18] HLA antibodies in particular can react with cognate antigens on transfused lymphocytes, granulocytes, or platelets.

Treatment

When an FNHTR is suspected, the transfusion should be discontinued and a transfusion reaction workup initiated. Antipyretics (eg, acetaminophen) may be administered. For more severe reactions that include rigors, meperidine may be administered, although its efficacy has not been rigorously studied.

When fever develops during transfusion, the remainder of the implicated component should not be transfused. Among the few situations in which transfusion of the remainder of the component should be considered is when the component is a medically indicated rare unit. If a portion of the component remains, the laboratory workup to exclude hemolysis must be completed and a discussion with the patient's clinical care team regarding the likelihood of transfusion-transmitted sepsis must be held before the transfusion is resumed.

Prevention

Prestorage leukocyte reduction decreases the frequency of FNHTRs.[19,20] Premedication with acetaminophen reduces the overall incidence of febrile reactions, without impairing the ability to detect other complications of transfusion such as acute hemolysis, sepsis, and TRALI.[21] Plasma reduction reduces the rate of FNHTRs to platelets.[22]

Allergic Reactions

Presentation

Most allergic transfusion reactions (ATRs) are mild, but their spectrum can range from a simple allergic reaction (urticaria or hives) to life-threatening anaphylaxis. Symptoms generally occur within minutes after the start of the transfusion. If symptoms do not appear until >4 hours later, they may represent an allergic reaction that is unrelated to the blood transfusion.

Hives are usually associated with itching (pruritus) but may also burn or sting. Hives can appear anywhere on the body and can coalesce over large areas. They can last from hours to several days before fading, but most respond quickly to treatment with antihistamines. More extensive cases may be accompanied by angioedema, which is a deep tissue swelling, often around the eyes and lips. Angioedema can involve the throat, tongue, or lungs, causing respiratory distress, although feeling throat fullness or dyspnea without respiratory insufficiency is more common.

Anaphylactic transfusion reactions can be generally defined as the presentation of mucocutaneous signs of urticaria and angioedema in combination with other organ system involvement (cardiovascular, respiratory, gastrointestinal).[23] Manifestations of anaphylaxis are hypotension, loss of consciousness, dyspnea, wheezing, stridor, abdominal pain, and vomiting.

Differential Diagnosis

Initially it may be difficult to distinguish anaphylaxis from other reactions characterized by hypotension, dyspnea, and/or loss of consciousness. Reactions that may be mistaken for anaphylactic shock are vasovagal and hypotensive reactions. Urticaria, angioedema, pruritus, and respiratory symptoms, such as wheezing or stridor, are symptoms of anaphylaxis that do not occur in vasovagal or hypotensive reactions. The respiratory symptoms of anaphylaxis may be suggestive of asthma exacerbations or TRALI. However, the classic symptoms of allergy, including urticaria, angioedema, and pruritus, do not occur in asthma or TRALI. Fever, a prominent symptom of HTR and bacterial contamination, is not a feature of anaphylaxis. Patients who take angiotensin-converting enzyme (ACE) inhibitors and undergo plasma exchange sometimes develop hypotensive reactions that mimic anaphylaxis.

Pathophysiology

The pathophysiology of nearly all ATRs is not understood. Extrapolating from a small number of case reports, ATRs are attributed to hypersensitivity reactions to allergens in the component caused by preformed IgE antibody in the recipient. A combination of recipient and donor factors is likely involved, as recipients with an atopic predisposition appear to have a higher rate of ATRs, and certain donors' platelets are associated with an increased risk.[23,24] Clinical transfusion parameters (eg, infusion rate or volume, ABO mismatch, component age, premedication) have not been associated with ATRs.[25]

Selective protein deficiency, classically IgA deficiency, is a rare cause of ATRs. These reactions are caused by anti-IgA in the recipient.[26] Although IgA deficiency is present in approximately 1:700 people of European ancestry, only a small percentage of these people ever make antibodies against IgA. People with absolute IgA deficiency (<0.05 mg/dL) may form class-specific antibodies that are associated with anaphylactic reactions. Those with decreased but detectable amounts of IgA, or relative IgA deficiency, can form subclass-specific antibodies (eg, anti-IgA1 or anti-IgA2) that typically result in less severe reactions.[27]

Although precautions should be taken when transfusing an IgA-deficient patient, it must be kept in mind that the majority of ATRs are caused by substances other than IgA.[28] Most of these allergens are not identified but rarely may include haptoglobin[29] or the complement protein C4.[30] Transfusion can passively sensitize patients to donor antibodies, resulting in transient allergy (eg, to peanuts).[31]

Frequency

ATRs are common, with an overall frequency of approximately 2% with traditional platelet and plasma components.[32] The incidence is about 10-fold lower with RBCs.[33] Platelet additive solution platelets have lower rates of ATRs.[34] Life-threatening anaphylactic reactions account for <1% of all ATRs. Of the transfusion-associated fatalities reported to the FDA from 2012 to 2016, 6% (11 of 176) were caused by anaphylaxis, and most were not caused by IgA deficiency.[1,28]

Treatment

Urticaria is the only transfusion reaction in which the administration of the component may be routinely resumed after prompt treatment. When a patient develops symptoms, the transfusion should be paused so that an antihistamine may be administered. Once the symptoms have dissipated, the transfusion may be resumed, and a laboratory workup need not be initiated.

Severe urticarial reactions may be treated with H1 and H2 receptor antagonists and corticosteroids. Epinephrine is the consensus first-line treatment for anaphylaxis; the dose may be repeated up to every 5 minutes.[35]

Prevention

Evidence does not support routine premedication to prevent ATRs.[36] Antihistamines (diphenhydramine or a nonsedating antihistamine, eg, cetirizine) are useful to treat allergic symptoms once they arise. If H1 receptor antihistamines are not sufficient, an H2 receptor antagonist (eg, ranitidine) or corticosteroids may be considered. For patients whose reactions are severe or recurrent, washed RBCs or platelets, platelet-additive-solution platelets, or pooled solvent/detergent-treated plasma may be considered.

Recipient IgA or haptoglobin concentrations are often not available by the time a subsequent transfusion is needed; however, most cases of anaphylaxis are idiosyncratic to a specific unit and not the result of selective protein deficiency. Tolerance of prior plasma and platelet transfusions is a reasonable indicator that subsequent plasma transfusions may be acceptable from unselected donors. Pooled solvent/detergent-treated plasma has a lower risk of allergic reactions, but its value for prevention of recurrent anaphylactic reactions has not been established. At some institutions, the plasma from IgA-deficient donors is preferred for transfusions to patients with a history of severe ATRs and diagnosed IgA deficiency (<0.05 mg/dL). If IgA-deficient plasma is not available, desensitization with IgA-containing plasma may be possible.[37] Cellular components (RBCs and platelets) can be depleted of plasma proteins through washing. IgA deficiency without the presence of anti-IgA or without a history of an ATR does not clearly warrant the use of IgA-deficient or plasma-depleted components.

Transfusion-Related Acute Lung Injury

Presentation

TRALI is clinically similar to acute respiratory distress syndrome (ARDS) but usually resolves within 96 hours. Clinical signs and symptoms of TRALI include fever, chills, dyspnea, cyanosis, hypotension, hypoxia, and new-onset or worsening bilateral pulmonary edema.[38] A dramatic transient neutropenia or leukopenia may also be observed.[39] Symptoms arise within 6 hours of transfusion, with most cases becoming evident within 1 to 2 hours.

All plasma-containing components, including whole blood, RBCs, platelets, cryoprecipitate, and Fresh Frozen Plasma (FFP), have been implicated in TRALI. Transfusion volumes as small as 15 mL have led to TRALI.

TRALI is a form of ARDS. The Berlin definition[40] delineated various categories of ARDS, all of which were characterized by bilateral pulmonary edema on frontal chest radiograph but differed based on the degree of hypoxemia: mild defined as acute hypoxemia with a PaO_2/FiO_2 (partial pressure of oxygen in arterial blood/inspired oxygen concentration) ratio between 200 mm Hg and ≤300 mm Hg, moderate as between 100 mm Hg and ≤200 mm Hg, and severe as ≤100 mm Hg. In recognition of the difficulty in determining whether an underlying ARDS risk factor or the transfusion is the cause of the acute lung injury, a panel of experts recently proposed revision of the consensus definition for TRALI.[41] The revised diagnostic criteria for TRALI are as follows (see Table 22-2): 1) acute onset of symptoms within 6 hours of transfusion, 2) ARDS with hypoxemia and PaO_2/FiO_2 ≤300 mm Hg or SpO_2 (blood oxygen saturation) <90% on room air, 3) clear evidence of bilateral pulmonary edema on imaging, and 4) no evidence of left atrial hypertension (LAH) or, if present, deemed to not be the main contributor to hypoxemia. The panel further sub-

classified TRALI into Type I, with no temporal relationship with an alternative risk factor for ARDS, and Type II, with stable respiratory status in the 12 hours before transfusion, but with risk factors for ARDS or with mild ARDS,[40] but whose respiratory status deteriorates and is judged to be due to transfusion.

Although the lung injury in ARDS is often irreversible, the lung injury in TRALI is most often transient. Approximately 80% of patients with TRALI improve within 48 to 96 hours. The remaining 20% of patients who do not improve rapidly have either a protracted clinical course or a fatal outcome. In one TRALI study, 100% of the patients required oxygen support and 72% required mechanical ventilation.[42]

TABLE 22-2. Consensus TRALI Definition*

TRALI Type I
Patients who have no risk factors for ARDS and meet the following criteria:
1. Symptoms:
a. Acute onset
b. Hypoxemia (P/F ≤300[†] or SpO_2 <90% on room air)
c. Clear evidence of bilateral pulmonary edema on imaging (eg, chest radiograph, chest CT, or ultrasound)
d. No evidence of LAH[‡] or, if LAH is present, it is judged to not be the main contributor to the hypoxemia
2. Onset during or within 6 hours of transfusion[§]
3. No temporal relationship to an alternative risk factor for ARDS

TRALI Type II
Patients who have risk factors for ARDS (but who have not been diagnosed with ARDS) or who have existing mild ARDS (P/F of 200-300), but whose respiratory status deteriorates[◊] and is judged to be due to transfusion based on:
1. Findings as described in categories 1 *and* 2 of TRALI Type I, and
2. Stable respiratory status in the 12 hours before transfusion

*Modified with permission from Vlaar et al.[41]

[†]If altitude is higher than 1000 m, the correction factor should be calculated as follows: [(P/F) × (barometric pressure/760)].

[‡]Use objective evaluation when LAH is suspected (imaging, eg, echocardiography; or invasive measurement using, eg, pulmonary artery catheter).

[§]Onset of pulmonary symptoms (eg, hypoxemia—lower P/F ratio or SpO_2) should be within 6 hours of end of transfusion. The additional findings needed to diagnose TRALI (pulmonary edema on a lung imaging study and determination of lack of substantial LAH) would ideally be available at the same time but could be documented up to 24 hours after TRALI onset.

[◊]Use P/F ratio deterioration along with other respiratory parameters and clinical judgment to determine progression from mild to moderate or severe ARDS. See conversion table (Vlaar et al[41]) to convert nasal O_2 supplementation to FiO_2.

TRALI = transfusion-related acute lung injury; ARDS = acute respiratory distress syndrome; P/F = PaO_2/FiO_2 (partial pressure of oxygen in arterial blood/inspired oxygen concentration); CT = computerized tomography; LAH = left atrial hypertension.

Differential Diagnosis

The main complications that need to be distinguished from TRALI are 1) anaphylactic transfusion reactions, 2) TACO, 3) TRALI/TACO, 4) ARDS from underlying illness, 5) transfusion-associated dyspnea (TAD), and 6) transfusion-related sepsis. In anaphylactic transfusion reactions, bronchospasm, laryngeal edema, severe hypotension, erythema (often confluent), and urticaria are prominent symptoms. Fever and pulmonary edema are not associated with anaphylactic reactions. The clinical presentation of TACO is very similar to that of TRALI, with respiratory distress, tachypnea, and cyanosis as the most prominent features. Key distinctions between TACO and TRALI are that the pulmonary edema in TACO is cardiogenic and responsive to diuretics, whereas it is noncardiogenic and not responsive to diuretics in TRALI. The classification of TRALI/TACO is reserved for situations compatible with TRALI and TACO and/or with lack of data to establish whether or not significant LAH is present. Cases that meet the criteria for TRALI but without stable pulmonary status in the previous 12 hours should be considered ARDS, and if there is no documentation that $PaO_2/FiO_2 \leq 300$ mm Hg, then cases should be classified as TAD. High fever with hypotension and vascular collapse are prominent features of transfusion-related sepsis. Respiratory distress and ARDS are infrequently associated with septic transfusion reactions. Finally, other possible causes of ARDS should be considered, such as coincident sepsis, myocardial infarction, and pulmonary embolus.

Pathophysiology

Several mechanisms for the pulmonary manifestations of TRALI have been proposed. The primary effector cell is the neutrophil, with lung histology from fatal cases showing predominantly neutrophilic infiltrates and alveolar edema.[43] TRALI has been associated with the infusion of antibodies to leukocyte antigens and of biologic response modifiers (BRMs).[44] Infusions of these antibodies or BRMs are thought to initiate cellular activation and neutrophil-mediated damage of the endothelial basement membrane in the lungs, leading to leakage of protein-rich fluid into the alveolar space.

A two-event model of the mechanism of TRALI has been hypothesized.[45] In the first event, generation of biologically active compounds activates pulmonary vascular endothelial cells and primes neutrophils, resulting in sequestration of neutrophils in the pulmonary microvasculature. This first event predisposes the recipient to develop TRALI and can result from a variety of physiologic stressors, including sepsis, surgery, and massive transfusion. The infusion of BRMs or antibodies is the second event. BRMs consist of a mixture of lysophosphatidylcholines that accumulate in some cellular components during storage. The transfused antibodies may be to HLA Class I, HLA Class II, or human neutrophil antigens (HNAs). These stimuli are hypothesized to activate the primed neutrophils in the pulmonary microvasculature, resulting in pulmonary endothelial damage, capillary leakage, and pulmonary edema.

Frequency

TRALI occurs in about 1 in 10,000 units transfused.[44] TRALI was the leading cause of transfusion-related mortality reported to the FDA until 2016, when TACO supplanted it.[1] Because HLA or HNA antibodies are more common in multiparous women, efforts to reduce the risk of transfusing plasma from potentially alloimmunized female donors have been associated with decreased TRALI fatalities.[46] In 2006, the year before many blood centers implemented measures to reduce the risk of TRALI from plasma transfusions (eg, donor selection criteria and HLA-antibody screening of selected donors), 35 fatal cases of TRALI, 22 of which were associated with transfusion of FFP, were reported to the FDA. Since 2008, the year after many blood centers implemented such measures, the numbers of TRALI fatalities have decreased by over half.[1]

Treatment

Treatment of TRALI consists of respiratory and circulatory support. Oxygen supplementation with or without mechanical ventilation is required in almost all cases. Pressor agents may be needed to support blood pressure. Because TRALI is not associated with volume overload, diuretics are typically not indicated and may increase the risk of hypotension. Administration of corticosteroids has not been shown to improve clinical outcome in TRALI or ARDS.[47]

Prevention

There is no method to predict which patients will develop TRALI. Donors whose collections are linked to cases of TRALI are permanently deferred. Although approximately 10% of blood donations contain HLA and/or HNA antibodies, TRALI is much rarer. Nevertheless, an important mitigation strategy is to collect plasma components, whole blood, and platelets from male donors, never-pregnant female donors, or females who have been tested since their last pregnancy and found to be negative for HLA antibodies. Although these measures reduce the risk of TRALI, it is important to recognize that they do not eliminate TRALI completely because they do not address the risk of TRALI from RBC or cryoprecipitate components, and donor testing of previously pregnant females does not screen for HNA antibodies and BRMs.

Transfusion-Associated Circulatory Overload

Presentation

It is well known that transfusion can precipitate acute pulmonary edema caused by volume overload. Patients >70 years and infants are at greatest risk, as well as patients with compromised ability to regulate fluid balance (eg, those with congestive heart failure and end-stage renal disease), although all transfusion recipients are susceptible to some degree. Whereas large volumes of components and nonblood fluids are most frequently implicated, modest volumes can also precipitate TACO in susceptible patients. A high flow rate is frequently a cofactor.

TACO has no pathognomonic signs or symptoms. Within 1 to 2 hours of transfusion, patients may develop any or all of the following: S3 gallop, jugular venous distension, elevated central venous pressure, dyspnea, orthopnea, new ST-segment and T-wave changes on electrocardiogram, elevated serum troponin, and elevated brain natriuretic peptide (BNP).[48] Radiographs may show a widened cardiothoracic ratio in addition to pulmonary edema. Hemovigilance systems have reported cases of TACO beyond 6 hours of transfusion.[49] Additionally, it was realized that some reactions accepted clinically as TACO did not meet the 2011 surveillance definition from the International Society of Blood Transfusion (ISBT)/International Hemovigilance Network (IHN)/AABB. An international revision group composed of clinical, laboratory, blood bank, and hemovigilance experts published a revised and validated TACO definition in 2019.[50] The revised surveillance definition (see Table 22-3) classifies cases as TACO during or up to 12 hours after transfusion when they meet a total of three or more of the following criteria, with at least one from the required criteria (1 and 2): 1) acute or worsening respiratory compromise, 2) evidence of pulmonary edema, 3) evidence of cardiovascular system changes not explained by the patient's underlying medical condition, 4) evidence of fluid overload, and 5) supportive result of a relevant biomarker [eg, an increase of BNP or N-terminal-propeptide BNP (NT-proBNP)].[51]

Differential Diagnosis

TACO is frequently confused with TRALI because both types of reactions produce pulmonary edema. It is also possible for TACO and TRALI to occur concurrently in the same patient. The timelines and the clinical presentation are similar, but hypertension is a more typical feature of TACO, whereas it is only an infrequent and transient manifestation of TRALI. Furthermore, rapid improvement with diuresis is consistent with TACO.

In congestive heart failure, BNP levels are elevated. A posttransfusion-to-pretransfusion BNP ratio of 1.5 with a posttransfusion level of at least 100 pg/mL as a cutoff yields a sensitivity and specificity >80% in TACO.[48] However, in the intensive care setting, BNP is only of moderate value for distinguishing TACO from TRALI.[52] Some clinical laboratories measure the NT-proBNP, which has a longer half-life than BNP. NT-proBNP is also predictive of TACO.[53] With

TABLE 22-3. TACO Reporting Criteria*†

Patients classified with TACO (surveillance diagnosis) should have acute or worsening respiratory compromise and/or evidence of pulmonary edema (A and/or B below) during or up to 12 hours after transfusion and presence of a total of 3 or more of the criteria below:

A. Acute or worsening respiratory compromise.

B. Evidence of acute or worsening pulmonary edema based on:

• Clinical physical examination, *and/or*

• Radiographic chest imaging and/or other noninvasive assessment of cardiac function (eg, echocardiogram).

C. Evidence for cardiovascular system changes not explained by the patient's underlying medical condition, including development of tachycardia, hypertension, widened pulse pressure, jugular venous distension, enlarged cardiac silhouette, and/or peripheral oedema.

D. Evidence of fluid overload, including any of the following: a positive fluid balance; response to diuretic therapy, eg, from diuretic therapy or dialysis combined with clinical improvement; and change in the patient's weight in the peritransfusion period.

E. Supportive result of a relevant biomarker, eg, an increase of B-type natriuretic peptide level (eg, BNP or NT-proBNP) above the age-group-specific reference range and greater than 1.5 times the pretransfusion value. A normal posttransfusion NP level is not consistent with a diagnosis of TACO; serial testing of NP levels in the peritransfusion period may be helpful in identifying TACO.

*Modified from ISBT et al.[51]

†These criteria establish a surveillance case definition based on a complete description of an event, including information that becomes available well after onset. This is for reporting and tracking purposes and the criteria do not constitute clinical diagnosis for the purpose of real-time clinical interventions. If a case could be TACO according to clinical judgment but fewer than three criteria are met based on available information, the listed criteria can guide collection of additional details, eg, from case notes or discussion with clinical staff.

TACO = transfusion-associated circulatory overload; NT-proBNP = N-terminal-propeptide BNP.

rapid onset of respiratory distress, possible causes of ARDS, such as coincident myocardial infarction, pulmonary embolus, and others, should be considered in addition to TACO and TRALI.

Frequency

TACO is an underreported adverse reaction to transfusion, and hemovigilance and retrospective studies underestimate the incidence. Furthermore, the incidence differs across patient populations with different comorbidities.[54] In aggregate, from 2013 to 2017, the highest number (32%) of transfusion-associated fatalities reported to the FDA (59 patients) were a consequence of TACO, with TACO-related fatalities surpassing those from TRALI after 2015.[1] Platelet and plasma components are associated with a TACO incidence of approximately 1%,[55,56] and RBCs, with an incidence of up to 2.7%.[54]

Treatment

As soon as symptoms suggest TACO, the transfusion should be stopped. The symptoms should be treated by placing the patient in a seated position (if possible), providing supplementary oxygen, and reducing the intravascular volume with diuretics. If symptoms persist in confirmed TACO, administration of additional diuretics or therapeutic phlebotomy is appropriate.

Prevention

In the absence of ongoing and rapid blood loss, components should be administered slowly, particularly in patients at risk of TACO (ie, pediatric and elderly patients, patients with severe anemia, and patients with congestive heart failure). Rates of 2 to 4 mL/minute and 1 mL/kg of body weight per hour are the most frequently cited, despite a paucity of data on appropriate infusion rates. Total fluid input and output must be monitored.

Hypotensive Reactions

Presentation

Hypotensive transfusion reactions (HyTRs) are defined as the sudden and unexpected onset of clinically significant hypotension associated with the transfusion of blood or blood components that resolves shortly after the transfusion is stopped. Systolic blood pressure (SBP) declines by >30 mm Hg or to <80 mm Hg in adults. In children, an SBP decrease of >25% is consistent with a HyTR. Another characteristic is that HyTRs usually start within the first 15 minutes of transfusion. All types of patients can be affected, with any blood component.[57] The HyTR rate per blood component has been reported as 0.019% for platelets, 0.015% for RBCs, and 0.006% for plasma.[57] Another study found 1% of platelet transfusions can be complicated by HyTRs.[58]

Differential Diagnosis

Hypotension can be a primary manifestation of HyTR, anaphylaxis, septic transfusion reaction, AHTR, TRALI, or an underlying disease/medication. All may present within the first 15 minutes of transfusion, but the absence of concomitant signs and symptoms and the prompt resolution of hypotension upon discontinuation of transfusion distinguish HyTRs from other reactions. Anaphylactic shock usually is accompanied by mucocutaneous allergic manifestations

(eg, flushing, angioedema, urticaria). Septic shock from transfusion is often accompanied by fever. AHTRs are associated with hemoglobinuria, pain, and fever. A minority of TRALI cases involve clinically significant hypotension, but TRALI cases have acute pulmonary insufficiency, a finding that is atypical for HyTRs.

Pathophysiology

Bradykinin is thought to have a causal role in HyTRs.[59] Bradykinin is a vasoactive peptide generated via activation of the kinin-kallikrein system from its precursor, high-molecular-weight kininogen. Factors that increase concentrations of bradykinin in blood components include storage, filtration, and ACE activity in donors and recipients. ACE activity can be affected by ACE-inhibitor medication and cardiopulmonary bypass circuits, because the lungs are a primary site of ACE activity.[60] Recent prostatectomy may increase bradykinin concentrations in patients as a result of kallikreins released from the prostate.

Treatment

The primary treatment intervention is to stop the transfusion. Blood pressure usually increases within minutes after cessation of transfusion, but circulatory support with intravenous fluids and vasopressors may be needed. With acute onset of hypotension, the etiology is often not immediately clear. Treatments for anaphylaxis and sepsis may be initiated as the clinical presentation unfolds.

Prevention

If a patient who experienced a HyTR is taking ACE-inhibitor medication that is not discontinued, subsequent transfusions should be given as slowly as is feasible to prevent a recurrence. Because HyTRs are typically idiosyncratic to a specific unit, patients without risk factors for a HyTR typically tolerate subsequent transfusions well. Washing cellular blood components will reduce accumulated bradykinin, but washed component protocols are seldom needed, as most cases are not recurrent.

Complications of Massive Transfusion

The potential complications of massive transfusion, usually defined as the receipt of >10 RBC units within 24 hours, include metabolic and hemostatic abnormalities, immune hemolysis, and air embolism. Metabolic abnormalities can depress cardiac function. Hypothermia from refrigerated blood, citrate toxicity, and lactic acidosis from underperfusion and tissue ischemia, which are often complicated by hyperkalemia, can contribute to this effect. Although metabolic alkalosis caused by citrate metabolism may occur, it is not likely to be clinically significant. Patients who lose blood rapidly may have preexisting or coexisting hemostatic abnormalities or develop them during resuscitation. Hemostatic abnormalities may include dilutional coagulopathy, DIC, and liver and platelet dysfunction.[61]

Citrate Toxicity

Pathophysiology and Manifestations. When large volumes of citrated blood components are transfused rapidly, particularly in the presence of liver disease, plasma citrate levels may rise, binding calcium, resulting in hypocalcemia. In patients with a normally functioning liver, citrate is rapidly metabolized; thus, these symptoms are transient.[62] Hypocalcemia is more likely to cause manifestations in patients who are hypothermic or in shock.

A decrease in ionized calcium levels increases neuronal excitability, which in the conscious patient leads to symptoms of perioral and peripheral tingling, shivering, and lightheadedness, followed by a diffuse sense of vibration, muscle cramps, fasciculations, spasm, and nausea. In the central nervous system, hypocalcemia is thought to increase the respiratory center sensitivity to carbon dioxide, causing hyperventilation. Because myocardial contraction is dependent on the intracellular movement of ionized calcium, hypocalcemia depresses cardiac function.

Treatment and Prevention. Unless the patient has a predisposing condition that hinders citrate metabolism, hypocalcemia caused by citrate overload during massive transfusion can usually be treated by slowing the infusion. Intra-venous calcium replacement with calcium gluconate or calcium chloride should be considered early, as hypocalcemia contributes to a hypocoagulable state in massive transfusion.[63]

Hyperkalemia and Hypokalemia

Pathophysiology. When red cells are stored at 1 to 6 C, the intracellular potassium gradually leaks into the supernatant plasma or additive solution. Although the concentration in the supernatant may be high, because of the small volume, the total extracellular potassium load is <0.5 mEq for fresh RBC units and only 5 to 7 mEq for units at expiration. These potassium concentrations rarely cause problems in the recipient because rapid dilution, redistribution into cells, and excretion blunt the effect.[64] However, irradiation followed by prolonged storage may increase supernatant potassium to unacceptable levels. Furthermore, hyperkalemia can be a problem in patients with renal failure, in premature infants, and in newborns receiving large transfusions, such as in cardiac surgery or exchange transfusion; otherwise, hyperkalemia is typically a transient effect during very rapid transfusions.[65]

Hypokalemia occurs more frequently than hyperkalemia after transfusion because potassium-depleted donor red cells reaccumulate this ion intracellularly, and citrate metabolism causes further movement of potassium into the cells in response to the consumption of protons. Catecholamine release and aldosterone-induced urinary loss can also trigger hypokalemia in the setting of massive transfusion.[64]

Treatment and Prevention. Usually, no treatment or preventive strategy for hypokalemia and hyperkalemia, aside from appropriate monitoring, is necessary provided that the patient is adequately resuscitated from the underlying condition that required massive transfusion. For infants receiving routine transfusions, units infused up to 0.5 cc/kg/minute may be used safely until the expiration date.[66] Although washing of RBC units results in very low levels of potassium, there is no evidence that this is indicated for routine RBC transfusions, even in patients with impaired renal function,[67] and it may even cause increased hemolysis and higher potassium levels in the component with time after washing.[68]

Hemostatic Abnormalities in Massive Transfusion

Pathophysiology. Coagulopathy can occur in massive transfusion, particularly when the lost blood is initially replaced with RBCs and crystalloids. Coagulopathy in massive transfusion is frequently ascribed to the dilution of platelets and clotting factors as patients lose hemostatically active blood, and enzymatic activity is reduced as the core body temperature lowers if a blood warmer is not used. Mortality rates associated with hemostatic abnormalities range from 20% to 50%.[69] The high rate of mortality results from hypothermia, metabolic acidosis, and coagulopathy.[70]

Studies of military and civilian trauma patients, before wide acceptance of transfusions with a more balanced ratio of RBCs to platelets to plasma, demonstrated a progressive increase in the incidence of microvascular bleeding (MVB) characteristic of a coagulopathy with increasing transfusion volumes that typically occurs after replacement of 2 to 3 blood volumes (20 to 30 units).[71] Although platelet counts, coagulation parameters, and levels of selected clotting parameters correlate with the volume transfused, contrary to expectations from a simple dilutional model, the relationship is marked by tremendous variability. Moreover, there is frequently discordance between the laboratory assessment and the clinical evidence of bleeding.

MVB increases with platelet counts below ~50,000/µL; however, no simple relationship can be determined between a patient's coagulation test results and the onset of bleeding. The etiology of bleeding (elective surgery vs massive trauma) may play a role as well.[72]

Subsequent studies have refined these observations. Significant platelet dysfunction has been demonstrated in recipients of massive transfusion.[73] Low fibrinogen and platelet counts are better predictors of hemostatic failure than elevations of prothrombin time (PT) and partial thromboplastin time (PTT), suggesting that consumptive coagulopathy is an important factor in MVB in addition to dilution.[74] The degree of platelet and clotting abnormalities correlates with the length of time that the patient is hypotensive, suggesting that shock is the most important cause of DIC. In aggregate, hypoperfusion is a major risk factor for coagulopathy in recipients of heavy transfusion.[75]

These data may not be generalizable to patients undergoing massive transfusion in the controlled setting of the operating room, where hypotension caused by volume loss is prevented. In this context, coagulation factor levels may be more significant than platelet problems. Murray and colleagues documented that excessive bleeding in elective surgery patients who received >1 blood volume (RBCs and crystalloid) corresponded to a prolongation in PT and PTT compared to patients with normal hemostasis.[72]

Treatment and Prevention. The dilutional model of coagulopathy in massive transfusion suggests that prophylactic replacement of hemostatic components based on the volume of RBCs or whole blood transfused prevents the development of a bleeding diathesis. No specific regimen has yet been shown to be superior to any other in prospective studies. Although there was no statistically significant difference in mortality, the Pragmatic Randomized Optimal Platelet and Plasma Ratios (PROPPR) trial indicated improvement in hemorrhage control using a 1:1:1 plasma/platelet/RBC unit ratio vs a 1:1:2 ratio.[76] Furthermore, in injured patients at risk for hemorrhagic shock, early administration of thawed plasma results in lower mortality.[77]

Although the optimal transfusion ratio in trauma resuscitation is still debated, institutions should develop a massive transfusion protocol. Replacement of platelets and coagulation factors in the surgical or trauma patient receiving massive transfusion should be based on the identification of a specific abnormality using platelet counts, PT, activated PTT, and fibrinogen levels, as clinically indicated. Frequent monitoring of these laboratory values serves to avoid overuse of platelets and plasma components by anticipating the specific components needed while avoiding dilutional coagulopathy. It is imperative that the laboratory provide results of these tests rapidly. Intraoperative and postoperative laboratory testing, such as thromboelastography, may be useful.

Antifibrinolytics have a role in controlling massive bleeding from trauma. The Clinical Randomization of an Antifibrinolytic in Significant Hemorrhage 2 (CRASH-2) and other studies conclude that tranexamic acid should be given as early as possible in trauma patients.[78] Activated clotting factors do not have a defined role in massive transfusion.

Air Embolism

Air embolism can occur if blood in an open system is infused under pressure or if air enters a central catheter while containers or blood administration sets are being changed. Air embolism has been reported in association with intraoperative and perioperative blood recovery systems that allow air into the blood infusion bag. The minimum volume of air embolism that is potentially fatal for an adult is approximately 100 mL.[79] Symptoms include cough, dyspnea, chest pain, and shock. If air embolism is suspected, the patient should be placed on the left side with the head down to displace the air bubble from the pulmonic valve. Aspiration of the air is sometimes attempted.[80]

Hypothermia

Blood warmers may be used to prevent hypothermia. Proper procedures for the use of blood warmers should be followed because overheating may induce hemolysis and serious transfusion reactions, including fatalities.

DELAYED TRANSFUSION REACTIONS

Delayed Hemolytic Transfusion Reactions

Presentation

Development of an alloantibody following transfusion can result in an asymptomatic delayed serologic transfusion reaction (DSTR) or in a delayed HTR (DHTR). Fever and anemia occurring days to weeks after transfusion of an RBC component are characteristic of a DHTR. The hemolysis associated with a DHTR is more protracted than an AHTR and typically does not precipitate the acute signs and symptoms of an AHTR, although some patients may develop jaundice and leukocytosis. In a DHTR, the hemolysis is primarily extravascular, so although hemoglobinuria may occur in rare cases, acute renal failure and DIC are not generally present. In some cases, the hemolysis occurs without causing clinical symptoms. These patients present with unexplained anemia or do not experience the expected sustained increase in hemoglobin concentrations following transfusion.

Differential Diagnosis

Fever with hemolysis may also occur well after transfusion when the component has been contaminated with an intracellular red cell parasite, such as malaria or babesia. Fever without hemolysis may be an indication of graft-vs-host disease (GVHD) [described in the section on transfusion-associated (TA)-GVHD, below] or transfusion-transmitted viral disease (eg, cytomegalovirus). Hemolysis resulting from antibody production by donor passenger lymphocytes may occur after transplantation of a minor-ABO-incompatible organ (eg, transplantation of a group O liver in a group A patient).

In a DHTR/DSTR, antibodies may be found in the serum, on transfused red cells, or both. Diagnosis by routine antibody screening and antibody identification should be possible. If transfused red cells are still present in the patient's circulation, the DAT result may be positive. When the DAT result is positive, an eluate should be performed and the antibody identified. If a segment from the unit is available, antigen typing may confirm the diagnosis.

Pathophysiology

After transfusion, transplantation, or pregnancy, a patient may make an antibody to a red cell antigen that he or she lacks. Red cell antibodies, missed during pretransfusion testing due to waning of their peak levels with time (ie, evanescence), may cause a delayed transfusion reaction if the patient subsequently receives a unit of blood expressing the corresponding red cell antigen. Primary alloimmunization occurs anywhere from days to months after a transfusion of antigen-positive red cells, depending on the immunogenicity and dose of the antigen.

Approximately 1% to 1.6% of RBC transfusions are associated with antibody formation, excluding antibodies to antigens in the Rh system. D-negative blood is usually transfused to D-negative patients, so the frequency attributable to anti-D is relatively low. Newly formed alloantibodies are routinely detected during pretransfusion screening. (See Chapters 13 and 17.) Recipients of recent transfusion or pregnant patients must have samples drawn for compatibility testing within 3 days of the scheduled transfusion to ensure identification of any potential new alloantibodies. A 5-year retrospective study of alloimmunization showed that 11 of 2932 patients (0.4%) had developed new antibodies, including anti-E, anti-K, and anti-Jk^a, within 3 days after transfusion.[81]

DHTRs and DSTRs rarely, if ever, occur as a result of primary immunization and are generally associated with subsequent transfusions. Because of evanescence (described above),[82] as many as 30% to 60% of alloantibodies become undetectable over months to years. Antibodies against antigens of some blood group systems, such as the JK system, frequently exhibit this behavior. Subsequent transfusion of an antigen-positive unit triggers an anamnestic response, with production of antibody occurring over the next several days to weeks after the transfusion. The rapidity of antibody production and the hemolytic potential of the antibody both combine to influence the clinical presentation. Blood group antibodies most commonly associated with DHTRs/DSTRs include those targeting antigens of the JK, FY, KEL, and MNS systems.

Frequency

As with AHTRs, the estimated rate of DHTRs varies widely from study to study. Some of this variation is the result of the practice of considering DSTRs and DHTRs as one category. Also, improvements in laboratory techniques have contributed to an increased number of DSTRs detected. Nonetheless, delayed reactions occur much more frequently than AHTRs, with estimates of approximately 1:2500 for either type of delayed reaction, and DSTRs being twice as

common as DHTRs.[83] These reactions are likely to be greatly underrecognized because most patients do not undergo red cell antibody screening following transfusion.[84]

Treatment

The treatment of DHTRs consists of monitoring the patient and providing supportive care. Correction of the anemia by transfusing antigen-negative RBCs may be needed. In addition a case report has shown some benefit of eculizumab in the treatment of DHTRs.[85]

Prevention

DHTRs/DSTRs caused by known antibody specificities can be prevented by the transfusion of antigen-negative RBCs. It is essential to obtain prior transfusion records for the recipient because of antibody evanescence. Many institutions have programs to provide prophylactic, partial phenotype-matching of blood for patients with sickle cell disease or other chronic anemias to prevent alloimmunization. Patients with sickle cell disease may develop a life-threatening complication known as hyperhemolysis, even after crossmatch-compatible RBC transfusion, in which autologous and allogeneic cells are destroyed. (See Chapter 19.)

Transfusion-Associated Graft-vs-Host Disease

Presentation

TA-GVHD occurs in <1 per million transfusions. The clinical manifestations of TA-GVHD typically begin 8 to 10 days after transfusion, although symptoms can occur as early as 3 days and as late as 30 days. Signs and symptoms include rash, fever, enterocolitis with watery diarrhea, elevated liver function test results, and pancytopenia. The rash begins on the trunk and progresses to the extremities. In severe cases, bullae may develop.[86] Unlike GVHD after allogeneic hematopoietic stem cell transplantation, TA-GVHD leads to profound marrow aplasia, with a mortality rate higher than 90%. The time course of the reaction is very rapid; death typically occurs within 1 to 3 weeks of the first symptoms.

Differential Diagnosis

Because the clinical manifestations of TA-GVHD appear several days after a transfusion, it may be difficult to associate the patient's symptoms with the transfusion. The symptoms can easily be attributed to other conditions, including drug reactions and viral illness. In cases of TA-GVHD, a skin biopsy reveals a superficial perivascular lymphocytic infiltrate, necrotic keratinocytes, compact orthokeratosis, and bullae formation. Molecular techniques, including HLA typing, cytogenetics, and chimerism assessment, can be used to make the diagnosis.

Pathophysiology

There are three requirements for GVHD to develop in a patient. First, there must be differences in the HLA antigens expressed between the donor and the recipient. Second, immunocompetent cells must be present in the component. Finally, the host must be incapable of rejecting the immunocompetent cells. The three primary factors that determine the risk of developing TA-GVHD are the degree of recipient cellular immunodeficiency, number of viable T lymphocytes in the transfusion, and degree of a population's genetic diversity. The number of viable lymphocytes in a transfusion can be affected by the age, leukocyte reduction status, and irradiation status of the component.[87] Although current leukocyte-reduction technologies significantly reduce the number of lymphocytes in a component, leukocyte reduction does not eliminate the risk of TA-GVHD.

Clinical risk factors for developing TA-GVHD include leukemia, lymphoma, use of immunosuppressive drugs administered for transplantation or myeloablative chemotherapy, congenital immunodeficiency disorders, and neonatal age, although immunodeficiency is not required for TA-GVHD.[88] TA-GVHD can occur after a transfusion from a donor who is homozygous for an HLA haplotype to a heterozygous recipient (one-way haplotype match). In this circumstance, the recipient's immune system does not reject the HLA-homozygous transfused lymphocytes as foreign. The transfused lymphocytes are able to recognize the host cells as foreign and are able to mount an immunologic attack on the host. As mentioned, the degree of genetic diversity in a population affects the risk of developing TA-GVHD.

Treatment

Treatment of TA-GVHD has been attempted with a variety of immunosuppressive agents. Unfortunately, the disorder is almost uniformly fatal; only rare cases of successful treatment, many involving stem cell transplantation, have been reported. Therefore, emphasis is placed on prevention of the disorder.

Prevention

TA-GVHD can be prevented by irradiation of cellular blood components. AABB *Standards* requires a minimum dose of 25 Gy (2500 cGy) delivered to the central portion of the container and a minimum of 15 Gy (1500 cGy) elsewhere.[14(p27)] The *Standards* requires blood banks and transfusion services to apply methods known to prevent TA-GVHD, including irradiation, to cellular blood components when 1) the patient is identified as being at risk of TA-GVHD, 2) the donor is a blood relative of the recipient, and 3) the donor is selected for HLA compatibility by typing or crossmatching.[14(pp44-45)] These standards are minimum requirements for irradiation of cellular blood components, and institutions may choose to administer irradiated components to other categories of patients. (See Table 22-4.) Finally, pathogen inactivation technologies are also effective against proliferating T cells and offer an alternative to irradiation.[89]

Posttransfusion Purpura

Presentation

Posttransfusion purpura (PTP) is an uncommon complication of transfusion, and its true incidence is therefore difficult to estimate. Nonetheless, >200 cases have been reported in the literature, and data from the Serious Hazards of Transfusion (SHOT) program in the United

TABLE 22-4. Well-Documented Indications for Irradiated Components

Intrauterine transfusions
Prematurity, low birthweight, or erythroblastosis fetalis in newborns
Congenital immunodeficiencies
Hematologic malignancies or solid tumors (neuroblastoma, sarcoma, Hodgkin disease)
Peripheral blood stem cell/marrow transplantation
Components that are crossmatched or HLA matched, or donations from family members (blood relatives)
Fludarabine therapy
Granulocyte components

Kingdom suggest that the disorder may be more common than previously believed.[90]

Patients typically present with wet purpura and thrombocytopenia within 2 weeks after a transfusion. The thrombocytopenia is often profound, with platelet counts of <10,000/µL.[91] Bleeding from mucous membranes and the gastrointestinal and urinary tract is common. Mortality rates in large case series range up to 16%, primarily due to intracranial hemorrhage.[92]

PTP has most commonly been associated with transfusions of RBCs or whole blood; however, the disorder has also been associated with transfusions of platelets or plasma.

Differential Diagnosis

The differential diagnosis of PTP includes alternative causes of thrombocytopenia, such as autoimmune thrombocytopenic purpura, thrombotic thrombocytopenic purpura, heparin-induced thrombocytopenia, DIC, and drug-induced thrombocytopenia. Although the diagnosis of PTP can be obvious in patients with previously normal platelet counts and no other significant medical abnormalities, it can be a challenge in patients with multiple medical problems. Platelet serology studies may aid in the diagnosis.

Pathophysiology

The pathogenesis of PTP is related to the presence of platelet-specific alloantibodies in a patient who has previously been exposed to platelet antigens via pregnancy or transfusion. The female-to-male ratio of affected patients is 5 to 1. Antibodies against human platelet antigen 1a (HPA-1a), located on glycoprotein IIIa, are identified in about 70% of PTP cases. Antibodies to HPA-1b, other platelet antigens, and HLA antigens have also been implicated in PTP.[93]

The reason for the concomitant destruction of autologous platelets in this disorder is unknown. The theory that the platelet alloantibody has autoreactivity that develops when a patient is re-exposed to a foreign platelet-specific antigen currently has the most support.

Treatment

Because the duration of thrombocytopenia in untreated patients is about 2 weeks, it can be difficult to assess the effectiveness of therapies for PTP. Steroids, whole-blood exchange, and plasma exchange have all been used to treat PTP. The current treatment of choice for PTP is IVIG.[94] Patients respond within 4 days, on average, and some respond within hours. HPA-1a-negative platelet transfusions have been useful in some cases.[95]

Prevention

The use of prestorage leukocyte reduction may decrease the incidence of PTP. In the 3 years before the implementation of universal leukocyte reduction in the United Kingdom, there were 10.3 cases of PTP per year, compared to 2.3 cases per year after universal leukocyte reduction (p <0.001).[90]

PTP typically does not recur with subsequent transfusions. However, there are case reports of PTP recurrence. Therefore, for patients with previously documented PTP, efforts should be made to obtain components from antigen-matched donors.[96] Autologous donations and directed donations from antigen-matched donors and family members may also be appropriate. Because PTP has also occurred after transfusions of deglycerolized, rejuvenated, or washed RBCs, such manipulations are not indicated to prevent recurrence.

Iron Overload

A unit of RBCs contains approximately 200 to 250 mg of iron. Because humans lack a physiologic means to excrete excess iron, persistent increase in iron influx from transfusions can result in iron overload. When the accumulation of iron overwhelms the capacity for safe storage, tissue damage can ensue. As iron accumulates in the reticuloendothelial system, liver, heart, spleen, and endocrine organs, tissue damage leading to heart failure, liver failure, diabetes, and hypothyroidism may occur. Patients who chronically receive transfusion for diseases such as thalassemia, sickle cell disease, and other chronic anemias are at greatest risk for iron overload. Cumulative doses of as few as 20 or more RBC units are associated with increased morbidity and mortality.[97,98] Preventing the accumulation of toxic iron levels by reducing iron stores through the use of exchange transfusions, iron chelators, or therapeutic phlebotomy can reduce these complications.

FATALITY REPORTING REQUIREMENTS

When the death of a patient results from a reaction to or complication of a transfusion, current regulations require that the fatality be reported to the FDA by the facility that performed the compatibility testing. The director of the Office of Compliance and Biologics Quality at the FDA Center for Biologics Evaluation and Research must be notified as soon as possible, followed by the submission of a written report within 7 days. Table 22-5 lists the contact information for the FDA. The report should contain the pertinent medical record, including laboratory reports, and the autopsy results when available.

TABLE 22-5. How to Contact the FDA[99]

Method	Contact Details
E-mail	fatalities2@fda.hhs.gov
Telephone/voicemail	240-402-9160
Fax	301-827-0333, Attn: CBER Fatality Program Manager
Express mail	US Food and Drug Administration CBER Office of Compliance and Biologics Quality Document Control Center 10903 New Hampshire Avenue WO71, G112 Silver Spring, MD 20993-0002

FDA = Food and Drug Administration; CBER = Center for Biologics Evaluation and Research.

The patient's underlying illness may make determination of the cause of death difficult. If there is any clinical suspicion that the transfusion may have contributed to the patient's death, that possibility should be investigated. Most transfusion-associated fatalities are caused by acute hemolysis, TRALI, or TACO. Investigations of these cases must attempt to rule out errors made in the areas of the laboratory, the transfusion service, or during blood administration.

KEY POINTS

1. The greatest risks associated with transfusion are noninfectious complications.
2. Many transfusion reactions have signs or symptoms that may be present in more than one type of reaction. Early recognition of the reaction, prompt cessation of the transfusion, and further evaluation are key to the successful resolution of a reaction.
3. Acute intravascular hemolytic reactions are often caused by sample or patient misidentification and are therefore usually preventable.
4. Allergic reactions range from urticaria (hives) to anaphylaxis. Most severe reactions are idiosyncratic and not due to selective protein deficiencies (eg, IgA and haptoglobin).
5. TRALI is often caused by HLA and HNA antibodies in donor components. Recognition of TRALI requires diagnosis by exclusion. Most patients recover from TRALI with supportive care.
6. TACO can be confused with TRALI because both feature pulmonary edema. TACO should be suspected in patients with positive fluid balance and patients who have difficulty regulating fluid balance; for example, those with congestive heart failure and end-stage renal disease.
7. Recently, TACO has surpassed TRALI as the leading cause of transfusion-related mortality reported to the FDA.
8. Massive transfusion can cause metabolic and hemostatic abnormalities. Each institution should develop its own massive transfusion protocol that takes into account the availability of appropriate laboratory testing.
9. TA-GVHD has a much more acute and severe course than GVHD after marrow or stem cell transplantation. TA-GVHD is fatal in >90% of cases and can be prevented by irradiation of blood components.
10. PTP is a serious but rare complication in which antibodies to human platelet antigens result in destruction of autologous and allogeneic platelets.
11. Iron overload is a noninfectious complication of chronic transfusion. Chelation and therapeutic phlebotomy are the primary treatments.
12. Recipient fatalities must be reported to the FDA by the compatibility testing facility as soon as possible after a fatal complication of transfusion has been confirmed.

REFERENCES

1. Food and Drug Administration. Transfusion/donation fatalities (annual summaries). Silver Spring, MD: CBER Office of Communication, Outreach, and Development, 2019. [Available at https://www.fda.gov/vaccines-blood-biologics/report-problem-center-biologics-evaluation-research/transfusiondonation-fatalities.]
2. Centers for Disease Control and Prevention. National Healthcare Safety Network manual: Biovigilance Component v2.5.2 Hemovigilance Module surveillance protocol. Atlanta, GA: Division of Healthcare Quality Promotion, National Center for Emerging and Zoonotic Infectious Diseases, 2018. [Available at https://www.cdc.gov/nhsn/pdfs/biovigilance/bv-hv-protocol-current.pdf.]
3. Berseus O, Boman K, Nessen SC, Westerberg LA. Risks of hemolysis due to anti-A and anti-B caused by the transfusion of blood or blood components containing ABO-incompatible plasma. Transfusion 2013;53(Suppl 1):114S-23S.

4. Stowell SR, Winkler AM, Maier CL, et al. Initiation and regulation of complement during hemolytic transfusion reactions. Clin Dev Immunol 2012;2012:307093.

5. Brodsky RA. Complement in hemolytic anemia. Blood 2015;126:2459-65.

6. Hod EA, Cadwell CM, Liepkalns JS, et al. Cytokine storm in a mouse model of IgG-mediated hemolytic transfusion reactions. Blood 2008;112:891-4.

7. Long AT, Kenne E, Jung R, et al. Contact system revisited: An interface between inflammation, coagulation, and innate immunity. J Thromb Haemost 2016;14:427-37.

8. Vamvakas EC, Blajchman MA. Transfusion-related mortality: The ongoing risks of allogeneic blood transfusion and the available strategies for their prevention. Blood 2009;113:3406-17.

9. Weinstock C, Mohle R, Dorn C, et al. Successful use of eculizumab for treatment of an acute hemolytic reaction after ABO-incompatible red blood cell transfusion. Transfusion 2015;55:605-10.

10. Maskens C, Downie H, Wendt A, et al. Hospital-based transfusion error tracking from 2005 to 2010: Identifying the key errors threatening patient transfusion safety. Transfusion 2014;54:66-73; quiz, 65.

11. Heddle NM, Fung M, Hervig T, et al. Challenges and opportunities to prevent transfusion errors: A Qualitative Evaluation for Safer Transfusion (QUEST). Transfusion 2012;52:1687-95.

12. Dunbar NM, Ornstein DL, Dumont LJ. ABO incompatible platelets: Risks versus benefit. Curr Opin Hematol 2012;19:475-9.

13. Rapido F, Brittenham GM, Bandyopadhyay S, et al. Prolonged red cell storage before transfusion increases extravascular hemolysis. J Clin Invest 2017;127:375-82.

14. Gammon R, ed. Standards for blood banks and transfusion services. 32nd ed. Bethesda, MD: AABB, 2020.

15. Francis RO, Jhang J, Hendrickson JE, et al. Frequency of glucose-6-phosphate dehydrogenase-deficiency red blood cell units in a metropolitan transfusion service. Transfusion 2013;53:606-11.

16. Eder AF, Meena-Leist CE, Hapip CA, et al. Clostridium perfringens in apheresis platelets: An unusual contaminant underscores the importance of clinical vigilance for septic transfusion reactions (CME). Transfusion 2014;54:857-62; quiz, 6.

17. Heddle NM, Klama L, Singer J, et al. The role of the plasma from platelet concentrates in transfusion reactions. N Eng J Med 1994;331:625-8.

18. Brubaker DB. Clinical significance of white cell antibodies in febrile nonhemolytic transfusion reactions. Transfusion 1990;30:733-7.

19. King KE, Shirey RS, Thoman SK, et al. Universal leukoreduction decreases the incidence of febrile nonhemolytic transfusion reactions to RBCs. Transfusion 2004;44:25-9.

20. Paglino JC, Pomper GJ, Fisch GS, et al. Reduction of febrile but not allergic reactions to RBCs and platelets after conversion to universal prestorage leukoreduction. Transfusion 2004;44:16-24.

21. Ezidiegwu CN, Lauenstein KJ, Rosales LG, et al. Febrile nonhemolytic transfusion reactions. Management by premedication and cost implications in adult patients. Arch Pathol Lab Med 2004;128:991-5.

22. Heddle NM, Blajchman MA, Meyer RM, et al. A randomized controlled trial comparing the frequency of acute reactions to plasma-removed platelets and prestorage WBC-reduced platelets. Transfusion 2002;42:556-66.

23. Savage WJ, Tobian AA, Fuller AK, et al. Allergic transfusion reactions to platelets are associated more with recipient and donor factors than with product attributes. Transfusion 2011;51:1716-22.

24. Savage WJ, Hamilton RG, Tobian AA, et al. Defining risk factors and presentations of allergic reactions to platelet transfusion. J Allergy Clin Immunol 2014;133:1772-5.e9.

25. Savage WJ, Tobian AA, Savage JH, et al. Transfusion and component characteristics are not associated with allergic transfusion reactions to apheresis platelets. Transfusion 2015;55:296-300.

26. Vyas GN, Fudenberg HH. Isoimmune anti-IgA causing anaphylactoid transfusion reactions. N Engl J Med 1969;280:1073-4.

27. Vyas GN, Holmdahl L, Perkins HA, Fudenberg HH. Serologic specificity of human anti-IgA and its significance in transfusion. Blood 1969;34:573-81.

28. Sandler SG, Eder AF, Goldman M, Winters JL. The entity of immunoglobulin A-related anaphylactic transfusion reactions is not evidence based. Transfusion 2015;55:199-204.

29. Shimada E, Tadokoro K, Watanabe Y, et al. Anaphylactic transfusion reactions in haptoglobin-deficient patients with IgE and IgG haptoglobin antibodies. Transfusion 2002;42:766-73.

30. Westhoff CM, Sipherd BD, Wylie DE, Toalson LD. Severe anaphylactic reactions following transfusions of platelets to a patient with anti-Ch. Transfusion 1992;32:576-9.

31. Poisson JL, Riedo FX, AuBuchon JP. Acquired peanut hypersensitivity after transfusion. Transfusion 2014;54:256-7.

32. Kaufman RM, Assmann SF, Triulzi DJ, et al. Transfusion-related adverse events in the Platelet Dose study. Transfusion 2015;55:144-53.

33. Kleinman S, Chan P, Robillard P. Risks associated with transfusion of cellular blood components in Canada. Transfus Med Rev 2003;17:120-62.

34. Tobian AA, Fuller AK, Uglik K, et al. The impact of platelet additive solution apheresis platelets on allergic transfusion reactions and corrected count increment. Transfusion 2014;54:1523-9.

35. Kemp SF, Lockey RF, Simons FE. Epinephrine: The drug of choice for anaphylaxis. A statement of the World Allergy Organization. Allergy 2008;63:1061-70.

36. Tobian AA, King KE, Ness PM. Transfusion premedications: A growing practice not based on evidence. Transfusion 2007;47:1089-96.

37. Kiani-Alikhan S, Yong PF, Grosse-Kreul D, et al. Successful desensitization to immunoglobulin A in a case of transfusion-related anaphylaxis. Transfusion 2010;50:1897-901.

38. Popovsky MA, Haley NR. Further characterization of transfusion-related acute lung injury: Demographics, clinical and laboratory features, and morbidity. Immunohematology 2000;16:157-9.

39. Nakagawa M, Toy P. Acute and transient decrease in neutrophil count in transfusion-related acute lung injury: Cases at one hospital. Transfusion 2004;44:1689-94.

40. Ferguson ND, Fan E, Camporota L, et al. The Berlin definition of ARDS: An expanded rationale, justification, and supplementary material. Intensive Care Med 2012;38:1573-82.

41. Vlaar APJ, Toy P, Fung M, et al. A consensus redefinition of transfusion-related acute lung injury. Transfusion 2019;59:2465-76.

42. Popovsky MA, Moore SB. Diagnostic and pathogenetic considerations in transfusion-related acute lung injury. Transfusion 1985;25:573-7.

43. Cherry T, Steciuk M, Reddy VV, Marques MB. Transfusion-related acute lung injury: Past, present, and future. Am J Clin Pathol 2008;129:287-97.

44. Toy P, Gajic O, Bacchetti P, et al. Transfusion-related acute lung injury: Incidence and risk factors. Blood 2012;119:1757-67.

45. Silliman CC, Boshkov LK, Mehdizadehkashi Z, et al. Transfusion-related acute lung injury: Epidemiology and a prospective analysis of etiologic factors. Blood 2003;101:454-62.

46. Eder AF, Dy BA, Perez JM, et al. The residual risk of transfusion-related acute lung injury at the American Red Cross (2008-2011): Limitations of a predominantly male-donor plasma mitigation strategy. Transfusion 2013;53:1442-9.

47. Steinberg KP, Hudson LD, Goodman RB, et al. Efficacy and safety of corticosteroids for persistent acute respiratory distress syndrome. N Engl J Med 2006;354:1671-84.

48. Zhou L, Giacherio D, Cooling L, Davenport RD. Use of B-natriuretic peptide as a diagnostic marker in the differential diagnosis of transfusion-associated circulatory overload. Transfusion 2005;45:1056-63.

49. Bolton-Maggs P, Poles D, et al for the Serious Hazards of Transfusion (SHOT) Steering Group. The 2017 Annual SHOT Report. Manchester, UK: SHOT, 2018. [Available at https://www.shotuk.org/shot-reports/.]

50. Wiersum-Osselton JC, Whitaker B, Grey S, et al. Revised international surveillance case definition of transfusion-associated circulatory overload: A classification agreement validation study. Lancet Haematol 2019;6(7):e350-e358.

51. International Society of Blood Transfusion Working Party on Haemovigilance, International Haemovigilance Network, AABB. Transfusion-associated circulatory overload (TACO) definition (2018). [Available at http://www.aabb.org/research/hemovigilance/Documents/TACO-2018-Definition.pdf (accessed December 3, 2019).]

52. Li G, Daniels CE, Kojicic M, et al. The accuracy of natriuretic peptides (brain natriuretic peptide and N-terminal pro-brain natriuretic) in the differentiation between transfusion-related acute lung injury and transfusion-related circulatory overload in the critically ill. Transfusion 2009;49:13-20.

53. Tobian A, Sokoll L, Tisch D, et al. N-terminal pro-brain natriuretic peptide is a useful diagnostic marker for transfusion-associated circulatory overload. Transfusion 2008;48:1143-50.

54. Clifford L, Jia Q, Yadav H, et al. Characterizing the epidemiology of perioperative transfusion-associated circulatory overload. Anesthesiology 2015;122:21-8.

55. Narick C, Triulzi DJ, Yazer MH. Transfusion-associated circulatory overload after plasma transfusion. Transfusion 2012;52:160-5.

56. Raval JS, Mazepa MA, Russell SL, et al. Passive reporting greatly underestimates the rate of transfusion-associated circulatory overload after platelet transfusion. Vox Sang 2015;108:387-92.

57. Pagano M, Ness P, Chajewski O, et al. Hypotensive transfusion reactions in the era of prestorage leukoreduction. Transfusion 2015;55:1668-74.

58. Li N, Williams L, Zhou Z, Wu Y. Incidence of acute transfusion reactions to platelets in hospitalized pediatric patients based on the US hemovigilance reporting system. Transfusion 2014;54:1666-72.

59. Cyr M, Hume H, Champagne M, et al. Anomaly of the des-Arg9-bradykinin metabolism associated with severe hypotensive reactions during blood transfusions: A preliminary study. Transfusion 1999;39:1084-8.

60. Cugno M, Nussberger J, Biglioli P, et al. Increase of bradykinin in plasma of patients undergoing cardiopulmonary bypass: The importance of lung exclusion. Chest 2001;120:1776-82.

61. Sihler KC, Napolitano LM. Complications of massive transfusion. Chest 2010;137:209-20.

62. Dzik WH, Kirkley SA. Citrate toxicity during massive blood transfusion. Transfus Med Rev 1988;2:76-94.

63. Spinella PC, Holcomb JB. Resuscitation and transfusion principles for traumatic hemorrhagic shock. Blood Rev 2009;23:231-40.

64. Wilson RF, Binkley LE, Sabo FM Jr, et al. Electrolyte and acid-base changes with massive blood transfusions. Am Surg 1992;58:535-44; discussion, 44-5.

65. Strauss RG. RBC storage and avoiding hyperkalemia from transfusions to neonates and infants. Transfusion 2010;50:1862-5.

66. Liu EA, Mannino FL, Lane TA. Prospective, randomized trial of the safety and efficacy of a limited donor exposure transfusion program for premature neonates. J Pediatr 1994;125:92-6.

67. Bansal I, Calhoun BW, Joseph C, et al. A comparative study of reducing the extracellular potassium concentration in red blood cells by washing and by reduction of additive solution. Transfusion 2007;47:248-50.

68. O'Leary MF, Szklarski P, Klein TM, et al. Hemolysis of red blood cells after washing with different automated technologies: Clinical implications in a neonatal cardiac surgery population.

69. Malone DL, Hess JR, Fingerhut A. Massive transfusion practices around the globe and a suggestion for a common massive transfusion protocol. J Trauma 2006;60:S91-6.

70. Engstrom M, Schott U, Romner B, Reinstrup P. Acidosis impairs the coagulation: A thromboelastographic study. J Trauma 2006;61:624-8.

71. Counts RB, Haisch C, Simon TL, et al. Hemostasis in massively transfused trauma patients. Ann Surg 1979;190:91-9.

72. Murray DJ, Pennell BJ, Weinstein SL, Olson JD. Packed red cells in acute blood loss: Dilutional coagulopathy as a cause of surgical bleeding. Anesth Analg 1995;80:336-42.

73. Harrigan C, Lucas CE, Ledgerwood AM, et al. Serial changes in primary hemostasis after massive transfusion. Surgery 1985;98:836-44.

74. Martini WZ. Coagulopathy by hypothermia and acidosis: Mechanisms of thrombin generation and fibrinogen availability. J Trauma 2009;67:202-8; discussion, 8-9.

75. Collins JA. Recent developments in the area of massive transfusion. World J Surg 1987;11:75-81.

76. Holcomb JB, Tilley BC, Baraniuk S, et al. Transfusion of plasma, platelets, and red blood cells in a 1:1:1 vs a 1:1:2 ratio and mortality in patients with severe trauma: The PROPPR randomized clinical trial. JAMA 2015;313:471-82.

77. Sperry JL, Guyette FX, Brown JB, et al. Prehospital plasma during air medical transport in trauma patients at risk for hemorrhagic shock. N Engl J Med 2018;379:315-26.

78. Roberts I, Shakur H, Ker K, et al. Antifibrinolytic drugs for acute traumatic injury. Cochrane Database Syst Rev 2012;12:CD004896.

79. O'Quin RJ, Lakshminarayan S. Venous air embolism. Arch Intern Med 1982;142:2173-6.

80. Mirski MA, Lele AV, Fitzsimmons L, Toung TJ. Diagnosis and treatment of vascular air embolism. Anesthesiology 2007;106:164-77.

81. Schonewille H, van de Watering LM, Loomans DS, Brand A. Red blood cell alloantibodies after transfusion: Factors influencing incidence and specificity. Transfusion 2006;46:250-6.

82. Tormey CA, Stack G. The persistence and evanescence of blood group alloantibodies in men. Transfusion 2009;49:505-12.

83. Vamvakas EC, Pineda AA, Reisner R, et al. The differentiation of delayed hemolytic and delayed serologic transfusion reactions: Incidence and predictors of hemolysis. Transfusion 1995;35:26-32.

84. Schonewille H, van de Watering LM, Brand A. Additional red blood cell alloantibodies after blood transfusions in a nonhematologic alloimmunized patient cohort: Is it time to take precautionary measures? Transfusion 2006;46:630-5.

85. Dumas G, Habibi A, Onimus T, et al. Eculizumab salvage therapy for delayed hemolysis transfusion reaction in sickle cell disease patients. Blood 2016;127:1062-4.

86. Ruhl H, Bein G, Sachs UJ. Transfusion-associated graft-versus-host disease. Transfus Med Rev 2009;23:62-71.

87. Klein HG. Transfusion-associated graft-versus-host disease: Less fresh blood and more gray (Gy) for an aging population. Transfusion 2006; 46:878-80.

88. Kopolovic I, Ostro J, Tsubota H, et al. A systematic review of transfusion-associated graft-versus-host disease. Blood 2015;126:406-14.

89. Castro G, Merkel PA, Giclas HE, et al. Amotosalen/UVA treatment inactivates T cells more effectively than the recommended gamma dose for prevention of transfusion-associated graft-versus-host disease. Transfusion 2018;58:1506-15.

90. Williamson LM, Stainsby D, Jones H, et al. The impact of universal leukodepletion of the blood supply on hemovigilance reports of posttransfusion purpura and transfusion-associated graft-versus-host disease. Transfusion 2007;47:1455-67.

91. Taaning E, Svejgaard A. Post-transfusion purpura: A survey of 12 Danish cases with special reference to immunoglobulin G subclasses of the platelet antibodies. Transfus Med 1994;4:1-8.

92. Shtalrid M, Shvidel L, Vorst E, et al. Posttransfusion purpura: A challenging diagnosis. Isr Med Assoc J 2006;8:672-4.

93. Hayashi T, Hirayama F. Advances in alloimmune thrombocytopenia: Perspectives on current concepts of human platelet antigens, antibody detection strategies, and genotyping. Blood Transfus 2015;13:380-90.

94. Ziman A, Klapper E, Pepkowitz S, et al. A second case of post-transfusion purpura caused by HPA-5a antibodies: Successful treatment with intravenous immunoglobulin. Vox Sang 2002; 83:165-6.

95. Loren AW, Abrams CS. Efficacy of HPA-1a (PlA1)-negative platelets in a patient with post-transfusion purpura. Am J Hematol 2004;76: 258-62.

96. Vu K, Leavitt AD. Posttransfusion purpura with antibodies against human platelet antigen-4a following checkpoint inhibitor therapy: A case report and review of the literature. Transfusion 2018;58;2265-9.

97. Alessandrino EP, Della Porta MG, Bacigalupo A, et al. Prognostic impact of pre-transplantation transfusion history and secondary iron overload in patients with myelodysplastic syndrome undergoing allogeneic stem cell transplantation: A GITMO study. Haematologica 2010;95:476-84.

98. Fung EB, Harmatz P, Milet M, et al. Morbidity and mortality in chronically transfused subjects with thalassemia and sickle cell disease: A report from the multi-center study of iron overload. Am J Hematol 2007;82:255-65.

99. Food and Drug Administration. Notification process for transfusion related fatalities and donation related deaths. Silver Spring, MD: CBER Office of Communication, Outreach, and Development, 2019. [Available at https://www.fda.gov/vaccines-blood-biologics/report-problem-center-biologics-evaluation-research/transfusiondonation-fatalities.]

CHAPTER 23

Perinatal Issues in Transfusion Practice

Lani Lieberman, MD; Gwen Clarke, MD; and Annika M. Svensson, MD, PhD

23

HEMOLYTIC DISEASE OF THE FETUS and newborn (HDFN), fetal/neonatal alloimmune thrombocytopenia (FNAIT), and immune thrombocytopenia (ITP) affect pregnant women, their fetuses, and newborns. The blood bank and transfusion service play critical roles in supporting the diagnosis and treatment of these conditions, including the appropriate provision of Rh Immune Globulin (RhIG).

HEMOLYTIC DISEASE OF THE FETUS AND NEWBORN

HDFN refers to the destruction of fetal and newborn red cells by maternal red cell antibodies specific for paternally inherited antigens on fetal red cells or erythroid precursors. HDFN can range from an isolated serologic finding with a clinically unaffected newborn and a positive direct antiglobulin test (DAT) result to severe anemia and occasionally fetal demise.

Pathophysiology

Maternal immunoglobulin G (IgG) antibody crosses the placenta into the fetal circulation, where it binds to fetal red cells or erythroid precursors. The immunoglobulin subclasses IgG1 and IgG3 are more likely than IgG2 or IgG4 to cause early and/or severe hemolytic disease.[1,2] The resulting increased hematopoietic drive causes a condition termed erythroblastosis fetalis, with liver and spleen enlargement secondary to extramedullary hematopoiesis, and portal hypertension. Liver enlargement can lead to decreased production of albumin and associated decreased plasma oncotic pressure, with generalized edema, ascites, and effusions known as hydrops fetalis. Severe HDFN can occur as early as 18 to 20 weeks' gestation or earlier with antibodies to K1 (of the KEL system), but may be difficult to detect; severity usually increases in subsequent pregnancies. Untreated, hydrops fetalis, with its associated high-output cardiovascular failure secondary to anemia, can lead to fetal death. The destruction of red cells also leads to elevated bilirubin levels. The maternal liver clears the bilirubin, preventing the accumulation of bilirubin in the fetus. After birth, the infant's immature liver enzymatic pathways cannot metabolize the unconjugated bilirubin, which can increase to dangerous levels. The hyperbilirubinemia can cause permanent brain damage, known as kernicterus.[3] The maternal antibody typically decreases in the neonate over 12 weeks, with a half-life of about 25 days. Some antibodies may cause more prolonged anemia or delayed-onset anemia. Al-Alaiyan et al found that prolonged (mean postnatal age of

Lani Lieberman, MD, Assistant Professor, Department of Laboratory Medicine and Pathobiology, University of Toronto, and Department of Clinical Pathology, University Health Network, Toronto, Ontario, Canada; Gwen Clarke, MD, Clinical Professor, Department of Laboratory Medicine and Pathology, University of Alberta, and Associate Medical Director, Clinical Services, Canadian Blood Services, Edmonton, Alberta, Canada; and Annika M. Svensson, MD, PhD, Transfusion Medicine Consultant, Denver, Colorado
The authors have disclosed no conflicts of interest.

43.3 ± 15.7 days) hyporegenerative anemia (hemoglobin <8 g/dL) is common among Rh-isoimmunized infants, regardless of the use of intravascular intrauterine transfusion (IUT), in term and late-preterm infants.[4] Other antibodies that cause anemia through erythropoietic suppression (anti-K1, anti-Jr[a], anti-Ge, and rare cases of high-titer IgG anti-M antibodies) may also contribute to prolonged anemia.[5-9]

Because of the widespread prophylactic use of RhIG in high-development-index nations, ABO incompatibility is currently the most common cause of HDFN. When present, ABO HDFN is typically mild.[10] ABO HDFN is defined by maternal/fetal ABO incompatibility, an elevated bilirubin (corrected for gestational age), and a positive DAT result. If treatment is needed, phototherapy is usually sufficient, and the need for neonatal exchange transfusion is uncommon. The incidence of ABO HDFN ranges from 1% to 4%, depending on the ethnicity of the population. It develops when naturally occurring IgG anti-A and/or -B are transported across the placenta and bind to fetal A and/or B antigens on red cells. Group O mothers of European or Asian ancestry with group A infants are most commonly affected; in populations of African ancestry, group B infants with group O mothers are most likely to be affected. ABO HDFN rarely leads to severe anemia, because fetal ABO antigens are poorly developed and isohemagglutinins are neutralized by tissue and soluble antigens. If a cord blood DAT result is negative, clinically significant ABO HDFN is unlikely, and titration of these antibodies is not typically required.

Maternal Alloimmunization

The biological characteristics that make certain individuals responsive to immunogenic stimuli have not been clearly elucidated. Females can be alloimmunized to red cell antigens by pregnancy, blood transfusion, transplantation, or from unknown stimuli.[11] Minor fetomaternal hemorrhage (FMH) occurs spontaneously in a high proportion of women during gestation. The likelihood of FMH increases with gestational age (from 3% in trimester 1 to 12% and 45% in trimesters 2 and 3, respectively) and is at the high-

est risk at delivery. After exposure, the maternal immune system must form the red cell antibody and switch class from IgM to IgG before HDFN becomes a clinically significant risk. For all of these reasons, the first pregnancy is rarely affected by HDFN.[12,13] Rick factors for FMH include the following: abdominal trauma, placenta previa, abruptio placentae, ectopic pregnancy, threatened termination, or fetal death, as well as procedures such as amniocentesis, fetal blood sampling (FBS), intrauterine manipulation, or abortion.[14]

RhD is the most potent immunogenic red cell antigen. It remains the most important cause of HDFN in nations without robust access to prenatal care.[15,16] As little as 0.1 to 1 mL of D-positive red cells can stimulate alloantibody production.[17] In ABO-incompatible, D-negative mothers, the alloimmunization rate for the D antigen is markedly diminished, thus demonstrating a partially protective effect of ABO incompatibility.[18,19] Anti-K1 is also an important cause of HDFN, and a potent immunogen. The level of hemolysis caused by the presence of anti-K1 is less than that caused by anti-D, because the K1 antigen is expressed on the early red cell precursors leading to reticulocytopenia and significant anemia.[5] Other antibodies that have been less commonly reported to cause moderate or severe disease include antibodies against E, c, C, k, Kp[a], Kp[b], Ku, Js[a], Js[b], Jk[a], Fy[a], Fy[b], S, s, and U.[20,21] (See Table 13-5 in Chapter 13.) The presence of multiple antibodies may lead to more severe HDFN.[22]

Diagnosis and Monitoring

The diagnosis of HDFN and ongoing laboratory assessments involve the cooperation of the patient, health-care provider, and blood bank/transfusion laboratory personnel. The patient's obstetric and transfusion history are important; a previously affected pregnancy predicts the potential for future HDFN.[23] During the first prenatal visit, the maternal ABO and RhD type and an antibody screen to detect IgG-phase antibodies [37 C with antihuman globulin (AHG)] should be performed. If a D-negative woman does not have anti-D, she is a candidate for RhIG administration to prevent RhD alloimmunization (see below). A positive antibody screen requires antibody identification and titration. Antibodies against minor carbohydrate blood group antigens such as anti-I, -P1, -Le^a, and -Le^b, whether IgM or IgG, do not cause HDFN and may be ignored because these antigens are poorly developed at birth. Treatment of the mother's plasma with dithiothreitol (DTT) preferentially destroys IgM antibodies and can help distinguish IgG from IgM antibodies for cases of anti-M with increasing titer.[24,25] After identifying a clinically significant red cell antibody, the father should be tested for the corresponding red cell antigen, if possible, to stratify risk of fetal inheritance. Homozygous fathers have a 100% chance of offspring expressing the red cell antigen; heterozygous fathers portend a 50% chance. For women sensitized to RhD, serologic methods cannot readily determine paternal zygosity; when possible, a predicted genotype using paternal DNA testing is indicated.[26] Alternatively, fetal risk stratification through prediction of the fetal red cell antigen type can be accomplished by genotyping fetal DNA, either using amniocytes or noninvasively with cell-free fetal DNA (cffDNA) present in maternal plasma.[27,28]

During an alloimmunized pregnancy, monthly to biweekly maternal antibody titers can be used to deduce if the fetus is the source of ongoing maternal immune stimulation and is at risk for clinically significant HDFN. Once an antibody titer reaches a level above which clinically significant HDFN could occur (the critical titer), further titration may not be of benefit and noninvasive clinical monitoring for fetal anemia should commence.[23] The AABB-recommended method for titration is a saline AHG test incubated for 60 minutes at 37 C ("tube" method; see Method 5-3). Other methods, such as albumin or gel, may result in higher titers than the recommended method and should be validated with clinical findings and laboratory data to ensure appropriate interpretation. Because of the potential for poor reproducibility of red cell antibody titers, individual blood banks should validate their testing internally and keep previous specimens for subsequent comparison.[29] The critical titer for anti-D is usually 8 to 32 in the AHG phase. Because sensitization to the K1 antigen may lead to hypoproliferative anemia, a ti-

ter of 8 or lower may be accepted as the critical level, although some centers regard any K1 sensitization as critical. The critical titer for other antibody specificities is typically 16 to 32, and for all antibodies a "two tube" increase in titer level is also considered important.[30-32] Once a critical titer is reached, Doppler fetal ultrasound of the middle cerebral artery (MCA) is a noninvasive way to assess fetal anemia.[23] Decisions about when to intervene with fetal transfusion or delivery are based on the degree of fetal anemia and gestational age; an increase in the velocity of the end systolic MCA blood flow to >1.5 multiples of the mean (MoM) on the ultrasound denotes moderate to severe anemia.

Treatment

In cases of severe anemia, if it is too early in gestation for delivery, fetal transfusion is indicated to treat the anemia. The transfusion will suppress the fetal erythropoiesis and thus the production of red cells with the antigen corresponding to the maternal alloantibody. After birth, neonatal therapies such as phototherapy, simple transfusion, and exchange transfusion may be indicated.

Fetal Transfusion

Red Blood Cell (RBC) units for IUT should be 1) group O (in most cases) and crossmatch compatible with maternal plasma, 2) irradiated to prevent transfusion-associated graft-vs-host disease (TA-GVHD), 3) cytomegalovirus (CMV) reduced-risk (leukocyte reduced or from a CMV-seronegative donor), and 4) known to lack hemoglobin S to prevent sickling under low oxygen tension. RBC units collected within 5 to 7 days are preferred, if available, because of the large transfusion volume and to prolong the circulation of transfused red cells. RBC units may be washed or concentrated to a hematocrit of 70% to 85%. Most institutions will routinely use group O, D-negative units for IUT, but type-specific (D-positive) units may be used if anti-D is not causative and/or if the fetus is known to be D positive. If the maternal antibody is directed at a high-prevalence antigen and no other compatible blood is available, the mother's washed, irradiated red cells or compatible, irradiated red cells from maternal siblings or rare donor registries can be used.[33]

The volume of blood to be transfused can be calculated by 1) multiplying the ultrasound-estimated fetal weight in grams by the factor 0.14 mL/g to determine the fetal and placental total blood volume, 2) multiplying this amount by the difference in posttransfusion (desired) and pretransfusion hematocrit, and 3) dividing the resulting amount by the hematocrit of the RBC unit to be transfused.[34] For example: with an estimated fetal weight of 1000 g, a desired posttransfusion hematocrit of 40% (0.4), a pre-transfusion hematocrit of 15% (0.15), and a measured hematocrit of the RBC unit of 85% (0.85), the volume to transfuse is 41.2 mL, as shown below.

$$[1000 \text{ g} \times 0.14 \text{ mL/g} \times (0.40 - 0.15)]/0.85 = 41.2 \text{ mL}$$

The volume and rate of the transfusion should be adjusted to accommodate the clinical status of the fetus. Because these calculations are based on estimates and the fetal placental volume can vary for any estimated fetal weight, the hemoglobin or hematocrit should be checked after transfusion to confirm that the desired posttransfusion hemoglobin level has been achieved.[35] When delivery is not imminent, IUT is repeated according to the severity of the disease or based on an estimated decline in hematocrit of 1% per day. Generally, the strategy is to raise the hematocrit to >40% with transfusion and to repeat transfusion when the calculated hematocrit has declined to 30% or below.[36] Transfusion into the peritoneal cavity can be used in cases where the umbilical cord artery cannot be accessed, particularly when IUT is required in early pregnancy. In the absence of hydrops fetalis, the outcome of a successful IUT treatment is generally good, with a low incidence of neurodevelopmental impairment and a low risk of fetal loss.[37]

Maternal Treatment

During pregnancy, alternative or adjunctive therapies to IUT have been recommended, including maternal plasma exchange and the ad-

ministration of intravenous immune globulin (IVIG). Both have been used in small studies, early in gestation before IUT can be accomplished, or as alternatives to IUT, with the goal of blunting the effect of the maternal antibody.[4] In small case series, IVIG infusion has been shown to stabilize anti-D titers, and results were best when the procedure was started before 28 weeks' gestation.[38] Plasma exchange can temporarily reduce antibody levels by as much as 75% and has been shown to reduce the risk of fetal death and/or morbidity in a mother with a previous severe course of HDFN in one case series.[39] The American Society for Apheresis classifies HDFN as a Category III indication [based on weak (grade 2) evidence] for the use of plasma exchange before commencement of IUT.[40]

Neonatal Treatment

After delivery, hemoglobin and bilirubin must be closely monitored. The threat of kernicterus can be high in HDFN, especially in premature neonates.[41] Phototherapy oxidizes elevated unconjugated bilirubin, allowing the oxidation products to be excreted in the urine. For severe jaundice unresponsive to phototherapy, most experts recommend IVIG with the goal to avoid an exchange transfusion (American Academy of Pediatrics), although other studies question its efficacy, particularly given side effects such as hemolysis and necrotizing enterocolitis.[42-44] In neonates who are unresponsive to phototherapy and IVIG, a double-volume exchange transfusion replaces approximately 85% to 90% of the blood volume and removes 50% of the bilirubin. Exchange transfusion with reconstituted whole blood (Chapter 24) is generally unnecessary if the infant received IUTs; however, small-volume "top-up" transfusions may be required until the neonate's erythropoiesis is able to support the hemoglobin requirement and residual maternal antibodies have disappeared.

Prevention

Rh Immune Globulin

D-negative and some variant D-positive females are candidates for RhIG prophylaxis during pregnancy to prevent RhD alloimmunization. RhIG is made from pooled human plasma from individuals either naturally or intentionally immunized to the D antigen; recombinant products are in development. The product contains IgG-subtype anti-D. It is available in 300-, 120-, and 50-μg doses. Appropriate ante- and postpartum administration of RhIG reduces the risk of a D-negative mother becoming immunized by a D-positive fetus from about 16% to <0.1%. The American College of Obstetricians and Gynecologists recommends the first dose of RhIG be given at 28 weeks' gestation because 92% of women who develop anti-D during pregnancy do so at or after 28 weeks.[45-47] RhIG is indicated after any event that increases the risk for FMH. D-negative females who have been previously immunized to the D antigen, D-positive females, and D-negative females whose infants are known to be D negative are not candidates for RhIG. Women with apparent antibodies to both D and C should be investigated for presence of anti-G before determining their candidacy for RhIG. Unless specific reactivity to D is demonstrated, a pregnant D-negative female with anti-G should receive RhIG. Outside of the United States, RhIG prophylactic protocols may differ. Antenatal RhIG may be targeted to those women who have a D-positive fetus determined by cffDNA testing. cffDNA obtained from maternal blood samples can identify pregnancies with D-negative fetuses and avoid RhIG administration.[46,47]

Administration of RhIG during pregnancy typically leads to a positive antibody screening result in the mother, but the anti-D titer is low and thus poses no risk to the fetus. Occasionally, RhIG will cause a positive DAT result in the newborn. The mechanism of action of RhIG has not been completely elucidated. D-positive red cells are opsonized by RhIG and cleared by macrophages in the spleen, which results in cytokine secretion and immunomodulation.[48,49] Similar antigen-specific suppression of the immune response has been observed in a murine system where anti-K1 prevented immunization against transfused K1-positive cells but not against other antigens.[50]

Historically, pregnant women with serologic weak D (see Chapter 11) were treated as D negative and deemed eligible for RhIG.[51] However,

in populations of European ancestry, a majority of individuals with the serologic weak D phenotype may not benefit from the administration of RhIG, because most have underlying *RHD* genotypes of weak D types 1, 2, or 3. Individuals with these genotypes have not been reported to form D alloantibody after exposure to conventional D epitopes.[52,53] Genotyping pregnant women with serologic weak D phenotype early in pregnancy to identify weak D genotypes 1, 2, or 3 allows for selective administration of RhIG to those who will benefit and avoids unnecessary treatment of women who will not. The practice of weak D genotyping in this population is becoming standard. If a woman is found to have serologic weak D phenotype for the first time at the time of delivery, *RHD* genotyping often cannot practically be completed before the 72-hour window for RhIG administration. In such cases, administration of RhIG is the prudent choice, with subsequent *RHD* genotyping for weak D types to guide care for future pregnancies. Women proven to have weak D types 1, 2, or 3 can be managed as D-positive for the purpose of transfusion, thus conserving the supply of D-negative blood.[52,54-56] Counseling female patients found to have weak D genotypes 1, 2, or 3 about their *RHD* status is important for their peace of mind and to minimize confusion. These females should be made aware that their serologic RhD status may be designated differently by different laboratories, and reassured that they do not need RhIG in the future. At this time, there is not enough experience to determine if other variant *RHD* genotypes can form anti-D; thus, women with *RHD* genotypes other than weak D types 1, 2, or 3 should be considered D negative for the purposes of transfusion and RhIG administration.

After delivery of a D-positive infant, D-negative mothers without alloanti-D should receive RhIG. About 10% of the RhIG dose given at 28 weeks' gestation will be present in the mother when the infant is delivered at term. (The half-life of IgG is about 25 days.) To determine the correct RhIG dose for postpartum administration, a maternal blood sample is screened for FMH. Three tests are available to test for FMH: the rosette screening test, the Kleihauer-Betke (KB) test, and the flow cytometry test.

The rosette test (Method 5-1) is a semiquantitative screen that is positive when more than 10 mL of D-positive fetal red cells are present in the maternal circulation. The maternal specimen should be collected 1 to 2 hours after all of the products of conception are delivered.[57-59] The test is performed by incubating the D-negative maternal blood sample with D antisera and subsequently adding D-positive indicator red cells, which form agglutinates (rosettes) with any fetal D-positive red cells in the maternal sample. The sample is read microscopically and rosettes (agglutinates) are counted. If the screening test result is negative, a standard dose of 300-µg RhIG is given. This is sufficient to prevent immunization by 15 mL of fetal red cells or 30 mL of whole blood. A positive screening test result indicates that the FMH may be >15 mL of fetal red cells (30 mL of whole blood) and requires further testing to quantify FMH and determine the appropriate dose of RHIG. Mothers with variant *RHD* genes may have false-positive rosette screening results. A positive DAT result may also reflect a false-positive result. To quantify the volume of the FMH, a quantitative assay, such as the KB test or flow cytometric assessment, is used. The risk of FMH >30 mL at the time of delivery is approximately 1 in 1250.[12]

The KB test capitalizes on the resistance of fetal hemoglobin to acid treatment (Method 5-2). A thin smear of maternal blood is placed on a slide, treated with acid, rinsed, counterstained, and read microscopically by counting 1000 to 2000 cells to estimate the ratio of fetal to maternal red cells. The maternal red cells appear as pale "ghost" cells, and the fetal red cells are pink. KB results can be confounded by the presence of fetal hemoglobin in the maternal cells due to hereditary persistence of fetal hemoglobin (HbF), elevated maternal HbF cells that increase during pregnancy, or hemoglobinopathies such as sickle cell disease or thalassemia. In such cases, flow cytometry can help to differentiate between FMH and alternate causes. Flow cytometry measures fetal hemoglobin and/or D-positive red cells. It has higher precision than the KB test, although the requirement for rapid turnaround time and lack of availability of flow cytometry or related expertise leads many laboratories to continue using the KB method.[60,61] If assessment of the FMH by flow cytometry is used, a more precise dose of RhIG can be calculated. The volume of fetal red cells is estimated as follows:

(Fetal cells/total cells counted) × maternal blood volume (mL) = FMH, whole blood (mL)

For example: For 6 fetal cells counted out of 2000 cells, and an estimated maternal blood volume of 5000 mL, the FMH is calculated to be 15 mL. Females with very high body mass indices may have a total blood volume significantly higher than 5000 mL, which needs to be considered in the calculation.[62,63]

The estimated FMH volume is used to calculate the dose of RhIG. A 300-µg dose of RhIG will suppress alloimmunization by 30 mL of fetal whole blood. In the above example, the FMH is 15 mL, so the number of 300-µg RhIG vials to administer can be calculated as 15 mL/ 30 mL RhIG/vial = 0.5 vial. If the KB test is used, due to the subjective nature of the test performance and interpretation, the RhIG dose is rounded up to the next whole number if the number to the right of the decimal point is ≥5 (if <5, it is rounded down). An additional vial should be added to all calculations. (See Table 23-1.) For example, the dose is calculated as follows: 0.5 vial is rounded up to 1 vial, then 1 extra vial is added, resulting in a total of 2 vials to be administered.

1.6 vials calculated from formula = 2 (rounded up) + 1 (one vial added) = 3 vials

1.4 vials calculated from formula = 1 (rounded down) + 1 (one vial added) = 2 vials

Postpartum RhIG should be given to the mother within 72 hours of delivery. If prophylaxis is delayed, the American College of Obstetricians and Gynecologists recommends that RhIG treatment should still be provided.[45] RhIG should also be administered if the RhD type of the newborn is unknown or undetermined (eg, for a stillborn infant). RhIG is given by the intramuscular (IM) or intravenous (IV) route. Some

TABLE 23-1. Examples of RhIG Dose Selection Based on Differing Volumes of Fetomaternal Hemorrhage in a 70-kg Female Using Vial Size of 300 μg

% Fetal Cells	Vials to Inject	Dose	
		μg (mcg)	IU
0.3-0.8	2	600	3000
0.9-1.4	3	900	4500
1.5-2.0	4	1200	6000
2.1-2.6	5	1500	7500

Notes:

1. Table reflects calculations based on an example maternal blood volume of 5000 mL.

2. In the United States, 1 vial of 300 μg (1500 IU) is needed for each 15 mL of fetal red cells or 30 mL of fetal whole blood. Other vial sizes are available.

preparations are for IM administration only. RhIG consists almost entirely of IgG, with only small amounts of other immunoglobulins. Active D immunization has a significant IgM component; thus, new anti-D produced by the mother is often detected in the saline phase and can be completely or partially inactivated by 2-mercaptoethanol or DTT treatment, whereas reactivity passively acquired from RhIG IgG remains. Passively acquired anti-D rarely achieves a titer >4. Failure of RhIG to prevent immunization to D may result from a number of factors such as increased FMH volumes and high maternal body weight, leading to inadequate IM injection.[63] However, in many cases, a cause for D immunization despite administration of RhIG cannot be determined.[64]

Red Cell Selection

Prevention of HDFN aims to reduce exposure of females of childbearing age to red cell alloantigens. In life-threatening hemorrhage when uncrossmatched RBCs are needed, it is standard to use D-negative RBCs initially for such females until the blood type can be determined.[65] In some countries, more extensive matching (K, C, c, E, or e) is undertaken for transfusion to these females.[9] RBC units that are antigenically similar to the mother may be selected in an attempt to

decrease the risk for additional alloimmunization.[66] Decreased alloimmunization in women who received IUT strictly matched for Fy, Jk, and S antigens was shown in one study.[67]

PREGNANCY-RELATED THROMBOCYTOPENIA

Maternal thrombocytopenia (platelet counts <150,000/μL) occurs in 5% to 10% of pregnant women.[68] The causes of the thrombocytopenia include incidental thrombocytopenia of pregnancy or gestational thrombocytopenia (74%), thrombocytopenia complicating hypertensive disorders in pregnancy (21%), and immunologic disorders of pregnancy (4%).[69] Regardless of the etiology, it is rare for maternal platelet counts to decrease below 80,000/μL, in any trimester.[68] When the cause is immunologic, maternal IgG antibodies to platelets can cross the placenta and cause fetal thrombocytopenia. Two categories of immune-mediated thrombocytopenia are recognized: cases caused by alloantibodies (FNAIT) and those caused by autoantibodies, such as ITP and systemic lupus erythematosus (SLE). The diagnostic distinction between these conditions is important for therapy selection.

Fetal and Neonatal Alloimmune Thrombocytopenia

Pathophysiology

FNAIT occurs when the maternal immune system forms platelet-specific antibodies that cross the placenta and destroy fetal platelets. Platelet antigens represent specific polymorphisms in platelet membrane glycoproteins. (See Chapter 15.) In people of European ancestry, approximately 79% of FNAIT cases are caused by antibodies to human platelet antigen (HPA)-1a, which is present in about 98% of the US population. About 9% of cases are caused by anti-HPA-5b, 4% by anti-HPA-1b, 2% by anti-HPA-3a, and 6% by other antibodies (including multiple antibodies).[70] In people of Asian ancestry, HPA-4b and HPA-5b are more often implicated than HPA-1a.[71]

The reported incidence of affected pregnancies ranges from 0.3 to 1 in 1000.[72,73] In 25% of FNAIT cases, the platelet antibody develops during the first pregnancy and affects the first pregnancy. In fact, the maternal antibody has been detected as early as 17 weeks' gestation, and the fetus may develop thrombocytopenia as early as 20 weeks' gestation. However, because FNAIT is often not discovered until birth, when the newborn presents with petechiae, ecchymoses, gastrointestinal bleeding, and/or intracranial hemorrhage (ICH), the focus has been on prevention in subsequent pregnancies. FNAIT-related ICH occurs in 0.02 to 0.1 in 1000 live births.[74-76] More than 50% of ICHs occur in utero, often before 28 weeks' gestation.[77,78] Thirty-five percent of ICH events are fatal; nonfatal events are often associated with significant neurologic consequences.[77,79]

Diagnosis

A history of antenatal ICH or FNAIT in a sibling is one of the most important predictors of thrombocytopenia in a fetus.[80] The mother and father should be typed for platelet antigens, and the mother should be screened for alloantibodies. DNA testing of the father can determine the zygosity of the antigen involved. Direct fetal platelet genotyping can be determined via amniotic fluid (18-20 weeks), chorionic villus material (8-10 weeks), or fetal DNA present in a maternal blood sample.[81,82] Amniocentesis has an associated risk of pregnancy loss of 0.5% to 1.0%.[83] Chorionic villus sampling increases the risk of alloimmunization and is not recommended. Noninvasive prenatal testing uses cffDNA techniques but is available only in some centers.[81,82] Genetic counseling of maternal siblings should be considered.

Treatment

Antenatal intervention should be offered to all mothers of affected fetuses who have had a previous pregnancy with FNAIT. The goal of treatment is to avoid a fetal or neonatal ICH. Assessment of the fetus should begin at or before 20 weeks' gestation. Mainstay antenatal treatment includes close monitoring at a high-risk obstetrical center, with or without IVIG, and with or without corticosteroids. The optimal dose, schedule, and gestational age to initiate IVIG is not known. In most reports, IVIG is administered at a dose of 1 g/kg per week; however, reported doses include 0.4 g/kg per day for 5 days, 0.5 g/kg per week, 0.8 g/kg per week, 1 g/kg every 2 weeks, and 2 g/kg per week.[76,84,85]

There are no trials that have evaluated the most appropriate mode of delivery; both routes, cesarean section and vaginal delivery, are offered.[86,87] The mode of delivery should be based on obstetrician and patient preference. Furthermore, procedures used to measure the infant's platelet count before delivery, such as FBS with intrauterine platelet transfusions, are not recommended, because the risk of morbidity and mortality from the procedure (11%) is greater than or equal to the risk of severe bleeding in utero or at delivery.[76] If FBS is performed, an irradiated, CMV-reduced-risk, antigen-negative platelet transfusion should be administered at the same time. Procedures during labor associated with increased hemorrhagic risk to the fetus (eg, fetal scalp electrodes, forceps) should be avoided.

After delivery, the greatest risk of infant bleeding is present during the first few days of life. The primary goal of management is to prevent major hemorrhage such as ICH or death. Expert opinions propose a wide range of platelet counts as a safe transfusion threshold. To date, no randomized controlled studies have addressed this question. For nonbleeding, asymptomatic newborns, 30,000/μL is suggested as an appropriate threshold. For neonates with bleeding symptoms, such as ICH or gastrointestinal bleeding, platelets should be transfused to maintain their platelet counts initially above 100,000/μL and then above 50,000/μL for at least 7 days.[85] HPA-selected platelet transfusions (maternal or donor), if available, are considered first-line therapy because they lead to higher platelet increments and longer response durations when compared to unselected platelet transfusions. If HPA-selected platelets are not immediately available, HPA-unselected platelets should be ordered.[88] Maternal platelets may cause a delay in providing the transfusion, as they are often logistically challenging to obtain in terms of collection and component manipulation. The typical platelet nadir occurs within 48 hours of delivery,[89,90] and the majority of infants improve within 1 to 5 weeks.[91] In rare cases, thrombocytopenia may persist for up to 8 to 12 weeks.[85]

Immune Thrombocytopenia

Infants of mothers with thrombocytopenia from ITP, SLE, or other autoimmune disorders may be thrombocytopenic because of placental transfer of maternal autoantibodies. In general, thrombocytopenia and sequelae in neonates born to mothers with these conditions is less severe than in FNAIT. Although clinically significant bleeding episodes are rare, newborns should be followed closely, as platelet counts can decrease after birth.

ITP is estimated to occur in 1 in 1000 to 1 in 10,000 pregnant women.[92] Fortunately, bleeding symptoms during pregnancy or at the time of delivery are uncommon.[93] The management of pregnant patients with ITP is similar to that in nonpregnant women. Recommendations are based on expert consensus. American Society of Hematology (ASH) guidelines state that there is no evidence to support obtaining intrapartum fetal platelet counts routinely and that data are limited in support of specific platelet count thresholds that are safe in the ante- or peripartum period.[94] An international panel with expertise in ITP management suggested that, during the first two trimesters, treatment should be initiated when the patient is symptomatic, when platelet counts are <20,000 to 30,000/μL, or to increase the platelet count before a procedure. For women who require treatment, both IVIG and oral corticosteroids provide a good response.[95]

Prospective studies report an incidence of severe neonatal thrombocytopenia (<50,000/μL) in 9% to 15% and ICH in 0 to 1.5% of infants.[95] Although maternal platelet counts do not predict neonatal thrombocytopenia, mothers with a previous history of delivering a thrombocytopenic infant are at a greater risk of delivering another thrombocytopenic infant.[93,96] The mode of delivery should be based on obstetrician and patient preference, similar to FNAIT management noted above.

In all infants born to mothers with a history of ITP, an early postnatal platelet count should be performed. IM injections such as vitamin K should be avoided until the platelet count is known to be normal. A head ultrasound should be performed to rule out ICH in thrombocytopenic infants (platelet counts <50,000/μL). Although treatment of the neonate is rarely needed, most hemorrhagic events in neonates occur 24 to 48 hours after delivery. Platelet counts should be repeated daily, as the nadir is frequently seen 2 to 5 days after birth. In those with clinical hemorrhage or if the platelet count remains <30,000/μL, IVIG and/or platelet transfusion should be considered.[97] Neonatal counts should be monitored until normalized because thrombocytopenia can persist and could represent an inherited form of thrombocytopenia.

Literature and recommendations are available for ITP management, but less so for other autoimmune conditions. Maternal thrombocytopenia secondary to SLE is usually less severe than thrombocytopenia of ITP. Treatment of thrombocytopenia related to these autoimmune conditions is similar to the approach for an ITP patient.[97]

KEY POINTS

1. HDFN is caused by maternal red cell antibodies that are specific to a paternally derived red cell antigen. The maternal IgG antibody is transported across the placenta, where it destroys fetal red cells, causing fetal anemia and hyperbilirubinemia.

2. The most common clinically significant antibodies that cause HDFN are anti-D and anti-K1; anti-C, -c, and -E, along with others, are significant but less common. ABO HDFN is common but usually causes only mild to moderate symptoms. Some antibodies, such as anti-I, -P1, -Le^a, and -Le^b, can be ignored during pregnancy.

3. Molecular typing of cffDNA can be performed on maternal plasma to determine the fetal red cell antigens. Paternal testing can also predict fetal inheritance. Molecular methods are required to determine paternal *RHD* zygosity.

4. For IUT, the RBCs should be irradiated, CMV reduced-risk, hemoglobin S negative, group O (in most cases), and <7 days old.

5. The rosette test is a sensitive method for detecting FMH of approximately 10 mL or more. The KB test is used to quantify the size of the FMH levels. Flow cytometry can more precisely measure fetal hemoglobin and/or D-positive red cells compared to KB testing.

6. The calculated RhIG dose should be rounded up if the number to the right of the decimal point is ≥0.5, or rounded down if the number is <0.5. In either case, an additional vial should be added to the result.

7. In FNAIT, the maternal platelet antibody may develop as early as 17 weeks of gestation in the first pregnancy, and fetal thrombocytopenia may develop as early as 20 weeks. Previous pregnancy outcomes predict future outcomes.

8. Irradiated, CMV-reduced-risk platelets should be given to treat neonatal thrombocytopenia and avoid hemorrhage. Corresponding-HPA antigen-negative platelets (if available) will produce greater posttransfusion platelet count increments.

9. HPA-selected platelet transfusions, if available, are considered first-line therapy for FNAIT. If HPA-selected platelets are not immediately available, HPA-unselected platelets should be ordered.

10. Thrombocytopenia in neonates born to mothers with autoimmune conditions tends to be less severe than thrombocytopenia in neonates born with FNAIT.

REFERENCES

1. Firan M, Bawdon R, Radu C, et al. The MHC class I-related receptor, FcRn, plays an essential role in the maternofetal transfer of gamma-globulin in humans. Int Immunol 2001;13:993-1002.

2. Pollock JM, Bowman JM. Anti-Rh(D) IgG subclasses and severity of Rh hemolytic disease of the newborn. Vox Sang 1990;59:176-9.

3. Dennery PA, Seidman DS, Stevenson DK. Neonatal hyperbilirubinemia. N Engl J Med 2001; 344:581-90.

4. Al-Alaiyan S, al Omran A. Late hyporegenerative anemia in neonates with Rhesus hemolytic disease. J Perinat Med 1999;27:112-15.

5. Vaughan JI, Manning M, Warwick RM, et al. Inhibition of erythroid progenitor cells by anti-Kell antibodies in fetal alloimmune anemia. N Engl J Med 1998;338:798-803.

6. Endo Y, Ito S, Ogiyama Y. Suspected anemia caused by maternal anti Jr^a antibodies: A case report. Biomark Res 2015;3:23.

7. Yasuda H, Ohto H, Nollet KE, et al. Hemolytic disease of the newborn with late onset anemia due to anti M: A case report and review of the Japanese literature. Transfus Med Rev 2014;28: 1-6.

8. Blackall DP, Pesek GD, Montgomery MM, et al. Hemolytic disease of fetus and newborn due to anti-Ge3: Combined antibody-dependent hemolysis and erythroid precursor cell growth inhibition. Am J Perinatol 2008;25(9):541-5.

9. Arndt PA, Garratty G, Daniels G, et al. Late on-set neonatal anaemia due to maternal anti-Ge: Possible association with destruction of erythroid progenitors. Transfus Med 2005;15(2):125-32.

10. Ping L, Pang LH, Liang HF, et al. Maternal IgG anti-A and anti-B titer levels screening in predicting ABO hemolytic disease of the newborn: A meta-analysis. Fetal Pediatr Pathol 2015; 34:341-50.

11. Delaney M, Wikman A, van de Watering L, et al. Blood Group Antigen Matching Influence on Gestational Outcomes (AMIGO) study. Transfusion 2017;57:525-32.

12. Bowman JM, Pollock JM, Penston LE. Fetomaternal transplacental hemorrhage during pregnancy and after delivery. Vox Sang 1986;51: 117-21.

13. Sebring ES, Polesky HF. Fetomaternal hemorrhage: Incidence, risk factors, time of occurrence, and clinical effects. Transfusion 1990;30: 344-57.

14. Zipursky A, Pollock J, Chown B, Israels LG. Transplacental foetal hemorrhage after placental injury during delivery or amniocentesis. Lancet 1963;7:493-4.

15. Bhutani VK, Zipursky A, Blencowe H, et al. Neonatal hyperbilirubinemia and Rhesus disease of the newborn: Incidence and impairment estimates for 2010 at regional and global levels. Pediatr Res 2013;74(Suppl 1):86-100.

16. Zipursky A, Paul VK. The global burden of Rh disease. Arch Dis Child Fetal Neonatal Ed 2011; 96(2):F84-5.

17. Bowman JM. The prevention of Rh immunization. Transfus Med Rev 1988;2:129-50.

18. Bowman JM. Controversies in Rh prophylaxis. Who needs Rh immune globulin and when should it be given? Am J Obstet Gynecol 1985;151:289-94.

19. Ayache S, Herman JH. Prevention of D sensitization after mismatched transfusion of blood components: Toward optimal use of RhIG. Transfusion 2008;48:1990-9.

20. Reid ME, Lomas-Francis C, Olsson ML. The blood group antigen factsbook. 3rd ed. San Diego, CA: Academic Press, 2012.

21. Koelewijn JM, Vrijkotte TG, van der Schoot CE, et al. Effect of screening for red cell antibodies, other than anti-D, to detect hemolytic disease of the fetus and newborn: A population study in the Netherlands. Transfusion 2008;48:941.

22. Markham KB, Rossi KQ, Nagaraja HN, O'Shaughnessy RW. Hemolytic disease of the fetus and newborn due to multiple maternal antibodies. Am J Obstet Gynecol 2015;213:68.e61-5.

23. Moise KJ Jr, Argoti PS. Management and prevention of red cell alloimmunization in pregnancy: A systematic review. Obstet Gynecol 2012; 120:1132-9.

24. De Young-Owens A, Kennedy M, Rose RL, et al. Anti-M isoimmunization: Management and outcome at the Ohio State University from 1969 to 1995. Obstet Gynecol 1997;90:962-6.

25. Stetson B, Scrape S, Markham KB. Anti-M alloimmunization: Management and outcome at a single institution. AJP Rep 2017;7:e205-10.

26. Wagner FF, Flegel WA. RHD gene deletion occurred in the Rhesus box. Blood 2000;95:3662.

27. Finning KM, Martin PG, Soothill PW, Avent ND. Prediction of fetal D status from maternal plasma: Introduction of a new noninvasive fetal RHD genotyping service. Transfusion 2002;42: 1079.

28. Van der Schoot E, De Haas M, Clausen FB. Genotyping to prevent Rh disease: Has the time come? Curr Opin Hematol 2017;24:544-50.

29. Bachegowda LS, Cheng YH, Long T, Shaz BH. Impact of uniform methods on interlaboratory antibody titration variability: Antibody titration and uniform methods. Arch Pathol Lab Med 2017;141:131-8.

30. Zwingerman R, Jain V, Hannon J, et al. Alloimmune red blood cell antibodies: Prevalence and pathogenicity in a Canadian prenatal population. J Obstet Gynaecol Can 2015;37(9):784-90.

31. Judd WJ for the Scientific Section Coordinating Committee. Guidelines for prenatal and perinatal immunohematology. Bethesda, MD: AABB, 2005.

32. Slootweg YM, Lindenburg IT, Koelewijn JM, et al. Predicting anti-Kell-mediated hemolytic disease of the fetus and newborn: Diagnostic accuracy of laboratory management. Am J Obstet Gynecol 2018;219(4):393.e1-8.

33. Biale Y, Dvilansky A. Management of pregnancies with rare blood types. Acta Obstet Gynecol Scand 1982;61:219.

34. Mandelbrot L, Daffos F, Forestier F. Assessment of fetal blood volume for computer-assisted management of in utero transfusion. Fetal Ther 1988;3:60-6.

35. Radunovic N, Lockwood CJ, Alvarez M, et al. The severely anemic and hydropic isoimmune fetus: Changes in fetal hematocrit associated

with intrauterine death. Obstet Gynecol 1992;
79:390-3.

36. Mari G, Norton ME, Stone J, et al. Society for Maternal-Fetal Medicine (SMFM) clinical guideline #8: The fetus at risk for anemia—Diagnosis and management. Am J Obstet Gynecol 2015; 212(6):697.

37. Lindenburg IT, Smits-Wintjens VE, van Klink JM, et al. Long-term neurodevelopmental outcome after intrauterine transfusion for hemolytic disease of the fetus/newborn: The LOTUS study. Am J Obstet Gynecol 2012;206:141. e141-8.

38. Margulies M, Voto LS, Mathet E, Margulies M. High-dose intravenous IgG for the treatment of severe Rhesus alloimmunization. Vox Sang 1991;61:181-9.

39. Ruma MS, Moise KJ Jr, Kim E, et al. Combined plasmapheresis and intravenous immune globulin for the treatment of severe maternal red cell alloimmunization. Am J Obstet Gynecol 2007; 196:138.e131-6.

40. Padmanabhan A, Connelly-Smith L, Aqui N, et al. Guidelines on the use of therapeutic apheresis in clinical practice - Evidence-based approach from the Writing Committee of the American Society for Apheresis: The eighth special issue. J Clin Apher 2019;34(3):171-354.

41. American Academy of Pediatrics Subcommittee on Hyperbilirubinemia. Management of hyperbilirubinemia in the newborn infant 35 or more weeks of gestation. Pediatrics 2004;114:297-316.

42. Smits-Wintjens VE, Walther FJ, Rath ME, et al. Intravenous immunoglobulin in neonates with Rhesus hemolytic disease: A randomized controlled trial. Pediatrics 2011;127:680-6.

43. Figueras-Aloy J, Rodriguez-Miguelez JM, Iriondo-Sanz M, et al. Intravenous immunoglobulin and necrotizing enterocolitis in newborns with hemolytic disease. Pediatrics 2010;125: 139-44.

44. Christensen RD, Ilstrup SJ, Baer VL, Lambert DK. Increased hemolysis after administering intravenous immunoglobulin to a neonate with erythroblastosis fetalis due to Rh hemolytic disease. Transfusion 2015;55:1365-6.

45. ACOG practice bulletin. Prevention of Rh D alloimmunization. Number 4, May 1999 (replaces educational bulletin Number 147, October 1990). Clinical management guidelines for obstetrician-gynecologists. American College of Obstetrics and Gynecology. Int J Gynaecol Obstet 1999;66:63-70.

46. Daniels G, Finning K, Martin P, Massey E. Noninvasive prenatal diagnosis of fetal blood group phenotypes: Current practice and future prospects. Prenat Diagn 2009;29:101-7.

47. Clausen FB. Integration of noninvasive prenatal prediction of fetal blood group into clinical prenatal care. Prenat Diagn 2014;34:409-15.

48. Kumpel BM. On the immunologic basis of Rh immune globulin (anti-D) prophylaxis. Transfusion 2006;46:1652-6.

49. Brinc D, Lazarus AH. Mechanisms of anti-D action in the prevention of hemolytic disease of the fetus and newborn. Hematology Am Soc Hematol Educ Program 2009:185-91.

50. Stowell SR, Arthur CM, Girard-Pierce KR, et al. Anti-KEL sera prevents alloimmunization to transfused KEL RBCs in a murine model. Haematologica 2015;100:e394-7.

51. Sandler SG, Roseff SD, Domen RE, et al. Policies and procedures related to testing for weak D phenotypes and administration of Rh immune globulin: Results and recommendations related to supplemental questions in the Comprehensive Transfusion Medicine survey of the College of American Pathologists. Arch Pathol Lab Med 2014;138:620-5.

52. Sandler SG, Flegel WA, Westhoff CM, et al. It's time to phase in RHD genotyping for patients with a serologic weak D phenotype. Transfusion 2015;55:680-9.

53. Pham BN, Roussel M, Peyrard T, et al. Anti-D investigations in individuals expressing weak D Type 1 or weak D Type 2: Allo- or autoantibodies? Transfusion 2011;51:2679-85.

54. Kacker S, Vassallo R, Keller MA, et al. Financial implications of RHD genotyping of pregnant women with a serologic weak D phenotype. Transfusion 2015;55:2095-103.

55. Haspel RL, Westhoff CM. How do I manage Rh typing in obstetric patients? Transfusion 2015; 55:470-4.

56. Sandler SG, Chen LN, Flegel WA. Serological weak D phenotypes: A review and guidance for interpreting the RhD blood type using the RHD genotype. Br J Haematol 2017;179:10-19.

57. Qureshi H, Massey E, Kirwan D, et al. BCSH guideline for the use of anti-D immunoglobulin for the prevention of haemolytic disease of the fetus and newborn. Transfus Med 2014;24:8-20.

58. Judd WJ, Luban NLC, Ness PM, et al. Prenatal and perinatal immunohematology: Recommendations for serologic management of the fetus,

newborn infant, and obstetric patient. Transfusion 1990;30:175-83.

59. Kelsey P, Reilly JT, Chapman JF, et al for the working party of the BCSH Blood Transfusion and General Haematology Task Forces. The estimation of fetomaternal haemorrhage. Transfus Med 1999;9:87-92.

60. Sandler SG, Delaney M, Gottschall JL. Proficiency tests reveal the need to improve laboratory assays for fetomaternal hemorrhage for Rh immunoprophylaxis. Transfusion 2013;53:2098-102.

61. Chen JC, Davis BH, Wood B, Warzynski MJ. Multicenter clinical experience with flow cytometric method for fetomaternal hemorrhage detection. Cytometry 2002;50:285-90.

62. Pham HP, Marques MB, Williams LA 3rd. Rhesus Immune Globulin dosing in the obesity epidemic era (letter). Arch Pathol Lab Med 2015;139:1084.

63. Woo EJ, Kaushal M. Rhesus Immunoglobulin dosage and administration in obese individuals (comment). Arch Pathol Lab Med 2017;141:17.

64. Koelewijn JM, de Haas M, Vrijkotte TG, et al. Risk factors for RhD immunisation despite antenatal and postnatal anti-D prophylaxis. BJOG 2009;116:1307-14.

65. Callum JL, Waters JH, Shaz BH, et al. The AABB recommendations for the Choosing Wisely campaign of the American Board of Internal Medicine. Transfusion 2014;54:2344.

66. Schonewille H, Klumper FJ, van de Watering LM, et al. High additional maternal red cell alloimmunization after Rhesus- and K-matched intrauterine intravascular transfusions for hemolytic disease of the fetus. Am J Obstet Gynecol 2007;196:143.e141.

67. Schonewille H, Prinsen-Zander KJ, Reijnart M, et al. Extended matched intrauterine transfusions reduce maternal Duffy, Kidd, and S antibody formation. Transfusion 2015;55:2912-19.

68. Reese JA, Peck JD, Deschamps DR, et al. Platelet counts during pregnancy. N Engl J Med 2018;379(1):32-43.

69. Kelton JG. Idiopathic thrombocytopenic purpura complicating pregnancy. Blood Rev 2002;16:43-6.

70. Davoren A, Curtis BR, Aster RH, McFarland JG. Human platelet antigen-specific alloantibodies implicated in 1162 cases of neonatal alloimmune thrombocytopenia. Transfusion 2004;44:1220-5.

71. Ohto H, Miura S, Ariga H, et al. The natural history of maternal immunization against foetal platelet alloantigens. Transfus Med 2004;14(6):399-408.

72. Turner ML, Bessos H, Fagge T, et al. Prospective epidemiologic study of the outcome and cost-effectiveness of antenatal screening to detect neonatal alloimmune thrombocytopenia due to anti-HPA-1a. Transfusion 2005;45:1945-56.

73. Williamson LM, Hackett G, Rennie J, et al. The natural history of fetomaternal alloimmunization to the platelet-specific antigen HPA-1a (PlA1, Zwa) as determined by antenatal screening. Blood 1998;92:2280-7.

74. Kamphuis MM, Paridaans N, Porcelijn L, et al. Screening in pregnancy for fetal or neonatal alloimmune thrombocytopenia: Systematic review. BJOG 2010;117(11):1335-43.

75. Kjeldsen-Kragh J, Killie MK, Tomter G, et al. A screening and intervention program aimed to reduce mortality and serious morbidity associated with severe neonatal alloimmune thrombocytopenia. Blood 2007;110(3):833-9.

76. Winklehorst D, Murphy MF, Greinacher A, et al. Antenatal management in fetal and neonatal alloimmune thrombocytopenia: A systematic review. Blood 2017;129(11):1538-47.

77. Tiller H, Kamphuis MM, Flodmark O, et al. Fetal intracranial haemorrhages caused by fetal and neonatal alloimmune thrombocytopenia: An observational cohort study of 43 cases from an international multicentre registry. BMJ Open 2013;3:3.

78. Bussel JB, Berkowitz RL, Hung C, et al. Intracranial hemorrhage in alloimmune thrombocytopenia: Stratified management to prevent recurrence in the subsequent affected fetus. Am J Obstet Gynecol 2010;203(2):135e13-14.

79. Winkelhorst D, Kamphuis MM, Steggerda SJ, et al. Perinatal outcome and long-term neurodevelopment after intracranial haemorrhage due to fetal and neonatal alloimmune thrombocytopenia. Fetal Diagn Ther 2019;45(3):184-91.

80. Bussel JB, Zabusky MR, Berkowitz RL, McFarland JG. Fetal alloimmune thrombocytopenia. N Engl J Med 1997;337:22-6.

81. Le Toriellec E, Chenet C, Kaplan C. Safe fetal platelet genotyping: New developments. Transfusion 2013;53:1755-62.

82. Scheffer PG, Ait Soussan A, Verhagen OJ, et al. Noninvasive fetal genotyping of human platelet antigen-1a. BJOG 2011;118:1392-5.

83. Wilson RD, Gagnon A, Audibert F, et al. Prenatal diagnosis procedures and techniques to obtain a diagnostic fetal specimen or tissue:

Maternal and fetal risks and benefits. J Obstet Gynaecol Can 2015;37(7):656-68.

84. Lakkaraja M, Berkowitz RL, Vinograd CA, et al. Omission of fetal sampling in treatment of subsequent pregnancies in fetal-neonatal alloimmune thrombocytopenia. Am J Obstet Gynecol 2016;215(4):471.e1-9.

85. Lieberman L, Greinacher A, Murphy MF, et al. Fetal and neonatal alloimmune thrombocytopenia: Recommendations for evidence-based practice, an international approach. Br J Haematol 2019;185(3):549-62.

86. van den Akker ES, Oepkes D, Lopriore E, et al. Vaginal delivery for fetuses at risk of alloimmune thrombocytopenia? Br J Obstet Gynaecol 2006; 113:781-3.

87. Ghevaert C, Campbell K, Walton J, et al. Management and outcome of 200 cases of fetomaternal alloimmune thrombocytopenia. Transfusion 2007;47:901-10.

88. Chakravorty S, Roberts I. How I manage neonatal thrombocytopenia. Br J Haematol 2012;156: 155-62.

89. Allen D, Verjee S, Rees S, et al. Platelet transfusion in neonatal alloimmune thrombocytopenia. Blood 2007;109(1):388-9.

90. Kiefel V, Bassler D, Kroll H, et al. Antigen-positive platelet transfusion in neonatal alloimmune thrombocytopenia (NAIT). Blood 2006; 107(9):3761-3.

91. Galea P, Patrick MJ, Goel KM. Isoimmune neonatal thrombocytopenic purpura. Arch Dis Child 1981;56(2):112-15.

92. Gill KK, Kelton JG. Management of idiopathic thrombocytopenic purpura in pregnancy. Semin Hematol 2000;37:275-89.

93. Webert KE, Mittal R, Sigouin C, et al. A retrospective 11-year analysis of obstetric patients with idiopathic thrombocytopenic purpura. Blood 2003;102:4306-11.

94. Neunert C, Lim W, Crowther M, et al. The American Society of Hematology 2011 evidence-based practice guideline for immune thrombocytopenia. Blood 2011;117:4190-207.

95. Provan D, Stasi R, Newland AC, et al. International consensus report on the investigation and management of primary immune thrombocytopenia. Blood 2010;115:68.

96. Koyama S, Tomimatsu T, Kanagawa T, et al. Reliable predictors of neonatal immune thrombocytopenia in pregnant women with idiopathic thrombocytopenic purpura. Am J Hematol 2012;87:15-21.

97. Gernsheimer T, James A, Stasis R. How I treat thrombocytopenia in pregnancy. Blood 2013; 121(1):38-47.

CHAPTER 24

Neonatal and Pediatric Transfusion Practice

Edward C.C. Wong, MD, and Rowena C. Punzalan, MD

TRANSFUSION PRACTICE IN PEDIATric patients, particularly in neonates, differs from that in adults.[1] The differences are related to physiologic changes occurring during the transition from fetus to adolescent, blood volume, development of hematopoiesis and coagulation, immune system maturity, and physiologic response to hypovolemia and hypoxia that are variable in this heterogeneous population. All of these factors contribute to the complexity and intricacies of pediatric transfusion practice. Advances in neonatology now permit the survival of extremely premature infants, and most neonatal transfusions are given to very low-birthweight (VLBW) infants.[2] This chapter discusses neonatal and pediatric transfusion practice during two distinct periods: the newborn period (birth to 4 months), and infancy (after 4 months) through childhood. Transfusion practices relevant to special pediatric populations are also described.

HEMATOPOIESIS, COAGULATION, AND PHYSIOLOGY

Neonates

Patients younger than 4 months have small blood/plasma volumes and immature organ sys-tem function that necessitate special approaches to component therapy. This is especially important for VLBW infants (<1500 g) and extremely low-birthweight infants (<1000 g). The mean cord blood hemoglobin level of healthy neonates is 16.9 ± 1.6 g/dL, whereas that of preterm neonates is 15.9 ± 2.4 g/dL. The hemoglobin concentration normally declines during the first few weeks of life, resulting in physiologic anemia of infancy, a condition that is self-limited and usually tolerated without harmful effects in term infants but is potentially more worrisome in preterm infants.[3]

The rate of decline in hemoglobin levels is a function of gestational age at birth. At 4 to 8 weeks after birth, hemoglobin decreases to as low as 8.0 g/dL in preterm infants weighing 1000 to 1500 g, and 7.0 g/dL in neonates weighing <1000 g at birth.[4] The physiologic decrease in hemoglobin concentration is caused by several factors: 1) a decrease in erythropoietin (EPO) that is more prolonged in preterm infants, resulting in diminished red cell production; 2) decreased survival of fetal red cells; and 3) increasing blood volume due to rapid growth. Reduced EPO production results from increased oxygen delivery to tissues because of increased pulmonary blood flow, elevated arterial pO_2 (partial pressure of oxygen) levels, increased red

Edward C.C. Wong, MD, Medical Director, Coagulation, Quest Diagnostics Nichols Institute, Chantilly, Virginia and Adjunct Associate Professor, Pediatrics and Pathology, George Washington School of Medicine and Health Sciences, and formerly Associate Director of Transfusion Medicine, Children's National Health System, Washington, District of Columbia; and Rowena C. Punzalan, MD, Medical Director, Transfusion Service, Versiti Blood Center of Wisconsin and Children's Hospital of Wisconsin, and Associate Professor, Pediatrics (Hematology), Medical College of Wisconsin, Milwaukee, Wisconsin
The authors have disclosed no conflicts of interest.

cell 2,3-diphosphoglycerate (2,3-DPG), and increased hemoglobin A levels.[5]

Platelet counts in term and preterm neonates are similar to those in children and adults. Thrombopoietin is found in fetal liver as early as 6 weeks of gestation. Nevertheless, for various reasons, thrombocytopenia (platelet count <150,000/μL) occurs in up to 25% of admissions to neonatal intensive care units (ICUs).[6]

In neonates, low levels of vitamin-K-dependent factors (Factors II, VII, IX, and X) and contact factors (Factor XI, Factor XII, prekallikrein, and high-molecular-weight kininogen) contribute to altered coagulation test results.[7,8] (See Table 24-1.) The naturally occurring anticoagulants (proteins C and S and antithrombin) are also decreased.[8] In spite of these issues, the procoagulant and anticoagulant systems are usually in balance in healthy newborns, so spontaneous bleeding and thrombosis are rare.[9] However, the reserve capacity for both systems is limited. Platelet function is likely different between VLBW preterm and full-term infants. An in-vitro arterial shear model using surface immobilized von Willebrand factor (vWF) found that platelets from VLBW preterm infants had increased interaction with vWF, and increased platelet glycoprotein Ibα (GPIbα) expression compared to platelets from full-term infants. Despite this increased interaction, no significant differences were observed in the number of platelets that adhered in a stationary fashion to vWF, comparing platelets from these neonatal populations.[10] Whether this reflects a compensatory mechanism to a higher risk of bleeding in VLBW preterm infants or contributes to the higher risk in VLBW preterm infants is unclear. A study of premature infants aged 33 weeks or less, having platelet counts <100,000/μL, showed that those with high bleeding scores had higher adenosine diphosphate (ADP) closure times using the platelet function analyzer (PFA)-100.[11] However, given the large amount of blood needed for testing, it remains to be seen whether this approach will be acceptable to neonatology specialists to guide platelet transfusions in patients with high ADP closure times. Regardless of these findings, serious bleeding and, less commonly, thrombosis may occur in sick premature infants during the first week of life.

Preterm infants and neonates have underdeveloped immune function. It is not well under-

TABLE 24-1. Screening Laboratory Tests for Hemostasis: Neonates vs Adults*

	Preterm Neonates vs Full-Term Neonates	Neonates vs Older Children/Adults	Approximate Age Adult Values Are Reached[†]
aPTT	Longer	Longer	16 years
Prothrombin time	Longer	Same or longer	16 years
Thrombin time	Longer	Same or longer	5 years
Bleeding time	Longer[‡]	Shorter	1 month
PFA-100	Longer[‡]	Shorter	1 month
ROTEM/TEG			
Clotting time	Same	Shorter	3 months
Clot formation time	Same	Shorter	3 months
Maximal clot firmness	Stronger	Stronger	3 months

*Modified with permission from Revel-Vilk.[9]
[†]Maximum age reported.
[‡]In samples drawn in the first 7 to 10 days of life.
aPTT = activated partial thromboplastin time; PFA = platelet function analyzer; ROTEM = rotational thromboelastometry; TEG = thromboelastography (both ROTEM and TEG are viscoelastic methods for hemostasis testing in whole blood).

stood why unexpected red cell alloantibodies of either immunoglobulin M (IgM) or IgG class are rarely produced during this time. Possible explanations include deficient T-helper-cell function, enhanced T-suppressor-cell activity, and poor antigen-presenting-cell function.[12] Cellular immune responses are also incompletely developed during this period and may make infants susceptible to transfusion-associated graft-vs-host disease (TA-GVHD).

Infants younger than 4 months of age have decreased ability for liver metabolism of the anticoagulant citrate, making them vulnerable to acidosis and/or hypocalcemia. Immature kidneys also have lower glomerular filtration rates and concentrating ability than in older children, leading to difficulties in excreting excess potassium, acid, and/or calcium. In addition, very young infants <3 days old have blunted parathyroid hormone secretion in response to decreased ionized calcium, especially resulting from citrate exposure during whole blood exchange.[13]

Children Older Than 4 Months

Hemoglobin continues to increase after the neonatal period until typical adult levels are achieved after adolescence. Levels of most procoagulant and anticoagulant factors are not significantly different from those in adults by 6 months of age.[14]

RBC TRANSFUSION IN NEONATES

This section reviews several general aspects of transfusion practice to highlight situations that warrant special attention in caring for the neonate. In addition to the issues listed in the first section below, sections that follow address indications, thresholds, exchange transfusion, and conditions specific to neonates.

Considerations for Transfusion

Body Size and Blood Volume

Full-term newborns have a blood volume of approximately 85 mL/kg; in contrast, preterm newborns have about 100 mL/kg.[15] To avoid waste, blood banks must be capable of providing appropriately sized blood components.[16] The vast majority of preterm infants weighing <1.0 kg or at <28 weeks' gestational age need at least one transfusion.[17]

Many factors, including iatrogenic blood loss from repeated phlebotomy, can lead to frequent transfusions in sick newborns. Hypovolemia (>10% blood volume loss) is not tolerated well in newborns because of their limited ability to compensate with increased heart rate. In such situations, the decreased cardiac output (along with increased peripheral vascular resistance to maintain blood pressure) ultimately results in poor tissue perfusion and oxygenation, and metabolic acidosis.[18] As described later in more detail, Red Blood Cell (RBC) transfusions are often administered to maintain a target hemoglobin level in certain clinical situations and for symptomatic anemia.[2,19,20]

Erythropoietin Physiology and Therapy

In contrast to older children and adults, newborns have decreased EPO production in response to hypoxia, likely to prevent polycythemia in the hypoxic intrauterine environment. Most premature infants produce the smallest amount of EPO expected for any degree of anemia.[21,22] The reduction in EPO production is greatest in preterm infants because of persistent liver-based EPO production, which is normally regulated in the more hypoxic in-utero state. Kidney-based EPO production, which is regulated at higher pO$_2$ levels, does not normally occur until after term delivery.[5]

As an alternative to transfusion, the early administration of erythropoiesis-stimulating agents (ESAs) such as recombinant human EPO or the longer-acting darbepoetin have been used to decrease transfusions in at-risk neonates. However, a recent meta-analysis (3643 infants in 34 studies) showed that early administration of ESA (vs no treatment or placebo) in preterm or low-birthweight infants minimally reduced the total amount of transfusion but did not reduce the number of donor exposures. There was decreased incidence of necrotizing enterocolitis [NEC: relative risk, 0.62; 95% confidence interval (CI), 0.48-0.80] and a trend toward improved neurodevelopmental outcome in the ESA group.[23] In contrast, earlier studies showed possible increased severity of retinopathy of prematurity[24] and increased incidence of infantile hemangiomas[25] with use of ESAs in preterm and low-birthweight infants. As compliance with strict transfusion threshold criteria has improved, clinicians have decreased phlebotomy rates and volumes and used point-of-care testing in VLBW infants, resulting in a decrease in the rates of iatrogenic anemia and need for transfusions.[26,27] Thus, in most cases, this approach combined with the use of aliquots from a single-donor blood component unit for multiple transfusions achieves the same goal (ie, decreases number of transfusions and donor exposures) without the need for EPO therapy.

Cold Stress

Hypothermia in the neonate can trigger or exaggerate several responses, including 1) increased metabolic rate, 2) hypoglycemia, 3) metabolic acidosis, and 4) potential apneic events that may lead to hypoxia, hypotension, and cardiac arrest.[28] In-line blood warmers are recommended for large-volume transfusions, including red cell exchange transfusions, to combat the effects of hypothermia. A radiant heater should never be used to warm the blood being transfused because of the risk of hemolysis. Furthermore, to prevent hemolysis in neonates undergoing phototherapy, the blood-administration tubing should be positioned to minimize exposure to phototherapy light.[29]

RBC Additive Solutions

Historically, RBCs transfused to children contained only citrate-phosphate-dextrose-adenine (CPDA)-1 anticoagulant-preservative solution.[30,31] However, as the use of additive solutions (AS) containing adenine and mannitol evolved to extend the shelf life of RBCs, many experts began to question their safety in neonates. One concern is the dose of adenine in AS and its relation to renal toxicity. Mannitol is a potent diuretic with effects on fluid dynamics that can result in fluctuations in the cerebral blood flow of preterm infants. However, because the use of AS extends shelf life, the number of aliquots that

can be used from a single RBC unit is increased, which may reduce the overall donor exposure to a patient.

Luban and colleagues used theoretical calculations in a variety of clinical settings to demonstrate that red cells preserved in extended storage media present no major risk when used for small-volume transfusions.[32] Prospective randomized controlled trials to assess the outcomes of longer vs shorter storage times of RBCs have been performed in this population and found that small-volume transfusion comparing older AS-1 or AS-3 units to fresher CPDA units were equivalent in terms of safety and efficacy.[30,31] (See next section.)

Because it is unknown whether these theoretical concerns for AS are significant for patients with renal or hepatic insufficiency, some facilities may remove the AS from RBC units, particularly if multiple transfusions from the same unit are expected; however, this is technically challenging and not possible in many facilities. The safety of AS-preserved RBCs in trauma-related massive transfusions, extracorporeal membrane oxygenation (ECMO), cardiac surgery, or exchange transfusions has not been studied. In a recent hospital survey in the United States about large-volume transfusions in neonates, 43% of responders used RBC units stored in AS-3, 29% used RBCs stored in AS-1, and 28% used RBCs stored in CPD or CPDA.[33] AS-preserved RBC units should be used with caution in settings where large volumes are being transfused.[32,34,35]

Ionized calcium and potassium levels should be monitored frequently during large-volume transfusions. A blood warmer should be used to avoid hypothermia.[36] These principles should be applied to infants and small children as well.

RBC Age and the Storage Lesion

Small-volume, simple transfusions administered slowly have been shown to have little effect on serum potassium concentrations in infants younger than 4 months despite the high potassium levels in the supernatant of stored RBCs. In calculating levels of infused potassium, Strauss mathematically determined that transfusion of an aliquot from an RBC unit that is sedimented by gravity (80% hematocrit) and stored in an extended storage medium for 42 days would deliver 2 mL of plasma containing only 0.1 mmol/L of potassium when transfused at 10 mL/kg.[37,38] This amount of potassium is much less than the daily requirement of 2 to 3 mmol/L for a patient weighing 1 kg. It must be stressed that this calculation does not apply to the transfusion of large volumes of RBCs (>20 mL/kg), such as during surgery, exchange transfusion, or ECMO.[39,40]

The type of anticoagulant-preservative solution used to store RBCs at collection determines the amount of potassium delivered.[37,41] In addition, special component processing, such as irradiation, can potentiate potassium leakage from the red cell membrane. If irradiated components are stored for more than 24 hours, washing may be required to remove the excess potassium before transfusion to vulnerable patients.[42] There are reports of severe adverse effects, including cardiac arrest and death, in infants who received either older RBC units or those that had been irradiated (>1 day before transfusion) via central or intracardiac line.[43,44] Alternatively, and more practically, several institutions accept AS units for low-volume neonatal transfusions without washing as long as these units do not exceed a certain storage age or time after irradiation.[45]

Levels of 2,3-DPG in red cells are known to decline rapidly after 1 to 2 weeks of storage. Older children and adult recipients are able to replenish the missing 2,3-DPG in vivo and compensate for hypoxia by increasing heart rate. Infants younger than 4 months are not able to compensate as effectively because of low levels of intracellular 2,3-DPG that further decrease with respiratory distress syndrome or septic shock. Thus, if a large proportion of the neonate's blood volume is composed of transfused, 2,3-DPG-depleted blood, the resulting shift in the hemoglobin oxygen dissociation curve further increases oxygen affinity for hemoglobin and reduces oxygen availability to the tissues.[46] However, this shift in the hemoglobin dissociation curve might be minimized by opposing shifts to the curve from decreased pH and increased pCO_2 that is associated with hypoxia. The usual recommendation for newborns re-

quiring red cell exchange and large-volume transfusion is that the RBC units selected should be <14 days old, although this practice is variable and dependent on institutional policy.

The impact of RBC age and the "storage lesion" is seen in in-vitro and retrospective studies, but clinical confirmation has not been found in prospective studies. A randomized controlled trial conducted in Canada, Age of Red Blood Cells in Premature Infants (ARIPI), randomly assigned low-birthweight infants to receive RBCs that were 7 days old (mean = 5.1 days; n = 188) or standard-issue RBCs divided into aliquots and stored for 2 to 42 days (mean = 14.6 days; n = 189).[47] The primary composite endpoints included NEC, intraventricular hemorrhage (IVH), and bronchopulmonary dysplasia. The study found no differences in the primary endpoints between infants in the two arms, suggesting that in the study population, the age of RBCs does not affect these common morbidities of prematurity. ARIPI's generalizability has been questioned because of the study's liberal transfusion strategy (hemoglobin threshold of 10 g/dL), use of SAGM (saline, adenine, glucose, and mannitol) units, and average duration of blood storage. These practices do not reflect the transfusion practices, storage solution, and age of RBCs used in many centers in the United States.[48]

Compatibility Testing

AABB *Standards for Blood Banks and Transfusion Services* (*Standards*) allows pretransfusion serologic testing for infants younger than 4 months to be limited.[49(pp39-40)] Initial patient testing must include ABO and D typing of the patient's red cells and screening for unexpected red cell antibodies using either plasma or serum from the infant or mother. During any hospitalization, crossmatch-compatibility testing and repeat ABO and D typing need not be conducted as long as all of the following criteria are met: 1) the antibody screening result is negative; 2) transfused RBCs are group O, ABO identical, or ABO compatible; and 3) transfused cells are either D negative or the same D type as the patient. Testing the infant's reverse type for anti-A and/or anti-B is not necessary. However, before non-group-O RBCs can be issued, testing of the infant's plasma or serum is required to detect passively acquired maternal anti-A or anti-B and should include an antiglobulin phase. If ABO antibody is present, maternally ABO-compatible RBCs are transfused until the acquired antibody is no longer detected.

If an unexpected non-ABO alloantibody is detected in the infant's or mother's specimen, RBC units provided for the infant must lack the corresponding antigen(s) or be compatible by antiglobulin crossmatch. This regimen should continue until the maternal antibody is no longer detected in the infant's plasma or serum. The policy of the hospital transfusion service determines the frequency for reevaluating the patient's antibodies. Once a negative antibody screening result is obtained, crossmatches and use of antigen-negative blood are no longer required in infants younger than 4 months because of their immature immunologic status.

Multiple observational studies have shown that alloimmunization to red cell antigens is rare during the neonatal period.[12,50,51] For this reason, repeated typing and screening, which is required for adults and children older than 4 months and contributes to significant iatrogenic blood loss, is unnecessary in younger infants. Also, the transfusion service should avoid transfusing any components that may passively transfer high-titer alloantibodies to recipients.[52]

Indications and Thresholds for Transfusion

Sick neonates are more likely to receive RBC transfusions than any other patient age group, and RBCs are the component most often transfused during the neonatal period.[2] Symptoms of anemia in neonates include tachycardia and/or tachypnea, increased episodes of bradycardia and/or apnea, poor weight gain despite adequate feeding, increased oxygen requirement, and increased blood lactate. Because of the poor specificity of the signs and symptoms of anemia, prophylaxis for anemia is a major reason for simple transfusion. Specifically, a venous hemoglobin <13 g/dL in the first 24 hours of life necessitates consideration of RBC transfusion.[19,20,36] Red cell replacement is considered for sick neonates when approximately 10% of blood volume has been lost or they have symptomatic anemia.

Several guidelines have been published over the past 15 years regarding the indications for RBC transfusions in neonates.[19,20,36,53,54] Most of the recommendations are based on experience acquired in clinical practice rather than published evidence. To this end, a critical need exists for clinical studies in this area. Table 24-2 lists the indications from one of these guidelines.[19]

When 10 mL/kg of RBCs with a hematocrit of >80% (achieved by allowing an RBC unit to sediment by gravity undisturbed with aliquot ports on the bottom) is transfused, the expected increase in hemoglobin concentration in a neonate is approximately 3 g/dL. A similar volume of RBCs with AS usually has a hematocrit of 65%, and its transfusion results in a projected posttransfusion hemoglobin increase of 2 g/dL. (See Table 24-3 for blood component dosing recommendations and the expected results.[55])

Two randomized controlled trials have compared the outcomes of restrictive (hemoglobin = 7 g/dL) vs liberal (hemoglobin = 10 g/dL) RBC transfusion thresholds in VLBW infants. The Iowa trial revealed a lower rate of transfusion events (3.3 vs 5.2; p = 0.025) with a restrictive compared to a liberal strategy.[56] However, rates of periventricular leukomalacia and death were higher in the restrictive arm. The Premature Infants in Need of Transfusion (PINT) study from Canada found no significant difference between the two arms, which had similar thresholds as the Iowa study, in the composite endpoint of death or bronchopulmonary dysplasia, retinopathy of prematurity (stage >3), or brain injury (periventricular leukomalacia, intracranial hemorrhage Grade 4, or ventriculomegaly).[57] The follow-up of the PINT study revealed that at 18 to 24 months after birth, infants in the restrictive arm had more cognitive delay than those in the liberal arm.[58] On the other hand, follow-up studies on the patients in the Iowa trial showed decreased brain structure and function at ages 7 to 10 years in the liberal arm, suggesting an opposite effect in long-term neurocognitive outcomes.[59,60] However, these follow-up studies were post-hoc analyses and not powered to detect differences.

TABLE 24-2. Transfusion Guidelines for RBCs in Infants Younger than 4 Months[19]

1.	Hematocrit <20% with low reticulocyte count and symptomatic anemia (tachycardia, tachypnea, poor feeding).
2.	Hematocrit <30% and any of the following:
a.	On <35% oxygen hood.
b.	On oxygen by nasal cannula.
c.	On continuous positive airway pressure and/or intermittent mandatory ventilation or mechanical ventilation with mean airway pressure <6 cm of water.
d.	With significant tachycardia or tachypnea (heart rate >180 beats/minute for 24 hours, respiratory rate >80 beats/minute for 24 hours).
e.	With significant apnea or bradycardia (>6 episodes in 12 hours or 2 episodes in 24 hours requiring bag and mask ventilation while receiving therapeutic doses of methylxanthines).
f.	With low weight gain (<10 g/day observed over 4 days while receiving ≥100 kcal/kg/day).
3.	Hematocrit <35% and either of the following:
a.	On >35% oxygen hood.
b.	On continuous positive airway pressure/intermittent mandatory ventilation with mean airway pressure ≥6-8 cm of water.
4.	Hematocrit <45% and either of the following:
a.	On extracorporeal membrane oxygenation.
b.	With congenital cyanotic heart disease.

A recent meta-analysis of 16 randomized and 45 nonrandomized studies in neonates showed no significant difference between liberal and restrictive transfusion strategies in terms of mortality, NEC, retinopathy of prematurity, chronic lung disease, and intraventricular hemorrhage, although many studies had a high risk of bias.[61] Therefore, there is still no definitive answer to the question of appropriate threshold for prophylactic RBC transfusion in neonates.

Despite the lack of difference between liberal and restrictive transfusion thresholds in outcomes for neonates in general, neonates undergoing surgery may have different risk profiles. In a recent analysis of the pediatric database of the American College of Surgeons national quality program, the prevalence of in-hospital mortality among neonates with preoperative hematocrit <40% was 7.5%, compared to 1.4% among those with hematocrit ≥40%.[62]

There are two ongoing studies looking at transfusion thresholds in premature and low-birthweight infants. The Transfusion of Premature Infants Study (TOPS), currently being conducted in the United States, is examining whether death and neurodevelopmental outcome at 22 to 26 months corrected age is less common among premature infants who received transfusion at high hemoglobin thresholds.[63] In Europe, the ETTNO trial will be randomly assigning 920 VLBW infants to receive RBC transfusions based on a restrictive or liberal threshold, and evaluating death rates and neurodevelopmental outcome at 24 months.[64]

TABLE 24-3. Blood Components and Dosing of Small Volumes in Neonatal and Pediatric Patients[55]

Component	Dose	Expected Increment
Red Blood Cells	10-15 mL/kg	Hemoglobin increase: 2-3 g/dL*
Fresh Frozen Plasma	10-15 mL/kg	15%-20% rise in factor levels (assuming 100% recovery)
Platelets [whole-blood-derived (WBD) or apheresis]	5-10 mL/kg or 1 WBD unit/10 kg (patients ≥10 kg)	50,000/µL rise in platelet count (assuming 100% recovery)[†]
Cryoprecipitated AHF	1-2 units/10 kg	60-100 mg/dL rise in fibrinogen (assuming 100% recovery)

*Dependent on anticoagulant-preservative solution, with 3 g/dL increment for CPD and CPDA-1, and 2 g/dL for AS-1, AS-3, AS-5, AS-7, and SAGM.

[†]Assumes ≥5.5×10^{10} platelets in 50 mL of plasma (WBD) and 3.0×10^{11} platelets in 250 to 300 mL plasma (apheresis).

AHF = antihemophilic factor; CPD = citrate-phosphate-dextrose; CPDA-1 = citrate-phosphate-dextrose-adenine-1; AS = additive solution; SAGM = saline-adenine-glucose-mannitol.

Neonatal Exchange Transfusion

The most common indication for exchange transfusion in neonates is hyperbilirubinemia caused by hemolytic disease of the fetus and newborn, discussed in detail in Chapter 23. Occasionally, it is used to eliminate toxins, drugs, or chemicals administered to the mother near the time of delivery. Exchange transfusion is also used when toxic doses of drugs have been administered to the infant or accumulate at high levels as a result of prematurity and/or an inborn error of metabolism.[65,66]

Physiology

In neonates, excessively high levels of unconjugated bilirubin may cross the blood-brain barrier, concentrate in the basal ganglia and cerebellum and cause irreversible damage, known as kernicterus. Infants are susceptible to hyperbilirubinemia because their immature liver conjugates bilirubin poorly and because their incompletely developed blood-brain barrier allows bilirubin transit. Phototherapy (blue/green light in the range of 460-490 nm, which converts unconjugated bilirubin into a water-soluble isomer, aiding excretion) is the current treatment of choice for hyperbilirubinemia; exchange transfusion is reserved for patients who fail phototherapy.[67]

Two critical objectives of exchange transfusion are the removal of unconjugated bilirubin and maximization of albumin-binding of residual bilirubin. In addition, in antibody-mediated hemolytic processes, exchange transfusion removes both free antibody and antibody-coated red cells, replacing these with antigen-negative red cells.

Exchange transfusion needs to be performed before the development of kernicterus. In full-term infants, kernicterus rarely develops at bilirubin levels <25 mg/dL. However, in sick VLBW infants, kernicterus can occur at bilirubin levels as low as 8 to 12 mg/dL.[68]

A double-volume exchange transfusion (two 85-mL/kg transfusions for full-term infants and two 100-mL/kg transfusions for VLBW infants) removes approximately 70% to 90% of circulating red cells and approximately 50% of total bilirubin.[69] After the first exchange transfusion, bilirubin may reequilibrate between extravascular tissue and plasma, which may necessitate another exchange transfusion.

Component Choice

Typically, RBCs are resuspended in ABO-compatible, thawed Fresh Frozen Plasma (FFP) for an exchange transfusion. No single method of combining components has been shown to be superior to another. RBCs <5 to 7 days old and stored in CPDA-1 have been used to avoid high levels of potassium and to maximize red cell survival.[70] When using AS-RBC units, some blood banks elect to remove the additive-containing plasma to reduce the volume transfused.

Most transfusion services provide RBC units that are hemoglobin S negative, cytomegalovirus (CMV) reduced-risk (leukocyte reduced or CMV seronegative), and irradiated. Irradiation should be performed just before the exchange to prevent potentiation of the potassium storage lesion. If units are not irradiated immediately before use, some experts recommend removing the supernatant of red cells or washing the unit to avoid the complications of hyperkalemic cardiac arrhythmias.[71]

The glucose load administered during exchange transfusion can be high in some cases, which stimulates the infant's pancreas to release insulin and results in rebound hypoglycemia.[72] Therefore, infant plasma glucose levels should be monitored during the first few hours following exchange transfusion. Because resuspended RBCs do not include platelets, the platelet count should be assessed after completion of the exchange transfusion.

A double-volume exchange transfusion in neonates rarely necessitates the infusion of >1 RBC unit. The unit's hematocrit should be approximately 45% to 60%, and the unit should have sufficient plasma (based on estimated blood volume) to provide clotting factors.[71] If the neonate's condition requires a higher postexchange transfusion hematocrit, a small-volume RBC transfusion may be given or a unit with a higher hematocrit can be used for the initial exchange transfusion. The reconstituted blood should be well mixed to sustain the intended hematocrit throughout the exchange.

Postexchange transfusion hematocrit, platelet count, and bilirubin should be measured. This can be performed by using the last portion of blood removed for the exchange. Complications have been reviewed in detail elsewhere.[70]

Vascular Access and Technique

Umbilical venous catheters are used for exchange transfusions in preterm and full-term in-fants just after birth. If umbilical venous catheters are not available, small saphenous catheters may be used. Two exchange transfusion techniques are commonly employed: isovolumetric and manual push-pull. In isovolumetric exchange transfusion, two catheters of identical size provide vascular access. The catheters allow simultaneous withdrawal and infusion of blood and are regulated by a single peristaltic pump. The umbilical vein is typically used for infusion, and the umbilical artery is used for withdrawal. The manual push-pull technique uses a single vascular access portal with a three-way stopcock attached to the unit of blood, the patient, and a graduated discard container. A standard filter and in-line blood warmer are recommended.

With both techniques, the absolute maximum volume of each withdrawal and infusion depends on the infant's body weight and hemodynamic status. Usually, no more than 5 mL/kg body weight or 5% of the infant's blood volume is removed and replaced during a 3- to 5-minute cycle.[70] The exchange transfusion should not be performed rapidly because sudden hemodynamic changes may affect cerebral blood flow and shift intracranial pressure, contributing to IVH.[73] A total double-volume exchange transfusion typically takes 90 to 120 minutes.[70]

Conditions Specific to Neonates

Hemolytic disease of the fetus and newborn and neonatal alloimmune thrombocytopenia are discussed in Chapter 23.

Polycythemia

Neonatal polycythemia is defined as venous hematocrit >65% or hemoglobin >22 g/dL at any time during the first week after birth. Approximately 5% of all newborns develop polycythemia for a variety of reasons, most commonly intrauterine growth restriction and gestational diabetes. Once the hematocrit rises above 65%, viscosity increases and oxygen transport decreases. However, in neonates, the exponential rise in viscosity can occur at a hematocrit as low as 40%.[74] Congestive heart failure can result because infants have limited capability to increase their cardiac output to compensate for hyperviscosity. Central nervous system abnormalities, pulmonary and renal failure, and NEC can occur from the resultant decreased blood flow.

A partial exchange is used to normalize the hematocrit to between 55% and 60% and improve tissue perfusion while maintaining blood volume. This exchange is accomplished by removing whole blood and replacing it with normal saline or other crystalloid solutions. Plasma is not used to replace whole blood because NEC has been reported as a complication of plasma transfusion.[75]

The formula below can be used to approximate the volume of replacement fluid required and the volume of whole blood that must be withdrawn for the partial exchange:

$$\text{Volume of replacement fluid} = \frac{\text{Blood volume} \times (\text{Observed Hct} - \text{Desired Hct})}{\text{Observed Hct}}$$

Necrotizing Enterocolitis

NEC, a serious condition in neonates, is characterized by ischemic necrosis of the intestinal mucosa, associated with inflammation, invasion of enteric-gas-forming organisms, and dissection of gas into the abdominal cavity. Small studies have suggested the possibility of RBC transfusion as an independent risk factor for development of NEC in neonates, and a previous meta-analysis showed an increased risk of NEC (odds ratio = 2) in neonatal transfusion recipients.[76] However, a recent, prospective, multicenter, observational cohort study of VLBW infants found that severe anemia itself, rather than transfusion, was independently associated with NEC.[77]

RBC TRANSFUSION IN INFANTS OLDER THAN 4 MONTHS AND CHILDREN

The most significant differences between RBC transfusions in infants older than 4 months and adults are 1) blood volume, 2) the ability to tolerate blood loss, and 3) age-appropriate hemoglobin and hematocrit levels. In this age group, the most common indication for RBC transfusion is treatment or prevention of tissue hypoxia

caused by decreased red cell mass, typically because of surgery, anemia from underlying chronic disease, or hematologic malignancies. Chronic RBC transfusions are administered to combat tissue hypoxia and suppress endogenous hemoglobin production in children with hemoglobinopathies. Table 24-4 can help guide transfusion decisions in patients older than 4 months.

Before receiving any RBC transfusion, all pediatric patients older than 4 months require ABO and Rh testing and screening for the presence of clinically significant antibodies in the same frequency as adult patients. Compatibility testing should be performed according to AABB *Standards*.[49(40)]

Special Populations

Sickle Cell Disease

Chronic transfusion in patients with sickle cell disease (SCD) decreases the proportion of red cells containing hemoglobin S, reduces sickling, and prevents blood viscosity increase. The main indication for chronic transfusion is primary and secondary prevention of stroke. It has been shown that the risk of recurrent stroke is reduced to <10% if hemoglobin levels are maintained between 8 and 9 g/dL and the percentage of hemoglobin S stays <30%.[78,79] In children with SCD and silent cerebral infarcts (SCIs), transfusion therapy is more effective at preventing stroke and SCI recurrence than hydroxyurea and phlebotomy[80] or observation.[81,82]

Simple or partial manual exchange transfusions can be administered every 3 to 4 weeks. Automated red cell exchange has also been used to prevent iron overload in patients with SCD who require chronic transfusion.[83] See Table 24-4 for a list of other indications for simple or chronic RBC transfusion in SCD. RBCs for patients with SCD should be screened for hemoglobin S and, ideally, leukocyte reduced to prevent HLA alloimmunization and platelet refractoriness in preparation for possible hematopoietic progenitor cell transplantation.

Red Cell Alloimmunization in SCD. Although the benefits of chronic transfusion therapy in patients with SCD have been demonstrated, it is not without risks. Patients with SCD have the highest rates of red cell alloimmunization of

TABLE 24-4. Transfusion Guidelines for RBCs in Patients Older than 4 Months[19,20]

1.	Emergency surgical procedure in patient with significant postoperative anemia.
2.	Preoperative anemia when other corrective therapy is not available.
3.	Intraoperative blood loss >15% total blood volume.
4.	Hematocrit <24% and:
a.	In perioperative period, with signs and symptoms of anemia.
b.	While on chemotherapy/radiotherapy.
c.	Chronic congenital or acquired symptomatic anemia.
5.	Acute blood loss with hypovolemia not responsive to other therapy.
6.	Hematocrit <40% and:
a.	With severe pulmonary disease.
b.	On extracorporeal membrane oxygenation.
7.	Sickle cell disease and:
a.	Cerebrovascular accident.
b.	Acute chest syndrome.
c.	Splenic sequestration.
d.	Aplastic crisis.
e.	Recurrent priapism.
f.	Preoperatively when general anesthesia is planned (target hemoglobin = 10 g/dL).
8.	Chronic transfusion programs for disorders of red cell production (eg, β-thalassemia major and Diamond-Blackfan syndrome unresponsive to therapy).

any patient group.[84,85] Antibodies are produced against common RH, KEL, FY, and JK system antigens. Many SCD treatment centers perform an extended red cell phenotype or genotype analysis of a patient's red cells before beginning transfusion therapy, and preferentially transfuse red cell antigen-matched (RH and KEL) units to reduce the rate of red cell alloimmunization.[86,87] Red cell genotyping can identify extended phenotype, provide information about variant Rh alleles that may appear phenotypically negative but form antibodies against Rh antigens, and provide results about common silencing mutations.[88] However, particularly for patients who are not yet alloimmunized, this process of matching for red cell antigens is not uniformly practiced because phenotypically compatible

units are considerably more costly[89] and may be difficult to obtain.[90]

In academic institutions in the United States and Canada, the most common protocol for prevention of red cell alloimmunization in nonalloimmunized patients with SCD is transfusion of ABO/Rh-compatible units that are additionally matched for C, E, and K antigens.[91] Once patients have developed a red cell antibody, extension of matching to additional red cell antigens (Fy^a/Fy^b, Jk^a/Jk^b, S) is often used to prevent further alloimmunization.[92]

Other Complications of RBC Transfusions in SCD. SCD transfusion recipients also face risks such as iron overload (which can cause hepatic and cardiac dysfunction)[93] and the risks of increased donor exposure during red cell exchange. In addition, patients with SCD may be at risk of life-threatening, delayed hemolytic transfusion reactions. If a patient's hemoglobin level decreases after transfusion, the patient might have developed "hyperhemolytic" syndrome. This poorly understood phenomenon is characterized by destruction of the patient's own red cells along with transfused cells and may or may not display allo- or autoantibodies. If hyperhemolytic syndrome is suspected, case reports suggest that stopping and withholding transfusion and administering corticosteroids in combination with intravenous immune globulin may be beneficial.[94,95] These patients should also be monitored closely for the formation of autoantibodies.[87,88]

Alternatives to Transfusion in SCD. Early hydroxyurea therapy has been shown to decrease transfusions, hospitalizations, vaso-occlusive pain crises, and acute chest syndrome. This is now standard-of-care in children with hemoglobin SS or Sβ⁰-thalassemia.[91,96] The optimal clinical circumstances for hematopoietic progenitor cell transplantation in SCD have not been determined.[97]

Thalassemia

Thalassemia with severe anemia is treated with transfusion to improve tissue oxygenation and suppress extramedullary erythropoiesis in the liver, spleen, and marrow, decreasing long-term associated complications. Most transfusion protocols aim for target hemoglobin between 8 to 10 g/dL to allow normal growth and development. Iron overload can occur due to the patient's underlying physiology even without transfusion. If this occurs, it is treated with chelation therapy beginning early in childhood.[98]

Besides iron overload, alloimmunization can cause significant problems in patients receiving chronic transfusions for thalassemia. The incidence of alloantibody formation in this population ranges from 5.6% to 24.7% worldwide,[99-101] and is 19% in the United States.[102] However, among those who received RBCs matched for C, c, E, e, and K, alloimmunization rates were reported as 0 to 3.5%,[100-103] with another study noting there was not a statistically significant trend toward decreased red cell alloimmunization when patients received RBCs matched for C, c, E, e, and K1.[104] Recently, an international expert panel made a recommendation to provide RBCs matched for C, c, E, e, and K to thalassemia patients without alloantibodies, and RBCs matched for C, c, E, e, K, Fyᵃ, Fyᵇ, Jkᵃ, Jkᵇ, S, and s to those with one or more alloantibodies; however, evidence to support their recommendation was weak.[105]

Age of RBCs

To avoid hyperkalemia in patients with renal failure or anuria or patients who receive RBCs rapidly (ie, for ECMO), RBCs <7 days old may be provided. The practice of providing fresh RBCs for all pediatric patients is based on less evidence than for adults, in whom the evidence from randomized controlled trials is weak.

In the TOTAL randomized noninferiority trial of 290 children (aged 6-60 months), most with malaria or SCD, with hemoglobin ≤5 g/dL and lactate ≥5 mmol/L, older RBCs (25 to 35 days) did not result in statistically different worsening of lactate levels 24 hours after transfusion compared to fresher RBCs (1 to 10 days). There were also no differences in clinical assessment, cerebral oxygen saturation, electrolyte abnormalities, adverse events, survival, and 30-day recovery between the groups.[106] Although data are being analyzed from a multicenter trial (ABC PICU study) comparing clinical outcomes in children in the ICU who receive RBCs stored <7 days or those of standard age,[107] there is currently no evidence to support the transfusion of fresh RBCs in the pediatric population.

Whole Blood

There are limited indications for transfusion of whole blood in children. Since the early 1990s, after Manno et al[108] studied the hemostatic effects of fresh whole blood vs reconstituted whole blood following open-heart surgery in children for 24 hours after surgery, fresh whole blood has been advocated in order to improve hemostasis and decrease systemic inflammation. In that study, children <2 years undergoing cardiopulmonary bypass (CPB) surgery who received whole blood <48 hours old had significantly decreased mean 24-hour postoperative blood loss compared to children who received reconstituted whole blood. Of note, children >2 years of age undergoing simpler defect repairs did not have a greater benefit from fresh whole blood <48 hours old over reconstituted whole blood. Improved hemostasis was attributed to better platelet function in fresh whole blood. In 2004, Mou et al[109] examined fresh whole blood (<48 hours old) vs reconstituted blood (RBCs and FFP) for priming of the CPB circuit in children <1 year old. Neither postoperative bleeding nor inflammatory markers were significantly different between groups. Interestingly, circuit priming with whole blood was associated with a longer ICU stay and increased fluid overload. Thus, the use of fresh whole blood after CPB may be warranted if it can be obtained from the local blood center or hospital blood center to use in the postoperative setting, but it may not be as useful for the CPB prime.

Recently, a large US pediatric hospital reported on the experience of using fresh whole blood in both pediatric cardiac and pediatric craniofacial reconstructive surgeries.[110,111] In both studies, donor exposure, compared to either published studies (cardiac surgery) or a historical control group before the implementation of whole blood (reconstructive surgery), was significantly decreased; other outcomes were not assessed. However, logistical issues in obtaining whole blood vs the process of providing reconstituted whole blood need to be considered in the decision to use this product.

PLATELET TRANSFUSION IN NEONATES AND CHILDREN

Mild-to-moderate thrombocytopenia (platelet count <150,000/µL) is the most common hemostatic abnormality in ill preterm and full-term infants, affecting approximately 20% to 25% of infants in neonatal ICUs.[6,112] The most common cause is increased destruction of platelets that is generally associated with a variety of self-limited conditions.[113] Other causes of thrombocytopenia include impaired platelet production, abnormal platelet distribution, and/or platelet dilution secondary to massive transfusion. In rare instances, thrombocytopenia may be the result of in-utero destruction associated with maternal

alloimmunization to paternally inherited platelet antigens. (See Chapter 23.)

Indications

Most platelet transfusions in preterm and full-term infants are performed for platelet counts <50,000/µL to treat active bleeding or prevent occurrence or extension of IVH.[114,115] Prophylactic platelet transfusions in this population are controversial.[116,117] (See Table 24-5 for transfusion indications and thresholds.) Unlike adult patients who rarely have severe bleeding complications until platelet counts decline to <10,000/µL, preterm infants with other complicating illnesses may bleed at higher platelet counts.[114] This increased risk may be attributable to 1) lower concentrations of plasma coagulation factors, 2) circulation of an anticoagulant that potentiates thrombin inhibition, 3) intrinsic or extrinsic platelet dysfunction/hyperreactivity, or 4) increased vascular fragility, especially intracranial vessels.

A severe complication of prematurity is IVH, which occurs in approximately 40% of preterm neonates in the first 72 hours after birth. Although prophylactic platelet transfusions may increase platelet counts and shorten bleeding times, this approach has not been shown to reduce the incidence of IVH, and the severity of thrombocytopenia appears to be independent of the risk of IVH Grade >2.[118] Hence, the use of platelets in this situation and the appropriate platelet dose remain controversial.[119]

In the PlaNeT2 study, a European multicenter randomized controlled trial in 660 preterm neonates, there was a higher rate of new major bleeding or death within 28 days in those who received transfusion for a platelet count threshold of 50,000/µL than in those treated using a platelet count threshold of 25,000/µL, with 88% of transfusions apparently occurring within protocol. Although the reason for improved survival in the lower-threshold group is unclear, this study indicates that platelet transfusion for a threshold of 25,000/µL is at least as safe as for a threshold of 50,000/µL.[120]

In older infants and children, platelets are most often prophylactically administered for chemotherapy-induced thrombocytopenia. The

TABLE 24-5. Transfusion Guidelines for Platelets in Neonates and Older Children[19,20]

With Thrombocytopenia
1. Platelet count <10,000/µL with failure of platelet production.
2. Platelet count <30,000/µL in neonate with failure of platelet production.
3. Platelet count <50,000/µL in stable premature infant:
a. With active bleeding, or
b. Before an invasive procedure, with failure of platelet production.
4. Platelet count <100,000/µL in sick premature infant:
a. With active bleeding, or
b. Before an invasive procedure in patient with DIC.
Without Thrombocytopenia
1. Active bleeding in association with qualitative platelet defect.
2. Unexplained excessive bleeding in a patient undergoing cardiopulmonary bypass.
3. Patient undergoing ECMO with:
a. A platelet count of <100,000/µL, or
b. Higher platelet counts and bleeding.

DIC = disseminated intravascular coagulation; ECMO = extracorporeal membrane oxygenation.

transfusion threshold for these patients is usually a platelet count between 10,000 and 20,000/µL, although the platelet count should not be the sole determinant for transfusion. The PLADO study, which focused on prophylactic platelet dose, showed that in children and adults with hypoproliferative thrombocytopenia, prophylactic platelet transfusions for platelet counts ≤10,000/µL, in concert with different doses of platelets, had no effect on the incidence of moderate to severe bleeding.[121] However, subgroup analysis of the 198 children in this study showed that children were at a higher risk of bleeding over a wider range of platelet counts compared to adults. In the pediatric patients, the rate of Grade 2 or greater bleeding was highest in the youngest patient cohorts—86% in patients aged 0 to 5 years, 88% in 6- to 12-year-olds, and 77% in 13- to 18-year-olds, compared to 67% in adults—suggesting other measures may be needed to prevent thrombocytopenic bleeding in pediatric cancer patients.[122]

Components and Dose

The use of whole-blood-derived platelets at doses of 5 to 10 mL/kg body weight have been demonstrated to raise the platelet count of an average full-term newborn by 50,000 to 100,000/µL, depending on the concentration of the platelet component used.[38,112] A similar dosing regimen is typically used for apheresis platelets and older children. (See Table 24-3 for platelet dosing for desired increment, and Table 24-5 for indications for platelet transfusion.) Although 15- to 60-minute posttransfusion platelet counts can help evaluate platelet survival, these counts are not necessarily good predictors of hemostatic efficacy.

When possible, the platelet component should be ABO group specific or compatible. Transfusion of ABO-incompatible plasma should be avoided in children, and especially in infants, because of their small blood and plasma volumes.[52] If it becomes necessary to administer ABO-incompatible platelets to an infant, plasma

TABLE 24-6. Transfusion Guidelines for Plasma Components in Neonates and Older Children[19,20]

Fresh Frozen Plasma (FFP)	
1.	Support during treatment of disseminated intravascular dissemination.
2.	Replacement therapy.
	a. When specific factor concentrates are not available, including, but not limited to, antithrombin; protein C or S; and Factor II, Factor V, Factor X, and Factor XI.
	b. During therapeutic plasma exchange when FFP is indicated (cryopoor plasma, plasma from which the cryoprecipitate has been removed).
3.	Reversal of warfarin in an emergency situation may also be an alternative, such as before an invasive procedure with active bleeding.

Note: FFP is not indicated for volume expansion or enhancement of wound healing.

Cryoprecipitated AHF	
1.	Hypofibrinogenemia or dysfibrinogenemia with active bleeding.
2.	Hypofibrinogenemia or dysfibrinogenemia while undergoing an invasive procedure.
3.	Factor XIII deficiency with active bleeding or while undergoing an invasive procedure in the absence of Factor XIII concentrate.
4.	Limited directed-donor cryoprecipitate for bleeding episodes in small children with hemophilia A (when recombinant and plasma-derived Factor VIII products are not available).
5.	In the preparation of fibrin sealant.
6.	Von Willebrand disease with active bleeding, but only when both of the following are true:
	a. Deamino-D-arginine vasopressin (DDAVP) is contraindicated, not available, or does not elicit response.
	b. Virus-inactivated plasma-derived Factor VIII concentrate (which contains von Willebrand factor) or von Willebrand recombinant concentrate is not available.

may be removed either by volume reduction or washing with saline resuspension. (Refer to local protocols.) However, routine centrifugation to remove plasma from the platelets should be avoided because it has been shown to decrease the posttransfusion platelet count increment.[123]

In addition, when platelets are stored in a syringe, the pH has been shown to decrease rapidly, a potential problem for an already ill and acidotic recipient.[124,125] Therefore, when volume reduction in an open system is used and the component is placed in a syringe, the processing should be performed as close to the time of issuance as possible, and the component should be infused within 4 hours from the start of processing.

PLASMA AND CRYOPRECIPITATE TRANSFUSION IN NEONATES AND CHILDREN

Plasma

Plasma is frequently used to replace coagulation factors in preterm and full-term infants with hemorrhage or before surgery, particularly if multiple factor deficiencies are present, such as in hemorrhagic disease of the newborn due to vitamin K deficiency. It is occasionally used to replace anticoagulant factors when anticoagulation is contraindicated in infants with life-threatening thrombosis. Table 24-6 provides the indications for the transfusion of plasma, which are similar in older infants, children, and adults.

FFP is plasma that was frozen within 8 hours of collection and is used within 24 hours of thawing. Twenty-four hours after being thawed, the plasma can be relabeled as Thawed Plasma, which is considered an acceptable substitute that can be used over the next 4 days. (See Chapter 6.) Another form of plasma used in children is Plasma Frozen Within 24 Hours After Phlebotomy (PF24), used within 24 hours of thawing. The usual dose of plasma is 10 to 15 mL/kg, which is expected to increase all factor activity levels by 15% to 20% unless there is a marked consumptive coagulopathy.[117] The evidence for use of plasma to correct coagulopathy without bleeding is weak.[117,126]

To limit donor exposure for each recipient while minimizing plasma waste, blood can be collected into a system with multiple, integrally attached bags that create ready-to-freeze aliquots.[70] Once thawed, the aliquots can be subdivided further for several patients if they can be used within a 24-hour period. A common practice at some institutions is to use group AB plasma because a single unit can provide multiple small-volume doses for several neonates. However this can be difficult to maintain, as AB plasma is usually not in plentiful supply. A plasma product that is being increasingly used is solvent/detergent-treated plasma (SD plasma). SD plasma is plasma pooled from many donors that has undergone processing to remove lipid-enveloped viruses. A recent study showed decreased mortality in children in the ICU who received SD plasma compared to those who received FFP or PF24.[127] In addition, the risk of allergic reactions and transfusion-related acute lung injury (TRALI) appears reduced due to the process of filitration to remove cellular debris, as well as the dilution of individual donor plasma proteins. Use of this type of plasma will depend on the risk/benefit analysis performed by transfusion services.

A recent prospective observational study showed that plasma transfusions were independently associated with an increased risk of new or progressive multiple-organ dysfunction, nosocomial infections, and prolonged length of stay in 831 children admitted to one institution's pediatric critical care unit.[128] Plasma transfusions should be considered with caution in this population.

Cryoprecipitated Antihemophilic Factor

Cryoprecipitate transfusions are primarily used to treat conditions resulting from 1) decreased or dysfunctional fibrinogen (congenital or acquired) or 2) Factor XIII deficiency, if Factor XIII concentrate [eg, Corifact (CSL Behring)] is not available. Cryoprecipitate is also given in conjunction with platelets and FFP to treat disseminated intravascular coagulation (DIC). Typically, 1 unit is sufficient to achieve hemostatic levels in an infant.

ABO-compatible cryoprecipitate is preferred in neonates because transfusion of a large volume of ABO-incompatible cryoprecipitate may result in a positive direct antiglobulin test result and, in very rare cases, mild hemolysis.[129,130]

Cryoprecipitate transfusion is not recommended for patients with Factor VIII deficiency because standard therapy for this condition is infusion of recombinant or virus-inactivated, monoclonal-antibody-purified, plasma-derived Factor VIII products.[131] In the United States, cryoprecipitate should be used to treat von Willebrand disease only if plasma-derived, virus-inactivated concentrates or recombinant products containing vWF are not available.[75] Recombinant vWF [Vonvendi (Baxalta Inc)] was recently approved in the United States for treatment and prevention of bleeding in adults with von Willebrand disease; there is currently an open study in children aged 6 years and above. See Tables 24-3 and 24-6 for dosing and guidelines regarding plasma and cryoprecipitate use.[117,131]

GRANULOCYTE TRANSFUSION IN NEONATES AND CHILDREN

The role of granulocyte transfusion for sepsis in neonates is unclear, and this treatment is rarely used, although dosage appears to correlate with efficacy. For patients of any age, it is important to establish the following factors before the transfusion of granulocytes: 1) evidence of bacterial or fungal septicemia; 2) absolute neutrophil count <500/µL, chronic granulomatous disease, or leukocyte adhesion deficiency; and 3) diminishing storage pool (such that 7% of nucleated cells in the marrow are granulocytes that are metamyelocytes or more mature).[132,133]

Granulocyte concentrates are produced by standard apheresis techniques or by pooling buffy coats from whole blood. A typical dose for infants is 10 to 15 mL/kg body weight, which is approximately 1×10^9 to 2×10^9 polymorphonuclear cells/kg.[19,132] For larger children and adults, a minimum dose of 1×10^{10} is suggested.[19,131,132] If a patient weighs over 20 kg, either one-half of a unit or the whole unit can be transfused, depending on its volume and the volume status of the patient.

Treatment is usually administered daily until an adequate neutrophil count is maintained and/or the patient shows clinical improvement. Granulocytes must be irradiated, given that recipients are either neonates with immature T-cell function or older immunosuppressed individuals, both groups that are at increased risk for TA-GVHD. Because granulocytes cannot be leukocyte reduced, if the recipient is CMV seronegative, the component should be obtained from CMV-seronegative donors to prevent virus transmission.[2] Granulocytes should be ABO compatible with the red cells of the recipient because of the significant red cell content in these components.[49(p35)] Many institutions also provide D-compatible components to decrease Rh alloimmunization.

To obtain higher doses of granulocytes for larger patients, donors can receive mobilizers such as steroids, granulocyte colony-stimulating factor (G-CSF), or a combination. A multicenter study that randomly assigned neutropenic adults and children with systemic bacterial or fungal infection to receive standard antimicrobials with or without granulocytes (from donors stimulated with G-CSF and steroid) showed no benefit in mortality or microbial response in the granulocyte group. However, the study closed early because of poor accrual and was insufficiently powered to adequately address the efficacy of granulocyte transfusions.[132] Therefore, there remains no definitive evidence for the benefit (or lack thereof) of granulocyte transfusions.

OTHER CONSIDERATIONS COMMON TO TRANSFUSION OF NEONATES AND CHILDREN

Vascular Access

Vascular access is the most difficult aspect of transfusion administration in patients younger than 4 months old, particularly preterm infants who require long-term or continuous intravenous infusions. The umbilical vein is most frequently cannulated after birth to facilitate administration of fluids and transfusions and to monitor central venous pressure. Vascular catheters (24-gauge) and small needles (25-gauge) generally can be safely used for RBC transfusions without causing hemolysis if constant flow rates are applied. The outcomes of transfusions using smaller-gauge needles and catheters or intra-osseous catheters in neonates have not been evaluated.

Filters and Transfusion Sets

The plastic tubing in the administration sets can add a significant amount of dead-space volume to the transfusion and should be accounted for when preparing a transfusion dose. Pediatric infusion sets created for platelets and other small-volume components have less dead space than standard sets. When using normal saline to flush blood components into the patient, ceasing the flush before the normal saline reaches the patient may decrease the risk of dilution. For standard filter requirements, see Chapter 18.

Rate of Administration

The rate of blood component administration is dictated by the clinical needs of the patient, whether neonate or older child. Therefore, administering a simple transfusion over 2 to 4 hours is adequate in nonemergent situations. However, in states of shock or severe bleeding, a rapid infusion is often required. Rapid infusion devices should be used with caution; in neonates, syringe push can be used instead. In small infants, despite concerns from neonatologists that rapid blood infusion rates may adversely affect intravascular volume and electrolyte levels, an increased risk of IVH in these small and fragile patients has not been clearly demonstrated and remains a theoretical risk.[134]

Aliquoting for Small-Volume Transfusion

The purpose of creating small-volume aliquots is to limit donor exposures, prevent circulatory overload, and decrease blood waste.[30,135-138] Several technical approaches can be used.[54]

Small-volume RBC transfusion aliquots are commonly prepared with a multiple-pack system.[54,139] Quad packs, employed mostly by blood centers, are produced from a single unit of whole blood that is diverted into a primary bag with three integrally attached smaller bags. The plasma is then separated and diverted into one bag during component preparation. The remaining red cells are drawn into the smaller bags as needed for transfusion. Each of the smaller units has the same expiration date as the original unit because the system's original seal has remained intact and a "closed system" is maintained. A hospital transfusion service can then remove (either by heat sealer or metal clips) each aliquot as needed. For hospital transfusion services that do not have a sterile connection device (Fig 24-1), this method provides three aliquots from a single unit.[36] However, some blood components may still be wasted when used in aliquots that are larger than the dose selected for each patient based on body weight.

Hospital transfusion services that have a sterile connection device have multiple options to produce aliquots, such as transfer packs [eg, T3000 (Charter Medical), Fig 24-2], small-volume bags, or tubing that has integrally attached syringes. Syringe sets (Fig 24-3) offer the greatest accuracy for obtaining the desired volume to be transfused based on volume-per-weight calculations. Some syringe sets have an attached 150-micron in-line filter for use during the aliquoting process so that, when issued by the blood bank, the cells are ready to be placed on a syringe pump without further manipulation of the component or filtration at the bedside. This process eliminates the need for the nurse to transfer blood from the pack to a syringe at the bedside for delivery by a syringe pump. Removing this additional step reduces the risk of contamination, mislabeling, or damage to the unit that results in blood loss or spillage.[55]

Reducing donor exposures is readily accomplished by aliquoting, which enables a recipient to receive multiple small-volume transfusions from a single unit until it reaches its expiration date.[31,140] Some hospital transfusion services assign a single unit of RBCs to one or more infants based on their weight.[137-139]

Once an aliquot is produced at either the blood center or hospital blood bank, it must be labeled with the expiration date and the origin and disposition of each smaller unit, and often the parent unit must be recorded. Aliquot expiration dates vary from institution to institution and depending on the oversight authority; thus, the local standard and standard operating procedures should always be followed.

Extracorporeal Membrane Oxygenation

ECMO is a prolonged treatment whereby blood is removed from the patient's venous circulation, circulated through a machine to remove CO_2 and replenish O_2, and then returned to the patient. In neonates and children, ECMO has become a lifesaving treatment for meconium aspiration syndrome, persistent pulmonary hypertension of the newborn, congenital diaphragmatic hernia, and respiratory failure due to sepsis. It is also used for postoperative support following cardiac surgery. Because standardized guidelines for transfusion practice in ECMO have not been established, centers typically establish their own criteria. Table 24-7 provides some guidelines for ECMO.[141]

Bleeding complications are frequent during ECMO treatment and are usually multifactorial. Causes include 1) systemic heparinization, 2) platelet dysfunction, 3) thrombocytopenia, 4) other coagulation defects, and/or 5) the nonendothelial ECMO circuit. Thrombotic complications are also common. Hospital blood banks and transfusion services must be in close com-

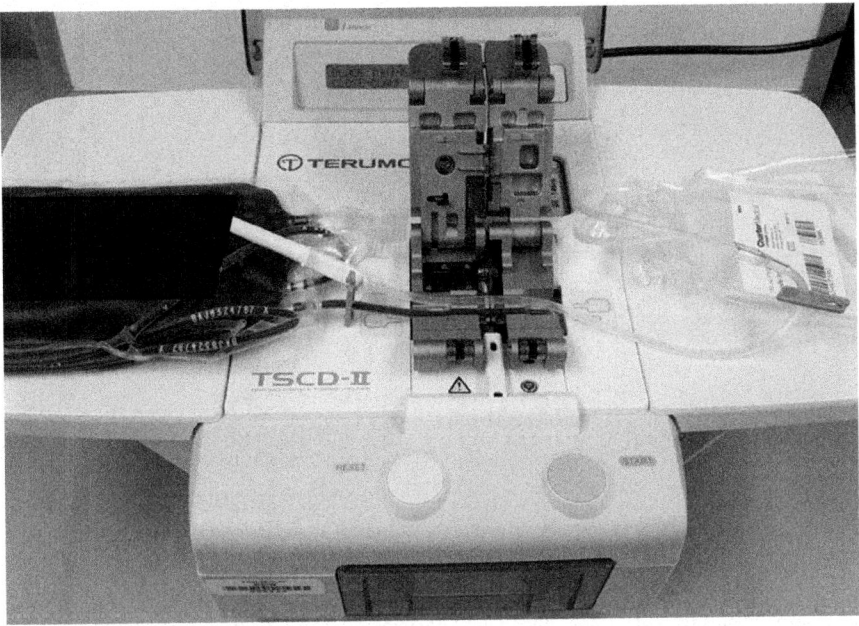

FIGURE 24-1. A sterile tubing welder. (Courtesy of R. Punzalan, Versiti Blood Center of Wisconsin and Children's Hospital of Wisconsin.)

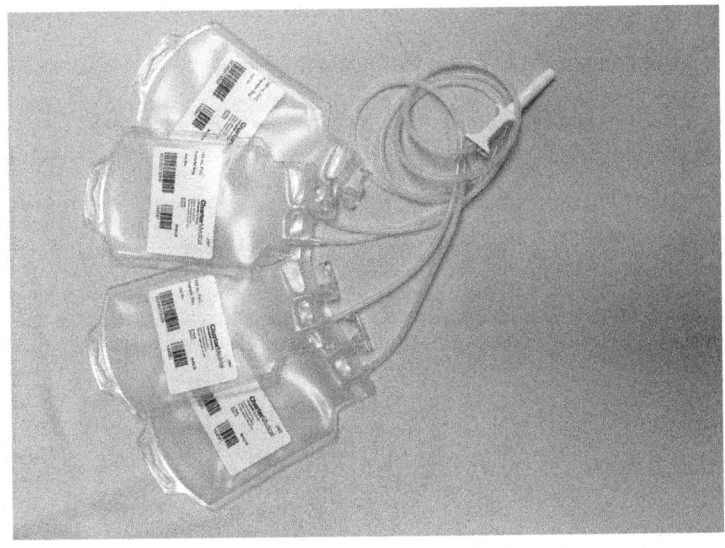

FIGURE 24-2. T3000 neonatal/pediatric 150-mL aliquot system. (Courtesy of P. Niston, Charter Medical, Ltd.)

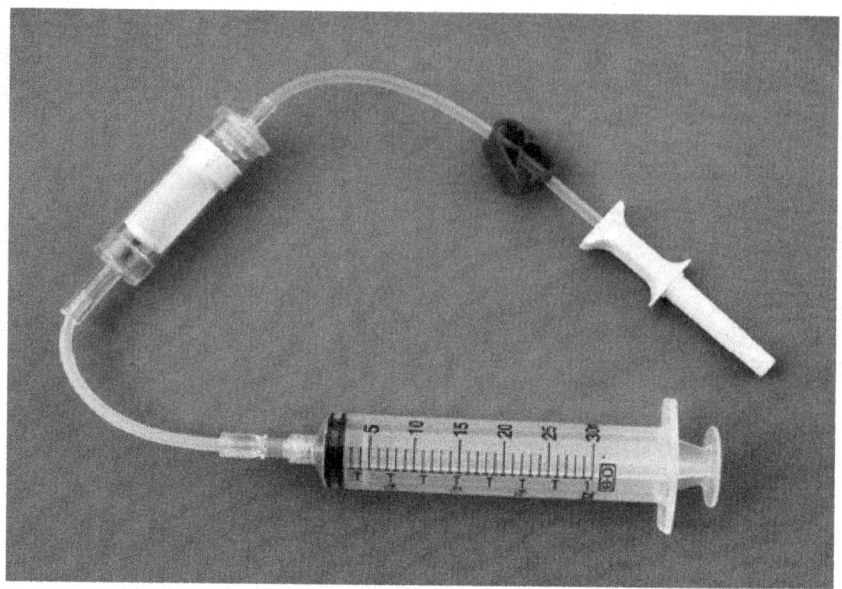

FIGURE 24-3. Neonatal syringe set. (Reproduced with permission from Charter Medical, Ltd.)

munication with the ECMO staff and observe local protocols to ensure safe, efficient, and consistent care.

There has been increased use of antithrombin infusion during ECMO, prophylactically or to manage resistance to heparin, without strong data to support the practice.[142] A retrospective cohort study showed tighter control of heparin and decreased incidence of thrombosis without increased bleeding when antithrombin was giv-

TABLE 24-7. Blood Component Preparation Protocols for ECMO[141]

Clinical Scenario	Urgency	Components	Blood Groups	Storage
Cardiac arrest	5-10 min	2 units RBCs	O-neg RBCs	<14 days, AS
ECMO circuit disruption	5-10 min	2 units RBCs	O-neg RBCs	<14 days, AS
Progressive septic shock (nonneonate)	30 min	2 units RBCs	O-neg RBCs or type specific	<10 days, any preservative
Neonate transferred for ECMO	1-2 hours	2 units RBCs 1 unit FFP 1 unit platelets	O-neg RBCs AB plasma	<10 days, CPD or CPDA
Cardiac ICU	30-60 min	2 units RBCs	Type specific	<7 days, AS
Gradual respiratory or cardiac failure on conventional support	Hours to days	2 units RBCs	Type specific	<10 days, CPD

ECMO = extracorporeal membrane oxygenation; RBCs = Red Blood Cells; AS = additive solution; FFP = Fresh Frozen Plasma; CPD = citrate-phosphate-dextrose; CPDA = citrate-phosphate-dextrose-adenine; ICU = intensive care unit.

en prophylactically to neonates on ECMO.[143] However, a retrospective review of the US Pediatric Health Information Systems database showed that children who received at least 1 dose of antithrombin during ECMO had more bleeding and thrombotic events than those who did not.[144] Therefore, studies on the role of antithrombin replacement during ECMO are needed.

ECMO initiation typically requires 1 to 2 units of ABO and Rh group-compatible and cross-match-compatible RBCs for blood priming. In emergencies, uncrossmatched blood may be used. In addition, a single unit of group-compatible FFP should be allocated to the ECMO patient. RBC units are usually negative for hemoglobin S, relatively fresh (<5 to 7 days old), irradiated (many patients requiring ECMO are neonates and/or potential transplant recipients), and CMV seronegative or leukocyte reduced.[71] Because the ECMO circuit consumes platelets, higher platelet counts are often maintained. However, there are no evidence-based guidelines for transfusion in patients on ECMO.

Ventricular Assist Devices

The use of ventricular assist devices (VADs) in children is increasing, especially with the US Food and Drug Administration (FDA) approval of the first long-term VAD (Berlin Heart EXCOR VAD) in children, in 2011, as a bridge to cardiac transplantation or as a bridge from ECMO for cardiac support.[145] In children, the most concerning complications include stroke and device-related thromboembolism. These occur in large part due to activation of the endothelium, hemostatic proteins, and the fibrinolytic system, as well as platelets and leukocytes, resulting in increased thrombin generation necessitating thromboprophylaxis.[146] Therefore, 8 to 24 hours after implantation of a VAD, aggressive anticoagulation and antiplatelet treatment are initiated, with close monitoring of anticoagulant levels, including use of viscoelastic testing. Oral anticoagulant drugs (eg, warfarin) are considered in children older than 12 months when oral or enteral feeding is optimized. Because of the very small extracorporeal size of the device, priming is typically not required. However, the pediatric

transfusion medicine specialist and the coagulation laboratory should be aware of unusual hemostatic monitoring requirements of these devices.[146]

Massive Transfusion

Trauma is the leading cause of death in infants, children, and young adults aged 1 to 21 years. Although trauma rarely leads to hemorrhagic shock and massive transfusion, resuscitation after trauma can be challenging.

The evidence to support a pediatric massive transfusion protocol (MTP) is limited, but several pediatric institutions use MTPs to improve the outcomes of patients who have massive bleeding with trauma.[147] Although studies indicate that an MTP in the pediatric setting is feasible not only for providing rapid and balanced blood component support but also for decreasing the risk of thromboembolic events, the role of the MTP and the optimal ratio of components has not been studied in the pediatric setting.[148-150] A large pediatric trauma trial has not been undertaken and, given the rarity of patients, would be difficult to accomplish.[148-152] In a recently published multicenter trial, adults with severe trauma and major bleeding who received early administration of plasma, platelets, and RBCs in a 1:1:1 ratio compared with a 1:1:2 ratio did not have significant difference in mortality at 24 hours or at 30 days. However, there were fewer deaths from bleeding at 24 hours in the 1:1:1 group, so this ratio has been adopted by many trauma centers, including for older children.[153]

Tranexamic acid has been used for massive trauma-associated bleeding in adults. In the CRASH-2 study, a multicenter randomized controlled trial in >7500 massively bleeding patients, early (within 1-3 hours) treatment with tranexamic acid was associated with decreased bleeding-associated mortality (5.3% vs 7.7% in the placebo group; p <0.0001). However, late (>3 hours) treatment with tranexamic acid was associated with *increased* bleeding-associated mortality (4.4% vs 3.1% in the placebo group; p = 0.004). No patients <16 years old were enrolled in that study.[154] The use of tranexamic acid in pediatric trauma has not been studied.

TABLE 24-8. Irradiation Guidelines for Children Who Require Cellular Blood Components[19,20,131]

1.	Premature neonates weighing <1200 g at birth.
2.	Any patient with:
	a. Known or suspected cellular immune deficiency.
	b. Significant immunosuppression related to chemotherapy or radiation treatment.
3.	Any patient receiving:
	a. Components from blood relatives.
	b. HLA-matched or crossmatched platelet components.
	c. Granulocyte transfusion.

ADVERSE EFFECTS AND PREVENTION

Acute Transfusion Reactions

In general, acute transfusion reactions are more commonly reported in children than in adults.[155] In particular, there is increased incidence of febrile nonhemolytic, allergic, and hypotensive reactions in pediatric patients.[155,156]

CMV Prevention

The manifestation of CMV infection in susceptible individuals (eg, neonates, immunocompromised patients) is variable, ranging from asymptomatic seroconversion to multiorgan involvement, viremia, and death. CMV may be transmitted transplacentally, during the birth process, during breastfeeding, as a result of personal contact with infected persons, or from transfusion. With current technologies, the risk of acquiring CMV from transfusion is likely lower than the historically reported 1% to 3%.[157] In a recent study, it was found that breast milk was the main source of CMV transmission in neonates.[158] The risk of transfusion-transmitted CMV infection may be higher in low-birthweight infants (<1200 g) who were born to seronegative mothers and have received multiple transfusions.[37,159]

Reduction of CMV transmission from transfusion is achieved by leukocyte reduction or provision of blood from CMV-seronegative donors, as evidenced by similar efficacy in adults.[157] Using both approaches has been shown in a non-randomized study to completely prevent CMV transmission by transfusion in VLBW neonates.[158] However, in the absence of superior benefit for using both approaches, providing leukocyte-reduced components is generally felt to be adequate to prevent transfusion-transmitted CMV.[160]

Leukocyte Reduction

The benefits of transfusing leukocyte-reduced components include reducing the risk of transfusion-transmitted CMV, preventing febrile nonhemolytic transfusion reactions, and decreasing the risk of HLA alloimmunization.[161]

Irradiation

TA-GVHD has been reported most frequently in newborns with confirmed or suspected congenital immunodeficiency. The majority of TA-GVHD cases reported in nonimmunocompromised infants have occurred after intrauterine transfusion and subsequent postnatal exchange transfusion, and were almost always associated with transfusion from maternal directed donation.[162,163] There have also been rare cases of TA-GVHD in extremely premature infants, infants with neonatal alloimmune thrombocytopenia, or infants on ECMO.[42,162] Mortality from TA-GVHD is >90%.

Cellular blood components are irradiated to prevent TA-GVHD in immunocompromised recipients and for situations when the patient may share an HLA haplotype with the blood donor. (See Table 24-8.) Expert opinion and practices differ on this topic. Therefore, protocols should be based on the patient populations served, equipment available, and procedures that have the highest likelihood of ensuring that a patient who needs irradiated blood receives it. The processes of irradiation, irradiator quality control, and quality assurance are addressed in Chapters 1, 2, 6, and 17.

Volume Reduction and Washing

The plasma volume of the component (usually platelets, because RBCs have little plasma) is usually reduced in transfusions to patients who cannot tolerate increased intravascular volume (eg, patients with renal ischemia or compromised cardiac function). In 1993, the AABB Committee on Pediatric Hemotherapy stated that volume reduction of platelet concentrates should be reserved for infants who have total body fluid restrictions.[164] Methods for platelet volume reduction have been published.[165] However, there is no optimal centrifugation rate and preparation method. As with any platelet modification, the total number of platelets typically decreases, and platelet activation may occur with these procedures.[166]

Saline-washed RBCs and platelets are administered to reduce the risk of recurrence of severe allergic reactions from plasma. Other uses of washing may include removal of anticoagulant-preservative solutions and removal of high levels of potassium in RBCs, although centrifugation and volume reduction alone may be adequate. Maternal cells should be washed to remove maternal antibodies and irradiated if these are being used for fetal or neonatal transfusion.

Pathogen Inactivation

One pathogen inactivation technique for platelets and plasma has been approved by the FDA [INTERCEPT (Cerus Corp)]. Other systems [Mirasol (Terumo BCT) and Theraflex (MacoPharma)] have been used in several European countries for many years, including in children.[167,168] In a recent meta-analysis of randomized controlled trials (only some of which include children), the use of pathogen-reduced platelets was associated with increased risk of platelet refractoriness and platelet transfusion requirement, but was not associated with increased mortality, clinically significant bleeding, or other adverse events.[169] There are very few studies describing the use of pathogen-reduced platelets in pediatric patients. Seven years of European hemovigilance data, including in children, showed minimal adverse events, usually mild, and no increase in TRALI, TA-GVHD, transfusion-transmitted infection, or death after transfusion of pathogen-reduced platelets.[170]

In an Austrian study that examined RBC and plasma utilization (as a marker of significant bleeding before and after implementation of pathogen-reduced platelets), there was no statistically significant difference in RBC and FFP transfusion or transfusion-related adverse events among children and neonates.[171] In a retrospective review, posttransfusion platelet count increments in children with cancer who received pathogen-reduced platelets using riboflavin were not as increased as in those who received untreated platelets, but there was no difference in bleeding outcomes.[172]

KEY POINTS

1. RBCs are the most frequently transfused blood component in neonates.
2. Frequent blood loss, including iatrogenic losses from repeated phlebotomy, contributes to the need for RBC transfusions in neonates.
3. A full-term newborn has a blood volume of approximately 85 mL/kg; a preterm infant has a total approximate blood volume of 100 mL/kg.
4. In infants <4 months of age, initial patient testing must include ABO and D typing of the infant's red cells and a screen for unexpected red cell antibodies, using either plasma or serum from the infant or mother. During any one hospitalization, crossmatch-compatibility testing and repeat ABO and D typing may be omitted as long as all of the following criteria are met: the antibody screen is negative; transfused RBCs are group O, ABO identical, or ABO compati-

ble; and transfused cells are either D negative or the same D type as the patient. Testing the infant's reverse type for anti-A and/or anti-B is not necessary.

5. Small-volume (10-15 mL/kg) simple transfusions of RBCs (regardless of storage solution), when administered slowly, have been shown to have little effect on serum potassium concentrations in infants <4 months of age despite elevated potassium levels in the plasma of stored RBCs.

6. During component preparation, if aliquots are made with a sterile connection device, they are considered to have been prepared within a "closed system," and the original unit's expiration date can be used for the new aliquot.

7. Transfusion of ABO-incompatible plasma should be avoided in infants and children because of their small blood and plasma volumes. If ABO out-of-group platelet transfusion becomes necessary, plasma may be removed by volume reduction.

8. Chronic RBC transfusion therapy of indefinite duration to maintain hemoglobin S levels below 30% is the therapy of choice to reduce the risk of stroke recurrence in patients with SCD. SCD patients have the highest rates of alloimmunization to red cell minor antigens of any patient group. The most commonly formed antibodies are to RH, KEL, FY, and JK system antigens. Many SCD treatment centers try to prevent red cell alloimmunization by matching components and recipients for phenotypically similar antigen profiles. This strategy is not the same at all centers and is controversial because obtaining enough phenotypically similar units may be difficult and costly.

9. To decrease the risk of transfusion-transmitted CMV infection in susceptible populations such as low-birthweight neonates and immunocompromised children, these patients should receive blood components that either have been leukocyte reduced or are from CMV-seronegative donors.

REFERENCES

1. Hillyer CD, Mondoro TH, Josephson CD, et al. Pediatric transfusion medicine: Development of a critical mass. Transfusion 2009;49:596-601.

2. Hume H, Bard H. Small volume red blood cell transfusions for neonatal patients. Transfus Med Rev 1995;9:187-99.

3. Blanchette V, Doyle J, Schmidt B, et al. Hematology. In: Avery G, Fletcher M, MacDonald M, eds. Neonatology: Pathophysiology and management of the newborn. 4th ed. Philadelphia: JB Lippincott, 1994:952-99.

4. Brugnara C, Platt OS. The neonatal erythrocyte and its disorders. In: Nathan DG, Orkin SH, eds. Nathan and Oski's hematology of infancy and childhood. 7th ed. Philadelphia: WB Saunders, 2009:21-66.

5. Dame C, Fahnenstich H, Freitag P, et al. Erythropoietin mRNA expression in human fetal and neonatal tissue. Blood 1998;92:3218-25.

6. Roberts I, Stanworth S, Murray NA. Thrombocytopenia in the neonate. Blood Rev 2008;22:173-86.

7. Andrew M, Paes B, Johnston M. Development of the hemostatic system in the neonate and young infant. Am J Pediatr Hematol 1990;12:95-104.

8. Monagle P, Barnes C, Ignjatovic V, et al. Developmental haemostasis: Impact for clinical haemostasis laboratories. Thromb Haemost 2006;95:362-72.

9. Revel-Vilk S. The conundrum of neonatal coagulopathy. Hematology Am Soc Hematol Educ Program 2012;2012:450-4.

10. Cowman J, Quinn N, Geoghegan S, et al. Dynamic platelet function on von Willebrand factor is different in preterm neonates and full-term neonates: Changes in neonatal platelet function. J Thromb Haemost 2016;14:2027-35.

11. Deschmann E, Saxonhouse MA, Feldman HA, et al. Association between in vitro bleeding time and bleeding in preterm infants with thrombocytopenia. JAMA Pediatr 2019;173(4):393-4.

12. DePalma L. Review: Red cell alloantibody formation in the neonate and infant: Considerations for current immunohematologic practice. Immunohematology 1992;8:33-7.

13. Dincsoy MY, Tsang RC, Laskarzewski P, et al. The role of postnatal age and magnesium on

parathyroid hormone responses during "exchange" blood transfusion in the newborn period. J Pediatr 1982;100:277-83.

14. Monagle P, Barnes C, Ignjatovic V, et al. Developmental haemostasis. Impact for clinical haemostasis laboratories. Thromb Haemost 2006; 95:362-72.

15. Sisson TR, Whalen LE, Telek A. The blood volume of infants. II. The premature infant during the first year of life. J Pediatr 1959;55:430-46.

16. Fabres J, Wehrli G, Marques MB, et al. Estimating blood needs for very-low-birth-weight infants. Transfusion 2006;46:1915-20.

17. Lin JC, Strauss R, Kulhavy JC, et al. Phlebotomy overdraw in the neonatal intensive care nursery. Pedatrics 2000;106:E19.

18. Wallgren G, Hanson JS, Lind J. Quantitative studies of the human neonatal circulation. 3. Observations on the newborn infants central circulatory responses to moderate hypovolemia. Acta Paediatr Scand 1967;(Suppl 179):45.

19. Roseff SD, Luban NL, Manno CS. Guidelines for assessing appropriateness of pediatric transfusion. Transfusion 2002;42:1398-413.

20. Saifee NH, Lau W, Keir A. Intrauterine, neonatal, and pediatric transfusion. In: Marques MB, Schwartz J, Wu Y, eds. Transfusion therapy: Clinical principles and practice. 4th ed. Bethesda, MD: AABB Press, 2019:291-341.

21. Ohls RK. Evaluation and treatment of anemia in the neonate. In: Christensen RD, ed. Hematologic problems of the neonate. Philadelphia: WB Saunders, 2000:137-69.

22. Halvorsen S, Bechensteen AG. Physiology of erythropoietin during mammalian development. Acta Paediatr Suppl 2002;91:17-26.

23. Ohlsson A, Aher SM. Early erythropoiesis-stimulating agents in preterm or low birth weight infants. Cochrane Database Syst Rev 2017;11: CD004863.

24. Kandasamy Y, Kumar P, Hartley L. The effect of erythropoietin on the severity of retinopathy of prematurity. Eye 2014;28:814-18.

25. Doege C, Pritsch M, Fruhwald MC, et al. An association between infantile haemangiomas and erythropoietin treatment in preterm infants. Arch Dis Child Fetal Neonatal Ed 2012;97:F45-9.

26. Henry E, Christensen RD, Sheffield MJ, et al. Why do four NICUs using identical RBC transfusion guidelines have different gestational age-adjusted RBC transfusion rates? J Perinatol 2015;35:132-6.

27. Carroll PD, Widness JA. Nonpharmacological, blood conservation techniques for preventing neonatal anemia—Effective and promising strategies for reducing transfusion. Semin Perinatol 2012;36:232-43.

28. Barcelona SL, Cote CJ. Pediatric resuscitation in the operating room. Anesthesiol Clin North Am 2001;19:339-65.

29. Luban NL, Mikesell G, Sacher RA. Techniques for warming red blood cells packaged in different containers for neonatal use. Clin Pediatr 1985;24:642-4.

30. Strauss RG, Burmeister LF, Johnson K, et al. AS-1 red cells for neonatal transfusions: A randomized trial assessing donor exposure and safety. Transfusion 1996;36:873-8.

31. Strauss RG, Burmeister LF, Johnson K, et al. Feasibility and safety of AS-3 red blood cells for neonatal transfusions. J Pediatr 2000;136:215-19.

32. Luban NL, Strauss RG, Hume HA. Commentary on the safety of red cells preserved in extended-storage media for neonatal transfusions. Transfusion 1991;31:229-35.

33. Pyles R, Lowery J, Delaney M. The use of red cell units containing additives in large volume neonatal transfusion in neonatology units in the USA (letter). ISBT Science Series 2017;12:322-3.

34. Rock G, Poon A, Haddad S, et al. Nutricel as an additive solution for neonatal transfusion. Transfus Sci 1999;20:29-36.

35. Tuchschmid P, Mieth D, Burger R, et al. Potential hazard of hypoalbuminemia in newborn babies after exchange transfusions with ADSOL red blood cell concentrates. Pediatrics 1990;85: 234-5.

36. New HV, Berryman J, Bolton-Maggs PHB, et al. Guidelines on transfusion for fetuses, neonates and older children. Br J Haematol 2016;175: 784-828.

37. Strauss RG. Data-driven blood banking practices for neonatal RBC transfusions. Transfusion 2000;40:1528-40.

38. Strauss RG. Transfusion therapy in neonates. Am J Dis Child 1991;145:904-11.

39. Strauss RG. Neonatal transfusion. In: Anderson KC, Ness PN, eds. Scientific basis of transfusion medicine: Implications for clinical practice. 2nd ed. Philadelphia: WB Saunders, 2000:321-6.

40. Strauss RG. Routinely washing irradiated red cells before transfusion seems unwarranted. Transfusion 1990;30:675-7.

41. McDonald TB, Berkowitz RA. Massive transfusion in children. In: Jefferies LC, Brecher ME,

eds. Massive transfusion. Bethesda, MD: AABB, 1994:97-119.

42. Ohto H, Anderson KC. Posttransfusion graft-versus-host disease in Japanese newborns. Transfusion 1996;36:117-23.

43. Lee AC, Reduque LL, Luban NLC, et al. Transfusion-associated hyperkalemic cardiac arrest in pediatric patients receiving massive transfusion. Transfusion 2014;54:244-54.

44. Hall TL, Barnes A, Miller JR, et al. Neonatal mortality following transfusion of red cells with high plasma potassium levels. Transfusion 1993; 33:606-9.

45. Fung MK, Roseff SD, Vermoch KL. Blood component preferences of transfusion services supporting infant transfusions: A University HealthSystem Consortium benchmarking study. Transfusion 2010;50:1921-5.

46. Wong EC, Luban NL. Hematology and oncology. In: Slonim AD, Pollack MM, eds. Pediatric critical care medicine. Philadelphia: Lippincott, Williams and Wilkins, 2006:157-95.

47. Fergusson DA, Hébert P, Hogan DL, et al. Effect of fresh red blood cell transfusions on clinical outcomes in premature, very low-birth-weight infants: The ARIPI randomized trial. JAMA 2012;308:1443-51.

48. Patel RM, Josephson CD. Storage age of red blood cells for transfusion of premature infants. JAMA 2013;309:544-5.

49. Gammon R, ed. Standards for blood banks and transfusion services. 32nd ed. Bethesda, MD: AABB, 2020.

50. Strauss RG. Selection of white cell-reduced blood components for transfusions during early infancy. Transfusion 1993;33:352-7.

51. Turkmen T, Qiu D, Cooper N, et al. Red blood cell alloimmunization in neonates and children up to 3 years of age. Transfusion 2017;57:2720-6.

52. Josephson CD, Castillejo M, Grima K, et al. ABO-mismatched platelet transfusions: Strategies to mitigate patient exposure to naturally occurring hemolytic antibodies. Transfus Apher Sci 2010;42:83-8.

53. Girelli G, Antoncecchi S, Casadei AM, et al. Recommendations for transfusion therapy in neonatology. Blood Transfus 2015;13:484-97.

54. Roseff SD. Pediatric blood collection and transfusion technology. In: Herman JK, Manno CS, eds. Pediatric transfusion therapy. Bethesda, MD: AABB Press, 2002:217-47.

55. Wong E, Roseff SD, eds. Pediatric hemotherapy data card. Bethesda, MD: AABB, 2015.

56. Bell EF, Strauss RG, Widness JA, et al. Randomized trial of liberal versus restrictive guidelines for red blood cell transfusion in preterm infants. Pediatrics 2005;115:1685-91.

57. Kirpalani H, Whyte RK, Andersen C, et al. The premature infants in need of transfusion (PINT) study: A randomized, controlled trial of a restrictive (low) versus liberal (high) transfusion threshold for extremely low birth weight infants. J Pediatr 2006;149:301-7.

58. Whyte RK, Kirpalani H, Asztalos EV, et al. Neurodevelopmental outcome of extremely low birth weight infants randomly assigned to restrictive or liberal hemoglobin thresholds for blood transfusion. Pediatrics 2009;123:207-13.

59. McCoy TE, Conrad AL, Richman LC, et al. Neurocognitive profiles of preterm infants randomly assigned to lower or higher hematocrit thresholds for transfusion. Child Neuropsychol 2011; 17:347-67.

60. Nopoulos PC, Conrad AL, Bell EF, et al. Long-term outcome of brain structure in premature infants: Effects of liberal vs restricted red blood cell transfusions. Arch Pediatr Adolesc Med 2011;165:443-50.

61. Keir A, Pal S, Trivella M, et al. Adverse effects of red blood cell transfusions in neonates: A systematic review and meta-analysis. Transfusion 2016;56:2773-80.

62. Goobie SM, Faraoni D, Zurakowski D, et al. Association of preoperative anemia with postoperative mortality in neonates. JAMA Pediatr 2016; 170:855-62.

63. Kirpalani H, Bell E, D'Angio C, et al. Transfusion of prematures (TOP) trial: Does a liberal red blood cell transfusion strategy improve neurologically-intact survival of extremely-low-birth-weight infants as compared to a restrictive strategy? Version 1.0 (October 8, 2012). Bethesda, MD: National Institute of Child Health and Human Development, 2012. [Available at https://www.nichd.nih.gov/sites/default/files/about/Documents/TOP_Protocol.pdf.]

64. ETTNO Investigators. The 'Effects of Transfusion Thresholds on Neurocognitive Outcome of Extremely Low Birth-Weight Infants (ETTNO)' Study: Background, aims, and study protocol. Neonatology 2012;101:301-5.

65. Ballard RA, Vinocur B, Reynolds JW, et al. Transient hyperammonemia of the preterm infant. N Engl J Med 1978;299:920-5.

66. Leonard JV. The early detection and management of inborn errors presenting acutely in the neonatal period. Eur J Pediatr 1985;143:253-7.

67. American Academy of Pediatrics Subcommittee on Hyperbilirubinemia. Management of hyperbilirubinemia in the newborn infant 35 or more weeks of gestation. Pediatrics 2004;114:297-316.

68. Kliegman RM, Stanton BMD, St. Geme J, Schor NF, eds. Nelson's textbook of pediatrics. 20th ed. Philadelphia: WB Saunders, 2016.

69. Valaes T. Bilirubin distribution and dynamics of bilirubin removal by exchange transfusion. Acta Paediatr Scand 1963;52:604.

70. Wong EC, Pisciotto PT. Technical considerations/mechanical devices. In: Hillyer CD, Strauss RG, Luban NLC, eds. Handbook of pediatric transfusion medicine. London: Elsevier Academic Press, 2004:121-8.

71. Luban NL. Massive transfusion in the neonate. Transfus Med Rev 1995;9:200-14.

72. Weisz B, Belson A, Milbauer B, et al. [Complications of exchange transfusion in term and preterm newborns]. Harefuah 1996;130:170-3.

73. Bada HS, Chua C, Salmon JH, et al. Changes in intracranial pressure during exchange transfusion. J Pediatr 1979;94:129-32.

74. Maheshwari A, Carlo WA. Plethora in the newborn infant (polycythemia). In: Kliegman RM, Stanton BF, Schor NF, et al, eds. Nelson textbook of pediatrics. 20th ed. Philadelphia: Elsevier, 2015:887-8.

75. Black VD, Rumack CM, Lubchenko LD, Koops BL. Gastrointestinal injury in polycythemic infants. Pediatrics 1985;76:225-31.

76. Mohamed A, Shah PS. Transfusion associated necrotizing enterocolitis: A meta-analysis of observational data. Pediatrics 2012;129:529-40.

77. Patel RM, Knezevic A, Shenvi N, et al. Association of red blood cell transfusion, anemia, and necrotizing enterocolitis in very low-birthweight infants. JAMA 2016;315:889-97.

78. Ware RE, Helms RW, SWiTCH Investigators. Stroke with transfusions changing to hydroxyurea (SWiTCH). Blood 2012;119:3925-32.

79. Estcourt LJ, Fortin PM, Hopewell S, et al. Blood transfusion for preventing primary and secondary stroke in people with sickle cell disease. Cochrane Database Syst Rev 2017;1:003146.

80. Ware RE, Davis BR, Schultz WH, et al. Hydroxycarbamide versus chronic transfusion for maintenance of transcranial doppler flow velocities in children with sickle cell anaemia—TCD with transfusions changing to hydroxyurea (TWiTCH): A multicentre, open-label, phase 3, non-inferiority trial. Lancet 2016;387:661-70.

81. DeBaun MR, Gordon M, McKinstry RC, et al. Controlled trial of transfusions for silent cerebral infarcts in sickle cell anemia. N Engl J Med 2014;371:699-710.

82. Adams RJ, McKie VC, Hsu L, et al. Prevention of a first stroke by transfusions in children with sickle cell anemia and abnormal results on transcranial doppler ultrasonography. N Engl J Med 1998;339:5-11.

83. Kelly S, Quirolo K, Marsh A, et al. Erythrocytapheresis for chronic transfusion therapy in sickle cell disease: Survey of current practices and review of the literature. Transfusion 2016;56:2877-88.

84. Rosse WF, Gallagher D, Kinney TR, et al. Transfusion and alloimmunization in sickle cell disease: The cooperative study of sickle cell disease. Blood 1990;76:1431-7.

85. Rosse WF, Telen M, Ware RE. Transfusion support for patients with sickle cell disease. Bethesda, MD: AABB Press, 1998.

86. Vichinsky EP, Luban NL, Wright E, et al. Prospective RBC phenotype matching in a stroke-prevention trial in sickle cell anemia: A multicenter transfusion trial. Transfusion 2001;41:1086-92.

87. Yazdanbakhsh K, Ware RE, Noizat-Pirenne F. Red blood cell alloimmunization in sickle cell disease: Pathophysiology, risk factors, and transfusion management. Blood 2012;120:528-37.

88. Chou ST, Jackson T, Vege S, et al. High prevalence of red blood cell alloimmunization in sickle cell disease despite transfusion from Rh-matched minority donors. Blood 2013;122:1062-71.

89. Kacker S, Ness PM, Savage WJ, et al. Cost-effectiveness of prospective red blood cell antigen matching to prevent alloimmunization among sickle cell patients. Transfusion 2014;54:86-97.

90. Hillyer KL, Hare VW, Josephson CD, et al. Partners for life: The transfusion program for patients with sickle cell disease offered at the American Red Cross Blood Services, Southern Region, Atlanta, Georgia. Immunohematology 2006;22:108-11.

91. Yawn BP, Buchanan GR, Afenyi-Annan AN, et al. Management of sickle cell disease: Summary of the 2014 evidence-based report by expert panel members. JAMA 2014;312:1033-48.

92. Tahhan HR, Holbrook CT, Braddy LR, et al. Antigen-matched donor blood in the transfusion management of patients with sickle cell disease. Transfusion 1994;34:562-9.

93. Wood JC, Cohen AR, Pressel SL, et al. Organ iron accumulation in chronically transfused children with sickle cell anaemia: Baseline results from the TWiTCH trial. Br J Haematol 2016; 172:122-30.

94. Petz LD, Calhoun L, Shulman IA, et al. The sickle cell hemolytic transfusion reaction syndrome. Transfusion 1997;37:382-92.

95. Win N, Doughty H, Telfer P, et al. Hyperhemolytic transfusion reaction in sickle cell disease. Transfusion 2001;41:323-8.

96. Wong TE, Brandow AM, Lim W, et al. Update on the use of hydroxyurea therapy in sickle cell disease. Blood 2014;124:3850-7.

97. Arnold SD, Bhatia M, Horan J, et al. Haematopoietic stem cell transplantation for sickle cell disease—Current practice and new approaches. Br J Haematol 2016;174:515-25.

98. Olivieri NF, Brittenham GM. Iron-chelating therapy and the treatment of thalassemia. Blood 1997;89:739-61.

99. Dhawan HK, Kumawat V, Marwaha N, et al. Alloimmunization and autoimmunization in transfusion dependent thalassemia major patients: Study on 319 patients. Asian J Transfus Sci 2014;8:84-8.

100. Romphruk AV, Simtong P, Butryojantho C, et al. The prevalence, alloimmunization risk factors, antigenic exposure, and evaluation of antigen-matched red blood cells for thalassemia transfusions: A 10-year experience at a tertiary care hospital. Transfusion 2019;59:177-84.

101. Davoudi-Kiakalayeh A, Mohammadi R, Pourfathollah AA, et al. Alloimmunization in thalassemia patients: New insight for healthcare. Int J Prev Med 2017;8:101.

102. Vichinsky E, Neumayr L, Trimble S, et al. Transfusion complications in thalassemia patients: A report from the Centers for Disease Control and Prevention. Transfusion 2014;54:972-81.

103. Pujani M, Pahuja S, Dhingra B, et al. Alloimmunisation in thalassaemics: A comparison between recipients of usual matched and partial better matched blood. An evaluation at a tertiary care centre in India. Blood Transfus 2014; 12(Suppl 1):s100-4.

104. Michail-Merianou V, Pamphili-Panousopoulou L, Piperi-Lowes L, et al. Alloimmunization to red cell antigens in thalassemia: Comparative study of usual versus better-match transfusion programmes. Vox Sang 1987;52:95-8.

105. Compernolle V, Chou ST, Tanael S, et al. Red blood cell specifications for patients with hemoglobinopathies: A systematic review and guideline. Transfusion 2018;58:1555-66.

106. Dhabangi A, Ainomugisha B, Cserti-Gazdewich C, et al. Effect of transfusion of red blood cells with longer vs shorter storage duration on elevated blood lactate levels in children with severe anemia: The TOTAL randomized clinical trial. JAMA 2015;314:2514-23.

107. Age of blood in children in pediatric intensive care units (ABC PICU). St. Louis, MO: Washington University School of Medicine, 2015. [Available at https://clinicaltrials.gov/ct2/show/NCT01977547.]

108. Manno CS, Hedberg KW, Kim HC, et al. Comparison of the hemostatic effects of fresh whole blood, stored whole blood, and components after open heart surgery in children. Blood 1991; 77:930-6.

109. Mou SS, Giroir BP, Molitor-Kirsch EA, et al. Fresh whole blood versus reconstituted blood for pump priming in heart surgery in infants. N Engl J Med 2004;351:1635-44.

110. Jobes DR, Sesok-Pizzini D, Friedman D. Reduced transfusion requirement with use of fresh whole blood in pediatric cardiac surgical procedures. Ann Thorac Surg 2015;99:1706-11.

111. Thottathil P, Sesok-Pizzini D, Taylor JA, et al. Whole blood in pediatric craniofacial reconstruction surgery. J Craniofac Surg 2017;28: 1175-8.

112. Blanchette VS, Kuhne T, Hume H, et al. Platelet transfusion therapy in newborn infants. Transfus Med Rev 1995;9:215-30.

113. Castle V, Andrew M, Kelton J, et al. Frequency and mechanism of neonatal thrombocytopenia. J Pediatr 1986;108:749-55.

114. Andrew M, Vegh P, Caco C, et al. A randomized, controlled trial of platelet transfusions in thrombocytopenic premature infants. J Pediatr 1993;123:285-91.

115. Honohan A, van't Ende E, Hulzebos C, et al. Posttransfusion platelet increments after different platelet products in neonates: A retrospective cohort study. Transfusion 2013;53:3100-9.

116. New HV, Stanworth SJ, Engelfriet CP, et al. Neonatal transfusions. Vox Sang 2009;96:62-85.

117. Poterjoy BS, Josephson CD. Platelets, frozen plasma, and cryoprecipitate: What is the clinical evidence for their use in the neonatal intensive care unit? Semin Perinatol 2009;33:66-74.

118. von Lindern JS, van den Bruele T, Lopriore E, et al. Thrombocytopenia in neonates and the risk of intraventricular hemorrhage: A retrospective cohort study. BMC Pediatrics 2011;11:16.

119. Josephson CD, Su LL, Christensen RD, et al. Platelet transfusion practices among neonatologists in the United States and Canada: Results of a survey. Pediatrics 2009;123:278-85.

120. Curley A, Stanworth SJ, Willoughby K, et al. Randomized Trial of Platelet-Transfusion Thresholds in Neonates. N Engl J Med 2019; 380(3):242-51.

121. Slichter SJ, Kaufman RM, Assmann SF, et al. Dose of prophylactic platelet transfusions and prevention of hemorrhage. N Engl J Med 2010; 362:600-13.

122. Josephson CD, Granger S, Assmann SF, et al. Bleeding risks are higher in children versus adults given prophylactic platelet transfusions for treatment-induced hypoproliferative thrombocytopenia. Blood 2012;120:748-60.

123. Honohan A, Tomson B, van der Bom J, et al. A comparison of volume-reduced versus standard HLA/HPA-matched apheresis platelets in allo-immunized adult patients. Transfusion 2012;52: 742-51.

124. Pisciotto PT, Snyder EL, Snyder JA, et al. In-vitro characteristics of white cell-reduced single-unit platelet concentrates stored in syringes. Transfusion 1994;34:407-11.

125. Diab Y, Wong E, Criss VR, et al. Storage of aliquots of apheresis platelets for neonatal use in syringes with and without agitation. Transfusion 2011;51:2642-6.

126. Motta M, Del Vecchio A, Radicioni M. Clinical use of fresh-frozen plasma and cryoprecipitate in neonatal intensive care unit. J Matern Fetal Neonatal Med 2011;24:129-31.

127. Camazine MN, Karam O, Colvin R, et al. Outcomes related to the use of frozen plasma or pooled solvent/detergent treated plasma in critically ill children. Pediatr Crit Care Med 2017; 18:e215-23.

128. Karam O, Lacroix J, Robitaille N, et al. Association between plasma transfusions and clinical outcome in critically ill children: A prospective observational study. Vox Sang 2013;104:342-9.

129. AABB, America's Blood Centers, American Red Cross, Armed Services Blood Program. Circular of information for the use of human blood and blood components. Bethesda, MD: AABB, 2017.

130. Cushing M, Bandarenko N, eds. Blood transfusion therapy: A handbook. 13th ed. Bethesda, MD: AABB, 2020 (in press).

131. Wong ECC, Roseff SD, Bandarenko N, eds. Pediatric transfusion: A handbook. 5th ed. Bethesda, MD: AABB, 2020 (in press).

132. Price TH, Boeckh M, Harrison RW, et al. Efficacy of transfusion with granulocytes from G-CSF/dexamethasone-treated donors in neutropenic patients with infection. Blood 2015; 126:2153-61.

133. Marfin AA, Price TH. Granulocyte transfusion therapy. J Intensive Care Med 2015;30:79-88.

134. Ballabh P. Intraventricular hemorrhage in premature infants: Mechanism of disease. Pediatr Res 2010;67(1):1-8.

135. Wang-Rodriguez J, Mannino FL, Liu E, et al. A novel strategy to limit blood donor exposure and blood waste in multiply transfused premature infants. Transfusion 1996;36:64-70.

136. Liu EA, Mannino FL, Lane TA. Prospective, randomized trial of the safety and efficacy of a limited donor exposure transfusion program for premature neonates. J Pediatr 1994;125:92-6.

137. Bednarek FJ, Weisberger S, Richardson DK, et al. Variations in blood transfusions among newborn intensive care units. SNAP II study group. J Pediatr 1998;133:601-7.

138. Maier RF, Sonntag J, Walka MM, et al. Changing practices of red blood cell transfusions in infants with birth weights less than 1000 g. J Pediatr 2000;136:220-4.

139. Levy GJ, Strauss RG, Hume H, et al. National survey of neonatal transfusion practices: I. Red blood cell therapy. Pediatrics 1993;91:523-9.

140. Goodstein MH, Herman JH, Smith JF, et al. Metabolic consequences in very low birth weight infants transfused with older AS-1 preserved erythrocytes. Pediatr Pathol Lab Med 1999;18: 173-85.

141. Friedman DF, Montenegro LM. Extracorporeal membrane oxygenation and cardiopulmonary bypass. In: Hillyer CD, Strauss RG, Luban NLC, eds. Handbook of pediatric transfusion medicine. London: Elsevier Academic Press, 2004: 181-9.

142. Wong TE, Huang YS, Weiser J, et al. Antithrombin concentrate use in children: A multicenter cohort study. J Pediatr 2013;163:1329-34.

143. Stansfield BK, Wise L, Ham PB 3rd, et al. Outcomes following routine antithrombin III replacement during neonatal extracorporeal membrane oxygenation. J Pediatr Surg 2017;52:609-13.

144. Wong TE, Nguyen T, Shah SS, et al. Antithrombin concentrate use in pediatric extracorporeal membrane oxygenation: A multicenter cohort study. Pediatr Crit Care Med 2016;17:1170-8.

145. Eghtesady P, Almond CS, Tjossem C, et al; Berlin Heart Investigators. Post-transplant out-

comes of children bridged to transplant with the Berlin Heart EXCOR Pediatric ventricular assist device. Circulation 2013;128(11 Suppl 1):S24-31.

146. Massicotte MP, Bauman ME, Murray J, Almond CS. Antithrombotic therapy for ventricular assist devices in children: Do we really know what to do? J Thromb Haemost 2015;13(Suppl 1):S343-50.

147. Horst J, Leonard JC, Vogel A, et al. A survey of US and Canadian hospitals' paediatric massive transfusion protocol policies. Transfus Med 2016;26:49-56.

148. Hendrickson JE, Shaz BH, Pereira G, et al. Implementation of a pediatric trauma massive transfusion protocol: One institution's experience. Transfusion 2012;52:1228-36.

149. Nosanov L, Inaba K, Okoye O, et al. The impact of blood product ratios in massively transfused pediatric trauma patients. Am J Surg 2013;206:655-60.

150. Hwu RS, Spinella PC, Keller MS, et al. The effect of massive transfusion protocol implementation on pediatric trauma care. Transfusion 2016;56:2712-19.

151. Chidester SJ, Williams N, Wang W, et al. A pediatric massive transfusion protocol. J Trauma Acute Care Surg 2012;73:1273-7.

152. Dehmer JJ, Adamson WT. Massive transfusion and blood product use in the pediatric trauma patient. Semin Pediatr Surg 2010;19:286-91.

153. Holcomb JB, Tilley BC, Baraniuk S, et al. Transfusion of plasma, platelets, and red blood cells in a 1:1:1 vs a 1:1:2 ratio and mortality in patients with severe trauma: The PROPPR randomized clinical trial. JAMA 2015;313:471-82.

154. The CRASH-2 collaborators. The importance of early treatment with tranexamic acid in bleeding trauma patients: An exploratory analysis of the CRASH-2 randomised controlled trial. Lancet 2011;377(9771):1096-101, 1101.e1-2.

155. Oakley FD, Woods M, Arnold S, Young PP. Transfusion reactions in pediatric compared with adult patients: A look at rate, reaction type, and associated products. Transfusion 2015;55:563-70.

156. Bolton-Maggs PHB, ed, et al on behalf of the Serious Hazards of Transfusion (SHOT) Steering Group. The 2017 annual SHOT report. Manchester, UK: SHOT Office, 2018. [Available at https://www.shotuk.org/shot-reports/ (accessed December 5, 2019).]

157. Bowden RA, Slichter SJ, Sayers M, et al. A comparison of filtered leukocyte-reduced and cyto-megalovirus (CMV) seronegative blood products for the prevention of transfusion-associated CMV infection after marrow transplant. Blood 1995;86:3598-603.

158. Josephson CD, Caliendo AM, Easley KA, et al. Blood transfusion and breast milk transmission of cytomegalovirus in very low-birth-weight infants: A prospective cohort study. JAMA Pediatr 2014;168:1054-62.

159. Brady MT, Milam JD, Anderson DC, et al. Use of deglycerolized red blood cells to prevent post-transfusion infection with cytomegalovirus in neonates. J Infect Dis 1984;150:334-9.

160. Heddle NM, Boeckh M, Grossman B, et al for the Clinical Transfusion Medicine Committee. AABB committee report: Reducing transfusion-transmitted cytomegalovirus infections. Transfusion 2016;56:1581-7.

161. Trial to Reduce Alloimmunization to Platelets study group. Leukocyte reduction and ultraviolet B irradiation of platelets to prevent alloimmunization and refractoriness to platelet transfusions. N Engl J Med 1997;337:1861-9.

162. Sanders MR, Graeber JE. Posttransfusion graft-versus-host disease in infancy. J Pediatr 1990;117:159-63.

163. Rühl H, Bein G, Sachs UJH. Transfusion-associated graft-versus-host disease. Transfus Med Rev 2009;23:62-71.

164. Strauss RG, Levy GJ, Sotelo-Avila C, et al. National survey of neonatal transfusion practices: II. Blood component therapy. Pediatrics 1993;91(3):530-6.

165. Moroff G, Friedman A, Robkin-Kline L, et al. Reduction of the volume of stored platelet concentrates for use in neonatal patients. Transfusion 1984;24:144-6.

166. Schoenfeld H, Muhm M, Doepfmer UR, et al. The functional integrity of platelets in volume-reduced platelet concentrates. Anesth Analg 2005;100:78-81.

167. Knutson F, Osselaer J, Pierelli L, et al. A prospective, active haemovigilance study with combined cohort analysis of 19,175 transfusions of platelet components prepared with amotosalen-UVA photochemical treatment. Vox Sang 2015;109:343-52.

168. McCullough J, Vesole DH, Benjamin RJ, et al. Therapeutic efficacy and safety of platelets treated with a photochemical process for pathogen inactivation: The SPRINT trial. Blood 2004;104:1534-41.

169. Estcourt LJ, Malouf R, Hopewell S, et al. Pathogen-reduced platelets for the prevention of

bleeding. Cochrane Database Syst Rev 2017;7: CD009072.

170. Knutson F, Osselaer J, Pierelli L, et al. A prospective, active haemovigilance study with combined cohort analysis of 19,175 transfusions of platelet components prepared with amotosalen-UVA photochemical treatment. Vox Sang 2015; 109:343-52.

171. Amato M, Schennach H, Astl M, et al. Impact of platelet pathogen inactivation on blood component utilization and patient safety in a large Austrian Regional Medical Centre. Vox Sang 2017; 112:47-55.

172. Trakhtman P, Karpova O, Balashov D, et al. Efficacy and safety of pathogen-reduced platelet concentrates in children with cancer: A retrospective cohort study. Transfusion 2016;56(Suppl 1):S24-8.

CHAPTER 25

Therapeutic Apheresis

Jennifer Webb, MD, MSCE, and Chester Andrzejewski Jr, PhD, MD

THERAPEUTIC APHERESIS (TA) IS AN extracorporeal therapy used in the treatment and management of various diseases and is accomplished either through the removal and discard of selected blood constituents or via the collection of selected blood elements and subsequent ex-vivo manipulation and return of those elements to the patient. It is related to but distinct from "preparative apheresis," in which blood components are collected from blood donors for therapeutic uses (covered in Chapter 6). Standards and guidelines for TA performance, health-care provider education, qualifications and clinical privileging, and procedural documentation have been promulgated by AABB, the American Society for Apheresis (ASFA), and the College of American Pathologists (CAP).[1-7] In 2012, the National Heart, Lung, and Blood Institute (NHLBI) sponsored a National Institutes of Health (NIH) State of the Science Symposium in Therapeutic Apheresis exploring various aspects related to TA, including scientific opportunities in TA, what challenges/barriers exist to increasing TA research, and prioritization of TA research activities.[8-10]

GENERAL PRINCIPLES

The major goals of TA are 1) to remove a pathologic cellular and/or humoral element(s) from a patient's blood; 2) to replace a deficient substance(s), typically in the context of the removal of a pathologic constituent; 3) to modulate cellular functionality (eg, via further extracorporeal manipulations and the return of those cellular elements, such as performed with the use of ultraviolet light exposure in photopheresis); and/or 4) to collect various autologous nonpathologic cellular populations for further manipulation and therapeutic uses (eg, cellular therapies involving stem cells, dendritic cells, and chimeric antigen receptor T-cell production).

The various types of apheresis procedures are listed in Table 25-1. In the most commonly performed clinical apheresis procedure, therapeutic plasma exchange (TPE), 1.0 to 1.5 plasma volumes are typically removed in a single session. A series of treatments may be necessary to achieve the desired clinical effect. Targeting of larger volumes for removal increases the risk of coagulopathy, citrate toxicity, or electrolyte

Jennifer Webb, MD, MSCE, Assistant Professor of Pediatrics, Division of Pediatric Hematology, George Washington University, School of Medicine and Health Sciences, and Director of the Therapeutic Apheresis Program, Children's National Hospital, Washington, DC; and Chester Andrzejewski Jr, PhD, MD, Medical Director, System Blood Banking/Transfusion and Apheresis Medicine Services, Baystate Health, Assistant Professor, Department of Pathology, University of Massachusetts Medical School-Baystate, Springfield, Massachusetts, and Adjunct Assistant Professor, Department of Pathology, Tufts University School of Medicine, Boston, Massachusetts

J. Webb has disclosed no conflicts of interest. C. Andrzejewski has disclosed financial relationships with Amgen and Haemonetics.

TABLE 25-1. Therapeutic Apheresis Modalities

Procedure	Blood Component Removed	Typical Indication	Replacement Fluid
Therapeutic plasma exchange	Plasma	Reduction of an abnormal plasma protein (eg, autoantibody)	Albumin, crystalloid, or plasma
Red cell exchange	Red cells	Sickle-cell-disease-related complications	Red Blood Cells
Leukocytapheresis	Buffy coat	Leukemia with leukostasis	As needed
Thrombocytapheresis	Buffy coat	Thrombocytosis	As needed
Erythrocytapheresis	Red cells	Erythrocytosis	As needed
Extracorporeal photopheresis	Buffy coat (reinfused)	Graft-vs-host disease, Cutaneous T-cell lymphoma	None
Selective adsorption	Specific plasma protein, antibody, or lipid	Hypercholesterolemia	None
Adsorptive cytapheresis	Activated monocytes or granulocytes	Inflammatory bowel disease	None
Rheopheresis	High-molecular-weight plasma proteins	Age-related macular degeneration	None
Double-filtration plasmapheresis	Pathogenic substances of a particular size or molecular weight	Atopic dermatitis	None

imbalances, depending on the replacement fluids used.[11] In plasmapheresis, used generally in the donor setting although the term is often used interchangeably with TPE, lesser volumes of plasma (≤ 1 L) are removed, resulting in little to no need for fluid replacement.

The effectiveness of apheresis in removing pathologic substances depends on the concentration of the substance in the blood, its volume of distribution into the extravascular space, the degree of protein-binding of the targeted substance, the volume of blood processed and plasma removed, and the equilibrium between the substance's blood and extravascular concentrations. Most efficient at the procedure's beginning stages, component removal decreases exponentially and asymptotically with time because of the required addition of replacement fluids needed to maintain physiologic stability in the patient. Continued production of the substance, mobilization from the extravascular

space, or recirculation at the openings of a double-lumen catheter will result in a less-than-predicted decrease. In a 1.0-plasma-volume exchange, approximately two-thirds of a targeted "idealized substance,"[12] such as immunoglobulin M (IgM) or fibrinogen, is typically removed, provided that the constituent does not diffuse significantly from the extravascular to the intravascular compartments.

DEVICE MODALITIES

Several technological platforms for performing apheresis exist. The most commonly available ones are described below.

Continuous-flow centrifugation apheresis devices have a rotating channel designed to introduce whole blood at one site. The blood elements will subsequently separate largely by density as blood flows through the channel. The resulting layers of plasma, platelets, leukocytes, and red cells can be selectively removed. The targeted constituent is diverted into a collection bag, while the remaining blood components are returned to the patient with appropriate replacement fluids. To achieve optimal separation and treatment blood volume, modern apheresis devices calculate and control blood-withdrawal flow rates, amounts of anticoagulant solution and replacement fluids needed, as well as centrifuge speed.

Intermittent-flow centrifugation devices process smaller volumes of blood in cycles, where a cycle consists of whole blood being drawn and separated, and then components are reinfused or diverted. Multiple cycles are often required to achieve the goals of treatment. The volume of whole blood drawn in a cycle is targeted to achieve a specific red cell threshold. This leads to larger extracorporeal volumes achieved than in continuous-flow devices.

Filtration-based apheresis devices also operate by continuous flow. Anticoagulated whole blood is passed through a microporous filter that allows plasma to pass through while retaining the blood cells. The separated plasma can then be diverted into a waste bag or, as with selective adsorption, further processed and returned to the patient. This type of device is not suitable for the removal of select cellular components in circulation (cytapheresis). Variants of this technique are rheopheresis or double-filtration plasmapheresis (DFPP), which further processes the separated plasma through a secondary filter that removes high-molecular-weight molecules, thereby reducing plasma viscosity, or targets a specific component. Secondary filters of different pore sizes remove different pathogenic substances, such as immune complexes, autoantibodies, or lipoproteins.

In selective adsorption, blood or plasma is passed over a column or matrix that has a high affinity for a specific component, such as immunoglobulin G (IgG) in immunoadsorption (IA) or lipoproteins in lipoprotein apheresis (LA). The effluent is returned to the patient after being reunited with cellular components. This approach has the advantage of highly specific removal of the target of interest. However, it is restricted to the few conditions for which affinity adsorbents are available. In adsorptive cytapheresis, also known as granulocyte-monocyte apheresis (GMA), monocytes and granulocytes are selectively removed from whole blood through adhesion or filtration. Inactivated leukocytes and the remaining blood components are returned to the patient. This technique has been used to treat autoimmune, inflammatory conditions such as ulcerative colitis and psoriasis.

PATIENT EVALUATION AND MANAGEMENT

All patients should be evaluated by a physician familiar with apheresis before beginning any course of TA. General considerations in formulating an overall therapy plan are identified in Table 25-2. A more comprehensive evaluation of the patient is typically performed in this setting, with the clinical evaluation focusing on select elements at subsequent TPE encounters in stable patients receiving an extended series of treatments, unless changes in the patient's clinical status dictate otherwise.

The indication, type of procedure, choice of replacement fluid (Table 25-3), vascular access, frequency and number of treatments, and the treatment goal or endpoint should be documented in the patient's record. During the initial evaluation, the nature of the procedure and its expected benefits, possible risks, and available alternatives must be explained to the patient, and informed consent must be documented. Depending on institution-specific policies, these informed consent discussions should be repeated periodically (eg, annually) and documented in the medical record. Procedures should be performed only in settings where there is ready access to care for untoward reactions, including equipment, medications, and personnel trained in managing serious adverse events, such as anaphylaxis, metabolic alkalosis, air embolus, and hypotensive reactions. Comorbidities that may affect the patient's ability to tolerate apheresis and concurrent medication reconciliation should be noted. Other specific points to consider when evaluating a patient include the following:

TABLE 25-2. Elements* in a Comprehensive Evaluation and Treatment Plan for Patients Being Considered for TA Interventions

Clinical diagnosis and differential diagnosis / chief complaint / clinical objective / reason for referral
History of the pertinent present illness
Patient's past / family medical histories, including prior TA and hemotherapies (eg, blood transfusions and IVIG infusions) and history of reactions, comorbidities
Pertinent review of systems and medication reconciliation
Pertinent physical examination, including vascular access assessment
TA indication / rationale / outcome objectives
Selection of apheresis modality and equipment
Volume / duration / frequency targets / fluid balance
• Per procedure
• For entire series
Vascular access device considerations as needed
Choice of replacement fluids
• Blood prime, if required
• Specially prepared units (eg, antigen negative, phenotyped), if applicable
Physiologic / adverse reaction / clinical outcomes monitoring
Coordination of pre- / intra- / post- / and interprocedural laboratory testing, drug / blood component administration, and other procedures (eg, dialysis)
Use of ancillary equipment prn
• Blood warmers
• Fetal monitors
• Ventilatory support devices
• Separate IV access for calcium infusion
Patient educational materials and discharge instructions
Need for initial series extension / concurrent immunosuppressive therapies
Coagulopathies / anticoagulation medication when relevant

*Identified elements are typically considered in the clinical evaluation at the time of the initial consultation of all patients being assessed for TA. In stable individuals undergoing an extended series of TA, apheresis medicine specialists may elect to exclude select aspects from the patient's evaluation at each subsequent apheresis session (if such elements were obtained at time of initial consultation) unless changes in the clinical status of the patient warrant otherwise.
TA = therapeutic apheresis; IVIG = intravenous immune globulin; prn = as needed.

• **Transfusion/apheresis history:** Notation of prior transfusion/apheresis interventions and reactions, outcomes from such therapies, and special blood component requirements.

• **Neurologic status:** Mental status and the ability to consent and cooperate.

• **Cardiorespiratory status:** Adequate ventilation and oxygenation capabilities, presence

TABLE 25-3. Comparison of Replacement Fluids

Replacement Solution	Advantages	Disadvantages
Crystalloids	Low cost Nonallergenic No viral risk	Two- to threefold more volume required Hypo-oncotic Lacking coagulation factors and immunoglobulins
Albumin	Iso-oncotic Low risk of reactions	Higher cost Lacking coagulation factors and immunoglobulins
Plasma	Iso-oncotic Normal levels of coagulation factors, immunoglobulins, and other plasma proteins	Viral transmission risk Increased citrate load ABO compatibility required Higher risk of allergic reactions
Cryoprecipitate-poor plasma	Iso-oncotic Reduced high-molecular-weight von Willebrand factor and fibrinogen Normal levels of most other plasma proteins	Same as plasma

of hyper- or hypovolemia, and any cardiac arrhythmias.

- **Renal and metabolic status:** Fluid balance, alkalosis, and electrolyte abnormalities, including hypocalcemia, hypokalemia, and hypomagnesemia.
- **Hematologic status:** Presence of clinically significant anemia, thrombocytopenia, coagulopathy, bleeding, or thrombosis.
- **Medications:** Recently administered intravenous immunoglobulin (IVIG) and antibody biologics, angiotensin-converting enzyme (ACE) inhibitors, drugs with high albumin-binding properties, and anticoagulants.

Appropriate laboratory monitoring is guided by the TA indication, type and frequency of procedures, duration of therapeutic course, and concomitant medical conditions. In general, it is wise to obtain test results, including a complete blood cell count, blood type and antibody detection test (antibody screen), coagulation profile, and electrolytes, before starting treatment. Other diagnostic study results, such as tests for infectious diseases and pertinent specific disease markers, should be collected before the first treatment. Coagulation monitoring may be appropriate when albumin is used as the primary replacement fluid during frequently repeated procedures. The collection of an "archive specimen" before the initial apheresis session should also be considered, because concentrations of plasma constituents are altered by TA. Similarly, apheresis medicine practitioners should make colleagues and patients aware that diagnostic testing after apheresis can be differentially affected depending on the analyte of interest, the replacement fluids used, and the frequency of TPE sessions.

VASCULAR ACCESS

TA requires excellent vascular access to achieve adequate flow rates.[13] Peripheral access is preferred and generally requires at least a 17-gauge needle for blood withdrawal and at least an 18-gauge catheter for return. Patients without adequate peripheral veins, those who require multiple frequent procedures, and those unable to provide hand compressions to maintain vascular flow may require placement of central venous catheters (CVCs). CVCs for apheresis must have rigid walls to accommodate the negative pressure generated in the withdrawal line. Dual-lumen catheters similar to the types used in hemodialysis are preferred, although single-lumen catheters can be used for intermittent-flow procedures. For a short series of procedures, a nontunneled catheter may be adequate; however, for long-term access, tunneled and cuffed CVCs allow for stable, safe, durable points of apheresis access.[14,15] Compared to nontunneled catheters, tunneled CVCs have lower rates of infection and may be suitable for outpatient procedures over months to years.

Peripherally inserted central catheters (ie, PICC lines) typically do not support the high flow rates used in adult apheresis; however, for single points of access or pediatric patients who typically use slower flow rates, PICC lines have been successfully used as an alternative CVC option. One device that has been successfully used in pediatric patients receiving extracorporeal photopheresis (ECP) is the 5-fr, single-lumen, Turbo-flo (Cook Medical) PICC.[16] It offers a single point of access of moderate duration (6-12 months). Like other dual-lumen CVCs, there is no needlestick when connecting to the apheresis equipment because the hub is external; however, there are additional home-care needs with a PICC line, as many require daily flushing and frequent cap changes.

Implanted subcutaneous ports, also known as totally implantable venous access devices (TIVADs), may provide an option for some patients requiring long-term treatment, such as chronic red cell exchange for complications of sickle cell anemia. Procedures using double-lumen ports tend to be longer, often last for years, and can provide stable access with few lifestyle limitations; however, they have more procedural complications than procedures using other CVCs.[17] An arteriovenous (AV) fistula may also be used for apheresis, but personnel should be suitably trained before attempting to access an AV fistula. AV fistulas increase demand on cardiac output and should therefore be performed only in selected patients with sufficient cardiovascular reserve.[18,19]

The choice of placement site for a CVC is influenced by the anticipated duration of treatment. Subclavian or internal jugular access is generally preferable for TPE courses lasting up to several weeks. Femoral vein access should be used only temporarily because of the higher risk of infection. Patients requiring extended treatment courses usually have tunneled CVC placement. With proper care, tunneled catheters can be used for prolonged periods. Confirmation of CVC placement, usually performed radiographically, should be obtained before initiation of the first apheresis session and whenever a CVC replacement occurs.

Good catheter care is very important for patient safety and to maintain CVC patency. Responsibility for CVC maintenance needs to be clearly defined, and apheresis medicine services need to be actively involved in either directly providing this care or in its coordination with other parties involved in treating the patient. Catheters need to be flushed regularly. Heparin (10-1000 U/mL) or 4% trisodium citrate is usually placed in each lumen after each use to prevent occlusion by clots. If a port becomes clotted, instillation of a fibrinolytic agent, such as urokinase or recombinant tissue plasminogen activator, may restore patency. Routine dressing care is essential to prevent insertion-site infections.

Venous access devices may cause thrombosis. Infrequently, their placement may result in severe complications, such as pneumothorax, arrhythmia, or perforation of the heart or great vessels, occurring with up to 1% of procedures.[20] Other complications such as arterial puncture, deep hematomas, and AV formation are more frequent, occurring with 1% to 3% of procedures.[21] Bacterial colonization may lead to catheter-associated bloodstream infection, especially in immunosuppressed patients. Inadvertent disconnection of catheters may produce hemorrhage or an air embolism.

ANTICOAGULATION

Acid-citrate-dextrose solution A (ACD-A) is the most commonly used anticoagulant, although heparin combined with ACD-A is also used, particularly in the setting of large-volume leukocytapheresis for hematopoietic progenitor cell or mononuclear cell collection in small patients who may not be able to metabolize large volumes of citrate.[22,23] Heparin anticoagulation is necessary for LA and may be desirable for selected patients undergoing TPE who are particularly susceptible to hypocalcemia, such as small children, or in the setting of severe metabolic alkalosis, liver failure, or renal failure. Heparin is also the standard anticoagulant for ECP. With citrate anticoagulation, coagulation monitoring is generally not necessary, although knowledge and monitoring of ionized calcium levels may be helpful in selected patients. In patients with normal hepatic function, the infused citrate is rapidly metabolized and rarely causes systemic anticoagulation.

ADVERSE EFFECTS

Although TA is very safe, complications do occur; adverse events, mostly mild, occur in approximately 4% to 6% of procedures (Table 25-4).[24-27] Other than adverse events related to vascular access, symptomatic hypocalcemia due to citrate anticoagulation is the most common adverse effect, typically characterized by perioral and digital paresthesiae. Nausea or other gastrointestinal symptoms may also occur, although tetany is rare. Cardiac arrhythmia is very rare, but patients with preexisting hypocalcemia or significant prolongation of the QT interval should be monitored carefully. Calcium supplementation may alleviate symptoms of citrate toxicity; a typical dose is 1 g of calcium gluconate per liter of albumin infused. Citrate also chelates ionized magnesium, so it is possible that hypomagnesemia contributes to the symptoms of citrate toxicity; however, one randomized clinical trial showed no benefit of adding magnesium during leukocytapheresis with con-

TABLE 25-4. Reported Frequency of Adverse Reactions to Apheresis*

Reaction	Frequency (%)
Paresthesia	1.95
Access/device	1.56
Hypotension	0.77
Urticaria	0.63
Nausea/vomiting	0.23
Shivering	0.11
Flushing	0.09
Arrhythmia	0.03
Anaphylaxis	0.022
Vertigo	0.01
Abdominal pain	0.008
Other (includes seizures, back pain, hypertension, etc)	0.39
Total	5.8

*Adapted from Mörtzell-Henriksson et al.[27]

tinuous intravenous (IV) calcium supplementation.[28] Metabolism of citrate to bicarbonate leads to a mild metabolic alkalosis, which can exacerbate hypocalcemia and may cause hypokalemia.[29]

Allergic reactions are most common with plasma replacement, although they may also occur with albumin.[30] Most reactions are mild, characterized by urticaria or cutaneous flushing. Severe allergic reactions can involve the respiratory tract with dyspnea, wheezing, and (rarely) stridor. Most allergic reactions respond quickly to IV diphenhydramine. Anaphylaxis is very rare but can occur. Patients receiving large volumes of plasma, such as those with thrombotic thrombocytopenic purpura (TTP), may be most at risk for allergic reactions.[31] Premedication with an antihistamine, or possibly steroids, is not necessary for routine apheresis but may be indicated for patients with repeated or previous severe reactions.   Solvent/detergent-treated, pooled donor plasma has also been used as replacement fluid successfully in patients with a history of severe allergic reactions to conventional plasma, though experience is limited.[32,33]

Respiratory difficulty during or immediately following apheresis can have many causes, such as pulmonary edema, pulmonary embolism, air embolism, or leukostasis. If using plasma as the replacement fluid, transfusion reactions such as transfusion-related acute lung injury (TRALI), anaphylaxis, or transfusion-associated circulatory overload (TACO) are possible.[34] Hemothorax or hemopericardium resulting from vascular erosion from a CVC is rare but may be fatal.[35] Pulmonary edema due to volume overload or cardiac failure is usually associated with dyspnea, an increase in diastolic blood pressure, and characteristic chest radiograph findings. Predominantly ocular reactions (periorbital edema, conjunctival swelling, and tearing) have occurred in individuals sensitized to the ethylene-oxide gas used to sterilize disposable plastic apheresis kits.[36,37]

Hypotension during apheresis can be a sign of citrate toxicity, hypovolemia, or a vasovagal, allergic, drug, or transfusion reaction. Hypovolemia can occur early in treatments of small patients when the return fluid consists of the saline used to prime the apheresis circuit. Vasovagal reactions are characterized by bradycardia and hypotension. Such reactions usually respond well to a fluid bolus and placing the patient in the Trendelenburg position.

When hypotension occurs during plasma or red cell exchanges, potential transfusion reactions such as acute hemolysis, bacterial contamination, or anaphylaxis should be considered. Hypotension is more frequent in children, the elderly, neurology patients, anemic patients, and those treated with intermittent-flow devices that have large extracorporeal volumes. Continuous-flow devices typically do not have large extracorporeal volumes but can produce hypovolemia if return flow is inadvertently diverted to a waste collection bag, either through operator oversight or device malfunction. Hypovolemia may also be secondary to inadequate volume or protein replacement. During all procedures, it is essential to carefully document and maintain records of the volumes processed, removed, and returned.

When plasma is exposed to foreign surfaces such as plastic tubing or filtration devices, the kinin system can be activated, resulting in production of bradykinin. Infusion of plasma containing bradykinin can cause abrupt hypotension. Patients taking ACE inhibitors are more susceptible to these hypotensive reactions because these drugs block the enzymatic degradation of bradykinin.[38] Hypotensive reactions are more likely during selective adsorption procedures because these devices expose plasma to a very large surface area. Holding ACE inhibitors for 24 to 48 hours ahead of procedures or transitioning the patient to an angiotensin-receptor blocker may decrease the frequency of reaction; however, because some ACE inhibitors have a long duration of action, medications should be reviewed to ensure they are stopped with enough time to avoid unnecessary adverse reactions.[39]

Intensive TPE without plasma replacement depletes coagulation factors. A 1.0-plasma-volume exchange typically reduces coagulation factor levels by 25% to 50%, although most factor levels recover quickly[40]; levels of fibrinogen, a large intravascular molecule, are reduced by ~66%. If the patient has normal hepatic synthetic function, coagulation factor levels typically return to near normal within 1 to 2 days.[41] Thus, many patients can tolerate TPE every other day for 1 to 2 weeks without developing significant coagulopathies requiring plasma replacement.

Bleeding due to coagulation factor depletion is rare. For patients at risk, plasma may be used for replacement at the end of the procedure. Apheresis can also cause thrombocytopenia. Intensive TPE can cause hypogammaglobulinemia, which may affect the accuracy of subsequent serologic testing. Serum levels of IgG and IgM recover to 40% to 50% of the preapheresis level by 48 hours.[40] In addition, IVIG or subcutaneous IgG is often used to treat conditions that respond to TPE and is often administered following completion of a series of TPE procedures. The absolute immunoglobulin level at which a patient becomes at risk for infection has not been established.

Albumin-bound drugs are removed by TPE. This can produce subtherapeutic levels of medications unless dosages are adjusted. Biologic therapeutics, such as IVIG, antithymocyte globulin, and monoclonal antibodies, have a long intravascular half-life and are readily removed by apheresis. Drugs should be administered following a TPE procedure to avoid impairing their effectiveness.

Collapsed or kinked tubing, malfunctioning pinch valves, or improper threading of tubing may damage red cells in the extracorporeal circuit. Instrument-related hemolysis occurs in 0.06% of TA procedures.[25] Hemolysis can also occur with the use of hypotonic replacement fluids or ABO-incompatible plasma. The operator should carefully observe plasma collection lines for pink discoloration suggestive of hemolysis. Other types of equipment failure, such as problems with the rotating seal, leaks in plasticware, and roller pump failure, are rare.

Fatalities during apheresis are rare and are reportable to the Food and Drug Administration (FDA).[42] Venous thromboembolism (VTE), including pulmonary emboli (PE), shortly after or during ECP has been reported to the FDA, and an investigation is ongoing.[43] Historically, death has been reported in 0.006% to 0.09% of therapeutic procedures, with most fatalities attributable to underlying medical conditions.[25,44,45]

PEDIATRIC APHERESIS

Although apheresis is safe and generally well tolerated in pediatric patients, special attention should be paid to this population. Given the relatively small total blood volumes (TBVs) of children, priming of the machine with blood or albumin may be necessary to avoid excessive, unsafe extracorporeal volume. In addition, pediatric patients may be sensitive to rapid fluid shifts, so significantly slower flow rates are used. Vascular access devices are often necessary due to inadequate peripheral access or inability to tolerate the duration of the procedure peripherally because of the requirement to stay still. Because of the slow flow rates, devices and configurations may differ from CVC use in adults, although generally they must be apheresis or hemodialysis capable. Often, empiric calcium and/or magnesium supplementation is used to avoid toxicity from citrate anticoagulation.[46,47]

Few randomized studies have been performed in pediatric patients receiving therapeutic apheresis, and much of the evidence is extrapolated from adult data, single-center experiences, anecdotal reports, or expert opinion, thus highlighting the need for future research in this field.[48]

THERAPEUTIC APHERESIS INDICATIONS

Although there are many case reports of successful treatment of various diseases and conditions by apheresis, there are few high-quality, prospective, clinical trials. ASFA has published evidence-based clinical guidelines categorizing treatment indications.[5] The classifications used in the guidelines are defined as follows:

- **Category I:** Disorders for which apheresis is accepted as first-line therapy, either as a primary stand-alone treatment or in conjunction with other modes of treatment.
- **Category II:** Disorders for which apheresis is accepted as second-line therapy, either as a stand-alone treatment or in conjunction with other modes of treatment.
- **Category III:** Disorders in which the optimal role of apheresis therapy is not established. Decision-making for patients should be individualized.
- **Category IV:** Disorders in which published evidence demonstrates or suggests that apheresis is ineffective or harmful. Institutional review board approval is desirable if apheresis treatment is undertaken in these circumstances.

Fuller discussions of the conditions treated with TA may be found by consulting more comprehensive medical texts on the respective disorders. An overview of some of the more commonly encountered diseases treated by TA is provided below.

Therapeutic Plasma Exchange

In both alloimmune and autoimmune disorders, pathogenic factors that are circulating in the blood are targets for removal by TPE. Autoantibody-mediated diseases include acute and chronic inflammatory demyelinating polyradiculoneuropathies (AIDP and CIDP), antiglomerular basement membrane disease, and myasthenia gravis. Examples of conditions where the goal is to remove problematic alloantibodies include renal transplantation with presensitization and antibody-mediated organ transplant rejection. Diseases in which immune complexes may be pathogenic and can be removed by apheresis include rapidly progressive glomerulonephritis, cryoglobulinemia, and vasculitis. Other indications include conditions treated by removing protein-bound drugs, toxins, or high concentrations of lipoproteins. In addition, there is emerging evidence on the immunomodulatory effects of TPE, which may be partially responsible for the clinical effects seen in autoimmune disorders.[11] Indications for TPE are listed in Table 25-5.

In TTP, an absolute or functional deficiency of the von Willebrand factor (vWF)-cleaving metalloprotease ADAMTS13 results in the accumulation of high-molecular-weight vWF multimers, with subsequent intravascular platelet activation and platelet-rich thrombi formation in the microvasculature.[49] In many cases, an inhibitor of ADAMTS13 can be demonstrated. TPE is first-line treatment for TTP, with the goal of removing both the inhibitor and large vWF multimers while simultaneously replacing the deficient enzyme through replacement with Fresh Frozen Plasma (FFP). Early identification and treatment of patients with severe ADAMTS13 deficiency is critical in this illness, which has a 90% mortality rate when left untreated. Early initiation of TPE reduces mortality to <15%.[50] The PLASMIC score, a validated tool based on readily available clinical parameters, has been shown to discriminate between TTP and other thrombotic microangiopathies with high sensitivity and reliability, and may serve as a useful tool in clinical practice.[51-54] TPE is typically performed daily until the platelet count and lactate dehydrogenase level normalize, often with the former being >150,000/μL for 48 hours, but treatment duration should be guided by the individual patient's course. After response has been achieved, intermittent apheresis or plasma infusion tapers may be instituted, but the efficacy of these approaches in preventing relapse has

not been established.[55] TPE results in greatly improved survival in TTP patients; however, treatment failures do occur.[56,57] The use of cryoprecipitate-poor plasma, which is deficient in vWF, for replacement fluid has not been shown to improve clinical response or outcomes,[58] although it is often tried in refractory TTP cases. Adjunctive therapies including rituximab and immunosuppression are often used to augment treatment and prevent relapse. In a Phase III trial, caplacizumab, an anti-vWF immunoglobulin fragment (nanobody) in conjunction with TPE increased the rate of recovery, decreased recurrence rates, and decreased mortality in patients with acquired TTP when compared to placebo, leading to its approval by the FDA.[59]

Hemolytic uremic syndrome (HUS), also called infection-associated thrombotic microangiopathy (TMA), is a similar condition that occurs more commonly in children than in adults and is often confused for TTP. HUS may follow diarrheal infections with verotoxin-secreting strains of *Escherichia coli* (strain 0157:H7) or *Shigella*. Compared to patients with classic TTP, those with HUS have more renal dysfunction and less prominent neurologic and hematologic findings. Although diarrhea-associated HUS rarely responds to TPE, atypical HUS (aHUS) may respond (also called complement-mediated TMA, caused by complement factor deficiencies or autoantibodies to Factor H); however, patients with aHUS caused by membrane cofactor protein (MCP or CD46) mutations may not respond to TPE. Eculizumab, a monoclonal antibody directed against C5a, thereby inhibiting terminal complement activation, has been shown to be effective in treating individuals with aHUS.[60] Treatment with eculizumab has been shown to prevent progression to renal transplantation and dialysis dependence in patients with aHUS and is the preferred therapy instead of prolonged TPE without signs of renal recovery.[61,62]

Secondary forms of microangiopathic hemolytic anemia (MAHA), associated with systemic lupus erythematosus, cancer, hematopoietic progenitor/stem cell transplantation, chemotherapy, or immunosuppressive medications, may be clinically indistinguishable from classical TTP. In many of these cases, however, ADAMTS13

TABLE 25-5. Indications for Therapeutic Plasma Exchange[5]

Indication	Modifying Conditions	Category	Typical Course (number of treatments)
Acute disseminated encephalomyelitis	Steroid refractory	II	QOD (3-6)
Acute inflammatory demyelinating polyradiculoneuropathy (Guillain-Barré syndrome)	Primary treatment	I	QOD (5-6)
Acute liver failure	High-volume TPE	I	QD (3)
	Routine TPE	III	QD (variable)
Amyloidosis, systemic		IV	
Antiglomerular basement membrane disease (Goodpasture syndrome)	DAH	I	QD or QOD (variable)
	Dialysis independence	I	
	Dialysis dependence, no DAH	III	
Atopic (neuro-) dermatitis (atopic eczema), recalcitrant		III	Weekly (variable)
Autoimmune hemolytic anemia, severe	Severe cold agglutinin disease	II	QD or QOD (variable)
	Severe WAIHA	III	
Burn shock resuscitation		III	1-3 within 24-36 hours
Cardiac neonatal lupus		III	3/week to monthly
Catastrophic antiphospholipid syndrome		I	QD or QOD (variable)
Chronic focal encephalitis (Rasmussen encephalitis)		III	QOD (3-6)
Chronic inflammatory demyelinating polyradiculoneuropathy		I	2-3/week
Coagulation factor inhibitors		III	QD (variable)
Complex regional pain syndrome	Chronic	III	QOD (5-7)
Cryoglobulinemia	Symptomatic/severe	II	QOD (3-8)
Dilated cardiomyopathy, idiopathic	NYHA II-IV	III	QOD (5)
Erythropoietic protoporphyria, liver disease		III	QOD (variable)
Familial hypercholesterolemia	Homozygotes/heterozygotes	II	Every 1-2 weeks

(Continued)

TABLE 25-5.   Indications for Therapeutic Plasma Exchange[5] (Continued)

Indication	Modifying Conditions	Category	Typical Course (number of treatments)
Focal segmental glomerulosclerosis	Recurrent in transplanted kidney	I	QD or QOD (variable)
	Steroid resistant in native kidney	III	
HELLP syndrome	Postpartum	III	QD (variable)
	Antepartum	IV	
Hemophagocytic lymphohistiocytosis; hemophagocytic syndrome; macrophage-activating syndrome		III	QD (variable)
Heparin-induced thrombocytopenia and thrombosis (HIT/HITT)	Before cardiopulmonary bypass	III	QD or QOD (variable)
	Thrombosis	III	
Hypertriglyceridemic pancreatitis	Severe	III	QD (1-3)
	Prevention of relapse	III	
Hyperviscosity in hypergammaglobulinemia	Symptomatic	I	QD (1-3)
	Prophylaxis for rituximab	I	QD (1-2)
Immune thrombocytopenia	Refractory	III	QOD (6)
IgA nephropathy (Berger disease)	Crescentic	III	QOD (6-9)
	Chronic progressive	III	
Lambert-Eaton myasthenic syndrome		II	QD or QOD (variable)
Multiple sclerosis	Acute attack/relapse	II	QOD (5-7)
	Chronic	III	Variable
Myasthenia gravis	Acute, short-term treatment	I	QD or QOD (variable)
	Long-term treatment	II	
Myeloma cast nephropathy		II	QOD (10-12)
Nephrogenic systemic fibrosis		III	QD or QOD (5-14)
Neuromyelitis optica spectrum disorders	Acute attack/relapse	II	QOD (5-10)
	Maintenance	III	
N-methyl-D-aspartate receptor antibody encephalitis		I	QOD (5-6)

TABLE 25-5. Indications for Therapeutic Plasma Exchange[5] (Continued)

Indication	Modifying Conditions	Category	Typical Course (number of treatments)
Overdose, envenomation, and poisoning	Mushroom poisoning	II	QD (variable)
	Envenomation	III	
	Drug overdose/poisoning	III	
Paraneoplastic neurologic syndromes		III	QD or QOD (5-6)
Paraproteinemic demyelinating neuropathies/chronic acquired demyelinating polyneuropathies	IgG/IgA/IgM	I	QOD (5-6)
	Multiple myeloma	III	
	Anti-MAG neuropathy	III	
	Multifocal motor neuropathy	IV	
Pediatric autoimmune neuropsychiatric disorders associated with streptococcal infections (PANDAS); Sydenham chorea	PANDAS exacerbation	II	QD or QOD (3-6)
	Sydenham chorea, severe	III	
Pemphigus vulgaris	Severe	III	QD or QOD (variable)
Phytanic acid storage disease (Refsum disease)		II	QD (variable)
Posttransfusion purpura		III	QD (variable)
Progressive multifocal leukoencephalopathy associated with natalizumab		III	QOD (variable)
Pruritus due to hepatobiliary diseases	Treatment resistant	III	Weekly (3) (variable)
Psoriasis	Disseminated pustular	IV	
Red cell alloimmunization	Pregnancy, GA <20 weeks	III	1-3/week
Scleroderma (systemic sclerosis)		III	1-3/week
Sepsis with multiorgan failure		III	QD (variable)
Steroid-responsive encephalopathy associated with autoimmune thyroiditis (Hashimoto encephalopathy)		II	QD or QOD (3-9)
Stiff-person syndrome		III	QOD (3-5)
Sudden sensorineural hearing loss		III	QD or QOD (1-3)
Systemic lupus erythematosus	Severe complications	II	QD or QOD (3-6)
Thrombotic microangiopathy, coagulation mediated	*THBD, DGKE* and *PLG* mutations	III	QD or QOD (variable)

(Continued)

TABLE 25-5. Indications for Therapeutic Plasma Exchange[5] (Continued)

Indication	Modifying Conditions	Category	Typical Course (number of treatments)
Thrombotic microangiopathy, complement mediated	Factor H autoantibodies	I	QD (variable)
	Complement factor gene mutations	III	
Thrombotic microangiopathy, drug associated	Ticlopidine	I	QD or QOD (variable)
	Clopidogrel	III	
	Gemcitabine/quinine	IV	
Thrombotic microangiopathy, infection associated	STEC-HUS, severe	III	QD (variable)
	pHUS	III	
Thrombotic microangiopathy, thrombotic thrombocytopenic purpura		I	QD (variable)
Thrombotic microangiopathy, transplantation associated		III	QD (variable)
Thyroid storm		II	QD or QOD (variable)
Toxic epidermal necrolysis	Refractory	III	QD or QOD (variable)
Transplantation, cardiac	Desensitization	II	QD or QOD (variable)
	Antibody-mediated rejection	III	
Transplantation, hematopoietic stem cell, ABOi	Major—HPC(M), HPC(A)	II	QD (variable)
	Major/Minor ABOi with pure red cell aplasia	III	
Transplantation, hematopoietic stem cell, HLA sensitization		III	QOD (4-5)
Transplantation, liver	Desensitization, ABOi LD	I	QD or QOD (variable)
	Desensitization, ABOi DD or antibody-mediated rejection	III	
Transplantation, lung	Antibody-mediated rejection or desensitization	III	QOD (variable)
Transplantation, renal, ABO compatible	Antibody-mediated rejection	I	QD or QOD (variable)
	Desensitization, LD	I	
	Desensitization, DD	III	
Transplantation, renal, ABO incompatible	Desensitization, LD	I	QD or QOD (variable)
	Antibody-mediated rejection	II	

TABLE 25-5. Indications for Therapeutic Plasma Exchange[5] (Continued)

Indication	Modifying Conditions	Category	Typical Course (number of treatments)
Vasculitis, ANCA associated	RPGN, Cr ≥5.7 mg/dL	I	QD or QOD (7-12)
	DAH	I	
	RPGN, Cr ≤5.7 mg/dL	III	
	EGPA	III	
Vasculitis, IgA (Henoch-Schönlein purpura)	Crescentic RPGN	III	QD or QOD (4-11)
	Severe extrarenal disease	III	
Vasculitis, other	HBV-PAN	II	QOD (9-12)
	Behçet disease	III	
	Idiopathic PAN	IV	
Voltage-gated potassium channel antibody related diseases		II	QOD (5-7)
Wilson disease	Fulminant	I	QD or QOD (variable)

QOD = every other day; TPE = therapeutic plasma exchange; QD = daily; DAH = diffuse alveolar hemorrhage; WAIHA = warm autoimmune hemolytic anemia; NYHA = New York Heart Association (class); HELLP = hemolysis, elevated liver enzymes, low platelet count (syndrome); IgA = immunoglobulin A; MAG = myelin-associated glycoprotein; GA = gestational age; THBD = thrombomodulin; DGKE = diacylglycerol kinase epsilon; PLG = plasminogen; STEC-HUS = Shiga-like toxin hemolytic uremic syndrome; pHUS = *S. pneumoniae* hemolytic uremic syndrome; LD = living donor; DD = deceased donor; ABOi = ABO incompatible; HPC(M) = hematopoietic progenitor cells collected from marrow; HPC(A) = HPCs from apheresis; ANCA = antineutrophil cytoplasmic antibodies; RPGN = rapidly progressive glomerulonephritis; EGPA = eosinophilic granulomatosis with polyangiitis; HBV = hepatitis B virus; PAN = polyarteritis nodosa; Cr = creatinine.

activity is normal or only moderately reduced, and the response to TPE is typically poor. Transplant-associated microangiopathic hemolysis responds to eculizumab, but rarely apheresis, due to the different pathophysiologic mechanism of endothelial injury and complement activation.[63,64] HELLP syndrome (hemolysis, elevated liver enzymes, low platelet count), a pregnancy-associated TMA, responds to TPE in the postpartum period, but TPE has not been as effective antenatally.[65]

In multiple myeloma, where patients may exhibit hyperviscosity-related adverse sequelae, the goal is to remove excessive amounts of the tumor-associated paraprotein (M protein). Plasma viscosity measurements may not be useful in guiding therapy in some patients because they may not correlate with symptoms. Normal plasma viscosity is 1.4 to 1.8 centipoise (cP). Because most patients are asymptomatic until plasma viscosity is >6.0 to 7.0 cP, those with mild elevations may not require treatment. In general, hyperviscosity becomes a concern when M protein concentrations reach 3 g/dL for IgM, 4 g/dL for IgG, and 6 g/dL for IgA.[66] Nonetheless, symptomatic patients, regardless of plasma viscosity levels, especially those with visual and neurologic symptoms, are candidates for urgent apheresis treatments.

Conflicting data exist regarding the efficacy of TPE for treating acute renal failure in myeloma. A randomized controlled trial of TPE vs conventional care showed no difference in mortality or renal function at 6 months[67]; however, among dialysis-dependent patients, 43% in the TPE group and none in the control group recovered renal function. Another randomized clinical trial showed no benefit of TPE in a composite outcome measure of death, dialysis dependence, and glomerular filtration rate[68]; however, biopsy confirmation of the renal diagnosis was not required in this trial. Similarly, a retrospective cohort study showed no benefit of TPE in either reducing mortality or preserving renal function.[69] If TPE is to be undertaken, biopsy confirmation of cast nephropathy may be advisable. With the advent of new drugs to treat multiple-myeloma patients, including proteosome inhibitors and monoclonal antibodies, the role for TPE in this setting continues to evolve, as effects are often transient and overall survival clearly depends on patient response to chemotherapy.[70]

Patients receiving rituximab (anti-CD20) for IgM Waldenström macroglobulinemia may experience a transient increase in M protein levels after drug initiation, and a short TPE series before starting this medication may be indicated in select patients. Patients with pretreatment IgM levels >4 g/dL may benefit from TPE to avoid developing symptomatic hyperviscosity.[5,71]

TPE has been evaluated as a therapeutic treatment for acute liver failure and shown to be efficacious in treating liver failure due to Wilson disease.[5] High-volume plasma filtration was superior to standard medical therapy at improving transplant-free survival in patients with liver failure.[72] Molecular Adsorbent Recirculating System (MARS) therapy (beyond the scope of this chapter) is another extracorporeal technique that may bridge patients with liver failure to transplantation.[73]

TPE may be used to treat central nervous system (CNS) acute disseminated encephalomyelitis. Experience in treating chronic progressive multiple sclerosis with TPE has been discouraging. However, for acute CNS inflammatory demyelinating diseases unresponsive to steroids, TPE may be beneficial.[74] Early initiation of TPE may facilitate response, and some clinical responses may not manifest until later in followup.[75] TPE may also be effective in neuromyelitis optica (NMO), also called Devic disease, even in the absence of NMO antibodies.[76]

TPE to treat select peripheral nervous system diseases [eg, AIDPs such as Guillain-Barré syndrome (GBS)] is well established, with randomized controlled clinical trials substantiating its efficacy in GBS patients not exhibiting spontaneous recovery.[5] IVIG infusions alone or following a course of TPE appear equally effective.[77] No biomarkers are currently known to predict response to upfront therapeutic strategy. As a result of concomitant autonomic nervous system involvement, patients often exhibit blood pressure and pulse variability that can complicate initial sessions of TPE but typically becomes less pronounced during later TPE sessions. Given equivalent efficacy and similar severity and frequencies of adverse events with either TPE or IVIG, TPE appears to be a less expensive firstline therapy option for treating patients with GBS.[78]

In focal segmental glomerulosclerosis (FSGS), a circulating factor that increases glomerular permeability with resultant proteinuria has been hypothesized, as FSGS frequently recurs after renal transplantation and can produce allograft failure.[79,80] TPE may effectively remove the permeability factor and induce remission in recurrent FSGS following renal transplantation. However, response to TPE in primary FSGS has not been well studied.

TPE may provide adjunctive immunosuppression in treating or preventing antibody-mediated rejection (AMR) of solid-organ transplants. AMR presenting in the early posttransplantation period may respond better to TPE than later AMR.[81] TPE before transplantation of an ABO-incompatible kidney may prevent hyperacute rejection, and TPE following implantation is often used to treat AMR in this setting.[82,83] TPE in conjunction with immunomodulatory therapies, such as IVIG, rituximab, or bortezomib, before transplantation can reduce the risk of rejection in HLA-alloimmunized patients.[84,85]

Cytapheresis

The goal of cytapheresis is to remove excessive or pathogenic leukocytes, platelets, or red cells. Indications for cytapheresis are listed in Table 25-6.

In leukemia, high cell counts (typically >100,000/µL) can produce microvascular stasis with headache, mental status changes, visual disturbances, or dyspnea. The leukocyte count at which a patient becomes symptomatic is variable but occurs more often in myelomonocytic and monocytic leukemias. Typically, patients with acute or chronic lymphocytic leukemia are asymptomatic at higher cell counts, and cytapheresis may not be required. Cytapheresis commonly results in a less-than-predicted reduction in leukocyte count, despite excellent collection, because of mobilization and reequilibration of marginalized intravascular cells and cells from extravascular sites. Myelogenous leukemia cells commonly have a higher density than lymphocytic cells and can be difficult to separate from red cells by centrifugation. Use of hydroxyethyl starch enhances red cell sedimentation by rouleaux formation and can improve cytapheresis efficiency in acute myelogenous leukemia. In a typical leukocyte-reduction procedure, 2.0 blood volumes are processed and the collection rate is determined by the white cell count and inlet flow rate, removing up to 20% of TBV into the collection bag. Many patients with hyperleukocytosis are receiving hyperhydration with crystalloid during their apheresis procedures to mitigate tumor lysis complications; however, pediatric patients may benefit from FFP or albumin replacement due to the risk of hypovolemia caused by the procedure. Advances in the available automated

TABLE 25-6. Indications for Therapeutic Cytapheresis[5]

Indication	Modifying Conditions	Procedure	Category	Typical Course (number of treatments)
Hereditary hemochromatosis		Erythrocytapheresis	I	Every 2-3 weeks (variable)
Hyperleukocytosis	Symptomatic	Leukocytapheresis	II	QD (variable)
	Prophylactic or secondary		III	
Inflammatory bowel disease	Ulcerative colitis/ Crohn disease	Adsorptive cytapheresis	III	Weekly (5-10)
Polycythemia vera; erythrocytosis	Polycythemia vera	Erythrocytapheresis	I	Variable
	Secondary erythrocytosis		III	
Psoriasis	Disseminated pustular	Adsorptive cytapheresis	III	Weekly (5)
Thrombocytosis	Symptomatic	Thrombocytapheresis	II	QD (variable)
	Prophylactic or secondary		III	
Vasculitis	Behçet disease	Adsorptive cytapheresis	II	Weekly (5)

QD = daily.

apheresis platforms may further improve fluid management in these critically ill patients.[86]

Massive thrombocytosis, typically >1,000,000/µL, can occur in essential thrombocythemia, in polycythemia vera, or as a reactive phenomenon. Such patients may be at risk of both thrombosis and hemorrhage. Hemorrhage risk is partly due to acquired von Willebrand disease secondary to the very high platelet count. Reduction in platelet count is commonly less than predicted because of mobilization of platelets to the peripheral blood, primarily from the spleen.

Red Cell Exchange

Indications for red cell exchange are listed in Table 25-7. Red cell exchange is most commonly performed in sickle cell disease (SCD). The goal is to reduce the burden of hemoglobin-S-containing red cells, provide donor red cells containing hemoglobin A, and restore oxygen-carrying capacity in the setting of severe anemia. A common goal is to reduce hemoglobin S to <30%, with a final hematocrit not to exceed ~30% to avoid hyperviscosity in patients with

TABLE 25-7. Indications for Therapeutic Red Cell Exchange[5]

Indication	Modifying Conditions	Procedure	Category	Typical Course (number of treatments)
Babesiosis	Severe	Red cell exchange	II	Once
Erythropoietic protoporphyria, liver disease		Red cell exchange	III	3/week
Hematopoietic stem cell transplantation, ABOi	Minor—HPC(A)	Red cell exchange	III	Once
Malaria	Severe	Red cell exchange	III	1-2 treatments
Red cell alloimmunization, prevention and treatment	Exposure to RhD+ red cells	Red cell exchange	III	Once
Sickle cell disease, acute	Acute stroke	Red cell exchange	I	Once
	Acute chest syndrome, severe		II	
	Other complications		III	
Sickle cell disease, nonacute	Stroke prophylaxis	Red cell exchange	I	As needed to maintain target HbS
	Recurrent vaso-occlusive pain crisis		II	
	Pregnancy		II	
	Preoperative management		III	Once

HPC(A) = hematopoietic progenitor cells collected from apheresis; HbS = hemoglobin S; ABOi = ABO incompatible.

chronic anemia. Prevention or treatment of acute stroke is an indication for red cell exchange in patients with SCD. Retrospective data has shown that patients with SCD who received red cell exchange as their treatment for acute stroke had fewer episodes of recurrent stroke. For patients with elevated cerebral blood flow velocity, determined by transcranial Doppler imaging, transfusion reduces the risk of stroke.[87,88] Chronic red cell exchange, typically every 4 to 6 weeks, can normalize cerebral blood flow while minimizing iron overload. Acute chest syndrome, another serious complication of SCD, presents as dyspnea, chest pain, and cough, often accompanied by fever, leukocytosis, decreasing hematocrit, hypoxia, and pulmonary infiltrates. Respiratory failure can develop, and death occurs in ~3% of cases.[89] Red cell exchange is indicated for progressive infiltrates and hypoxemia refractory to conventional therapy and simple transfusion, and there is some evidence supporting early intervention with exchange in pediatric patients with acute chest syndrome.[90,91] Red cell exchange may have a role in other sickle cell syndromes, including multiorgan failure, hepatic/splenic sequestration, priapism, and intrahepatic cholestasis. In addition, it may be used for preventing iron overload and for preventing or managing vaso-occlusive pain crises. AABB and the American Society of Hematology (ASH) have developed consensus statements on transfusion for sickle cell disease that include guidance on the utility and goals of red cell exchange in this population, both for acute and chronic complications.[92]

Red Blood Cells (RBCs) for replacement must be ABO compatible and negative for antigen(s) to known, clinically significant alloantibodies present in the recipient. For patients with SCD, RBCs should also be phenotype-matched for C, E, and K, if possible.[93] Units for these patients should also be tested for hemoglobin S and found to be negative before including them as part of the RBC replacement. It is desirable to use relatively fresh units to maximize posttransfusion red cell survival. RBC units containing either citrate-phosphate-dextrose-adenine (CPDA)-1 or additive solutions (AS) may be used. It is desirable that all units used in a given procedure contain the same anticoagulant solution so that they have similar hematocrits. Chronic red cell exchange may carry a lower risk of alloimmunization than simple transfusion in SCD patients, despite the increased donor exposures associated with the procedure.[94]

Isovolemic hemodilution, an optional modification to automated red cell exchange, involves initial depletion of the patient's red cells to a predetermined hematocrit, and replacement with saline or albumin. This can reduce donor exposures by reducing the volume of RBCs needed for exchange.[95] Although it is generally well tolerated, patient volume status, preprocedure hematocrit, and cerebral vascular autoregulation should be considered before undertaking this modification. In general, isovolemic hemodilution may be performed in patients who are hemodynamically stable and who maintain a preprocedure hematocrit >23% to 26%. Studies have shown that decreasing the patient's hematocrit by 6% to 8% may be safe and well tolerated; however, this should be modified based on the individual patient's needs and tolerance of procedure.[92,96]

In addition, red cell exchange may be used in severely ill patients to decrease parasite burden in bloodborne infections, such as malaria and babesiosis. Red cell exchange may also be used following large-volume transfusion of Rh-positive RBCs to an Rh-negative female of childbearing potential, to limit Rh sensitization.

Extracorporeal Photopheresis

In ECP, the buffy-coat layer is collected from peripheral blood, treated with 8-methoxypsoralen and ultraviolet A light, and reinfused into the patient. The treatment causes crosslinking of leukocyte DNA, which prevents replication and induces apoptosis. ECP was developed to treat cutaneous T-cell lymphoma, although it is increasingly used for other indications (Table 25-8). ECP has complex immunomodulatory effects, including induction of monocyte differentiation into dendritic cells, alteration of T-cell subsets, and changes in cytokine profiles.[97,98] ECP has been shown to be effective in acute and chronic skin-associated graft-vs-host disease (GVHD), although response rates are lower in non-skin-associated GVHD. ECP often offers a

TABLE 25-8. Indications for Photopheresis[5]

Indication	Modifying Conditions	Category	Typical Course* (duration)
Atopic (neuro-) dermatitis (atopic eczema), recalcitrant		III	Every 2 weeks (12 weeks)
Cutaneous T-cell lymphoma; Mycosis fungoides; Sézary syndrome	Erythrodermic	I	Every 2-4 weeks (variable)
	Nonerythrodermic	III	
Graft-vs-host disease	Acute	II	Weekly, tapering to every 2 weeks
	Chronic	II	Weekly (4), then every 2 weeks (8-12 weeks)
Inflammatory bowel disease	Crohn disease	III	Weekly (4), every 2 weeks (8)
Nephrogenic systemic fibrosis		III	Every 2-4 weeks (5)
Pemphigus vulgaris	Severe	III	Every 2-4 weeks (variable)
Psoriasis	Disseminated pustular	III	Weekly (4 months)
Scleroderma (systemic sclerosis)		III	Every 4-6 weeks (6-12 months)
Transplantation, cardiac	Cellular/recurrent rejection	II	Weekly or every other week (several months)
	Rejection prophylaxis	II	
Transplantation, liver	Desensitization, ABOi	III	Weekly or every 2-8 weeks (several months)
	Acute rejection/immune suppression withdrawal	III	
Transplantation, lung	Bronchiolitis obliterans syndrome	II	Weekly (5), every 2 weeks (4), every month (3)

*One cycle typically consists of extracorporeal photopheresis on 2 consecutive days.
ABOi = ABO incompatible.

steroid-sparing approach to management of GVHD.[99,100]

ECP for solid-organ transplant rejection has been carefully studied in cardiac and lung transplantation. In a randomized clinical trial, prophylactic ECP, in conjunction with previous-generation immunosuppression (ie, not including calcineurin inhibitors or mycophenolate), resulted in fewer rejection episodes, decreased HLA antibodies, and reduced coronary artery intimal thickness; but no difference was found in time to first rejection episode, incidence of hemodynamic compromise, or survival at 6 or 12 months.[101,102] In cardiac rejection, ECP may de-crease rejection severity and allow for reduced immunosuppressive dosages, even in the setting of hemodynamic compromise.[103,104] ECP may have a role in stabilizing lung function in bronchiolitis obliterans syndrome after lung transplantation.[105,106]

Selective Adsorption

The currently established indications for selective adsorption of plasma proteins are listed in Table 25-9, although in general these are not widely used, as they require specialized equipment.

TABLE 25-9. Indications for Selective Adsorption[5]

Indication	Modifying Conditions	Treatment Modality	Category	Typical Course (number of treatments)
Acute inflammatory demyelinating polyradiculoneuropathy (Guillain-Barré syndrome)	Primary treatment	IA	I	QD or QOD (5-6)
Age-related macular degeneration, dry	High-risk	Rheopheresis	II	8-10 (2/week) over 8-21 weeks
Amyloidosis, systemic	Dialysis-related	β_2-microglobulin column	II	3/week with dialysis
Atopic (neuro-) dermatitis (atopic eczema), recalcitrant		IA	III	10-12 treatments over 4-6 weeks
		DFPP	III	Weekly
Chronic inflammatory demyelinating polyradiculoneuropathy		IA	I	2-3/week, then tapered
Coagulation factor inhibitors		IA	III	QD
Cryoglobulinemia	Symptomatic/ severe	IA	II	Every 1-3 days (3-8)
Dilated cardiomyopathy, idiopathic	NYHA II-IV	IA	II	QD or QOD (5)
Familial hypercholesterolemia	Homozygotes	LA	I	Once every 1-2 weeks (indefinite)
	Heterozygotes		II	
Focal segmental glomerulosclerosis	Recurrent in kidney transplant	IA	I	QD or QOD at initiation, wean based on response
	Recurrent in kidney transplant/ steroid-resistant in native kidney	LA	II	Twice per week (3), once per week (6)
Hypertriglyceridemic pancreatitis	Severe	LA	III	QD (1-3)
	Prevention of relapse		III	
Immune thrombocytopenia	Refractory	IA	III	1-3/week (variable)
Lipoprotein (a) hyperlipoproteinemia	Progressive atherosclerotic cardiovascular disease	LA	II	Once every 1-2 weeks (indefinite)
Multiple sclerosis	Acute attack/ relapse	IA	II	QOD (5-7)
	Chronic		III	Variable

(Continued)

TABLE 25-9. Indications for Selective Adsorption[5] (Continued)

Indication	Modifying Conditions	Treatment Modality	Category	Typical Course (number of treatments)
Myasthenia gravis	Acute, short-term treatment	IA	I	QD or QOD (3-6)
	Long-term treatment		II	Every 1-2 weeks
Neuromyelitis optica spectrum disorders	Acute attack/relapse	IA	II	QD or QOD (variable)
N-methyl-D-aspartate receptor antibody encephalitis		IA	I	QD or QOD (5-12)
Paraneoplastic neurologic syndromes		IA	III	2/week (6)
Pemphigus vulgaris	Severe	IA	III	QD (3), then weekly and tapering (variable)
Peripheral vascular disease		LA	II	1-2/week (variable)
Phytanic acid storage disease (Refsum disease)		LA	II	QD (variable)
Sudden sensorineural hearing loss		Rheopheresis/LA	III	QD (1-2)
Thrombotic microangiopathy, infection associated	STEC-HUS, severe	IA	III	QD (variable)
Transplantation, renal, ABO compatible	Antibody-mediated rejection	IA	I	QD or QOD (5-6)
	Desensitization, LD		I	
	Desensitization, DD		III	
Renal transplantation, ABO incompatible	Desensitization, LD	IA	I	QD or QOD (variable)
	Antibody-mediated rejection		II	
Voltage-gated potassium channel antibody related diseases		IA	II	QD or QOD (5-10)

IA = immunoadsorption; QD = daily; QOD = every other day; DFPP = double-filtration plasmapheresis; NYHA = New York Heart Association (class); LA = lipoprotein apheresis; STEC-HUS = Shiga-like toxin hemolytic uremic syndrome; LD = living donor; DD = deceased donor.

Selective removal of low-density lipoprotein (LDL) can be accomplished by passing heparinized plasma over a dextran-sulfate column or beads coated with anionic polyacrylate ligands, or by precipitation of heparin-LDL complexes in acidified plasma. LA treatments need to be repeated indefinitely, typically at 2-week intervals. There is evidence that LA reduces the incidence of major coronary events and stroke.[107] In addition, atherosclerotic plaque regression may occur in some patients.[24] Potentially beneficial, secondary effects of LA include reduction in levels of C-reactive protein, fibrinogen, tissue factor, and soluble adhesion molecules.[108,109] LA is also used to treat primary or recurrent FSGS, although the mechanism of action is not well defined.[110] LA may also be performed with DFPP techniques, as described earlier in this chapter.

IgG can be selectively removed by passing plasma over a column of staphylococcal protein A bound to silica. The putative mechanism of action is the removal of pathogenic autoantibodies or immune complexes, although an alternative mechanism has been proposed in immune thrombocytopenia (ITP).[111] Staphylococcal protein A adsorption treatment can be performed manually or in conjunction with automated TPE. Affinity columns containing IgG antibodies, IgE monoclonal antibodies, or ABO blood group carbohydrate ligands have been tested in clinical trials but are not currently approved for use in the United States.

THERAPEUTIC APHERESIS PROCEDURE DOCUMENTATION, PAYMENT, AND PROVIDER CREDENTIALING

Pertinent clinical documentation is essential for ensuring patient safety, health-care team communications, adherence to regulatory and accreditation agency requirements, monetary reimbursement of hospitals and providers, and medicolegal protections. Although no specific formats are mandated, certain items should be included in practitioners' written/electronic communications. Some of these items related to the direct clinical care of the patient have been highlighted in earlier sections of this chapter (see "Patient Evaluation and Management"). Other information regarding specific aspects of the apheresis intervention itself should be documented in nursing procedure records. Lot numbers of disposables, identification numbers of apheresis devices and related equipment (eg, blood warmers, medications, and blood components given during the procedure), and patient educational materials are some items that should be noted. Checklist approaches to such documentation are useful (Fig 25-1). Using an electronic medical record to document all fluids and medications administered during an apheresis intervention can enhance patient care by contributing more accurate data for the calculation of a patient's total fluid status, thus potentially averting fluid-related adverse consequences (Fig 25-2). It also facilitates investigation of any adverse events. Additionally, electronic medical alerts that highlight a patient's recent apheresis procedure may provide useful guidance at the time of test ordering and test interpretation for clinicians who may be less familiar with how therapeutic apheresis procedures may impact results from laboratory testing performed in the periapheresis interval (Fig 25-3).[112]

Navigating payment systems for apheresis services in today's diverse health-care insurer environment can be challenging. Readers are referred to an annually updated reimbursement guide from ASFA detailed information in this area.[113]

Apheresis medicine is a professionally diverse discipline involving specialists across a broad clinical spectrum. Hospital clinical privileging of both physicians and nurses involved in the delivery of apheresis medicine services is a topic of interest and discussion within professional societies and health-care institutions. Although no uniform approach has been mandated regarding practitioners' professional requirements, institutions interested in more formally addressing this subject may wish to review an ASFA commentary on the topic.[3]

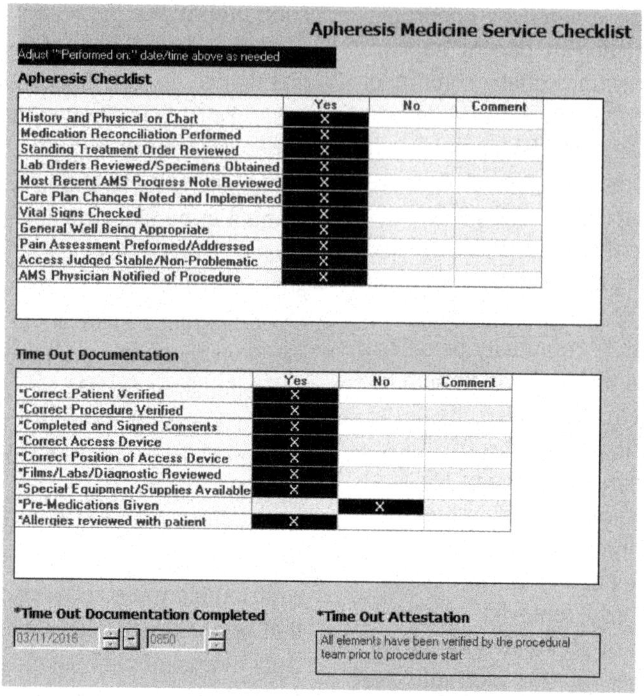

(A)

(B)

FIGURE 25-1. Computer-screen displays of select sections of an apheresis procedural note documented in a patient's electronic medical record used at Baystate Medical Center, Springfield, MA. Note checklist format and time-out review features incorporating various patient safety and regulatory/accreditation agencies' required documentation items (A) and information regarding disposables used in the procedure (B).

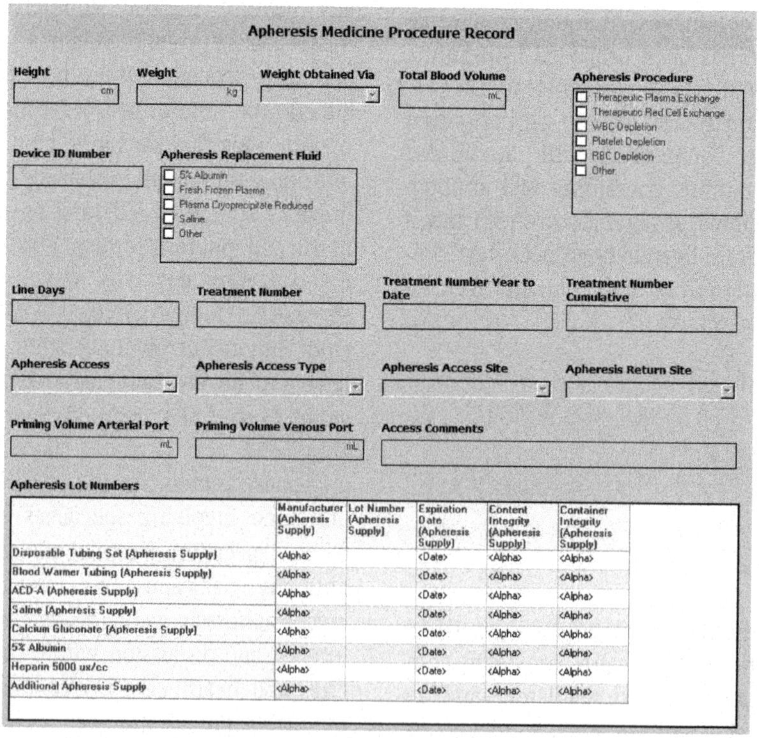

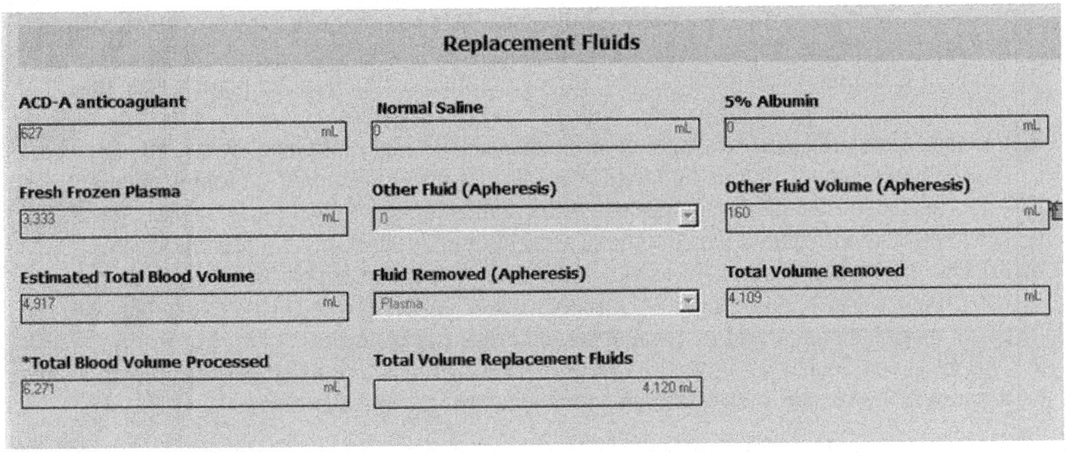

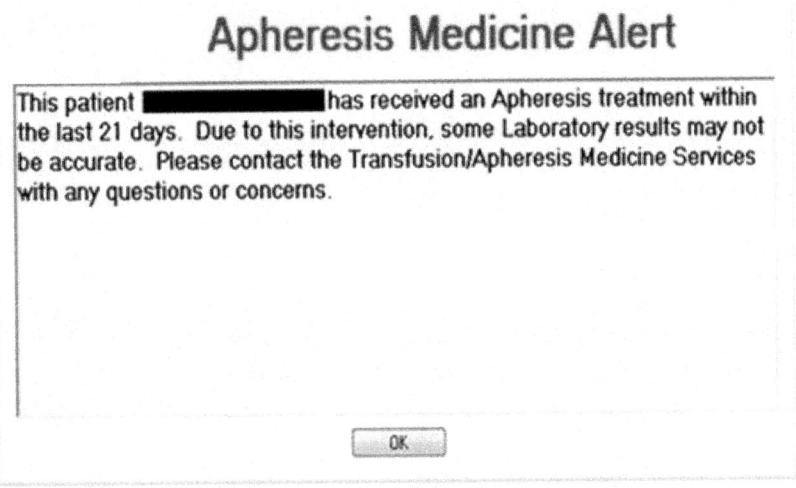

Replacement Fluids

ACD-A anticoagulant	**Normal Saline**	**5% Albumin**
627 mL	0 mL	0 mL
Fresh Frozen Plasma	**Other Fluid (Apheresis)**	**Other Fluid Volume (Apheresis)**
3,333 mL	0 ▾	160 mL
Estimated Total Blood Volume	**Fluid Removed (Apheresis)**	**Total Volume Removed**
4,917 mL	Plasma ▾	4,109 mL
***Total Blood Volume Processed**	**Total Volume Replacement Fluids**	
8,271 mL	4,120 mL	

FIGURE 25-2. Computer-screen display of a select section of an apheresis procedural note detailing volumes and identities of fluids processed, removed, and replaced during a therapeutic plasma exchange for a patient with thrombotic thrombocytopenic purpura; these details are documented in the patient's electronic medical record used at Baystate Medical Center, Springfield, MA.

Apheresis Medicine Alert

This patient ███████████ has received an Apheresis treatment within the last 21 days. Due to this intervention, some Laboratory results may not be accurate. Please contact the Transfusion/Apheresis Medicine Services with any questions or concerns.

[OK]

FIGURE 25-3. Electronic medical alert used at Baystate Medical Center, Springfield, MA.

KEY POINTS

1. Therapeutic apheresis treats diseases by removal or extracorporeal manipulation of pathologic plasma constituents, white cells, platelets, or red cells and may be accomplished by centrifugation, filtration, selective adsorption, or photopheresis.
2. Medical evaluation of the apheresis patient should focus on the disease indication; type of procedure; frequency, number, and duration of treatments; therapeutic goal; tolerance of the patient for apheresis; vascular access; replacement fluids; and medications. Appropriate laborato-

ry monitoring is guided by the disease indication, type and frequency of procedures, duration of therapy, and concomitant medical conditions.

3. Albumin is the most commonly used replacement fluid for therapeutic plasma exchange, but plasma may be indicated for patients with TTP or coagulopathy.

4. Vascular access for apheresis may be accomplished through peripheral veins, but large-bore double-lumen central venous catheters or AV fistulas may be required for some patients.

5. Anticoagulation is usually accomplished with citrate, although heparin may be used, particularly for selective adsorption, hematopoietic progenitor cell collection, and photopheresis.

6. Adverse effects of apheresis are usually mild but may include symptomatic hypocalcemia, hypotension, urticaria, and nausea. Consequences of apheresis can include coagulopathy, hypogammaglobulinemia, and removal of certain drugs and biologics.

7. The American Society for Apheresis (ASFA) publishes updated guidelines and recommendations every 3 years for the use of therapeutic apheresis in clinical practice.

REFERENCES

1. Gammon R, ed. Standards for blood banks and transfusion services. 32nd ed. Bethesda, MD: AABB, 2020.

2. College of American Pathologists Commission on Laboratory Accreditation. Transfusion medicine checklist. Northfield, IL: CAP, 2019.

3. Andrzejewski C, Linz W, Hofmann J, et al. American Society for Apheresis white paper: Considerations for medical staff apheresis medicine physician credentialing and privileging. J Clin Apher 2012;27(6):330-5.

4. Marshall CS, Andrzejewski C, Carey PM, et al. Milestones for apheresis education. J Clin Apher 2012;27(5):242-6.

5. Padmanabhan A, Connelly-Smith L, Aqui N, et al. Guidelines on the use of therapeutic apheresis in clinical practice - Evidence-based approach from the Writing Committee of the American Society for Apheresis: The eighth special issue. J Clin Apher 2019;34(3):171-354.

6. American Society for Apheresis. Guidelines for therapeutic apheresis clinical privileges. J Clin Apher 2007;22(3):181-2.

7. American Society for Apheresis. Guidelines for documentation of therapeutic apheresis procedures in the medical record by apheresis physicians. J Clin Apher 2007;22(3):183.

8. National Institutes of Health. Therapeutic apheresis: Recap from an NHLBI working group, November 28-29, 2012. Bethesda, MD: National Heart, Lung, and Blood Institute, 2012. [Available at https://www.nhlbi.nih.gov/events/2012/therapeutic-apheresis (accessed January 27, 2020).]

9. Karafin MS, Sachais BS, Connelly-Smith L, et al. NHLBI state of the science symposium in therapeutic apheresis: Knowledge gaps and research opportunities in the area of hematology-oncology. J Clin Apher 2015;31(1):38-47.

10. Winters JL, Cooper LT, Ratcliffe NR, et al. National Heart, Lung, and Blood Institute state of the science symposium in therapeutic apheresis-Therapeutic apheresis in cardiovascular disease. J Clin Apher 2015;30(3):183-7.

11. Winters JL. Plasma exchange: Concepts, mechanisms, and an overview of the American Society for Apheresis guidelines. Hematology Am Soc Hematol Educ Program 2012;2012:7-12.

12. Chopek M, McCullough J. Protein and biochemical changes during plasma exchange. In: Ulmas J Berkman E, eds. Therapeutic hemapheresis: A technical workshop. Bethesda, MD: AABB, 1980:13-24.

13. Kaufman RM, ed. Special issue: Strategies for long-term intravenous access for apheresis procedures: History, applications and challenges. Transfusion 2018; 58(S1):545-613.

14. Adamski J. Vascular access considerations for extracorporeal photopheresis. Transfusion 2018;58(Suppl 1):590-7.

15. Kalantari K. The choice of vascular access for therapeutic apheresis. J Clin Apher 2012;27(3):153-9.

16. Kapadia E, Wong E, Perez-Albuerne E, Jacobsohn D. Extracorporeal photopheresis performed on the CELLEX(R) compared with the UVAR-XTS(R) instrument is more efficient and better tolerated in children with steroid-refractory graft-versus-host disease. Pediatr Blood Cancer 2015;62(8):1485-8.

17. Shrestha A, Jawa Z, Koch KL, et al. Use of a dual lumen port for automated red cell exchange in

adults with sickle cell disease. J Clin Apher 2015;30(6):353-8.

18. Agarwal AK. Systemic effects of hemodialysis access. Adv Chronic Kidney Dis 2015;22(6): 459-65.

19. Rao NN, Dundon BK, Worthley MI, Faull RJ. The impact of arteriovenous fistulae for hemodialysis on the cardiovascular system. Semin Dial 2016;29(3):214-21.

20. Dariushnia SR, Wallace MJ, Siddiqi NH, et al. Quality improvement guidelines for central venous access. J Vasc Interv Radiol 2010;21(7): 976-81.

21. Lee KA, Ramaswamy RS. Intravascular access devices from an interventional radiology perspective: Indications, implantation techniques, and optimizing patency. Transfusion 2018; 58(S1):549-57.

22. Ceppi F, Rivers J, Annesley C, et al. Lymphocyte apheresis for chimeric antigen receptor T-cell manufacturing in children and young adults with leukemia and neuroblastoma. Transfusion 2018;58(6):1414-20.

23. Mandal S, Baron BW, Mischeaux M, et al. Collection of peripheral blood stem cells from a 7 month-old girl weighing 7 kg with the use of combined heparin and citrate anticoagulation. J Clin Apher 2013;28(4):309-10.

24. Matsuzaki M, Hiramori K, Imaizumi T, et al. Intravascular ultrasound evaluation of coronary plaque regression by low density lipoprotein-apheresis in familial hypercholesterolemia. J Am Coll Cardiol 2002;40(2):220-7.

25. McLeod BC, Sniecinski I, Ciavarella D, et al. Frequency of immediate adverse effects associated with therapeutic apheresis. Transfusion 1999;39(3):282-8.

26. Norda R, Berséus O, Stegmayr B. Adverse events and problems in therapeutic hemapheresis. A report from the Swedish registry. Transfus Apher Sci 2001;25(1):33-41.

27. Mörtzell Henriksson M, Newman E, Witt V, et al. Adverse events in apheresis: An update of the WAA registry data. Transfus Apher Sci 2016; 54(1):2-15.

28. Haddad S, Leitman SF, Wesley RA, et al. Placebo-controlled study of intravenous magnesium supplementation during large-volume leukapheresis in healthy allogeneic donors. Transfusion 2005; 45(6):934-44.

29. Marques MB, Huang ST. Patients with thrombotic thrombocytopenic purpura commonly develop metabolic alkalosis during therapeutic plasma exchange. J Clin Apher 2001;16(3):120-4.

30. Wang KY, Friedman DF, DaVeiga SP. Immediate hypersensitivity reaction to human serum albumin in a child undergoing plasmapheresis. Transfusion 2019;59(6):1921-3.

31. Reutter JC, Sanders KF, Brecher ME, et al. Incidence of allergic reactions with fresh frozen plasma or cryo-supernatant plasma in the treatment of thrombotic thrombocytopenic purpura. J Clin Apher 2001;16(3):134-8.

32. Lee LJ, Roland KJ, Sreenivasan GM, et al. Solvent-detergent plasma for the treatment of thrombotic microangiopathies: A Canadian tertiary care centre experience. Transfus Apher Sci 2018;57(2):233-5.

33. Sidhu D, Snyder EL, Tormey CA. Two approaches to the clinical dilemma of treating TTP with therapeutic plasma exchange in patients with a history of anaphylactic reactions to plasma. J Clin Apher 2017;32(3):158-62.

34. Askari S, Nollet K, Debol SM, et al. Transfusion-related acute lung injury during plasma exchange: Suspecting the unsuspected. J Clin Apher 2002;17(2):93-6.

35. Duntley P, Siever J, Korwes ML, et al. Vascular erosion by central venous catheters. Chest 1992;101(6):1633-8.

36. Leitman SF, Boltansky H, Alter HJ, et al. Allergic reactions in healthy platelet-pheresis donors caused by sensitization to ethylene oxide gas. N Engl J Med 1986;315(19):1192-6.

37. Purello D'Ambrosio F, Savica V, Gangemi S, et al. Ethylene oxide allergy in dialysis patients. Nephrol Dial Transplant 1997;12(7):1461-3.

38. Owen HG, Brecher ME. Atypical reactions associated with use of angiotensin-converting enzyme inhibitors and apheresis. Transfusion 2003;34(10):891-4.

39. Perkins KA. Contraindication of angiotensin-converting enzyme (ACE) inhibitors for patients receiving therapeutic plasma exchanges. Nephrol Nurs J 2008;35(6):571-4.

40. Orlin JB, Berkman EM. Partial plasma exchange using albumin replacement: Removal and recovery of normal plasma constituents. Blood 1980; 56(6):1055-9.

41. Flaum MA, Cuneo RA, Appelbaum FR, et al. The hemostatic imbalance of plasma-exchange transfusion. Blood 1979;54(3):694-702.

42. Food and Drug Administration. Transfusion/donation fatalities. Silver Spring, MD: CBER Office of Communication, Outreach, and Development, 2019. [Available at https://www.fda.

gov/vaccines-blood-biologics/report-problem-center-biologics-evaluation-research/transfu siondonation-fatalities (accessed January 27, 2020).]

43. Food and Drug Administration. Death and pulmonary embolism related to extracorporeal photopheresis (ecp) treatment - Letter to health care providers. (February 5, 2018) Silver Spring, MD: Division of Industry and Consumer Education, 2018. [Available at https://www.fda.gov/medical-devices/letters-health-care-providers/death-and-pulmonary-embolism-related-extra corporeal-photopheresis-ecp-treatment-letter-health-care (accessed January 27, 2020).]

44. Kiprov DD, Golden P, Rohe R, et al. Adverse reactions associated with mobile therapeutic apheresis: Analysis of 17,940 procedures. J Clin Apher 2001;16(3):130-3.

45. Food and Drug Administration. FDA executive summary (prepared for the February 26, 2016 meeting of the Gastroenterology-Urology Devices Panel): Classification of centrifuge-type therapeutic apheresis devices. Silver Spring, MD: FDA, 2016. [Available at https://www.fda.gov/media/96112/download (accessed January 27, 2020).]

46. Kim HC. Therapeutic pediatric apheresis. J Clin Apher 2000;15(1-2):129-57.

47. Kim YA, Sloan SR. Pediatric therapeutic apheresis: Rationale and indications for plasmapheresis, cytapheresis, extracorporeal photopheresis, and LDL apheresis. Pediatr Clin North Am 2013;60(6):1569-80.

48. Meyer EK, Wong EC. Pediatric therapeutic apheresis: A critical appraisal of evidence. Transfus Med Rev 2016;30(4):217-22.

49. Terrell DR, Williams LA, Vesely SK, et al. The incidence of thrombotic thrombocytopenic purpura-hemolytic uremic syndrome: All patients, idiopathic patients, and patients with severe ADAMTS-13 deficiency. J Thromb Haemost 2005;3(7):1432-6.

50. Lara PN Jr, Coe TL, Zhou H, et al. Improved survival with plasma exchange in patients with thrombotic thrombocytopenic purpura-hemolytic uremic syndrome. Am J Med 1999; 107(6):573-9.

51. Bendapudi PK, Hurwitz S, Fry A, et al. Derivation and external validation of the PLASMIC score for rapid assessment of adults with thrombotic microangiopathies: A cohort study. Lancet Haematol 2017;4(4):e157-e64.

52. Jajosky R, Floyd M, Thompson T, Shikle J. Validation of the PLASMIC score at a University Medical Center. Transfus Apher Sci 2017; 56(4):591-4.

53. Li A, Khalighi PR, Wu Q, Garcia DA. External validation of the PLASMIC score: A clinical prediction tool for thrombotic thrombocytopenic purpura diagnosis and treatment. J Thromb Haemost 2018;16(1):164-9.

54. Tiscia GL, Ostuni A, Cascavilla N, et al. Validation of PLASMIC score and follow-up data in a cohort of patients with suspected microangiopathies from Southern Italy. J Thromb Thrombolysis 2018;46(2):174-9.

55. Bandarenko N, Brecher ME. United States thrombotic thrombocytopenic purpura apheresis study group (US TTP ASG): Multicenter survey and retrospective analysis of current efficacy of therapeutic plasma exchange. J Clin Apher 1998;13(3):133-41.

56. Howard MA, Williams LA, Terrell DR, et al. Complications of plasma exchange in patients treated for clinically suspected thrombotic thrombocytopenic purpura-hemolytic uremic syndrome. Transfusion 2006;46(1):154-6.

57. Page EE, Kremer Hovinga JA, Terrell DR, et al. Thrombotic thrombocytopenic purpura: Diagnostic criteria, clinical features, and long-term outcomes from 1995 through 2015. Blood Adv 2017;1(10):590-600.

58. Zeigler ZR, Shadduck RK, Gryn JF, et al. Cryoprecipitate poor plasma does not improve early response in primary adult thrombotic thrombocytopenic purpura (TTP). J Clin Apher 2001; 16(1):19-22.

59. Scully M, Cataland SR, Peyvandi F, et al. Caplacizumab treatment for acquired thrombotic thrombocytopenic purpura. N Engl J Med 2019; 380(4):335-46.

60. Legendre CM, Licht C, Muus P, et al. Terminal complement inhibitor eculizumab in atypical hemolytic-uremic syndrome. N Engl J Med 2013;368(23):2169-81.

61. Fakhouri F, Hourmant M, Campistol JM, et al. Terminal complement inhibitor eculizumab in adult patients with atypical hemolytic uremic syndrome: A single-arm, open-label trial. Am J Kidney Dis 2016;68(1):84-93.

62. Legendre CM, Licht C, Loirat C. Eculizumab in atypical hemolytic-uremic syndrome. N Engl J Med 2013;369(14):1379-80.

63. Jodele S, Dandoy CE, Myers KC, et al. New approaches in the diagnosis, pathophysiology, and treatment of pediatric hematopoietic stem cell transplantation-associated thrombotic microan-

giopathy. Transfus Apher Sci 2016;54(2):181-90.

64. Jodele S, Laskin BL, Dandoy CE, et al. A new paradigm: Diagnosis and management of HSCT-associated thrombotic microangiopathy as multisystem endothelial injury. Blood Rev 2015; 29(3):191-204.

65. Simetka O, Klat J, Gumulec J, et al. Early identification of women with HELLP syndrome who need plasma exchange after delivery. Transfus Apher Sci 2015;52(1):54-9.

66. Somer T. Rheology of paraproteinaemias and the plasma hyperviscosity syndrome. Baillières Clin Haematol 1987;1(3):695-723.

67. Johnson WJ. Treatment of renal failure associated with multiple myeloma. Arch Intern Med 1990;150(4):863.

68. Clark WF, Stewart AK, Rock GA, et al. Plasma exchange when myeloma presents as acute renal failure. Ann Intern Med 2005;143(11):777.

69. Movilli E, Guido J, Silvia T, et al. Plasma exchange in the treatment of acute renal failure of myeloma. Nephrol Dial Transplant 2007; 22(4):1270-1.

70. Abramson HN. The multiple myeloma drug pipeline-2018: A review of small molecules and their therapeutic targets. Clin Lymphoma Myeloma Leuk 2018;18(9):611-27.

71. Treon SP, Branagan AR, Hunter Z, et al. Paradoxical increases in serum IgM and viscosity levels following rituximab in Waldenstrom's macroglobulinemia. Ann Oncol 2004;15(10): 1481-3.

72. Larsen FS, Schmidt LE, Bernsmeier C, et al. High-volume plasma exchange in patients with acute liver failure: An open randomised controlled trial. J Hepatol 2016;64(1):69-78.

73. Gerth HU, Pohlen M, Tholking G, et al. Molecular adsorbent recirculating system can reduce short-term mortality among patients with acute-on-chronic liver failure-a retrospective analysis. Crit Care Med 2017;45(10):1616-24.

74. Gwathmey K, Balogun RA, Burns T. Neurologic indications for therapeutic plasma exchange: 2013 update. J Clin Apher 2014;29(4):211-19.

75. Llufriu S, Castillo J, Blanco Y, et al. Plasma exchange for acute attacks of CNS demyelination: Predictors of improvement at 6 months. Neurology 2009;73(12):949-53.

76. Bonnan M, Valentino R, Olindo S, et al. Plasma exchange in severe spinal attacks associated with neuromyelitis optica spectrum disorder. Mult Scler 2009;15(4):487-92.

77. Randomised trial of plasma exchange, intravenous immunoglobulin, and combined treatments in Guillain-Barre syndrome. Plasma Exchange/Sandoglobulin Guillain-Barre Syndrome Trial Group. Lancet 1997;349(9047):225-30.

78. Winters JL, Brown D, Hazard E, et al. Cost-minimization analysis of the direct costs of TPE and IVIg in the treatment of Guillain-Barré syndrome. BMC Health Serv Res 2011;11:101.

79. De Vriese AS, Sethi S, Nath KA, et al. Differentiating primary, genetic, and secondary FSGS in adults: A clinicopathologic approach. J Am Soc Nephrol 2018;29(3):759-74.

80. Wada T, Nangaku M. A circulating permeability factor in focal segmental glomerulosclerosis: The hunt continues. Clin Kidney J 2015;8(6): 708-15.

81. Al-Badr W, Kallogjeri D, Madaraty K, et al. A retrospective review of the outcome of plasma exchange and aggressive medical therapy in antibody mediated rejection of renal allografts: A single center experience. J Clin Apher 2008; 23(6):178-82.

82. Sivakumaran P, Vo AA, Villicana R, et al. Therapeutic plasma exchange for desensitization prior to transplantation in ABO-incompatible renal allografts. J Clin Apher 2009;24:155-60.

83. Tobian AAR, Shirey RS, Montgomery RA, et al. Therapeutic plasma exchange reduces ABO titers to permit ABO-incompatible renal transplantation. Transfusion 2009;49(6):1248-54.

84. Padmanabhan A, Ratner LE, Jhang JS, et al. Comparative outcome analysis of ABO-incompatible and positive crossmatch renal transplantation: A single-center experience. Transplantation 2009;87(12):1889-96.

85. Jordan SC, Choi J, Kahwaji J, Vo A. Progress in desensitization of the highly HLA sensitized patient. Transplant Proc 2016;48(3):802-5.

86. Schulz M, Bug G, Bialleck H, et al. Leucodepletion for hyperleucocytosis—First report on a novel technology featuring electronic interphase management. Vox Sang 2013;105(1):47-53.

87. Adams RJ, McKie VC, Hsu L, et al. Prevention of a first stroke by transfusions in children with sickle cell anemia and abnormal results on transcranial doppler ultrasonography. N Engl J Med 1998;339(1):5-11.

88. Lee MT. Stroke Prevention Trial in Sickle Cell Anemia (STOP): Extended follow-up and final results. Blood 2006;108(3):847-52.

89. Vichinsky EP, Neumayr LD, Earles AN, et al. Causes and outcomes of the acute chest syn-

drome in sickle cell disease. N Engl J Med 2000;
342(25):1855-65.

90. Saylors RL, Watkins B, Saccente S, Tang X. Comparison of automated red cell exchange transfusion and simple transfusion for the treatment of children with sickle cell disease acute chest syndrome. Pediatr Blood Cancer 2013; 60(12):1952-6.

91. Turner JM, Kaplan JB, Cohen HW, Billett HH. Exchange versus simple transfusion for acute chest syndrome in sickle cell anemia adults. Transfusion 2009;49(5):863-8.

92. Biller E, Zhao Y, Berg M, et al. Red blood cell exchange in patients with sickle cell disease-Indications and management: A review and consensus report by the therapeutic apheresis subsection of the AABB. Transfusion 2018; 58(8):1965-72.

93. Vichinsky EP, Luban NLC, Wright E, et al. Prospective RBC phenotype matching in a stroke-prevention trial in sickle cell anemia: A multicenter transfusion trial. Transfusion 2001;41(9): 1086-92.

94. Wahl SK, Garcia A, Hagar W, et al. Lower alloimmunization rates in pediatric sickle cell patients on chronic erythrocytapheresis compared to chronic simple transfusions. Transfusion 2012;52(12):2671-6.

95. Sarode R, Matevosyan K, Rogers ZR, et al. Advantages of isovolemic hemodilution-red cell exchange therapy to prevent recurrent stroke in sickle cell anemia patients. J Clin Apher 2011; 26(4):200-7.

96. Kim J, Joseph R, Matevosyan K, Sarode R. Comparison of Spectra Optia and COBE Spectra apheresis systems' performances for red blood cell exchange procedures. Transfus Apher Sci 2016;55(3):368-70.

97. Bladon J, Taylor PC. Extracorporeal photopheresis: A focus on apoptosis and cytokines. J Dermatol Sci 2006;43(2):85-94.

98. Morelli AE, Larregina AT. Concise review: Mechanisms behind apoptotic cell-based therapies against transplant rejection and graft versus host disease. Stem Cells 2016;34(5):1142-50.

99. Del Fante C, Scudeller L, Viarengo G, et al. Response and survival of patients with chronic graft-versus-host disease treated by extracorporeal photochemotherapy: A retrospective study according to classical and National Institutes of Health classifications. Transfusion 2012;52(9): 2007-15.

100. Zhang H, Chen R, Cheng J, et al. Systematic review and meta-analysis of prospective studies for ECP treatment in patients with steroid-refractory acute GVHD. Patient Prefer Adherence 2015;9:105-11.

101. Barr ML, Baker CJ, Schenkel FA, et al. Prophylactic photopheresis and chronic rejection: Effects on graft intimal hyperplasia in cardiac transplantation. Clin Transplant 2000;14(2): 162-6.

102. Barr ML, Meiser BM, Eisen HJ, et al. Photopheresis for the prevention of rejection in cardiac transplantation. N Engl J Med 1998;339(24): 1744-51.

103. Dall'Amico R, Montini G, Murer L, et al. Extracorporeal photochemotherapy after cardiac transplantation: A new therapeutic approach to allograft rejection. Int J Artif Org 2000;23(1): 49-54.

104. Colvin MM, Cook JL, Chang P, et al. Antibody-mediated rejection in cardiac transplantation: Emerging knowledge in diagnosis and management: A scientific statement from the American Heart Association. Circulation 2015;131(18): 1608-39.

105. Hachem R, Corris P. Extracorporeal photopheresis for bronchiolitis obliterans syndrome after lung transplantation. Transplantation 2018; 102(7):1059-65.

106. Jaksch P, Scheed A, Keplinger M, et al. A prospective interventional study on the use of extracorporeal photopheresis in patients with bronchiolitis obliterans syndrome after lung transplantation. J Heart Lung Transplant 2012; 31(9):950-7.

107. Masaki N, Tatami R, Kumamoto T, et al. Ten-year follow-up of familial hypercholesterolemia patients after intensive cholesterol-lowering therapy. Int Heart J 2005;46(5):833-43.

108. Kobayashi S, Oka M, Moriya H, et al. LDL-apheresis reduces P-selectin, CRP and fibrinogen—Possible important implications for improving atherosclerosis. Ther Apher Dial 2006; 10(3):219-23.

109. Wang Y. Effects of heparin-mediated extracorporeal low-density lipoprotein precipitation beyond lowering proatherogenic lipoproteins—Reduction of circulating proinflammatory and procoagulatory markers. Atherosclerosis 2004; 175(1):145-50.

110. Muso E, Mune M, Yorioka N, et al. Beneficial effect of low-density lipoprotein apheresis (LDL-A) on refractory nephrotic syndrome (NS) due to focal glomerulosclerois (FGS). Clin Nephrol 2007;67(06):341-5.

111. Silverman GJ, Goodyear CS, Siegel DL. On the mechanism of staphylococcal protein A immunomodulation. Transfusion 2005;45(2):274-80.

112. Levy R, Pantanowitz L, Cloutier D, et al. Development of electronic medical record charting for hospital-based transfusion and apheresis medicine services: Early adoption perspectives. J Pathol Inform 2010;1:8.

113. Berman K. Therapeutic apheresis: A guide to billing and securing appropriate reimbursement. 2019 ed. Vancouver, Canada: American Society for Apheresis, 2019. [Available at https://www.apheresis.org/page/ApheresisReimbursem (accessed December 6, 2019).]

CHAPTER 26

The Collection and Processing of Hematopoietic Progenitor Cells

Laura S. Connelly-Smith, MBBCh, DM, and Michael L. Linenberger, MD, FACP

PLURIPOTENT HEMATOPOIETIC STEM cells, capable of self-renewal and differentiation, and committed lineage-restricted progenitor cells are collectively referred to as hematopoietic progenitor cells (HPCs). These cells are capable of reconstituting marrow function when transplanted into conditioned recipients. HPCs for clinical use can be collected either from marrow [HPC(M)], from peripheral blood after mobilization [HPC(A)], or from umbilical cord blood (UCB) collected at birth [HPC(CB)].[1,2] HPCs tend to reside with mesenchymal elements within the marrow microenvironment, their interaction generating a niche that supports and regulates hematopoiesis.[3] Cytoadhesive interactions between membrane receptors and ligands expressed on the microenvironment stromal cells and within the extracellular matrix ensure that HPCs mostly situate within the marrow.[4] Disruption of these cellular and microenvironmental interactions allows mobilization of the HPCs into the peripheral blood from where they can be collected. Mobilization can be accelerated with an increase in progenitor cells into the bloodstream following treatment with chemotherapy and by the administration of certain exogenous cytokines such as granulocyte colony-stimulating factor (G-CSF), granulocyte-macrophage colony-stimulating factor (GM-CSF), and stem cell factor (SCF). Plerixafor, a C-X-C chemokine receptor type 4 (CXCR4) receptor antagonist, allows for rapid mobilization of HPCs into the blood.[5] UCB contains HPCs that may be sufficient to reconstitute hematopoiesis.[6]

CD34 is a cell-surface antigen that is expressed on progenitor cells. Even though its exact function is undefined and is not specific to HPCs, CD34 is used for identifying and quantifying HPCs and can be used to select and enrich HPCs for transplantation.[7]

CLINICAL UTILITY

Hematopoietic progenitor/stem cell transplantation (HSCT) is an established procedure to treat many acquired and congenital disorders of the hematopoietic system ranging from hematologic malignancies to nonneoplastic immune disorders and hemoglobinopathies to disorders of enzyme metabolism. Several nonhematologic malignant and nonmalignant disorders are also selected indications for HSCT (Table 26-1). Certain indications for HSCT occur more frequently and are dependent on patient age. For instance, immunodeficiency and inborn errors of metabolism are

Laura S. Connelly-Smith, MBBCh, DM, Assistant Medical Director, Apheresis and Cellular Therapy, Seattle Cancer Care Alliance, Associate Professor, Division of Hematology, Department of Medicine, University of Washington, and Assistant Member, Clinical Research Division, Fred Hutchinson Cancer Research Center; and Michael L. Linenberger, MD, FACP, Medical Director, Apheresis and Cellular Therapy, Seattle Cancer Care Alliance, Professor, Division of Hematology, Department of Medicine, University of Washington, and Member, Clinical Research Division, Fred Hutchinson Cancer Research Center, Seattle, Washington
The authors have disclosed no conflicts of interest.

26

TABLE 26-1. Diseases Treated with Autologous or Allogeneic HSCT

Hematologic Malignancies
Leukemia
Multiple myeloma
Myelodysplasia
Non-Hodgkin lymphoma
Hodgkin disease
Myeloproliferative neoplasms (MPN)
Other Clonal Disorders of Marrow/Marrow Failure Syndromes
Severe aplastic anemia
Paroxysmal nocturnal hemoglobinuria
Fanconi anemia
Diamond-Blackfan anemia
Pure red cell aplasia
Amegakaryocytic thrombocytopenia
Inherited Metabolic Disorders
Mucopolysaccharidoses
Leukodystrophies
Gaucher disease
Lysosomal storage disorders
Congenital Immunodeficiency
Severe combined immunodeficiency (SCID)
Wiskott-Aldrich syndrome
Omenn syndrome
X-linked lymphoproliferative syndrome
Chronic granulomatous disease
Leukocyte adhesion deficiency
DiGeorge syndrome
Hemoglobinopathies
Sickle cell disease
Thalassemia
Other Nonhematologic Malignancies
Germ cell tumors
Neuroblastoma

TABLE 26-1. Diseases Treated with Autologous or Allogeneic HSCT (Continued)

Medulloblastoma
Ewing sarcoma
Wilms tumor
Autoimmune Diseases
Systemic sclerosis
Multiple sclerosis

more common in children, whereas adults more commonly have clonal disorders of their marrow or hematologic malignancies. The decision to perform any HSCT requires careful consideration with the complex integration of numerous variables framing a treatment plan. These include patient-specific goals, age, prognosis, disease progression, previous therapy, comorbidities, availability of a suitable HPC source, and the type of transplant being considered (eg, autologous vs allogeneic, myeloablative vs nonmyeloablative therapy).

Autologous Transplantation

Autologous HSCT refers to the donor and recipient being the same person. In autologous transplantation, the reinfusion of the patient's stem cells allows for the recovery of the marrow following the provision of high-dose therapy. The antitumor effect comes from the chemotherapy and radiotherapy used during the conditioning phase of transplantation. Chemotherapy received by patients can be associated with significant toxicity but requires less immune suppression than allogeneic transplantation. Autologous transplantation is most successful for patients whose marrow is not actively affected with the disease. For patients with marrow involvement in their malignant disease, there is always concern over the collection and reinfusion of cancer cells. Peripheral blood has, for the most part, replaced marrow as a graft source in the majority of the autologous HSCTs performed in the United States.[8] For autologous transplantation, the collected HPC product is cryopreserved until the patient has been deemed ready for preconditioning with high-dose preparative therapy be-

fore receiving the stored HPC(A) product. Notably, some resource-limited transplantation centers have successfully used short-term storage of HPC(A) products without cryopreservation for autologous transplantation.[9]

Autologous patients must be medically well enough to undergo mobilization and HPC procurement, and should be assessed for their suitability. Significant levels of prior chemotherapy or radiation or ongoing marrow disease involvement may make HPC mobilization and collection difficult because of reduced HPC quality or number. Patients must undergo a full medical evaluation with history and physical evaluation per institutional policies and procedures, accreditation standards, and regulatory requirements.[10,11] Unlike allogeneic transplantation, eligibility requirements are not mandated by the Food and Drug Administration (FDA) for autologous HSCT, so screening questionnaires to identify relevant infectious disease risk factors are not required. Similarly laboratory testing for human immunodeficiency virus types 1 and 2 (HIV-1/2), hepatitis B virus, hepatitis C virus, syphilis, and human T-cell lymphotropic virus types I and II (HTLV-I/II) is not mandated but should be assessed, because autologous products are cryopreserved and stored with other products; thus, the presence of these viruses is a cross-contamination risk.[11] (For discussion of infectious disease testing, see Chapter 7.) Autologous patients can still proceed to transplantation if tested positive for one of the relevant infectious diseases, but the apheresis product should be quarantined and stored in such a way as to minimize contamination risks (see "Cryopreservation"). All autologous HPC products must, however, be labeled to indicate that they are for autologous use only and that they have not been evaluated for infectious substances, unless all otherwise-applicable screening and testing has been performed as for allogeneic products.[11]

Allogeneic Transplantation

The aim of allogeneic transplantation is to replace a diseased or nonfunctioning hematopoietic and/or immune system with normal HPCs from a healthy related or unrelated donor. When allogeneic transplantation is used to treat malignant conditions, patients may receive aggressive conditioning with radiotherapy and/or chemotherapy regimens. Myeloablative regimens induce cytotoxicity and prevent rejection of the new graft. Posttransplantation immunosuppression is required to prevent graft-vs-host disease (GVHD). In allogeneic transplantation, the transplanted cells are also seen as therapeutic in view of the anticipated graft-vs-neoplasm (GVN) effect. For patients with inborn errors of metabolism, congenital immunodeficiency, or other diseases and conditions in which germline mutations are present in the patient's cells, the goal of allogeneic HSCT is to reconstitute a healthy lymphohematopoietic system while avoiding GVHD.

In the allogeneic setting, the healthy donor undergoes the HPC collection. Screening and testing for infectious diseases are mandated in the United States to determine whether transplantation of mobilized peripheral blood or UCB poses a risk for transmitting a relevant infectious disease to the recipient. US federal regulations are laid out in Title 21 of the *Code of Federal Regulations* (CFR), Part 1271 [covering human cells, tissues, and cellular and tissue-based products (HCT/Ps)].[11] Screening and testing include a standardized health questionnaire, a physical examination, a review of the relevant medical records, and applicable testing for relevant infectious diseases. Although marrow products are administered under Sections 375 and 379 of the Public Health Service Act and are not subject to CFR Part 1271, marrow donors are screened and tested similarly to mobilized peripheral blood and UCB donors, because all three products are treated similarly under the standards of various accrediting bodies, such as AABB and the Foundation for the Accreditation of Cellular Therapy (FACT), and by the National Marrow Donor Program (NMDP). For HPC(CB) transplantation, the screening and testing process involves the mother and her samples. In the United States, there are currently no donor tests that have been approved for UCB samples; therefore, infectious disease testing is performed on a maternal sample. The maternal blood samples serve as a surrogate for the UCB unit, and testing should reflect the health of the mother at the time the unit is collected, ideally having been taken within 7 days of UCB collection.

Relevant infectious disease agents that can be transmitted by HPCs to the transplant recipient, and for which there is an FDA-licensed screening test, include HIV, hepatitis B and C viruses, *Treponema pallidum*, HTLV-I/II, *Trypanosoma cruzi*, West Nile virus, and cytomegalovirus (CMV). Appropriate screening measures have been developed for Zika virus (ZIKV), such as review of medical and travel history. Two FDA-licensed ZIKV assays are available to screen whole blood and blood components for transfusion. One is also FDA-approved for use in testing plasma or serum specimens from HPC donors. However, the FDA does not consider this test appropriate for preventing transmission of ZIKV through HCT/Ps, because ZIKV is readily detected in HCT/Ps after viral RNA is no longer detectable in plasma.[12]

If donor screening or testing detects a risk of transmitting a relevant infectious disease, the potential HPC donor is considered ineligible. The donor, recipient, and their physicians are informed of the donor's ineligible status, and a risk/benefit analysis is performed to determine whether the donor's HPCs might still be considered safe to use. If a decision is made to proceed with transplantation using the ineligible donor's HPCs, justification must be documented under "urgent medical need" criteria, as defined by the FDA. Finally, in addition to screening and testing for infectious diseases, the donor's medical fitness is evaluated to determine whether the donor is healthy enough to safely undergo HPC mobilization and collection.

HISTOCOMPATIBILITY, DONOR TYPE, AND GRAFT SOURCE

Histocompatibility

One of the major barriers influencing the clinical success of allogeneic HSCT is compatibility across the highly polymorphic classical HLA system. The transplantation physician preferably selects an HLA-compatible donor in order to reduce the risk of graft failure, GVHD, and mortality.[13-15] The HLA alleles that are important for HSCT compatibility are the Class I genes *HLA-A*, *-B*, and *-C*, and the Class II genes *HLA-DRB1*, *-DQB1*, and *-DPB1*. Other HLA genes are less important either because they have low levels of polymorphism (because they are pseudogenes) or because they are minimally or not expressed. The human major histocompatibility complex (MHC), where HLA genes are found, displays "linkage disequilibrium," where certain alleles are inherited together more frequently than would occur by chance. This inheritance pattern is not random and explains why an HLA-identical sibling is more likely to be an exact match and thus preferred as the optimal donor. Unfortunately, ~70% of patients will not have a suitable sibling match.

Molecular techniques (high-resolution DNA-based tissue typing) have supplanted serologic methods for HLA typing. This has led to a significant improvement in resolution and matching at the allele level. Allogeneic transplantation using either HPC(A) or HPC(M) that are mismatched at *HLA-A*, *-B*, *-C*, and *-DRB1* loci (by high-resolution typing) are associated with a 5% to 10% decrease in survival with each mismatch.[16] Thus, patients should be typed using high-resolution techniques at the *HLA-A*, *-B*, *-C*, and *-DRB1* loci to facilitate finding an optimal donor. The matching process considers both of the inherited alleles for each of these four loci, for a total of eight possible matches; alternatively, if *DQB1* and *DPB1* are also considered, 10 or 12 alleles are examined. Because two large studies failed to show an individual impact of *DQB1* on survival, it is common practice in US centers to consider an 8/8-matched donor as "fully matched." Other studies, however, have shown

a lower survival with *DQB1* mismatching, and in particular if this mismatch is added to a mismatch at *HLA-A*, *-B*, *-C*, and *-DRB1*. As a result, *HLA-DQB1*, *-DPB1*, and *-DRB3/4/5* may be added to prioritize donors with minimal or permissible mismatching at these loci, especially if a 10/10 or 12/12 match is being considered.[17] High-resolution 8/8- and 10/10-matched transplants of HPCs from unrelated donors are, at least in part, responsible for recently improved survival outcomes of matched unrelated-donor transplantations for several diseases.[18-25] The great diversity of HLA alleles and haplotypes makes identifying an unrelated donor matched at allelic resolutions a major challenge for most patients.[26,27] The likelihood of finding an optimally HLA-matched unrelated donor (MUD) ranges from 75% for patients of European ancestry to 16% for South or Central Americans of African ancestry.[28] In addition, the time needed to procure a graft from an unrelated donor may be up to 8 weeks.[29] With these ongoing limitations to donor availability, alternate sources of stem cells have been identified and include UCB, as well as haploidentical and mismatched related donors or mismatched unrelated donors.

Studies show that survival after UCB transplantation is similar to other graft sources, and emerging data demonstrate acceptable outcomes with haploidentical donor transplantation.[30-37] Due to the immaturity of UCB T cells, the HLA matching requirements for UCB are less stringent than those for marrow and mobilized peripheral blood HPCs, but HLA matching is still an important factor for engraftment. Conventionally, HLA matching of UCB for HSCT has used low-/intermediate-resolution typing for HLA-A and HLA-B (antigenic level) and high-resolution typing for *HLA-DRB1* (allelic level). HLA matching for UCB units is generally based on three loci, and a maximum of 2/6 HLA mismatches is considered acceptable, with a very high transplant-related mortality (TRM) associated with greater mismatch.[38] Provided that sufficient cell dose is achieved, the outcomes of 4/6-matched UCB transplants are comparable to that of HLA- matched unrelated donors, albeit with an increased risk of nonrelapse mortality (NRM).[1] In a study analyzing the role of HLA-C on UCB transplantation, Eurocord and NMDP/

CIBMTR (Center for International Blood and Marrow Transplant Research) reported higher TRM in patients receiving a UCB unit with an HLA-C mismatch; also, contemporary mismatching at HLA-C and HLA-DRB1 was associated with the highest risk of mortality.[39] When using a single unit of HPC(CB), HLA-C antigen mismatching was shown to increase TRM, particularly if combined with HLA-DRB1 mismatching. When using double HPC(CB) units (as in most adult patients), there are no guidelines for HLA matching between the two units other than the minimum requirement, for each unit, of 4/6 HLA matches with the patient's HLA specificities. Nevertheless, some centers prefer to use at least a 4/6 match between the two units. With UCB, it is also possible to select permissible HLA mismatches with reduced immunogenicity, such as the noninherited maternal antigens (NIMA). NIMA matching is not essential, although in patients with hematologic malignancies, NIMA-matched grafts have been associated with a lower TRM and improved engraftment, leading to reduced overall mortality compared with HLA-mismatched, non-NIMA-matched grafts.[40]

Haploidentical transplantation, using an HPC donor who is a parent, a child, or a sibling matched at only half of the HLA loci with the recipient, is becoming more common as a result of advances in GVHD prevention. A major component of success with haploidentical transplantation is the use of posttransplantation cyclophosphamide.[41] Advantages of haploidentical HPC transplants include faster procurement and near-universal donor availability because the majority of patients needing an allogeneic HPC transplant have access to one first-degree relative.[29,42] Haploidentical HSCT presents unique challenges, including overcoming immunologic barriers between donor and recipient with chemotherapy or HPC product manipulation. HSCT in recipients with antibodies against donor HLA determinants have a higher risk of primary graft failure and associated adverse outcomes.[43] It is essential to test the recipient for preformed donor-specific antibodies (DSAs) for HLA. The antibody level at which DSAs have a significant impact is not clear, nor is the appropriate course of action when DSAs are detected; however, when an alternative donor is lacking, reduction of strong-reacting DSAs must be attempted.[44]

Other Considerations for Donor Selection

Donor selection for allogeneic transplantation is determined largely by histocompatibility. However, several other variables are taken into consideration, especially when more than one equivalent HLA-matched unrelated donor is available and eligible. These include the underlying disease and the disease stage, the clinical stability of the patient, CMV status of the patient and donor, ABO blood group matching with the patient, donor gender and age, weight discrepancy between donor and patient, and, in some institutions, killer cell immunoglobulin-like receptor (KIR) status of the donor.[1] Male gender, younger age, nulliparity, matching of ABO and CMV status, and greater size of the donor relative to the recipient may have positive effects. For example, survival is greater for recipients of grafts from younger, unrelated donors aged 18-32 years compared to grafts from older donors, after controlling for HLA compatibility.[45] Other variables specific to HPC(CB) donation include maternal history as well as UCB collection, processing, and unit storage conditions.[46] A scoring system, the "cord blood apgar," has been derived to determine the utility of the HPC(CB) unit by considering the total nucleated cell (TNC) count, CD34+ cell count, colony-forming-unit (CFU) count, mononuclear cell (MNC) content, and product volume.[47]

Graft Source

Graft sources include HPC(A), HPC(M) and HPC(CB). The choice of graft source is determined mostly by the transplantation center's preference and experience. Donor preference should also be considered. The three sources of grafts have biologic differences related to their different cellular composition. HPC(A) products, the preferred source for autologous and allogeneic transplantation in adults, engraft faster, reconstitute immunity more quickly, and may exert a greater GVN effect when compared to HPC(M) and HPC(CB). These features make

HPC(A) attractive for patients undergoing non-myeloablative (NMA) and reduced-intensity conditioning (RIC) regimens and may offer an advantage in overall and disease-free survival for selected patients with late-stage hematologic malignancies.[48] Chronic GVHD (cGVHD) continues to be a major long-term complication of HPC(A) grafts.

HPC(M) was the primary source of HPCs before the availability of mobilized peripheral blood grafts collected by leukocytapheresis, and allogeneic HPC(M) from pediatric sibling donors continues to be used predominantly in children. HPC(M) products have significantly fewer T cells than HPC(A) products, and as a result have a higher risk of engraftment failure and delayed immune reconstitution, as well as a potential risk of disease relapse (ie, less GVN effect). However, HPC(M) grafts are associated with lower risk of cGVHD. In recipients of myeloablative transplants from unrelated donors for hematologic malignancies, a randomized controlled trial indicated that HPC(M) and mobilized HPC(A) grafts yield equivalent effects on survival. However, marrow grafts were associated with less cGVHD but more graft failure.[49] In children, the risk of engraftment failure is lower with HPC(M), as they usually receive adequate CD34+ cells due to their smaller body weight. Children may also better tolerate infectious complications when immune reconstitution is delayed, compared to adults, who also often have more serious medical comorbidities. The risk of relapse of neoplastic diseases with HPC(M) (by virtue of lesser GVN effect) may be mitigated by myeloablative regimens, which children can tolerate better than adults.

HPC(CB) units are cryopreserved and usually readily available from cord blood banks after acceptable matched units are identified. They are typically of small volume with 1-log-fewer TNCs and CD34+ cells/recipient weight, compared to HPC(A) and HPC(M) grafts. For most adults, 2 units [double cord transplantation or double HPC(CB) transplants] are required in order to constitute an adequate dose for a successful transplantation. When double cord units are used, eventually only one HPC(CB) unit engrafts and the other one disappears after contributing to cellular immune support during the early posttransplantation period. HPC(CB) grafts have more immature T cells and, thus, are less immunologically reactive. Consequently, they are associated with higher risk of engraftment failure (particularly with NMA regimens) and delayed immune reconstitution. By comparison, the potential for neoplastic disease relapse may be lower for patients receiving HPC(CB) grafts for malignancy and minimal residual disease at the time of transplantation.[34] The risk of GVHD with UCB depends on the degree of HLA disparity with the recipient.

HPC COLLECTION

Patients undergoing HPC collection for a future autologous transplantation are evaluated for their medical fitness and ability to tolerate either marrow harvest or mobilization treatment with G-CSF and leukocytapheresis. Allogeneic donors, once selected, also require evaluations to ensure the safety of the donation process (ie, donor suitability) for them, in addition to assessments to minimize the risk of transmission of infectious disease agents (ie, donor eligibility). Allogeneic donor eligibility is determined through compliance with the screening requirements mandated by FDA regulations (21 CFR 1271). Suitability determination and risk assessment for related and unrelated donors are based on accreditation standards and published consensus guidelines and criteria.[50-53] After screening results are available, the donor is documented to be either: eligible and suitable; acceptable as a donor despite ineligibility (and justified through urgent medical need criteria); or declared ineligible or medically unsuitable and deferred from donation.

Informed consent must be obtained from all autologous patients and allogeneic donors or their designated representatives before any collection procedure. The consent process includes providing the donor with information regarding the risks and benefits of the selected procedure, any tests required to protect the recipient, alternative collection methods, and protection of donor health information. In the case of allogeneic transplantation, the donor should be made aware of any potential consequences of not proceeding with the donation once the recipient has started conditioning therapy. The donor is always given the opportunity to ask questions and to refuse donation. Consent must be obtained from the maternal donor for UCB collection, processing, testing, storage, and medical use.[54] A medical order is required for procurement and must include collection goals.[50(p59)]

Facilities that collect HPCs are required to ensure donor access to medical care based on the risks and clinical situation associated with each type of donation. Licensed providers, nurses, and allied health professionals must be trained and experienced in HPC procurement and product handling. They must be competent to manage any potential adverse events (AEs) incurred by donors and patients and any technical variances that might affect the integrity or quality of the HPC product.

Marrow HPC Collection

Marrow harvest is an invasive operative procedure performed under sterile conditions and typically under general anesthesia. In addition to undergoing relevant donor screening, infectious disease testing, and HLA compatibility testing, marrow donors must also be physically suitable for donation and be able to tolerate the type of anesthesia required to perform the harvest successfully. The donor's preoperative physical status can be assessed using the American Society of Anesthesiologists Physical Status (ASA-PS) classification system.[55] Donors with preexisting ischemic heart disease, cardiac failure, cerebrovascular disease, insulin-dependent diabetes mellitus, or liver or renal dysfunction are at higher risk of AEs with general anesthesia.[56] Donors with serious oropharyngeal, neck, back, spine, or hip conditions; abnormal platelet function or coagulopathy; or history of malignant hyperthermia should be precluded due to the risks of anesthesia. Donors should be counseled about potential bone, nerve, or vessel damage and bleeding during or after the marrow harvest. Autologous donors may have had previous radiation therapy to the pelvis, which will limit the amount of marrow nucleated cells available in the posterior iliac crests.

A high recipient-to-donor weight ratio may require a relatively high volume of marrow to be collected from a small donor who has limited total blood volume. In such cases, preoperative autologous blood storage can be considered to avoid the potential need for allogeneic red cell transfusion. The NMDP guidelines suggest removing no more than 20 mL of marrow per kilogram of donor weight.[57] The volume of the harvest is dictated by the recipient's weight, the underlying diagnosis, and by treatment protocol. Usually a minimum of 2 to 3×10^8 nucleated cells/kg recipient weight are needed to facilitate efficient engraftment. Checking the nucleated cell concentration of an aliquot from the marrow product midway through the harvest can help estimate the total volume of marrow needed to reach the TNC goal and will prevent unnecessary blood loss. Determination of CD34+ cell concentration midway through the procedure is not practical, given the slow turnaround time for this assay and the high priority to minimize the procedure and anesthesia time.

Marrow harvest techniques vary considerably, depending on institutional practice; however, a standard approach by experienced operators optimizes donor safety and product quality.[57] At least two individuals are required to perform the procedure, one of whom is the senior surgeon. After the induction of anesthesia, the donor is placed in the prone position and the posterior iliac crests are aseptically prepared and draped with sterile barriers. An 11- to 14-gauge needle with attached syringe flushed with anticoagulant is inserted into each posterior iliac crest, and approximately 5 mL of marrow is aspirated. The needle and syringe are then rotated up to 180 degrees, and the aspiration is repeated. Large-volume aspiration is avoided to prevent significant peripheral blood contamination of the product. The aspirated marrow is then collected into a large collection bag containing heparin anticoagulant mixed with acid-citrate-dextrose formula A (ACD-A) anticoagulant, tissue culture medium, or physiologic buffer. Approved collection systems incorporate in-line filters to remove bone spicules, aggregates, and debris. The process is repeated at different bone sites (aiming to minimize the number of skin puncture sites) until the target TNC count or maximum safe donor-volume limit is reached.

Marrow donation is generally considered a safe procedure in healthy donors, and serious complications of marrow harvest are rare. Minor complications, such as pain at the site of harvest, fatigue, insomnia, nausea, dizziness, and anorexia, occur frequently but resolve in most donors by 1 month after the procedure.[58] A large study of unrelated marrow donors observed a 3% prevalence of persistent discomfort compared to baseline at 6 months.[59] Not surprisingly, marrow donors suffer more immediate postdonation physical side effects compared to donors of HPC(A) products; however, their overall experience over the long term is equivalent.[60,61] Marrow donors often have significant decreases in hemoglobin concentration after the procedure. Depending on the marrow volume to be collected, marrow donors may be advised to store an autologous unit of Red Blood Cells (RBCs) before the procedure. Historically, up to 70% to 76% of marrow donors received at least 1 autologous RBC unit during or shortly after marrow harvest.[58,59,62] More recently, the utility of autologous blood storage and transfusion in this setting has been questioned.[63] If the donor requires an allogeneic RBC or platelet transfusion before or during the procedure, the units should be irradiated to prevent contamination of the graft by viable leukocytes from these blood components. Marrow donors should be made aware during the informed consent process that they might need a transfusion.

Peripheral Blood HPC Collection

Over the last few decades, HPC(A) products containing mobilized peripheral blood HPCs have been the most frequently used graft source of CD34+ cells for autologous and allogeneic transplantation. Collection of HPC(A) is performed mostly as an outpatient procedure because of the ease of the procedure and limited side effects. Adequate vascular access is required to accommodate the high flow rates necessary for efficient blood processing. In patients undergoing HPC(A) collection for autologous transplantation, a semipermanent (tunneled) apheresis central venous catheter (CVC) is com-

monly placed and used for both HPC(A) collection and longer-term intravenous (IV) fluid/ medication administration during the transplantation process. Peripheral venous access is usually sufficient for adult allogeneic donors who can tolerate one or two procedures using two large-bore needles (16/17 gauge). Nevertheless, 7% to 10% of healthy volunteer donors overall and approximately 20% of female donors require a temporary central venous catheter.[59] CVCs are usually placed in the internal jugular veins, and less commonly in the subclavian, avoiding femoral access because of the higher risk of infection and discomfort. CVCs are associated with additional risks such as bleeding, thrombosis, and pneumothorax. Correct placement of the line needs to be confirmed before apheresis for HPC(A) collection.[50(p58)]

For patients undergoing autologous transplantation, HPCs are mobilized into the peripheral circulation using hematopoietic growth factors, most commonly G-CSF (filgrastim) with or without mobilization chemotherapeutic agents.[64-68] More recently, HPC mobilization in patients has been augmented with adjunctive use of plerixafor, the reversible CXCR4 receptor antagonist.[69-72] Long-acting, pegylated G-CSF (pegfilgrastim) and biosimilar forms of G-CSF are also now available as alternative mobilizing agents, with efficacy equivalent to filgrastim.[66,73] Other hematopoietic growth factors, such as GM-CSF, are rarely used for HPC mobilization. Adult allogeneic donors undergo HPC mobilization with G-CSF alone. Chemotherapy is never used to mobilize stem cells in healthy donors, and plerixafor is still an experimental agent for this indication.[74] Mobilized HPC(A) collections using G-CSF have been safely performed in sibling pediatric donors, but this is not a uniform practice in all pediatric transplantation centers.[75]

Myeloid hematopoietic growth factors, such as G-CSF, cause expansion of the granulocytic population in the marrow and the release of proteases that disrupt several cytoadhesive "anchors" that retain HPCs within the hematopoietic niche. This includes the binding of CXCR4 on the HPC membrane with stromal-cell-derived factor 1 (SDF1) in the marrow stroma. When used alone, G-CSF is administered daily over at least 4 to 5 days to achieve a major mobilization effect and significant increase in circulating CD34+ stem/progenitor cells. As monotherapy or after mobilization chemotherapy, G-CSF is typically dosed at 10 µg/kg/day; however, higher daily doses (up to 16 µg/kg/day in two divided doses) have been given.[65,66,68] For practical purposes, G-CSF doses are often rounded to the nearest vial size, and effective dosing may be based on adjusted ideal body weight in obese patients.[66,68] When mobilizing HPCs from "steady state" (ie, without prior chemotherapy), apheresis is usually initiated 96-120 hours after the start of G-CSF administration, when the peripheral CD34+ cell concentration is peaking. Leukocytapheresis is optimized for collection of MNCs and will yield a product rich in CD34+ cells. Daily G-CSF administration and leukocytapheresis continues until the desired number of CD34+ cells are obtained.

The time course of HPC mobilization and apheresis after chemotherapy plus G-CSF varies based on the treatment regimen and the patient's baseline clinical and hematologic status.[66,68] Certain chemotherapy agents at specific doses will cause significant but transient marrow suppression. During the recovery from marrow suppression, there is a substantial increase in the number of circulating CD34+ cells, and this effect can be magnified by the daily administration of G-CSF. This chemo-mobilization approach leads to a sharp increase in circulating CD34+ cells, typically at 9 to 11 days from the administration of chemotherapy, at which time daily leukocytapheresis is initiated.[65,66,68] The threshold for starting leukocytapheresis is typically when the CD34+ cell count is at 10/µL or greater. Side effects of G-CSF are common, mild, and transient. These include bone pain, myalgia, headache, insomnia, and flu-like symptoms; less frequently, sweating, anorexia, fever, chills, and nausea occur.[58-62,68,75] Potentially serious complications, such as splenic rupture, severe thrombocytopenia, and acute lung injury are rare.

For some autologous patients and, rarely, allogeneic donors, mobilization of HPCs can be challenging and result in inadequate collections. Cases of poor mobilization may require additional pharmacotherapy or repeat attempts at mobilization in order to achieve an adequate

number of CD34+ cells for efficient engraftment. The minimum number of cells needed for transplantation is commonly cited as 2×10^6 CD34+ cells/kg recipient weight, although 5×10^6 CD34+ cells/kg is more desirable.[76-79] Patients with poor mobilization may benefit from higher-dose G-CSF and/or the addition of plerixafor in combination with G-CSF. Various clinical studies have demonstrated that plerixafor in combination with G-CSF significantly increases HPC collection yields compared to G-CSF alone.[69-72] Several clinical scenarios where plerixafor was used as a salvage agent have been described.[66,72] Randomized clinical trials in patients with multiple myeloma or lymphoma have demonstrated that the addition of plerixafor to G-CSF can double the circulating CD34+ cell HPCs, allowing fewer apheresis procedures to collect a sufficient quantity of HPCs.[70,71,80]

Procurement of HPC(A) from a patient or donor by leukocytapheresis typically involves processing two to three times the total blood volume (TBV). This translates to processing 10-12 L for an adult in accordance with the instrument hardware, software programming, and manufacturer's instructions. Large-volume leukocytapheresis (LVL), which involves processing between three and six times the TBV, is frequently performed to collect higher numbers of CD34+ cells in children and adults undergoing autologous HSCT.[81]

Anticoagulation used for HPC(A) collection varies according to local institutional practices and instrument requirements. The standard anticoagulant is ACD-A, either alone or in combination with heparin.[82] Toxicities and side effects of ACD-A are related to hypocalcemia, with symptoms of paresthesias, muscle irritability, and, less commonly, muscle spasm and cardiac arrhythmia. For LVL procedures, the requirement for high volumes of ACD-A over the course of treatment can lead to a large net-positive fluid balance and potential fluid overload complications. Up to 20% of donors experience minor apheresis/collection-related AEs, such as citrate toxicity, nausea, fatigue, chills, hypertension, hypotension, allergic reactions, or syncope.[59,62,75] Use of heparin results in modest systemic anticoagulation for a short time after completion of the procedure, with mild bleeding risks in patients with severe thrombocytopenia. Adjunctive use of heparin also carries a small risk of heparin-induced thrombocytopenia (HIT).[82] The benefit of heparin-based anticoagulation during HPC(A) collection is that the total volume of anticoagulant can be two to three times smaller, thereby decreasing risk of volume overload and citrate toxicity.

Once HPC collection starts, daily apheresis continues until the target CD34+ cell goal is reached. Prediction algorithms can be used to estimate the required processed blood volume to achieve a desired CD34+ cell yield. The algorithms use a precollection CD34+ count along with the expected collection efficiency for the standard or large-volume leukocytapheresis procedure.[83,84] Institutions vary in their practice in terms of when to commence HPC(A) collections, with some centers measuring CD34+ cell levels before collection in each patient, and others using this approach only in patients with known risk factors of mobilization failure. For most allogeneic donors, sufficient numbers of HPCs can be obtained in one to two collections commencing on day 4 or 5 of G-CSF administration. A complete blood count, including platelet count, is required within 24 hours before leukocytapheresis. This is especially important for autologous patients recovering from mobilization chemotherapy, because they may still be thrombocytopenic at the time of collection, and the apheresis procedure itself reduces the blood platelet count by 30% to 50%.[51,59,75,81]

Some studies have demonstrated that the absolute lymphocyte count on day 15 after transplantation (ALC-15) is an independent prognostic factor for improved survival after autologous HSCT for certain hematologic malignancies.[85] In addition, increasing the number of apheresis collections to achieve an absolute count of >0.5 × 10^9 lymphocytes/kg has been associated with early ALC recovery and improved outcomes.[85-88] Although it may be possible to perform additional lymphocyte collections without mobilization, the costs of additional days of collection and processing are not inconsequential. More data, including randomized clinical trials, need to be obtained and analyzed to confirm the applicability of these observations in other populations to define the potential financial and survival benefits.

Umbilical Cord Blood HPC Collection

UCB can be collected either before delivery of the placenta (in utero) or after delivery of the placenta (ex utero) in either a vaginal or cesarean birth. Several reports have suggested higher collection volumes with cesarean deliveries and when UCB is collected in utero.[89,90] Both in- and ex-utero collection methods continue to be routinely used, but in-utero collections are more common.[90] UCB is collected by cannulating the umbilical vein and allowing the placental blood to be removed by gravity into collection containers to which anticoagulation, most commonly citrate-phosphate-dextrose (CPD), has been added. Closed systems using collection bags have reduced the incidence of bacterial contamination.[91] The collection bag is weighed to estimate the collection volume. The volume collected varies but usually ranges from 50 to 200 mL. There is a close correlation between the weight of the bag and the TNC count, and often cord blood banks will have a minimum volume threshold for the UCB to be shipped to the processing laboratory. Some cord blood banks establish thresholds for banking based on TNC and will measure the TNC at the collection site. Factors associated with higher UCB volumes and greater yield of nucleated cells include birthweight, placental weight, gestational age, induction of labor, prolonged labor, cesarean section, early cord clamping, firstborn infants, European ancestry, and female infant gender.[92] The training and experience of the UCB collector will often also have an effect on the volumes obtained.

All studies focused on HPC(CB) have demonstrated the impact that infused TNCs, CFUs, and CD34+ cells have on engraftment, transplant-related events, and survival.[93,94] Sometimes, and particularly in adults, there is an insufficient cell dose in a single HPC(CB) for transplantation. This cell dose limitation has been overcome by the development of double HPC(CB) transplantations.[95] A large CIBMTR study demonstrated that double HPC(CB) transplants had similar outcomes to single HPC(CB) transplants in patients with acute myelogenous leukemia.[96] This has been confirmed by other studies in patients with hematologic malignancies.[97,98] According to several different reports, a minimum TNC count of 3×10^7/kg at cryopreservation needs to be obtained for engraftment.[94,95] For double HPC(CB) transplants, some centers require that each HPC(CB) unit has a minimum TNC count of 1.5×10^7/kg at cryopreservation.[99] A cryopreserved TNC dose of 2.5×10^7 cells/kg, however, has typically been accepted as the minimum cell dose for successful engraftment in single HPC(CB) transplants.[99] In double HPC(CB) transplants, an arbitrary precryopreservation CD34+ cell dose of $\geq 1 \times 10^5$/kg has been used by several transplantation centers as the minimum accepted cell doses for each unit.[99]

PROCESSING HUMAN PROGENITOR CELLS

After collection, HPC products are transferred from the operating room or apheresis center to the processing facility either at room temperature or at 2 to 8 C, depending on the type of product and anticipated duration of transportation and storage. The HPC product may subsequently undergo quality control (QC) testing that may include cell enumeration, flow cytometric immunophenotypic studies, sterility testing, and viability studies. Some products will require further processing, cryopreservation, and storage. Cryopreserved HPC products that are anticipated to be stored for many years should be maintained under conditions that retain cell viability and function as demonstrated by stability studies. Processing refers to all aspects of manipulation, cryopreservation, packaging, and labeling of cellular therapy products. During processing, steps are taken to guarantee the potency and purity of the product for transplantation and/or storage.

HPC processing methods are often divided into basic/routine (minimal manipulation) procedures that are commonly used in clinical cell processing laboratories, and more specialized manipulations that involve complex technologies and more than minimal manipulation of the product (see next section).[100] Centrifuged-based processing is commonly used for plasma reduction, red cell reduction, and buffy-coat preparation before cryopreservation and storage. For clinical indications, plasma or volume reduction may be required for a minor-ABO-mismatched allograft (marrow or peripheral blood) with high titers of anti-A and/or anti-B to reduce the amount of donor isoagglutinins and risks of recipient hemolysis.[101] Plasma volume reduction might also be required to prevent fluid overload in recipients with small body weight or those with renal disease or cardiac failure. Before storage, product volume reduction is often necessary to concentrate the cells and reduce the volume before addition of cryopreservative and freezing. The smaller volumes following plasma reduction allow for a smaller number of bags that require storage, thawing, and infusing. Smaller volume translates into reduced risk of dimethylsulfoxide (DMSO) toxicity at the time of infusion.

Red Cell and Plasma Reduction

Red cell reduction may be required to prevent hemolysis of donor cells in major-ABO-mismatched allografts that contain an unacceptable volume of red cells for a recipient with anti-A and/or anti-B isoagglutinin titers >16.[101] The amount of acceptable incompatible red cells in the final product is defined by institutional policy but is usually in the range of 20 to 30 mL or 0.2 to 0.4 mL/kg (for pediatric recipients).[101] Most HPC(A) products have low hematocrits and smaller product volumes such that the risk of a hemolytic transfusion reaction is minimal. By comparison, HPC(M) products have high hematocrits and larger total volume and red cell volume such that red cell reduction is frequently required. Cord blood banks often reduce red cells from products before cryopreservation.[102] This minimizes unwanted red cells that lyse on thawing and reduces the final volume to optimize storage space and limit costs.

Classically, HPC product red cell reduction employs sedimentation agents such as hydroxyethyl starch (HES) and centrifugation to pellet the red cells, or gravity, where hanging the bag allows for sedimentation.[100] If both major and minor ABO mismatches exist (termed bidirectional ABO incompatibility), red cells and plasma may need to be reduced from the product. For larger marrow volumes, buffy-coat concentration of marrow may be achieved by centrifugation and harvesting using an apheresis or cell-washing device.[100,103] Newer apheresis instruments can efficiently reduce red cells from larger-volume marrow products with excellent CD34+ cell recovery.[104] Regardless of the method used, both volume and red cell reduction procedures must be weighed against the potential loss of HPC numbers and viability and increased risk of contamination during the additional manipulations.

Storage Preparation

Most allogeneic HPC(M) and HPC(A) products are infused fresh within 48 to 72 hours after collection. If the fresh products are not intended to be infused within that time, they are cryopreserved.[105] HPC(A) that are transported or stored for more than a few hours should be maintained at 2 to 8 C and, ideally, diluted to a cell concentration that minimizes metabolic stress. By comparison, HPC(M) products do not require dilution and may be stored and transported at room temperature for up to 48 to 72 hours without significant loss of CD34+ cell viability or numbers.[106] Autologous HPC(A) products are concentrated and cryopreserved until the patient has undergone preconditioning therapy and is ready for transplantation.

Washing

Washing the thawed HPC product after cryopreservation removes lysed red cells, hemoglobin, and the cryoprotectant (ie, DMSO). Because some HPCs may be lost with postthaw manipulation and washing of cryopreserved HPC(M) and HPC(A) products, this processing step is not routinely performed. By comparison, cryopreserved HPC(CB) products are routinely processed after thawing even if they have undergone red cell reduction before storage.[102] Historically, most institutions based their HPC(CB) processing methods, including the thawing/washing process, on the procedure adopted by the New York Placental Blood Program.[107] This involves slow, sequential addition of a wash solution (eg, 10% dextran followed by 5% albumin), transfer into an appropriately sized bag for centrifugation, and resuspension of the cell pellet(s) before delivery to the patient-care unit for infusion. Some laboratories perform two centrifugation steps—removing the supernatant from the first spin and centrifuging that portion a second time before combining the two cell pellets; this optimizes cell recovery.[108] In order to minimize cell loss, several processing laboratories are now thawing and diluting the HPC(CB) product without washing the cells.[102,108-111] With these no-wash methods, studies have demonstrated a high rate of engraftment with a low incidence of serious adverse reactions following HPC(CB) infusion.[109,110]

In selected circumstances, such as for patients with a documented severe DMSO allergy, washing thawed HPC products may be the safer choice. Washing to remove DMSO and other additives raises concerns over loss of HPCs due to additional manipulation and increased exposure time of cells to DMSO. Various procedures have been developed to remove DMSO through manual or automated methods, and some of these have been associated with reduced infusion-related AEs.[112-114] Importantly, the cellular component of thawed HPC(A) products, particularly granulocytes, may also contribute to toxicities during or shortly after reinfusion.[115] Separating out these cellular components and debris after thawing to mitigate toxicity is technically challenging; however, limiting the number of infused nucleated cells can reduce severe infusion-related complications.[116] In most settings, it is safe to infuse the cryopreserved HPC(A) product directly into the patient after the thawing process is completed at the bedside.

Thawing

Cryopreserved HPC(A) or HPC(M) products are usually thawed at the time and place of the planned infusion—typically at the bedside. This is done to minimize the amount of time cells are exposed to DMSO in the liquid state after thawing and before infusion. Rapid thawing in a 37 C waterbath followed by infusion as quickly and safely as possible is recommended to avoid DMSO-mediated cytotoxicity.[117] Caution must be used, however, because frozen plastic containers are prone to breakage.[118] The cryopreserved product is usually brought to the bedside in a liquid-nitrogen dry shipper. After removal, the product must be handled with care while it is verified to determine the product's identity and ensure the integrity of the bag. The product is then placed into a clean or sterile plastic overwrap bag and submerged in a 37 C waterbath. While the bags are in the waterbath, the product is gently massaged to achieve an icy slush consistency. If the product bag breaks, the cells may be recovered from the outer bag; however, a risk/benefit discussion should occur regarding the need for infusing potentially contaminated cells. The same risk applies when the washing of a cellular component is required. If bag leakage occurs, a hemostat should be used to prevent loss of the product, and the contents should be aseptically diverted into a transfer bag.[112] A sample should also be sent for culture. Local hospital and laboratory policies must be followed for recipients with multiple products to be infused at a given time. Many facilities thaw and infuse products sequentially to ensure that the previous unit was infused safely and without major AEs before thawing and infusing the next bag.

SPECIALIZED CELL-PROCESSING METHODS

Specialized processing of HPC products can optimize product purity and potency beyond levels obtained by routine methods. More-specialized manipulations require unique reagents and instrumentation, and these are discussed elsewhere. Therefore, the descriptions of methods in this chapter are brief and focus on their application to HPCs.

Elutriation

Counterflow centrifugal elutriation separates cell populations based on two physical characteristics—size and density (sedimentation coefficient)—and uses a stream of fluid/media flowing in a direction usually opposite to the direction of gravity sedimentation. A centrifuge

separates the cell populations of a cell product based on density alone. However, as the liquids are passed through the chamber housing the cells in the direction opposite (counterflow) to the centrifugal force, adjustment of flow rate and/or centrifugation speed also allows separation of cell populations based on size.[119,120] Through this process, cells with specific size and density profiles can be separated from other cells. This method has been successfully used to isolate monocytes from apheresis products for vaccine applications and lymphocytes for adoptive immunotherapy. This method was also historically used for T-cell depletion of HPC grafts.

Cell-Selection Systems

In positive cell selection, strategies are employed to mark and isolate a target cell population of interest that becomes the desired HPC product. Immunomagnetic cell-selection systems such as the CliniMACS system (Miltenyi Biotec Bergisch) incorporate monoclonal antibody-based technologies to target cell-surface antigens. For positive cell selection of CD34+ cells or CD34+ enrichment, a magnetically labeled CD34 monoclonal antibody reagent is mixed with the HPC product to first tag the cells. Magnetically labeled target cells are retained as the cell suspension passes through a column in which a magnetic field is generated. Unlabeled cells pass through the column and are collected in a negative-fraction bag. Once the column has been washed to ensure that only the CD34+ cells are retained, bound cells are then released from the column by removal of the magnetic field. The CD34+ cells pass into a separate collection bag as the HPC product. Target cell recovery has been reported to be 50% to 100% when successfully performed.[121,122] This strategy is very effective at enriching the product for CD34+ cells, with purities of 90% to 99% commonly obtained. Other cellular constituents of the original product are removed from the HPC product, and thereby the procedure also becomes a method for passive T-cell reduction or depletion.

In negative-selection procedures, the undesirable target cell population(s) is actively removed from the HPC product.[122] Negative-selection methods have been used to remove CD3+/CD19+ cells as the target in HPC products in an effort to reduce the risk of severe GVHD. However, in order to reduce the incidence of graft rejection, some investigators supplement the HPC graft by adding back a smaller fixed dose of CD3+/CD19+ cells.[123] One major benefit to negative selection is the retention of other cell populations such as natural killer cells in the HPC graft, which could aid in providing an antitumor effect. Newer targets for negative "specific" selection include T-cell receptor (TcR) α/β, and CD45RA+ cells.[124,125] Historically, negative selection was achieved through physical methods such as soybean lectin agglutination followed by sheep erythrocyte-rosette depletion (E-rosetting), or counterflow elutriation. More recently, immunologic approaches to T-cell depletion have used monoclonal antibodies, such as anti-CD3 monoclonal antibodyconjugated immunomagnetic beads.

Cell Expansion

Because the infused dose of nucleated, CD34+, and colony-forming cells in an HPC product is positively correlated with the speed of engraftment and patient outcomes, much effort has been focused on the ability to expand HPCs and other progenitors ex vivo. Ex-vivo expansion has the potential to increase the number of lymphocytes, committed progenitors, and long-term repopulating hematopoietic stem cells. In recent years, HPC(CB) products have been the focus of expansion trials because UCB HPCs possess higher proliferative and self-renewal capacity, and the use of these products is limited by the relatively small quantity of nucleated and CD34+ cells.[126,127] Ex-vivo expansion could increase the hematopoietic stem cell content and improve the availability of adequately sized and matched UCB units for transplantation. It may also eliminate the need for double HPC(CB) transplants for those without an adequately sized single HPC(CB) graft.[126,127] Ex-vivo expanded HPC(CB) products that lack significant numbers of T cells and contain more committed progenitors might also provide a bridge to early granulocyte recovery after aggressive treatment

for leukemia or other disorders associated with an expected prolonged period of neutropenia.[128] Most expansion cultures contain a cytokine cocktail that includes SCF, Fms-like tyrosine kinase 3 (FLT-3) ligand, and thrombopoietin, along with novel and/or proprietary ingredients. The media, culture vessels, and culture duration vary from protocol to protocol.

CRYOPRESERVATION

Cryopreservation allows for long-term storage of HPC products and is used predominantly for HPC(CB) and autologous HPC(A) products that have been collected for future hematopoietic rescue following high-dose therapy. Allogeneic products may be cryopreserved if the transplantation is unexpectedly delayed (eg, due to the recipient's medical condition), if the donor will not be available at the time of transplantation, or in situations where more donor cells are obtained than needed (and excess cells are stored for future use). During HPC product cryopreservation, a cryoprotectant agent is required to prevent ice crystal formation within and outside of cells. The freezing process must also be slow, ideally using an automated step-wise method (controlled rate). Ice crystal formation can result in cell injury and death, resulting in reduced viable cell recovery at thawing and potential slow engraftment after transplantation. The concentration of cryoprotectant and the steps in the cryopreservation protocol must be validated by each HPC processing facility for each product type. Standard protocols are used, but consensus is lacking on a universally accepted method. Similarly, the maximum acceptable duration of cryopreserved storage for HPC products remains undefined.[129-131]

DMSO is the most frequently used cryoprotectant for HPC product cryopreservation. This highly polar solvent penetrates the cell membrane, reduces intracellular ice formation, and prevents cell damage due to dehydration during freezing.[132] The most common additives for cryopreservation of HPC(A) or HPC(M) are plasma in saline, human albumin in saline, dextran, and HES. HES and dextran are the preferred and optimal additives for cryopreserving

HPC(CB) products.[133-135] Because of concern about adverse reactions to DMSO (see "Patient Care"), newer cryoprotectants, such as trehalose, are currently being assessed as alternate cryoprotectants for HPCs.[136] Laboratories vary in their final concentration of DMSO. A final concentration of 10% (volume/volume) is most frequent, but lower concentrations (to <5%) have been reported as equally effective.[137-139] Using low DMSO concentrations could decrease cell toxicity, as well as reduce the risk of AEs at the time of infusion, but might also affect cell recovery due to poor cryopreservation. Each processing facility should validate the freezing solution and the DMSO concentration for optimal viable cell recovery of the target population. Some laboratories use HES as a way to decrease the concentration of DMSO (eg, 5% DMSO plus 6% HES).[140] HES is a nonpenetrating (extracellular), macromolecular cryoprotectant; it likely functions by forming a glassy shell, or membrane, around the cells, retarding the extrusion of water out of the cell and into the extracellular ice crystals.

After addition of cryoprotectant, the HPC product must be cooled slowly to preserve post-thaw viability and function. Automated controlled-rate freezing, using an instrument with computer programming capability, decreases HPC product temperature incrementally and in a closely monitored fashion. The HPC product is cooled at a rate of 1 C/minute until the transition temperature from liquid to solid. At this point, when the solution starts to freeze, there is a release of latent heat of fusion. The freezer program then triggers a period of supercooling to counteract this heat release. Following solidification of the HPC product, cooling resumes at the rate of 1 C/minute until the product has reached −60 C. From this point on, the product is cooled at a controlled rate determined by facility policy until it reaches −100 C.

HPC products may also be frozen at a manual "noncontrolled rate." For this approach, the HPC product with additives and cryoprotectant is transferred into metal freezing cassettes and placed horizontally on shelves in a −80 C mechanical freezer. The metal cassette can be wrapped in disposable absorbent pads or styrofoam insulation to adjust the cooling rate to the desired 1 to 2 C/minute. The freezing rate can be monitored by placing the probe of an electronic temperature monitor inside the cassette, against the cryopreservation bag. Cell viability, recovery, and engraftment are generally comparable to controlled-rate freezing.[141] Following both controlled-rate and noncontrolled-rate freezing, the HPC product is transferred to a storage freezer. Most clinical facilities store HPC products in the liquid or vapor phase of liquid nitrogen (LN_2; −195 C or −150 to −125 C, respectively). Some processing laboratories may also place cassettes directly into LN_2 vapor storage without slow cooling to −80 C first. It has not been determined if viability and engraftment potential are increased by storage in the liquid phase vs the vapor phase; however, cryopreserved HPC(A) and HPC(CB) have been evaluated in both phases, and they remain viable and function for at least 15 and 23.5 years, respectively.[142,143] In theory, storage in the liquid phase would avoid the risk of transient warming events when the freezer is entered. HPC cryopreserved products requiring quarantine can be stored in the vapor phase of LN_2 in an attempt to minimize contamination risk. Other methods may include overwrap of collection bags or physical segregation during storage.

QUALITY CONTROL

HPC product collection, transport, receipt, processing, storage, and release are significant processes for QC monitoring in any quality management program involving HPCs. Policies and procedures related to these issues include the operational techniques and activities that determine the accuracy and reliability of the institution's personnel, equipment, reagents, and operations, along with the handling and manipulation of HPC products. Quality standards used in QC address testing and characterization of the product to ensure its safety, purity, and potency, as well as the requirements for release and distribution of the product for infusion. The extent of QC testing primarily depends on the complexity of the manufacturing process and the nature of the planned treatment, and whether the HPC product is within the scope of standard practice or in the context of a clinical trial. Testing requirements for the release of cellular therapy products from the processing facility must be clearly defined and must comply with local, state, and federal regulations. Voluntary standards are provided by AABB, FACT, the College of American Pathologists (CAP), The Joint Commission, and the International Organization for Standardization (ISO). These standards define the requirements for QC, and accreditation mandates compliance.

Commonly performed QC tests for HPCs include TNC count and differential, cell viability, CD34+ cell count and viability, sterility testing, and, for allogeneic products, T-cell content. CFU assays are performed in some centers; however, these are not uniformly validated for standard clinical practice or release criteria. Several of these tests may be performed during in-process manipulations, such as red cell reduction, plasma/volume reduction, MNC and/or cell subset enrichment, cell depletion, and selection of target cells. Cell count (or TNC count) and differential are commonly performed on a validated hematology analyzer. CD34+ cell enumeration is performed by flow cytometry. Most CD34+ cell-enumeration strategies are based on guidelines of the International Society for Cellular Therapy (ISCT).[144] TNC and CD34+ counts are general measures of product quantity but do not provide information about viability. Cell viability may be determined using various methods, including trypan blue, acridine orange, and 7-aminoactinomycin D (7-AAD). The use of 7-AAD, a fluorescent chemical compound with DNA affinity, in flow-cytometric analyses offers advantages over traditional trypan blue staining. These include decreased subjectivity, increased accuracy (particularly with thawed HPC products), and the ability to combine with CD34+ assessment. Because turnaround times for flow-based assays may limit the laboratory's ability to release a product for fresh infusion, microscope-based methods using vital dyes or fluorescent stains may be particularly useful for quick assessment of overall nucleated cell viability.

The colony-formation assay, or clonogenic assay with the counting of CFUs, has been considered the in-vitro "gold standard" for measuring progenitor potency. The practical application of the CFU assay is limited by the 2-week culture period and poor interlaboratory standardization. The results of this assay correlate with the speed and likelihood of engraftment of HPCs from marrow, peripheral blood, or UCB.[145-149] A reasonable correlation between engraftment speed and the more rapidly available CD34+ cell count (flow cytometry) has made this assay the accepted surrogate QC test for graft potency. The clonogenic assay is still useful, despite difficulties in standardization, for HPC(CB) products that are stored for long periods.

Sterility testing of the product assesses for aerobic and anaerobic bacteria and fungi. In US laboratories, culture-based methods are the most common tests, and these must be validated by each processing laboratory for their products and reagents. Other rapid methods are needed for products that undergo more extensive manipulation, and these may include Gram staining, endotoxin measurement, and mycoplasma testing.

Additional considerations for release testing include labeling and assessment of product appearance (eg, color, turbidity, and container integrity). Cell composition, storage conditions, product expiration, patient identification, product identification, processing laboratory name and address, warnings, and precautions are common labeling elements required for HPC product release. The implementation of labeling standards by the International Society of Blood Transfusion (ISBT) has helped to move standardization forward in this matter.[150] ISBT 128 is a coding and labeling system that was developed for blood and blood components to improve quality, safety, and traceability in blood banking. The goal of ISBT 128 for HPC products is to globally standardize terminology, coding, labeling, and identification of medical products of human origin. Today the standard is managed by the International Council for Commonality in Blood Banking Automation (ICCBBA). Full implementation of ISBT 128 improves traceability, transparency, vigilance and surveillance, and interoperability.

SHIPPING AND TRANSPORTING HPC CELLULAR PRODUCTS

Shipping and transportation refer to the physical act of transferring a product within or between facilities. Transplantations requiring unrelated-donor allogeneic HPC products, and some related-donor allogeneic transplantations that occur when the donor and recipient are not located together, require the cellular therapy products to be shipped and transported between different geographic locations. Less frequently, cryopreserved autologous HPC products need to be transported to a different location from the original collection site. Standards for safe and effective shipping and transportation are defined by accreditation organizations.[50(pp42-44),150] *Shipping* involves the HPC product leaving the control of trained personnel in the facility that collected, received, stored, and/or distributed the product after collection. *Transporting* refers to the transfer of a product between or within facilities when the product remains under the control of a facility's trained personnel.

The necessary conditions for shipping and transport vary depending on the type of product, its state (fresh or cryopreserved), and the distance involved.[151] HPC products may be shipped on public roads and/or on aircraft. All procedures involved in the transportation or shipment should be compliant with applicable regulations and standards. Shipping and transporting HPC products is tightly regulated by the FDA, Department of Transportation, International Air Transport Association, International Civil Aviation Organization, AABB, and FACT. The requirements for continuous temperature monitoring and the procedures for packaging, labeling, and documentation are all designed to maintain the integrity of the HPC product while protecting the health and safety of personnel involved in the transfer process.

During shipment, products must be placed in secondary containers that are sealed to prevent leakage and that have been validated to maintain the temperature range required for the integrity of the product under the shipping conditions.[50(p43),152] Containers should be made of durable material that is able to withstand shocks, pressure changes, and extremes of temperature. Unrelated allogeneic fresh products that are shipped directly to a transplantation center are typically intended for immediate infusion into a patient who has already undergone preparative chemoradiotherapy. These products generally travel in the custody of a qualified representative or properly trained courier who has direct control of the product at all times. The NMDP standards and guidelines provided by cellular therapy accreditation programs recommend that HPC(A) products be infused within 48 hours of collection. Several studies have shown that maintaining a product temperature between 2 and 8 C throughout the shipment retains optimal product integrity and potency at the time of infusion.[105,106,153] This temperature can maintain CD34+ cell viability more effectively than shipment at room temperature, particularly for HPC(A) and shipping times of 24 to 72 hours. Shipment at cold temperature is particularly important for products with higher nucleated-cell concentrations.

Cryopreserved products are shipped in dry shippers charged with LN_2. These containers maintain temperatures below −150 C for up to 2 weeks, and their temperatures are continuously monitored with electronic data loggers.[151] The HPC product should not be exposed to gamma irradiation or x-ray devices; instead, it should be manually inspected, if necessary. Appropriate records must accompany the product, and the chain of custody of the HPC product must be clearly documented as the product is transferred from the transfer facility to the receiving facility via the courier. Upon receipt of the product, trained personnel at the receiving facility should promptly follow the instructions for opening the container and inspecting the HPC product. At that point, a decision is made to accept, reject, or quarantine the HPC product.[50(pp44-45)]

PATIENT CARE

For fresh HPC products, once the physician caring for the patient has ordered and approved the HPC product for infusion, the product should be delivered to the patient-care area without delay. The cell product is usually handled by the clinical staff caring directly for the patient and infused by personnel who are trained in monitoring and management of infusion-related events. The procedure for infusion is similar to that used for most blood components.[153,154] After patient and product identification procedures are performed in accordance with local institutional guidelines and policies, the product is usually infused by IV gravity drip directly through a CVC, and typically without a pump, although some centers may use pumps. HPC products should never be leukocyte reduced or irradiated. Even though the practice is not universal, some institutions use a standard blood filter at the bedside. One group found no clear disadvantage to filtration as they demonstrated no difference in any markers of viability or potency for products after routine filtration.[155] Because HPC(M) products are routinely filtered in the operating room, filtration at the bedside (eg, using a standard blood filter that excludes >170 microns) is often not performed; however, including this practice is at the discretion of institutional policy. The pore size of the standard blood filter is many times larger than the typical white cell or red cell (5-10 microns), and filtration should remove unwanted clotted cells or macroaggregates without removal of the intended transfused product. If a standard blood filter is used, the laboratory should validate this process. Normal saline is usually the only fluid administered concomitantly with the HPC product, and it may be used to flush the product bag and IV tubing after the bag empties to maximize the cell dose infused. It may also be added directly to the bag if the flow rate becomes too slow.

At the time of infusion of cryopreserved HPC(A) products, they are thawed in a 37 C waterbath at the patient's bedside. Thawing of the product is usually completed by trained cellular therapy technicians before immediately handing over to the clinical staff for infusion. The preparation of any HPC product that requires washing and/or dilution before infusion, including HPC(CB) products after thawing, is usually completed in the processing laboratory before the final product is delivered to the patient's bedside for infusion. Thawed products are infused slowly to start and with sufficient observation to detect symptoms. After ensuring that there is no immediate AE with the initial volume, the product can be infused more quickly, based on patient tolerability.[154] The number of bags of cryopreserved product to be infused is determined by the number of cells collected and the maximum dose of DMSO that can be given in one day (1 g/kg/day or 1 mL/kg/day of HPC product cryopreserved in final 10% DMSO concentration).[113,153,156] Bags with the highest CD34+ cell content are often infused first, followed by bags with a lower number of CD34+ cells. Some centers limit the total number of TNCs to be infused per day due to AEs attributed to a high number of granulocytes in the HPC product.[115,116,157,158]

Infusion-related AEs associated with HPC products may be similar to those that occur with transfusion of blood components. These include allergic, hemolytic, and febrile reactions, as well as fluid overload. Certain AEs have been attributed specifically to DMSO, including nausea, vomiting, headache, changes in blood pressure and pulse, and cough. The incidence of AEs following infusion of cryopreserved HPC products ranges from 6% up to 70%, with variable degrees of severity.[113,159] The variability probably reflects differences in processing, premedication, patient monitoring, and the classification of AEs. Additional AEs include facial flushing, skin rashes, nausea, vomiting, fever, chills, abdominal pain, hypotension, hypertension, bradycardia, and tachycardia.[113,160] In one study of 1191 adult patients, hypoxia requiring oxygen was noted in 29% of infusions, chest tightness in 16.7%, and shortness of breath in 8.3%.[160] Neurologic toxicities have also been reported, including amnesia, encephalopathy, seizures, and stroke.[115,161-163] Fortunately, severe infusion-related AEs are uncommon.

Many patients may receive premedication in an attempt to prevent allergic, DMSO-related, and febrile nonhemolytic reactions, along with a combination of hydration, antihistamines, antipyretics, and anti-inflammatory agents.[154,159] Intravenous hydration (eg, for 2-6 hours before and up to 6 hours after infusion) along with diuretics may be needed with DMSO-containing HPCs. Patients' vital signs and oxygen saturation should be closely monitored during and up to several hours after infusion of cryopreserved HPC products. After infusion of HPC(CB), monitoring for AEs is required for 24 hours. All monitoring information should be captured on an accompanying infusion form. When completed, this form is returned to the laboratory.

The transplantation physician and the medical director of the cell therapy laboratory should be notified immediately of any unexpected or moderate-to-severe infusion-related AE. An investigation into whether the AE is HPC product related and whether it might represent transmission of infectious disease from the product should be carried out and guided by the signs or symptoms of the reaction. Important data include laboratory test results (eg, direct antiglobulin test, antibody titer, Gram stain, or blood cultures), imaging (eg, chest x-ray), and echocardiogram results. Product and infusion-related AEs may be reduced by certain cell-processing techniques, such as red cell or plasma reduction, postthaw washing, or dilution. Some transplantation centers routinely wash cryopreserved products after thawing and before infusion in order to reduce the DMSO content.[112,115] DMSO depletion has been shown to reduce the frequency of AEs but could result in loss of CD34+ cells and introduction of bacterial contamination.[111,164] For these reasons, most transplantation centers avoid postthaw washing or other manipulations.

Clinical outcome data, including delayed or failed engraftment and infusion-related AEs, should be reviewed regularly and discussed with the institutional quality management group. The medical director's review should include assessment of the HPC product's quality indicators (eg, dose, viability, and, if available, CFUs), any associated deviations, and the presence of infusion reactions. Particular attention is paid to any potential laboratory-related issues that could contribute to less-than-optimal outcomes.

REGULATORY AND ACCREDITATION CONSIDERATIONS

The collection and provision of HPCs are regulated in the United States both at the state and federal levels to ensure the safety, purity, and potency of cellular therapy products. The FDA and the Centers for Medicare and Medicaid Services (CMS) are the main governing bodies that provide federal oversight. State health departments may also enforce local regulations for collection centers and processing laboratories/manufacturing facilities. Individuals and organizations or institutions involved in cellular therapy processing must be familiar with the requirements of these agencies as regulated by force of law. The FDA was granted authority to establish regulations for all HCT/Ps, including hematopoietic stem/progenitor cells derived from peripheral blood and UCB, by Section 361 of the Public Health Service (PHS) Act. FDA requirements are aimed at protecting the public health by preventing the introduction, transmission, and spread of infectious disease. The general and permanent rules published in the *Federal Register* by the departments and agencies of the federal government are codified in the CFR. The FDA's Center for Biologics Evaluation and Research (CBER) regulates HCT/Ps under Title 21 CFR 1270 and 1271.[165]

HPCs that are minimally manipulated and collected for transplantation in an autologous fashion or transplanted into a first- or second-degree relative are regulated solely under Section 361 of the PHS Act and are subject to the jurisdiction of CBER under 21 CFR 1271.[166] If, in the manufacturing process, the relevant biologic or functional characteristics of an HPC product are altered (eg, genetically modified, expanded ex vivo, or combined with a drug, device, or biologic), or the cells are intended for transplantation into a non-first-or-second-degree relative (unrelated donors), the HPC product is subject to regulation under Section 351 and 361 of the PHS Act and 21 CFR 1271 as a drug and/or biologic product. These products require licensing or an exemption from licensing from the FDA as part of an IND application. Issuance of HPCs from unrelated donors facilitated through the NMDP/Be The Match Registry may be administered under the registry's IND or an institutionally held IND protocol. Similarly, minimally manipulated, unrelated UCB intended for hematopoietic or immunologic reconstitution in patients with disorders affecting the hematopoietic system must be FDA licensed or used under an IND. Minimally manipulated marrow that is not combined with another regulated article (with some exceptions) and is intended for homologous use is not considered an HCT/P.

Manufacturers of HCT/Ps are required by FDA regulations to use a tracking and labeling system that enables each product to be tracked from the donor to the recipient and from the recipient back to the donor. The FDA requires institutions that manufacture HCT/Ps to register with the agency and list their HCT/Ps.[167] The FDA also inspects laboratories that manufacture or process FDA-regulated products, such as HCT/P processing laboratories, to verify that they comply with relevant regulations.[168] The CMS regulates all laboratory testing (except research) performed on humans in the United States through the Clinical Laboratory Improvement Amendments (CLIA).[169] Regulations require that laboratories be certified under CLIA as both a general requirement and a prerequisite for receiving Medicare and Medicaid reimbursement. They provide minimal standards for facilities, equipment, and personnel.[170] CMS can revoke certification or impose fines on laboratories that fail to comply with its regulations.

In the United States, cellular therapy collection centers and processing facilities may also be accredited by organizations such as FACT,[171] CAP,[172] or AABB.[173] Accreditation through these organizations is voluntary; however, they allow institutions and facilities to be officially recognized as having operations of high quality that meet federal and local state regulations.

Maintaining standards and compliance with regulations is verified through institutional and laboratory inspections. Having sufficient personnel that are highly trained and competent, adequate facilities and equipment, and a solid quality-management plan are essential for a successful program.

CONCLUSION

HSCT is an established lifesaving treatment, especially for patients with hematologic malignancies. Use of HSCT has more recently expanded to nonmalignant disorders, such as thalassemia, sickle cell disease, and autoimmune conditions. As HPC biology becomes better understood and the ability to engineer HPC grafts evolves, clinical applications will continue to grow. New processing techniques, technology, mobilization methods, and ex-vivo manipulations add to this complex, developing field. To maintain a high-quality product that ensures safe engraftment and optimal patient outcomes, each step of the procedure from donor qualification through product infusion must be performed appropriately by collection facilities, processing laboratories, and transplantation centers. Transplantation logistics and care are overseen by accreditation organizations and regulatory agencies, which require updates and modifications to their applicable rules, regulations, and standards to maintain high-quality care.

Additional focused descriptions on HPC procurement and cellular processing, including UCB banking and UCB use, may be found in other AABB publications.

KEY POINTS

1. HSCT is a widely accepted treatment strategy for most hematologic malignancies and for some nonhematologic malignancies and nonmalignant conditions.
2. HPCs for transplantation can be collected either from marrow [HPC(M)], peripheral blood after mobilization [HPC(A)], or umbilical cord blood collected at birth [HPC(CB)].
3. Autologous HPC transplants are used for the recovery of marrow following the provision of high-dose radiotherapy and/or chemotherapy. Autografting re-establishes normal hematopoiesis and resets immunity within a relatively short period of time.
4. For several diseases, high-resolution HLA typing is responsible, at least in part, for the improved survival outcomes of unrelated-donor transplantations as compared with HLA-identical sibling-donor transplantations.

5. Allogeneic HPC products have the ability to replace defective hematopoiesis and cellular and humoral immunologic functions, thereby providing a graft-vs-neoplasm effect.

6. Screening and testing for relevant infectious diseases in allogeneic HPC donors is mandated by the FDA. The donor is declared ineligible if risk for such disease is discovered. The donor may still donate if there is an urgent medical need and justification criteria are met.

7. HPC processing techniques that reduce product volume, plasma, red cells, and (postthaw) cryoprotectant are used based on graft specification and the recipient's clinical needs. Specialized processing or more-than-minimal manipulation involves special instruments and reagents for cell selection, depletion, expansion, or further modification.

8. HPCs for autologous transplantation are cryopreserved with DMSO. Cryopreservation, thawing, infusion, and infusion-related adverse-event monitoring require personnel and standard operating procedures that maximize patient safety and minimize toxicity.

9. QC is an important component of any quality management program and includes testing and characterization of the product to ensure a safe and effective product for infusion. Common QC testing includes TNC count and viability, CD34+ cell count and viability, microbiologic testing, and T-cell content for allogeneic products.

10. Regulatory and accreditation standards outline requirements for product procurement, handling, and processing; labeling, storage, transportation, and shipping; recipient outcomes, tracking, and reporting; document and record control; and facility safety and operational controls.

REFERENCES

1. Saad A, Marques MB, Mineishi S. Donor and graft selection strategy. In: Abutalib S, Hari P, eds. Clinical manual of blood and bone marrow transplantation. Hoboken, NJ: John Wiley & Sons Ltd, 2017:1-8.

2. Panch SR, Szymanski J, Savani BN, et al. Sources of hematopoietic stem and progenitor cells and methods to optimize yields for clinical cell therapy. Biol Blood Marrow Transplant 2017;23:1241-9.

3. Bianco P. Bone and the hematopoietic niche: A tale of two stem cells. Blood 2011;117:5281-8.

4. Yu VW, Scadden DT. Hematopoietic stem cell and its bone marrow niche. Curr Top Dev Biol 2016;118:21-44.

5. Devine SM, Flomenberg N, Vesole DH, et al. Rapid mobilization of CD34+ cells following administration of the CXCR4 antagonist AMD3100 to patients with multiple myeloma and non-Hodgkin's lymphoma. J Clin Oncol 2004;22:1095-102.

6. Broxmeyer HE, Hangoc G, Cooper S, et al. Growth characteristics and expansion of human umbilical cord blood and estimation of its potential for transplantation in adults. Proc Natl Acad Sci U S A 1992;89:4109-13.

7. Sidney LE, Branch MJ, Dunphy SE, et al. Concise review: Evidence for CD34 as a common marker for diverse progenitors. Stem Cells 2014;32:1380-9.

8. D'Souza A, Fretham C. Current uses and outcomes of hematopoietic cell transplantation (HCT): CIBMTR summary slides, 2018. Milwaukee, WI: Center for International Blood and Marrow Transplant Research, 2018. [Available at https://www.cibmtr.org/ReferenceCenter/SlidesReports/SummarySlides/Pages/index.aspx (accessed December 8, 2019).]

9. Kardduss-Urueta A, Gale RP, Gutierrez-Aguirre CH, et al. Freezing the graft is not necessary for autotransplants for plasma cell myeloma and lymphomas. Bone Marrow Transplant 2018;53:457-60.

10. Donor history questionnaire—HPC, Apheresis and HPC, Marrow. Version 2.0. Bethesda, MD: AABB, 2019. [Available at http://www.aabb.org/tm/questionnaires/Pages/dhqhpc.aspx (accessed December 12, 2019).]

11. Food and Drug Administration. Human cells, tissues, and cellular and tissue-based products; donor screening and testing, and related labeling. Fed Regist 2005;70(100):29949-52.

12. Food and Drug Administration. Guidance for industry: Donor screening recommendations to reduce the risk of transmission of Zika virus by human cells, tissues, and cellular and tissue-

based products. (May 2018) Silver Spring, MD: CBER Office of Communication, Outreach, and Development, 2018. [Available at https://www.fda.gov/downloads/BiologicsBloodVaccines/GuidanceComplianceRegulatoryInformation/Guidances/Tissue/UCM488582.pdf.]

13. Lee SJ, Klein J, Haagenson M, et al. High-resolution donor-recipient HLA matching contributes to the success of unrelated donor marrow transplantation. Blood 2007;110:4576-83.

14. Loiseau P, Busson M, Balere ML, et al. HLA association with hematopoietic stem cell transplantation outcome: The number of mismatches at HLA-A, -B, -C, -DRB1, or -DQB1 is strongly associated with overall survival. Biol Blood Marrow Transplant 2007;13:965-74.

15. Spellman S, Setterholm M, Maiers M, et al. Advances in the selection of HLA-compatible donors: Refinements in HLA typing and matching over the first 20 years of the National Marrow Donor Program Registry. Biol Blood Marrow Transplant 2008;14(9 Suppl):37-44.

16. Spellman SR, Eapen M, Logan BR, et al. A perspective on the selection of unrelated donors and cord blood units for transplantation. Blood 2012;120:256-65.

17. Shaw BS, Spellman SR. HLA typing and implications. In: Abutalib S, Hari P, eds. Clinical manual of blood and bone marrow transplantation. Hoboken, NJ: John Wiley & Sons Ltd, 2017:9-18.

18. National Marrow Donor Program/Be The Match. HLA typing and matching. Minneapolis, MN: NMDP, 2018. [Available at https://bethematchclinical.org/Transplant-Therapy-and-Donor-Matching/HLA-Typing-and-Matching/ (accessed December 8, 2019).]

19. Zhang MJ, Davies SM, Camitta BM, et al. Comparison of outcomes after HLA-matched sibling and unrelated donor transplantation for children with high-risk acute lymphoblastic leukemia. Biol Blood Marrow Transplant 2012;18:1204-10.

20. Saber W, Opie S, Rizzo JD, et al. Outcomes after matched unrelated donor versus identical sibling hematopoietic cell transplantation in adults with acute myelogenous leukemia. Blood 2012;119:3908-16.

21. Saber W, Cutler CS, Nakamura R, et al. Impact of donor source on hematopoietic cell transplantation outcomes for patients with myelodysplastic syndromes (MDS). Blood 2013;122:1974-82.

22. Schetelig J, Bornhauser M, Schmid C, et al. Matched unrelated or matched sibling donors result in comparable survival after allogeneic stem-cell transplantation in elderly patients with acute myeloid leukemia: A report from the cooperative German Transplant Study Group. J Clin Oncol 2008;26:5183-91.

23. Gupta V, Tallman MS, He W, et al. Comparable survival after HLA-well-matched unrelated or matched sibling donor transplantation for acute myeloid leukemia in first remission with unfavorable cytogenetics at diagnosis. Blood 2010;116:1839-48.

24. Walter RB, Pagel JM, Gooley TA, et al. Comparison of matched unrelated and matched related donor myeloablative hematopoietic cell transplantation for adults with acute myeloid leukemia in first remission. Leukemia 2010;24:1276-82.

25. Peters C, Schrappe M, von Stackelberg A, et al. Stem-cell transplantation in children with acute lymphoblastic leukemia: A prospective international multicenter trial comparing sibling donors with matched unrelated donors-The ALL-SCT-BFM-2003 trial. J Clin Oncol 2015;33:1265-74.

26. Marsh SGE, Albert ED, Bodmer WF, et al. Nomenclature for factors of the HLA system, 2004. Tissue Antigens 2005;65:301-69.

27. Robinson J, Halliwell JA, McWilliam H, et al. The IMGT/HLA database. Nucleic Acids Res 2013;41:1013-17.

28. Gragert L, Eapen M, Williams E, et al. HLA match likelihoods for hematopoietic stem-cell grafts in the U.S. registry. N Engl J Med 2014;371:339-48.

29. Barker JN, Krepski TP, DeFor TE, et al. Searching for unrelated donor hematopoietic stem cells: Availability and speed of umbilical cord blood versus bone marrow. Biol Blood Marrow Transplant 2002;8:257-60.

30. Weisdorf D, Eapen M, Ruggeri A, et al. Alternative donor transplantation for older patients with acute myeloid leukemia in first complete remission: A Center for International Blood and Marrow Transplant Research-Eurocord analysis. Biol Blood Marrow Transplant 2014;20:816-22.

31. Marks DI, Woo KA, Zhong X, et al. Unrelated umbilical cord blood transplant for adult acute lymphoblastic leukemia in first and second complete remission: A comparison with allografts from adult unrelated donors. Haematologica 2014;99:322-8.

32. Eapen M, Rubinstein P, Zhang MJ, et al. Outcomes of transplantation of unrelated donor um-

bilical cord blood and bone marrow in children with acute leukaemia: A comparison study. Lancet 2007;369:1947-54.

33. Laughlin MJ, Eapen M, Rubinstein P, et al. Outcomes after transplantation of cord blood or bone marrow from unrelated donors in adults with leukemia. N Engl J Med 2004;351:2265-75.

34. Milano F, Gooley T, Wood B, et al. Cord-blood transplantation in patients with minimal residual disease. N Engl J Med 2016;375:944-53.

35. Luo Y, Xiao H, Lai X, et al. T-cell-replete haploidentical HSCT with low-dose anti-T-lymphocyte globulin compared with matched sibling HSCT and unrelated HSCT. Blood 2014; 124: 2735-43.

36. Wang Y, Liu QF, Xu LP, et al. Haploidentical vs identical-sibling transplant for AML in remission: A multicenter, prospective study. Blood 2015;125:3956-62.

37. Solomon SR, Sizemore CA, Sanacore M, et al. Total body irradiation-based myeloablative haploidentical stem cell transplantation is a safe and effective alternative to unrelated donor transplantation in patients without matched sibling donors. Biol Blood Marrow Transplant 2015;21: 1299-307.

38. Barker JN, Scaradavou A, Stevens CE. Combined effect of total nucleated cell dose and HLA match on transplantation outcome in 1061 cord blood recipients with hematologic malignancies. Blood 2010;115:1843-9.

39. Eapen M, Klein JP, Sanz GF, et al. Effect of donor-recipient HLA matching at HLA A, B, C, and DRB1 on outcomes after umbilical-cord blood transplantation for leukaemia and myelodysplastic syndrome: A retrospective analysis by Eurocord-European Group for Blood and Marrow Transplantation; Netcord; Center for International Blood and Marrow Transplant Research. Lancet Oncol 2011;13:1214-21.

40. Van Rood JJ, Stevens CE, Smits J, et al. Reexposure of cord blood to noninherited maternal HLA antigens improves transplant outcome in hematological malignancies. Proc Natl Acad Sci U S A 2009;106:19952-7.

41. Bashey A, Zhang MJ, McCurdy SR, et al. mobilized peripheral blood stem cells versus unstimulated bone marrow as a graft source for T-cell-replete haploidentical donor transplantation using post-transplant cyclophosphamide. J Clin Oncol 2017;35:3002-9.

42. Ciurea SO, Bayraktar UD. "No donor"? Consider a haploidentical transplant. Blood Rev 2015; 29:63-70.

43. Spellman S, Bray R, Rosen-Bronson S, et al. The detection of donor-directed, HLA-specific alloantibodies in recipients of unrelated hematopoietic cell transplantation is predictive of graft failure. Blood 2010;115:2704-8.

44. Brand A, Doxiadis IN, Roelen DL. On the role of HLA antibodies in hematopoietic stem cell transplantation. Tissue Antigens 2013;81:1-11.

45. Kollman C, Spellman SR, Zhang M, et al. The effect of donor characteristics on survival after unrelated donor transplantation for hematologic malignancy. Blood 2016;127:260-7.

46. McCullough J, McKenna D, Kadidlo D, et al. Issues in the quality of umbilical cord blood stem cells for transplantation. Transfusion 2005;45: 832-41.

47. Page KM, Zhang L, Medizabal A, et al. The cord blood apgar: A novel scoring system to optimize the selection of banked cord blood grafts for transplantation. Transfusion 2012;52:272-83.

48. Stem Cell Trialists' Collaborative Group. Allogeneic peripheral blood stem-cell compared with bone marrow transplantation for hematologic malignancies: An individual patient data meta-analysis of nine randomized trials. J Clin Oncol 2005;23:5074-87.

49. Anasetti C, Logan BR, Lee SJ, et al. Peripheral-blood stem cells versus bone marrow from unrelated donors. N Engl J Med 2012;367:1487-96.

50. Haspel RL, ed. Standards for cellular therapy services. 9th ed. Bethesda, MD: AABB, 2019.

51. Lown RN, Philippe J, Navarro W, et al. Unrelated adult stem cell donor medical suitability: Recommendations from the World Marrow Donor Association Clinical Working Group Committee. Bone Marrow Transplant 2014;49(7):880-6.

52. Worel N, Buser A, Greinix HT, et al. Suitability criteria for adult related donors: A consensus statement from the Worldwide Network for Blood and Marrow Transplantation Standing Committee on Donor Issues. Biol Blood Marrow Transplant 2015;21:2052-60.

53. Bitan M, van Walraven SM, Worel N, et al. Determination of eligibility in related pediatric hematopoietic cell donors: Ethical and clinical considerations. Recommendations from a Working Group of the Worldwide Network for Blood and Marrow Transplant Association. Biol Blood Marrow Transplant 2016;22:96-103.

54. Babic AM, Regan DM. Umbilical cord blood banking. In: Fung MK, Grossman BJ, Hillyer

CD, Westhoff CM, eds. Technical manual. 18th ed. Bethesda, MD: AABB, 2014:729-52.

55. Hackett NJ, De Oliveira GS, Jain UK, Kim JY. ASA class is a reliable independent predictor of medical complications and mortality following surgery. Int J Surg 2015;18:184-90.

56. Fleisher LA, Fleischmann KE, Auerbach AD, et al. 2014 ACC/AHA guideline on perioperative cardiovascular evaluation and management of patients undergoing noncardiac surgery: A report of the American College of Cardiology/American Heart Association Task Force on practice guidelines. J Am Coll Cardiol 2014;64:e77-137.

57. Spitzer TR. Bone marrow collection. In: Loper K, Areman EM, eds. Cellular therapy: Principles, methods, and regulations. 2nd ed. Bethesda, MD: AABB, 2016:294-305.

58. Miller JP, Perry EH, Price TH, et al. Recovery and safety profile of marrow and PBSC donors: Experience of the National Marrow Donor Program. Biol Blood Marrow Transplant 2008;14:29-36.

59. Pulsipher MA, Chitphakdithai P, Logan BR, et al. Acute toxicities of unrelated bone marrow versus peripheral blood stem cell donation: Results of a prospective trial from the National Marrow Donor Program. Blood 2013;121(1):197-206.

60. Switzer GE, Bruce JG, Harrington D, et al. Health-related quality of life of bone marrow versus peripheral blood stem cell donors: A prespecified subgroup analysis from a Phase III RCT-BMTCTN protocol 0201. Biol Blood Marrow Transplant 2014;20(1):118-27.

61. Burns LJ, Logan BR, Chitphakdithai P, et al. Recovery of unrelated donors of peripheral blood stem cells versus recovery of unrelated donors of bone marrow: A prespecified analysis from the Phase III Blood and Marrow Transplant Clinical Trials Network Protocol 0201. Biol Blood Marrow Transplant 2016;22(6):1108-16.

62. Pulsipher MA, Chitphakdithai P, Miller JP, et al. Adverse events among 2408 unrelated donors of peripheral blood stem cells: Results of a prospective trial from the National Marrow Donor Program. Blood 2009;113:3604-11.

63. Spitzer TR, Sugrue MW, Gonzalez C, et al. Transfusion practices for bone marrow harvests: A survey analysis from the AABB Bone Marrow Quality Improvement Initiative Working Group (letter). Bone Marrow Transplant 2017;52:1199-200.

64. Narayanasami U, Kanteti R, Morelli J, et al. Randomized trial of G-CSF versus chemotherapy and G-CSF mobilization of hematopoietic progenitor cells for rescue in autologous transplantation. Blood 2001;98:2059-64.

65. Kroger N, Zeller W, Fehse N, et al. Mobilizing peripheral blood stem cells with high-dose G-CSF alone is as effective as Dexa-BEAM plus G-CSF in lymphoma patients. Br J Haematol 1998;102:1101-6.

66. Yuan S, Wang S. How do we mobilize and collect autologous peripheral blood stem cells? Transfusion 2017;57:13-23.

67. Sung AD, Grima DT, Bernard LM, et al. Outcomes and costs of autologous stem cell mobilization with chemotherapy plus filgrastim vs filgrastim alone. Bone Marrow Transplant 2013;48:1444-9.

68. Gertz MA. Review: Current status of stem cell mobilization. Br J Haematol 2010;150:647-62.

69. DiPersio JF, Stadtmauer EA, Nademanee A, et al, for the 3102 Investigators. Plerixafor and filgrastim versus placebo and filgrastim to mobilize hematopoietic stem cells for autologous stem cell transplantation in patients with multiple myeloma. Blood 2009;113:5720-6.

70. DiPersio JF, Micallef IN, Stiff PJ, et al. Phase III prospective randomized double-blind placebo-controlled trial of plerixafor plus granulocyte colony-stimulating factor compared with placebo plus granulocyte colony-stimulating factor for autologous stem-cell mobilization and transplantation for patients with non-Hodgkin's lymphoma. J Clin Oncol 2009;27:4767-73.

71. Smith VR, Popat U, Ciurea S, et al. Just-in-time rescue plerixafor in combination with chemotherapy and granulocyte-colony stimulating factor for peripheral blood progenitor cell mobilization. Am J Hematol 2013;88:754-7.

72. Costa LJ, Abbas J, Hogan KR, et al. Growth factor plus preemptive ('just-in-time') plerixafor successfully mobilizes hematopoietic stem cells in multiple myeloma patients despite prior lenalidomide exposure. Bone Marrow Transplant 2012;47:1403-8.

73. Becker P, Schwebig A, Brauninger S, et al. Healthy donor hematopoietic stem cell mobilization with biosimilar granulocyte-colony-stimulating factor: safety, efficacy, and graft performance. Transfusion 2016;56:3055-64.

74. Schroeder MA, Rettig MP, Lopez S, et al. Mobilization of allogeneic peripheral blood stem cell donors with intravenous plerixafor mobilizes a unique graft. Blood 2017;129:2680-92.

75. Pulsipher MA, Levine JE, Hayashi RJ, et al. Safety and efficacy of allogeneic PBSC collection in normal pediatric donors: The pediatric blood and marrow transplant consortium experience (PBMTC) 1996-2003. Bone Marrow Transplant 2005;35:361-7.

76. Weaver CH, Hazelton B, Birch R, et al. An analysis of engraftment kinetics as a function of the CD34 content of peripheral blood progenitor cell collections in 692 patients after the administration of myeloablative chemotherapy. Blood 1995;86:3961-9.

77. Reiffers J, Faberes C, Boiron JM, et al. Peripheral blood progenitor cell transplantation in 118 patients with hematological malignancies: Analysis of factors affecting the rate of engraftment. J Hematother 1994;3:185-91.

78. Pulsipher MA, Chitphakdithai P, Logan BR, et al. Donor, recipient, and transplant characteristics as risk factors after unrelated donor PBSC transplantation: Beneficial effects of higher CD34 + cell dose. Blood 2009;114:2606-16.

79. Baron F, Maris MB, Storer BE, et al. High doses of transplanted CD34 + cells are associated with rapid T-cell engraftment and lessened risk of graft rejection, but not more graft-versus-host disease after nonmyeloablative conditioning and unrelated hematopoietic cell transplantation. Leukemia 2005;19:822-8.

80. Keating GM. Plerixafor. Drugs 2011;71:1623-47.

81. Abrahamsen JF, Stamnesfet S, Liseth K, et al. Large-volume leukapheresis yields more viable CD34+ cells and colony-forming units than normal-volume leukapheresis, especially in patients who mobilize low numbers of CD34+ cells. Transfusion 2005;45:248-53.

82. Lee G, Arepally GM. Anticoagulation techniques in apheresis: From heparin to citrate and beyond. J Clin Apher 2012;27:117-25.

83. Lefrère F, Zohar S, Beaudier S, et al. Evaluation of an algorithm based on peripheral blood hematopoietic progenitor cell and CD34+ cell concentrations to optimize peripheral blood progenitor cell collection by apheresis. Transfusion 2007;47:1851-7.

84. Leberfinger DL, Badman KL, Roig JM, Loos T. Improved planning of leukapheresis endpoint with customized prediction algorithm: Minimizing collection days, volume of blood processed, procedure time, and citrate toxicity. Transfusion 2017;57:685-93.

85. Porrata LF, Inwards DJ, Ansell SM, et al. Early lymphocyte recovery predicts superior survival after autologous stem cell transplantation in non-Hodgkin Lymphoma: A prospective study. Biol Blood Marrow Transplant 2008;14;807-16.

86. Porrata LF, Litzow MR, Inwards DJ, et al. Infused peripheral blood autograft absolute lymphocyte count correlates with day 15 absolute lymphocyte count and clinical outcome after autologous peripheral hematopoietic stem cell transplantation in non-Hodgkin's lymphoma. Bone Marrow Transplant 2004;33:291-8.

87. Porrata LF, Burgstaler EA, Winters JL, et al. Immunologic autograft engineering and survival in non-Hodgkin lymphoma. Biol Bood Marrow Transplant 2016;22:1017-23.

88. Hiwase DK, Hiwase S, Bailey M, et al. Higher infused lymphocyte dose predicts higher lymphocyte recovery, which in turn, predicts superior overall survival following autologous hematopoietic stem cell transplantation for multiple myeloma. Biol Blood Marrow Transplant 2008; 14:116-24.

89. Page KM, Kurtzberg J. Current cord blood banking concepts and practices. In: Horwitz M, Chao N, eds. Cord blood transplantations. In: Abutalib SA, Armitage JO, series eds. Advances and controversies in hematopoietic transplantation and cell therapy. Cham, Switzerland: Springer, 2017:13-34.

90. Armson BA, Allan DS, Casper RF. Umbilical cord blood: Counselling, collection, and banking. J Obstet Gynaecol Can 2015;37:832-44.

91. Bertolini F, Lazzari L, Lauri E, et al. Comparative study of different procedures for the collection and banking of umbilical cord blood. J Hematother 1995;4:29-36.

92. Jones J, Stevens CE, Rubinstein P, et al. Obstetric predictors of placental/umbilical cord blood volume for transplantation. Am J Obstet Gynecol 2003;188:503-9.

93. Wagner JE, Barker JN, DeFor TE, et al. Transplantation of unrelated donor umbilical cord blood in 102 patients with malignant and nonmalignant diseases: Influence of CD34 cell dose and HLA disparity on treatment-related mortality and survival. Blood 2002;100:1611-18.

94. Gluckman E, Rocha V, Arcese W, et al. Factors associated with outcomes of unrelated cord blood transplant: Guidelines for donor choice. Exp Hematol 2004;32:397-407.

95. Barker JN, Weisdorf DJ, DeFor TE, et al. Transplantation of 2 partially HLA-matched umbilical cord blood units to enhance engraftment in adults with hematologic malignancy. Blood 2005;105:1343-7.

96. Scaradavou A, Brunstein CG, Eapen M, et al. Double unit grafts successfully extend the application of umbilical cord blood transplantation in adults with acute leukemia. Blood 2013;121: 752-8.

97. Wagner JE Jr, Eapen M, Carter S, et al, for the Blood and Marrow Transplant Clinical Trials Network. One-unit versus two-unit cord-blood transplantation for hematologic cancers. N Engl J Med 2014;371:1685-94.

98. Michel G, Galambrun C, Sirvent A, et al. Single versus double-unit cord blood transplantation for children and young adults with acute leukemia or myelodysplastic syndrome. Blood 2016; 127:3450-7.

99. Politikos I, Barker JN. Cell dose and immunogenetic considerations in cord blood transplantation. In: Horwitz M, Chao N, eds. Cord blood transplantations. In: Abutalib SA, Armitage JO, series eds. Advances and controversies in hematopoietic transplantation and cell therapy. Cham, Switzerland: Springer, 2017:47-69.

100. McKenna DH. Basic cellular therapy manufacturing procedures. In: Loper K, Areman EM, eds. Cellular therapy: Principles, methods, and regulations. 2nd ed. Bethesda, MD: AABB, 2016:361-7.

101. Staley EM, Schwartz J, Pham HP. An update on ABO incompatible hematopoietic progenitor cell transplantation. Transfus Apher Sci 2016;54: 337-44.

102. Coelho PH, Kadidlo D, Chapman J. Umbilical cord blood processing. In: Loper K, Areman EM, eds. Cellular therapy: Principles, methods, and regulations. 2nd ed. Bethesda, MD: AABB, 2016:368-75.

103. Sorg N, Poppe C, Bunos M, et al. Red blood cell depletion from bone marrow and peripheral blood buffy coat: A comparison of two new and three established technologies. Transfusion 2015;55:1275-82.

104. Kim-Wanner SZ, Bug G, Steinmann J, et al. Erythrocyte depletion from bone marrow: Performance evaluation after 50 clinical-scale depletions with Spectra Optia BMC. J Transl Med 2017;15:174.

105. Antonenas V, Garvin F, Webb M, et al. Fresh PBSC harvests, but not BM, show temperature-related loss of CD34 viability during storage and transport. Cytotherapy 2006;8:158-65.

106. Kao GS, Kim HT, Daley H, et al. Validation of short-term handling and storage conditions for marrow and peripheral blood stem cell products. Transfusion 2011;51(1):137-47.

107. Rubinstein P, Dobrila L, Rosenfield R, et al. Processing and cryopreservation of placental/umbilical cord blood for unrelated bone marrow reconstitution. Proc Natl Acad Sci U S A 1995; 92:10119-22.

108. Laroche V, McKenna D, Moroff G, et al. Cell loss and recovery in umbilical cord blood processing: A comparison of post-thaw and post-wash samples. Transfusion 2005;45:1909-16.

109. Barker JN, Abboud M, Rice RD, et al. A "no-wash" albumin-dextran dilution strategy for cord blood unit thaw: High rate of engraftment and a low incidence of serious infusion reactions. Biol Blood Marrow Transplant 2009;15: 1596-602.

110. Regan DM, Wofford JD, Wall DA. Comparison of cord blood thawing methods on cell recovery, potency, and infusion. Transfusion 2010;50: 2670-5.

111. Pasha R, Elmoazzen H, Pineault N. Development and testing of a stepwise thaw and dilute protocol for cryopreserved umbilical cord blood units. Transfusion 2017;57:1744-54.

112. Haspel RL. Thawing and infusing cellular therapy products. In: Loper K, Areman EM, eds. Cellular therapy: Principles, methods, and regulations. 2nd ed. Bethesda, MD: AABB, 2016: 459-67.

113. Shu Z, Heimfeld S, Gao D. Hematopoietic SCT with cryopreserved grafts: Adverse reactions after transplantation and cryoprotectant removal before infusion. Bone Marrow Transplant 2014; 49:469-76.

114. Sánchez-Salinas A, Cabañas-Perianes V, Blanquer M, et al. An automatic wash method for dimethyl sulfoxide removal in autologous hematopoietic stem cell transplantation decreases the adverse effects related to infusion. Transplantation 2012;52:2382-6.

115. Calmels B, Lemarie C, Esterni B, et al. Occurrence and severity of adverse events after autologous hematopoietic progenitor cell infusion are related to the amount of granulocytes in the apheresis product. Transfusion 2007;47:1268-75.

116. Khera N, Jinneman J, Storer BE, et al. Limiting the daily total nucleated cell dose of cryopreserved peripheral blood stem cell products for autologous transplantation improves infusion-related safety with no adverse impact on hematopoietic engraftment. Biol Blood Marrow Transplant 2012;18:220-8.

117. Cameron G, Filer K, Hall A, Hogge D. Evaluation of post-thaw blood progenitor product in-

tegrity and viability over time at room temperature and 4°C. Cytotherapy 2013;15:S27.

118. Khuu HM, Cowley H, David-Ocampo V, et al. Catastrophic failures of freezing bags for cellular therapy products: Description, cause, and consequences. Cytotherapy 2002;4:539-49.

119. Tran CA, Torres-Coronado M, Gardner A, et al. Optimized processing of growth factor mobilized peripheral blood CD34+ products by counterflow centrifugal elutriation. Stem Cells Transl Med 2012;1:422-9.

120. Edwards J. Cell separation by counterflow centrifugal elutration. In: Loper K, Areman EM, eds. Cellular therapy: Principles, methods, and regulations. 2nd ed. Bethesda, MD: AABB, 2016:381-3.

121. Keever-Taylor CA, Devine SM, Soiffer RJ, et al. Characteristics of CliniMACS®System CD34-enriched T cell-depleted grafts in a multi-center trial for acute myeloid leukemia-Blood and Marrow Transplant Clinical Trials Network (BMT CTN) Protocol 0303. Biol Blood Marrow Transplant 2012;8:690-7.

122. Kadidlo D. Hematopoietic progenitor cell graft modification: Cell enrichment or depletion. In: Loper K, Areman EM, eds. Cellular therapy: Principles, methods, and regulations. 2nd ed. Bethesda, MD: AABB, 2016:376-80.

123. Geyer MB, Ricci AM, Jacobson JS, et al. T cell depletion utilizing CD34(+) stem cell selection and CD3(+) addback from unrelated adult donors in paediatric allogeneic stem cell transplantation recipients. Br J Haematol 2012;157:205-19.

124. Aversa F. T-cell depletion: From positive selection to negative depletion in adult patients. Bone Marrow Transplant 2015;50(Suppl 2):S11-13.

125. Bleakley M, Heimfeld S, Loeb KR, et al. Outcomes of acute leukemia patients transplanted with naive T cell-depleted stem cell grafts. J Clin Invest 2015;125:2677-89.

126. Horwitz ME. Ex vivo expansion or manipulation of stem cells to improve outcome of umbilical cord blood transplantation. Curr Hematol Malig Rep 2016;11:12-18.

127. Horwitz ME, Frassoni F. Improving the outcome of umbilical cord blood transplantation through ex vivo expansion or graft manipulation. Cytotherapy 2015;17:730-8.

128. Delaney C, Milano F, Cicconi L, et al. Infusion of a non-HLA-matched ex-vivo expanded cord blood progenitor cell product after intensive acute myeloid leukaemia chemotherapy: A

Phase 1 trial. Lancet Haematol 2016;3(7):e330-9.

129. Veeraputhiran M, Theus JW, Pesek G, et al. Viability and engraftment of hematopoietic progenitor cells after long-term cryopreservation: Effect of diagnosis and percentage dimethyl sulfoxide concentration. Cytotherapy 2010;12:764-6.

130. Mitchell R, Wagner JE, Brunstein CG, et al. Impact of long-term cryopreservation on single umbilical cord blood transplantation outcomes. Biol Blood Marrow Transplant 2015;21:50-4.

131. Lecchi L, Giovanelli S, Gagliardi B, et al. An update on methods for cryopreservation and thawing of hemopoietic stem cells. Transfus Apher Sci 2016;54:324-36.

132. Smagur A, Mitrus I, Ciomber A, et al. Comparison of the cryoprotective solutions based on human albumin vs. autologous plasma: Its effect on cell recovery, clonogenic potential of peripheral blood hematopoietic progenitor cells and engraftment after autologous transplantation. Vox Sang 2015;108:417-24.

133. Chen G, Yue A, Ruan Z, et al. Comparison of the effects of different cryoprotectants on stem cells from umbilical cord blood. Stem Cells Int 2016;2016:1396783.

134. Kozlowska-Skrzypczak M, Kubiak A, Bembnista E, et al. Analysis of the effect of cryoprotectant medium composition to viability of autologous hematopoietic cells collected by leukapheresis. Transplant Proc 2014;46:2535-8.

135. Rowley SD, Feng Z, Chen L, et al. A randomized phase III clinical trial of autologous blood stem cell transplantation comparing cryopreservation using dimethylsulfoxide vs dimethylsulfoxide with hydroxyethylstarch. Bone Marrow Transplant 2003;31:1043-51.

136. Rodrigues JP, Paraguassú-Braga FH, Carvalho L, et al. Evaluation of trehalose and sucrose as cryoprotectants for hematopoietic stem cells of umbilical cord blood. Cryobiology 2008;56:144-51.

137. Smagur A, Mitrus I, Giebel S, et al. Impact of different dimethyl sulphoxide concentrations on cell recovery, viability and clonogenic potential of cryopreserved peripheral blood hematopoietic stem and progenitor cells. Vox Sang 2013;104:240-7.

138. Windrum P, Morris TCM, Drake MB, et al, for the EBMT Chronic Leukaemia Working Party Complications Subcommittee. Variation in dimethyl sulfoxide use in stem cell transplantation: A survey of EBMT centres. Bone Marrow Transplant 2005;36:601-3.

139. Bakken AM, Bruserud O, Abrahamsen JF. No differences in colony formation of peripheral blood stem cells frozen with 5% or 10% dimethyl sulfoxide. J Hematother Stem Cell Res 2003; 12:351-8.

140. Stiff PJ, Koester AR, Weidner MK, et al. Autologous bone marrow transplantation using unfractionated cells cryopreserved in dimethylsulfoxide and hydroxyethyl starch without controlled-rate freezing. Blood 1987;70:974-8.

141. Weinberg RS. Cryopreservation techniques and freezing solutions. In: Schwartz J, Shaz BH, eds. Best practices in processing and storage for hematopoietic cell transplantation. In: Abutalib SA, Armitage JO, series eds. Advances and controversies in hematopoietic transplantation and cell therapy. Cham, Switzerland: Springer, 2018:63-72.

142. Broxmeyer HE, Lee M-R, Hangoc G, et al. Hematopoietic stem/progenitor cells, generation of induced pluripotent stem cells and isolation of endothelial progenitors from 21- to 23.5-year cryopreserved cord blood. Blood 2011;117: 4774-7.

143. Winter JM, Jacobson P, Bullough B, et al. Long-term effects of cryopreservation on clinically prepared hematopoietic progenitor cell products. Cytotherapy 2014;16:965-75.

144. Sutherland DR, Keeney M. Enumeration of CD34+ cells by flow cytometry. In: Loper K, Areman EM, eds. Cellular therapy: Principles, methods, and regulations. 2nd ed. Bethesda, MD: AABB, 2016:558-69.

145. Spitzer G, Verma DS, Fisher R, et al. The myeloid progenitor cell: Its value in predicting hematopoietic recovery after autologous bone marrow transplantation. Blood 1980;55:317-23.

146. Douay L, Gorin NC, Mary JY, et al. Recovery of CFU-GM from cryopreserved marrow and in vivo evaluation after autologous bone marrow transplantation are predictive of engraftment. Exp Hematol 1986;14:358-65.

147. Schwartzberg L, Birch R, Blanco R, et al. Rapid and sustained hematopoietic reconstitution by peripheral blood stem cell infusion alone following high-dose chemotherapy. Bone Marrow Transplant 1993;11:360-74.

148. Migliaccio AR, Adamson JW, Stevens CE, et al. Cell dose and speed of engraftment in placental/umbilical cord blood transplantation: Graft progenitor cell content is a better predictor than nucleated cell quantity. Blood 2000;96:2717-22.

149. Pamphilon D, Selogie E, McKenna D, et al. Current practices and prospects for standardization of the hematopoietic colony-forming unit assay: A report by the cellular therapy team of the Biomedical Excellence for Safer transfusion (BEST) collaborative. Cytotherapy 2013;15:255-62.

150. Slaper-Cortenbach I. ISBT 128 coding and labeling for cellular therapy products. Cell Tissue Bank 2010;11:375-8.

151. Regan D, Yost A. Transportation and shipping of cellular therapy products. In: Loper K, Areman EM, eds. Cellular therapy: Principles, methods, and regulations. 2nd ed. Bethesda, MD: AABB, 2016:483-93.

152. Jansen J, Nolan P, Reeves M, et al. Transportation of peripheral blood progenitor cell products: Effects of time, temperature and cell concentration. Cytotherapy 2009;11:79-85.

153. AABB, America's Blood Centers, American Red Cross, American Society for Apheresis, American Society for Blood and Marrow Transplantation, College of American Pathologists, Cord Blood Association, Foundation for the Accreditation of Cellular Therapy, ICCBBA, International Society for Cellular Therapy, Joint Accreditation Committee of ISCT and EBMT, National Marrow Donor Program, World Marrow Donor Association. Circular of information for the use of cellular therapy products. Bethesda, MD: AABB, 2018. [Available at http://www.aabb.org/aabbcct/coi/Documents/CT-Circular-of-Information.pdf (accessed December 9, 2019).]

154. Sauer-Heilborn A, Kadidlo D, McCullough J. Patient care during infusion of hematopoietic progenitor cells. Transfusion 2004;44:907-16.

155. Paulson K, Gilpin SG, Shpiruk TA, et al. Routine filtration of hematopoietic stem cell products: The time has arrived. Transfusion 2015;55: 1980-4.

156. Júnior AM, Arrais CA, Saboya R, et al. Neurotoxicity associated with dimethylsulfoxide-preserved hematopoietic progenitor cell infusion. Bone Marrow Transplant 2008;41:95-6.

157. Cordoba R, Arrieta R, Kerguelen A, et al. The occurrence of adverse events during the infusion of autologous peripheral blood stem cells is related to the number of granulocytes in the leukapheresis product. Bone Marrow Transplant 2007;40:1063-7.

158. Rowley SD, Feng Z, Yadock D, et al. Post-thaw removal of DMSO does not completely abrogate infusional toxicity or the need for pre-infusion histamine blockade. Cytotherapy 1999;1:439-46.

159. Milone G, Mercurio S, Strano A, et al. Adverse events after infusions of cryopreserved hematopoietic stem cells depend on non-mononuclear cells in the infused suspension and patient age. Cytotherapy 2007;9:348-55.

160. Otrock ZK, Sempek DS, Carey S, Grossman BJ. Adverse events of cryopreserved hematopoietic stem cell infusions in adults: A single-center observational study. Transfusion 2017;57:1522-6.

161. Hoyt R, Szer J, Grigg A. Neurological events associated with the infusion of cryopreserved bone marrow and/or peripheral blood progenitor cells. Bone Marrow Transplant 2000;25:1285-7.

162. Rowley S, MacLeod B, Heimfeld S, et al. Severe central nervous system toxicity associated with the infusion of cryopreserved PBSC components. Cytotherapy 1999;1:311-17.

163. Otrock ZK, Beydoun A, Barada WM, et al. Transient global amnesia associated with the infusion of DMSO-cryopreserved autologous peripheral blood stem cells. Haematologica 2008;93:e36-7.

164. Akkök CA, Liseth K, Melve GK, et al. Is there a scientific basis for a recommended standardization of collection and cryopreservation of peripheral blood stem cell grafts? Cytotherapy 2011;13:1013-24.

165. Food and Drug Administration. Tissue and tissue products. Silver Spring, MD: CBER Office of Communication, Outreach, and Development, 2019. [Available at https://www.fda.gov/Bio logicsBloodVaccines/TissueTissueProducts/de fault.htm.]

166. Food and Drug Administration. Draft guidance for industry and Food and Drug Administration staff: Minimal manipulation of human cells, tissues, and cellular and tissue-based products. (December 2014) Silver Spring, MD: CBER Office of Communication, Outreach, and Develop-

ment, 2014. [Available at https://bioinfor mant.com/wp-content/uploads/2016/09/FDA-Regulation-of-Stem-Cells-Draft-Guidances.pdf].

167. Food and Drug Administration. Registration and listing. Silver Spring, MD: CBER Office of Communication, Outreach, and Development, 2019. [Available at https://www.fda.gov/For Industry/FDABasicsforIndustry/ucm234625.htm.]

168. Food and Drug Administration. What does FDA inspect? Silver Spring, MD: CBER Office of Communication, Outreach, and Development, 2018. [Available at https://www.fda.gov/about-fda/fda-basics/what-does-fda-inspect.]

169. Centers for Medicare and Medicaid Services. Clinical Laboratory Improvement Amendments (CLIA). Baltimore, MD: CMS, 2019. [Available at https://www.cms.gov/Regulations-and-Guidance/Legislation/CLIA/index.html.]

170. Centers for Medicare and Medicaid Services. Proficiency testing programs. Baltimore, MD: CMS, 2019. [Available at https://www.cms.gov/Regulations-and-Guidance/Legislation/CLIA/Proficiency_Testing_Providers.html.]

171. Process overview. Omaha, NE: Foundation for the Accreditation of Cellular Therapy, 2014. [Available at http://www.factwebsite.org/accreditationprocess/(accessed December 9, 2019).]

172. Laboratory accreditation program. Northfield, IL: College of American Pathologists, 2019. [Available at http://www.cap.org/web/home/lab/accreditation/laboratory-accreditation-pro gram (accessed December 9, 2019).]

173. Accreditation program. Bethesda, MD: AABB, 2019. [Available at http://www.aabb.org/sa/overview/Pages/program.aspx (accessed December 9, 2019).]

CHAPTER 27

Transfusion Support for Hematopoietic Stem Cell Transplant Recipients

James M. Kelley, MD, PhD, and Melissa M. Cushing, MD

HEMATOPOIETIC STEM CELL TRANS-plantation (HSCT) involves infusing hema-topoietic progenitor cells (HPCs) to replace or restore the cellular components within a pa-tient's marrow and for reconstitution of the im-mune system. HSCT is often performed for pa-tients with hematologic malignancies, marrow failure states, primary immunodeficiencies, and congenital blood disorders, or following treat-ment with chemotherapy regimens. Over 200 hospitals offer the approximately 20,000 HSCT procedures performed each year in the United States, demonstrating the widespread use of this procedure.[1] HSCT patients often pre-sent to com-munity hospitals for follow-up care, and thus a broader base of the medical community needs to understand their transfusion needs.

Two main categories of HSCT exist: autolo-gous and allogeneic. The majority of HSCTs are autologous (58%).[1] Autologous HSCTs occur when a patient receives stored HPCs he or she previously donated. Such patients undergo HPC collection and storage and are subsequently treated with high-dose chemotherapy, which targets their underlying cancer but also ablates their marrow. Patients then receive their autolo-gous HPCs to circumvent the myeloablation af-ter completing chemotherapy. Allogeneic HSCTs occur when a patient receives HPCs from anoth-er individual. Allogeneic HPCs can be donated from matched related donors (MRDs), who are typically siblings or other family members; matched or single-antigen-mismatched unrelat-ed donors (MUDs) recruited by organizations such as the National Marrow Donor Program (NMDP); or related haploidentical donors, who are typically parents or children. "Matching" re-fers to the degree of similarity between specific HLA alleles of the donor and recipient and pre-dicts the likelihood of tissue compatibility. Hap-loidentical HPCs match only half the HLA loci evaluated, as they derive from a parent or child who shares half the genes with the recipient. (See Chapter 16 for discussion of HLA.)

HPCs can be harvested directly by using a wide-bore needle inserted into the donor's marrow, or through apheresis collection after stimulating a donor with granulocyte colony-stimulating factor [G-CSF (filgrastim)] or plerixa-for to mobilize stem cells from the marrow into the peripheral circulation (ie, peripheral blood stem cells). They can also be derived from do-nated umbilical cords/placenta after a birth (ie, cord blood). Given the low cell count of a cord blood donation, HPCs from two cord blood donations are often used for adult patients, al-though a single donation is sufficient for smaller pediatric patients.

Appropriate transfusion support for patients receiving an HSCT is both critical (as this pa-

James M. Kelley, MD, PhD, Assistant Professor of Laboratory Medicine, The University of Texas MD Anderson Cancer Center, Houston, Texas; and Melissa M. Cushing, MD, Professor of Pathology and Laboratory Medicine, Weill Cornell Medicine, Medical Director, Transfusion Medicine and Cellular Therapy, and Associate Director of the Clinical Laboratories, NewYork-Presbyterian/Weill Cornell Medical Campus, New York, New York

J. Kelley has disclosed no conflicts of interest. M. Cushing is a consultant for Cerus Corporation and Octapharma.

tient population often lacks the ability to produce blood cells effectively) and challenging (as their blood types can transition if receiving HPCs from an allogeneic donor with a different blood type). Complexities such as the patient's underlying condition, level of immunosuppression, additional medications, existing alloantibodies, rate of engraftment, adverse events related to transplantation, the type of HPC transplant, and the presence of donor passenger lymphocytes affect the need for and the expected response to transfusion. This chapter offers an introduction to navigating some of these complexities when providing transfusion for this unique patient population.

ABO COMPATIBILITY FOR BLOOD COMPONENT SELECTION FOLLOWING HSCT

ABO matching of blood components to the HSCT recipient is not essential when selecting allogeneic HPC donors. Unlike solid-organ transplants, HPCs do not express ABO antigens and will not activate an immediate humoral immune response leading to rapid rejection. Therefore, it is possible (and common) to select an HPC donor with a different ABO group than the recipient—meaning that samples from HSCT patients can simultaneously express more than one ABO group during immunohematology testing.

Interpreting such potentially complex immunohematology results and selecting appropriate blood components for HSCT patients requires medical record investigation. The following data help transfusion service staff determine the patient's stage of transplantation (eg, pretransplantation, immediate posttransplantation, or postengraftment): the original ABO group of the HSCT patient; the ABO group, type of product, and date of infusion of all HPC products; any ABO titer results; molecular engraftment study results (if available); and the pre- and posttransplantation transfusion histories from all centers at which the patient received care. Once obtained, these data should be documented in a hospital's blood bank information system because HSCT patients frequently receive transfusion. Such histories can become complex: pa-

tients may receive multiple HPC products at one time, such as through a cord blood transplantation, or undergo HSCTs of different ABO groups following disease relapse or incomplete engraftment.

ABO-Compatible Blood Components

Patients in the pretransplantation or postengraftment phase of HSCT can be given transfusion based on their current forward- and reverse-typing results, as the composition of their blood should derive completely from one progenitor source. That is, they can be assigned blood components based on a hospital's standard procedures for general patients. Figure 27-1 illustrates that in the pretransplantation and postengraftment phases of HSCT, the patient produces blood from one progenitor source. The exception to this is in the setting of nonmyeloablative HSCT, where patients will occasionally have sustained mixed chimerism, with existing erythrocytes of both donor and recipient origin.

Patients in the immediate posttransplantation period, between HPC infusion and engraftment (see Fig 27-1), require more careful attention to ABO compatibility and selection of blood components. Blood circulating during this time can consist of a shifting composition of cells that transitions from cells arising from the patient's original marrow to those of the donor. Often this can lead to identification of ABO discrepancies during pretransfusion testing in the blood bank, which can cause delays in test result reporting. Each sample will require manual review by blood bank staff, rather than immediate reporting and interfacing with the electronic medical record through blood bank automation. During the posttransplantation phase, or if complete engraftment is not achieved, the ABO groups of both the donor and recipient should be considered in selecting components for transfusion because it is common for an HPC donor and HSCT patient to have different ABO groupings.[2,3] Selecting components with ABO compatibility for both the donor and recipient is ideal for transfusion in such cases. Suggestions for ABO selection are listed in Table 27-1, but specific recommendations vary by center, particularly with platelets.

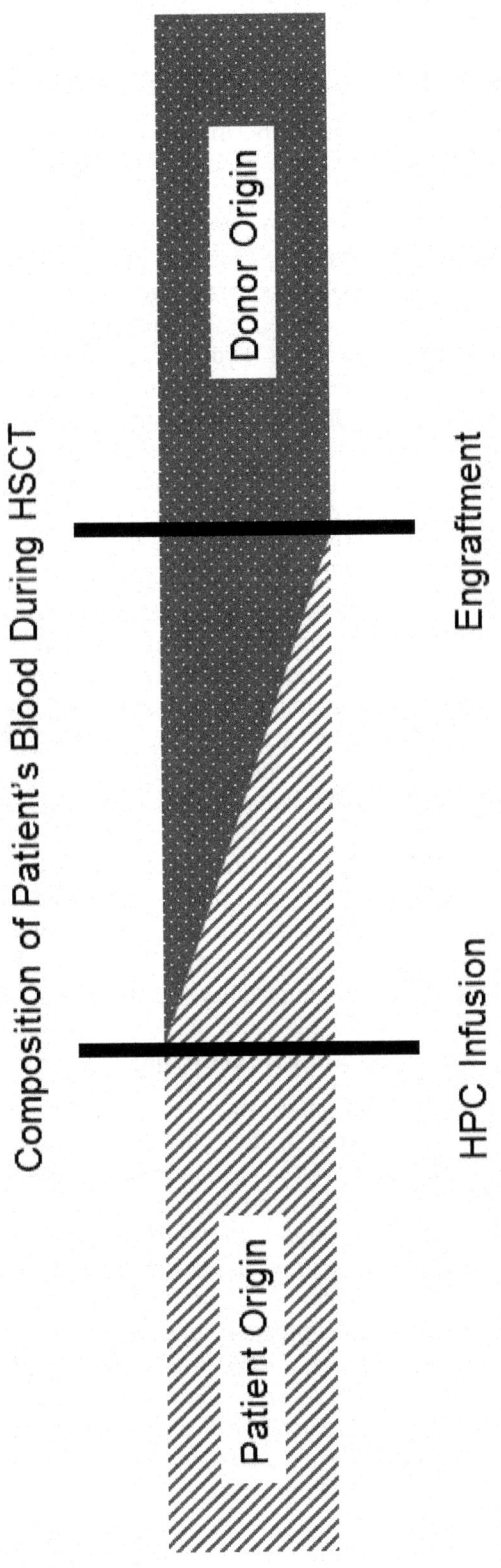

FIGURE 27-1. The shifting composition of the origin of blood in a recipient of hematopoietic stem cell transplantation (HSCT), from infusion of hematopoietic progenitor cells (HPCs) until engraftment. Although this is presented as a linear transition for graphic simplicity, many factors influence the rate of engraftment. During the period between HPC infusion and engraftment, care should be taken in selecting the ABO compatibility of blood components. For suggestions, see Table 27-1.

Although the time point of infusion is clear, engraftment is evaluated by laboratory testing and defined at each center. After an expected period has passed, the patient's blood counts (eg, white cell count, platelet count) should recover in a predictable manner as engraftment occurs. The definition of engraftment is usually based on the patient's absolute neutrophil count (ANC), but it can also include an assessment of ABO typing results (to determine whether the ABO type consistently matches that of the donor on multiple occasions) or molecular chimerism assays (to look for a sufficient percentage of lymphoid/myeloid cells arising from the donor).

Compatible Blood Components for Non-ABO Antigens

A corresponding approach of providing components compatible with both the HPC donor and recipient is applicable to other antigens. For example, if either the donor or the recipient has an alloantibody to another blood group, such as RH or KEL, antigen-negative Red Blood Cell (RBC) units should be provided for transfusion. With regard to RhD, the recipient can continue to receive the same type of components transfused before transplantation as long as the HSCT donor and recipient match. The benefit of providing RhD-negative RBCs if either the recipient or the donor is RhD negative, to prevent alloimmunization to the highly immunogenic D antigen, has not been well studied but leads to significant depletion of the RhD-negative RBC inventory. RhD-negative patients with an RhD-negative donor generally receive RhD-negative RBCs.[4] In one study, 7% of RhD-negative patients with hematologic malignancies formed anti-D when given RhD-positive RBCs for transfusion.[5] Given the minimal risk of RhD alloimmunization from red cells contained in RhD-positive platelet units, selection of RhD-negative platelets is not mandatory.

The degree of ABO matching between HPC donor and HSCT recipient is grouped into four categories, as shown in Table 27-1: ABO compatibility, major ABO incompatibility, minor ABO incompatibility, and bidirectional ABO incompatibility. Transfusion management of ABO-compatible HSCT is more easily accomplished, but challenges exist for the other categories.[3]

Major ABO Incompatibility

Major ABO incompatibility may lead to acute intravascular hemolysis if residual donor red cells in the HPC product are infused into a patient with high ABO antibody titers. This risk is mitigated by reducing the red cell content in the HPC products (to generally less than 10-30 mL of red cells), using one of a number of methods, such as hydroxyethyl starch sedimentation. Most peripheral blood stem cell products and cord blood units contain few red cells, but marrow-derived products will frequently require red cell depletion. If the recipient ABO antibody titer is high, plasmapheresis may be used before HPC infusion, to reduce the titer of circulating ABO antibodies. Hemolysis or delay of engraftment can occur if residual host immune cells continue to produce antibodies against the erythroid progenitors and red cells arising from the donor HPCs. This can continue for several months after infusion, leaving HSCT patients transfusion dependent for long periods after transplantation. Pure red cell aplasia (PRCA) can develop in severe cases. Although no standard treatment for PRCA is established, corticosteroids, rituximab, bortezomib, alemtuzumab, rapid tapering of calcineurin inhibitors, plasma exchange, donor lymphocyte infusions, and daratumumab have been used.

Minor ABO Incompatibility

In minor ABO incompatibility, cells in the HPC product from the donor produce antibodies against the patient's original blood type. This occurs when preformed antibodies from the donor are present in the HPC product or when plasma cells from the donor continue to produce antibodies after infusion. Plasma reduction of the HPC product can decrease this effect before infusion. Donor-origin lymphocytes can produce anti-A and anti-B that attack the patient's residual red cells, typically 5 to 16 days after infusion, creating a passenger lymphocyte syndrome. The resulting acute, immune-mediated hemolysis can range from subclinical to severe and usually resolves once all the patient's original red cells

TABLE 27-1. ABO Compatibility during HSCT*

| | ABO Group | | Preferred ABO to Transfuse | | | |
Category	Recipient ABO	Donor ABO	RBCs	Platelets/Plasma	Clinical Challenges	Possible Interventions
ABO compatibility	O	O	O	O, A, B, AB	None due to ABO	None
	A	A	A, O	A, AB		
	B	B	B, O	B, AB		
	AB	AB	AB, A, B, O	AB		
Major ABO incompatibility	O	A	O	A, AB	Acute hemolysis Delayed engraftment PRCA	Red cell depletion of HPC product Plasmapheresis
	O	B	O	B, AB		
	O	AB	O	AB		
	A	AB	A, O	AB		
	B	AB	B, O	AB		
Minor ABO incompatibility	A	O	O	A, AB	Acute hemolysis Passenger lymphocyte syndrome	Plasma reduction of HPC product Monitoring HSCT patient for hemolysis
	B	O	O	B, AB		
	AB	O	O	AB		
	AB	A	A, O	AB		
	AB	B	B, O	AB		
Bidirectional ABO incompatibility	A	B	O	AB	Combination of major and minor ABO incompatibilities	
	B	A	O	AB		

*This table suggests possible guidelines for selecting blood components for each category and ABO group combination of recipient and donor. Challenges related to preparing the HPC and during engraftment are listed. Appropriate component selection should be determined by each center and is often more liberal than listed here, particularly for platelet components.
HSCT = hematopoietic stem cell transplantation; RBCs = Red Blood Cells; PRCA = pure red cell aplasia; HPC = hematopoietic progenitor cell.

are cleared. In extreme and life-threatening cases, red cell exchange with compatible units (eg, group O) is possible.

Bidirectional ABO Incompatibility

Bidirectional ABO incompatibility leads to the complexities of both major and minor ABO incompatibilities described above.

HSCT in Non-Oncologic Patients

Extra care should be taken if the allogeneic HSCT is provided for sickle cell disease or other serious blood disorders. These patients often have red cell alloantibodies due to frequent transfusion, including antibodies against antigens potentially expressed by the HPC donor. Their HSCT preparation may also use a reduced-intensity conditioning regimen that leaves a long-term mixed chimerism of red cells. Careful attention to red cell phenotypes of the donor and patient is needed to guide selection of the best-matched components. Additional discussion of sickle cell patient management is included in Chapter 19.

BLOOD COMPONENT SUPPORT FOR HSCT PATIENTS

Red Blood Cells

The need to transfuse RBCs after HSCT is common, as symptomatic anemia can occur in this patient population. The need for transfusion can be influenced by the patient's gender, underlying disease, source of HPCs, and degree of myeloablation.[6,7] Transfusion decisions are typically guided by standard institutional transfusion guidelines. Although AABB clinical practice guidelines recommend restricting RBC transfusion to those with a hemoglobin level <7 g/dL for the general patient population, the evidence supporting these guidelines is not sufficient to recommend a threshold for hematology/oncology patients with severe anemia.[8] Transfusion-associated iron overload is a significant concern in HSCT patients because increased serum ferritin has been associated with decreased

survival,[9] acute graft-vs-host disease (GVHD), propensity for bloodstream infections,[10] and development of veno-occlusive disease.[11] Given the challenges with ABO compatibility, it is essential that transfusion services maintain a sufficient supply of group O RBCs, as these will be required for many allogeneic HSCT patients.

Platelets

The timing of platelet engraftment has been associated with many factors, including relationship to donor (eg, MRD transplants engraft faster than MUD transplants), conditioning regimen, lack of transplantation complications such as infection or onset of GVHD, and the source and dose of CD34+ progenitor cells in the HPC product (eg, apheresis stem cell or marrow-harvested products engraft faster than cord-blood-derived products).[12,13]

Platelets are often stored in plasma, which exposes recipients to isohemagglutinins. Although the small quantity of antibodies typically present in platelet components is rarely clinically relevant, the total volume of ABO-incompatible plasma given should be carefully considered. Some centers transfuse platelets suspended in platelet additive solution (PAS) rather than plasma to reduce isohemagglutinins exposure. Suggestions for selecting components for transfusion based on ABO groups are listed in Table 27-1. Antibodies other than those against ABO groups, such as those targeting HLA or platelet antigens may occur in HSCT patients, contributing to platelet refractoriness. This clinical situation is described in Chapters 15, 16, and 19.

The transfusion threshold for platelets in HSCT is determined by each center. For most uncomplicated cases, a platelet count of 10,000/μL is sufficient to prevent spontaneous bleeding, but higher thresholds are needed for those undergoing procedures or experiencing sepsis or active bleeding.[14] Patients receiving defibrotide, a drug that enhances the fibrinolytic activity of plasmin, used to treat veno-occlusive disease or sinusoidal obstruction syndrome during HSCT, may require a higher platelet threshold.[15] Dosing of platelets for HSCT patients should follow guidelines similar to those for the general patient population. Much work in recent years has evaluated standard- vs low-dose platelet transfusion strategies,[16,17] with evidence suggesting that low-dose platelets for prophylaxis does not affect the incidence of bleeding.

There is also an ongoing discussion on the appropriateness of transfusing platelets only for therapeutic intent rather than for prophylaxis before potential bleeding is present. Although a therapeutic-only strategy may be appropriate for autologous HSCT patients, data in patients with acute myelogenous leukemia (AML), a condition frequently leading to HSCT, indicate a need to maintain prophylactic transfusions.[18] The Trial of Prophylactic Platelets (TOPPS) also indicated benefit for prophylactic transfusion in patients with hematologic malignancies.[19] Recent systematic reviews support these conclusions specifically in HSCT patients.[20]

Plasma, Cryoprecipitate, and Other Blood Derivatives

There are no standard guidelines related to the use of plasma, cryoprecipitate, or other factors in HSCT patients.[21] Issues related to ABO compatibility should be addressed as discussed above.

Granulocytes

Granulocytes have been used to treat neutropenic patients, typically with ANCs <500/μL and with bacterial or fungal infections that are refractory to standard treatment. The Resolving Infection in Neutropenia with Granulocytes (RING) trial, although underpowered, showed that granulocyte therapy did not confer benefit beyond standard antimicrobial therapy.[22] A Cochrane review found insufficient evidence to determine an effect of granulocyte transfusion on all-cause mortality in HSCT patients.[23]

Processing of Blood Components for HSCT Recipients

Given the immunocompromised nature of HSCT patients, care must be taken to mitigate risks of transfusion-related adverse events. Specifically, these patients are susceptible to viral infections, such as cytomegalovirus (CMV), that can be transmitted through blood components. CMV-reduced-risk cellular blood components (from a CMV-seronegative donor or leukocyte reduced) should be used. Irradiating components to prevent transfusion-associated GVHD (TA-GVHD), an almost universally fatal but rare complication, is also recommended for this immunocompromised population. Providing pathogen-reduced components is an alternative option for providing CMV-reduced-risk blood and preventing TA-GVHD. These component modifications are discussed elsewhere in this manual.

PEDIATRIC CONSIDERATIONS

Transfusion support of pediatric HSCT recipients is similar to that for adults, as standard-of-care has often been extrapolated from published data in adult HSCT patients.[24] Recommendations by one expert group for RBC transfusion support in children following HSCT who are critically ill but hemodynamically stable suggests a transfusion threshold hemoglobin level of 7 to 8 g/dL.[25]

Clinical decisions related to donor selection and HPC product type may differ based on the patient's age and size. For example, children commonly receive one cord-blood-derived HPC product compared to the two usually infused in adults. Children may also be conditioned with reduced-intensity chemotherapy that allows residual production of some recipient red cells.

Additional indications for HSCT include congenital diseases (eg, sickle cell disease, β-thalassemia major, certain marrow failure states); some childhood malignancies (eg, neuroblastoma) are treated with high-dose chemotherapy followed by autologous HSCT rescue. Managing these patients following HSCT includes addressing transfusion considerations related to their underlying disease. For example, in sickle cell or thalassemia patients, determining from molecular methods the red-cell-antigen predicted phenotype of both the donor and recipient, as well as documenting and addressing any history of existing red cell alloantibodies, is useful when providing transfusion support and when selecting HPC donors. In addition, avoiding iron overload and maintaining a higher platelet count than in other HSCT recipients

to prevent cerebrovascular bleeding may be warranted.[24]

KEY POINTS

1. HSCT offers the ability to replace or restore marrow function following destruction by disease or treatment.
2. HSCT is increasingly being performed in numerous centers, with patients seeking follow-up in community/regional hospitals.
3. HSCT patients present unique challenges, as these immunocompromised patients can possess blood cells and immune effector cells from multiple individuals (recipient, multiple allogeneic donors, cord blood donors, etc). These patients can experience complications due to their underlying condition, treatment regimens, and the transplant itself.
4. Although ABO compatibility is not essential for selection of an HPC donor, providing acceptable blood components from HPC infusion to engraftment requires consideration of the original blood group of the patient and the blood group(s) of all HPC products received. Extensive record-keeping of the transplantation and transfusion history aids in selecting ABO-compatible blood components.
5. Transfusion guidelines and thresholds should be carefully considered by each center for this patient population.
6. These immunocompromised patients require blood components that are irradiated or pathogen reduced and CMV reduced risk (ie, leukocyte reduced or CMV seronegative) to mitigate the risks of transfusion-associated graft-vs-host disease and CMV infection.

REFERENCES

1. Health Resources and Services Administration. Transplant activity report. Rockville, MD: HRSA, 2018. [Available at https://bloodstemcell.hrsa.gov/data/donation-and-transplantation-statistics/transplant-activity-report (accessed February 24, 2020).]
2. Bolan CD, Leitman SF, Griffith LM, et al. Delayed donor red cell chimerism and pure red cell aplasia following major ABO-incompatible nonmyeloablative hematopoietic stem cell transplantation. Blood 2001;98:1687-94.
3. Kim JG, Sohn SK, Kim DH, et al. Impact of ABO incompatibility on outcome after allogeneic peripheral blood stem cell transplantation. Bone Marrow Transplant 2005;35:489-95.
4. Cid J, Lozano M, Klein HG, Flegel WA. Matching for the D antigen in haematopoietic progenitor cell transplantation: Definition and clinical outcomes. Blood Transfus 2014;12:301-6.
5. Arora K, Kelley J, Sui D, et al. Cancer type predicts alloimmunization following RhD-incompatible RBC transfusions. Transfusion 2017;57:952-8.

6. Le Viellez A, P'Ng S, Buffery S, et al. Red cell and platelet transfusion burden following myeloablative allogeneic haemopoietic stem cell transplantation. Intern Med J 2015;45:1286-92.
7. Kekre N, Christou G, Mallick R, et al. Factors associated with the avoidance of red blood cell transfusion after hematopoietic stem cell transplantation. Transfusion 2012;52:2049-54.
8. Carson JL, Guyatt G, Heddle NM, et al. Clinical practice guidelines from the AABB: Red blood cell transfusion thresholds and storage. JAMA 2016;316:2025-35.
9. Meyer SC, O'Meara A, Buser AS, et al. Prognostic impact of posttransplantation iron overload after allogeneic stem cell transplantation. Biol Blood Marrow Transplant 2013;19:440-4.
10. Pullarkat V, Blanchard S, Tegtmeier B, et al. Iron overload adversely affects outcome of allogeneic hematopoietic cell transplantation. Bone Marrow Transplant 2008;42:799-805.
11. Maradei SC, Maiolino A, de Azevedo AM, et al. Serum ferritin as risk factor for sinusoidal obstruction syndrome of the liver in patients un-

dergoing hematopoietic stem cell transplantation. Blood 2009;114:1270-5.

12. Chang YJ, Xu LP, Liu DH, et al. The impact of CD34+ cell dose on platelet engraftment in pediatric patients following unmanipulated haploidentical blood and marrow transplantation. Pediatr Blood Cancer 2009;53:1100-6.

13. Pulsipher MA, Chitphakdithai P, Logan BR, et al. Donor, recipient, and transplant characteristics as risk factors after unrelated donor PBSC transplantation: Beneficial effects of higher CD34+ cell dose. Blood 2009;114:2606-16.

14. Kaufman RM, Djulbegovic B, Gernsheimer T, et al. Platelet transfusion: A clinical practice guideline from the AABB. Ann Intern Med 2015;162:205-13.

15. Richardson PG, Smith AR, Triplett BM, et al, for the Defibrotide Study Group. Defibrotide for patients with hepatic veno-occlusive disease/sinusoidal obstruction syndrome: Interim results from a treatment IND study. Biol Blood Marrow Transplant 2017;23:997-1004.

16. Heddle NM, Cook RJ, Tinmouth A, et al. A randomized controlled trial comparing standard- and low-dose strategies for transfusion of platelets (SToP) to patients with thrombocytopenia. Blood 2009;113:1564-73.

17. Slichter SJ, Kaufman RM, Assmann SF, et al. Dose of prophylactic platelet transfusions and prevention of hemorrhage. N Engl J Med 2010;362:600-13.

18. Wandt H, Schaefer-Eckart K, Wendelin K, et al. Therapeutic platelet transfusion versus routine prophylactic transfusion in patients with haematological malignancies: An open-label, multicentre, randomised study. Lancet 2012;380:1309-16.

19. Stanworth SJ, Estcourt LJ, Powter G, et al. A no-prophylaxis platelet-transfusion strategy for hematologic cancers. N Engl J Med 2013;368:1771-80.

20. Christou G, Iyengar A, Shorr R, et al. Optimal transfusion practices after allogeneic hematopoietic cell transplantation: A systematic scoping review of evidence from randomized controlled trials. Transfusion 2016;56:2607-14.

21. Roback JD, Caldwell S, Carson J, et al. Evidence-based practice guidelines for plasma transfusion. Transfusion 2010;50:1227-39.

22. Price TH, Boeckh M, Harrison RW, et al. Efficacy of transfusion with granulocytes from G-CSF/dexamethasone-treated donors in neutropenic patients with infection. Blood 2015;126:2153-61.

23. Estcourt LJ, Stanworth SJ, Hopewell S, et al. Granulocyte transfusions for treating infections in people with neutropenia or neutrophil dysfunction. Cochrane Database Syst Rev 2016;4:CD005339.

24. Webb J, Abraham A. Complex transfusion issues in pediatric heamtopoietic stem cell transplantation. Transfus Med Rev 2016;30(4):202-8.

25. Steiner ME, Zantek ND, Standworth SJ, et al. Recommendations on RBC transfusion support in children with hematologic and oncologic diagnoses from the Pediatric Critical Care Transfusion and Anemia Expertise Initiative. Pediatr Crit Care Med 2018;19:S149-56.

CHAPTER 28

Human Tissue Allografts and the Hospital Transfusion Service

Annette J. Schlueter, MD, PhD; Fran Rabe, MS; and Cassandra D. Josephson, MD

THE SURGICAL USE OF HUMAN CELLS, tissues, and cellular and tissue-based products (HCT/Ps) continues to expand. Every year, member organizations of the American Association of Tissue Banks (AATB) recover tissue from more than 39,000 donors and provide more than 3.2 million tissue grafts for transplantation.[1] These activities are increasing, in part because of the successful clinical application of tissue allografts from living donors (eg, delivery mothers donating the placenta for grafts derived from the amniotic/chorionic membranes). Many surgical specialties use human tissue allografts: orthopedic surgery, neurosurgery, cardiothoracic surgery, plastic surgery, vascular surgery, urology, ophthalmology, burn and other skin wound care, podiatry, sports medicine, trauma, and cranio/maxillofacial surgery. Increasingly sophisticated HCT/Ps continue to be developed by tissue suppliers to meet diverse clinical needs.

Oversight of activities of a tissue service may be managed by an individual, a diverse group, or a department within a hospital, and various departments or surgical specialties may prefer to manage only the tissue their service handles.

However, because ordering, receiving, storing, dispensing (issuing), tracking, tracing, investigating adverse events, and managing recalls are functions performed by both transfusion and tissue services, AABB recommends using a centralized tissue service model located within the transfusion service.[2]

TISSUE DONATION AND TRANSPLANTATION

Allografts are selected for transplantation based on intrinsic qualities that meet the surgeon's functional requirements for the patient. Bone, tendons/ligaments, and corneas are the most frequently implanted human tissues. Others include skin and associated adipose; amniotic/chorionic membranes; cartilage/meniscus (with or without bone); certain veins/arteries; soft tissue, such as fascia, pericardium, nerves, rotator cuff, and dura mater; semilunar heart valves; and cardiac conduit grafts. Tissue recovery from deceased donors occurs within 24 hours of death after appropriate consent (also known as "authorization") is obtained from a designated

28

Annette J. Schlueter, MD, PhD, Clinical Professor of Pathology and Medical Director, DeGowin Blood Center Patient Services and Tissue and Cellular Therapies, Department of Pathology, University of Iowa, Iowa City, Iowa; Fran Rabe, MS, Quality Assurance Director, Molecular and Cellular Therapeutics, University of Minnesota, Minneapolis, Minnesota; and Cassandra D. Josephson, MD, Professor, Pathology and Pediatrics, Emory University School of Medicine, Director of Clinical Research, Center for Transfusion and Cellular Therapies, and Program Director and Medical Director, Children's Healthcare of Atlanta Blood, Tissue, and Apheresis Services, Atlanta, Georgia

C. Josephson has disclosed financial relationships with Octapharma, Immucor, Medtronic, and Terumo. A. Schlueter and F. Rabe have disclosed no conflicts of interest.

legal authority (eg, the donor's next of kin) or by first-person authorization, if the donor registered his or her wishes before death. Steps taken to minimize tissue contamination include planning for body cooling after death; use of aseptic surgical recovery techniques, instruments, and supplies; and control of the site where recovery takes place.

Tissue bank personnel responsible for determining donor eligibility do so based on an evaluation of 1) the validity of the document of authorization (or informed consent for a living donor); 2) answers provided by the donor or other knowledgeable person to questions about the donor's travel, medical history, and behavior that could indicate increased risk of disease transmission; 3) available relevant medical records, including circumstances surrounding death; 4) a physical assessment or physical examination of the donor to identify evidence of high-risk behavior or active infectious disease; 5) relevant infusion and transfusion information to evaluate for potential plasma dilution of any blood samples collected for infectious disease testing, as well as infectious disease test results; and 6) the autopsy report (if an autopsy was performed). High-risk behavior that is considered to increase the possibility of disease transmission

leads to a determination that the donor is not eligible. Allografts, similar to blood components and cellular therapy products, are released for use in patients only after the donor has been screened and tested for relevant infectious diseases and the results are determined to be acceptable. (See Table 28-1.)

Types of Transplantable Tissue

Allografts, sometimes referred to as *homografts*, are grafts transferred between members of the same species. Human allograft tissue may be processed (including activities such as disinfecting, sterilizing, packaging, labeling, testing, and/or preservation) to prevent or retard biologic or physical deterioration and maintain tissue quality for its intended use. Tissue allografts can be derived from a single tissue or multiple tissues acting as a functional unit. During processing, they may be combined with other biocompatible agents to achieve desired handling and functional characteristics. Depending on the extent of processing and the intended use and effect, human tissue allografts can be regulated by the US Food and Drug Administration (FDA) as human tissue, biological products, drugs, or medical devices.[3]

TABLE 28-1. Required Infectious Disease Testing for Donors of Allograft Tissue[3]

Infectious Agent	Test Performed—FDA Licensed or Cleared
Cytomegalovirus*	FDA-cleared donor screening test for anti-CMV (total IgG and IgM)
Hepatitis B virus (HBV)	HBV surface antigen HBV core antibody (IgM and IgG) HBV nucleic acid testing
Hepatitis C virus (HCV)	HCV antibody HCV nucleic acid testing
Human immunodeficiency virus (HIV)	HIV-1 and HIV-2 antibodies HIV-1 nucleic acid testing
Human T-cell lymphotropic virus (HTLV)*	HTLV-I and HTLV-II antibodies
Treponema pallidum	FDA-cleared donor screening test for syphilis
West Nile virus (WNV)†	WNV nucleic acid testing

*Required only for tissues that are rich in viable leukocytes.
†Required only for tissues from living donors.
IgM = immunoglobulin M.

Autografts are implanted into the individual from whom they were removed. Some examples of autograft tissue are bone that has been surgically removed from a patient's ilium, shaped to desired dimensions, and implanted into the vertebral disk space of the same patient; skull flaps surgically removed after cranial trauma, then reimplanted when cerebral edema recedes; and parathyroid fragments cryopreserved after parathyroidectomy that may be reimplanted if the patient later experiences hypoparathyroidism.

Xenografts are transplanted from one species to another. Many medical products have been developed from highly processed, nonviable tissue from nonhuman animals and are regulated as medical devices. For example, porcine cardiac valves are xenografts used in certain valve-replacement surgeries.

Xenotransplantation products, often confused with xenografts, contain live cells, tissues, or organs from a nonhuman animal, or the products have been exposed during manufacture to live cells, tissues, or organs from a nonhuman animal. Depending on its classification by the FDA, a xenotransplantation product can be a biological product, a drug, or a medical device. For example, xenogeneic cells contained in a device used for extracorporeal hemoperfusion would be considered a xenotransplantation product.

Information concerning certain allografts, such as reproductive tissues (eg, gametes) and cellular therapy products, as well as xenografts and xenotransplantation products, is not provided in this chapter; nonetheless, such allografts might be handled by a transfusion service and tracked and maintained using procedures established for tissue allografts.

Tissue Processing

After tissue has been recovered from a donor, various levels of tissue processing and preservation may be accomplished. The tissue-processing facility and the processing steps (ie, manufacturing) are designed to prevent tissue contamination and cross-contamination. Similar to current good manufacturing practice requirements, current good tissue practice (cGTP) regulations promote the expectation that temperature, humidity, ventilation, and air filtration will be controlled in critical manufacturing areas to the extent deemed necessary by the tissue establishment and supported by data.

During bone, soft tissue, and connective tissue processing, various solutions may be used to reduce or eliminate bacterial contamination (the bioburden) and to remove lipids and other cellular material. Antibiotics alone or in combination with chemicals such as alcohol, peroxide, and surfactants can be used, and some methods are patented or proprietary. Depending on the type of tissue and its clinical utility or the biomechanical expectations for it, treatment with chemicals and/or graft sterilization may or may not be possible. Allografts containing viable cells or a fragile matrix (eg, fresh or cryopreserved vessels or cardiac grafts) cannot be subjected to chemicals or sterilization without an adverse affect on cellular or matrix integrity. Low-dose electron beam and gamma irradiation are the most frequently used sterilization treatments in the United States; however, the tissue is first treated using proprietary solutions and methods. Claims regarding allograft sterility must be supported by validation, and although some methods inactivate viruses, claims of sterility do not include viruses.

Various tissue preservation methods can be used to extend storage of tissue allografts so an inventory (ie, a "bank") can be readily available. Tissue integrity can be maintained through simple freezing or through cryopreservation, a process in which tissues are preserved using a cryoprotectant, such as glycerol or dimethylsulfoxide (DMSO), and frozen at a controlled rate to lower subzero temperatures that allow for long-term storage (ie, several years). Refrigerated storage can also be used to preserve cellular viability or slow matrix degradation, but only for short-term storage (days to weeks); examples include corneas and osteochondral or osteoarticular allografts. The latter two grafts provide bone with a small or large articulating cartilage surface. If the clinical utility of the tissue allows, allografts can be preserved by removing intrinsic water using dehydration, dessication, or, if a very low residual moisture level is desired, lyophilization (ie, freeze-drying). The storage potential (the expiry) is often predicated on the ability of the packaging configuration to maintain a low level of moisture over time (a year or more).

Clinical Uses of Allografts

Various human tissues are used for transplantation.[4] Examples are listed in Table 28-2. Cadaveric human bone can replace bone lost to degenerative disease, trauma, or malignancy. Allogeneic bone has unique healing characteristics, including osteoconductive and osteoinductive properties. In vivo, it acts as a scaffold that allows recipient capillary growth into the graft (osteoconductivity) and provides stimulation for the production of new bone (osteoinductivity) by exposing the patient's osteogenic progenitor cells to bone morphogenetic proteins (BMPs), which are growth factors in bone that induce new bone formation. The result is creeping substitution, in which bone remodeling occurs through osteoclastic resorption of the implanted tissue and osteoblastic generation of new bone. Crushed bone, subjected to acid demineralization, can be used alone or suspended in a biologically compatible carrier and applied to exposed bone surfaces. BMPs in demineralized bone stimulate osteogenesis, the fusion of adjacent bones, and healing. Precision bone grafts, including a growing array of spinal implants, are shaped using sophisticated, computer-aided cutting devices to fit snugly into surgical instrumentation designed to allow surgeons to place the grafts delicately in the defect. Bone-tendon (eg, Achilles tendon) or bone-ligament-bone (eg, patellar-tibia ligament) grafts are routinely used for anterior cruciate ligament (ACL) repair. The implanted tendon or ligament spans the joint space, and the bone provides an anchor into the femur and/or tibia, thereby restoring joint stability. Surgical techniques for ACL repair were developed using alternative fixation methods with a combination of tendons (without a bony attachment), such as the anterior or posterior tibialis tendons, gracilis, semitendinosus, and peroneus longus. Meniscus and joint allografts are also used to regain mobility after disease or trauma. Skin from a deceased donor can be used as a temporary wound dressing for a severely burned patient, protecting the underlying tissues from dehydration and infection. Human skin and amniotic/chorionic membranes can be preserved and frozen, or processed to remove cellular elements, producing an acellular matrix that provides a scaffold for revascularization and cellular incorporation in soft tissue reconstructive surgery and wound care. In addition, donor corneal tissues can treat various ocular surface diseases, such as keratoconus, other eye pathologies, and trauma. Scleral, pericardial, and amnion-derived allografts can treat glaucoma, scleral ulcers, and other eye damage.

Although some tissue allografts may provoke an immune response resulting in sterile inflammation, these do not usually result in failure of the allograft, presumably because of a lack of abundant residual cellular material in processed grafts.[5,6] Therefore, it is not necessary to match most allografts to the recipient's HLA or ABO type. This is in distinct contrast to organ allografts, where donor-specific HLA or ABO blood group antibodies can pose significant challenges to organ function.[7,8] HLA antibodies have been associated with corneal transplant rejection, but HLA matching of these allografts is not commonly performed.[9] Although they may not affect the function of the tissue graft, HLA antibodies that develop as the result of a bone or skin graft may affect the patient's subsequent ability to receive an organ allograft.[10,11]

Some surgeons request ABO compatibility for cardiovascular grafts, including cryopreserved heart valves, veins, or arteries, although the significance of this practice is unproven. Development of RhD, Fy^a, and Jk^b antibodies in recipients following transplantation of unprocessed bone allografts has been documented in case reports[12]; however, unprocessed allograft bone is no longer provided in the United States. If unprocessed bone contains marrow elements that cannot be removed mechanically and is intended for use in an RhD-negative female of childbearing potential, her future offspring may be at risk of hemolytic disease of the fetus and newborn. Thus, Rh Immune Globulin prophylaxis can be considered if the Rh type of the allograft donor is positive or unknown.

TABLE 28-2. Examples for Clinical Use of Human Tissue Allografts

Allograft Tissue	Clinical Use
Amniotic/chorionic membranes	Leg and foot ulcer/wound care Conjunctiva surface repair Corneal repair Neurosurgery and spine surgery Orthopedic surgery Dental/periodontal surgery Burns
Bone (cortical, corticocancellous, cancellous; powders, pastes, putties, gels, and moldable strips)	Skeletal reconstruction Spinal fusion Dental implant placement Bony defect filler
Bone-tendon (Achilles tendon) Bone-ligament-bone (patellar ligament) Tendons (anterior and posterior tibialis, semitendinosus, gracilis, and peroneus longus)	Anterior cruciate ligament repair Posterior cruciate ligament repair Rotator cuff restoration Biceps tendon rupture repair
Cardiac valves (aortic and pulmonary) and conduits	Replacement for reversal of valvular insufficiency Congenital cardiac defect repairs
Cartilage (costal)	Facial reconstruction
Cornea	Keratoconus correction Fuchs dystrophy repair Traumatic scarring repair Corneal-scleral fistula repair
Decellularized skin (dermal matrix)	Hernia repair Soft tissue reconstruction Gingival restoration
Demineralized bone	Dental implant placement Spinal fusion Bony defect filler
Dura mater	Dural defect/cerebrospinal leak repair
Fascia lata	Soft tissue reconstruction Pelvic floor support
Meniscus	Meniscus replacement
Osteoarticular/osteochondral graft (bone and joint cartilage)	Joint restoration
Pericardium	Dura patch Eyelid reconstruction Soft tissue reconstruction
Sclera	Eye enucleation Scleral ulcer repair Eyelid repair

(Continued)

TABLE 28-2. Examples for Clinical Use of Human Tissue Allografts (Continued)

Allograft Tissue	Clinical Use
Skin	Treatment of burns
	Leg and foot ulcer/wound care
	Plastic surgery reconstruction
Veins/arteries	Coronary artery bypass grafting
	Tissue revascularization
	Aneurysm repair
	Dialysis access shunts

Disease Transmission through Tissue

In the past, rare, sporadic transmission of infectious diseases, including human immunodeficiency virus (HIV), hepatitis C virus (HCV), hepatitis B virus (HBV), and Creutzfeldt-Jakob disease (CJD), was documented following tissue implantation.[13] In addition, bacterial and fungal infections from allograft transmission resulted in morbidity and mortality. Potential sources of contaminating agents included those that were donor derived or from environmental contaminants introduced at the processing facility. Malignancy was also rarely reported to be transmitted from tissue grafts and is limited to corneal allografts.[13] Currently, disease transmission from transplanted tissue is rare, but vigilance and surveillance are necessary to maintain confidence that controls, such as cGTP measures, are working. Advances in donor screening, such as for Zika virus, effectively reduce the risk of a donation from an infected donor.[14] Additionally, the application of newly validated donor testing and tissue culture and treatment methods, as well as the application of quality assurance and quality control measures, continue to improve the safety profiles of human tissue.

FEDERAL REGULATIONS, STATE LAWS, AND PROFESSIONAL STANDARDS

The FDA regulates the activities of tissue establishments (tissue banks) under Title 21, Parts 1270 and 1271, of the *Code of Federal Regulations* (CFR).[3] Tissue banks engage in one or more manufacturing functions, such as donor screening and testing and tissue recovery, packaging, labeling, processing, storage, and/or distribution for clinical use. These entities manufacture what the FDA classifies as HCT/Ps. Table 28-2 lists examples of common nonhematopoietic HCT/Ps. Although a tissue distribution intermediary might perform limited manufacturing functions (eg, storage, distribution), it must follow applicable regulations. By default, an allogeneic HCT/P is regulated as a drug, device, and/or biologic product under the Food, Drug, and Cosmetic Act and/or Section 351 of the Public Health Service (PHS) Act. If it meets the four criteria in Table 28-3, it is regulated solely under section 361 of the PHS Act, and regulations in 21 CFR Part 1271.[15]

Three subparts of 21 CFR Part 1271 concern 1) registration of tissue establishments, 2) donor eligibility, and 3) cGTP requirements related to handling of HCT/Ps. Compliance with these regulations is required of tissue establishments to control contamination and cross-contamination and avoid disease transmission. Tissue-dispensing institutions, such as hospitals, dental offices, and surgical centers that provide and use tissue within their own facility, are not subject to this oversight except under certain circumstances (eg, routine redistribution of allografts or autografts to other institutions, including an affiliate located at a different address; application of certain manufacturing steps that could contaminate the tissue).

TABLE 28-3. Criteria from 21 CFR 1271.10(a) for Regulation of an HCT/P under Section 361 of the PHS Act

1. The HCT/P is minimally manipulated, and
2. The HCT/P is intended for homologous use only, and
3. The HCT/P is not combined with another article (with some limited exceptions), and
4. The HCT/P does not have a systemic effect and is not dependent upon the metabolic activity of living cells for its primary function   Or   The HCT/P has a systemic effect or is dependent upon the metabolic activity of living cells for its primary function and is for autologous use; for allogeneic use in a first- or second-degree blood relative; or for reproductive use

21 CFR 1271.10(a) = *Code of Federal Regulations*, Title 21, Part 1271.10(a); HCT/P = human cells, tissues, and cellular and tissue-based products; PHS = Public Health Service.

For a hospital-based tissue service that does not also qualify as a tissue establishment, compliance oversight may be provided by state laws and/or accrediting organizations. The Joint Commission, AABB, the College of American Pathologists (CAP), the Association of periOperative Registered Nurses (AORN), the AATB, and the Eye Bank Association of America (EBAA) all publish standards or guidelines that apply to the practices of tissue services.[16-21] The location of a tissue service in a hospital or medical facility and the scope of its operations dictate which standards are applicable. These standards are updated regularly; therefore, periodic review of the most recent versions is important to guarantee ongoing compliance and to maintain best practices.

Both the AATB and EBAA are voluntary accrediting organizations dedicated to ensuring that human tissues intended for transplantation are safe, available, and of high quality. The AATB's standards pertain to institutional and quality program requirements; donor authorization/informed consent; donor screening and testing; and tissue recovery/acquisition, storage, processing, release, distribution, and dispensing.[20] EBAA's scope encompasses all aspects of eye banking.[21] Accreditation by these organizations is based on verified compliance with established standards and periodic inspections. Both organizations serve as scientific and educational resources for the donation and transplantation communities. A tissue service may find AATB and EBAA accreditation of a supplier to be valuable in assessing that supplier's qualifications. The Joint Commission, CAP, AABB, and AORN all have standards/guidelines that are directed specifically at the activities performed by hospital-based tissue services.

Several states have requirements for tissue banking performed within the state, and these statutes can affect the tissue service of a transfusion service. For example, New York State requires tissue bank licensure when a "tissue service" meets the definition of a "tissue storage facility" or a "tissue transplantation service" as described in Part 52 of Title 10 (Health) of the *Official Compilation of Codes, Rules and Regulations of the State of New York*. In the *California Health and Safety Code*, Section 1635, a tissue bank licensing provision is included, but for a transfusion service that handles tissue, it depends, in part, on meeting criteria involving the storage of certain tissues.

Finally, other organizations that advise or accredit specific health-care services provide direction that may affect the functions performed by a hospital-based tissue service. For example, the United Network for Organ Sharing (UNOS) has policies for organ-donor vessel packaging, labeling, storage, shipping, tracking, and reporting.[22]

HOSPITAL TISSUE SERVICES

There is no requirement for a tissue service to be managed in any particular department or by a specific individual. A tissue service located within a transfusion service can be accredited by AABB through adherence to AABB *Standards for Blood Banks and Transfusion Services*,[17] which is based on expertise in providing human-derived products that are perishable, potentially infectious, and sometimes in short supply, and that require bidirectional traceability between donor and recipient. Ordering, receiving, storing, distributing (issuing), tracking, and tracing products, as well as investigating adverse events, including complaints, recalls, and lookback investigations, are activities that are common to a transfusion service and a tissue service.

Responsibility for Hospital-Based Tissue Services

The Joint Commission requires organizations to assign oversight responsibility for their tissue program, use standardized procedures in tissue handling, maintain traceability of all tissues, and have a process for investigating and reporting adverse events.[16] Either a centralized or a decentralized process is permitted to manage these activities. In either model, designated oversight is required to coordinate tissue-related activities and ensure standardization of practices throughout the organization. The Joint Commission's requirements apply to human and nonhuman cellular-based transplantable and implantable products, including tissue allografts and certain medical devices, as classified by the FDA. Table 28-4 lists the controls a tissue service could support.

Standard Operating Procedures and Policies

Hospital tissue services must have written standard operating procedures (SOPs), either printed or electronic, for all functions pertaining to the acquisition, receipt, storage, issuance, and tracing of tissue grafts, as well as procedures for investigating adverse events and handling recalls. Manufacturers' instructions for handling tissues must be followed. When the blood bank or transfusion service is responsible, AABB requires the medical director to approve all medical and technical policies and procedures.[17(p2)] Establishing policies that address the provision

---

TABLE 28-4. Overview of Controls a Tissue Service Could Support

1. Tissue supplier (vendor) qualification
2. Tissue graft receipt and inspection
3. Maintenance of graft storage and monitoring, including alarms
4. Promotion of tissue recipient informed consent
5. Assurance that allograft tissue preparation steps (ie, instructions for use) are followed
6. Maintenance of traceability of tissue grafts from receipt through storage, issue (or reissue), and final disposition, including timely tracking to specific tissue recipients
7. Prompt handling of allograft tissue recalls or market withdrawals
8. Recognition and reporting of adverse events in tissue recipients, and participation in investigations
9. Compliance with applicable regulations, statutes, and/or professional standards
10. Oversight of a tissue utilization and safety committee
11. Promotion of cost-effective tissue use
12. Documentation of the above controls

of quality services to support the satisfaction and safety of patients is also helpful.

Tissue Supplier (Vendor) Qualifications and Certification

In contrast to blood banks, tissue processors and distributors often specialize in particular types of products (eg, allografts). Therefore, a hospital tissue service may acquire human tissue products from more vendors than are commonly used by a transfusion service to obtain blood components.

Tissue suppliers should be selected based on their ability to reliably provide high-quality tissues that meet expectations for availability, safety, and effectiveness. The tissue service should establish the minimal criteria for qualifying prospective suppliers. According to The Joint Commission's standards, accredited health-care facilities must confirm annually that tissue suppliers are registered with the FDA as tissue establishments and that they maintain a state license when required.[16] A written process for review and approval of suppliers is expected and may contain the elements listed in Table 28-5. A list of approved suppliers that includes documentation of each supplier's qualifications, certifications, and appropriate licenses or permits should be developed and maintained. Tissue services should establish procedures to receive or monitor evidence of compliance or noncompliance, such as reviewing FDA warning letters, tissue allograft recalls, and market withdrawals. Accreditation by AATB and/or EBAA may be desirable.

Qualification information for each supplier should be reviewed and approved annually by the hospital tissue service. During these reviews, the performance of suppliers in meeting the transplantation facility's needs should be evaluated. Each year, the tissue service should determine whether the supplier remains registered with the FDA. Whether AATB and/or EBAA accreditation is current can also be confirmed; it is best practice to confirm the status of this accreditation by accessing the websites of AATB and EBAA to perform a real-time search. PDF copies or photocopies of accreditation certificates might provide outdated information if the tissue establishment's accreditation has been suspended or withdrawn. FDA web postings should be reviewed for information related to closures, recalls, or MedWatch reports. Inspection reports can be requested from the FDA through the Freedom of Information Act. Complaints from transplanting surgeons concerning the supplier's tissue should be reviewed, along with any report of infection that might have been caused by a tissue allograft. Hospital management may consider establishing a committee of internal stakeholders, including physicians who implant tissue, to provide oversight of the approval of tissue suppliers, as well as tissue utilization and safety monitoring.

Inspection of Incoming Tissue Allografts

Before being placed into inventory, tissue allografts must be inspected upon receipt from a tissue supplier to ensure that packaging remains intact and the label is complete, appears to be accurate, and is adequately affixed and legible. The incoming inspection results should be recorded along with the date, time, and name of the staff person conducting the inspection.

The Joint Commission requires hospitals to verify package integrity and ensure that transport temperature was controlled and acceptable (if applicable).[16] Inspecting the shipping container for evidence of residual coolant (eg, wet ice for refrigerated grafts or dry ice for frozen grafts) may help determine that the required tissue-specific storage environment was maintained during transport.

Many tissue distributors use validated shipping containers that are tested to maintain required temperatures for a specified period. If such a container was used, the receiver of the tissue needs to verify only that there is no damage to the container and that it was received and opened within the specified time frame posted on the outside of the shipping container.

Tissues requiring "ambient temperature" (defined as the temperature of the immediate environment) for storage and shipping do not need to have the temperature verified upon receipt. However, the temperature of tissues requiring "room-temperature" storage should be verified and documented if the manufacturer has specified

TABLE 28-5. Suggested Vendor Qualification Criteria for Suppliers of Human Tissue Allografts

Criterion	Documentation/Performance
FDA registration	Perform an eHCTERS query (https://www.access-data.fda.gov/scripts/cber/CFAppsPub/tiss/index.cfm) for each tissue supplier and print the report
FDA inspection findings	FDA Form 483 findings, if any
	Warning letters and responses, if any
Voluntary accreditation, if available	Proof of current AATB accreditation (as applicable): access www.aatb.org and perform a search for accredited institutions for real-time information and produce a printout dated the day of the search
	Proof of current EBAA accreditation for ocular tissues: access http://restoresight.org/who-we-are/find-an-eye-bank/ to perform a search for real-time information
State license, permit, or registration, if required by state laws	Proof of current status (to be reviewed annually)
Reliable supply of tissue types	Adequate notification of tissue shortages
	Ability to meet special requests
	Suitable expiration dates for tissue products
Transparency of the organization	Willingness to provide information regarding donor selection criteria and tissue treatment methods
Medical consultation	Accessibility of the tissue supplier's medical director
Quality assurance/regulatory resources	Accessibility of the tissue supplier's quality program staff
New or trial tissue product support	Willingness to provide information on newly released tissue products
Professionalism of sales representatives	Approval sought by representatives through designated channels before promoting or providing tissue within the hospital

FDA = Food and Drug Administration; AATB = American Association of Tissue Banks; EBAA = Eye Bank Association of America; eHCTERS = electronic Human Cell and Tissue Establishment Registration System.

a temperature storage range on the allograft label or in the package insert.

Tissue Storage

As with blood components, tissue grafts are stored under various conditions. (See Table 28-6.) The appropriate storage conditions depend on the nature of the tissue, method of preservation, and type of packaging.

Hospital tissue services should store tissue allografts according to the processor's instructions on the allograft's label or package insert. Storage devices can include ambient- and/or room-temperature cabinets, refrigerators, mechanical freezers, and liquid-nitrogen storage units. Per The Joint Commission standards,[16] continuous temperature monitoring of refrigerators and freezers is required. Room-temperature storage

TABLE 28-6. Storage Conditions for Commonly Transplanted Human Tissue[20]

Human Tissue	Storage Conditions	Temperature*
Cardiac and vascular	Frozen, cryopreserved	−100 C or colder
Musculoskeletal and osteoarticular	Refrigerated	Above freezing (0 C) to 10 C
	Frozen, cryopreserved (temporary storage for 6 months or less)	−20 C or colder to −40 C (this is warmer than −40 C but colder than −20 C)
	Frozen, cryopreserved (long-term storage)	−40 C or colder
	Lyophilized, dehydrated	Ambient†
Birth tissue	Refrigerated, frozen, cryopreserved, lyophilized, dehydrated	As established and validated by the tissue bank
Skin and adipose	Refrigerated	Above freezing (0 C) to 10 C
	Frozen, cryopreserved	−40 C or colder
	Lyophilized, dehydrated	Ambient†

*Warmest target temperature unless a range is listed.
†Ambient temperature monitoring not required for lyophilized tissue.

equipment must be monitored if the allograft's package insert specifies a storage temperature range. Storage equipment for tissues held at refrigerated or frozen temperatures must have functional alarms, and there should be emergency backup capability in case of malfunction or damage to a storage unit. Storage SOPs should address steps to be taken in the case of excursions from allowable temperature limits or in the event of an equipment or power failure. Lyophilized tissues with package insert instructions specifying storage at ambient temperature or colder can tolerate a very broad temperature range, and monitoring during storage is not required.

Tissue Allograft Traceability and Record-Keeping

Proper management of human allografts requires that the hospital tissue service document all the steps taken in tissue handling as they occur and maintain comprehensive records of these steps. According to The Joint Commission standards,[16] staff members who have handled the tissue must be identifiable, along with dates and times when the tissue was accepted, issued, and prepared. Records should provide a clear history of all the actions performed. Documentation of the tissue supplier, the unique numeric or alphanumeric identifier(s) of the allograft, its expiration date, and the recipient's name must be maintained for all tissue grafts used. The Joint Commission also requires that documentation of the tissue type and its unique identifier be placed into the recipient's medical record.[16]

Tissue service records need to permit bidirectional traceability of all tissues from the donor and tissue supplier to the recipient(s) or other final disposition, including the discard of tissue. Records must be retained for 10 years, or longer if required by state or federal law, after distribution, transplantation, discard, or expiration (whichever occurs last).

Tissue usage information cards or other systems supplied with the allograft by the tissue bank must be completed and returned to the tissue source facility, although the identity of the recipient does not need to be disclosed. This information helps maintain the traceability of the allograft and expedites market withdrawals or recalls should they occur. The tissue supplier may also use this information to understand allograft utilization, obtain positive or negative feedback, and meet customer needs and expectations.

Recognizing and Reporting Adverse Events Possibly Caused by Allografts

Human-derived medical products, such as tissue allografts, carry some risks that must be balanced with clinical benefits. Albeit rarely, human tissue allografts have transmitted disease by bacteria, viruses, and fungi, and one tissue type (dura mater) transmitted a prion disease. In addition, an allograft may have a structural weakness that can lead to an unsuccessful outcome. (See Method 7-3.)

Hospital tissue services are required to have procedures to investigate in a timely fashion any adverse outcome suspected to be caused by a tissue allograft. The Joint Commission requires that allograft-transmitted infections and other severe adverse events be reported immediately to the tissue supplier.[16]

Surgeons play a critical role in identifying allograft-associated adverse outcomes and need to notify the hospital tissue service immediately when they suspect such events. Prompt notification of adverse events enables the hospital tissue service to investigate the cause, report the issue to the tissue supplier, and institute corrective action, including sequestration of any other suspect allografts. Tissue-associated adverse events may also be voluntarily reported directly to the FDA via MedWatch, but the reporter should be aware that FDA regulation is focused on whether an infection is suspected to have been caused by the tissue allograft. The investigation of infections and other adverse events requires cooperation between the tissue service, clinicians, and tissue supplier. Inclusion of the serial number of the graft with the report is essential for further investigation by the tissue bank. Consultation with the hospital infection-control department or an infectious disease specialist may be beneficial. Early notification can prevent complica-

tions for potential recipients of other allografts affected by the incident.

State health departments have lists of infectious diseases that must be reported when they are newly diagnosed. For example, a new diagnosis of HIV or viral hepatitis in a tissue allograft recipient where the allograft is suspected as a possible source may need to be reported to the relevant state department of health. An epidemiologic investigation may be needed to establish whether the tissue allograft was the source of the recipient's infection.

Recalls and Look-Back Investigations

A tissue product recall or market withdrawal can occur when a tissue allograft is determined by the tissue supplier to be compromised. The supplier may sequester tissues in inventory not yet distributed, recall all tissues from a specific donor or processing lot, and notify hospitals that received affected allografts. Depending on the nature of the recall, it may be prudent for the hospital to quarantine allografts in inventory, identify recipients, and/or notify the transplanting surgeon(s) of the notification. Surgeons should evaluate the circumstances and notify, if appropriate, each recipient who received a tissue graft that is being recalled.

Look-back investigation can be triggered when a tissue donor is found, after donation, to have been infected with HIV, human T-cell lymphotropic virus type I or II, HBV, HCV, or other infectious disease known to be transmitted by tissue grafts. Look-back investigations involving tissue grafts are uncommon.

Tissue Autograft Collection, Storage, and Use

Surgical reconstruction using the patient's own tissues has advantages and disadvantages when compared to the use of a tissue allograft. Advantages include faster incorporation/healing and relative safety from transmission of viral disease or immunologic rejection. Disadvantages include morbidity associated with an additional surgical procedure for the patient, including pain and potential surgical-site infection. In addition, the quality (eg, strength) and quantity of autologous tissue may not be adequate for the intended use, and removing the patient's tissue may adversely affect function at the site from which it was removed.

The collection, storage, and use of autologous tissues are exempted from regulation by the FDA as long as the autograft is used in the *same surgical procedure.*[3] The same-surgical-procedure rule allows for removal of the tissue and subsequent use in the same patient within a single operation or staged follow-up surgery. Hence, the removal and implantation may be several days apart and still be considered part of the same surgical procedure. Examples include skin grafting, coronary artery bypass surgery using autologous vessels, cranioplasty, and parathyroidectomy with implantation. Minimal manipulation allows exceptions for tissues that are maintained in their original form, which generally includes steps such as rinsing, cleansing, sizing, and shaping. A facility that removes autologous tissue that is intended to be shipped to a different facility for autologous use does not qualify for the FDA exemption, except under limited circumstances in order to accommodate the medical needs of an individual patient, which commonly occurs with cranial flaps and (less commonly) parathyroid tissue that may be removed at one facility and implanted in the patient at another facility.[23]

Written procedures should address the collection, microbial testing, packaging, storage, and issuance of tissue autografts for reimplantation. Appropriate cultures may be obtained after surgical removal and before packaging. Autografts should not be collected from patients with systemic infections or if the tissue is in close proximity to an infected area. Autografts may be stored at the medical facility where they are collected or at an off-site, FDA-registered tissue bank. Procedural recommendations have been published by the AATB and AORN.[19,20]

KEY POINTS

1. Human tissue allografts are obtained from living or deceased donors, who must meet stringent donor screening criteria and donor testing requirements similar to those applied to blood donors.

2. Not all tissue allografts are sterile. Depending on the type of allograft, sterilization may not be possible because treatment methods could compromise viability of cellular elements or the structural matrix of the graft and adversely affect performance after transplantation. Methods to mitigate contamination include the use of antibiotics, proprietary/patented processes, and ionizing radiation.

3. Human tissue allografts are used for various surgical applications to treat acquired disease, trauma, and other defects.

4. Rarely, viral, bacterial, fungal, and prion-associated diseases have been transmitted by allografts. Like blood components, allografts are released for use only after donor eligibility criteria are met and relevant infectious disease test results are deemed acceptable.

5. In general, bone and soft tissue allografts do not need to be matched for HLA, ABO, or Rh type.

6. Tissue banks are engaged in donor screening and testing and recovery, labeling, processing, storage, and distribution of human tissue for transplantation. They are regulated by the FDA under Title 21, CFR Parts 1270 and 1271 as manufacturers of HCT/Ps; may have a license or permit or be registered in certain states; and may seek voluntary accreditation from the AATB or EBAA.

7. Hospital-based tissue services are not subject to FDA regulatory oversight if their activities are limited to receiving, storing, and dispensing tissue for use within their own facilities. However, The Joint Commission, AABB, CAP, and AORN publish standards and guidelines that apply to tissue services.

8. Functions performed by tissue services that mimic transfusion services include vendor qualification; ordering, receiving, storing, distributing, and tracing products; and investigating adverse events, including complaints, recalls or withdrawals, and look-back investigations.

9. Additional controls that can be undertaken by a hospital tissue service include promoting tissue recipient informed consent and oversight of a tissue utilization and safety committee.

REFERENCES

1. American Association of Tissue Banks. About us. McLean, VA: AATB, 2018. [Available at http://www.aatb.org/?q=about-us (accessed July 30, 2018).]

2. Eastlund DT, Eisenbrey AB, for the Tissue Committee. Guidelines for managing tissue allografts in hospitals. Bethesda, MD: AABB, 2006.

3. Code of federal regulations. Title 21, CFR Parts 1270 and 1271. Washington, DC: US Government Publishing Office, 2019 (revised annually).

4. Warwick RM, Brubaker SA, eds. Tissue and cell clinical use: An essential guide. West Sussex, UK: Wiley-Blackwell, 2012.

5. Malini TI. Preparation and banking of bone and tendon allografts. In: Sherman OH, Minkoff J, eds. Arthroscopic surgery. Baltimore, MD: Williams and Wilkins, 1990:65-86.

6. Fehily D, Brubaker SA, Kearney JN, Wolfinbarger W, eds. Tissue and cell processing: An essential guide. West Sussex, UK: Wiley-Blackwell, 2012.

7. McCaughan JA, Tinckam KJ. Donor specific HLA antibodies and allograft injury: Mechanisms, methods of detection, manifestations and management. Transplant Int 2018;31:1059-70.

8. Subramanian V, Ramachandran S, Klein C, et al. ABO-incompatible organ transplantation. Int J Immunogenet 2012;39:282-90.

9. Sel S, Schlaf G, Schurat O, Altermann WW. A novel ELISA-based crossmatch procedure to detect donor-specific anti-HLA antibodies responsible for corneal allograft rejections. J Immunol Methods 2012;381:23-31.

10. Mosconi G, Baraldi O, Fantinati C, et al. Donor-specific anti-HLA antibodies after bone-graft transplantation. Impact on a subsequent renal transplantation: A case report. Transplant Proc 2009;41:1138-41.

11. Duhamel P, Suberbielle C, Grimbert P, et al. Anti-HLA sensitization in extensively burned patients: Extent, associated factors, and reduction in potential access to vascularized composite allotransplantation. Transpl Int 2015;28:582-93.

12. Cheek RF, Harmon JV, Stowell CP. Red cell alloimmunization after a bone allograft. Transfusion 1995;35:507-9.

13. Eastland T, Warwick, RM. Diseases transmitted by transplantation of tissue and cell allografts. In: Warwick RM, Brubaker SA, eds. Tissue and cell clinical use: An essential guide. West Sussex, UK: Wiley-Blackwell, 2012:72-113.

14. Silveira FP, Campos SV. The Zika epidemics and transplantation. J Heart Lung Transplant 2016; 35:560-3.

15. Food and Drug Administration. Guidance for industry: Regulatory considerations for human cells, tissues, and cellular and tissue-based products: Minimal manipulation and homologous use. (December 2017) Silver Spring, MD: CBER Office of Communication, Outreach, and Development, 2017. [Available at https://www.fda.gov/downloads/biologicsbloodvaccines/guidancecomplianceregulatoryinformation/guidances/cellularandgenetherapy/ucm585403.pdf.]

16. Transplant safety (TS). In: Comprehensive accreditation manual for hospitals. Oakbrook Terrace, IL: The Joint Commission, 2018:TS03.

17. Gammon R, ed. Standards for blood banks and transfusion services. 32nd ed. Bethesda, MD: AABB, 2020.

18. Standards for laboratory accreditation. Northfield, IL: College of American Pathologists, 2017.

19. Association of periOperative Registered Nurses. Standards of perioperative nursing. In: 2015 Guidelines for perioperative practice. Denver, CO: AORN, 2015. [Available at http://aorn.org/guidelines/clinical-resources/aorn-standards (accessed December 10, 2019).]

20. Osborne JC, Norman KG, Maye T, et al, eds. Standards for tissue banking. 14th ed. McLean, VA: American Association of Tissue Banks, 2016.

21. Medical standards. Washington, DC: Eye Bank Association of America, 2017.

22. Organ Procurement and Transplantation Network. Policy 16: Organ and vessel packaging,

labeling, shipping, and storage. Rockville, MD: Health Resources and Services Administration, 2018. [Available at https://optn.transplant.hrsa. gov/governance/policies/.]

23. Food and Drug Administration. Guidance for industry: Same surgical procedure exception under 21 CFR 1271.15(b): Questions and answers regarding the scope of the exception. (November 2017) Silver Spring, MD: CBER Office of Communication, Outreach, and Development, 2017. [Available at https://www.fda.gov/down loads/biologicsbloodvaccines/guidancecompli anceregulatoryinformation/guidances/tissue/ ucm419926.pdf.]

Index

*Page references in italics
refer to figures or tables.*

A

A/anti-A, 298-299, *298*, 305-306, 389
    peripheral core chain variants, *301*
    serologic reactions, *303*
A,B/anti-A,B, 305, 306
    plasma, 572
ABCB6, 380
ABCG2, 380
ABH, 299, *300, 301, 311*
ABO blood group systems, 297-327
    antibodies, 305-306
    blood component requirements, *507*
    carbohydrate epitopes, 297-327
    compatibility, 523-524, 768-772, *771, 769*
    development and aging, 299-300, 302
    discrepancies, 306-310, *308-309*
    genetics/genotyping, 289, 302-303, 507
    grouping, *299*
    HDFN, 305
    HPAs, 461-462
    HSCT, 768-772, *771, 769*
    incompatibility, 297-298, 770, 772
    key points, 323-324
    matching, *557*
    phenotypes, 298
    platelets, 564-565
    solid-organ donors, 289
    subgroups, 303-304
    titers, 300, 302
    typing, *299, 303*, 306
    see also individual blood groups
Accidents, reporting, 38-39
Accreditation, 21-22, 85-86, 756-757
    organizations, 2
    regulation vs, 77, *78*
    see also Regulations and recommendations
ACE inhibitors, in therapeutic apheresis, 712
ACHE, 373
Acid-citrate-dextrose solution A (ACD-A), 711
ACKR1, 370
Acute lung injury, transfusion-related, 96, 100, 128, 156, 162, 472, 492, 640-643
ADAMTS13, 714
Adenosine diphosphate (ADP), 674

Adsorption, 418-419
    allogeneic red cells, 437-438
    autologous red cells, 437
    -elution, 420
    protein, nonimmunologic, 447
    red cells
        allogeneic, 437-438, *438*
        autologous, 437
    selective, 707, 724-727, *726-727*
    serum, 438-439
Adverse events/reactions
    donor, 106, *107, 108-110*, 143-144
    hemovigilance, 100-103, *101-102*
    hospital reporting to blood suppliers, *116-123*
    MERS-TM, 99
    monitoring, CT, 99
    near-miss events, 26
    nonconforming events, 5, 17-20, *19*, 24
    reporting, 103
    severity grading tool for blood donor, *124-125*
    transfusion-related, 98
    see also Transfusion reactions
A4GALT, 321-322
Agglutination
    antigen and antibody concentrations, *239*
    mixed-field, 273
Agglutinin syndrome, cold (CAS), 318, 442-443
    alloantibodies, 443
    autoantibodies, 318
        cold-reactive, 443
        specificity, 442
    serologic characteristics, 442-443
Agreements, 10
AHA. *See* Anemia, autoimmune hemolytic
AHG testing, 318
AHTR. *See* Transfusion reactions, hemolytic immune-mediated acute
AIHA. *See* Hemolytic anemia, autoimmune
AIN. *See* Neutropenia, autoimmune
Air embolism, 648
Alarm fatigue, 600
Albumin-bound drugs, in therapeutic apheresis, 712-713
Aliquoting, 521-522
Alleles. *See* Genes/genetics
Allergic reactions, in therapeutic apheresis, 711-712
Alloantibodies, 389, 437
    autoantibody vs, 285-286

I

development, 250
H, 312
ALT, *174*
Amniocytes, 287
Amotosalen, 216
Amplification products
    detection of, 234-238
    DNA arrays, 235, 237
    next-generation sequencing, 237-238
    PCR, real-time, 234-235
Anemia, 598
    anemia, hemolytic autoimmune (AIHA), 283,
        285, 318, 434-445
        adsorption, 437-439
        autoantibody specificity, 439, 444
        blood selection for transfusion, 439-441
        DAT-negative, 440-441
        mixed-type, 443-444
        patient history, 432-434
        RBC transfusion, 559-560
        serologic characteristics and problems, 435-
            437, *435*, 443-444
        transfusion for patients, 444
        types, 434
    anemia, hemolytic immune, drug-induced
        (DIIHA), 445-449, *452-455*
        classification, 446-447
        mechanisms, 445, *445*
        protein adsorption, nonimmunologic, 447
    anemia, hemolytic warm (WAIHA), 435-442
        autoantibodies, DAT-negative, 441-442
        RBC transfusion, 560
        transfusion of patients, 441
    classification, *554*
    microangiopathic hemolytic (MAHA), 714, 719
    preoperative diagnosis and treatment, 591
ANH. *See* Hemodilution, acute normovolemic
Ankylosing spondylitis, HLA-B27 and, 496
Antibodies, 229
    agglutination reactions, *239*
    alloantibodies, 389, 437
        autoantibody vs, 285-286
        development, 250
        H, 312
    autoantibodies, 389, 436-437, 439
        AIHA, mixed type, 444
        alloantibody vs, 285-286
        CAS, 443
        DAT-negative, 441-442
        H, 313
        HI, 313
        PCH, 444-445
        specificity, 439, 440, 444
    binding, red cell destruction, *247*

blood group systems and antigens
    clinical significance, *356-358*
    key points, 384-385
donor-specific (DSAs), 742
drug-dependent
    autoantibody production, 447
    drug-treated red cells and, 446-447
    laboratory investigation, 448-449
    untreated red cells in the presence of drug, 447
exclusion, 398-401, *399-400*
HLA, 490
identification, 420-421
    Luminex-based, 472
    panel, 391-392, *393*, 396-397
    red cells, 391-392, *393*
insignificant, 250
interpretation, 509
isotypes, 244-245
monoclonal (MoAbs), 285
multiple, *393*, 402, 406-407, 421
receptors (FcγRs) in target clearance, 246
red cells, 391-392, *393*
serologic reactivity, *405-406*
unexpected, 507-508, 524
Antibodies to red cell antigens, 389-428
    additive solutions, 392, 394
    adults vs neonates, 390, *390*
    antigens
        alterations, *412*
        high-prevalence, 410-413, *411-412*
        low-prevalence, 413
    antiglobulin reagents, 394
    autoantibodies
        cold, 409
        warm, 408-409, 410
    biologic therapies, 395
    diagnosis and disease, 395
    dosage, 390
    drug-dependent, 413-414
    exclusion, 398-401, *399-400*
    identification, 391-402, *393*
        complex, 402-*414, 403, 404*
        considerations following, 421-424
    immunization to, 389
    incubation time, 416
    interpretation of results, 397-402
    key points, 424-425
    medications, 395
    patient history, 394-395
    pregnancy, 413
    procedures, 414-421
    reactivity
        positive and negative, 397
        specificity, without, 407-408

reagents, 391-394, *393*
    components, 414
red cells
    exclusion and confirmation, 401
    exposure, prior, 394-395
rouleaux formation, 414
serologic reactions, *405-406*
    anomalous, 414
serum-to-cell ratio, 415-416
specificity assessment, 398, 401
specimen requirements, 391
storage, 390-391
temperature reduction, 415
test methods, 392
transfusion reactions, delayed serologic/
    hemolytic, 409
zygosity, 390
Anticoagulation, in therapeutic apheresis,
  711
Antifibrinolytic drugs, 595-596, 606
Antigens, 280
    absence, 487
    agglutination reactions, *239*
    antithetical, 265, 281-282
    blood groups, 382-383
        without, 342-384
    Class I/II MHC
        characteristics, 479-481, *480*
        configuration, 481, *481*
    density, 265
    dose, *265*
    expressed, 265
    high-prevalence (901 series), 383, *383*
    low-prevalence (700 series), 383
    negative
        donors, molecular testing, 288
        phenotypes, 276
    phenotype prediction, molecular methods, 282-
      283, 288
    public, 482
    red cells, 390-391, *390*
Antigen capture assays (ACAs), 468
Antiglobulin testing
    direct (DAT), 285, 390, 395-396, 430-435
        elution, 433-434, *434*
        evaluation, 432
        key points, 449
        patient history, 432-434
        positive, *430*
        principles, 431-432
        serologic investigation, 433
    false-negative results, *534*
    false-positive results, *533*
    indirect (IAT), 285

Antihemophilic factor (AHF), 688
    cryoprecipitated, 157-158
    pooled, 160
Antihuman globulin (AHG) reaction, *506*
APACHE. *See* Evaluation
Apheresis, 141
    blood components, 149-150
    cytapheresis, 721-722, *721*
    devices, 150-153
        filtration-based, 707
        selective adsorption, 707
        QC, 31
    granulocyte-monocyte (GMA), 707
    key points, 165-166
    medicine, 727
    pediatric, 713
    plasma, 150
    platelet, 149
    red cell, 149
    therapeutic (TA), 705-735
        adverse effects, 711-713
        anticoagulation, 711
        cardiorespiratory status, 708-709
        classification, 713
        device modalities, 706-707
        documentation, 727-729
        evaluation and treatment, *708*
        granulocyte-monocyte, 707
        hematologic status, 709
        indications, 713-714, 719-727
        key points, 729-730
        medications, 709
        neurologic status, 708
        patient evaluation and management, 707-
          711
        pediatric, 713
        principles, 705-706
        renal and metabolic status, 709
        replacement fluids, *709*
        transfusion/apheresis history, 708
        vascular access, 709-711
Arboviruses, screening, 208-209
ARDS. *See* Respiratory distress syndrome, acute
Arterial puncture, 143
Assays
    ACA, 468
    antibodies to red cell antigens, 240, *240*
    ChLIAs, 181
    colony-formation, 753
    EIAs, 181
    ELISA, 240-242, *241*, *467*, 490
    NAT, 209, 212
    phenotyping red cells, 239, *240*
    platelets, 240, 467-468

protein, 238-242
solid-phase, 239-242, 490
Assessments, external, 21-22
ATAM, 381
ATML, 381
ATRs. *See* Transfusion reactions, allergic
Auditing
blood utilization
criteria, 615-617
guidelines, 614
process, 614-615 g
review items, *615*
review types, 617-620, *615*
provider feedback, 600, *603*
see also Monitoring
AUG (Augustine) system (036), 381
Aurora Plasmapheresis System, 151-152
Autoimmune hemolytic anemia. *See* Anemia,
hemolytic autoimmune
Autosomes, 256

B

B/anti-B, 305-306, 389
antigen, 298-299, *298*
phenotype, acquired, 305
serologic reactions, *303*
B(A) phenotype, 304-305
Babesia, 176, 179, 188, 210-212
donor testing regulations and standards, *193*
transfusion-transmitted (TTB), 211
Bacteria, screening, *193*, 204-205
BECs. *See* Computer systems, blood establishment
Benchmarking, 621-623
PBM metrics, *622*
Best practice advisory (BPA), *600*
Bg, 383-384
Biohazard waste and disposal, 46-48
Biologics
license application (BLA), 81
product deviation (BPD), 19-20, 84
safety cabinets (BSCs), 34, 42, *43-44*
Biovigilance, 26, 99
elements of, 99-100
reporting, 99-100
task force on, 99
US, 112
Bleeding
donors, 134
plasma transfusions, 567-568
platelet transfusions, 563-564
in therapeutic apheresis, 712
WHO scale, *562*
Blood
administration, 543-547

bags, 145
bloodless care, 605
collection
equipment, QC, 31
systems, 158-159
delivery, 606
devices, 82-83
irradiators, QC, 30
loss
intraoperative, 594-595
phlebotomy, 597, *598*
ordering, surgical practices, 528-529
order schedule, maximum surgical (MSBOS),
528, 591-592, *592*, 605
rare needed, 423-424
recovery
intraoperative autologous, 594
postoperative, 596-597
selection for transfusion, 439-441
spill cleanup, *47*
supply, zero risk, 1-2
volume, neonates, 675
warmers, 540-541
QC, 30
wrong blood in tube (WBIT), 539
Blood banks, inventory, 527-528, 623
Blood components, 141-172
ABO, 768-772
administration, 537-551
collection, 149-153
mobile sites, 35
defined, 78
discard, 4
dispensing, 537-543
equipment, 540-542
documentation, 4, 547-548
dosing, *680*
frozen, shipping, 522-523
HSCT, 772-773
infectious disease screening, 173
irradiation, 161-162, *651*
issuing, 523-527
key points, 165-166, 549-550
labeling, 164-165
leukocyte-reduced, 159
manufacturers' licensure, 81-82
non-ABO, 771
nonemergent settings, *546*
pooled, 159-160
preparation, 146-148, *147*
processing and modification, 158-164
production, automated, 148-149
quarantine, 4, 164
RBC ratio, 606

return and reissue, 529

storage, 153-158, 509-518, *510-516*

 expiration, *510-516*

 irradiation, 519-520

 monitoring, 509-518, *510-516*

 temperature, 509, 517

testing, 523

thawing devices, QC, 30

transportation and dispensing, 509, *510-516*, 542-543

transfusion settings, unique, 548-549

volume reduced, 162

washing, 162

Blood donors. *See* Donors

Blood group systems, 255, *259-262*, 279, 280

antigens, 355-385

 databases, 283

 naming, 280

function, *359*

history, 255

SNV, 279

terminology, 280-281, *281*

See also Genetics; particular system

Blood pressure

cuffs, QC, 31

donors, 130

Blood utilization, 20-21

auditing, 613-626

big data, 621-623

CPOE, 620-621

criteria, 615-617

high-risk patients, 620

key points, 623-624

monitoring, 623

PBM, 600, 604

process, 614-615

review items, *615*

review types, 617-620

Body size, neonates, 675

Bombay (Oh) phenotype, 310, 312

Bone

morphogenetic proteins (BMPs), 780

replacement, 780

Bruise, 143

BSCs. *See* Safety, biological safety cabinets

Buffy-coat preparation, *147*, 148

C

C3, 246-247

C3b, 250

C/c antigens, 344, 346, *346*

Calcium, 606

Calibration, 26

Cancer, donors, 133-134

Carbohydrates

blood group systems, 297-327

epitopes, 297

Cardiac. *See* Heart conditions

CAS. *See* Agglutinin syndrome, cold

Catheter, central venous (CVC), 710

Cautery, 595

CCIs. *See* Corrected count increments

CD11a/b, antigens, 471

CD34+, 746, 747

HPC, 750-751

CD38, 285, 395

monoclonal antibodies, RBC transfusion, 560-561

CD47, 285

monoclonal antibodies, RBC transfusion, 560-561

CD59 system (035), 381

CD109, HPAs, 461

CD177, 470-471

Cells

assays, 490

counters/hemoglobinometers, QC, 31

division, 257-258

donor testing, 195

enzyme-treated, 416-417

expansion, HPC, 751

processing methods, 750-751

selection systems, HPC, 750-751

separation methods, 283

somatic, 256

washing/washers, 29, 520-521, 695

see also particular cell type

Cellular therapies (CT), 99

accreditation, *89*

FDA, 78-84

key points, *90*

regulations, 77-93

Centrifuges/centrifugation, 146

continuous-flow, 706-707

intermittent-flow, 707

microhematocrit, 31

QC, 29, 31

Centromere, 256, *257*

Certification, PBM, 585, 606

Cesium irradiators, 56

CFR. *See Code of Federal Regulations*

CH/RG (Chido/Rodgers) system (017), 377, 417-418

Change control, 26

see also Patient blood management

Chemicals

fume hoods, 34, 51

hazardous, 39, 48-49, list, *67-68*

hygiene plan (CHP), 48, 50

modification, 417

signage, 50
spills
    categorization, 52
    managing, 52, *74-75*
    work safety, *69-70*
Chemical safety, 48-53
    emergency response plan, 52
    engineering controls and PPE, 51
    hazard identification and communication,
      50
    labeling, 50
    training, 49-50
    waste disposal, 52-53
    work practices, 51-52
Chikungunya virus (CHIKV), 208, 209
Chimerism, 273-274, 289
    TA-GVHD and, 492-493, *493*
    twin, 273-274
Chlamydia trachomatis, 196
ChLIAs. *See* Assays, chemiluminescent
  immunoassays
Chlorine, spill response, *71*
Choosing Wisely campaign, 587, 598-599, *599*
Chromatids, 257, *257*
Chromosomes, 256, *257, 258*
    6, *486*
    homologous, 256
Circular of Information for the Use of Cellular
  Therapy Products, 87, 165
Circulatory overload, transfusion-associated (TACO),
  100, 643-645
cis, 274
cisAB phenotype, 305
Citrate
    reactions, 144
    toxicity, 646
Citrate-phosphate-dextrose-adenine (CPDA)-1,
  neonates, 676
Class I/II
    antigens, 566
    molecules, role, 483-484
Clinical decision support (CDS), 599-600
  system (CDSS), 621
Clinical Laboratory Improvement Amendments of
  1988 (CLIA), 2, 12, 84, 85
Clinics
    consultation, HLA, 497-498
    massive transfusion, 606
    outcome data, PBM, 604, *604*
    utility, 737-742
Clocks, QC, 30
CO (Colton) system (015), 375, *376*
Coagulation
    abnormalities, AHTR, 635

disseminated intravascular (DIC), AHTR, 636
    optimizing, 592
Code of Federal Regulations (CFR), 2, 78, 79, *80*
    HCT/Ps, 87
    HPC, 740
    HSCT, 743, 756
    quality-related references, 28
    RTTIs, 127-128
    tissue grafts, *783*
Cold agglutinin syndrome. *See* Agglutinin syndrome,
  cold
Cold stress, neonates, 676
College of American Pathologists (CAP), 2
    transfusion medicine checklist TRM, 86, 87
Colony-formation assay. *See* Assays
Compatibility testing, neonates, 677-678
Competency assessments, 7-8
Complement
    activation outcomes, 247, 635
    AHTR, 635, 636
    cascade, 636
    target cell opsonization and destruction, 246-
      247
Complications. *See* Transfusion reactions
Computer systems
    blood establishment (BECS), 111
    provider order entry (CPOE) system, 599-600,
      601, 620-621
    validation, 13
Confidentiality, records, 16
Connection devices, sterile, 30
Consanguineous mating, 268
Consent, recipient, 537-538
Contracts, 10
Controls
    chart, 26
    in-process, 4
Copper sulfate, QC, 31
Coronary syndromes. *See* Heart conditions
Corrected count increments for platelets, 565, 566
Corrosive compounds, work safety, *69*
COST collection, 382
CPOE. *See* Computer systems, provider order entry
Creutzfeldt-Jakob disease (CJD), 213, 214
CROM (Cromer) system (021), 378
Crossing over/crossovers, 258, 270, 271-272, *272,*
  487
Crossmatching, 490
    antiglobulin, 509
    compatibility testing, 677-678
    computer/electronic, 508
    HLA, 490
    immediate-spin (IS), 508
    interpretation, 509

Cryoprecipitate
   AHF, 688
   HSCT, 773
   neonatal and pediatric, 688
   shipping, 522
   storage, 518
   thawing, 518-519
   transfusion, 569-570
   see also Antihemophilic factor, cryoprecipitated
Cryopreservation, 751-752
   RBC components, 160-161
CTL2 system (039), 342
   antigens on, 471
Customer feedback, 4
   focus, 5, 6, 23
CVC. *See* Catheter, central venous, 710
Cytapheresis, 721-722, *721*
Cytogenetics, 256
Cytomegalovirus (CMV) testing, *196*
   immunocompromised recipients, 194-195
   prevention, pediatric, 694
Cytoskeleton, *360*

D

D/anti-D, 329, 337-342
   assay, 290-291
   clinical considerations, 343
   elevated, 340
   HDFN and, 663
   molecular testing, 288
   partial, 339-340
   phenotypes
      fetal, 286
      negative, 340, 342
      positive, 337-340
   pregnant women, 287
   reagent reactivity, *341*
   structure, *338*
   testing for, 342-343
   typing
      discrepancies, 343
      donors, 342
      patients, 342-343
   weak, 338-339
DAT. *See* Antiglobulin test, direct
Data
   benchmark, 604-605
   big data, 621-623
   blood utilization, 614
   collection, 600-605
Databases, blood group antigen, 283
Decontamination, 45
Deemed status partners, 85
Deferral list, 128

Del types, 340
Dengue virus (DENV), 208-209
Deoxyribonucleic acid. *See* DNA
Devices, 706-707
   adverse effects, 20, 82-83, 711-713, *711*
   anticoagulation, 711
   classification, 82
   modalities, 706-70*7, 706*
   patient evaluation and management, 707-711
   pediatric, 713
   pressure, 541
   sterile connection, 30
   vascular access, 709-711
   ventricular assist (VADs), 693
   see also Equipment
DHQ. *See* Donor History Questionnaire
DI (Diego) system (010), 372-373
   antigens, 373
   band 3, 372, *372*
Di$^{a/b}$ (DI1/2)/anti-Di$^{a/b}$, 372-373
Diagnosis-related groups, 605
DIC. *See* Coagulation, disseminated intravascular
DIIHA. *See* Anemia, hemolytic immune, drug-induced
Dimethylsulfoxide (DMSO), 748, 749, 751-752
Diploid (2N), 257
2,3-Diphosphoglycerate (2,3-DPG), neonates, 674, 677
Disaster plan, 23
Disinfectants, 45
Distribution, 4, 522-523
   see also Blood components, dispensing
Dithiothreitol (DTT), 244
DMAIC process, 22, *23*
DNA, 256, *257*
   analysis, 229-238
   assays, alloantibody vs autoantibody, 285-286
   chemistry and structure, 230-231, *230*
   nucleotides in, 230-231
DO (Dombrock) system (014), 374-375
Documentation/documents and records, 4, 5, 14-16, 24
   creation, 14
   donors, 128
   electronic health records (EHR; HER), 111, 621
   maintenance, 16
   QC, 13-14
   therapeutic apheresis, 727, *728, 729*
   see also Reporting/reports
Donath-Landsteiner test, 323
Donors/donations
   acknowledgment, 129-130
   allogeneic
      criteria, 128

identification, 128-129
key points, *137*
registration, 128-129
selection, 127-140
autologous, 136-137
contraindications, 137
control, 395-396
donations, 136-137
infectious disease testing, 195
key points, *137*
selection, 127-140
blood diseases, 134
blood donor room, biosafety, 46
cancer, 133-134
compatibility, 491
consent, 129-130
directed, 136
deferral, 128, 129, 133
accommodations, 129-130
directed, 136
educational material, 129-130, 133
qualification screening, 130-131
temporary, *183*
education, 129-130, 133, 217
eligibility, 79, 130-131, 133-135, 189
bleeding conditions and blood diseases, 134
cancer, 133-134
heart and lung conditions, 134-135
medications, 135
not eligible for reentry, *184, 187*
pregnancy, 135
reentry, *183-187*
exclusion, HIV, 177
hemovigilance, 99, 103-106, *105*
history evaluations, 177
identification number (DIN), 142
preoperative autologous (PAD), 592, 594
preparation and care, 141-153
adverse reactions, 143-144
consent, 141-142
eligibility, 142
fatalities, 144
identification, 142
postphlebotomy care, 142-143
vein selection and disinfection, 142
prior, 189, 194
recipient
outcomes, 556
-specific, 135-137
regulations, 128
repeat, 197
samples
retention and storage, 523
RBC unit selection, 523-525

screening/testing, 128-129, 133, 217
eligibility, 127-128
identification, 128-129
international variations, 195-196
registration, 128-129
regulations and standards, *190-193*
selection, 742
tests, 173, *174-176*, 177-196, *178-180, 179*
siblings, 743
unit selection
antigen-negative blood, 422-423, *424*
crossmatch for compatibility, 423
phenotype-matched blood, 423
Donor History Questionnaire (DHQ), 128, 132
abbreviated (aDHQ), 132-133
FDA and, 132
frequent donors, 132-133
Dosage, 390
Drug-dependent antibodies. *See* Antibodies, drug-dependent
DSAs. *See* Antibodies, donor-specific

E

ECMO. *See* Oxygenation, extracorporeal membrane
E/e antigens, 344, 346
EIR. *See* Reports, establishment inspection
Electrical safety, 40-41
emergency response plan, 41
engineering controls and PPE, 40
hazard ID and communication, 40
training, 40
work practices, 40
see also Safety; Work environment
Electronic health records. *See* Documentation
ELISA. *See* Enzyme-linked immunosorbent assay
Elution, 419-420, 433-434, *434*
Elutriation, HPC, 750
Emergencies
equipment, 541-542
exits, 39
showers, 34, 51
transfusion, 525-526
Emergency response plans, 38, 40
biosafety, 46
chemical, 52
electrical, 41
radiation, 55
see also Safety
Employee health services, 38
Encephalomyelitis, acute disseminated, TPE, 720
End-product testing and inspection, 4, 26
Engineering controls, 37
biosafety, 42
chemical safety, 51

electrical safety, 40
fire prevention, 39
guidance, *63-65*
radiation, 55
see also Safety; Work environment
ENT1. *See* Nucleoside transporter 1, equilibrative
Enterocolitis, necrotizing, 682
Enzyme immunosorbent assays (EIAs), 181
Enzyme-linked immunosorbent assay (ELISA), 240-242, *241, 467*
   donor screening, 490
   sandwich ELISA, 241-242, *241*
   technical problems, 242
Equipment
   identification, 9
   maintenance and control, 4
   management, 5, 8-9, 23
   selection, 8-9
   see also Devices
Ergonomics, 35
Erythrocyte membrane-associated protein (ERMAP), 374
Erythroid phenotypes, 384
Erythropoiesis-stimulating agents (ESAs), neonates, 675-676
Erythropoietin (EPO) physiology and therapy, neonates, 675-676
Ethnicity, 398, 401
Euchromatic regions, 256
Evaluation, 5, 554-555, *708*
   see also Monitoring; Testing
Events
   near-miss, 26
   nonconforming, 5, 17-20, *19*, 24
   see also Adverse events
Expiration, components, *510-516*
Eyewashes, guidance, *65*
Eyewash stations, 34

F

Facilities, 5, 22-23, 24, 33-35
   design and workflow, 33-34
   exits, 39-40
   key points, 57
   restricted areas, 34-35
   visitors, 35
   see also Safety; Work environment
Failure mode effects analysis (FMEA), 18
Fatalities, 19
   blood donation, 144
   FDA contact information, *652*
   reporting, 38-39, 82, 97, 99, 652-653
   in therapeutic apheresis, 713
FcγR, 246, 250, 251

FcγRIIIb, antigens, 469-470
FDA. *See* Food and Drug Administration
FFP. *See* Plasma, fresh frozen
Fibrinogen, 569, 570
Ficin, 416
Filters
   leukocyte reduction, 159
   microaggregate, 543
   pediatric, 689
   standard administration, 543-544
Fire prevention, 39-41
   alarm systems, 39
   emergency response plan, 40
   engineering controls, 39
   extinguishers, 39
   hazard identification and communication, 39
   PPE, 39
   training, 49
   work practices, 39-40
   see also Safety
Flaviviruses, 208
Floseal, 595
Flow cytometry, 243
Fluorescent in-situ hybridization (FISH), 257
FNAIT, 566, 567
FNHTR. *See* Transfusion reactions, febrile nonhemolytic
Food additives, indirect, 164-165
Food and Drug Administration (FDA), 1, 2, 173
   Amendments Act (FDAAA), 89
   DHQ, 132, 133
   donor eligibility, 128, 189-194, *190-193*
   fatality reporting, *652*
   guidance, 79
   inspections, 83-84
   labels, 164-165
   oversight, 78-84
   regulations and recommendations, 78-79
   see also Code of Federal Regulations
Food, Drug, and Cosmetic (FD&C) Act, 78-79
Formaldehyde, spill response, *72*
Forms, 15
FORS blood group system, 323
Freezers, QC, 29
Frequency, alleles and genes, 275-278
Furosemide, AHTR, 636
FUT, 310, 312, 313, *316*
Fy3/5/6, 369
Fyᵃ/ᵇ (FY1/2), 368-369
FY (Duffy) system (008), 279, 291, 368-370
   clinical significance of antibodies, 369-370
   glycoprotein, *369*
   phenotypes and genotypes, *369*

G

G antigen, 343-344
  bands, 256-257
Gametes, 256, 258, *264*
Gases
  compressed, work safety, *69*
  cryogenic, spill response, *71*
  flammable, spill response, *72*
GCNT2, 316, 317
Genes/genetics, 255, 256
  alleles, 256, 265, 282
    frequency, 276-278, *278*
    silenced, 268
  arms, 256, *257*
  blood group systems, 255-296
    chimerism, 273-274
    inheritance, 266-271
    key points, 292-293
    modifiers, 274-275
    population genetics, 275-278
    relationship testing, 278-279
    structural variation, 271-273
    terminology, 280-281
    variation, 262-266
  frequency, 276-278
  incidence, 275
  inheritance, 266-271
  mapping, 256-257, *258,* 279
  markers, 278
  modifiers, 274-275
  nomenclature, 280
  nonsense coding, 264
  nonsynonymous coding regions, 264
  phenotype, 276
  population, 275-278
  position effects, 274
  prevalence, 275
  products, sequential interaction, 275
  recombinants, 271, *272*
  regulations, 256-262
  silenced, 290, 291
  synonymous, gene-coding regions, 264
  synteny, 271
  therapy, 89
  transcription factor, erythroid phenotypes, 384
  unlinked, 274-275
  variation, 262-266
  see also Polymorphisms
Genome/genomics, 255, 281-292
  blood group systems, 281-292
  human, 230-231, 279, 280
  organization, 256-262
Genotyping, 264, *265,* 281-282
  discrepancies, 289-291, *290, 291*

  platforms, 237
  red cell antigens, 237
GE (Gerbich) system (020), 377-378
  antigens, 377
  phenotype prevalence, *377*
GIL (Gill) system (029), 380
GLOB blood group system, 318-323
  antibodies to, 322
  biochemistry, 319, 321
  blood-group-carrying molecules, *321*
  genetics, 321-322
  phenotypes, 319, *319*
  prevalence, *319*
  transfusion practice, 322-323
Glomerulosclerosis, focal segmental (FSGS), TPE,
  720
Glutaraldehyde, spill response, *72*
Glycerol, cryopreservation and, 160, 161
Glycosphingolipids, synthetic pathways, *320*
  blood-group-carrying molecules, *321*
Glycosyltransferase, 297, *298*
GMA. *See* Apheresis, granulocyte-monocyte
Good manufacturing practice, current (cGMP), 2
GPA, 359
GPB, 359
GPIa/IIa, HPAs, 460-461
GPIb/V/IX, HPAs, 460
GPIIb/III, HPAs, 459-460
GPIV/CD36, HPAs, *461,* 462
GPVI, HPAs, 462
Grafts, HSC, source, 742-743
Graft-vs-host disease, transfusion-associated
  (TA-GVHD), 649-650, *651*
  chimerism and, 492-493, *493*
  pediatric, 694-695
  prevention, 161
Granulocytes
  agglutination test, 472
  antigens and antibodies, 457, 469-478
  HSCT, 773
  immunofluorescence test, 472
  key points, 473
  neonatal and pediatric, 688-689
  shipping, 522
  storage, *513,* 518
  testing for, 472-473
  therapeutic, 571
  transfusion, 570-571
Guidance, *63-65*
  FDA, 79
  manual, 83
  PBM, 606
GYPA/B, 359, *361,* 362-363

H

H systems, 310-313
 alloantibodies, 312
 antibodies to, 312-313
 antigen, 298-299
 biochemistry and genetics, 310
 genes, 302
 null phenotypes, 310, 312
 transfusion practice, 313
H(FUT1/FUT2) genes, 302
Hand-washing, 35, *65*
Haploid, 257, *264*
Haplotype, 256, 273
Hardy-Weinberg equilibrium, 276-278
Hazards
 areas, 34-35
 biosafety, 42
 categories, *49*, 56
 chemicals, list, *67-68*
 communication program, chemical, 50
 electrical safety, 40
 fire prevention, 39
 hazards, *49*
 health and physical, *49*
 identification and communication, 36, 42
 shipping, 56
 storage, 45
 waste-reduction program, 56
HBc, *174, 183*
 donor testing regulations and standards, *191*
HBsAg. *See* Hepatitis B surface antigen
 donor testing, regulations, and standards, *191*
 screening for, 200
HBV. *See* Hepatitis B virus
HCT/Ps. *See* Human cells, tissues, and cellular and tissue-based products
HCV. *See* Hepatitis C virus
HDFN. *See* Hemolytic disease of the fetus and newborn
Health history, DHQ, 132
Heart conditions, 134-135
 cardiac surgery, 569-570
 cardiovascular disease, donors, 134
 coronary syndromes, acute, 555-556
Heating blocks, QC, 30
Heavy chains, 243-244, *244*
Helgeson phenotype, 378
HELLP syndrome (hemolysis, elevated liver enzymes, low platelet count), 719
Hematocrit, 130, 131, 154
Hematoma, 143
Hematopoietic growth factors, myeloid, 745-746
Hematopoietic progenitor cells (HPCs), 737, 767
 accreditation considerations, 756-757

allogeneic, *738*-739, 740, 767
autologous, *738-739*, 739-740, 745, 746, 767
cell-processing methods, 750-751
clinical utility, 737-742
collection, 743-748, 758-766, 767
 marrow, 744-745
 peripheral blood, 745-747
 UCB, 747-748
cryopreserved, 743, 751-752, 755
graft source, 742-743
histocompatibility, 741-742
indications, *738-739*
infectious disease agents, 740
infusion-related adverse events, 755
key points, 757-758
manufacturers' regulations, *88*
matching, 767, 768
mobilization, 739
patient care, 754-756
processing, 748-750, 758-766
QC, 752-753
regulatory considerations, 756-757
shipping and transportation, 754
storage, 749
thawing, 749-750
washing, 749
Hematopoietic stem cell transplantation (HSCT), 493-494, 737-740, 757-766
 ABO compatibility for blood component, 768-772
 blood component support, 772-773
 donor selection, 740, 742
 key points, 774
 non-HLA, 490
 non-oncologic patients, 772
 pediatrics, 773-774
 platelets, 772-773
 RBCs, 772
 recipients, 767-775
Hemizygous, 265
Hemochromatosis, 145
Hemodilution
 acute normovolemic (ANH), 595
 isovolemic red cell exchange, 722
Hemoglobin
 donors, 130-131, 154-155
 reports, *603*
 thresholds, 597-598, *602*
Hemoglobinuria, paroxysmal cold (PCH), 434-435, 444-445
Hemolysis
 autoimmune, 434-445
 classification, *435*
 drug-induced, 445-449
 extravascular, 247-248

hyperhemolysis, antibody-negative DHTRs and, 249
immune-mediated, 429-455
instrument-related, 713
intravascular, 248
nonimmune-mediated, 637
types, 434-435, *435*
Hemolytic disease of the fetus and newborn (HDFN), 286, 329, 355, 389-390, 434, 659-665
    ABO-associated, 305
    anti-D, 329
    DAT, 434
    diagnosis and monitoring, 660-661
    maternal alloimmunization, 660
    molecular testing, 286-287
    pathophysiology, 659-660
    prevention, 662-665
    Rh testing, 348
    thrombocytopenia, pregnancy-related, 665-667
    treatment, 661-665
Hemorrhage, 596, 620
Hemostasis
    abnormalities, 647-648
    laboratory tests, *674*
Hemotherapy, decisions and outcomes, 553-581
    cryoprecipitate, 569-570
    granulocyte, 570-571
    key points, 573
    massive transfusion, protocols, 571-573
    plasma, 567-569
    platelets, 561-567
    RBCs, 553-561
Hemovigilance, 95-126, 627
    adverse events, 100
    donor, 99, 103-106, *105*
    goal, 97
    international, 96-97
    key points, *112-113*
    modules, 100
    next steps, 106-112
    recipients, 100-103
    reporting, 100
    standards, 106
    US, 97-100, *105*
Hepatitis
    B virus (HBV), 173, *175, 179,* 182, *183-184, 190, 191,* 196-201
        donor testing, *196*
        exposure, 38
        regulations and standards, *190, 191*
        transmission, 200, 217
    B surface antigen (HBsAg), *183*
        prophylaxis, 38
        screening, 173, *174*

C virus (HCV), *174, 175, 179, 185,* 196
    donor testing, *196*
    exposure, 38
    regulations and standards, *191*
    screening for, 201
    transmission, 201, 217
E virus (HEV), 202-203
    non-A, non-B (NANB), 173
    posttransfusion (PTH), 173
Heredity, 255
Heterochromatic regions, 256
Heterozygous, 265
Hil, *361*, 363
Histocompatibility, 741-742
    determinants, non-HLA, 489-490
HIT. *See* Thrombocytopenia, heparin-induced
HIV/AIDS, 1, *175,* 177, *179, 185,* 196
    donor testing, *196*
    regulations and standards, *190*
    screening, 173, *174,* 177, 199-200
    transmission, 199
HLA-B27, ankylosing spondylitis and, 496
HLA system, 479-501
    alleles
        Class I region, 484
        hypersensitivity reactions, 496
        nomenclature, 482-483, *483*
    antibodies
        detection, 490
        development, 491
    antigens
        Class I region, 484
        nomenclature, 481-482
        public, 482
        red cells, 383-384
    biochemistry, tissue distribution, and structure, 479-484
    clinical aspects, 495-498
    complex, *485*
    crossmatching and antibody detection, 490
    disease association, *495,* 496
    exposure, 38
    function, 483-484
    future, 498
    HPAs, 462
    immune responses, 498
    key points, 499
    matched unrelated donor (MUD), 740
    MHC genetics, 484-488
    non-HLA histocompatibility determinants, 489-490
    platelet transfusion, 565-567
    regulatory aspects, 498
    role, 498

splits and cross-reactive groups, 482
testing, 493-495
transfusion and, 491-493
transplantation, 493-495
typing, 488-489, 741
HNA. *See* Neutrophil alloantigen, human
Homozygosity, 265, 290
Hospital regulations, 85-86
Housekeeping, 34
HPA. *See* Platelets, alloantigens, human
HPC. *See* Hematopoietic progenitor cells
HSCT. *See* Hematopoietic stem cell transplantation
HTLV. *See* Human T-cell lymphotropic virus
HTRs. *See* Transfusion reactions, hemolytic
Human cells, tissues, and cellular and tissue-based
  products (HCT/PS), 82, 86-89
    donors, 86, *86*, 195, *196*
    manufacture, 87
Human genome, 230-231
Human Resources, 5, 7-8, 23
    aids, 15
    competency assessments, 7-8
    hiring, 7
    jobs descriptions, 7
    see also Training; Work environment
Human T-cell lymphotropic virus, Types I and II
  (HTLV-I/II), *174, 175, 179, 187, 196*
    donor testing, *196*
    regulations and standards, *192*
    screening, 201-202
Hyperhemolysis, antibody-negative DHTRs and, 249
Hyperkalemia, 646-647
Hypersensitivity reactions, HLA alleles, 496
Hypokalemia, 646-647
Hypotension
    intraoperative blood loss, 595
    in therapeutic apheresis, 712
Hypothermia, 648
    neonates, 676
HyTRs. *See* Transfusion reactions, hypotensive

I

I system (027), 315-318
    antibodies to, 317-318, *317*
    genetics, 317
    transfusion practice, 318
IAT. *See* Antiglobulin test, indirect
Ii blood group collection, 315-318
Immune effector cells (IECs), 89
Immunization, alloimmunization, 389
Immunocompromised recipients, CMV testing, 194-
  195
Immunoglobulins
    AHTR, 635

denaturation, 418
IgA, 245, *245*, 246
IgD, *245*
IgE, 245, *245*
IgG, 244-245, *245*, 249, 303, 436
IgM, 244, *245*, 246, 248, 305-306, 436
intravenous (IVIG), 395
papain and, 244
Rh, 329, 395
Immunohematology reference laboratories (IRLs), 424
Immunology, 244-251
    key points, 251
    red cells and, 250-251
    transfusion medicine, 229-254
Immunomodulatory therapy, 429-430
Immunosuppression, adjunctive (AMR), TPE, 720
Immunotherapy, 355, *356-359*
    agents, 395
IN system (023), 379
Incubation time, 416
Infants. *See* Pediatrics
Infections/infectious diseases, 606
    emerging, 111
    markers, *197*
    rates, 198
    relevant transfusion-transmitted (RTTIs), 127-
      128, 129
    residual risks of transfusion, 196-199
      agents for which blood is tested, 196-198
      agents with no donor screening tests, 198-199
      unknown risks, 196
    sepsis, transfusion-related, 637-638
    threat, 111
    transfusion-transmitted, estimated risks, *198*
    vector-borne, 205-212
Infectious waste, 46-47
    disposal, 48
Infectious disease screening, 173-227, *174-176*
    donors, 177-199
    key points, 217-218
    overview, 173-177
    pathogen inactivation technology, 215-217
    residual risks of transfusion, 196-199
    screening, 199-217
    transmission risks, 217
Information management, 5, 17, 24
    see also Computer systems; Data
Information systems, laboratory (LIS), 617
Informed consent, HSCT, 743-744
Infusions
    pumps, 541
    rapid, 548
    sets, 542-543
    syringes, 541

Inheritance
  autosomal
    codominant, 266-267
    dominant, 266, *267*
    recessive, 267-268
  dominant, sex-linked, 269-270, *269*
  genetic traits, 266-270
  patterns of, 486-488, *486*
  recessive, 270, *271*
  sex-linked, 268-270
Injuries, 583-584
  reporting, 38-39, 82
Inspections
  blood component units, 522
  incoming supplies, 10
  shipping, 522-523
INTERCEPT, 163, 199, 216, 567
Intravenous access, 542
Intravenous solutions, compatible, 544
Inventory management, 527-529
Iron
  overload, 652
  supplementation, 131
Irradiation. *See* Radiation
Ischemia, decreased risk, 605
ITP. *See* Thrombocytopenia, immune
IVIG. *See* Immunoglobulins, intravenous

J

Jehovah's Witnesses, 584
JK (Kidd) system (009), 291, 370-372
  antibodies to, 371
  glycoprotein, *370*
  phenotypes, *371*
  urea transport, 371-372
JMH (John Milton Hagen) system (026), 379-380
Jobs. *See* Human Resources
JR system (032), 380

K

KANNO system (037), 382
Karyotype, 256
KEL system (006), 364-368
  antibodies/antigens, 365, 366-367, *367*
  glycoprotein and gene, 365
  null (K_0) phenotype, 367-368
  phenotype prevalence, *366*
  protein, *365*
Kidney transplants, 494-495
Kleihauer-Betke test, 664
KN (Knops) system (022), 378-379
K_{mod} phenotype, 367-368
Kx Antigen (XK1), 368

L

Labeling, 15
  blood components, 164-165
  HSCs, 754
  RBCs, 517
  whole blood, 145
Laboratories, 34
  biosafety, 46
  design, 39
  medical, legalities, 84-85
  see also Work environment
Laboratory coats, guidance, *63*
LAN system (033), 380-381
Landsteiner, Karl, 255, 297
Laser desorption/ionization time-of-flight, matrix-
  assisted (MALDI-TOF), 282
Latex allergy, 39
LE (Lewis) system, *311*, 313-315, 417
  biochemistry and synthesis, 314-315
  phenotypes, 314-315, *314*
  transfusion practice, 315
Lean Six Sigma, 22
Leukemia, myelogenous, cytapheresis, 721-722
Leukocytapheresis, 743
Leukocytes
  filtration, 159, 543-544
  pediatric, 694
  prestorage, 158-159
  reduction, 159, 520
Light chains, 243-244, *244*
Linkage, 270-272, *273*
  disequilibrium, 273, 487-488
Lipoprotein, low-density (LDL), 727
Liquids, flammable, spill response, *72*
LISS, 415
Liver failure, acute, TPE, 720
Locus, 256
  reference genomic (LRG) record, 280
LU (Lutheran) system (005), 363-364, *364*
  rare phenotypes, 364
LW (Landsteiner-Wiener) system (016), 375-377
Lyonization, 258, 262

M

M (MNS1), 361-362, *362*
MAHA. *See* Anemia, microangiopathic hemolytic
Malaria, transfusion-transmitted (TTM), 212-213
  FY system and, 370
MALDI-TOF. *See* Laser desorption/ionization time-
  of-flight, matrix-assisted
Management, 38
  change control, 26
  see also Work environment
Manufacturers, HCT/Ps, 757

Markers, 255
Marrow
    collection guidelines, 744
    donation, *89*
    harvesting, 744-745
Mass spectrometry, 282
Massive transfusion. *See* Transfusions, massive
Materials management, 5, 23
McLeod phenotype, 270, *271*, 368
Medical devices. *See* Devices
Medical event (incident) reporting system for
    transfusion medicine (MERS-TM), 99
Medical need, exceptional, 135-136
Medical waste, 46, 48
Medications, transfusion deferral, 135
Meiosis, 256, 257-258, 279, *272*
Membrane attack complex (MAC), 247, *247*, 250
MER2, 379
Mercury, spill response, *73*
MHC genetics, 484-488, *485*
    HLA genetic regions, 484, 486
    restriction, 483
Minisatellite, 279
MINY, *361*, 363
Mirasol, 163, 216
Mitosis, 256, 257, *263*-264
MNS system (002), 359-363, *360*
    antigens and antibodies, 362-363
    phenotype prevalence, *362*
Molecular biology, 229-254
    genetics, 255
    immunohematology, 283
    key points, 251
Molecular testing
    antigen-negative donors, 288
    blood groups, 283-291
    D type, 288
    discrepancies, 289-291, *290, 291*
    HDFN, 286-287
    paternal, 287-288
    prenatal, 286-288
    red cell antigens, *284*
    resolution 282-283
    Rh variant antigen, 288
Monitoring, 5, 20-22, 24
    blood ordering and usage, 614
    components, 509-518, *510-516*
    look-back, 189, 194
    radiation, 54
    see also Audits
MSBOS. *See* Blood order schedule, maximum surgical
MTPs. *See* Transfusions, massive, protocols
Mur antigen, 363
Mutations, 263

N

N (MNS2), 361-362, *362*
NANB. *See* Hepatitis, non-A, non-B
National Committee for Clinical Laboratory
    Standards (NCCLS), 2
National Electrical Code, 34
National Healthcare Safety Network (NHSN), 99,
    100
    adverse reactions, *101-102*
    incident codes, *104*
National Marrow Donor Program (NMDP), 88-89,
    89
NEC. *See* Enterocolitis, necrotizing
Neonates. *See* Pediatric transfusions; Perinatal issues
Nerve injury, local, 143
Neuromyelitis optica (NMO), TPE, 720
Neutropenia
    autoimmune (AIN), 472
    neonatal alloimmune (NAN), 471-472
Neutrophils
    alloantigen, human (HNA), 472-473
    antigens, human (HNA), 469-470, *470*, 471
    immune disorders, 471-472
NGS. *See* Sequencing, next-generation
Nitrogen, liquid, work safety, *70*
Nucleic acids
    analysis, 229
    chemistry and structure, 230-231, *230*
    isolation, 231
    testing (NAT), 181-182, 233
Nucleic acid sequence-based amplification (NASBA),
    233-234
Nucleoside transporter 1, equilibrative (ENT1), 381
Nucleotides, single nucleotide variants (SNVs), 263-
    264, 279
    blood group system, 279
    genotyping, red cell phenotypes, 289-291

O

O allele, 302-303
Octaplas, 163-164, 199
OK system (024), 379
Organization. *See* Work environment
Outcomes measurement, 4
Oxygenation, extracorporeal membrane (ECMO),
    690-691
    blood component preparation protocols, *692*

P

P1Pk system (003), 318
P1 substance, 417
PAD. *See* Blood donation, preoperative autologous
Papain, 416

Para-Bombay phenotype, 312
Parvovirus B19, *193*, 214-215
Paternity, 279
    zygosity testing, 287-288
Pathogens
    blood-borne, 41
    inactivation, 162-164, 199
        pediatric, 695
        technologies, 215-217, *216*
    reduction technology (PRT), 566
Patient blood management (PBM), 20-21, 583-612,
    613, 615-616
    certification, 585, 606
    data collection, 600-605
    definition and scope, 583-584
    education, 585, 587-588
    guidance, 606
    implementation, *588*, 606
    key points, 607
    methods, 585-600
    performance measures, 614
    program levels, *586-587*
    qualification/competence, 588
    resources, 584-585
    standards and certification, 585
    strategies
        intraoperative, 594-596
        postoperative, 596-598
        preoperative, 588, 591-592, 594
    transfusion extremes, 605-606
Patient care, 754-756
    controls chart, 26
    evaluation and management, 707-711
    high-risk patients, 620
    specimens, shipping, 56
    in therapeutic apheresis, 707-709, *708, 709*
PCR. *See* Polymerase chain reaction
Pediatric transfusions, 673-703, 713
    administration, rate of, 689-690
    adverse effects, 694-695
    body size and blood volume, 675
    cell washing, 695
    cold stress, 676
    compatibility testing, 677-678
    component choice, 680-681
    conditions specific to, 681-682
    cryoprecipitate, 688
    erythropoietin physiology and therapy, 675-676
    exchange, 680-681
    granulocytes, 688-689
    guidelines, 679
    hematopoiesis, coagulation, and physiology, 673-
        675, *674*
    HSCT, 773-774

indications and thresholds, 678-679
key points, 695-696
neonates, 687-688, *687*
orders to prepare and to transfuse blood and blood
    components, 538-539
        pretransfusion sample, 539
        prophylactic medications, 540
out-of-hospital, 548-549
thrombocytopenia, fetal and neonatal alloimmune
    (FNAIT), 464-465, 667-668
vascular access and technique, 681
ventricular assist devices (VADs), 693
WB, 684-685
Pedigrees, 266, *266*
PEG, 415
Peptide-binding specificity, vaccine development,
    496
Perinatal issues, 659-672
    HDFN, 659-665
    key points, 668
    thrombocytopenia, pregnancy-related, 665-
        667
    see also Neonatal and pediatric, transfusions,
Peripheral blood
    HPC collection, 745-747
    stem cells (PBSCs), 87
Peripheral nervous system diseases, TPE, 720
pH, 416
    meters, QC, 30
Phenotypes, 265-266, 275, 282
    ABO, 298, *299*
    antigen-negative, 276
    null, 310, 312
    prevalence, 276
    secretor, 297
Photopheresis, extracorporeal, 723-724, *724*
Phlebotomy, therapeutic, 144-145
Physical examination, donors, 130
Pipette recalibration, QC, 30
Plasma
    AB, 572
    AHF, cryoprecipitated, *687*
    apheresis, 150
    component storage, 155-158
    cryoprecipitate reduced, 158
    derivatives, screening, 214-215
    exchange, therapeutic (TPE), 705-720, *715-719*
    fresh frozen (FFP), 155-156, 568-569, 606, *687*
        cryoprecipitate-depleted, 158
        within 24 hours after phlebotomy (PF24),
        156-157
    HSCT, 773
    liquid, 157
    neonatal and pediatric, 687-688, *687*

platelet-rich (PRP), *147*, 148
pooled, 159-160
quarantined, 156
recovered, 158
reduction, HPC, 748-749
shipping, 522
storage, *513-515*, 518
testing problems, 307, 309
thawed, 157, 518-519
in therapeutic apheresis, 712
transfusions, 567-569
    bleeding, 567-568
    prophylaxis for invasive procedures, 567
    vitamin K antagonist reversal, 568
types, 568-569
usage, 616-617
whole blood, 572-573
Plasmodium spp., 212
Platelets
additive solution (PAS), 150, 155, 160
alloantigens, human (HPAs), 457-461, *458-459*, 566-567
    ABO and other blood groups, 461-462
    CD109, 461
    GPIa/IIa, 460-461
    GPIb/V/IX, 460
    GPIIb/III, 459-460
    GPIV/CD36, *461*, 462
    GPVI, 462
    HLA, 462
    nomenclature, 457
    testing, 466-469
antigens and antibodies, 457-469, 473-478
    drug-dependence, 469
    key points, 473
    testing, 466-469
apheresis, 149-150
    screening for bacteria, 204-205
assays, 240, 467-468
autoantibodies, 468
bacterial contamination, *175*
corrected count increment, 565-566
cryopreservation and cold storage, 161
disorders, alloimmune, 462-465
genotyping, 468
HSCT, 772-773
inventory shortage, 527-528
pooled, 159-160
shelf life, 154
storage, 154-155, *511-513*, 518
    gel production, 519
    QC, 29
    shipping, 522
    volume reduction, 520

transfusions, 561-567, 685-687
    ABO, 564-565
    bleeding, 563-564
    components, 686-687
    dose, 562-563, 686-687
    guidelines, *686*
    HLA, 565-567
    invasive procedures, 563
    neonatal and pediatric, 685-687
    prophylactic, 561-563, *564*
    RhD matching, 564-565
volume-reduced, 162
washing, 162
Pollution, minimizing, 56
Polycythemia, neonatal, 681-682
Polymerase chain reaction (PCR), 231-233, *232*, 279, 283
contamination, 233
inhibitors, 232
primer design, 232-233
real-time, *236*, 282
reverse transcriptase, 233
specimen processing and template degradation, 232
Polymorphisms, 262, 278
restriction fragment length (RFLP), 282
short tandem repeat (STR), 492, 496-497
single nucleotide (SNPs), 457
Pooling, 159-160, 521
PPE. *See* Protective equipment, personal
P1PK blood group system, 318-323
antibodies to, 322
biochemistry, 319, 321
blood-group-carrying molecules, *321*
genetics, 321-322
phenotypes, 319, *319*
prevalence, *319*
transfusion practice, 322-323
Pragmatic Randomized Optimal Platelet and Plasma Ratios (PROPPR) trial, 572
Prenatal practice/pregnancy, 420, 665-667
donors, 135
fibrinogen, 569
molecular testing, 286-288
see also Pediatric transfusions
Pressure devices, 541
Pretransfusion. *See* Transfusions, pretransfusion
Primer
design, 232-233
sequence-specific (SSP), *488*, 489
Prions, 213-214
Proband, 266
Process, 26
computer system, 13

control and management, 3, 5, 10-14, 23-24, 26
documents, 15
improvement, 22, 24
interaction, 4
protocols, 12
test methods, 13
validation, 10-13, *12*
Processing, 748-750
Proficiency testing (PT), 22, 84
Protective equipment, personal (PPE), *63-65*
biosafety, 42, 45
chemical safety, 51
electrical safety, 40
fire prevention, 39
laboratory coats, *63*
masks, *64-65*
PBM, 606
radiation, 55
see also Safety, 37; Work environment
Protein assays
flow cytometry, 243
fluid-phase, 238-239
less common, 242-243
protein microarrays, 242
solid-phase, 239-242
suspension array technology (SAT), 243
Western blotting (WB), 242-243
Proteins
analysis, 238-244
nomenclature, 280
PRT. *See* Pathogens, reduction technology
Public Health Service (PHS) Act, 78, 79, 82, 84, 86, 87
Purpura, posttransfusion (PTP), 465, 650-652

Q

Qualification, 26
Quality
assurance, 2, 26
factor (QF), 53
glossary, 26-27
indicators, 20, 26
planning, 3, 4-5, 27
Quality control (QC), 2-3, 13-14, 26, 752-753
documentation, 13-14
frequency, 13
intervals, 29–31
objectives, 614-615
Quality management systems (QMS), 1-31
approach, 4-5
concepts, 2-4
evaluation, 5
key points, 23-24
practice, 5-23
systems and processes, *3*, 27

Quarantine
blood components, 164
errors, 197
failure, 197

R

Radiation, 53-57, 519-520
biological effects, 53
cesium irradiators, 56
dose, 161
emergency response plan, 55
engineering controls and PPE, 55
exposure limits, 54
irradiators
QC, 30
replacement, 56
measurement units, 53
monitoring, 54
neonatal and pediatric, 694-695, *694*
regulations, 53-54
training, 54-55
waste management, 55
work practices, 55
RAPH system (025), 379
Reaction rates, *107, 108-110*
Reagents
high-/low-protein, 348
QC, 31
Recalls, managing, 84
Receipts, 10
Receiving, supplies, 523
Recipients
baseline assessment, 538
consent, 537-538
designated/directed donation, 135-137
hemovigilance, 100-103
history and education, 538
identification and labeling, 503-504, 525
prior, 189, 194
testing, pretransfusion, 504-509
transfusion risks, 111
verification at administration, 544
Records, 5, 16-17, 24
changes to, 16
confidentiality, 16
error correction, 17
locus reference genomic (LRG), 280
retention policy, 16-17
storage, 17
see also Documentation
Red Blood Cell (RBC) transfusions, 553-561, 598-599, 682-685
additive solutions, 676
age, 676-677, 684

AIHA, 559-560
alternatives, 676-677
components, 153-154
cryopreservation, 160-161
emergency, 556-557
HDFN, 665
HSCT, 772
infants and children, 682-685
irradiation, 162
neonates, 675-682
recipients of monoclonal antibodies, 560-561
shipping, 522
single-unit, 598-599
storage, *510-511*, 517, 556, 676-677
storage lesion, 676-677
thalassemia and sickle cell disease, 557-559
thawing and deglycerolizing, 519
thresholds, *589-590*
unit selection, 523-525
Red cells
   alloimmunization, 682-683
   anion exchanger, 372
   antibodies
      binding, *247*
      nonhemolytic, 249-250
   antigens, 255
      expression differences, 255
      molecular testing, *284*
   apheresis, 149
   autologous phenotype, 397
      adsorption, 418-419
      adsorption-elution, 420
      antibodies, 421-422
      chemical modification, 417
      donor unit selection, 422-423
      elution, 419-420
      enzyme modification, 416-417
      immunoglobulins, denaturation, 418
      inhibition techniques, 417-418
      obtaining, 415
      pH, 416
      reactivity, *405-406*
      serologic clues, 410
      titration, 420-421
   drugs, therapeutic, 285
   exchange, 722-723, *722*
   IgG, 285
   immunologic responses, 250-251
   membrane, *301*
   phenotypes
      molecular testing, 283-285, *284*
      SNV genotyping, 289-291
   reduction, HPC, 748-749

SCD, 682-683
survival, 389-390
testing problems, 307, 309
washing, 162
Refrigerators, QC, 29
Registration, blood establishments and device manufacturers, 79, 81
Regulations and recommendations, 21, *61-62*, 498, 756-757
   accreditation vs, 77, *78*
   allografts, 782-783, *783*
   clinical histocompatibility, 498
   donor eligibility, 128
   FDA, 81
   radiation, 53-54
   see also Standards
Relationship testing, 278-279
Relative risk (RR), HLA type and disease, 496
Renal failure, acute, TPE, 720
Replacement fluids, in therapeutic apheresis, *709*
Reporting/reports
   adverse events, 111
   biovigilance, 99-100
   establishment inspection (EIR), 83
   hemovigilance, 100
   SDS, 50
   transfusion-related adverse reaction, 103
   virus test results, 111
   see also Documentation/documents; Records
Requirements, 27
Respiratory distress syndrome, acute (ARDS), 640-641
Reviews. *See* Audits; Evaluation; Monitoring
RFLP. *See* Polymorphism, restriction fragment length
RHAG blood group system (030), 347, 380
RHCE, 332, 334, *335, 345*
RhCE, 347
   D epitopes, 340
RHD, 286, 290-291, 292, 334, *335,* 337, *345*
   genotyping, 287
   molecular testing, 288
   nonfunctional, 340
   zygosity, 287-288, 346
RhD, 347
   -like loops, *339*
   matching, platelets, 564-565
   model, *339*
   typing, 507, 524
RH_{NULL} syndrome, 347
Rh system, 329-354
   antibodies to, 347-348
   antigens, 329, *330-332,* 337-346
      high-prevalence, 348
      molecular testing, 288

antisera, *336-337*
chromosomal structure, 333-334
gene products, 334
genotyping, 346-347
    confirming, 346-347
    fetal, 346
    RHD zygosity testing, 346
    SCD patients, 347
    transfusion recipients, 346
glycoprotein, associated (RhAG), 380
haplotypes prevalence, *333*
immune globulin (RhIG), 329, 395
    HDFN, 662-665, *665*
key points, 349-350
locus, 333-334, *335*
phenotypes, 337-340, 342
proteins, 334
terminology332-333
typing
    discrepancies, resolving, 349
    false-positive and false-negative, 348-349
    technical considerations, 348-349
Riboflavin (vitamin B2), 216, 217
Risk assessment, 11, *12*
Rituximab, TPE, 720
Root cause analysis, 18, *19*
Rosette test, 664
Rouleaux formation, 414

S

S (MNS3)/s (MNS4), 361-362, *362*
    antibodies to, 362
Safety, 5, 22-24, 33
    acids, *69, 71*
    acrylamide, *69*
    alkalis, *69*
    bases, spill response, *71*
    biosafety, 41-48
    cabinets, 42, *43-44*
    caustics, spill response, *71*
    chemicals, 48-53
    data sheet (SDS), 49, 50, 51
    disaster plan, 23
    electrical, 40-41
    emergency response, 38, 46
    engineering controls and PPE, 37, 42
    eyewashes, *65*
    eyewash stations, 34
    face shields, *64-65*
    federal regulations and recommendations, 33
    fire prevention, 40-41
    goggles, *64*
    hazard identification and communication, 36, 42
    HBV, HCV, or HIV exposure, 38

    incidental spill response, *71-73*
    key points, 57
    levels, 41-42, *43-44, 66*
    mobile blood-collection sites, 35
    nitrogen, liquid, *70*
    plan, 35-38, 46
    precautions, 41-42, *66*
    program, 33, 35-39
    radiation, 53-57
    solvents, flammable, *70*
    training, 36, *37*, 42
    work practices, 37, 45-46
    see also Fire prevention; Protective equipment,
        personal; Work environment
"Safety Reporting Requirements for Human Drug and
    Biological Products," 97
Samples, 503-504
    donors, retention and storage, 523
    pretransfusion, 539
    recipients, 503-507, 523
SC (Scianna) system (013), 374
SCD, RH genotyping, 347
Screening
    infectious diseases, *174-176*
    specific agents, 199-217
Sd^a substance, 417
Secretor phenotype, 297
Sepsis. *See* Infections/infectious diseases
Sequencing, 489
    massively parallel (MPS), 283
    next-generation (NGS), 237-238, 279, 489
Serologic testing, 181, 504
    discrepancies, molecular testing, 288, 289-291,
        289, 290, 291
    principles, 504-505, *505, 506*
Serum
    testing problems, 307, 309
    -to-cell ratio, increasing, 415-416
Sex chromosomes, 256
    see also Genes/genetics
Shipping and transportation, 522-523, 754
    blood components, 509, *510-516*, 542-543
    containers, QC, 31
    hazardous materials, 56
    HSC, 754
Shock, AHTR, 635
Short tandem repeat (STR), 279
SHOT. *See* Transfusions, serious hazards of
Siblings, 268
Sickle cell disease (SCD), 286, 682-684
    RBC transfusion, 557-558, *559*
    red cell exchange, 722-723
    transfusion complications, 683-684
    WBC filtration, 159

SID system (038), 323, 382 (Sb[a])
Skin
    donors, lesions, 131
    uses, 780
SLC14A1, 371-372
SMIM1, 381
SNP. *See* Polymorphisms, single nucleotide
SNV. *See* Nucleotides, single gene
Solid-organ transplantation, 495
    consultation, 497-498
    donors, ABO genotyping, 289
    non-HLA, 490
Specification, 27
Spills
    bases, *71*
    blood, *47*
    caustics, *71*
    chlorine, *71*
    formaldehyde, *72*
    gases, *71, 72*
    glutaraldehyde, *72*
    incidental, *71-73*
    liquids, flammable, *72*
    mercury, *73*
SSP. *See* primer, sequence-specific
S–s–U– phenotype, 362
Standard operating procedures (SOPs), 10, 15
Standards
    clean spaces/rooms, 34
    hemovigilance, 106
    PBM, 585
    see also Regulations and recommendations
Staphylococcus aureus, contamination, 205
Statistical tools, 3
Storage
    antibody changes, 390-391
    bags, 156
    components, 153-158, 509-518, *510-516*
    hazardous materials, 45
    lesion, 517
    plasma, 156
    WB, 146
STR. *See* Polymorphisms, short tandem repeat
Structural variation, 263-264, 271-273
Sulfhydryl reagents, 418
Suppliers, 4, 5, 9-10, 23
    contracts and agreements, 10
    factors, *9*
    qualification, 9-10
    receipt and inspection of incoming supplies, 10
Surgery, minimally invasive, 595
    see also Blood, ordering
Surveillance terms, reconciled, 106

Suspension array technology (SAT), 243
Syphilis. *See Treponema pallidum*
Syringe set, neonatal, *692*
System, *27*

T

TACO. *See* Circulatory overload, transfusion-associated
TA-GVHD. *See* Graft-vs-host disease, transfusion-associated
Tandem repeats, variable number of (VNTR), 279
T cells, 483
Temperature reduction, 415
Templates, 15
    degradation, 232
Terminology, 106, 280-281
    Fisher-Race DCE, 333
Testing
    cases, 11-12
    logistics, 178
    method validation, 13
    molecular, 288, 289-291, *289, 290, 291*
    nucleic acid (NAT), 181-182, 233
    point-of-care, 596
    recipients, pretransfusion, 504-509
    relationship, 278-279
    results, reactive 182, 189
    RHD zygosity, 346
    rosette, 664
    serologic, 181, 504, 504-505, *505, 506*
    serum, 307, 309
    surrogate, 173-174
    see also Evaluation
Thalassemia, 286, 684
    RBC transfusion, 557, 558
Thermometers, QC, 30
Thrombocytopenia
    drug-induced, 465-464
    fetal and neonatal alloimmune (FNAIT), 464-465, 667-668
    heparin-induced (HIT), 465-466
    immune (ITP), 466, 667
    pregnancy-related, 665-667
    therapy-induced hypoproliferative, 561-563
    transfusion guidelines, *686*
Thrombocytopenic purpura, thrombotic (TTP), 567-568
    in therapeutic apheresis, 711-712
Thrombocytosis, massive, cytapheresis, 722
Thromboelastography (TEG), 21
Thromboelastometry (TEM), 21
Thrombosis, 606
Timers, QC, 30

Tissue
   allografts, 778
      clinical use, 780, *781-782*
      disease transmission, 782
      donation, 777-782
      donor eligibility, 778
      hospital tissue services, 784-790
      hospital transfusion service and, 777-791
      infectious disease testing, 778, *778*
      key points, 789-790
      laws, regulations, and standards, 782-783, *783*
      preservation, 779-780
      processing, 779
      transplantation, 777-782
   autografts, 788-789
   donor testing, 195
   homografts, 778
   processing, 779-780
   storage, *516*, 786-787, *787*
      adverse events, 788
      recalls and look-back investigations, 788
      record-keeping, 787-788
      traceability, 787-788
   transplantable, 778
   xenografts, 779
Tissue-based products, testing donors, 195
Tissue services, hospital-based, 784-789
   incoming tissue, inspection, 785-786
   responsibility for, 784, *784*
   standard operating procedures and policies, 784-785
   supplier qualifications and certification, 785, *786*
Titration, 420-421
Tracking, 9, 14
Training, 7
   biosafety, 42
   electrical safety, 40
   fire safety, 39
   new employees, 14
   nonconformances, 17
   radiation, 54-55
   restricted areas, 34
   safety program, 36, *37*
   see also Human Resources
Traits, 256
   recessive, 268
   see also Genes/genetics; Inheritance
TRALI. *See* acute lung injury, transfusion-related
Tranexamic acid, 596
trans, 274
Transcription-mediated amplification (TMA), 233-234, *234*
Transfusion medicine, 1
   FDA, 78-84

   key points, *90*
   regulatory considerations, 77-93
Transfusion reactions, 634-648
   allergic (ATRs), 639-640
   categories, *628-632*
   clinical evaluation and management, 633
   fatality reporting, 651-652
   hemolytic (HTRs), 355, 389-390, 434
      acute (AHTR), 247-248, 634-636
      antibody-negative (AN-DHTRs), 249
      delayed (DHTRs), 248, 286, 648-652
   hemovigilance, 627
   hypotensive (HyTRs), 645
   identification, 627, 632
   key points, 653
   laboratory investigation, standard, 633-634
   nonhemolytic, febrile (FNHTR), 491-492, 540, 638-639
   noninfectious, 627-657
   pediatric, 694
   purpura, posttransfusion (PTP), 465, 650-652
   surveillance, 623
   suspected, 547, 627-634
Transfusions
   blood selection, 439-441
   blood utilization, 613-626
   chain, 95
   completion, 547
   components, issuing, 523-527
   deferral list, 135
   distribution, 522-523
   documentation, 525, 547-548
   emergency, 525-527
   extremes, 605-606
   fetal, 661-662
   guidelines, 599-600
   hemoglobin, *602*
   HLA and, 491-493
   infections, transmitted (TTI), 100
      monitoring system (TTIMS), 111-112
      sepsis, transfusion-related, 637-638
   inventory management, 527-529
   key points, 529-530
   massive, 526-527, 571-573, 605-606
      complications, 647-648
      formula-based, 571
      hemostatic abnormalities, 647-648
      liberal vs restrictive strategies, 553-556
      pediatric, 693
      protocols (MTPs), 572
   monitoring, 509-518, *510-516*, 545, 547
   nonemergent, *546*
   pediatric, 693
   P1PK blood group system, 322-323

preparation of ordered units, 539-540
pretransfusion, 537
    processing, 518-522
    recipient's blood, 504-509, *505*
    testing, 504-509
    test results, positive, *535*
rate of, 545
readiness, 542
recent recipients, 283, 285
reduction, 177
refractoriness, 462-464, 491, 565-567
requests, 503
safety officer (TSO), 21
samples and requests, 503-504
second, 21, *21*
serious hazards of (SHOT), 96-97, *96*
service-related activities, 503-535
    FDA and, 81
    registration, 81
small-volume aliquoting, 690, *691*
starting, 545
storage, 509-518, *510-516*
threshold, 597-598
    platelets, HSCT, 772-773
    RBC, *589-590*
unique settings, 548-549
warm-reactive patients, 441
see also Plasma, transfusions; Platelets,
    transfusions; RBC transfusions
Transplantation
    haploidentical, 742
    HLA testing and, 493-495
    stage of, 768, *769*
Transportation. *See* Shipping
Trending, 14
Treponema pallidum, 180, 186, 196
    donor testing, *192*
    screening for, 203
Trypanosoma cruzi, 175, 180, 187, 209-210
    regulations and standards, *192*
    screening, 173, *174*
Trypsin, 416
Tubing welder, sterile, *691*
Typing, sequence-based, 489

U

Ultraviolet light
    A (UVA), 216, 217
    B (UVB), 216
Umbilical cord blood (UCB), 87, 737, 740, 741-742
    HPC collection, 747-748
Universal Protocol, preprocedure verification process,
    86
Utilization review, 617-620

V

Vaccine development, peptide-binding specificity
    and, 496
Validation, 10-13, 27
Variants of unknown significance (VUS), 283
Vascular access
    central catheters, 710
    pediatric, 689
    subcutaneous ports, 710
    in therapeutic apheresis, 709-711
Vasovagal reactions, 143-144
VEL (Vel) system (034), 270, 279, 381
Venipuncture site, 142
Venous access
    devices, 710
    HPC collection peripheral blood, 745
Ventilation, 34
Ventricular assist devices (VADs), pediatric, 693
Verification, 27, 544-545
View boxes, QC, 30
Vitamin K antagonist reversal, plasma, 568
VNTR. *See* Tandem repeats, variable number of
Volume reduction, 520
    pediatric, 695
von Willebrand factor (vWF)
    plasma and, 567-568
    TPE, 714

W

WAIHA. *See* Anemia, hemolytic warm
Waste disposal/management, 56-57
    biohazard, 46-48
    chemical, 52-53
    infectious, 46
    medical, 46
    radiation, 55
Waterbaths, QC, 30
West Nile virus (WNV), *180, 188*
    donor screening/testing, 195, *196*
    NAT, *175*
    regulations and standards, *193*
    screening for, 206
Western blotting, 242-243
Whole blood (WB), 141-172
    cold-stored, 153
    collection, 145-148, *147*
    filtration, *147,* 148
    key points, 165-166
    labeling, 145
    resuscitation, 572-573
    shipping, 522
    storage, 146, *510,* 518
    transfusion, pediatric, 684-685
    See also Blood components; Donors

Withdrawals, managing, 84
Work environment, 5, 22-23, 24, 33-75
    change control, 26
    ergonomics, 35
    gloves, *63-64*
    guidance, *63-65*
    hand-washing, 35, *65*
    instructions, 15
    inventory management, 527-529
    key points, 57
    leadership, 5, 6, 23
    management, 38
    organization, 5, 6, 7, 23
    radiation, 55
    uniforms, *63*
    see also Facilities; Human Resources; Safety
Wr$^{a/b}$, 373
Wrong blood in tube (WBIT), 539

X

XCFR, hemovigilance, 96, 99
X chromosome inactivation, 258, 262
Xenotransplantation products, 779
XG (Xg^a) system (012), 374
XK system (019), 364-368
    protein, *365*

Y

YTEG (YT3), 373
YTLI (YT4), 373
YTOT (YT5), 373
YT system (011), 373

Z

Zika virus (ZIKV), *176, 180, 188*
    donor testing, regulations and standards, *193*
    screening for, 206-208
Zygosity, *265*, 390
    paternal samples, 287-288